EMERGENCY MEDICINE
Just the Facts

EDITORS

O. John Ma, MD

Professor of Emergency Medicine
University of Missouri–Kansas City School of Medicine
Vice Chair
Department of Emergency Medicine
Truman Medical Center
Kansas City, Missouri

David M. Cline, MD

Associate Professor of Emergency Medicine
Research Director
Department of Emergency Medicine
Wake Forest University School of Medicine
Winston-Salem, North Carolina

Judith E. Tintinalli, MD, MS

Professor and Chair
Department of Emergency Medicine
Adjunct Professor
Department of Health Policy and Administration
University of North Carolina at Chapel Hill
Chapel Hill, North Carolina

Gabor D. Kelen, MD

Professor and Chair
Department of Emergency Medicine
Johns Hopkins University
Baltimore, Maryland

J. Stephan Stapczynski, MD

Professor and Former Chair
Department of Emergency Medicine
University of Kentucky College of Medicine
Lexington, Kentucky

EMERGENCY MEDICINE
Just the Facts

Second Edition

O. John Ma

David M. Cline

Judith E. Tintinalli

Gabor D. Kelen

J. Stephan Stapczynski

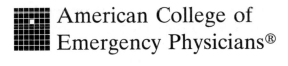 American College of
Emergency Physicians®

McGRAW-HILL
Medical Publishing Division

*New York   Chicago   San Francisco   Lisbon   London   Madrid   Mexico City   Milan
New Delhi   San Juan   Seoul   Singapore   Sydney   Toronto*

EMERGENCY MEDICINE: *Just the Facts, Second Edition*

1 2 3 4 5 6 7 8 9 0   QDP/QDP   0 9 8 7 6 5 4

ISBN 0-07-141024-4

Notice

Medicine is an ever-changing science. As new research and clinical experience broaden our knowledge, changes in treatment and drug therapy are required. The authors and the publisher of this work have checked with sources believed to be reliable in their efforts to provide information that is complete and generally in accord with the standards accepted at the time of publication. However, in view of the possibility of human error or changes in medical sciences, neither the authors nor the publisher nor any other party who has been involved in the preparation or publication of this work warrants that the information contained herein is in every respect accurate or complete, and they disclaim all responsibility for any errors or omissions or for the results obtained from use of the information contained in this work. Readers are encouraged to confirm the information contained herein with other sources. For example and in particular, readers are advised to check the product information sheet included in the package of each drug they plan to administer to be certain that the information contained in this work is accurate and that changes have not been made in the recommended dose or in the contraindications for administration. This recommendation is of particular importance in connection with new or infrequently used drugs.

This book was set in Times New Roman by ATLIS Graphics and Design.
The editors were Andrea Seils, Michelle Watt, and Mary E. Bele.
The production supervisor was Catherine Saggese.
The cover designer was Aimee Nordin.
The index was prepared by Andover Publishing Services.
Quebecor/Dubuque was printer and binder.

This book is printed on acid-free paper.

Library of Congress Cataloging-in-Publication Data

Emergency medicine : just the facts / edited by O. John Ma . . . [et al.].–2nd ed.
   p. ; cm.
  Rev. ed. of: Just the facts in emergency medicine / editors, David M. Cline, O. John Ma. c2001.
  Includes bibliographical references and index.
  ISBN 0-07-141024-4
   1. Emergency medicine. 2. Medical emergencies. 3. Emergency medical services.
I. Ma, O. John. II. Just the facts in emergency medicine.
  [DNLM: 1. Emergency Medicine. 2. Emergencies. WB 105 E555752 2004]
RD755.5.E448 2004
616.02′5–dc22

2003066640

CONTENTS

Contributors   xv
Preface   xxi

Section 1
TEST PREPARATION AND PLANNING   1

  1 Facts about Emergency Medicine Board Exams
     David M. Cline   1
  2 Test-Taking Techniques   *David M. Cline*   4

Section 2
RESUSCITATIVE PROBLEMS AND TECHNIQUES   7

  3 Advanced Airway Support   *Robert J. Vissers*   7
  4 Dysrhythmia Management and Cardiovascular
     Pharmacology   *James K. Takayesu*   11
  5 Resuscitation of Children and Neonates
     Douglas K. Holtzman   32
  6 Fluids, Electrolytes, and Acid-Base Disorders
     David M. Cline   36

Section 3
SHOCK   47

  7 Therapeutic Approach to the Hypotensive Patient
     John E. Gough   47
  8 Septic Shock   *John E. Gough*   49
  9 Cardiogenic Shock   *Rawle A. Seupaul*   51
  10 Anaphylaxis and Acute Allergic Reactions
     Damian F. McHugh   53

11   Neurogenic Shock   *Rawle A. Seupaul*   54

Section 4
ANALGESIA, ANESTHESIA, AND SEDATION   57

12   Acute Pain Management and Conscious Sedation
     Diamond Vrocher   57
13   Management of Patients with Chronic Pain
     David M. Cline   60

Section 5
EMERGENCY WOUND MANAGEMENT   65

14   Evaluating and Preparing Wounds   *Timothy Reeder*   65
15   Methods for Wound Closure   *David M. Cline*   67
16   Lacerations to the Face and Scalp
     Russell J. Karten   71
17   Injuries of the Arm, Hand, Fingertip, and Nail
     David M. Cline   74
18   Lacerations to the Leg and Foot   *David M. Cline*   79
19   Soft Tissue Foreign Bodies   *Rodney L. McCaskill*   81
20   Puncture Wounds and Mammalian Bites
     Chris Melton   83
21   Postrepair Wound Care   *Eugenia B. Smith*   87

Section 6
CARDIOVASCULAR DISEASE   91

22   Approach to Chest Pain   *Thomas Rebbecchi*   91
23   Acute Coronary Syndromes: Management of
     Myocardial Ischemia and Infarction
     Jim Edward Weber   94
24   Syncope   *Michael G. Mikhail*   97
25   Congestive Heart Failure and Acute
     Pulmonary Edema   *Chadwick Miller*   99
26   Valvular Heart Disease   *David M. Cline*   101
27   The Cardiomyopathies, Myocarditis,
     and Pericardial Disease   *N. Stuart Harris*   107
28   Pulmonary Embolism   *Christopher Kabrhel*   112
29   Hypertensive Emergencies   *Jonathan A. Maisel*   115
30   Aortic Dissection and Aneurysms
     David E. Manthey   118
31   Peripheral Vascular Disorders
     Christopher Kabrhel   121

Section 7
PULMONARY EMERGENCIES 125

32	Respiratory Distress *Matthew T. Keadey*	125
33	Bronchitis, Pneumonia, and SARS *David M. Cline*	129
34	Tuberculosis *Amy J. Behrman*	133
35	Pneumothorax *Rodney L. McCaskill*	136
36	Hemoptysis *James E. Winslow*	137
37	Asthma and Chronic Obstructive Pulmonary Disease *Monika Ahluwalia*	138

Section 8
GASTROINTESTINAL EMERGENCIES 143

38	Acute Abdominal Pain *Peggy E. Goodman*	143
39	Gastrointestinal Bleeding *Mitchell C. Sokolosky*	146
40	Esophageal Emergencies *Mitchell C. Sokolosky*	148
41	Swallowed Foreign Bodies *Patricia Baines*	150
42	Peptic Ulcer Disease and Gastritis *Mark R. Hess*	152
43	Appendicitis *Peggy E. Goodman*	154
44	Intestinal Obstruction *Roy L. Alson*	156
45	Hernia in Adults and Children *N. Heramba Prasad*	158
46	Ileitis, Colitis, and Diverticulitis *Jonathan A. Maisel*	159
47	Anorectal Disorders *N. Heramba Prasad*	165
48	Vomiting, Diarrhea, and Constipation *Jonathan A. Maisel*	169
49	Jaundice, Hepatic Disorders, and Hepatic Failure *Gregory S. Hall*	174
50	Cholecystitis and Biliary Colic *Gregory S. Hall*	180
51	Pancreatitis *Robert J. Vissers*	183
52	Complications of General Surgical Procedures *N. Heramba Prasad*	185

Section 9
RENAL AND GENITOURINARY DISORDERS 189

53	Acute Renal Failure *Marc D. Squillante*	189
54	Emergencies in Renal Failure and Dialysis Patients *Jonathan A. Maisel*	192
55	Urinary Tract Infections and Hematuria *Kama Guluma*	195
56	Male Genital Problems *Stephen H. Thomas*	199
57	Urologic Stone Disease *Geetika Gupta*	202
58	Complications of Urologic Devices *David M. Cline*	204

Section 10
GYNECOLOGY AND OBSTETRICS 207

59 Vaginal Bleeding and Pelvic Pain in the
Nonpregnant Patient *Cherri D. Hobgood* 207
60 Ectopic Pregnancy *David M. Cline* 212
61 Comorbid Diseases in Pregnancy
Sally S. Fuller 214
62 Emergencies During Pregnancy and the
Postpartum Period *Sally S. Fuller* 217
63 Emergency Delivery *David M. Cline* 220
64 Vulvovaginitis *David A. Krueger* 223
65 Pelvic Inflammatory Disease and
Tubo-Ovarian Abscess *Robert W. Shaffer* 225
66 Complications of Gynecologic
Procedures *Debra Houry* 227

Section 11
PEDIATRICS 229

67 Fever *Douglas K. Holtzman* 229
68 Bacteremia, Sepsis, and Meningitis
in Children *Milan D. Nadkarni* 231
69 Common Neonatal Problems *Lance Brown* 235
70 Pediatric Heart Disease *David M. Cline* 239
71 Otitis and Pharyngitis *David M. Cline* 243
72 Skin and Soft Tissue Infections *David M. Cline* 246
73 Pneumonia in Children *Lance Brown* 250
74 Asthma and Bronchiolitis *Douglas R. Trocinski* 252
75 Seizures and Status Epilepticus
in Children *Michael C. Plewa* 255
76 Vomiting and Diarrhea in Children
Debra G. Perina 259
77 Pediatric Abdominal Emergencies
Debra G. Perina 261
78 Diabetic Ketoacidosis in Children *David M. Cline* 264
79 Hypoglycemia in Children *Juan A. March* 266
80 Altered Mental Status and Headache
in Children *Debra G. Perina* 268
81 Syncope and Sudden Death in Children
and Adolescents *Debra G. Perina* 270
82 Fluid and Electrolyte Disorders in Children
Lance Brown 273
83 Upper Respiratory Emergencies *Juan A. March* 275
84 Pediatric Exanthems *Lance Brown* 281
85 Musculoskeletal Disorders in Children
David M. Cline 286

86 Sickle Cell Anemia in Children
Douglas R. Trocinski   292
87 Pediatric Urinary Tract Infections   *Lance Brown*   296

Section 12
INFECTIOUS DISEASES/IMMUNOLOGY   299

88 Sexually Transmitted Diseases   *Gregory S. Hall*   299
89 Toxic Shock   *Kevin J. Corcoran*   303
90 Common Viral Infections   *Matthew J. Scholer*   306
91 HIV Infections and AIDS   *David M. Cline*   308
92 Infective Endocarditis   *Chadwick Miller*   313
93 Tetanus and Rabies   *C. James Corrall*   315
94 Malaria   *Gregory S. Hall*   319
95 Infections from Helminths and Other
Parasitic Worms   *Phillip A. Clement*   322
96 Zoonotic Infections   *Gregory S. Hall*   326
97 Soft Tissue Infections   *Chris Melton*   333
98 Bioterrorism   *Roy L. Alson*   338
99 The Transplant Patient   *David M. Cline*   341

Section 13
TOXICOLOGY AND PHARMACOLOGY   347

100 General Management of the Poisoned Patient
Sandra L. Najarian   347
101 Anticholinergic Toxicity   *O. John Ma*   351
102 Psychopharmacologic Agents
C. Crawford Mechem   353
103 Sedatives-Hypnotics   *Keith L. Mausner*   360
104 Alcohols   *Michael P. Kefer*   364
105 Drugs of Abuse   *Jeffrey N. Glaspy*   368
106 Analgesics   *Keith L. Mausner*   373
107 Theophylline   *Mark B. Rogers*   379
108 Cardiac Medications   *C. Crawford Mechem*   380
109 Phenytoin and Fosphenytoin Toxicity
Mark B. Rogers   386
110 Iron   *O. John Ma*   388
111 Hydrocarbons and Volatile Substances
J. Christian Fox   390
112 Caustics   *Christian A. Tomaszewski*   392
113 Insecticides, Herbicides, and Rodenticides
Christian A. Tomaszewski   394
114 Metals and Metalloids   *Lance H. Hoffman*   398
115 Hazardous Materials   *Christian A. Tomaszewski*   400
116 Herbals and Vitamins   *Christian A. Tomaszewski*   403

117 Antimicrobials   *Christian A. Tomaszewski*   405
118 Cyanide   *Mark E. Hoffmann*   407
119 Dyshemoglobinemias   *Howard E. Jarvis III*   408
120 Hypoglycemic Agents   *Christian A. Tomaszewski*   410

Section 14
ENVIRONMENTAL INJURIES   413

121 Frostbite and Hypothermia   *Mark E. Hoffmann*   413
122 Heat Emergencies   *T. Paul Tran*   415
123 Bites and Stings   *Burton Bentley II*   418
124 Trauma and Envenomation from
Marine Fauna   *Christian A. Tomaszewski*   423
125 High Altitude Medical Problems
Keith L. Mausner   425
126 Dysbarism and Complications of Diving
Christian A. Tomaszewski   428
127 Near Drowning   *Richard A. Walker*   430
128 Thermal and Chemical Burns   *Robert J. French*   432
129 Electrical and Lightning Injuries
Howard E. Jarvis III   436
130 Carbon Monoxide   *Christian A. Tomaszewski*   439
131 Poisonous Plants and Mushrooms
Sandra L. Najarian   441

Section 15
ENDOCRINE EMERGENCIES   445

132 Diabetic Emergencies   *Michael P. Kefer*   445
133 Alcoholic Ketoacidosis   *Michael P. Kefer*   448
134 Thyroid Disease Emergencies
Matthew A. Bridges   450
135 Adrenal Insufficiency and Adrenal Crisis
Michael P. Kefer   452

Section 16
HEMATOLOGIC AND ONCOLOGIC EMERGENCIES   455

136 Evaluation of Anemia and the Bleeding Patient
Sandra L. Najarian   455
137 Acquired Bleeding Disorders   *Matthew A. Bridges*   458
138 Hemophilias and Von Willebrand's Disease
Jeffrey N. Glaspy   462
139 Hemolytic Anemias   *Sandra L. Najarian*   464
140 Transfusion Therapy   *Walter N. Simmons*   468

141 Exogenous Anticoagulants and
Antiplatelet Agents   *Robert A. Schwab*   472
142 Emergency Complications of Malignancy
T. Paul Tran   474

Section 17
NEUROLOGY   483

143 Headache and Facial Pain   *Jason Graham*   483
144 Stroke and Transient Ischemic Attack
J. Stephen Huff   487
145 Altered Mental Status and Coma
C. Crawford Mechem   491
146 Ataxia and Gait Disturbances
C. Crawford Mechem   495
147 Vertigo and Dizziness   *Andrew Chang*   496
148 Seizures and Status Epilepticus in Adults
C. Crawford Mechem   499
149 Acute Peripheral Neurologic Lesions
Howard E. Jarvis III   503
150 Chronic Neurologic Disorders   *Mark B. Rogers* 505
151 Meningitis, Encephalitis, and Brain Abscess
O. John Ma   509

Section 18
EYE, EAR, NOSE, THROAT, AND   515
ORAL EMERGENCIES

152 Ocular Emergencies   *Steven Go*   515
153 Face and Jaw Emergencies   *Robert J. French*   519
154 Ear and Nose Emergencies   *Jeffrey N. Glaspy*   522
155 Oral and Dental Emergencies   *Steven Go*   526
156 Neck and Upper Airway Disorders
Robert J. French   528

Section 19
DISORDERS OF THE SKIN   535

157 Dermatologic Emergencies   *Michael Blaivas*   535
158 Other Dermatologic Disorders   *Michael Blaivas* 540

Section 20
TRAUMA   545

159 Initial Approach to the Trauma Patient
J. Christian Fox   545

160 Pediatric Trauma   *Charles J. Havel, Jr.*   547

161 Geriatric Trauma   *O. John Ma*   548

162 Trauma in Pregnancy   *C. Crawford Mechem*   550

163 Head Injury   *O. John Ma*   553

164 Spine and Spinal Cord Injuries   *Jeffrey N. Glaspy*   556

165 Maxillofacial Trauma   *C. Crawford Mechem*   560

166 Neck Trauma   *Walter N. Simmons*   563

167 Cardiothoracic Trauma   *Jeffrey N. Glaspy*   565

168 Abdominal Trauma   *O. John Ma*   571

169 Flank and Buttock Trauma   *Robert A. Schwab*   574

170 Genitourinary Trauma   *C. Crawford Mechem*   576

171 Penetrating Trauma to the Extremities
C. Crawford Mechem   579

Section 21
INJURIES TO THE BONES, JOINTS, AND SOFT TISSUE   583

172 Initial Evaluation and Management
of Orthopedic Injuries   *Michael P. Kefer*   583

173 Hand and Wrist Injuries   *Michael P. Kefer*   584

174 Elbow and Forearm Injuries   *Sandra L. Najarian*   588

175 Shoulder and Humerus Injuries   *Robert J. French*   591

176 Pelvis, Hip, and Femur Injuries
E. Parker Hays, Jr.   594

177 Knee and Leg Injuries   *Jeffrey N. Glaspy*   598

178 Ankle and Foot Injuries   *Michael C. Wadman*   601

179 Compartment Syndromes   *Gary M. Gaddis*   604

180 Rhabdomyolysis   *Gary M. Gaddis*   606

Section 22
NONTRAUMATIC MUSCULOSKELETAL DISORDERS   609

181 Neck and Thoracolumbar Pain   *Thomas K. Swoboda*   609

182 Shoulder Pain   *Andrew D. Perron*   612

183 Acute Disorders of the Joints and Bursae
Andrew D. Perron   614

184 Emergencies in Systemic Rheumatic Diseases
Michael P. Kefer   616

185 Infectious and Noninfectious Disorders of the Hand
Michael P. Kefer   618

186 Soft Tissue Problems of the Foot
Mark B. Rogers   620

Section 23
PSYCHOSOCIAL DISORDERS   623

187 Clinical Features of Behavioral Disorders
Lance H. Hoffman   623
188 Emergency Assessment and Stabilization
of Behavioral Disorders   *Lance H. Hoffman*   625
189 Panic and Conversion Disorders
Lance H. Hoffman   627

Section 24
ABUSE AND ASSAULT   629

190 Child and Elder Abuse   *Kristine L. Bott*   629
191 Sexual Assault and Intimate Partner Violence
and Abuse   *Stefanie R. Ellison*   631

Section 25
IMAGING   635

192 Principles of Emergency Department Use of
Computed Tomography and Magnetic
Resonance Imaging   *Matthew C. Gratton*   635
193 Principles of Emergency Department
Ultrasonography   *J. Christian Fox*   637

Section 26
ADMINISTRATION   641

194 Emergency Medical Services   *Matthew C. Gratton*   641
195 Emergency Medicine Administration
David M. Cline   645

Index   649

CONTRIBUTORS

Monika Ahluwalia, MD, Assistant Professor of Emergency Medicine, Department of Emergency Medicine, Emory University School of Medicine, Atlanta, Georgia (Chapter 37)

Roy L. Alson, MD, PhD, Associate Professor of Emergency Medicine, Department of Emergency Medicine, Wake Forest University School of Medicine, Winston-Salem, North Carolina (Chapters 44, 98)

Patricia Baines, MD, Assistant Professor of Emergency Medicine, Department of Emergency Medicine, Emory University School of Medicine, Atlanta, Georgia (Chapter 41)

Amy J. Behrman, MD, Associate Professor of Emergency Medicine, Department of Emergency Medicine, University of Pennsylvania Health System, Philadelphia, Pennsylvania (Chapter 34)

Burton Bentley II, MD, Attending Staff Physician, Department of Emergency Medicine, Northwest Medical Center, Tucson, Arizona (Chapter 123)

Michael Blaivas, MD, RDMS, Associate Professor, Director of Emergency Ultrasound, Department of Emergency Medicine, Medical College of Georgia, Augusta, Georgia (Chapters 157, 158)

Kristine L. Bott, MD, Assistant Professor, Section of Emergency Medicine, University of Nebraska College of Medicine, Omaha, Nebraska (Chapter 190)

Matthew A. Bridges, MD, Assistant Professor, University of Missouri–Kansas City School of Medicine, Department of Emergency Medicine, Truman Medical Center, Kansas City, Missouri (Chapters 134, 137)

Lance Brown, MD, MPH, Associate Professor of Emergency Medicine, Department of Emergency Medicine, Loma Linda University Medical Center and Children's Hospital, Loma Linda, California (Chapters 69, 73, 82, 84, 87)

Andrew Chang, MD, Assistant Professor, Department of Emergency Medicine, Albert Einstein College of Medicine, Montefiore Medical Center, Bronx, New York (Chapter 147)

Phillip A. Clement, MD, Clinical Assistant Professor of Emergency Medicine, Department of Emergency Medicine, East Carolina University School of Medicine, Greenville, North Carolina (Chapter 95)

David M. Cline, MD, Associate Professor of Emergency Medicine, Research Director, Department of Emergency Medicine, Wake Forest University School of Medicine, Winston-Salem, North Carolina (Chapters 1, 2, 6, 13, 15, 17, 18, 26, 33, 58, 60, 63, 70–72, 78, 85, 91, 99, 195)

Kevin J. Corcoran, DO, Clinical Associate Professor of Emergency Medicine, Department of Emergency Medicine, East Carolina University School of Medicine, Greenville, North Carolina (Chapter 89)

C. James Corrall, MD, Staff Physician, Department of Emergency Medicine, Harrison Hospital, Bremerton, Washington (Chapter 93)

Stefanie R. Ellison, MD, Assistant Professor, University of Missouri–Kansas City School of Medicine, Department of Emergency Medicine, Truman Medical Center, Kansas City, Missouri (Chapter 191)

J. Christian Fox, MD, RDMS, Assistant Clinical Professor, Director, Emergency Ultrasound Program, Department of Emergency Medicine, University of California, Irvine School of Medicine, Irvine, California (Chapters 111, 159, 193)

Robert J. French, DO, Assistant Clinical Professor, Saint Luke's Hospital, Medical College of Wisconsin, Milwaukee, Wisconsin (Chapters 128, 153, 156, 175)

Sally S. Fuller, MD, Clinical Assistant Professor of Emergency Medicine, Department of Emergency Medicine, University of North Carolina, Chapel Hill, North Carolina, Staff Physician, WakeMed, Department of Emergency Medicine, Raleigh, North Carolina (Chapters 61, 62)

Gary M. Gaddis, MD, PhD, Clinical Associate Professor, Saint Luke's Hospital, University of Missouri–Kansas City School of Medicine, Kansas City, Missouri (Chapters 179, 180)

Jeffrey N. Glaspy, MD, Assistant Professor, University of Missouri–Kansas City School of Medicine, Associate Program Director, Department of Emergency Medicine, Truman Medical Center, Kansas City, Missouri (Chapters 105, 138, 154, 164, 167, 177)

Steven Go, MD, Assistant Professor, University of Missouri–Kansas City School of Medicine, Department of Emergency Medicine, Truman Medical Center, Kansas City, Missouri (Chapters 152, 155)

Peggy E. Goodman, MD, Associate Professor of Emergency Medicine, Department of Emergency Medicine, East Carolina School of Medicine, Greenville, North Carolina (Chapters 38, 43)

John E. Gough, MD, Associate Professor of Emergency Medicine, Department of Emergency Medicine, East Carolina School of Medicine, Greenville, North Carolina (Chapters 7, 8)

Jason Graham, MD, Assistant Professor, University of Missouri–Kansas City School of Medicine, Department of Emergency Medicine, Truman Medical Center, Kansas City, Missouri (Chapter 143)

Matthew C. Gratton, MD, Associate Professor, University of Missouri–Kansas City School of Medicine, EMS Director, Department of Emergency Medicine, Truman Medical Center, Kansas City, Missouri (Chapters 192, 194)

Kama Guluma, MD, Clinical Assistant Professor of Medicine, Division of Emergency Medicine, Department of Medicine, University of California, San Diego, San Diego, California (Chapter 55)

Geetika Gupta, MD, Clinical Instructor of Emergency Medicine, Department of Emergency Medicine, University of Michigan, Staff Physician, Department of Emergency Medicine, St. Joseph Mercy Hospital, Ann Arbor, Michigan (Chapter 57)

Gregory S. Hall, MD, Assistant Professor of Emergency Medicine, Department of Emergency Medicine, University of Arkansas for Medical Science, Little Rock, Arkansas (Chapters 49, 50, 88, 94, 96)

N. Stuart Harris, MD, Clinical Instructor, Department of Emergency Medicine, Massachusetts General Hospital, Boston, Massachusetts (Chapter 27)

Charles J. Havel, Jr., MD, Assistant Clinical Professor, Elmbrook Hospital, Medical College of Wisconsin, Milwaukee, Wisconsin (Chapter 160)

E. Parker Hays, Jr., MD, Residency Program Director, Department of Emergency Medicine, Carolinas Medical Center, Charlotte, North Carolina (Chapter 176)

Mark R. Hess, MD, Assistant Professor of Emergency Medicine, Department of Emergency Medicine, Wake Forest University School of Medicine, Winston-Salem, North Carolina (Chapter 42)

Cherri D. Hobgood, MD, Assistant Professor of Emergency Medicine, Department of Emergency Medicine, University of North Carolina, Chapel Hill, North Carolina (Chapter 59)

Lance H. Hoffman, MD, Assistant Professor, Section of Emergency Medicine, University of Nebraska College of Medicine, Omaha, Nebraska (Chapters 114, 187–189)

Mark E. Hoffmann, MD, Attending Staff Physician, Department of Emergency Medicine, St. Cloud Hospital, St. Cloud, Minnesota (Chapters 118, 121)

Douglas K. Holtzman, MD, Assistant Professor of Emergency Medicine, Department of Emergency Medicine, Wake Forest University School of Medicine, Winston-Salem, North Carolina (Chapters 5, 67)

Debra Houry, MD, MPH, Assistant Professor of Emergency Medicine, Department of Emergency Medicine, Emory University School of Medicine, Atlanta, Georgia (Chapter 66)

J. Stephen Huff, MD, Associate Professor, Departments of Emergency Medicine and Neurology, University of Virginia School of Medicine, Charlottesville, Virginia (Chapter 144)

Howard E. Jarvis III, MD, Attending Staff Physician, Department of Emergency Medicine, Cox Medical Center, Springfield, Missouri (Chapters 119, 129, 149)

Christopher Kabrhel, MD, Clinical Instructor, Department of Emergency Medicine, Massachusetts General Hospital, Boston, Massachusetts (Chapters 28, 31)

Russell J. Karten, MD, Assistant Professor of Emergency Medicine, Department of Emergency Medicine, University of Pennsylvania, Philadelphia, Pennsylvania (Chapter 16)

Matthew T. Keadey, MD, Assistant Professor of Emergency Medicine, Department of Emergency Medicine, Emory University School of Medicine, Atlanta, Georgia (Chapter 32)

Michael P. Kefer, MD, Attending Staff Physician, Department of Emergency Medicine, Oconomowoc Memorial Hospital, Oconomowoc, Wisconsin (Chapters 104, 132, 133, 135, 172, 173, 184, 185)

David A. Krueger, MD, Staff Physician, Department of Emergency Medicine, Appleton Medical Center, Appleton, Wisconsin (Chapter 64)

O. John Ma, MD, Professor of Emergency Medicine, University of Missouri–Kansas City School of Medicine, Vice Chair, Department of Emergency Medicine, Truman Medical Center, Kansas City, Missouri (Chapters 101, 110, 151, 161, 163, 168)

Jonathan A. Maisel, MD, Clinical Assistant Professor of Surgery, Yale University School of Medicine, New Haven, Connecticut, Associate Program Director for Emergency Medicine, Bridgeport Hospital, Bridgeport, Connecticut (Chapters 29, 46, 48, 54)

David E. Manthey, MD, Assistant Professor of Emergency Medicine, Department of Emergency Medicine, Wake Forest University School of Medicine, Winston-Salem, North Carolina (Chapter 30)

Juan A. March, MD, Professor of Emergency Medicine, Department of Emergency Medicine, East Carolina School of Medicine, Greenville, North Carolina (Chapters 79, 83)

Keith L. Mausner, MD, Attending Staff Physician, Waukesha Memorial Hospital, Waukesha, Wisconsin (Chapters 103, 106, 125)

Rodney L. McCaskill, MD, Clinical Assistant Professor of Emergency Medicine, Department of Emergency Medicine, University of North Carolina, Chapel Hill, North Carolina, Staff Physician, WakeMed, Department of Emergency Medicine, Raleigh, North Carolina (Chapters 19, 35)

Damian F. McHugh, MD, Staff Physician, Department of Emergency Medicine, Rex Hospital, Raleigh, North Carolina (Chapter 10)

C. Crawford Mechem, MD, Associate Professor, Department of Emergency Medicine, University of Pennsylvania School of Medicine, Philadelphia, Pennsylvania (Chapters 102, 108, 145, 146, 148, 162, 165, 170, 171)

Chris Melton, MD, Assistant Professor of Emergency Medicine, Department of Emergency Medicine, University of Arkansas for Medical Science, Little Rock, Arkansas (Chapters 20, 97)

Michael G. Mikhail, MD, Clinical Instructor of Emergency Medicine, Department of Emergency Medicine, University of Michigan, Chairman of Emergency Medicine, Department of Emergency Medicine, St. Joseph Mercy Hospital, Ann Arbor, Michigan (Chapter 24)

Chadwick Miller, MD, Assistant Professor of Emergency Medicine, Department of Emergency Medicine, Wake Forest University School of Medicine, Winston-Salem, North Carolina (Chapters 25, 92)

Milan D. Nadkarni, MD, Assistant Professor of Emergency Medicine and Pediatrics, Department of Emergency Medicine, Wake Forest University School of Medicine, Winston–Salem, North Carolina (Chapter 68)

Sandra L. Najarian, MD, Assistant Professor, Case Western Reserve University School of Medicine, Department of Emergency Medicine, MetroHealth Medical Center, Cleveland, Ohio (Chapters 100, 131, 136, 139, 174)

Debra G. Perina, MD, Associate Professor of Emergency Medicine, Department of Emergency Medicine, University of Virginia Health Sciences, Charlottesville, Virginia (Chapters 76, 77, 80, 81)

Andrew D. Perron, MD, Assistant Professor, Department of Emergency Medicine, Maine Medical Center, Portland, Maine (Chapters 182, 183)

Michael C. Plewa, MD, Clinical Assistant Professor, Department of Surgery, Medical College of Ohio, Director of Research, Department of Emergency Medicine, Saint Vincent Mercy Medical Center, Toledo, Ohio (Chapter 75)

N. Heramba Prasad, MD, Associate Professor of Emergency Medicine, Department of Emergency Medicine, State University of New York, Upstate Medical University, Syracuse, New York (Chapters 45, 47, 52)

Thomas Rebbecchi, MD, Assistant Professor of Emergency Medicine, University of Medicine and Dentistry of New Jersey, Robert Wood Johnson Medical School at Camden, Cooper Hospital/University Medical Center, Camden, New Jersey (Chapter 22)

Timothy Reeder, MD, MPH, Assistant Professor of Emergency Medicine, Department of Emergency Medicine, East Carolina University School of Medicine, Greenville, North Carolina (Chapter 14)

Mark B. Rogers, MD, Attending Physician, Breech Medical Center, Lebanon, Missouri (Chapters 107, 109, 150, 186)

Matthew J. Scholer, MD, PhD, Assistant Professor of Emergency Medicine, Department of Emergency Medicine, University of North Carolina, Chapel Hill, North Carolina (Chapter 90)

Robert A. Schwab, MD, Professor and Chair, University of Missouri–Kansas City School of Medicine, Department of Emergency Medicine, Truman Medical Center, Kansas City, Missouri (Chapters 141, 169)

Rawle A. Seupaul, MD, Assistant Professor of Emergency Medicine, Department of Emergency Medicine, Indiana University School of Medicine, Indianapolis, Indiana (Chapters 9, 11)

Robert W. Shaffer, MD, Staff Physician, Mount Auburn Hospital, Department of Emergency Medicine, Cambridge, Massachusetts (Chapter 65)

Walter N. Simmons, MD, MPH, Assistant Professor, Department of Emergency Medicine, Rhode Island Hospital, Brown University, Providence, Rhode Island (Chapters 140, 166)

Eugenia B. Smith, MD, Assistant Professor of Emergency Medicine, Department of Emergency Medicine, University of North Carolina, Chapel Hill, North Carolina (Chapter 21)

Mitchell C. Sokolosky, MD, Assistant Professor of Emergency Medicine, Department of Emergency Medicine, Wake Forest University School of Medicine, Winston-Salem, North Carolina (Chapters 39, 40)

Marc D. Squillante, DO, Program Director, Residency in Emergency Medicine, University of Illinois College of Medicine at Peoria, Peoria, Illinois (Chapter 53)

Thomas K. Swoboda, MD, MS, Assistant Professor, Louisiana State University Health Sciences Center, Department of Emergency Medicine, Shreveport, Louisiana (Chapter 181)

James K. Takayesu, MD, Clinical Instructor, Department of Emergency Medicine, Massachusetts General Hospital, Boston, Massachusetts (Chapter 4)

Stephen H. Thomas, MD, Assistant Professor, Department of Emergency Medicine, Massachusetts General Hospital, Boston, Massachusetts (Chapter 56)

Christian A. Tomaszewski, MD, Associate Professor, Department of Emergency Medicine, Carolinas Medical Center, Charlotte, North Carolina (Chapters 112, 113, 115–117, 120, 124, 126, 130)

T. Paul Tran, MD, Assistant Professor, Section of Emergency Medicine, University of Nebraska College of Medicine, Omaha, Nebraska (Chapters 122, 142)

Douglas R. Trocinski, MD, Clinical Assistant Professor of Emergency Medicine, Department of Emergency Medicine, University of North Carolina, Chapel Hill, North Carolina, Associate Residency Director, WakeMed, Department of Emergency Medicine, Raleigh, North Carolina (Chapters 74, 86)

Robert J. Vissers, MD, Assistant Professor of Emergency Medicine, Department of Emergency Medicine, University of North Carolina, Chapel Hill, North Carolina (Chapters 3, 51)

Diamond Vrocher, MD, Assistant Professor of Emergency Medicine, Department of Emergency Medicine, University of Alabama at Birmingham, Birmingham, Alabama (Chapter 12)

Michael C. Wadman, MD, Assistant Professor, Section of Emergency Medicine, University of Nebraska College of Medicine, Omaha, Nebraska (Chapter 178)

Richard A. Walker, MD, Associate Professor, Section of Emergency Medicine, University of Nebraska College of Medicine, Omaha, Nebraska (Chapter 127)

Jim Edward Weber, DO, Assistant Professor of Emergency Medicine, Department of Emergency Medicine, University of Michigan, Ann Arbor, Michigan, Director of Emergency Medicine Research, Hurley Medical Center, Flint, Michigan (Chapter 23)

James E. Winslow, MD, MPH, Assistant Professor of Emergency Medicine, Department of Emergency Medicine, Wake Forest University School of Medicine, Winston-Salem, North Carolina (Chapter 36)

PREFACE

In a crunch, when interviewing an eyewitness, Dragnet's Sgt. Joe Friday would implore, "Just the facts, ma'am, just the facts." Our textbook, *Emergency Medicine: Just the Facts,* aims to provide just that for emergency physicians who are studying for either the written board (re)certification examination in emergency medicine or the in-training written examination.

This book evolved from Judith Tintinalli's *Emergency Medicine: A Comprehensive Study Guide,* which has long been considered the premier source for board certification preparation. Dr. Tintinalli's first edition of the *Study Guide,* published in 1978, was designed to cover the core content of emergency medicine for physicians preparing for the written board examination. Since then, along with the explosive growth in the field of emergency medicine, the *Study Guide* expanded to the point where it may be too voluminous to serve as a rapid examination review source. The other book that evolved from the *Study Guide,* the *Emergency Medicine Manual,* was designed as a streamlined pocket reference guide for the practicing clinician and contained only the essential information that was pertinent to the clinical care of the patient in the emergency department.

Each chapter in this second edition of *Emergency Medicine: Just the Facts* emphasizes the key points in the Epidemiology, Pathophysiology, Clinical Features, Diagnosis and Differential, and Emergency Department Care and Disposition of the subject matter. The bulleted outline for each factual item is designed to enhance its use as a rapid study aid.

We would like to express our appreciation to the *Emergency Medicine: Just the Facts* contributors for their time and commitment in writing their respective chapters. Also, the staff of McGraw-Hill Medical Publishing made the process of producing this textbook a pleasure for us and we would like to thank them all: Andrea Seils, Michelle Watt, Mary Bele, and Martin Wonsiewicz.

Finally, without the love, support, and encouragement of our families, this book would not have been possible. OJM would like to thank Robert Schwab, Mark Steele, and Judy Tintinalli for providing him with the opportunity to engage in academic emergency medicine. He also would like to dedicate this book to the emergency medicine residents and emergency department nursing staff of Truman Medical Center. DMC would like to dedicate this book to the memory of Jane M. Cline.

O. John Ma, MD
David M. Cline, MD

EMERGENCY MEDICINE
Just the Facts

TEST PREPARATION AND PLANNING

1 FACTS ABOUT EMERGENCY MEDICINE BOARD EXAMS

David M. Cline

- Through the year 2003, the American Board of Emergency Medicine (ABEM) administered three written exams each year: the Certification Exam, the Recertification Exam, and the In-Training Exam. The year 2004 marked the beginning of Emergency Medicine Continuous Certification (ConCert) and the Lifelong Learning and Self-Assessment (LLSA) tests. The new ConCert examination replaces the recertification exam. For up-to-date information concerning these exams, review the ABEM web site: www.abem.org.
- The American Osteopathic Board of Emergency Medicine (AOBEM) administers one certification examination per year. AOBEM is in the process of implementing a Continuous Certification in Emergency Medicine process. See www.aobem.org for details.

ABEM WRITTEN CERTIFICATION EXAM

- The Certification Exam is given each year in early November at several locations throughout the country; check for test site information at www.abem.org.
- The Certification Exam is approximately 335 single-best-answer multiple choice questions and lasts a total of 6 hours and 15 minutes (1.1 minute per question). There is a 60-minute break for lunch.
- Of the test questions, approximately 15% include a pictorial stimulus, and these are traditionally given during the first portion of the exam.
- The pass/fail criterion is 75% correct of those test items that are included in the examination for the purpose of scoring.

- Typically, only two thirds of the test is scored, with one third of the test questions representing new trial content. These investigational questions are compared with standardized questions for reliability and may be included as scored items the following exam cycle. Typically, a question requires 2 years from the time of creation to use as a scored item.
- The pass rate for the Certification Exam during the 2002 exam cycle was 90% for first-time takers with emergency medicine residency training, and 78% overall.[1]
- Beginning with the 2002 examinations, the subject matter of the certification exam is based on *The Model of the Clinical Practice of Emergency Medicine.*[2]
- A percentage breakdown of the exam content compared to the chapters of this book is listed in Table 1-1. Although many of the questions are different, the content percentages are the same for all three ABEM written exams. *Just the Facts in Emergency Medicine* (2nd edition) includes several chapters that include multiple topics; therefore our chapters do not precisely correlate with the exam question content areas.
- Another consideration for physicians preparing for the written exams is the acuity breakdown. The questions on the exam are rated by patient acuity (or issues surrounding the care of patients in each acuity category) with 27% critical, 37% emergent, 27% lower acuity, and 9% unrelated to acuity. Therefore, when reviewing specific topic areas, the reader should focus on the issues surrounding the assessment and care of critical or emergent patient presentations, as this content represents 64% of the exam.
- Compared to the ConCert Exam (formerly the Recertification exam), the Certification Exam has more pathophysiology-based questions. Roughly 60% of the questions are management-based, many of which require a diagnosis be made from the clinical description. Diagnostic criteria are covered in 20% and 10%

TABLE 1-1 Percentage Distribution of Test Items by Core Content Category Compared to Chapter Listing of *Just the Facts in Emergency Medicine,* 2nd ed.

	WRITTEN EXAM PERCENTAGE DISTRIBUTION	NUMBER OF CHAPTERS (PERCENT)	*JUST THE FACTS IN EMERGENCY MEDICINE* CHAPTERS REPRESENTED
Signs, symptoms and presentations	9%	11 (5.6)	7, 22, 32, 38, 52, 58, 66, 67, 69, 100, 172, plus "Clinical Features"
Abdominal and gastrointestinal disorders	9%	15 (7.7)	39, 49, 41, 42, 43, 44, 45, 46, 47, 48, 49, 50, 51, 76, 77
Cardiovascular disorders	10%	15 (7.7)	4, 5, 9, 23, 24, 25, 26, 27, 28, 29, 30, 31, 70, 81, 92
Cutaneous disorders	2%	5 (2.6)	72, 84, 97, 157, 158
Endocrine, metabolic, and nutritional disorders	3%	8 (4.1)	6, 78, 79, 82, 132, 133, 134, 135
Environmental disorders	3%	11 (5.6)	121, 122, 123, 124, 125, 126, 127, 128, 129, 130, 131
Head, ear, eye, nose, and throat disorders	5%	7 (3.6)	71, 83, 152, 153, 154, 155, 156
Hematologic disorders	2%	8 (4.1)	86, 136, 137, 138, 139, 140, 141, 142
Immune system disorders	2%	3 (1.5)	10, 91, 99
Systemic infectious disorders	5%	9 (4.6)	8, 68, 88, 89, 90, 93, 94, 95, 96
Musculoskeletal disorders (nontraumatic)	3%	7 (3.6)	85, 181, 182, 183, 184, 185, 186
Nervous system disorders	5%	13 (6.6)	11, 75, 80, 143, 144, 145, 146, 147, 148, 149, 150, 151
Obstetrics and gynecology	4%	7 (3.6)	59, 60, 61, 62, 63, 64, 65
Psychobehavioral disorders	3%	6 (3.1)	13, 187, 188, 189, 190, 191
Renal and urogenital disorders	3%	6 (3.1)	53, 54, 55, 56, 57, 87
Thoracic-respiratory disorders	8%	7 (3.6)	33, 34, 35, 36, 37, 73, 74
Toxicology	4%	20 (10.2)	101, 102, 103, 104, 105, 106, 107, 108, 109, 110, 111, 112, 113, 114, 115, 116, 117, 118, 119, 120
Traumatic disorders	11%	20 (10.2)	159, 160, 162, 163, 164, 165, 166, 167, 168, 169, 170, 171, 172, 173, 174, 175, 176, 177, 178, 179, 180
Procedures and skills	6%	12 (6.1)	3, 12, 14, 15, 16, 17, 18 19, 20, 21, 192, 193
Other components (including administration and legal aspects)	3%	5 (2.6)	1, 2, 98, 194, 195

are pathophysiology based. The remaining 10% of questions relate to emergency department administration, emergency medical service (EMS), disaster medicine, and miscellaneous issues.

• Certification expires every 10 years. Recertification requires participation in the Continuous Certification process (see below).

ABEM CONTINUOUS CERTIFICATION (RECERTIFICATION)

• The recertification process has been renamed Continuous Certification and now requires four components: (1) updated licensure requirement, (2) yearly lifelong learning self-assessment tests that are based on journal articles, (3) expanded availability of the ConCert (recertification) exam, and (4) assessment of practice performance.

• All diplomates of the boards should check the web site for information concerning their requirements for recertification, which vary according to the year their current certification expires.

• Information concerning the updated licensure requirement can be found at the ABEM web site: www.abem.org.

• The yearly required readings for the LLSA tests can be found at the ABEM web site: www.abem.org. The LLSA tests are based on these readings.

• The new ConCert exam will be a half-day exam and will be available at over 200 computer-administered testing centers across the country. See the ABEM website for more details: www.abem.org.

• The ConCert exam consists of approximately 200 multiple-choice questions.

• Of the test questions, approximately 15% will include a pictorial stimulus, and these are generally during the first portion of the exam.

• The pass/fail criterion for the ConCert exam has not been announced. Traditionally the Recertification Exam pass/fail criterion has been 75% correct of those test items that are included in the examination for the purpose of scoring.

- Typically only two thirds of the test is scored, with one third of the test questions representing new trial content. These investigational questions are compared with standardized questions for reliability and may be included as scored items the following exam cycle.
- The pass rate for the Recertification Exam during the 2002 exam cycle was 87%.[1]
- Examination content will be split between two sources. Ultimately, between 60 and 75% will be based on *The Model of the Clinical Practice of Emergency Medicine*[2] and 25 to 40% will be based on the LLSA readings.[1] The actual percentage of LLSA-based questions on the ConCert examination will be phased in from none in 2004 to as much as 40% in later years.
- Compared to the Certification Exam, the ConCert exam is more clinically based and has fewer pathophysiology-based questions.
- The content of the LLSA readings is published on the ABEM website and is summarized in Table 1-2.
- A percentage breakdown of the exam content compared to the chapters of this book is listed in Table 1-1. Although many of the questions are different, the content percentages are the same for all three ABEM written exams. *Just the Facts in Emergency Medicine* includes several chapters that include multiple topics; therefore our chapters do not precisely correlate to the exam question content areas.
- Recertification must be accomplished every 10 years to maintain ABEM Board Certification.

TABLE 1-2 Nine-Year Cycle of the EM Model for Lifelong Learning and Self-Assessment

Year 1	2004	Thoracic-respiratory disorders Immune system disorders Musculoskeletal disorders
Year 2	2005	Nervous system disorders Toxicologic disorders
Year 3	2006	Traumatic disorders Cutaneous disorders
Year 4	2007	Signs, symptoms, and presentations Psychobehavioral disorders
Year 5	2008	Procedures and skills integral to the practice of EM Environmental disorders
Year 6	2009	Cardiovascular disorders Hematologic disorders
Year 7	2010	Abdominal and gastrointestinal disorders Other components of the practice of EM
Year 8	2011	Head, ear, eyes, nose, and throat disorders Endocrine, metabolic, and nutritional disorders Renal and urogenital disorders
Year 9	2012	Systemic infectious disorders Obstetrics and gynecology

ABBREVIATIONS: EM = emergency medicine.

ABEM IN-TRAINING EXAM

- The In-Training Exam is given to all emergency medicine residents each year in late February.
- The test consists of approximately 225 questions and lasts 4 hours and 15 minutes (1.1 minute per question), given in a single session.
- Unlike other ABEM exams, there is no pass/fail criterion; rather, residents are compared to other residents across the country at their same level of training. Scores for individual training programs are compared with other training programs across the country, and this information is provided to residency program directors.
- Subject matter of the exam is based on *The Model of the Clinical Practice of Emergency Medicine.*[1]
- The target at which all questions are aimed is the expected knowledge base and experience of an emergency medicine third-year resident.
- A percentage breakdown of the exam content compared to the chapters of this book is listed in Table 1-1. Although many of the questions are different, the content percentages are the same for all three ABEM written exams. *Just the Facts in Emergency Medicine* includes several chapters that include multiple topics; therefore our chapters do not precisely correlate to the exam question content areas.

AOBEM WRITTEN CERTIFICATION EXAM

- The certification exam is given the first Saturday of February each year.
- The subject matter of the exam comes from the Emergency Medicine Core Content.[3] However, AOBEM will likely revise this listing in 2003 or 2004. See the AOBEM web site for details.[4]
- The percentage breakdown of the exam content is similar to the topic areas listed in Table 1-1.
- Like ABEM, AOBEM uses a preset passing score, but it is not currently published. Also, each exam contains nonscored test items that are in the process of evaluation and standardization.

REFERENCES

1. www.abem.org
2. Hockberger RS, Binder LS, Graber MA, et al: The model of the clinical practice of emergency medicine. *Ann Emerg Med* 37:745, 2001.
3. Task Force on the Core Content for Emergency Medicine Revision: Core content for emergency medicine. *Ann Emerg Med* 29:792, 1997.
4. www.aobem.org

2 TEST-TAKING TECHNIQUES

David M. Cline

- Excellent test performance requires both well-planned study methods and carefully applied test-taking skills.

EXAM PREPARATION AND PHYSICIAN PERFORMANCE

- Exam preparation techniques and successful test completion have not been well studied within the specialty of emergency medicine. Studies from other medical specialties or professional disciplines may or may not pertain to emergency medicine board exams.
- There is little evidence to suggest that continuing medical education positively impacts clinical practice.[1,2]
- Interactive sessions that emphasize practice skills may have a positive impact on physician practice behaviors.[1]
- There is little evidence that routine didactic educational conferences improve test performance.[3]
- Magarian was able to show that an intensive conference series focused on exam content improved test scores of medical students.[4]
- Godellas and colleagues found that increased conference attendance could improve test performance for surgery residents with higher past performance histories.[5]
- Studies conducted in other specialties have shown several factors that correlate with better test performance: self directed study,[6,7] programmed textbook review,[8,9] and individual resident effort.[5,10]
- In the specialties of both neurology[11,12] and surgery,[13] past performances on the in-training exam predicted performance on the certification examination.
- For surgery residents, being on call the night before the exam did not affect in-training exam scores.[14]

STUDY TECHNIQUES

- The following techniques are recommended based on common sense rules of study methods. Supporting studies in emergency medicine have not been conducted.
- Begin by setting a schedule to accomplish your study goals and objectives in the time remaining prior to the test. Allow time for reading this book, using a question-and-answer book to uncover any gaps in your knowledge base and your final review. Your schedule should be written and checked often to document your progress.
- Find a place to study that facilitates concentration, not distraction. Hettich found that a single place of study improved test performance for college students.[15]
- Begin reading each chapter by glancing over the topic headings to get an overview of the material. Formulate questions in your mind such as:
  1. What etiologic information will help me to identify the patient at risk for the disease?
  2. What pathophysiologic concepts will help to treat the disease?
  3. What clinical features will help me to identify the disease?
  4. What criteria confirm the diagnosis of the disease?
  5. What are the recommended treatments for the disease?
- Reading should be an active experience. Don't turn the exercise into a coloring contest with your highlighter. Write in the margins, circle, underline, and identify key points.
- Review your notes and key points at the end. If you find the material confusing or your understanding incomplete, you will need to go to other sources for additional information, such as the parent textbook for this review book: *Emergency Medicine: A Comprehensive Study Guide,* 6th ed. Consider also reviewing a pictorial atlas of disease, an electrocardiogram atlas, and a radiology atlas.
- If you do not have time to read this book in its entirety, review the index to identify gaps in your knowledge. Look for unfamiliar topics or disease-specific treatments you have not previously reviewed.
- Last-minute cramming is an inefficient study method, taxes your energy, and creates anxiety.[16]

PREPARATION IMMEDIATELY BEFORE THE TEST

- Get plenty of sleep the night before the test.
- Arrive at the test site well in advance of the start time to make sure you know where the exam room is located and become familiar with the surroundings.
- Check the temperature of the exam room so that you can anticipate proper attire. Dress comfortably.
- Schedule enough time to wake up, dress, and eat an unhurried breakfast.
- Eat an adequate, but not heavy breakfast. Do the same for the lunch break.
- Bring a photo ID to identify yourself.
- Pencils are provided. No food (including candy) is allowed at the exam tables.
- Although anxiety reduction techniques have long been recommended, a certain degree of test anxiety has been shown to improve test performance.[6]

TAKING THE TEST

- Listen carefully to verbal instructions and read completely any written instructions.
- You have 1.1 minute per question on the test. Make sure that you maintain this schedule. For example, at the 1-hour mark, you should have answered approximately 60 questions. However, the pictorial stimulus portion of the test is usually first, and these questions take more time than the remaining questions for most test takers.
- There is no penalty for guessing on this multiple-choice exam.
- Fill in the answer sheet as you go. Some authors recommend skipping the hard questions and returning to them at the end. This practice may leave you without time to revisit the unanswered questions. Skipping items also increases the chances that you will key the answer sheet incorrectly. Study proctors will not allow you extra time to correct or fill in your answer sheet.
- Carefully read the question stem and anticipate the answer before you read the options listed. If you see the choice you anticipate, that answer is most likely correct.
- Read all the answers to check for a more complete or better answer than the one you anticipated.
- Don't waste excessive time on a single question that puzzles you. Simply make your best guess and move on. Make a note in the test booklet margin and return to the question at the end for further consideration.
- Remember that approximately one third of the test is not scored (see Chap. 1). If you don't know the answer or find the question confusing, it may be a trial question. Don't lose your confidence or your momentum.
- Identify the incorrect options quickly so if you are forced to guess, you have a better chance of being correct.
- On items that have "all of the above" as an option, if you are certain that two other answers are correct, you should chose "all of the above."
- Options that include broad generalizations are more likely to be incorrect.
- There is no evidence to support the idea that option "C" is more likely to be correct than others on ABEM exams.
- Use every minute of the test time. If you have time left over, review first the questions you have identified as difficult, and then use the remaining time to reread the questions, looking for any misinterpretations that may have occurred the first time through.
- Contrary to popular opinion, your first guess is no more likely to be correct than a carefully considered re-evaluation of the answer.[17,18] If during the review process, you find a better answer to a question stem, do not hesitate to change your choice. You have a 57.8% chance of changing a wrong answer to a correct one, a 22.2% chance of changing a wrong answer to another wrong answer, and only a 20.2% chance of changing a correct answer to an incorrect one.[17] However, students who have a past record of doing well on exams are more likely to make a correct change than those students who have a history of poor test performance.[18]
- Do not spend your lunch break discussing specific test questions with colleagues. This practice could disqualify you from the test, and creates more anxiety, further limiting your performance in the afternoon. Remember, only two thirds of the test is scored.
- Relax. The odds are in your favor, and now that you own this book, you have a concise means to review the practice of emergency medicine.

REFERENCES

1. Davis DA, O'Brien MAT, Freemantle N, et al: Impact of formal continuing medical education. *JAMA* 282:867, 1999.
2. Davis DA, Thomson MA, Oxman AD, et al: Changing physician performance: A systematic review of the effect of continuing medical education strategies. *JAMA* 274:900, 1995.
3. Shetler PL: Observations on the American Board of Surgery in-training examination, board results, and conference attendance. *Am J Surg* 144:292, 1982.
4. Magarian GJ: Influence of a medicine clerkship conference series on student's acquisition of knowledge. *Acad Med* 68:923, 1993.
5. Godellas CV, Hauge LS, Huang R: Factors affecting improvement on the American Board of Surgery in-training exam. *J Surg Res* 91:1, 2000.
6. Godellas CV, Huang R: Factors affecting performance on the American Board of Surgery in-training examination. *Am J Surg* 181294, 2001.
7. Nackman GB, Sutyak J, Lowry SF, Rettie C: Predictors of educational outcome: Factors impacting performance on a standardized clinical evaluation. *J Surg Res* 106:314, 2002.
8. Dean RE, Hanni CL, Pyle MJ, Nicholas WR: Influence of programmed textbook review on American Board of Surgery In-service Examination scores. *Am Surgeon* 50:345, 1984.
9. Hirvela ER, Becker DR: Impact of programmed reading on ABSITE performance. *Am J Surg* 162:487, 1991.
10. Itani KM, Miller CC, Church HM, McCollum CH: Impact of a problem based learning conference on surgery residents' in training exam scores. *J Surg Res* 70:66, 1997.
11. Juel VC, Johnston KC: Predict resident exam performance (PREP) study. *Neurology* 60:1385, 2003.
12. Goodman JC, Juul D, Westmoreland B, Burns R: RITE performance predicts outcome on the ABPN Part I examination. *Neurology* 58:1144, 2002.
13. Beister TW: The American Board of Surgery In-Training Examination as a predictor of success on the qualifying examination. *Curr Surg* 44:194, 1987.

14. Stone MD, Doyle J, Bosch RJ, et al: Effect of resident call status on ABSITE performance. *Surgery* 128:465, 2000.

15. Hettich PI: *Learning Skills for College and Career.* Pacific Grove, CA: Brooks/Cole, 1992.

16. Zechmeister EB, Nyberg SE: *Human Memory: An Introduction to Research and Theory.* Pacific Grove, CA: Brooks/Cole, 1982.

17. Benjamin LT, Covell TA, Shallenberger WR: Staying with initial answers on objective tests: Is it a myth? *Teaching Psychol* 11:133, 1984.

18. Ferguson KJ, Kreiter CD, Peterson MW, et al: Is that your final answer? Relationship of changed answers to overall performance on a computer-based medical school course examination. *Teach Learn Med* 14:20, 2002.

3 ADVANCED AIRWAY SUPPORT

Robert J. Vissers

INITIAL APPROACH

- Control of the airway is the single most important task for emergency resuscitation.
- Indications for the airway management techniques described in this chapter include oxygenation, ventilation, protection of the airway, facilitation of therapy, and anticipation of a clinical course that requires preventive management (ie, burn victims).

PATHOPHYSIOLOGY

- The upper anatomic airway includes the oral and nasal cavities down to the larynx. The lower airway includes the trachea, bronchi, and lungs.
- Potentially difficult intubations can be predicted by the following:
  1. External features suggestive of difficulty, such as a beard or obesity, or a short neck, receding chin, or tracheostomy scars.
  2. Inability to open the mouth three fingerbreadths or a thyromental distance less than three fingerbreadths.
  3. A relatively large tongue for the oral cavity as estimated by the inability to visualize more than the base of the uvula in a cooperative patient opening the mouth in a sniffing position (Fig. 3-1).[1]
  4. Evidence of upper airway obstruction.
  5. Lack of neck mobility. This should be assessed only in patients without potential C-spine injury.

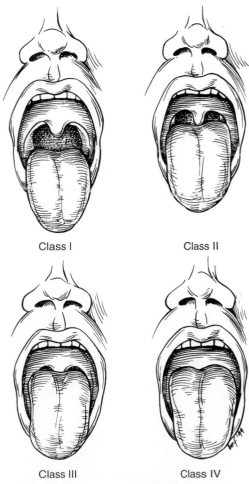

Class I   Class II

Class III   Class IV

FIG. 3-1. Classification of tongue size relative to the size of the oral cavity by Mallampati and colleagues.[1] Class I: Faucial pillars, soft palate, and uvula can be visualized. Class II: Faucial pillars and soft palate can be visualized. Class III: Only the base of the uvula can be visualized. Class IV: None of the three structures can be visualized.

EMERGENCY DEPARTMENT CARE AND DISPOSITION

- All patients who require airway management should be on a cardiac monitor, receive pulse oximetry with oxygen, and have IV access.
- The method of airway management is dependent upon the patient, the indications, and the perceived airway difficulty. Options for airway management include bag-valve-mask, tracheal intubation, alternative non-invasive airways, and surgical airways.
- If indicated on initial assessment, definitive airway management should not be delayed until the results of arterial blood gases are received.

TRACHEAL INTUBATION

- Tracheal intubation is the most common technique for definitive airway management.
- It is associated with a high success rate and a low complication rate and ensures airway protection, patency, and facilitation of ventilation and oxygenation.[2]
- Orotracheal intubation is associated with a higher success rate and lower complication rate than nasotracheal intubation.[2]

EMERGENCY DEPARTMENT CARE AND DISPOSITION

- Orotracheal intubation using rapid sequence intubation (RSI) techniques is the preferred method of tracheal intubation.[2,3]

- A laryngoscope using a number 3 or 4 Macintosh blade or a number 3 Miller (straight) blade is sufficient for most adults, depending on size and intubator preference.
- An endotracheal tube with an internal diameter of 7.5 to 8.0 mm and 8.0 to 8.5 mm is appropriate for most adult females and males, respectively.
- Endotracheal tubes with high-volume, low-pressure cuffs are preferred for the prevention of aspiration and to avoid ischemia of the tracheal mucosa.[4]
- The tube ideally is placed 2 cm above the carina. From the corner of the mouth, this is approximately 23 cm in men and 21 cm in women.[5]
- Patient positioning is critical to successful intubation. Flexion of the lower neck with extension at the atlanto-occipital joint aligns the oropharyngeolarygeal axes, allowing better glottic visualization.
- RSI involves the combined administration of an induction agent and a neuromuscular blocking agent to facilitate tracheal intubation.[2] The following steps are taken:
  1. Preparation of the patient and equipment and assessment of airway difficulty.
  2. Preoxygenation with 100% oxygen.
  3. Administration of pretreatment agents to blunt adverse responses to RSI in selected patients. The four most commonly used agents are lidocaine, opioids, defasciculating agents, and atropine.
  4. Administration of an induction agent (Table 3-1).[6]
  5. Administration of neuromuscular blockade. Succinylcholine is the most common agent used because of its rapid onset and short duration of action.[2] Some adverse effects are unique to depolarizing agents (Table 3-2).[7] Nondepolarizing agents

TABLE 3-1 Sedative Induction Agents

AGENT	DOSE	INDUCTION	DURATION	BENEFITS	CAVEATS
Thiopental	3–5 mg/kg IV	30–60 S	10–30 min	↓ ICP	↓ BP
Methohexital	1 mg/kg IV	<1 min	5–7 min	↓ ICP Short duration	↓ BP Seizures Laryngospasm
Ketamine	1–2 mg/kg IV	1 min	5 min	Bronchodilator "Dissociative" amnesia	↑ Secretions ↑ ICP Emergence phenomenon
Etomidate	0.3 mg/kg IV	<1 min	10–20 min	↓ ICP ↓ IOP Neutral BP	Myoclonic excitation Vomiting No analgesia
Propofol	0.5–1.5 mg/kg IV	20–40 s	8–15 min	Antiemetic Anticonvulsant ↓ ICP	Apnea ↓ BP No analgesia
Fentanyl	3–8 μg/kg IV	1–2 min	20–30 min	Reversible analgesia Neutral BP	Highly variable dose ICP: variable effects Chest wall rigidity

ABBREVIATIONS: ICP = intracranial pressure; IOP = intraocular pressure.

TABLE 3-2 Succinylcholine

Adult dose	1.0–1.5 mg/kg
Onset	45–60 s
Duration	5–9 min
Benefits	Rapid onset, short duration
Complications	Bradyarrhythmias
	Masseter spasm
	Increased intragastric, intraocular, and possibly intracranial pressure
	Malignant hyperthermia
	Hyperkalemia
	Prolonged apnea with pseudocholinesterase deficiency
	Fasciculation-induced musculoskeletal trauma
	Histamine release
	Cardiac arrest

can be used, but all have a much longer duration of action and a generally slower onset (Table 3-3).

6. Protection from passive reflux with cricoid pressure (Sellick's maneuver).
7. Insertion of the endotracheal tube.
8. Confirmation of tube placement.

• If the vocal cords are not visualized, manipulation of the thyroid cartilage using backwards, upwards, or rightwards pressure (the "burp" maneuver) may bring the cords into view. If unsuccessful, reoxygenation may need to be performed with a bag-valve-mask device. Consider changing the blade, the tube size, or the position of the patient prior to further attempts.

• Tracheal placement of the tube should be confirmed by clinical measures: visualization of the tube passing through the cords, tube condensation, chest and epigastric auscultation, and chest wall expansion.

• Clinical confirmation can be falsely positive and must be supplemented with either end-tidal CO_2 detectors or esophageal detection devices.[8,9]

• Several methods are available to assist with difficult orotracheal intubation: digital intubation, a semirigid stylet (gum-elastic bougie), transillumination with a lighted stylet, fiberoptic-assisted intubation, and retrograde tracheal intubation.[10,11]

• A failed airway is defined as three consecutive unsuccessful attempts at intubation attempted by the most experienced operator.

NASOTRACHEAL INTUBATION

• Nasotracheal intubation may be indicated when laryngoscopy is predicted to be difficult or neuromuscular blockade is contraindicated.

• The nares should be sprayed with a topical vasoconstrictor and anesthetic.

• Tube size is generally 1.0 mm smaller than that used for an oral intubation.

• The tube is inserted in a spontaneously breathing patient, ideally upon the initiation of inspiration.

• The optimal depth placement of a nasotracheal tube, measured from the nares, is 28 cm in men and 26 cm in women.[5]

• Nasotracheal intubation is associated with a lower success rate and a higher complication rate than RSI-assisted orotracheal intubation.[2]

ALTERNATIVE NONINVASIVE AIRWAY TECHNIQUES

• The primary alternative to tracheal intubation is bag-valve-mask (BVM) ventilation.

• BVM provides ventilation and oxygenation, but not airway protection from aspiration.

• The incidence of "can't intubate, can't ventilate" is estimated to be 1:1000 to 1:10,000 patients.

• Several airway rescue devices are available as alternatives to tracheal intubation.

EMERGENCY DEPARTMENT CARE AND DISPOSITION

• BVM is most effective using two-person technique, with positioning similar to that for intubation, and with nasal or oral airways in place.[12]

TABLE 3-3 Nondepolarizing Neuromuscular Relaxants

AGENT	ADULT INTUBATING IV DOSE	ONSET	DURATION	COMPLICATIONS
Vecuronium (intermediate/long)	0.08–0.15 mg/kg 0.15–0.28 mg/kg (high-dose protocol)	2–4 min	25–40 min 60–120 min	Prolonged recovery time in the obese or elderly, or if there is hepatorenal dysfunction
Rocuronium (intermediate/long)	0.6 mg/kg	1–3 min	30–45 min	Tachycardia
Doxacurium	0.05–0.08 mg/kg	3.5 min	80–100 min	Prolonged block
Atracurium (intermediate)	0.4–0.5 mg/kg	2–3 min	25–45 min	Hypotension Histamine release Bronchospasm

- Esophageal airways are devices used primarily in the prehospital setting when orotracheal intubation is not an option. The devices are inserted blindly in apneic unconscious patients.[13]
- Types of esophageal airways include the esophageal obturator airway, the pharyngotracheal lumen airway, the esophageal tracheal Combitube, and the tracheo-esophageal airway.
- A laryngeal mask airway (LMA) can be placed blindly without manipulation of the patient's head.[14] The LMA does not protect against aspiration and should be considered a temporizing device in the emergency setting.
- The intubating LMA (ILMA) provides a conduit to facilitate endotracheal intubation.[15] Blind intubation through the ILMA is over 90% successful and improves to almost 100% when a lighted stylet or fiberoptic bronchoscope is used to assist.[16]

SURGICAL AIRWAY TECHNIQUES

- The most common indication for a surgical airway is failure to intubate and ventilate. This may be secondary to acute airway obstruction, or rarely a failed intubation in a paralyzed patient.
- The incidence has been reported to be as high as 2%; however, recent studies suggest a rate less than 1%.[2,18]
- Most emergency surgical airway techniques access the airway through the cricothyroid membrane in the midline between the cricoid cartilage and the thyroid cartilage, approximately one third the distance from the manubrium to the mentum.

EMERGENCY DEPARTMENT CARE AND DISPOSITION

- An emergency cricothyrotomy requires a scalpel, a tracheal hook, and a dilator.
- Cricothyrotomy should be considered a blind technique. Success rates are only 70% for inexperienced clinicians.[17]
- A #4 Shiley tracheal tube is an adequate size for the majority of adults.
- Complications include bleeding, creation of a false passage outside the trachea, injury to structures of the neck, and pneumothorax. Delayed voice changes and stenosis may occur.[18]
- Cricothyrotomy is contraindicated in patients younger than 12 years of age because of the small size of the membrane, and needle cricothyrotomy should be used in these patients.
- Needle cricothyrotomy utilizes a large-gauge needle to access the cricothyroid membrane. Oxygenation can be performed with a BVM, or preferably with jet ventilation.
- Jet ventilation should be set at 50 psi for adults and 25 psi for children. Four seconds of expiration is allowed for each second of insufflation.

REFERENCES

1. Mallampati SR, Gatt SP, Gugino LD, et al: A clinical sign to predict difficult tracheal intubation: A prospective study. *Can Anaesth Soc J* 32:429, 1985.
2. Sackles JC, Laurin EG, Rantapaa AA, et al: Airway management in the emergency department: A one year study of 610 tracheal intubations. *Ann Emerg Med* 31:325, 1998.
3. Ma OJ, Bentley B II, Debehnke DJ: Airway management practices in emergency medicine residencies. *Am J Emerg Med* 13:501, 1995.
4. Barnhard WN, Cottrell JE, Sirakumarana C, et al: Adjustment of intracuff pressure to prevent aspiration. *Anesthesiology* 50:513, 1979.
5. Reed DB, Clinton JE: Proper depth of placement of nasotracheal tubes in adults prior to radiographic confirmation. *Acad Emerg Med* 4:1111, 1997.
6. Sivilotti MLA, Ducharme J: Randomized double-blind study on sedatives and hemodynamics during rapid-sequence intubation in the emergency department: The SHRED study. *Ann Emerg Med* 31:313, 1998.
7. Zink BJ, Snyder HS, Raccio-Robak N: Lack of a hyperkalemic response in emergency department patients receiving succinylcholine. *Acad Emerg Med* 2:974, 1995.
8. Ward KR, Yealy DM: End-tidal carbon dioxide monitoring in emergency medicine, part 2: Clinical applications. *Acad Emerg Med* 5:637, 1998.
9. Bozeman WP, Hexter D, Liang HK, Kelen GD: Esophageal detector device versus detection of end-tidal carbon dioxide level in emergency intubation. *Ann Emerg Med* 27:595, 1996.
10. Margolis GS, Menegazzi J, Abdlehak M, et al: The efficacy of a standard training program for transillumination-guided endotracheal intubation. *Acad Emerg Med* 3:371, 1996.
11. Van Stralen DW, Rogers M, Perkin RM, et al: Retrograde intubation training using a mannequin. *Am J Emerg Med* 13:50, 1995.
12. Jesudian MCS, Harrison BA, Keenan RL, et al: Bag-valve mask ventilation: Two rescuers better than one. *Crit Care* 13:122, 1985.
13. Hammargren Y, Clinton JE, Ruiz E: A standard comparison of esophageal obturator airway and endotracheal tube ventilation in cardiac arrest. *Ann Emerg Med* 14:953, 1985.
14. Calder I, Ordman AJ, Jackowski A, Crockard HA: The Brain laryngeal mask airway—An alternative to emergency tracheal intubation. *Anaesthesia* 45:137, 1990.
15. Levitan RM, Ochroch EA, Stuart S, et al: Use of intubating laryngeal mask airway by medical and non-medical personnel. *Am J Emerg Med* 18:12, 2000.
16. Ferson DZ, Rosenblatt WH, Johansen MJ, Osbom I, Ovassapian A: Use of the intubating LMA-Fastrach in 254 pa-

tients with difficult-to-manage airways. *Anesthesiology* 95: 1175, 2001.

17. Eisenburger P: Comparison of conventional surgical versus Seldinger technique emergency cricothyrotomy performed by inexperienced clinicians. *Anesthesiology* 92:687, 2000.

18. Erlandson MJ, Clinton JE, Ruiz E, Cohen J: Cricothyroidotomy in the emergency department revisited. *J Emerg Med* 7:115, 1989.

For further reading in *Emergency Medicine: A Comprehensive Study Guide*, 6th ed., see Chap. 18, "Noninvasive Airway Management," by A. Michael Roman; Chap. 19, "Tracheal Intubation and Mechanical Ventilation," by Daniel F. Danzl and Robert J. Vissers; and Chap. 20, "Surgical Airway Management," by David R. Gens.

4   DYSRHYTHMIA MANAGEMENT AND CARDIOVASCULAR PHARMACOLOGY

James K. Takayesu

THE NORMAL CARDIAC CONDUCTING SYSTEM

- The heart consists of three types of specialized tissue: (a) pacemaker cells that spontaneously depolarize and can initiate electrical impulses; (b) conductive cells that transmit electrical impulses more rapidly than other cardiac cells, causing rapid propagation of the impulse throughout the heart; and (c) myocardial cells that contract when electrically depolarized.
- The sinoatrial (SA) node is the dominant cardiac pacemaker. Its blood supply comes from the right coronary artery in 55% of individuals, and from the left circumflex artery in the remaining 45%. The normal rate for the SA node is 60 to 100 beats per minute (bpm).
- Normally, electrical impulses from the atria can reach the ventricles only by passing through the atrioventricular (AV) node and infranodal conduction system.
- The AV node receives its blood supply from the right coronary artery in 90% of individuals and from the left circumflex artery in the remaining 10%. This accounts for the common occurrence of AV conduction disturbances with acute inferior myocardial infarctions (MI).
- The AV node has two important electrophysiologic characteristics: it slows atrioventricular conduction and has a long refractory period, both of which allow time for atrial contraction to provide an additional

10% end-diastolic volume to the ventricles. This "atrial kick" is most important for patients with left ventricular failure.
- Electrical impulses leave the inferior pole of the AV node through the bundle of His, which consists of rapidly conducting Purkinje cells. The bundle of His divides into the right (RBB) and left bundle branches (LBB). The LBB divides into a narrow left anterior fascicle (LAF) and a broader left posterior fascicle (LPF).

THE NORMAL ELECTROCARDIOGRAM (ECG)

- In Fig. 4-1, depolarization starts on the left side of the ventricular septum and initially proceeds to the right; this is recorded as a small negative deflection in the recording electrode.
- Subsequent depolarization involves the free walls of both ventricles. Since the left ventricle (LV) has a greater mass compared to the right ventricle (RV), the net sum of electrical activity is directed toward the recording electrode (V_6) and a tall, positive deflection is recorded.

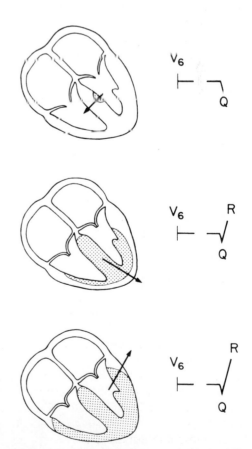

FIG. 4-1. Ventricular depolarization recorded in lead V_6.

- The P-QRS-T complex of the normal ECG represents electrical activity over one cardiac cycle (Fig. 4-2).
- The P wave is caused by atrial depolarization. The dominant QRS complex usually obscures atrial repolarization. The normal P-wave duration is less than 0.10 seconds (2.5 mm), and the normal amplitude is less than 0.3 mV (3 mm).
- The PR interval is the time between the onset of depolarization in the atria and the onset of depolarization in the ventricles. It is commonly used as an estimate of AV nodal conduction time because the AV node is the most common site for delay in atrioventricular conduction. For adults in sinus rhythm, the PR interval is 0.12 to 0.20 seconds (3 to 5 mm) at a velocity of 25 mm/s.
- The QRS complex represents ventricular depolarization, which in the normal heart, is performed by the His-Purkinje conduction system. These specialized cells rapidly propagate electrical impulses and coordinate myocardial depolarization. The normal QRS duration is 0.06 to 0.10 seconds (1.5 to 2.5 mm). Any delay in intraventricular conduction results in a widened QRS complex.
- Ectopic impulses that originate below the His bundle and impulses that arrive prior to repolarization of the bundle branches also result in a widened QRS because they do not use the Purkinje system.
- While small negative initial deflections (Q waves) are normal, large Q waves can be due to an electrically unexcitable area under the recording electrode. An abnormal Q wave has a width of 0.04 seconds or greater and an amplitude one third that of the QRS complex.
- The ST segment represents the plateau phase of ventricular depolarization. While the ST segment is usually isoelectric, a small deviation of less than 0.1 mV (1 mm) is not always pathologic.

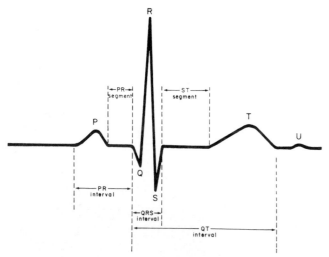

FIG. 4-2. Normal P-QRS-T ECG pattern.

- The T wave is caused by ventricular repolarization. While depolarization is a rapid, near-instantaneous process executed by the conduction system, repolarization is a slow, asynchronous event in which the metabolic machinery of each individual myocardial cell works to restore the transmembrane potential. Therefore, the T-wave duration is much longer and the amplitude much lower than those of the QRS complex.
- The QT interval represents the sum of ventricular depolarization and repolarization. While the QT interval is commonly between 0.33 and 0.42 seconds, it varies inversely with heart rate. The corrected QT interval (QTc) is obtained by dividing the measured QT interval (in seconds) by the square root of the R-R interval (in seconds). The normal QTc interval is less than 0.47 seconds.
- The U wave may be seen as a normal component of the surface ECG. The classic explanation is that the U wave represents the delayed repolarization of the Purkinje network. A pronounced U wave may be seen in patients with hypokalemia.

CARDIAC DYSRHYTHMIAS

MECHANISMS OF TACHYDYSRHYTHMIAS

- There are three accepted mechanisms for tachydysrhythmias: (1) increased automaticity in a normal or ectopic site, (2) reentry in a normal or accessory pathway, and (3) after-depolarizations triggering self-sustaining rhythms.
- An ectopic focus is an area of the heart away from the SA node pacemaker, that assumes independent pacemaker activity and usurps the SA node.
- These ectopic pacemakers can be the result of (1) enhanced automaticity of subsidiary pacemaker cells (ie, in the AV node or infranodal conducting system) or (2) abnormal automaticity of myocardial cells due to ischemia- or drug-induced spontaneous depolarization. Dysrhythmias due to an ectopic focus usually have a gradual onset ("warm-up period"). Their termination is also gradual, as opposed to the abrupt onset and termination seen with re-entrant or triggered mechanisms.
- Re-entry requires a temporary or permanent unidirectional block in one limb of a circuit and slower-than-normal conduction around the entire circuit. These conditions are secondary to disease, drugs, accessory pathways, or when tissue is stimulated during the relative refractory period (ie, before full repolarization), as with premature depolarizations.
- As indicated in Fig. 4-3, the inciting impulse traveling in the normal downward direction encounters the two

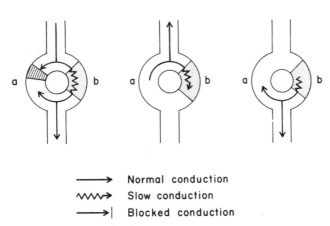

→ Normal conduction
〰→ Slow conduction
→| Blocked conduction

FIG. 4-3. Re-entry circuit.

limbs, and finding limb *a* blocked, travels down limb *b*. Upon reaching the bottom portion of the circuit where the two limbs rejoin, the impulse can then travel in a retrograde fashion back up limb *a*, reaching the upper connection of the circuit. Normally, conduction is so rapid that the impulse would encounter limb *b* still refractory to stimulation and no further propagation would occur. However, if conduction around the circuit were slow enough, limb *b* would be able to conduct the impulse again in the anterograde direction, completing the circular, or re-entrant, pathway.

- Re-entry can occur around anatomically defined circuits (eg, AV node or myocardial infarct scar tissue), resulting in a regular rapid rhythm such as paroxysmal supraventricular tachycardia (PSVT) or ventricular tachycardia (VT). Conversely, re-entry can also occur in a disorganized and chaotic fashion through a syncytium of myocardial tissue—as seen, for example, in atrial (AF) or ventricular fibrillation (VF).
- Triggered dysrhythmias are due to the oscillations of the transmembrane potential during or after repolarization (after-potentials). Under certain ideal conditions of rate, after-potentials reach threshold and trigger a complete depolarization (after-depolarization). Once triggered, this process may be self-sustaining.
- The urgency with which tachydysrhythmias require treatment is guided by two considerations: (1) evidence of hypoperfusion (eg, shock, altered mental status, anginal chest pain, or pulmonary edema) and (2) the potential to degenerate into a more serious dysrhythmia or cardiac arrest (eg, VT into VF).

MECHANISMS OF BRADYDYSRHYTHMIAS

- Bradydysrhythmias can be caused by two mechanisms: depression of SA nodal activity or conduction system blocks. In both situations, subsidiary

pacemakers take over pacing of the heart; and, provided the pacemaker is located above the bifurcation of the His bundle, the rate is generally adequate to maintain cardiac output.

- The need for emergent treatment of bradycardias is guided by two considerations: (1) evidence of hypoperfusion; or (2) the bradydysrhythmia is due to structural disease of the infranodal conducting system (either transient or permanent) that may degenerate into complete AV block or asystole.
- Two main interventions are currently available for emergent treatment of bradycardias: atropine and transcutaneous cardiac pacing. (Although isoproterenol has been used in the past, its use is currently not favored due to significant adverse effects compared to these other therapies.)
- Internal pacing is the definitive treatment for progressive or persistent bradycardias. Emergent internal pacing is possible with the use of balloon-tipped flotation catheters; however, it is often technically difficult to achieve stable internal placement in a patient with low cardiac output without fluoroscopic guidance.

SUPRAVENTRICULAR DYSRHYTHMIAS

SINUS DYSRHYTHMIA

CLINICAL FEATURES
- Some variation in the SA node discharge rate is common, but if the variation exceeds 0.12 seconds between the longest and shortest intervals, sinus dysrhythmia is present.
- The ECG characteristics of sinus dysrhythmia are: (1) normal sinus P waves and PR intervals; (2) 1:1 AV conduction; and (3) variation of at least 0.12 seconds between the shortest and longest P-P interval (Fig. 4-4).
- Sinus dysrhythmias are primarily affected by respiration and are most commonly found in children and young adults, disappearing with advancing age. Occasional junctional escape beats may be present during very long P-P intervals.

EMERGENCY DEPARTMENT CARE AND DISPOSITION
- No treatment is required.

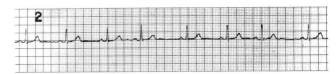

FIG. 4-4. Sinus dysrhythmia.

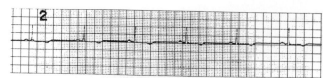

FIG. 4-5. Sinus bradycardia, rate 44.

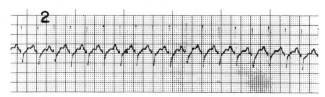

FIG. 4-6. Sinus tachycardia, rate 176.

SINUS BRADYCARDIA

CLINICAL FEATURES

- Sinus bradycardia occurs when the SA node rate falls below 60 bpm.
- The ECG characteristics of sinus bradycardia are: (1) normal sinus P waves and PR intervals, (2) 1:1 AV conduction, and (3) atrial rate below 60 bpm (Fig. 4-5).
- Sinus bradycardia represents a suppression of the sinus node discharge rate, usually in response to three categories of stimuli: (1) physiologic (vagal tone); (2) pharmacologic (calcium channel blockers, β-blockers, digoxin); and (3) pathologic (acute inferior myocardial infarction, increased intracranial pressure, carotid sinus hypersensitivity, hypothyroidism, sick sinus syndrome).

EMERGENCY DEPARTMENT CARE AND DISPOSITION

- Sinus bradycardia usually does not require specific treatment unless the heart rate is below 50 bpm and there is evidence of hypoperfusion.
- Initial therapy should begin with atropine 0.5 mg IV and may be repeated every 3 to 5 minutes up to a total of 3 mg IV.
- Transcutaneous cardiac pacing can be used in patients refractory to atropine.
- Epinephrine 2 to 10 μg/min IV or dopamine 3 to 10 μg/kg/min IV (moderate dose infusion causing β$_1$ stimulation with increased contractility) may be used if external pacing is not available.
- Internal pacing may be required in the patient with symptomatic recurrent or persistent sinus bradycardia due to sick sinus syndrome.

SINUS TACHYCARDIA

CLINICAL FEATURES

- The ECG characteristics of sinus tachycardia are (1) normal sinus P waves and PR intervals; (2) an atrial rate usually between 100 and 160 bpm, but occasionally may be higher; and (3) normally, 1:1 conduction between the atria and ventricles (although rapid rates can occur with AV blocks) (Fig. 4-6).
- Sinus tachycardia is in response to three categories of stimuli: (1) physiologic (pain, exertion); (2) pharmacologic (sympathomimetics, caffeine, bronchodilators); or (3) pathologic (fever, hypoxia, anemia, hypovolemia, pulmonary embolism, and hyperthyroidism).
- In many of these conditions, the increased heart rate is an effort to increase cardiac output to match increased circulatory needs.

EMERGENCY DEPARTMENT CARE AND DISPOSITION

- The underlying condition should be diagnosed and treated.

PREMATURE ATRIAL CONTRACTIONS (PACS)

CLINICAL FEATURES

- The ECG characteristics of premature atrial contractions are: (1) ectopic P wave appears sooner (premature) than the next expected sinus beat; (2) the ectopic P wave has a different shape and direction; and (3) the ectopic P wave may or may not be conducted through the AV node (Fig. 4-7).
- Most PACs are conducted with typical QRS complexes, but some may be conducted aberrantly through the infranodal system. When the PAC occurs during the absolute refractory period, it is not conducted. The sinus node is often depolarized and reset so that, while the interval following the PAC is often slightly longer than the previous cycle's length, the pause is less than fully compensatory.
- PACs are associated with stress, fatigue, alcohol use, tobacco, coffee, chronic obstructive pulmonary disease (COPD), digoxin toxicity, coronary artery disease (CAD), and may occur after adenosine-converted PSVT.
- PACs are common in all ages and are often seen in the absence of significant heart disease. Patients may present complaining of palpitations or an intermittent "sinking" or "fluttering" feeling in their chest.

EMERGENCY DEPARTMENT CARE AND DISPOSITION

- Any precipitating drugs (alcohol, tobacco, or coffee) or toxins should be discontinued.
- Underlying disorders should be treated (stress, fatigue).
- PACs that produce significant symptoms or initiate sustained tachycardias can be suppressed with various agents such as β-adrenergic antagonists (eg, metoprolol 25 to 50 mg PO tid), usually in consultation with a follow-up physician.

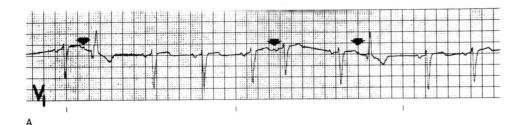

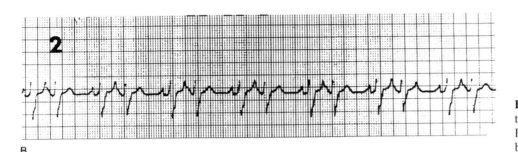

FIG. 4-7. Premature atrial contractions (PACs). **A.** Ectopic P' waves (arrows). **B.** Atrial bigeminy.

MULTIFOCAL ATRIAL TACHYCARDIA (MAT)

CLINICAL FEATURES
- Multifocal atrial tachycardia is caused by at least three different sites of atrial ectopy.
- The ECG characteristics of MAT are (1) three or more differently shaped P waves; (2) varying PP, PR, and R-R intervals; and (3) atrial rhythm usually between 100 and 180 bpm (Fig. 4-8). Because the rhythm is irregularly irregular, MAT can be confused with atrial flutter or fibrillation.
- MAT is most often found in elderly patients with decompensated COPD, but it also may be found in patients with congestive heart failure (CHF), sepsis, methylxanthine toxicity, or digoxin toxicity.

EMERGENCY DEPARTMENT CARE AND DISPOSITION
- Treatment is directed toward the underlying disorder.
- Specific antidysrhythmic treatment is uncommonly indicated.
- Magnesium sulfate 2 g IV over 60 seconds, followed by a constant infusion of 1 to 2 g/h, has been shown to decrease ectopy and convert MAT to sinus rhythm in many patients.
- Since COPD and CHF are relative contraindications to β-blockade, rate control may be achieved

with verapamil 5 to 10 mg IV or diltiazem 10 to 20 mg IV.
- Potassium levels should be raised to greater than 4 mEq/L to increase myocardial membrane stability (see Chap. 6).

ATRIAL FLUTTER

CLINICAL FEATURES
- Atrial flutter is a rhythm that originates from a small area within the atria. The exact mechanism is not known; however, possible mechanisms include re-entry, automatic focus, or triggered dysrhythmia.
- ECG characteristics of atrial flutter are (1) a regular atrial rate between 250 and 350 bpm (most commonly between 280 and 320 bpm); (2) "sawtooth" flutter waves directed superiorly and most visible in leads II, III, and aVF; and (3) AV block, usually 2:1, but occasionally greater or irregular (Fig. 4-9).
- Carotid sinus massage or Valsalva maneuvers are useful techniques to slow the ventricular response by increasing the degree of AV block, which can unmask flutter waves in uncertain cases.
- Atrial flutter is most commonly seen in patients with ischemic heart disease. Less common causes include

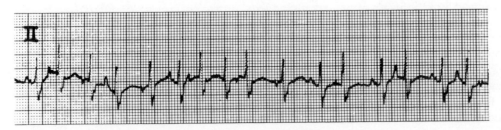

FIG. 4-8. Multifocal atrial tachycardia (MAT).

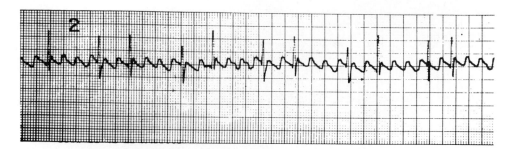

FIG. 4-9. Atrial flutter.

CHF, acute MI, pulmonary embolus, myocarditis, blunt chest trauma, and digoxin toxicity.

- Atrial flutter may be a transitional dysrhythmia between sinus rhythm and atrial fibrillation.
- Anticoagulation should be considered in patients with an unclear time of onset or duration greater than 48 hours prior to conversion to sinus rhythm, due to increased risk of atrial thrombus and embolization.

EMERGENCY DEPARTMENT CARE AND DISPOSITION

- For unstable patients or patients with onset less than 48 hours prior to presentation, low-energy synchronized cardioversion (25 to 50 J) can convert more than 90% of patients into sinus rhythm.
- Stable patients with atrial flutter for greater than 48 hours duration should be anticoagulated with heparin (80 U/kg IV followed by an infusion at 18 U/kg/h IV). A transesophageal echocardiogram (TEE) can be performed to rule out atrial thrombus prior to early cardioversion in these patients. If this cannot be performed, patients should be anticoagulated for a minimum of 3 weeks prior to chemical or electrical cardioversion.
- Rate control with diltiazem 20 mg (0.25 mg/kg) IV over 2 minutes is indicated for patients with both normal and impaired (defined by current Advanced Cardiac Life Support [ACLS] guidelines as ejection fraction less than 40% or CHF) cardiac systolic function. A second dose of 25 mg (0.35 mg/kg) IV can be given in 15 minutes if adequate rate control is not achieved. An infusion of 5 to 15 mg/h may be necessary after the initial dose to maintain rate control.
- Alternative rate control agents for patients with normal cardiac function include verapamil 5 to 10 mg IV, metoprolol 5 to 10 mg IV, and digoxin 0.5 mg IV.
- Alternative agents for patients with impaired cardiac function include digoxin 0.5 mg IV and amiodarone 150 mg IV over 10 minutes followed by an infusion of 900 mg IV at 1 mg/min for 6 hours, then 0.5 mg/min to a total of 2 g IV.
- Patients with atrial flutter for less than 48 hours' duration can be considered for chemical or electrical cardioversion in the emergency department. For patients with normal cardiac function, chemical cardioversion can be performed with amiodarone (as

above) or ibutilide 0.01 mg/kg IV up to 1 mg infused over 10 minutes. A second ibutilide dose may be given if there is no response in 20 minutes. Because of the possibility of provoking torsades de pointes, do not administer ibutilide to patients with known structural heart disease, hypokalemia, prolonged QTc intervals, hypomagnesemia, or CHF. Other chemical cardioversion agents include procainamide, flecainide, and propafenone (see cardiovascular pharmacology for details). Patients with impaired cardiac function may be cardioverted with amiodarone or electrically.

ATRIAL FIBRILLATION (AF)

CLINICAL FEATURES

- AF occurs when there are multiple small areas of atrial myocardium continuously discharging in a disorganized fashion. This results in loss of effective atrial contraction and decreases LV end-diastolic volume, which may precipitate CHF in patients with impaired cardiac function.
- The ECG characteristics of AF are (1) fibrillatory waves of atrial activity, best seen in leads V_1, V_2, V_3, and aVF; and (2) an irregularly irregular ventricular response, usually between 170 and 180 bpm in patients with a healthy AV node (Fig. 4-10).
- Predisposing factors for AF are increased atrial size and mass, increased vagal tone, and variation in refractory periods between different parts of the atrial myocardium.
- Atrial fibrillation can be idiopathic (lone AF) or may be found in association with long-standing hypertension, ischemic heart disease, rheumatic heart disease, alcohol use ("holiday heart"), COPD, or thyrotoxicosis.

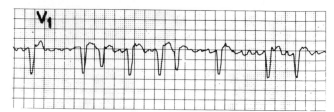

FIG. 4-10. Atrial fibrillation.

- Unanticoagulated patients with AF have a yearly embolic event rate as high as 5% and a lifetime risk of greater than 25%. Cardioversion from chronic AF to sinus rhythm carries a 1 to 2% risk of arterial embolism. Therefore one must consider anticoagulation with heparin prior to conversion to sinus rhythm in patients with AF for greater than 48 hours' duration and in those patients with an uncertain time of onset.

EMERGENCY DEPARTMENT CARE AND DISPOSITION
- Unstable patients should be treated with synchronized cardioversion (100 to 200 J). Over 60% can be converted with 100 J and over 80% with 200 J.
- Stable patients with AF for greater than 48 hours' duration should be anticoagulated with heparin (80 U/kg IV followed by infusion of 18 U/kg/h IV) prior to cardioversion. A TEE should be considered to rule out atrial thrombus prior to cardioversion.
- Rate control with diltiazem 20 mg (0.25 mg/kg) IV over 2 minutes is extremely effective for patients with both normal and impaired (ejection fraction less than 40% or CHF) cardiac systolic function. A second dose of 25 mg (0.35 mg/kg) IV can be given in 15 minutes if rate control is not achieved. An infusion of 5 to 15 mg/h may be started after the initial dose to maintain rate control.
- Alternative rate control agents for patients with normal cardiac function include verapamil 5 to 10 mg IV, metoprolol 5 to 10 mg IV, and digoxin 0.5 mg IV.
- Alternative agents for patients with impaired cardiac function include digoxin 0.5 mg IV and amiodarone 150 mg IV over 10 minutes followed by an infusion of 900 mg IV at 1 mg/min for 6 hours, then 0.5 mg/min to a total of 2 g IV.
- Patients with AF for less than 48 hours' duration can be considered for chemical or electrical cardioversion in the emergency department. For patients with normal cardiac function, chemical cardioversion can be performed with amiodarone, ibutilide (see comment earlier for atrial flutter), procainamide, flecainide, or propafenone. Patients with impaired cardiac function may be electrically cardioverted or chemically cardioverted with amiodarone.

SUPRAVENTRICULAR TACHYCARDIA (SVT)

CLINICAL FEATURES
- Supraventricular tachycardia is a regular, rapid rhythm that arises from either impulse re-entry or an ectopic pacemaker above the bifurcation of the His bundle.
- The re-entrant variety is the most common (Fig. 4-11). These patients often present with acute symptomatic

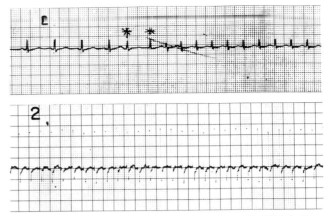

FIG. 4-11. Re-entrant supraventricular tachycardia (SVT). Top: 2nd (*) initiates run of PAT. Bottom: SVT, rate 286.

episodes termed paroxysmal supraventricular tachycardia (PSVT).
- In patients with atrioventricular bypass tracts, re-entry can occur in either direction. In 80 to 90% of patients, re-entry occurs in a direction that goes down the AV node and up the bypass tract, producing a narrow QRS complex (orthodromic conduction). In the remaining 10 to 20% of patients, re-entry occurs in the reverse direction (antidromic conduction).
- Re-entrant SVT can occur in a normal heart or in association with rheumatic heart disease, acute pericarditis, myocardial infarction, mitral valve prolapse, or one of the pre-excitation syndromes.
- Ectopic SVT usually originates in the atria with an atrial rate of 100 to 250 bpm (most commonly 140 to 200 bpm) (Fig. 4-12). This may be seen in patients with acute MI, chronic lung disease, pneumonia, alcohol intoxication, or digoxin toxicity.

EMERGENCY DEPARTMENT CARE AND DISPOSITION
- Synchronized cardioversion (25 to 50 J) should be done in any unstable patient (eg, hypotension, pulmonary edema, or severe chest pain).
- In stable patients, the first intervention should be vagal maneuvers, including:
- Carotid sinus massage: After listening to ensure that there is no carotid bruit, massage the carotid sinus against the transverse process of C6 for 10 seconds at a time, first on the side of the nondominant cerebral

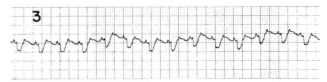

FIG. 4-12. Ectopic supraventricular tachycardia (SVT) with 2:1 AV conduction.

hemisphere. This should never be done simultaneously on both sides.

- Diving reflex: Have the patient immerse face in cold water or apply a bag of ice water to the face for 6 to 7 seconds. This maneuver is particularly effective in infants.
- Valsalva maneuver: While in the supine position, have the patient strain for at least 10 seconds. The legs may be lifted to increase venous return and augment the reflex.
- If vagal maneuvers fail, adenosine 6 mg rapid IV push followed by a 20-mL normal saline rapid flush may be used. If there is no effect within 2 minutes, a second dose of 12 mg IV can be given. Adenosine converts greater than 90% of PSVT to a sinus rhythm. Most patients experience distressing chest pain, flushing, or anxiety lasting less than 1 minute during treatment.
- In patients with narrow-complex SVT (orthodromic) and normal cardiac function, cardioversion can be achieved with nodal agents such as calcium channel blockade, β-adrenergic blockade, or digoxin:
- Diltiazem 20 mg (0.25 mg/kg) IV over 2 minutes or verapamil 0.075 to 0.15 mg/kg (3 to 10 mg) IV over 15 to 60 seconds with a repeat dose in 30 minutes if necessary. Verapamil may cause hypotension that can be treated and/or prevented with calcium chloride, 4 mL of a 10% solution.
- Esmolol 500 μg/kg initial dose, followed by an infusion of 50 μg/kg/min, metoprolol 5 to 10 mg IV, propranolol 0.5 to 1 mg IV.
- Digoxin 0.5 mg IV.
- Patients with impaired cardiac function may be cardioverted with digoxin, amiodarone 150 mg IV over 10 minutes, or diltiazem.
- In patients with digoxin toxicity, replete potassium to greater than 4.0 mEq/L and magnesium to greater than 2.0 mEq/L. Phenytoin (15 to 18 mg/kg IV infused at 50 mg/min) or lidocaine (1 to 1.5 mg/kg IV followed by an infusion at 1 to 4 mg/min) can be used. Patients unresponsive to these agents may require digoxin Fab fragments (empirically 10 vials IV).
- Patients with wide-complex SVT (antidromic) should be treated as presumed ventricular tachycardia (see section on ventricular tachycardia)

JUNCTIONAL RHYTHMS

CLINICAL FEATURES
- In patients with sinus bradycardia, SA node exit block, or AV block, junctional escape beats may occur, usually at a rate between 40 and 60 bpm, depending on the level of the rescue pacemaker within the conduction system. Junctional escape beats may conduct retrograde into the atria; however, the QRS complex will usually mask any retrograde P wave (Fig. 4-13).

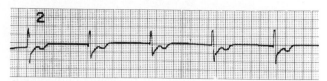

FIG. 4-13. Junctional escape rhythm, rate 42.

- When alternating rhythmically with the SA node, junctional escape beats may cause bigeminal or trigeminal rhythms.
- Sustained junctional escape rhythms may be seen with CHF, myocarditis, acute MI (especially inferior MI), hyperkalemia, or digoxin toxicity ("regularized AF"). If the ventricular rate is too slow, myocardial or cerebral ischemia may develop.
- In cases of enhanced junctional automaticity, junctional rhythms may be accelerated (60 to 100 bpm) or tachycardic (greater than 100 bpm), overriding the SA node rate.

EMERGENCY DEPARTMENT CARE AND DISPOSITION
- Isolated, infrequent junctional escape beats usually do not require specific treatment.
- If sustained junctional escape rhythms are producing symptoms, the underlying cause should be treated.
- Unstable patients with junctional rhythms can be given atropine 0.5 mg IV every 5 minutes to a total of 0.04 mg/kg to accelerate the SA node discharge rate and enhance AV nodal conduction.
- Transcutaneous or transvenous pacing is indicated in unstable patients not responsive to atropine.
- Patients with digoxin toxicity should be managed as previously discussed.

VENTRICULAR DYSRHYTHMIAS

ABERRANT VERSUS VENTRICULAR TACHYARRHYTHMIAS

- In general, most patients with wide complex tachycardia (WCT) have ventricular tachycardia (VT) and should be approached as VT until proven otherwise.
- A preceding ectopic P wave favors aberrancy, although coincidental atrial and ventricular ectopic beats or retrograde conduction can occur in VT. During a sustained run of WCT, AV dissociation favors VT.
- A varying bundle-branch block pattern suggests aberrancy. The right bundle is the slowest to repolarize within the conduction system; therefore aberrantly conducted beats tend to have a right bundle-branch block (RBBB) morphology.
- Coupling intervals are usually constant with ventricular ectopic beats, unless parasystole is present. Varying coupling intervals suggests aberrancy.

- Response to carotid sinus massage or other vagal maneuvers will slow conduction through the AV node and may abolish re-entrant SVT with aberrancy and slow the ventricular response in other supraventricular tachydysrhythmias. These maneuvers have essentially no effect on ventricular dysrhythmias.
- Fusion beats favor VT, but exceptions can occur.
- A QRS duration of longer than 0.14 seconds is usually only found in ventricular ectopy or VT.
- Historical criteria are also useful in predicting VT: age greater than 35 years old or a history of MI, CHF, or coronary artery bypass grafting in a patient with WCT strongly suggests VT.

EMERGENCY DEPARTMENT CARE AND DISPOSITION
- For pulseless patients, treat as presumed VT with unsynchronized cardioversion (200 to 360 J) followed by epinephrine or vasopressin and ACLS management (see VT and ventricular fibrillation sections).
- For stable WCT in patients with normal cardiac function, treat with procainamide or sotalol. Alternative agents include amiodarone. Patients with impaired cardiac function should be treated with amiodarone or lidocaine followed by synchronized cardioversion (see VT section).
- Adenosine 6 mg IV push may be tried prior to procainamide in stable patients with suspected SVT with aberrancy without any historical criteria indicative of possible VT (see PSVT section).

PREMATURE VENTRICULAR CONTRACTIONS (PVCS)

CLINICAL FEATURES
- Premature ventricular contractions are due to impulses originating from single or multiple areas in the ventricles.
- The ECG characteristics of PVCs are: (1) a premature and wide QRS complex; (2) no preceding P wave; (3) the ST segment and T wave of the PVC are directed opposite the preceding major QRS deflection; (4) most PVCs do not affect the sinus node, so there is usually a fully compensatory postectopic pause, or the PVC may be interpolated between two sinus beats; (5) many PVCs have a fixed coupling interval (within 0.04 second) from the preceding sinus beat; and (6) many PVCs are conducted into the atria, producing a retrograde P wave (Fig. 4-14).
- PVCs are very common, occurring in most patients with ischemic heart disease and acute MI. Other common causes of PVCs include digoxin toxicity, CHF, hypokalemia, alkalosis, hypoxia, and sympathomimetic drugs.

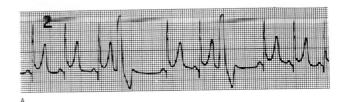

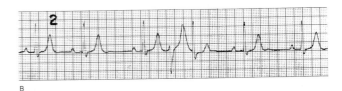

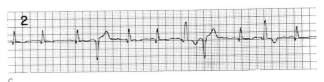

FIG. 4-14. Premature ventricular contractions (PVCs). **A.** Unifocal PVC. **B.** Interpolated PVC. **C.** Multifocal PVCs.

- Ventricular parasystole occurs when the ectopic ventricular focus fires frequently enough to compete with the SA node.

EMERGENCY DEPARTMENT CARE AND DISPOSITION
- Although single studies have suggested benefit, pooled data and meta analysis find no reduction in mortality from either suppressive or prophylactic treatment of PVCs. In fact, there has been a documented increased risk of mortality in MI patients treated with the antiarrhythmics flecainide and encainide due to their proarrhythmic effects.
- Hemodynamically unstable patients with PVCs will typically respond to lidocaine 1 to 1.5 mg/kg IV (up to 3 mg/kg), although some patients may require procainamide.
- Patients with acute coronary syndromes (ACS) and frequent PVCs should receive adequate β-adrenergic blockade to suppress ectopic rhythm generation with metoprolol 5 mg IV, up to three doses over 15 minutes.

ACCELERATED IDIOVENTRICULAR RHYTHM (AIVR)

CLINICAL FEATURES
- The ECG characteristics of accelerated idioventricular rhythm are (1) wide and regular QRS complexes not in a typical BBB pattern; (2) a rate between 40 and 100 bpm, often close to the preceding sinus rate; (3) runs short in duration (3 to 30 beats); and (4) the AIVR often begins with a fusion beat (Fig. 4-15).

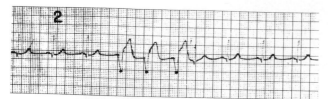

FIG. 4-15. Accelerated idioventricular rhythms (AIVR).

- This condition is found most commonly in acute myocardial ischemia and has been otherwise termed "slow VT." Rarely, normal patients may exhibit a stable AIVR.

EMERGENCY DEPARTMENT CARE AND DISPOSITION

- Treatment is not necessary. On occasion, AIVR may be the only functioning pacemaker, and suppression with lidocaine can lead to cardiac asystole.

VENTRICULAR TACHYCARDIA

CLINICAL FEATURES

- Ventricular tachycardia is the occurrence of three or more successive beats from a ventricular ectopic pacemaker at a rate greater than 100 bpm.
- The ECG characteristics of VT are: (1) a wide QRS complex; (2) a rate greater than 100 bpm (most commonly 150 to 200 bpm); (3) a regular rhythm, although there may be some beat-to-beat variation; and (4) a constant QRS axis (Fig. 4-16).
- Morphologic subtypes of VT include the following:
- Ventricular flutter: absence of any distinguishable QRS complex.
- Bidirectional VT: alternating polarity of ventricular depolarization (associated with digoxin toxicity).
- Alternating VT: alternating amplitude of the QRS complex (associated with digoxin toxicity).
- Polymorphic VT: alternating QRS morphology in at least one lead.
- Atypical VT (torsades de pointes): QRS axis swings between positive and negative axes due to spiraling ventricular depolarization (Fig. 4-17). Torsades de pointes is associated with long-QT syndrome and the Brugada syndrome (J point elevation in V_1 and V_3 with RBBB pattern). It can be provoked by procainamide, quinidine, phenothiazines, and tricyclic antidepressants (TCA) due to the QT-prolonging effects of these medications.

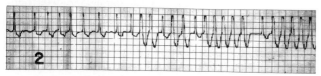

FIG. 4-16. Ventricular tachycardia.

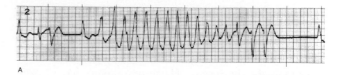

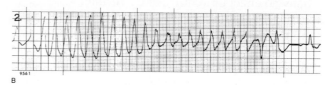

FIG. 4-17. Two examples of short runs of atypical ventricular tachycardia showing sinusoidal variation in amplitude and direction of the QRS complexes: "Le torsades de pointes" (twisting of the points). Note that example **A** is initiated by a late-occurring PVC (lead II).

- The most common causes of VT are ischemic heart disease and acute myocardial infarction. Other etiologies include hypertrophic cardiomyopathy, mitral valve prolapse, drug toxicity (digoxin, antiarrhythmics, and sympathomimetics), hypoxia, hypokalemia, and hyperkalemia.
- Adenosine appears to cause little harm in patients with VT; therefore stable patients with WCT due to suspected SVT with aberrancy (see previous section) may be treated safely with adenosine when the diagnosis is in doubt.

EMERGENCY DEPARTMENT CARE AND DISPOSITION

- Advanced Cardiac Life Support (ACLS) guidelines recommend that pulseless ventricular tachycardia be **defibrillated** with unsynchronized cardioversion starting at 200 J. Unstable patients who are not pulseless should be treated with synchronized cardioversion (200 to 360 J). VT can be converted with energies as low as 1 J and over 90% can be converted with less than 10 J; however, standard ACLS protocol begins at 200 J.
- Hemodynamically stable patients with monomorphic VT and normal cardiac function should be treated with IV procainamide at less than 20 mg/min until one of the following occur: (1) the dysrhythmia converts, (2) the total dose reaches 15 to 17 mg/kg in healthy patients (12 mg/kg in patients with CHF), or (3) early signs of toxicity develop with hypotension or QRS prolongation greater than 50%. The loading dose should be followed by a maintenance infusion of 1 to 4 mg/min in normal subjects. ACLS guidelines also recommend sotalol, amiodarone, and lidocaine as alternative agents.
- Hemodynamically stable patients with monomorphic VT and impaired cardiac function (ejection fraction less than 40% or CHF) should be treated with amiodarone 150 mg IV over 10 minutes followed by a 6-hour infusion at 1 mg/min. Alternative therapy with lidocaine 75 mg (1.0 to 1.5 mg/kg) IV over 60 to

90 seconds, followed by a constant infusion at 1 to 4 mg/min (10 to 40 μg/kg/min) is also acceptable. A repeat bolus dose of 50 mg of lidocaine may be required during the first 20 minutes to avoid a subtherapeutic dip in serum level due to the drug's early redistribution phase.

- In patients with torsades de pointes, overdrive pacing at 90 to 120 bpm may be therapeutic. Temporary pacing is the most effective and safest method to treat torsades de pointes and prevent its recurrence. Reports have shown that magnesium sulfate, 1 to 2 g IV over 60 to 90 seconds followed by an infusion of 1 to 2 g/h, is effective in abolishing torsades de pointes. These patients will require evaluation for permanent internal defibrillator placement.

VENTRICULAR FIBRILLATION (VF)

CLINICAL FEATURES

- Ventricular fibrillation is the totally disorganized depolarization and contraction of small areas of ventricular myocardium during which there is no effective ventricular pumping activity.
- The ECG shows a fine-to-coarse zigzag pattern without discernible P waves or QRS complexes (Fig. 4-18).
- Ventricular fibrillation is most commonly seen in patients with severe ischemic heart disease, with or without an acute myocardial infarction. It can also be caused by digoxin or quinidine toxicity, hypothermia, chest trauma, hypokalemia, hyperkalemia, or mechanical stimulation (eg, catheter wire).
- Primary VF occurs suddenly, without preceding hemodynamic deterioration, and usually is due to acute ischemia or peri-infarct scar re-entry. Secondary VF occurs after a prolonged period of hemodynamic deterioration due left ventricular failure or circulatory shock.

EMERGENCY DEPARTMENT CARE AND DISPOSITION

- Current ACLS guidelines recommend immediate electrical defibrillation (unsynchronized) starting at 200 J. If VF persists, defibrillation should be repeated immediately, with 200 to 300 J at the second attempt, and increased to 360 J at the third attempt. Defibrillation pads should be kept on the patient in the same location, since with successive countershocks, transthoracic impedance decreases. Defibrillation energies for biphasic shocks are lower.
- If the initial three attempts at defibrillation are unsuccessful, cardiopulmonary resuscitation (CPR) and in-

tubation should be initiated; further electrical defibrillations should be done after the administration of various intravenous drugs, including epinephrine 1 mg IV push or vasopressin 40 U IV push (one time only) followed by a 20-mL normal saline flush. Epinephrine dosing may be repeated every 3 to 5 minutes. If this is not successful, high-dose epinephrine (0.1 mg/kg) may be considered.

- Defibrillation should be attempted after each drug administration at 360 J unless lower energy levels have been previously successful.
- Between successive countershocks, antidysrhythmics should then be administered. Agents in order of current ACLS recommendation are: amiodarone 300 mg IV push, procainamide 100 mg IV push every 5 minutes, and lidocaine 1.5 mg/kg IV. Magnesium sulfate 2 g IV can be given in cases of presumed hypomagnesemia.

CONDUCTION DISTURBANCES

SINOATRIAL BLOCK

CLINICAL FEATURES

- Sinoatrial (SA) block occurs when there is a delay or failure in the conduction from the SA node to the atria (exit block).
- There are three subtypes of sinoatrial block:
  1. First-degree SA block: There is a delay of impulse conduction out of the SA node itself which is inapparent on the surface ECG.
  2. Second-degree SA block: Occasional impulses are blocked in the SA node. The variable type (Wenckebach) is caused by progressive lengthening of conduction time from the SA node to the atria, which on the surface ECG, can show shortening of successive P-P intervals until dropping of a P wave. In the constant type, SA conduction time is constant before and after the blocked sinus impulse; P-P intervals are constant multiples of each other on the ECG.
  3. Third-degree SA block: Complete blockade of the SA impulse leads to an absent P wave. This can also be seen in sinus arrest and atrial unresponsiveness.
- SA block is associated with rheumatic heart disease, MI, myocarditis, drug toxicity (digoxin, quinidine, aspirin, β-blockers, and calcium channel blockers), increased vagal tone, and sick sinus syndrome *(SSS)*.

EMERGENCY DEPARTMENT CARE AND DISPOSITION

- SA block is typically asymptomatic, requiring no treatment. However, if patients are symptomatic, treatment with atropine 0.5 mg IV can be given.
- External pacing can be performed for symptomatic patients unresponsive to atropine.

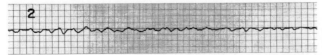

FIG. 4-18. Ventricular fibrillation.

SINUS PAUSE

CLINICAL FEATURES
- Sinus pause (arrest) is a failure of impulse formation from the SA node. The ECG shows no P-P relationship to baseline sinus cycle length.
- Sinus pause may be physiologic. It is also associated with rheumatic heart disease, MI, myocarditis, drug toxicity (digoxin, quinidine, aspirin, β-blockers, and calcium channel blockers), increased vagal tone, and sick sinus syndrome (SSS).

EMERGENCY DEPARTMENT CARE AND DISPOSITION
- Sinus pause is usually self-limited and asymptomatic, requiring no treatment. However, patients with prolonged pauses (greater than 3 to 5 seconds) may be symptomatic, requiring treatment with atropine 0.5 mg IV every 5 minutes to a maximum dose of 0.04 mg/kg.
- External pacing can be performed for symptomatic patients unresponsive to atropine.

ATRIOVENTRICULAR BLOCK

- First-degree AV block is characterized by a delay in AV conduction, manifested by a prolonged PR interval (greater than 0.2 second). It can be found in normal hearts as well as in association with increased vagal tone, digoxin toxicity, inferior MI, amyloid, and myocarditis. First-degree AV block needs no treatment and will not be discussed further.
- Second-degree AV block is characterized by intermittent AV conduction—some atrial impulses reach the ventricles while others are blocked, causing "grouped beating."
- Third-degree AV block is characterized by complete interruption in AV conduction with resulting AV dissociation.

SECOND-DEGREE MOBITZ I (WENCKEBACH) ATRIOVENTRICULAR BLOCK

CLINICAL FEATURES
- With this block there is progressive prolongation of conduction through the AV node itself until the atrial impulse is completely blocked. Usually, only a single atrial impulse is blocked at a time.
- After the dropped beat, the AV conduction returns to normal and the cycle usually repeats itself, with either the same conduction ratio (fixed ratio) or a different conduction ratio (variable ratio).
- The Wenckebach phenomenon has a seeming paradox. Although the PR intervals progressively lengthen

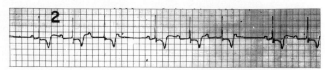

FIG. 4-19. Second-degree Mobitz I (Wenckebach) AV block 4:3 AV conduction.

prior to the dropped beat, the increments by which they lengthen **decrease** with successive beats. This produces a progressive **shortening** of each successive R-R interval prior to the dropped beat (Fig. 4-19).
- This block is often transient and usually is associated with an acute inferior MI, digoxin toxicity, myocarditis, or can be seen after cardiac surgery. Since the blockade occurs at the level of the AV node itself rather than the infranodal conducting system, this is usually a stable rhythm.

EMERGENCY DEPARTMENT CARE AND DISPOSITION
- Specific treatment is not necessary unless slow ventricular rates produce signs of hypoperfusion. In cases associated with acute inferior MI, adequate volume resuscitation should be ensured prior to initiating further interventions to correct hypotension.
- Atropine 0.5 mg IV repeated every 5 minutes as necessary may be given, titrated to the desired heart rate or until the total dose reaches 3.0 mg.
- Although rarely needed, transcutaneous pacing may be used.

SECOND-DEGREE MOBITZ II ATRIOVENTRICULAR BLOCK

CLINICAL FEATURES
- With this block, the PR interval remains constant before and after the nonconducted atrial beats (Fig. 4-20). One or more beats may be nonconducted at a single time.

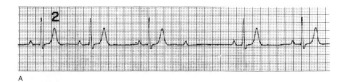

A

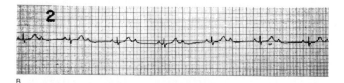

B

FIG. 4-20. A. Second-degree Mobitz II AV block. **B.** Second-degree AV block with 2:1 AV conduction.

- This block indicates significant damage or dysfunction of the infranodal conduction system, and therefore the QRS complexes are usually wide. Type II blocks are more dangerous than type I since they are usually permanent and may progress suddenly to complete heart block, especially in the setting of an acute anterior MI.
- When second-degree AV block occurs with a fixed conduction ratio of 2:1, it is not possible to differentiate between a Mobitz type I (Wenckebach) and Mobitz type II block.

EMERGENCY DEPARTMENT CARE AND DISPOSITION
- Atropine 0.5 to 1 mg IV push, repeated as needed up to 3.0 mg total dose, should be the first drug used, and pacing pads should be positioned on the patient ready for use in the case of further deterioration into complete heart block.
- Transcutaneous cardiac pacing (10 to 200 mA) is indicated in patients unresponsive to atropine.
- Transvenous pacing (0.2 to 20 mA at 40 to 140 bpm via a semi-floating or balloon-tipped pacing catheter) is indicated if transcutaneous pacing is unsuccessful. Balloon-tipped catheters are most common, and their placement into the right ventricle can be assisted by placing the patient in the right decubitus position.
- Most cases, especially in the setting of acute MI, will require permanent cardiac pacemaker placement.

THIRD-DEGREE (COMPLETE) ATRIOVENTRICULAR BLOCK

CLINICAL FEATURES
- In third-degree AV block, there is no AV conduction. The ventricles are paced by an escape pacemaker from the AV node or infranodal conduction system at a rate slower than the atrial rate (Fig. 4-21).
- When third-degree AV block occurs at the AV node, a junctional escape pacemaker takes over with a ventricular rate of 40 to 60 bpm, and since the rhythm originates from above the bifurcation of the His bundle, the QRS complexes are narrow. Nodal third-degree AV block may develop in up to 8% of acute inferior MIs and it is usually transient, although it may last for several days.
- When third-degree AV block occurs at the infranodal level, the ventricles are driven by a ventricular escape

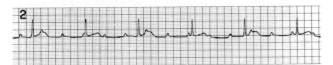

FIG. 4-21. Third-degree AV block.

rhythm at a rate less than 40 bpm. Third-degree AV block located in the bundle branch or the Purkinje system invariably has an escape rhythm with a wide QRS complex. Like Mobitz II block, this indicates structural damage to the infranodal conduction system and can be seen in acute anterior MIs. The ventricular escape pacemaker is usually inadequate to maintain cardiac output and is unstable with periods of ventricular asystole.

EMERGENCY DEPARTMENT CARE AND DISPOSITION
- Third-degree AV block should be treated the same as second-degree Mobitz II AV block, with atropine or a ventricular demand pacemaker as required.
- Transcutaneous cardiac pacing should be performed in unstable patients until a transvenous pacemaker can be placed.

BUNDLE-BRANCH AND FASCICULAR BLOCKS

- Bundle-branch and fascicular blocks are associated with ischemic heart disease, acute myocardial ischemia, post–cardiac surgery, valvular disease, myocarditis, and conduction system degeneration (Lenègre and Lev disease).
- Although unifascicular block is asymptomatic, patients presenting with syncope and bi or trifascicular block require evaluation for intermittent complete heart block requiring permanent pacemaker placement.

UNIFASCICULAR BLOCK

CLINICAL FEATURES
- Unifascicular blocks include right bundle-branch block (RBBB), left anterior fascicular block (LAFB), and left posterior fascicular block (LPFB).
- ECG findings in RBBB include: (1) left-to-right ventricular activation; (2) QRS greater than 0.12 seconds; (3) rSR' in leads V_1 and V_2; (4) wide S wave in leads I, V_5, and V_6; and (5) normal onset of ventricular activation in V_6.
- ECG findings in LAFB include: (1) inferior-to-superior and right-to-left ventricular activation; (2) normal QRS duration; (3) left axis deviation; (4) a qR complex in aVL; (5) R wave larger in lead I than leads II and III; and (6) deep S wave in the inferior leads.
- ECG findings in LPFB include: (1) superior-to-inferior and left-to-right ventricular activation; (2) normal QRS duration; (3) right axis deviation; (4) R wave in lead III larger than in lead II; and (5) qR complex in lead III.

EMERGENCY DEPARTMENT CARE AND DISPOSITION
- Although indicative of conduction system disease, these blocks are asymptomatic and require no treatment except to address the associated disorder(s).

BIFASCICULAR BLOCK

CLINICAL FEATURES
- Patients with bifascicular block are at risk for progression to complete heart block if the remaining fascicle is blocked; therefore symptomatic bifascicular block (eg, syncope) can be an indication for pacemaker placement.
- Patterns of bifascicular block: (1) RBBB and either LPFB or LAFB; or (2) left bundle-branch block (LBBB).
- ECG findings of LBBB include: (1) right-to-left and inferior-to-superior ventricular activation; (2) QRS greater than 0.12 seconds; (3) wide R wave in I, aVL, V_5, and V_6; (4) small R wave and deep S wave in II, III, aVF, V_1, V_2, and V_3; and (5) absent q in I, aVF, V_5, and V_6.

EMERGENCY DEPARTMENT CARE AND DISPOSITION
- Symptomatic patients should be admitted for monitoring and evaluated for permanent pacemaker placement.
- Patients presenting with acute MI require maximal ischemic therapy and early reperfusion with thrombolysis, percutaneous coronary intervention (PCI), or coronary artery bypass grafting (CABG).

TRIFASCICULAR BLOCK

CLINICAL FEATURES
- Patients with trifascicular block are at risk for progression to complete heart block; therefore symptomatic trifascicular block (eg, syncope) can be an indication for pacemaker placement.
- ECG findings are first-degree AV block with (1) RBBB and either LAFB or LPFB; (2) LBBB; or (3) alternating RBBB and LBBB.

EMERGENCY DEPARTMENT CARE AND DISPOSITION
- Symptomatic patients should be admitted for monitoring and evaluated for permanent pacemaker placement.
- Patients presenting with acute MI require maximal ischemic therapy and early reperfusion with thrombolysis, PCI, or CABG.

TACHYCARDIA-BRADYCARDIA SYNDROME

CLINICAL FEATURES
- Tachycardia-bradycardia syndrome, otherwise known as sick sinus syndrome (SSS), is a disorder caused by multiple abnormalities in supraventricular impulse generation and conduction, precipitating arrhythmogenic syncope and/or palpitations.
- Arrhythmias include both tachycardic (AF, junctional tachycardia, atrial flutter) and bradycardic (sinus bradycardia, sinus arrest, SA block) rhythms.
- Patients with SSS may have long-standing ischemic heart disease, rheumatic heart disease, myocarditis, rheumatologic disease, metastatic cancers, post–cardiac surgery, or cardiomyopathy.
- Exacerbations may occur in the setting of abdominal pain, hyperthyroidism, or drug therapy (digoxin, procainamide, nicotine, calcium channel blockade, or β-blockade).

EMERGENCY DEPARTMENT CARE AND DISPOSITION
- Treatment is specific to the presenting tachy- or bradycardia as discussed in previous sections.
- Symptomatic patients require permanent internal pacing. SSS is currently the most common indication for pacemaker implantation.

PACEMAKER MALFUNCTION

CLINICAL FEATURES
- Most pacemakers are demand mode pacers in which cardiac activity is sensed and pacing is initiated if no depolarization occurs within a preset sensing period.
- Pacemaker failure is due to one of four basic problems:
- Fail to sense: The pacemaker paces at a fixed rate due to a decrease in the QRS amplitude that prevents the pacemaker from sensing any intrinsic cardiac depolarizations.
- Fail to pace: The pacemaker leads fail to trigger depolarization due to fibrosis at the lead implant site.
- Over-sense: T-wave changes, external interference, or signals from other parts of the pacing system are sensed by the pacemaker as if they were spontaneous ventricular depolarizations.
- Fail to sense and pace: Lead fracture or battery failure causes complete failure of the pacing system (rare). Pacemaker batteries (lithium) have an 8- to 12-year lifespan.

EMERGENCY DEPARTMENT CARE AND DISPOSITION
- The magnetic toggle switch in pacemakers causes the pacemaker to change from demand mode to fixed pacing. This can be used in cases of malfunction to provide a fixed heart rate to the patient until the pacemaker can be interrogated. This carries a slight risk of triggering VT induced by pacing during the vulnerable period in the cardiac cycle (R on T phenomenon).
- In cases of pacer failure, transcutaneous pacing may be used with currents of 10 to 200 mA with appropriate sedation.

- Internal pacing is contraindicated due to the risk of ensnaring the pacer leads with the pacing catheter or wire, requiring surgical removal.

PRETERMINAL RHYTHMS

PULSELESS ELECTRICAL ACTIVITY

- Pulseless electrical activity (PEA) is the presence of electrical complexes without accompanying mechanical contraction of the heart.
- Potential mechanical causes should be diagnosed and treated, including severe hypovolemia, cardiac tamponade, tension pneumothorax, massive pulmonary embolus, MI, and rupture of the ventricular free wall. In addition, profound metabolic abnormalities such as acidosis, hypoxia, hypokalemia, hyperkalemia, and hypothermia should also be considered and treated.
- After intubation and initiating CPR, stabilizing treatment includes epinephrine 1 mg IV push repeated every 3 to 5 minutes. This may be followed by high-dose epinephrine at 0.1 mg/kg IV if no response is seen.
- Atropine 1 mg IV, up to 3 mg total, is also acceptable therapy if the rhythm is slow (less than 60 bpm).

IDIOVENTRICULAR RHYTHM

- Idioventricular rhythm is a ventricular escape rhythm at less than 40 bpm with a QRS wider than 0.16 second.
- It is associated with infranodal AV block, massive MI, cardiac tamponade, and exsanguinating hemorrhage.
- After intubation and initiating CPR, stabilizing treatment includes identifying contributing mechanical

factors (eg, volume resuscitation), and drug therapy with epinephrine 1 mg IV push every 3 to 5 minutes. One may also consider high-dose epinephrine at 0.1 mg/kg IV.
- Atropine has not been shown to be of benefit.

AGONAL RHYTHM

- Agonal rhythm is a wide irregular ventricular rhythm without contraction.

ASYSTOLE (CARDIAC STANDSTILL)

- Asystole is the complete absence of cardiac electrical activity.
- Treatment is the same as for pulseless electrical activity, with the addition of transcutaneous pacing if the preceding measures fail (although this is rarely successful).

PRE-EXCITATION SYNDROMES

CLINICAL FEATURES

- Pre-excitation occurs when an area of the ventricles is activated by an impulse from the atria sooner than would be expected if the impulse were transmitted down the normal conducting pathway.
- All forms of pre-excitation are felt to be due to accessory tracts that bypass part or all of the normal conducting system, the most common form being Wolff-Parkinson-White syndrome (WPW; Fig. 4-22).

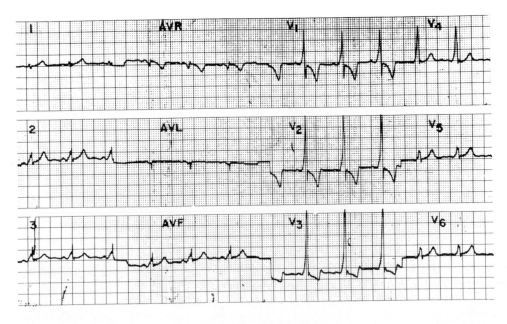

FIG. 4-22. Type A Wolff-Parkinson-White syndrome.

Activation via the AVN and myocardium causes initial fusion beat morphology with slurring of initial QRS complex, causing the pathognomonic delta wave.

- There is a high incidence of tachydysrhythmias in patients with WPW—atrial flutter (about 5%), atrial fibrillation (10 to 20%), and paroxysmal re-entrant SVT (40 to 80%). Among patients with WPW-PSVT, 80 to 90% will conduct in the orthodromic direction and the remaining 10 to 20% will conduct in the antidromic direction.
- ECG findings of AF or atrial flutter in patients with bypass tracts shows a wide QRS complex that is irregularly irregular with a rate greater than 180 to 200 bpm.

EMERGENCY DEPARTMENT CARE AND DISPOSITION

- Re-entrant SVT with a narrow QRS complex (orthodromic conduction) in the WPW syndrome can be treated like other cases of re-entrant SVT. Adenosine 6 mg IV or verapamil 5 to 10 mg IV are very successful at terminating this dysrhythmia in patients with WPW. β-Adrenergic antagonists are usually ineffective.
- Re-entrant SVT with a wide QRS complex in patients with WPW is usually associated with a bypass tract with a short refractory period that permits antidromic conduction. Patients with this type of tachycardia are at risk for rapid ventricular rates and degeneration into VF. Unstable patients should be cardioverted at 50 to 100 J. Stable patients should be treated with intravenous procainamide 100 mg IV push every 5 minutes or an infusion at 20 mg/min to a total dose of 15 to 17 mg/kg. β-Adrenergic blockers or calcium channel blockers (eg, verapamil) should be avoided.
- Atrial flutter or fibrillation with a rapid ventricular response and a wide QRS complex not known to be old is best treated with cardioversion at 50 to 100 J. Stable patients can be treated with procainamide as above.

CARDIOVASCULAR PHARMACOLOGY

- The Vaughan-Williams classification of antidysrhythmics classifies drugs based on their ability to block sodium channels (class I), block calcium channels (class IV), block β-adrenergic receptors (class II), or prolong the refractory period (class III). Digoxin and adenosine do not fit into this scheme.

CLASS I ANTIDYSRHYTHMIC AGENTS

PROCAINAMIDE

- Procainamide (IA) blocks fast sodium channels and depresses the speed of impulse conduction (phase 0) of the cardiac action potential. In so doing, it prolongs the PR interval, QT interval, and QRS complex duration. In large doses, it exerts anticholinergic activity. Rapid infusion can cause hemodynamically significant peripheral vasodilation and reflex tachycardia.
- These effects directly depress myocardial conduction, suppress fibrillatory activity in the atria and ventricles, and prevent ectopic or re-entrant dysrhythmias.
- Indications: WCT of unknown type, stable VT, stable PSVT not controlled by adenosine, and atrial fibrillation with rapid ventricular response in the setting of WPW.
- Dosing: 20 mg/min IV to a total of 15 to 17 mg/kg or until one of the following occurs: dysrhythmia conversion, QRS widening >50%, or hypotension. Maintenance infusion is at a rate of 1 to 4 mg/min. The dose must be decreased by half in patients with CHF, hypotension, and renal or hepatic failure.
- Contraindications include second- or third-degree AV block, prolonged QT interval, and torsades de pointes.
- Adverse effects of procainamide include myocardial depression, prolongation of the QRS and QT intervals, impairment of AV conduction, ventricular fibrillation, torsades de pointes, and hypotension.

LIDOCAINE

- Lidocaine (IB) preferentially depresses the automaticity (phase 4) of the distal conduction system and ischemic myocardial tissue; it does not affect normal myocardium and is not associated with peripheral vasodilation.
- Lidocaine is not effective against atrial dysrhythmias because it preferentially acts on the infranodal conduction system.
- Indications: lidocaine is a second-line treatment for ventricular dysrhythmias[1] after procainamide and amiodarone.[2]
- Dose: 1 to 1.5 mg/kg IV up to a total of 3 mg/kg. Maintenance infusions are at 1 to 4 mg/min. The dose should be reduced by 50% in patients with CHF or liver disease.
- Lidocaine is contraindicated in patients with known sensitivities to amide-type local anesthetics and in patients with second- or third-degree sinoatrial or AV block.
- Adverse effects from lidocaine usually occur when the drug is administered too rapidly in a conscious patient, when excessive doses are administered, or when a drug interaction potentiates toxicity.

- An abrupt change in mental status is a classic symptom of lidocaine toxicity. Symptoms of mild lidocaine toxicity that correlate with levels greater than 5 µg/mL include slurred speech, drowsiness, confusion, nausea, vertigo, ataxia, tinnitus, paresthesias, and muscle twitching. Serious symptoms occurring at plasma levels greater than 9 µg/mL may include psychosis, seizures, respiratory depression, and high degrees of sinoatrial or atrioventricular (AV) block.

CLASS II ANTIDYSRHYTHMICS: β BLOCKERS

METOPROLOL
- Metoprolol is a β_1 selective adrenergic antagonist that slows the sinus rate, depresses AV conduction, decreases cardiac output, and reduces blood pressure. It is a primary agent in the treatment of acute coronary ischemia for both rate control and suppression of ventricular ectopy.
- Indications: rate control and conversion of PSVT and atrial fibrillation; acute coronary ischemia.[3]
- Dose: in acute coronary syndromes and atrial tachyarrhythmias 2.5 to 5 mg IV every 5 to 15 minutes up to a total of 15 mg can be followed by 25 to 50 mg PO every 6 to 8 hours. The dose should be halved in patients with compensated heart failure.
- Adverse effects include asthma and COPD exacerbation, sinus bradycardia, AV block, and CHF.
- Decompensated CHF (New York Heart Association [NYHA] class IV) is a contraindication to its use.

PROPRANOLOL
- In therapeutic doses, the major effect of propranolol is its β-adrenergic blocking activity. The drug blocks the effects of catecholamines on β-receptors, inhibiting chronotropic, inotropic, and vasodilator responses to β-adrenergic stimulation.
- Propranolol slows the sinus rate, depresses AV conduction, decreases cardiac output, reduces blood pressure on exercise, and reduces both supine and standing blood pressures.
- Indications: rate control in supraventricular tachycardias and hyperthyroid emergencies.
- Dose: 0.5 to 1 mg IV up to 3 mg IV at a rate less than 1 mg/min.
- The drug is generally not given to patients with asthma or allergic rhinitis and is contraindicated in those with sinus bradycardia or advanced sinoatrial or AV block. Propranolol should also not be used in patients with congestive heart failure or cardiogenic shock, unless these conditions are due to tachyarrhythmias.

ESMOLOL
- Esmolol prevents excessive β-adrenergic stimulation of the myocardium by selectively blocking β_1 receptors, thus producing an increase in sinus cycle length, prolongation of SA nodal recovery time, and a prolongation in conduction through the AV node.
- Indications: rate control and conversion of PSVT and atrial fibrillation; rate control in combination with nitroprusside in acute vascular emergencies (eg, aortic dissection).
- Dose: a loading dose of 500 µg/kg IV over 1 minute is followed by an infusion starting at 50 µg/kg/min. Changes in the infusion require rebolus of 500 µg/kg IV followed by increases of 50 µg/kg/min every 5 minutes.
- The most common adverse effect associated with esmolol is hypotension, which occurs in approximately 20 to 50% of patients being treated for SVT.

LABETALOL
- Labetalol possesses membrane-stabilizing effects and thus has some antidysrhythmic action; however, the drug is often used as an antihypertensive agent because it blocks both α- and β-adrenergic receptors in a 1:7 ratio.
- Labetalol decreases heart rate, contractility, cardiac output, cardiac work, and total peripheral resistance.
- Indications: blood pressure control in acute vascular emergencies (eg, aortic dissection) and hypertensive crises.
- Dose: 20 mg IV can be given initially and the dose doubled every 10 minutes until blood pressure and heart rate control is achieved, or until a total dose of 300 mg IV is given. Infusions may be given at 0.5 to 2 mg/min IV.
- The most common adverse effect associated with labetalol use is orthostatic hypotension.
- Adverse central nervous system (CNS) effects that may occur include light-headedness, drowsiness, dizziness, fatigue, and lethargy.
- Avoid the use of IV labetalol in patients with risks for significant intracranial bleeding (eg, intraparenchymal hemorrhage, large subarachnoid hemorrhages, intracerebral lesions with mass effect), since a hypotensive episode can induce CNS infarction in patients with elevated intracranial pressure.

SOTALOL
- Sotalol is a nonselective β-adrenergic antagonist that prolongs ventricular repolarization and the absolute refractory period. It has a significant QT-prolonging effect.
- Indications: cardioversion of patients with stable ventricular and supraventricular tachycardia.

- Dose: 80 mg PO bid may be given with a time to on-set of 2 to 3 hours.
- Side effects include bradycardia, hypotension, hypoglycemia, and torsades de pointes due to QT prolongation.
- Contraindications to its use include CHF (NYHA class IV), known structural heart disease, prolonged QT interval, and second- or third-degree AV block.

CLASS III ANTIARRHYTHMIC AGENTS

AMIODARONE

- Amiodarone has a complex pharmacodynamic profile that includes class I, class II, and class IV properties, in addition to its predominant class III effects. The antifibrillatory effect of amiodarone is caused by inhibition of potassium ion fluxes that normally occur during phases 2 and 3 of the cardiac cycle.
- Amiodarone prolongs the action potential duration and the refractory period, slowing conduction through the SA node, AV node, His-Purkinje system, bypass tracts, and myocardial tissues. It suppresses automaticity in the His-Purkinje system.
- Indications: chemical cardioversion of ventricular and supraventricular dysrhythmias, including VT, VF, and atrial fibrillation/flutter in patients with a history of CHF.
- Dose: in patients with pulseless VT or VF, give 300 mg IV bolus; in patients with stable VT or supraventricular tachycardias, give 150 mg IV over 10 minutes, then 1 mg/min for 6 hours, followed by 0.5 mg/min IV for 18 hours.
- With parenteral use, hypotension is the most common side effect. Bradycardia may also occur. Long-term adverse effects include thyroid disorders, pulmonary fibrosis, and hepatic dysfunction.
- Amiodarone should not be used in patients with marked sinus bradycardia or second- and third-degree AV block unless emergent pacing is available. It is also contraindicated in patients with an allergy to shellfish due to the drug's iodine content.

IBUTILIDE

- This agent activates the slow inward potassium current in cardiomyocytes and the conduction system, increasing resting membrane potential and the effective refractory period.
- Indications: chemical cardioversion of atrial flutter and atrial fibrillation to sinus rhythm in patients with durations less than 48 hours, no known structural heart disease, and normal QT intervals.
- Dose: 0.01 mg/kg IV up to 1 mg IV over 10 minutes. Patients must have magnesium repletion to levels greater than 2.0 mEq/L prior to infusion to decrease

the likelihood of inducing torsades de pointes. A repeat dose of 0.01 mg/kg IV may be given in 20 minutes if no initial cardioversion occurs.
- Adverse effects include hypotension, bradycardia, sinus arrest, torsades de pointes, and VT. Patients must be observed for 4 hours postinfusion or until QTc normalization.
- Contraindications to ibutilide chemical cardioversion include CHF, known structural heart disease, and prolonged QT interval.

CLASS IV ANTIDYSRHYTHMIC AGENTS: CALCIUM CHANNEL BLOCKERS

- Some studies suggest an increased risk of adverse cardiovascular events with the administration of these agents, particularly in patients with left ventricular dysfunction;[4] other studies dispute these findings.[5] Currently, the American College of Cardiology/American Heart Association (ACC/AHA) Guidelines for the Management of Acute Myocardial Infarction do not recommend calcium channel blockers for routine use in the setting of acute MI since β-adrenergic antagonists are a more appropriate choice.
- However, if β-blockers are ineffective at rate control or contraindicated, verapamil or diltiazem may be given to patients with acute myocardial infarction without evidence of congestive heart failure, left ventricular dysfunction, or AV block.

VERAPAMIL

- Verapamil, a non-dihydropyridine calcium channel antagonist, decreases conduction velocity, prolongs the refractory period in the AV node, and decreases the discharge rate in the SA node. Verapamil interrupts AV nodal re-entrant pathways associated with PSVT, converting patients to normal sinus rhythm. In addition, verapamil can slow the ventricular response in patients with atrial fibrillation and/or flutter by its action on the AV node.
- Indications: rate control and conversion of narrow-complex PSVT and atrial fibrillation/flutter with rapid ventricular response.
- Dose: patients with PSVT should be given 5 to 10 mg IV every 20 minutes up to a total of 20 mg; pediatric dosing is 0.1 to 0.2 mg/kg IV over 2 to 3 minutes (in pediatric patients greater than 1 year old). Consider pretreatment with calcium gluconate 500 to 1000 mg IV to blunt verapamil's hypotensive effect (incidence of 5 to 10%).
- Adverse effects beside hypotension include conduction disturbances, such as bradycardia, AV block, and bundle-branch block. These complications occur in approximately 2% or fewer of patients and usually

respond to a dosage reduction or discontinuation of the drug.

- Verapamil is contraindicated in patients with WPW syndrome who present in atrial fibrillation or flutter since ventricular fibrillation may occur.[6]

DILTIAZEM

- Diltiazem slows AV nodal conduction time and prolongs AV nodal refractoriness. The ventricular rate is slowed in patients with a rapid ventricular response during atrial fibrillation or atrial flutter. PSVT is converted to normal sinus rhythm by interrupting the re-entry circuit in AV nodal re-entrant tachycardias and reciprocating tachycardias (eg, orthodromic SVT in WPW syndrome).
- Indications: rate control and conversion of narrow-complex PSVT and atrial fibrillation/flutter with rapid ventricular response.
- Dose: 0.25 mg/kg IV up to 20 mg should be given over 2 minutes; repeat dosing of 0.35 mg/kg IV up to 25 mg can be given if no initial effect is noted. For persistent tachycardia, continuous infusion at 5 to 15 mg/h may be necessary.
- Cardiovascular adverse effects of diltiazem may include angina, bradycardia, asystole, congestive heart failure, AV block, bundle-branch block, hypotension, and palpitations. Other side effects include nervousness, confusion, and rarely psychosis with high-dose infusions.
- Diltiazem is contraindicated in patients with WPW syndrome who present in atrial fibrillation or flutter since ventricular fibrillation may occur.[6]

OTHER ANTIARRHYTHMIC AGENTS

ADENOSINE

- The positive inotropic, chronotropic, and dromotropic response of catecholamines depends on cyclic adenosine monophosphate (cAMP). Adenosine exerts anti-adrenergic effects by inhibiting the adenyl cyclase-cAMP pathway.
- Adenosine terminates PSVT primarily via blockade of the AV node without altering conduction through accessory pathways, as is seen with the WPW syndrome. Re-entrant SVTs not involving the AV node are not terminated by adenosine.
- Indications: conversion of PSVT to sinus rhythm.
- Dose: 6 mg IV push should be followed by a 20-mL NS bolus. A repeat dose of 12 mg IV may be given if no initial response is noted. Onset of action is within approximately 30 seconds, with a duration of 60 to 90 seconds. The drug is rapidly metabolized in the blood, with a half-life of less than 7 seconds. Pediatric dose is 0.05 to 0.1 mg/kg over 1 to 2 seconds, and may be repeated to a maximum dose of 0.3 mg/kg.

- If infused too slowly, adenosine causes vasodilation with reflex tachycardia. In addition, methylxanthines competitively block adenosine's effects.
- When adverse effects occur, they are minor and well tolerated because of the drug's short half-life. The most common symptoms are dyspnea, cough, syncope, vertigo, paresthesias, numbness, nausea, and a metallic taste.
- Cardiovascular adverse effects may include facial flushing, palpitations, retrosternal chest pain, sinus bradyarrhythmias (ie, bradycardia, sinus arrest, AV block), atrial tachydysrhythmias (ie, atrial fibrillation or flutter), PVCs, and hypotension.
- Asthma is a relative contraindication to adenosine due to the potential for bronchospasm.

MAGNESIUM

- Magnesium affects skeletal and smooth muscle contractility, vasomotor tone, and neuronal transmission directly via the Na^+,K^+-ATPase pump and indirectly via calcium blocking activity.
- It increases membrane potential, prolongs AV conduction, and increases the absolute refractory period.
- Indications: torsades de pointes, second-line treatment of MAT, and suspected hypomagnesemia.
- Dose: magnesium sulfate 1 to 2 g IV bolus over 1 to 2 minutes; in stable patients, larger doses of 3 to 4 g can be given over 20 to 60 minutes.
- Hypotension is the predominant adverse effect. Other signs of hypermagnesemia include flushing, sweating, CNS depression, depression of reflexes, flaccid paralysis, depression of cardiac function, circulatory collapse, hypothermia, and fatal respiratory paralysis (usually at levels greater than 10 mEq/L).

VASOACTIVE DRUGS

ATROPINE

- Atropine sulfate, an antimuscarinic agent, enhances sinus node automaticity and AV conduction by blocking vagal activity; thus it has been termed a **parasympatholytic drug.** It has anticholinergic properties.
- Atropine is indicated as the treatment of choice for increasing heart rate in hemodynamically unstable bradycardias (eg, decreased heart rate with hypotension, altered mental status, escape beats, and/or chest pain).
- The dose of atropine for hemodynamically unstable bradycardias is 0.5 mg rapid IV push, repeated as necessary every 3 to 5 minutes until a desired heart rate is achieved (up to 3 mg). Bolus doses of 1 mg can be given for asystole or bradycardic PEA and repeated to a total dose of 3 mg (0.04 mg/kg), which results in full

vagolytic blockade. Atropine can be administered by IV push, IM, and via the endotracheal (ET) tube. When delivered via the ET tube, 2 to 2.5 times the IV dose is required and must be flushed into the bronchial tree with 20 mL NS.

- Atropine is not indicated for bradycardia in hemodynamically stable patients. If administered, marked increases in heart rate can increase myocardial oxygen consumption, possibly inducing ischemia and precipitating ventricular tachyarrhythmias (ventricular tachycardia and ventricular fibrillation). Other adverse effects include a paradoxical bradycardia if less than 0.4 mg IV is given, blurred vision, dry mouth, hallucinations, and mydriasis.

DOBUTAMINE

- Dobutamine exerts an inotropic effect, and to a lesser degree, a chronotropic effect via β_1 and β_2 stimulation. The drug's α_1 agonism is offset by its α_2 agonism, and therefore it has no significant vasopressor effect.
- Indications: moderate hypotension (70 to –100 mm Hg) with signs of cardiogenic shock.
- Dose: infusions of 2 to 20 μg/kg/min decrease peripheral vascular resistance and increase cardiac output. Infusions greater than 20 μg/kg/min increase heart rate and ectopy. Onset of effect after starting the infusion is within 1 to 2 minutes with a peak effect at 20 minutes. The duration of effect is 1 to 2 minutes, after which the drug is converted to inactive metabolites.
- Adverse effects include hypotension from skeletal muscle bed vasodilation, tachycardia, ectopy, headache, and paresthesias.

DOPAMINE

- Dopamine is a norepinephrine precursor which exerts its effects at dopaminergic, β-adrenergic, and α-adrenergic receptors. Tachyphylaxis can occur as endogenous norepinephrine stores are depleted with prolonged or high-dose infusions.
- Indications: moderate hypotension with signs of shock and symptomatic bradycardia.
- Dose: dopamine's effect is related to the dose of infusion. At low doses (1 to 2 μg/kg/min), increases in splanchnic and renal perfusion[7] are postulated to occur. Moderate infusions (3 to 10 μg/kg/min) cause β_1 stimulation with increased myocardial contractility. High doses (10 to 20 μg/kg/min) cause primarily α-adrenergic stimulation with a vasopressor effect. Onset of action after changing infusion dosing is approximately 5 minutes and it has a half-life of 2 minutes (longer in patients with hepatic and renal dysfunction).
- Adverse effects include myocardial ischemia, hypotension (at low doses), hypertension (at high doses),

headache, nausea, vomiting, and tachycardia. Prolonged infusions may cause peripheral ischemia and tissue necrosis. Augmented effect is seen in patients taking phosphodiesterase inhibitors, MAO inhibitors, halogenated anesthetics, and sympathomimetics.

EPINEPHRINE

- Epinephrine is a nonselective α- and β-adrenergic agonist that increases heart rate, contractility, and peripheral vascular resistance, resulting in blood volume redistribution centrally; additionally, epinephrine exerts mild histamine antagonism.
- Indications: shock resistant VT/VF, PEA, asystole, symptomatic bradycardia, anaphylaxis, and severe hypotension (<70 mm Hg).
- Dose: in cardiac arrest give 1 mg IV every 3 to 5 minutes or 2 to 2.5 mg via the ET tube in 10 to 20 mL NS. Patients with anaphylaxis, symptomatic bradycardia, or hypotension may be given 0.1 to 0.5 mL of a 1:1000 solution subcutaneously every 20 minutes until IV access is obtained, after which an infusion can be delivered at 2 to 10 μg/min. Onset of effect is approximately 1 to 2 minutes with a duration of 2 to 10 minutes as the drug is metabolized by the monoamine oxidase/ catecholamine O-methyl transferase (MAO/COMT) system.
- Adverse effects include myocardial ischemia, ventricular irritability, hypertension, tachycardia; prolonged infusions may cause peripheral ischemia.

NOREPINEPHRINE

- Like epinephrine, norepinephrine is an endogenous catecholamine causing α and β stimulation, which increases vascular tone and inotropy. It has a slightly more pronounced vasoconstrictive effect than epinephrine.
- Indications: severe cardiogenic or distributive (septic, anaphylactic) shock.
- Dose: infusions of 1 to 12 μg/min should be titrated to desired heart rate and mean arterial pressure. Onset is within 1 to 2 minutes with a duration of 5 to 10 minutes.
- Adverse effects include myocardial ischemia, ectopy, reflex bradycardia, hypertension (especially in patients using tricyclic antidepressants and MAO inhibitors). Prolonged infusions may cause peripheral ischemia. In cases of tissue extravasation, one may locally infiltrate 5 to 10 mg phentolamine to prevent tissue ischemia and necrosis.

VASOPRESSIN

- Vasopressin, or antidiuretic hormone (ADH), causes water reabsorption at the renal tubules (via vasopressin V_2 receptors), and central blood volume redistribution via calcium-mediated vasoconstriction (via V_1 receptors). It can augment other vasopressor effects in patients with refractory distributive shock, decreasing their pressor requirements and the possibility of peripheral ischemic injury.

- Indications: resuscitation of shock-refractory VT/VF; refractory hypotension, bleeding esophageal varices.
- Dose: for VT/VF give 40 U IV push once only; for refractory hypotension or bleeding esophageal varices, infuse at 0.2 to 0.4 U/min IV. Onset of action is within 1 minute, lasting 10 to 30 minutes. ADH is metabolized by the liver and kidney to inactive metabolites.
- Adverse effects include bradycardia, dysrhythmia (PACs, heart block), MI, hyponatremia, and mesenteric ischemia/thrombosis.

VASODILATOR AGENTS

NESIRITIDE
- Nesiritide, or b-type natriuretic peptide (BNP), is normally released from the myocardium in response to increased ventricular pressures. It acts via generation of cyclic guanosine monophosphate (cGMP), intracellularly triggering natriuresis, diuresis, and vasodilation.
- Indications: decompensated CHF.[8]
- Dose: patients with congestive heart failure should be given an initial 2 µg/kg IV bolus followed by infusion at 0.01 µg/kg/min; titrate 0.005 µg/kg upward every 20 minutes to a maximum dose of 0.03 µg/kg/min. Onset of effect is at 15 to 30 minutes and peak effect occurs by 60 minutes. The plasma half-life ranges from 30 to 120 minutes, depending on renal clearance.
- Adverse effects include hypotension (11%), headache, bradycardia, ectopy, and atrial fibrillation.
- Due to its vasodilatory effects, nesiritide is contraindicated in cardiogenic shock with systolic pressures less than 90 mm Hg.

NITROGLYCERIN
- Nitroglycerin is a direct vasodilator through the release of nitric oxide, that induces venodilation at low doses (<100 mg/min) and arteriolar vasodilation at high doses (>200 mg/min). Coronary artery vasodilation occurs throughout the dosage range.
- Nitroglycerin is approved for the prophylaxis, treatment, and management of angina pectoris and acute myocardial ischemia. Intravenous nitroglycerin can be used to control hypertension associated with surgery, but is most frequently used in congestive heart failure and in acute myocardial infarction.
- Nitroglycerin can be administered sublingually, lingually, intrabuccally, orally, topically, or by IV infusion.
- Sublingual tablets or sprays of 0.4 mg can be given every 5 minutes with immediate onset of action.
- Topical paste can be applied to the chest at a dose of 1 to 2 inches as needed every 4 to 8 hours, with onset of action in 15 to 20 minutes.

- Start IV infusion at 5 to 10 µg/min and titrate in increments of 5 to 10 µg/min to desired response. Most doses range between 50 and 200 µg/min.
- Complicated inferior MI (right ventricular involvement) is a relative contraindication to nitroglycerin due to the preload-dependence of these patients.

NITROPRUSSIDE
- Nitroprusside is an arteriolar vasodilator that acts through nitric oxide release along the vascular endothelium. Its metabolism yields thiocyanate, which can rise to toxic levels in prolonged infusions.
- Indications: hypertensive crisis, intracranial hemorrhage, and afterload reduction in CHF.
- Dose: 0.1 µg/kg/min titrated upward every 3 to 5 minutes to desired effect, up to a total of 5 µg/kg/min. Both the drug and the tubing must be covered from light with opaque material to prevent photodegradation.
- Adverse effects include hypotension, thiocyanate toxicity, carbon dioxide retention, pulmonary shunting, headaches, nausea, vomiting, and abdominal cramping.

REFERENCES

1. ECC Guidelines: Guidelines 2000 for Cardiopulmonary Resuscitation and Emergency Cardiovascular Care, International Consensus on Science. *Circulation* 102(Suppl 1):11, 2000.
2. Gorgels AP, van den Dool A, Hofs A, et al: Comparison of procainamide and lidocaine in terminating sustained monomorphic ventricular tachycardia [see comments]. *Am J Cardiol* 78:43, 1996.
3. Ryan TJ, Antman EM, Brooks NH, et al: 1999 Update: ACC/AHA Guidelines for the Management of Patients with Acute Myocardial Infarction: Executive Summary and Recommendations: A Report of the American College of Cardiology/American Heart Association Task Force on Practice Guidelines (Committee on Management of Acute Myocardial Infarction). *Circulation* 100:1016, 1999.
4. Kostis J, Lacy B, Cosgrove N, et al: Association of calcium channel blocker use with increased rate of acute myocardial infarction in patients with left ventricular dysfunction. *Am Heart J* 133:550, 1997.
5. Hagar WD, Davis B, Riba A, et al: Absence of a deleterious effect of calcium channel blockers in patients with left ventricular dysfunction after myocardial infarction: The SAVE study experience. *Am Heart J* 135:406, 1998.
6. Strasberg B, Sagie A, Rechavia E, et al: Deleterious effects of intravenous verapamil in Wolff-Parkinson-White patients and atrial fibrillation. *Cardiovasc Drugs Ther* 2:801, 1989.
7. Kellum JA, Decker J. Use of dopamine in acute renal failure: A meta-analysis. *Crit Care Med* 29:1638, 2001.
8. Silver MA, Horton DP, Ghali JK, Elkayam U: Effect of nesiritide versus dobutamine on short-term outcomes in the treatment of patients with acutely decompensated heart failure. *J Am Coll Cardiol* 39:798, 2002.

For further reading in *Emergency Medicine: A Comprehensive Study Guide,* 6th ed., see Chap. 28, "Disturbances of Cardiac Rhythm and Conduction," by Edmund Bolton; and Chap. 29, "Pharmacology of Antidysrhythmic and Vasoactive Medications," by Teresa M. Carlin.

5 RESUSCITATION OF CHILDREN AND NEONATES

Douglas K. Holtzman

EPIDEMIOLOGY

- Children have very poor survival rates from cardiac arrest, because it is often associated with prolonged hypoxia or shock.[1,2]
- In children who survive a cardiac arrest, about 98% have devastating neurologic sequelae.[3]

PATHOPHYSIOLOGY

- Children primarily develop cardiac arrest secondary to hypoxia from respiratory arrest or shock syndromes.[4]
- Infants younger than 6 months are obligate nose breathers (ie, primary nasal breathers).
- Because of age and size differences in children, drug dosages, compression and respiratory rates, and equipment sizes vary considerably (Table 5-1).

EMERGENCY DEPARTMENT CARE AND DISPOSITION

SECURING THE AIRWAY

- The airways of infants and children are much smaller than those of adults and have pronounced anatomic and functional differences.
- The prominent occiput and relatively large tongue may lead to obstruction, that may be relieved with mild extension of the head (sniffing position) and a chin lift or jaw thrust maneuver.
- The small nasal passages and hypertrophic adenoid tissue make nasopharyngeal airways less useful in children.
- In the unconscious child who requires continuous jaw thrust or chin lift, the oral airway may be useful. Oral airways are inserted by direct visualization using a tongue blade.

- Ventilation may be administered using a bag-valve-mask system. The minimum volume for ventilation bags for infants and children is 450 mL. Observe chest rise and auscultate breath sounds to ensure adequate ventilation.
- The large and flaccid epiglottis is best displaced using a straight (Miller) laryngoscope blade.
- Uncuffed endotracheal tubes are used for children up to 8 years of age.
- Resuscitation measuring tapes have been found to be more accurate than the age-based formula, which is more accurate than using the diameter of the patient's fifth digit.[5,6]
- The position of the tube at the lip is approximately 3 times the size of the tube (eg, $5.0 \times 3 = 15$ cm at the lip).
- Tidal volume for children is 10 to 15 mL/kg.
- If the child does not require hyperventilation, then the respiratory rate should be started at 20 breaths/minute for infants, 15 breaths/minute for young children, and 10 breaths/minute for adolescents.[4]
- Confirmation of endotracheal intubation is similar to that in adults: adequate chest rise, symmetric breath sounds, capnographic or capnometric readings,[7] improved oxygenation, and clinical improvement.
- The laryngeal mask airway (LMA) has been successfully utilized in the pediatric population.[8]
- Transtracheal jet ventilation using a catheter and high-pressure (50 psi) oxygen allows adequate ventilation and oxygenation. A 1-second jet of oxygen followed by a 4-second expiratory phase achieves satisfactory ventilation.[9]

RAPID SEQUENCE INDUCTION

- Rapid sequence induction (RSI) is the intravenous administration of an anesthetic and a neuromuscular blocking agent to facilitate endotracheal intubation.[10]
- Preoxygenate the patient with 100% oxygen.
- Head trauma patients may be premedicated with lidocaine (1 mg/kg IV) to prevent increased intracranial pressure (ICP).[11]
- Atropine (0.02 mg/kg, minimum dose 0.1 mg, maximum dose 1 mg) should be given to prevent reflex bradycardia in children less than 5 years old or in the older child or adolescent who requires a second dose of succinylcholine.
- Cricoid pressure should be applied before paralysis and continued until successful intubation is confirmed.
- Sedation is accomplished using a benzodiazepine (eg, midazolam, diazepam), barbiturate (thiopental), the nonbarbiturate sedative-hypnotic etomidate, the dissociative anesthetic ketamine, or the general anesthetic propofol, depending on the clinical situation and the experience of the physician.

TABLE 5-1 Length-Based Equipment Chart

ITEM	PATIENT LENGTH, CM						
	54–70	70–85	85–95	95–107	107–124	124–138	138–155
ET tube size, mm	3.5	4.0	4.5	5.0	5.5	6.0	6.5
Lip-tip length, mm	10.5	12.0	13.5	15.0	16.5	18.0	19.5
Laryngoscope	1 straight	1 straight	2 straight	2 straight or curved	2 straight or curved	2–3 straight or curved	3 straight or curved
Suction catheter	8F	8–10F	10F	10F	10F	10F	10F
Stylet	6F	6F	6F	6F	14F	14F	14F
Oral airway	Infant/small child	Small child	Child	Child	Child/small adult	Child/adult	Medium adult
Bag-valve-mask	Infant	Child	Child	Child	Child	Child/adult	Adult
Oxygen mask	Newborn	Pediatric	Pediatric	Pediatric	Pediatric	Adult	Adult
Vascular access catheter/butterfly	22–24/23–25, intraosseous	20–22/24–25, intraosseous	18–22/21–23, intraosseous	18–22/21–23, intraosseous	18–20/21–23	18–20/21–22	16–20/18–21
Nasogastric tube	5–8F	8–10F	10F	10–12F	12–14F	14–18F	18F
Urinary catheter	5–8F	8–10F	10F	10–12F	10–12F	12F	12F
Chest tube	12–16F	16–20F	20–24F	20–24F	24–32F	28–32F	32–40F
Blood pressure cuff	Newborn/infant	Infant/child	child	Child	Child	Child/adult	Adult

NOTE: Directions for use: (1) Measure patient length with centimeter tape; (2) Using measured length in centimeters, access appropriate equipment column.
SOURCE: Adapted from Luten et al.[5]

- Midazolam (0.1 to 0.2 mg/kg IV) has few side effects other than respiratory depression and no analgesic properties.
- Etomidate (0.2 to 0.4 mg/kg IV) is ultra short acting, decreases cerebral metabolic rate and ICP, and has minimal cardiovascular and respiratory depression. However, a single dose can suppress cortisol production.
- Thiopental (2 to 4 mg/kg IV) is also an ultra–short-acting agent which decreases cerebral metabolic rate and ICP. It also has a negative inotropic effect and causes hypotension.
- Ketamine (1 to 2 mg/kg IV) has little respiratory depression and a bronchodilator effect, but increases ICP, blood pressure, and secretions, and may cause laryngospasm.
- Propofol (2 to 3 mg/kg IV) is a rapid-acting, short-duration induction agent. Its disadvantages are hypotension (especially in patients with inadequate intravascular volume), pain on injection, and cost.
- Neuromuscular blockade is achieved using succinylcholine, vecuronium, or rocuronium.
- Succinylcholine (2 mg/kg for infants, 1 to 1.5 mg/kg for children) is a depolarizing, rapid-onset (45 seconds), short-duration (3 to 5 minutes) agent. It has numerous disadvantages, including hyperkalemia (may be life-threatening); hypertension; rises in intracranial, intraocular, and intragastric pressure; muscle fasciculations; rhabdomyolysis; and malignant hyperthermia. It is relatively contraindicated in patients with burns over 24 hours old, crush injuries, glau-

coma, open globe injuries, raised ICP, or conditions predisposing to hyperkalemia. It has also been known to cause bradycardia in young children, particularly infants.
- Vecuronium (0.1 to 0.2 mg/kg IV) is a nondepolarizing agent with an onset of 60 to 90 seconds and effects that last 30 to 90 minutes.
- Rocuronium (0.6 to 1.2 mg/kg IV) has a rapid onset of action equal to that of succinylcholine and lasts 30 to 60 minutes.

VASCULAR ACCESS

- Vascular access is performed in the quickest, least invasive manner possible; peripheral veins (antecubital, hand, foot, or scalp) are attempted first.
- Intraosseous cannulation is a rapid, safe, and reliable method and may be used for administration of fluids, resuscitation medications, colloids, and blood.
- Percutaneous central lines or saphenous vein cutdowns may also be used, but are more time consuming.
- The technique for insertion of intraosseous cannulation is as follows: the most common bony site is the proximal tibia. Other locations include the distal tibia and femur, as well as the iliac crest. Using sterile technique, the tibial tuberosity is identified by palpation. The cannulation site is 1 to 3 cm below this and in the middle of the anteromedial surface of the tibia. There are several types of needles available. The most

common and user friendly is the Jamshidi-type bone marrow needle. Support the tibia on a firm surface. Insert the needle in a slightly caudal direction using a firm twisting motion until the needle punctures the cortex (usually a decrease in resistance is felt). Remove the stylet and attempt to aspirate marrow. If marrow is aspirated, infuse fluids. If no marrow is aspirated, but you believe the needle is in the marrow, attempt to flush. Check for signs of increased resistance to injection, increased circumference of soft tissue of the calf, or increased firmness of the tissue. If the test injection is successful, secure the needle and connect to an infusion set.

FLUIDS

- In shock, intravenous isotonic fluid (ie, normal saline) boluses of 20 mL/kg should be given as rapidly as possible and should be repeated, depending on the clinical response[4] (see Chap. 82 for more details).
- If hypovolemia has been corrected and shock or hypotension still persists, a pressor agent should be considered.

DRUGS

- Proper drug dosages in children require knowledge of the patient's weight. The use of a length-based system such as the Broselow tape for estimating the weight of a child in an emergency situation reduces dosage errors.[5]
- Indications for resuscitation drugs are the same for children as they are for adults; the exception is epinephrine, which is considered first-line therapy in children with bradycardia.
- The rule of sixes may be used to quickly calculate continuous infusions of drugs such as dopamine and dobutamine. The amount of drug needed is 6 mg times the weight in kilograms added to a total volume of 100 mL D_5W. This produces an infusion rate in milliliters per hour that is equal to the micrograms per kilogram per minute rate (ie, an infusion of 1 mL/h = 1 μg/kg/min or 5 mL/h = 5 μg/kg/min).
- Epinephrine is the only drug proven effective in cardiac arrest. It is indicated in pulseless arrest and in hypoxia-induced slow pulse rates that are unresponsive to oxygenation and ventilation.
- The initial dose of epinephrine is 0.01 mg/kg (0.1 mL/kg of 1:10,000 solution) IV, intraosseous or 0.1 mg/kg (0.1 mL/kg of 1:1000 solution [high dose]) by the endotracheal route.
- Repeat dosing of epinephrine is recommended every 3 to 5 minutes for persistent arrest.

- The second and subsequent doses for epinephrine are the same (0.01 mg/kg [0.1 mL/kg] of 1:10,000 solution), but higher doses (0.1 to 0.2 mg/kg [0.1 to 0.2 mL/kg] of 1:1000 solution), the so-called "high-dose" epinephrine, may be considered.[4]
- Small infants and chronically ill children have limited stores of glycogen, which may be rapidly depleted during episodes of cardiopulmonary distress, leading to hypoglycemia.
- Glucose 25% given at 2 to 4 mL/kg or 5 to 10 mL/kg of 10% glucose will deliver 0.5 to 1 g/kg and generally corrects profound hypoglycemia.
- Sodium bicarbonate is no longer considered as a first-line resuscitation drug. It is recommended only after effective ventilation is established, epinephrine given, and chest compressions to ensure circulation are provided.
- Calcium is also not recommended in routine resuscitation, but may be useful in hyperkalemia, hypocalcemia, and calcium channel blocker overdoses.

DYSRHYTHMIAS

- Dysrhythmias in infants and children are most often secondary to respiratory insufficiency and hypoxia, not primary cardiac causes as in adults. Specific attention to oxygenation and ventilation are paramount to dysrhythmia management in pediatrics.
- The most common rhythm seen in a pediatric arrest is bradycardia progressing to asystole. Often, oxygenation and ventilation are sufficient to correct the situation. Epinephrine followed by atropine may be useful in bradycardia unresponsive to ventilation.
- Ventricular fibrillation as a cause of cardiac arrest is rare in children and even more rare in infants.[12]
- The most common dysrhythmia outside of the arrest situation is supraventricular tachycardia (SVT). It presents as a narrow complex tachycardia with rates typically between 250 and 350 beats per minute. The recommended treatment for stable SVT in children is adenosine (0.1 mg/kg) given simultaneously with a saline flush as rapidly as possible through a well-functioning IV. Treatment for the unstable SVT patient is synchronized cardioversion (one-quarter to one-half J/kg).
- It is often difficult to differentiate between sinus tachycardia (ST) and SVT. Small infants may have ST with rates above 200 beats per minute. Patients with ST may have a history of fever, dehydration, or shock. In ST, the heart rate typically varies with activity or stimulation.
- Transcutaneous pacing has not been associated with greatly improved survival rates, but it can be life saving if applied quickly in a child with sudden asystole

or bradycardia. Adult patches may be used in children weighing over 15 kg.[13]

DEFIBRILLATION AND CARDIOVERSION

- Ventricular fibrillation is rare in children. It is initially treated with defibrillation at 2 J/kg.[4] If unsuccessful, repeat defibrillation energy is doubled to 4 J/kg.
- If two attempts at defibrillation at 4 J/kg are unsuccessful, epinephrine should be given. Reassessment for treatable causes such as hypoxemia, hypovolemia, and metabolic acidosis should be performed.
- Unstable tachyarrhythmias are treated with cardioversion at a dose of one-quarter to one-half J/kg.
- The largest paddles that still allow contact of the entire paddle with the chest wall should be used. Electrode cream or paste is used to prevent burns. One paddle is placed on the right of the sternum at the second intercostal space, and the other is placed at the left midclavicular line at the level of the xiphoid.

NEONATAL RESUSCITATION

- Approximately 6% of all newborns require some form of resuscitation in the delivery room.
- The initial decision to resuscitate an infant should be made within the first 30 seconds of delivery.
- The first step is to maintain body temperature. The infant should be immediately dried and placed under a preheated radiant warmer.
- The mouth followed by the nose should be gently suctioned with either a bulb syringe or a mechanical suction device.
- The examiner should then assess heart rate, respiratory effort, color, and activity quickly over the next 5 to 10 seconds.
- Infants who are apneic, centrally cyanotic, or whose heart rate is less than 100 beats per minute should have positive pressure ventilation with 100% oxygen initiated.
- For infants who have not taken an initial breath, pressures over 30 cm H_2O may be required to initially expand the lungs.
- If no improvement is noted or if prolonged bagging is anticipated, endotracheal intubation should be performed.
- If the heart rate is still below 60 beats per minute after intubation and assisted ventilation, cardiac massage should be started at 120 compressions per minute and coordinated with assisted ventilation in a 3:1 ratio.
- If unsuccessful in restoring heart rate after approximately 30 seconds, drug therapy resuscitation should be initiated.

- Drugs may be administered via endotracheal tube, umbilical vein, or peripheral vein.
- Umbilical vein catheterization is a fast, reliable method of obtaining vascular access. The umbilical catheter is placed in the umbilical vein and advanced to 10 to 12 cm.
- Epinephrine (0.01 mg/kg of 1:10,000 solution) may be used for heart rates less than 60 beats per minute despite adequate ventilation and oxygenation.
- Sodium bicarbonate during neonatal resuscitation remains controversial. Adequate ventilation and circulation must be established prior to administration. Sodium bicarbonate (1 mEq/kg of a 4.2% solution, 0.5 mEq/L) should be given intravenously only.
- Naloxone (0.1 mg/kg IV) may be useful for respiratory depression caused by narcotics.

PREVENTION OF MECONIUM ASPIRATION

- Aspiration of meconium-stained amniotic fluid is associated with a high morbidity and mortality rate. With proper perinatal management, it is almost entirely preventable.
- Up to 20% of all births will have meconium staining of the amniotic fluid.
- If meconium is present, the infant's mouth, pharynx, and nose should be suctioned after delivery of the head and **before** delivery of the shoulders.
- If the infant is vigorous after delivery, the mouth and nose should be suctioned again with no further intervention necessary.
- If the infant is depressed after delivery, direct suctioning of the trachea should be performed by visualizing the trachea with a laryngoscope and suctioning via an endotracheal tube.
- If at any time during this procedure the heart rate drops below 100 beats per minute, positive pressure ventilation should be initiated.

REFERENCES

1. Schindler MB, Bohn D, Cox PN, et al: Outcome of out-of-hospital cardiac and respiratory arrest in children. *N Engl J Med* 335:1473, 1996.
2. Teach SJ, Moore PE, Fleisher GR: Death and resuscitation in the pediatric emergency department. *Ann Emerg Med* 25:799, 1995.
3. Ronco R, King W, Donley DK, et al: Outcome and cost at a children's hospital following resuscitation for out-of-hospital cardiopulmonary arrest. *Arch Pediatr Adolesc Med* 149:210, 1995.

4. Zaritsky AL, Nadkarni VM, Hazinski MF, et al: *Textbook of Pediatric Advanced Life Support.* Dallas: American Heart Association, 2002.

5. Luten RC, Wears RL, Broselow J, et al: Length-based endotracheal tube and emergency equipment in pediatrics. *Ann Emerg Med* 21:900, 1992.

6. King BR, Baker MD, Braitman LE: Endotracheal tube selection in children: A comparison of four methods. *Ann Emerg Med* 22:530, 1993.

7. Bhende MS, Thompson AE: Evaluation of an end-tidal CO_2 detector during pediatric cardiopulmonary resuscitation. *Pediatrics* 91:726, 1993.

8. Lopez-Gil M, Brimacombe J, Alvarez M: Safety and efficacy of the laryngeal mask airway: A prospective survey of 1400 pediatric patients. *Anesthesia* 51:969, 1996.

9. Benumof JC, Scheller MS: The importance of transtracheal jet ventilation in the management of the difficult airway. *Anesthesiology* 71:769, 1989.

10. Gerardi MJ, Sacchetti AD, Cantor RM, et al: Rapid-sequence intubation of the pediatric patient. *Ann Emerg Med* 28:55, 1996.

11. Walls RM: Rapid-sequence intubation comes of age. *Ann Emerg Med* 28:79, 1996.

12. Schoenfeld PS, Baker MD: Management of cardiopulmonary and trauma resuscitation in the pediatric emergency department. *Pediatrics* 91:726, 1993.

13. Beland MJ, Hesslein PS, Finlay CD, et al: Non-invasive transcutaneous cardiac pacing in children. *PACE* 10:1262, 1987.

For further reading in *Emergency Medicine: A Comprehensive Study Guide,* 6th ed., see Chap. 13, "Neonatal Resuscitation and Emergencies," by Eugene E. Cepeda and Mary P. Bedard; and Chap. 14, "Pediatric Cardiopulmonary Resuscitation," by William E. Hauda II.

6 FLUIDS, ELECTROLYTES, AND ACID-BASE DISORDERS
David M. Cline

FLUIDS

- When altered, fluids and electrolytes should be corrected in the following order: (1) volume; (2) pH; (3) potassium, calcium, magnesium; and (4) sodium and chloride. Re-establishment of tissue perfusion often re-equilibrates the fluid-electrolyte and acid-base balance.
- Because the osmolarity of normal saline (NS) matches that of the serum, it is an excellent fluid for volume replacement.
- Hypotonic fluids such as dextrose 5% in water (D_5W) should never be used to replace volume.

- Lactated Ringer's solution is commonly used for surgical patients or trauma patients; however, only NS can be given in the same line with blood components.
- Dextrose 5% in half normal saline ($D_5.45$ NS), with or without potassium, is given as a maintenance fluid.
- The more concentrated dextrose solutions, $D_{10}W$ or $D_{20}W$, are used for patients with compromised ability to mobilize glucose stores, such as patients with hepatic failure, or as part of total parenteral nutrition (TPN) solutions.

CLINICAL ASSESSMENT OF VOLUME STATUS

- Volume loss and dehydration can be inferred from the patient history. Historical features include vomiting, diarrhea, fever, adverse working conditions, decreased fluid intake, chronic disease, altered level of consciousness, and reduced urine output.
- Tachycardia and hypotension are most commonly late signs of dehydration.
- On physical exam, you may find dry mucosa, shrunken tongue (excellent indicator), and decreased skin turgor. In infants and children, sunken fontanelles, decreased capillary refill, lack of tears, and decreased wet diapers are typical signs and symptoms of dehydration (see Chap. 82).
- Lethargy and coma are more ominous signs and may indicate a significant comorbid condition.
- Laboratory values are not reliable indicators of fluid status. Plasma and urine osmolarity are perhaps the most reliable measures of dehydration. Blood urea nitrogen (BUN), creatinine, hematocrit, and other chemistries are insensitive.
- Volume overload is a purely clinical diagnosis and presents with edema (central or peripheral), respiratory distress (pulmonary edema), and jugular venous distention (in congestive heart failure).
- The significant risk factors for volume overload are renal, cardiovascular, and liver disease. Blood pressure (BP) does not necessarily correlate with volume status alone; patients with volume overload can present with hypotension or hypertension.

MAINTENANCE FLUIDS

- Adult: $D_5.45$ NS at 75 to 125 mL/h + 20 mEq/L of potassium chloride for an average adult (approximately 70 kg).
- Children: $D_5.45$ NS or $D_{10}.45$ NS, 100 mL/kg/day for the first 10 kg (of body weight), 50 mL/kg/day for the second 10 kg, and 20 mL/kg/day for every kilogram thereafter (see Chap. 82 for further discussion of pediatric fluid management).

ELECTROLYTE DISORDERS

- Correcting a single abnormality may not be the only intervention needed, as most electrolytes exist in equilibrium with others.
- Laboratory errors are common. Results should be double-checked when the clinical picture and the laboratory data conflict.
- Abnormalities should be corrected at the same rate they developed; however, slower correction is usually safe unless the condition warrants rapid and/or early intervention (ie, hypoglycemia, hyperkalemia).
- Evaluation of electrolyte disorders frequently requires a comparison of the measured and calculated osmolarity (number of particles per liter of solution). To calculate osmolarity, measured serum values in mEq/L are used:

$$\text{Osmolarity in mOsm/L} = 2[\text{Na}^+] + \frac{\text{glucose}}{18} + \frac{\text{BUN}}{2.8} + \frac{\text{ETOH}}{4.6}$$

HYPONATREMIA ([NA$^+$] <135 MEQ/L)

CLINICAL FINDINGS
- The clinical manifestations of hyponatremia occur when the [Na$^+$] drops below 120 mEq/L; they include abdominal pain, headache, agitation, hallucinations, cramps, confusion, lethargy, and seizures.

DIAGNOSIS AND DIFFERENTIAL
- The volume status is evaluated first, then the measured and calculated osmolarity.
- **True** hyponatremia presents with a reduced osmolarity. **Factitious** hyponatremia presents with a normal to high osmolarity (hypertonic or isotonic hyponatremia).
- The most common cause of true hyponatremia is loss of water with [Na$^+$] from diuretic therapy with disproportionate (hypotonic) water replacement (without electrolytes) through oral intake.
- Hypertonic hyponatremia presents with elevated osmolarity and the most common cause is hyperglycemia.
- Hypervolumic hyponatremia is commonly due to cardiac failure, cirrhosis, or renal failure.
- Isotonic hyponatremia may be due to hyperlipidemia, elevated protein or hyperglycemia.
- Extracellular fluid (ECF) or volume status and urine sodium level can classify true hyponatremia (low osmolarity). The syndrome of inappropriate secretion of antidiuretic hormone (SIADH) is a diagnosis made by exclusion. Causes of hyponatremia are listed in Table 6-1.

TABLE 6-1   Causes of Hyponatremia

Hypotonic (true) hyponatremia (P$_{osm}$ <275)
  Hypovolemic hyponatremia
    Extrarenal losses (urinary [Na$^+$] >20 mEq/L)
      Volume replacement with hypotonic fluids
      Sweating, vomiting, diarrhea
      Third-space sequestration (burns, peritonitis, pancreatitis)
    Renal losses (urinary [Na$^+$] >20 mEq/L)
      Loop or osmotic diuretics
      Aldosterone deficiency (Addison's disease)
      Ketonuria
      Salt-losing nephropathies; renal tubular acidosis
      Osmotic diuresis (mannitol, hyperglycemia, hyperuricemia)
    Euvolemic hyponatremia (urinary [Na$^+$] >20 mEq/L)
      Inappropriate ADH secretion (CNS, lung, or carcinoma disease)
      Physical and emotional stress or pain
      Myxedema, Addison's disease, Sheehan's syndrome
      Drugs, water intoxication
  Hypervolemic hyponatremia
    Urinary [Na$^+$] >20 mEq/L
      Renal failure (inability to excrete free water)
    Urinary [Na$^+$] <20 mEq/L
      Cirrhosis
      Cardiac failure
      Renal failure
Isotonic (pseudo) hyponatremia (P$_{osm}$ 275–295)
  Hyperproteinemia, hyperlipidemia, hyperglycemia
Hypertonic hyponatremia (P$_{osm}$ >295)
  Hyperglycemia, mannitol excess, and glycerol use

ABBREVIATIONS: ADH = antidiuretic hormone; CNS = central nervous system.

EMERGENCY DEPARTMENT CARE AND DISPOSITION
- The volume or perfusion deficit, if any, is corrected first, using normal saline.
- In stable normotensive patients, fluids are restricted (500 to 1500 mL of water daily).
- In severe hyponatremia ([Na$^+$] <120 mEq/L) with central nervous system (CNS) changes, hypertonic saline, 3% NS (513 mEq/L), is given at 25 to 100 mL/h. Concomitant use of furosemide in small doses of 20 to 40 mg has been shown to decrease the incidence of central pontine myelinolysis (CPM).[1]
- The sodium deficit can be calculated as follows:

Weight in kg 0.6 × (140 – measured [Na$^+$]) = sodium deficit in mEq

- Complications of rapid correction include congestive heart failure (CHF) and central pontine myelinolysis, which can cause alterations in consciousness, dysphagia, dysarthria, and paresis.

HYPERNATREMIA ([NA$^+$] >150 MEQ/L)

CLINICAL FEATURES
- The symptoms of hypernatremia usually begin when the osmolarity is greater than 350 mOsm/L. Irritability and

TABLE 6-2   Causes of Hypernatremia

Loss of water
  Reduced water intake
    Defective thirst
    Unconsciousness
    Inability to drink water
    Lack of access to water
  Water loss in excess of sodium
    Vomiting, diarrhea
    Sweating, fever
    Diabetes insipidus
    Drugs including lithium and phenytoin
    Dialysis
    Osmotic diuresis
    Thyrotoxicosis
    Severe burns

Gain of sodium
  Increased intake
    Increased salt use, salt pills
    Hypertonic saline ingestion or infusion
    Sodium bicarbonate administration
  Mineralocorticoid or glucocorticoid excess
    Primary aldosteronism
    Cushing's syndrome

ataxia occur at osmolarities above 375 mOsm/L. Lethargy, coma, and seizures occur with osmolarities above 400 mOsm/L.

- Brain hemorrhage can be seen in neonates after rapid infusion of $NaHCO_3$.
- An osmolarity increase of 2% sets off thirst to prevent hypernatremia. Morbidity and mortality are highest in infants and the elderly, who may be unable to respond to increased thirst.

DIAGNOSIS AND DIFFERENTIAL
- The most frequent cause of hypernatremia is a decrease in total body water due to decreased intake or excessive loss.
- Common causes are diarrhea, vomiting, hyperpyrexia, and excessive sweating.
- An important etiology of hypernatremia is diabetes insipidus (DI), which results from loss of hypotonic urine. It may be central (no ADH secreted) or nephrogenic (unresponsive to ADH.) The causes of hypernatremia are listed in Table 6-2.

EMERGENCY DEPARTMENT CARE AND DISPOSITION
- Treat any perfusion deficits with NS or lactated Ringer's (LR). Then switch to 0.5 NS after a urine output of 0.5 mL/kg/h is reached. Avoid lowering the $[Na^+]$ more than 10 mEq/L/day. Monitor central venous pressure and pulmonary capillary wedge pressure.
- Use the formula below to calculate the total body water deficit. As a rule, each liter of water deficit causes the $[Na^+]$ to increase 3 to 5 mEq/L.

- Water deficit in liters = TBW (1 − measured $[Na^+]$/ desired $[Na^+]$).
- If no urine output is observed after NS/LR rehydration, rapidly switch to 0.5 NS; unload the body of the extra sodium by using a diuretic (ie, furosemide, 20 to 40 mg IV).
- Central DI is treated using desmopressin (DDAVP) 0.05 mg PO every 12 hours (dose range is 0.1 to 1.0 mg/day divided 2 to 3 times daily).
- In children with a serum sodium level greater than 180 mEq/L, peritoneal dialysis using high glucose–low $[Na^+]$ dialysate should be considered in consultation with a pediatric nephrologist.

HYPOKALEMIA ($[K^+]$ <3.5 MEQ/L)

CLINICAL FEATURES
- The signs and symptoms of hypokalemia usually occur at levels below 2.5 mEq/L and affect the following body systems: the central nervous system (CNS) (weakness, cramps, hyporeflexia), gastrointestinal (GI) system (ileus), cardiovascular system (dysrhythmias, worsening of digoxin toxicity, hypotension or hypertension, U waves, ST-segment depression, and prolonged QT interval), and renal system (metabolic alkalosis and worsening hepatic encephalopathy); also, glucose intolerance can also develop.

DIAGNOSIS AND DIFFERENTIAL
- The most common cause is the use of loop diuretics. Table 6-3 lists the causes.

TABLE 6-3   Causes of Hypokalemia

Shift into the cell
  Alkalosis and sodium bicarbonate
  β-Adrenergics
  Administration of insulin and glucose

Reduced intake

Renal loss
  Diuretic therapy
  Osmotic diuresis
  Primary hyperaldosteronism
  Secondary hyperaldosteronism
  Renal artery stenosis
  Licorice use
  Excessive tobacco chewing
  Hypercalcemia
  Postobstructive diuresis
  Renal tubular acidosis

Drugs and toxins (PCN, lithium, L-dopa, theophylline)

GI loss (vomiting, diarrhea, fistulas)

Other causes (hypomagnesemia, acute leukemia)

ABBREVIATION: PCN = penicillin.

EMERGENCY DEPARTMENT CARE AND DISPOSITION

- Replacement of $[K^+]$ at 20 mEq/h will raise the $[K^+]$ by 0.25 mEq/L.
- Administer 10 to 15 mEq/h of potassium chloride (KCl) in 50 to 100 mL of dextrose in water (D_5W); piggyback into saline over 3 to 4 hours.[2] In general, up to 10 mEq/h of KCl can be given through a peripheral IV and up to 20 mEq/h can be given through a central line. Add no more than 40 mEq of KCl in 1 L of IV fluids. Patients should be monitored continuously for dysrhythmias.
- Oral replacement (in the awake asymptomatic patient) is rapid and safer than IV therapy. Use 20 to 40 mEq/L of KCl or similar agent.

HYPERKALEMIA ($[K^+]$ >5.5 MEQ/L)

CLINICAL FEATURES

- The most concerning and serious manifestations of hyperkalemia are the cardiac effects. At levels of 6.5 to 7.5 mEq/L the electrocardiogram (ECG) shows peaked T waves (precordial leads), prolonged PR intervals, and short QT intervals.
- At levels of 7.5 to 8.0 mEq/L, the QRS widens and the P wave flattens.
- At levels above 8 mEq/L, a sine-wave pattern, ventricular fibrillation, and heart blocks occur.
- Neuromuscular symptoms include weakness and paralysis. GI symptoms include vomiting, colic, and diarrhea.

DIAGNOSIS AND DIFFERENTIAL

- Beware of pseudohyperkalemia, which is commonly caused by hemolysis associated with blood draws.
- Renal failure with oliguria is the most common cause of true hyperkalemia.
- Appropriate tests for management include an ECG, electrolytes, calcium, magnesium, arterial blood gases (ABG) (check for acidosis), urinalysis (UA), and a digoxin level in appropriate patients.
- Causes of hyperkalemia are listed in Table 6-4.

EMERGENCY DEPARTMENT CARE AND DISPOSITION

- Symptomatic patients are treated in a stepwise approach: stabilize the cardiac membrane with $CaCl_2$, and then shift the $[K^+]$ into the cell using glucose and insulin and/or bicarbonate. Finally, excrete the potassium using sodium polystyrene sulfonate (Kayexalate), diuretics, and dialysis in severe cases.
- For levels over 7.0 mEq/L or if any ECG changes, give IV calcium chloride (5 mL of a 10% solution), or calcium gluconate (10 mL of a 10% solution); use caution in a digoxin-toxic patient (risk of dysrhythmias). In children, calcium gluconate (0.5 mL/kg of a 10% solution) is given.

TABLE 6-4   Causes of Hyperkalemia

Pseudohyperkalemia
  Hemolysis during blood draw
  Leukocytosis
  Thrombocytosis

Metabolic acidemia (acute)

Increased intake into the plasma
  Exogenous: diet, salt substitutes, low-sodium diet
  Endogenous: hemolysis, GI bleeding, catabolic states, crush injury

Oliguric renal failure

Impaired renin-aldosterone axis
  Addison's disease
  Primary hypoaldosteronism
  Other (heparin, β-blockers, prostaglandin inhibitors, captopril)

Primary renal tubular potassium secretory defect
  Sickle cell disease
  Systemic lupus erythematosus
  Post–renal transplantation
  Obstructive uropathy

Inhibition of renal tubular secretion of potassium
  Spironolactone
  Digitalis

Abnormal potassium distribution
  Insulin deficiency
  Hypertonicity (hyperglycemia)
  β-Adrenergic blockers
  Exercise
  Succinylcholine
  Digitalis

- The presence of digoxin toxicity with hyperkalemia is an indication for digoxin immune Fab (Digibind) therapy (see Chap. 108).
- For levels above 5.5 mEq/L (especially in acidotic patients), give 1 mEq/kg of sodium bicarbonate.
- Give 1 ampule of $D_{50}W$ with 10 U regular insulin IV (5 U in dialysis patients).
- Maintain diuresis with furosemide, 20 to 40 mg IV.
- Sodium polystyrene sulfonate (PO or rectally [PR]), 1 g binds 1 mEq of $[K^+]$ over 10 minutes. Administer 15 to 25 g of sodium polystyrene sulfonate PO with 50 mL of 20% sorbitol (sorbitol is used because sodium polystyrene sulfonate is constipating). Per rectum, give 20 g in 200 mL 20% sorbitol over 30 minutes. Sodium polystyrene sulfonate can exacerbate CHF.
- In patients with acute renal failure, consult a nephrologist for emergent dialysis.
- Albuterol (by nebulization), 0.5 mL of a 5% solution (2.5 mg) may also be used to lower $[K^+]$ (transient effect).

HYPOCALCEMIA ($[Ca^{2+}]$ <8.5 MEQ/L OR IONIZED LEVEL <2.0 MEQ/L)

CLINICAL FEATURES

- The signs and symptoms of hypocalcemia are usually seen with ionized $[Ca^{2+}]$ levels below 1.5 mEq/L.

Clinically patients have paresthesias, increased deep tendon reflexes (DTR), cramps, weakness, confusion, and seizures.

- Patients may also demonstrate Chvostek's sign (twitch of the corner of mouth on tapping with a finger over cranial nerve VII at the zygoma) or Trousseau's sign (more reliable, carpal spasm when the blood pressure cuff is left inflated at a pressure above the systolic BP for greater than 3 minutes).

DIAGNOSIS AND DIFFERENTIAL

- Common causes: shock, sepsis, renal failure, pancreatitis, drugs (cimetidine mostly), hypoparathyroidism, phosphate overload, vitamin D deficiency, fat embolism, strychnine poisoning, hypomagnesemia, and tetanus toxin.
- The ECG often shows prolonged QT interval.
- If the patient is alkalotic, ionized calcium (physiologically active) may be very low, even with normal total calcium.
- In refractory CHF, $[Ca^{2+}]$ can be low.

EMERGENCY DEPARTMENT CARE AND DISPOSITION

- If asymptomatic, use oral calcium gluconate tablets, 1 to 4 g/day divided every 6 hours, with or without vitamin D (calcitriol, 0.2 μg twice daily). Milk is not a good substitute (low $[Ca^{2+}]$).
- In more urgent situations with symptomatic patients, calcium gluconate or calcium chloride, 10 mL of a 10% solution, can be given over 10 minutes via slow IV.

HYPERCALCEMIA ([CA^{2+}] >10.5 OR IONIZED [CA^{2+}] >2.7 MEQ/L)

- Several factors affect the serum calcium level: parathyroid hormone (PTH) increases calcium and decreases phosphate; calcitonin and vitamin D metabolites decrease calcium.
- Decreased [H+] causes a decrease in ionized $[Ca^{2+}]$. Ionized $[Ca^{2+}]$ is the physiologically active form. Each rise in pH of 0.1 lowers $[Ca^{2+}]$ by 3 to 8%.
- A decrease in albumin causes a decrease in $[Ca^{2+}]$, but not in the ionized portion.
- Most cases of hypercalcemia are due to hyperparathyroidism or malignancies. A third of the patients develop hypokalemia.

CLINICAL FEATURES

- Clinical signs and symptoms develop at levels above 12 mg/dL.
- A mnemonic to aid recall common hypercalcemia symptoms is **stones** (renal calculi), **bones** (bone destruction secondary to malignancy), **psychic moans** (lethargy, weakness, fatigue, confusion), and **abdominal groans** (abdominal pain, constipation, polyuria, polydipsia).

DIAGNOSIS AND DIFFERENTIAL

- On the ECG you may see depressed ST segments, widened T waves, shortened QT intervals, and heart blocks. Levels above 20 mEq/L can cause cardiac arrest.
- A mnemonic to aid recall the common causes is **PAM P. SCHMIDT: P**arathyroid hormone, **A**ddison's disease, **M**ultiple myeloma, **P**aget's disease, **S**arcoidosis, **C**ancer, **H**yperthyroidism, **M**ilk-alkali syndrome, **I**mmobilization, excess vitamin **D,** and **T**hiazides.

EMERGENCY DEPARTMENT CARE AND DISPOSITION

- Emergency treatment is important in the following conditions: a calcium level above 12 mg/dL, a symptomatic patient, a patient who cannot tolerate PO fluids, or a patient with abnormal renal function.
- Correct dehydration with normal saline, 5 to 10 L, may be required over 1 to 2 days. Consider invasive monitoring.
- Administer furosemide, 40 mg IV; however, take care to avoid exacerbating the patient's dehydration if present. Correct the concurrent hypokalemia or hypomagnesemia. Do not use thiazide diuretics (worsen hypercalcemia).
- If the above treatments are not effective, administer calcitonin 0.5 to 4 IU/kg IV over 24 hours or IM divided every 6 hours, along with hydrocortisone 25 to 100 mg IV every 6 hours.

HYPOMAGNESEMIA

CLINICAL FEATURES

- $[Mg^{2+}]$, $[K^+]$, and $[PO_4^-]$ move together intra- and extracellularly. Hypomagnesemia can present with CNS symptoms (depression, vertigo, ataxia, seizures, increased DTR, tetany) or cardiac symptoms (arrhythmias, prolonged QT and PR intervals, worsening of digitalis effects).
- Also seen are anemia, hypotension, hypothermia, and dysphagia.

DIAGNOSIS AND DIFFERENTIAL

- The diagnosis should not be based on $[Mg^{2+}]$ levels, since total depletion can occur before any significant laboratory changes are seen; it must therefore be suspected clinically.
- In the U.S., the most common cause is alcoholism, followed by poor nutrition, cirrhosis, pancreatitis,

correction of diabetic ketoacidosis (DKA), or excessive GI losses

EMERGENCY DEPARTMENT CARE AND DISPOSITION

- First, correct volume deficits and any decreased potassium, calcium, or phosphate.
- If the patient is an alcoholic in delirium tremens (DTs) or pending DTs, administer 2 g magnesium sulfate in the first hour, then 6 g in the first 24 hours. Check DTR every 15 minutes. DTR disappear when the serum magnesium level rises above 3.5 mEq/L, at which time the magnesium infusion should be stopped.

HYPERMAGNESEMIA

CLINICAL FEATURES

- Signs and symptoms manifest progressively; DTR disappear with a serum magnesium level above 3.5 mEq/L, muscle weakness at a level above 4 mEq/L, hypotension at a level above 5 mEq/L, and respiratory paralysis at a level above 8 mEq/L.

DIAGNOSIS AND DIFFERENTIAL

- Hypermagnesemia is rare. Common causes are renal failure with concomitant ingestion of magnesium-containing preparations (antacids) and lithium ingestion. Serum levels are diagnostic. Suspect coexisting increased potassium and phosphate.

EMERGENCY DEPARTMENT CARE AND DISPOSITION

- Rehydrate with normal saline and furosemide 20 to 40 mg IV (in absence of renal failure).
- Correct acidosis with ventilation and sodium bicarbonate 50 to 100 mEq, if needed.
- In symptomatic patients, 5 mL (10% solution) of CaCl IV antagonizes the magnesium effects.

ACID-BASE DISORDERS

CLINICAL FEATURES

- Several conditions should alert the clinician to possible acid-base disorders: a history of renal, endocrine, or psychiatric disorders (drug ingestion), or signs of acute disease: tachypnea, cyanosis, Kussmaul's respiration, respiratory failure, shock, changes in mental status, vomiting, diarrhea, or other acute fluid losses.
- Acidosis is due to a gain of acid or a loss of alkali; causes may be metabolic (fall in serum $[HCO_3^-]$) or respiratory (rise in P_{CO_2}).
- Alkalosis is due to a loss of acid or an addition of base, and is either metabolic (rise in serum $[HCO_3^-]$) or respiratory (fall in P_{CO_2}).
- The lungs and kidneys primarily maintain the acid-base regulation. Metabolic disorders prompt an immediate compensatory change in ventilation, either venting CO_2 in cases of metabolic acidosis, or retaining it in cases of metabolic alkalosis.

DIAGNOSIS AND DIFFERENTIAL

- The diagnosis begins with measurement and analysis of serum $[HCO_3^-]$ from the electrolyte panel, and the pH and P_{CO_2} from the ABG.
- The effect of the kidneys in response to metabolic disorders is to excrete hydrogen ion (with chloride) and recuperate $[HCO_3^-]$, a process that requires hours to days. The compensatory mechanisms of the lungs and kidney will return the pH toward, but not to, normal.
- Diagnosis and differential must begin with defining the nature of the acid-base disorder (with the stepwise approach below), then determine the most likely etiology from the differential listings in each section that follows.
- In a mixed disorder the pH, P_{CO_2}, and $[HCO_3^-]$ may be normal, and the only clue to a metabolic acidosis is a widened anion gap (see step 4 below).

STEPWISE METHOD OF ACID-BASE CLINICAL PROBLEM SOLVING

1. If the patient's preillness values are known, use them as a baseline, otherwise use as normal: pH = 7.4, $[HCO_3^-]$ = 24 mm/L, P_{CO_2} = 40 mm Hg.
2. If the pH indicates acidosis (lower than 7.35), the primary (or predominant) mechanism can be ascertained by examining the $[HCO_3^-]$ and P_{CO_2}.
3. If the $[HCO_3^-]$ is low (implying a primary metabolic acidosis), then the anion gap (AG) should be examined and, if possible, compared with a known prior steady-state value.
4. The AG is measured as follows: anion gap = $[Na^+] - ([Cl^-] + [HCO_3^-])$ = approximately 10 to 12 mEq/L in the normal patient.
5. If the AG is increased compared to the known previous value, or is greater than 15, then by definition a wide-AG metabolic acidosis is present. If the AG is unchanged, then the disturbance is a

non-widened (sometimes termed unchanged AG or hyperchloremic) metabolic acidosis.

6. Next examine whether the ventilatory response is appropriate.
7. If the metabolic acidosis has been present for 24 hours or more, the expected P_{CO_2} can be calculated as $P_{CO_2} = (1.5 \times [HCO_3^-] + 8) \pm 2$. However, if the disorder is acute, then the relationship is simpler: the expected fall in P_{CO_2} in response to a fall in bicarbonate is the following: P_{CO_2} falls by 1 mm Hg for every 1 mEq/dL fall in bicarbonate. This relationship holds true provided the bicarbonate level is greater than 8 mEq/dL.
8. If the respiratory change is acute (judged by the history), use the following formula to calculate the expected change in pH when the P_{CO_2} changes: the change in $[H^+] = 0.8$ (change in P_{CO_2}). Thus a 10-mm Hg increment in P_{CO_2} produces an 8 mmol increase in hydrogen ion concentration.
9. If the decrease in the P_{CO_2} equals the decrease in the $[HCO_3^-]$ (or as expected), there is appropriate respiratory compensation.
10. If the decrease in the P_{CO_2} is greater than the decrease in the $[HCO_3^-]$, there is a concomitant respiratory alkalosis. If the decrease in the P_{CO_2} is less than the decrease in $[HCO_3^-]$, there is also a concomitant respiratory acidosis.
11. If the P_{CO_2} is elevated (rather than the $[HCO_3^-]$ decreased), the primary disturbance is respiratory acidosis. The next step is to figure out which type it is by examining the ratio of (the change in) $[H^+]$ to (the upward change in) the P_{CO_2}. If the ratio is 0.8, it is considered acute. If the ratio is 0.33, it is considered chronic.
12. If the pH is greater than 7.45, the primary or predominant disturbance is an alkalosis.
13. It is best to look at the $[HCO_3^-]$ first. If it is elevated, there is a primary metabolic alkalosis.
14. If the P_{CO_2} is low, there is a primary respiratory alkalosis.
15. See the sections below for determining the etiology and management.

METABOLIC ACIDOSIS

• When considering metabolic acidosis, causes should be further divided into wide (elevated) and normal anion-gap acidosis. The term **anion gap** is misleading because in serum, there is no gap between total positive and negative ions; however, we commonly measure more positive ions than negative ions.

CLINICAL FEATURES

• No matter what the etiology, acidosis can cause nausea and vomiting, abdominal pain, change in sensorium, and tachypnea, sometimes Kussmaul's respiratory pattern.
• Acidosis also leads to decreased muscle strength and force of cardiac contraction, arterial vasodilation, venous vasoconstriction, and pulmonary hypertension.
• Patients may present with nonspecific complaints or shock.

DIAGNOSIS AND DIFFERENTIAL

• Using clinical judgment to guide testing, helpful laboratory tests to consider after serum electrolytes and the ABG are BUN, creatinine, lactic acid, the ketoacids acetoacetate and β-hydroxybutyrate, and potential toxins such as salicylate, methanol, and ethylene glycol.
• Causes of metabolic acidosis can be divided into two main groups: (1) those associated with increased production of organic acids (increased anion-gap metabolic acidosis; see Table 6-5); and (2) those associated with a loss of bicarbonate or addition of chloride (normal anion-gap metabolic acidosis; see Table 6-6).
• Triglyceride levels greater than 600 mg/dL produce overestimation of chloride levels measured by colorimetric techniques and may result in underestimation of serum sodium, resulting in an apparently narrow or even negative anion gap.[3]
• Although an anion gap greater than 30 mEq/L is usually caused by lactic acidosis or ketoacidosis, these conditions may exist even when the anion gap is normal.

TABLE 6-5 Causes of High Anion-Gap Metabolic Acidosis

Lactic acidosis
  Type A: Decrease in tissue oxygenation
  Type B: No decrease in tissue oxygenation

Renal failure (acute or chronic)

Ketoacidosis
  Diabetes
  Alcoholism
  Prolonged starvation (mild acidosis)
  High-fat diet (mild acidosis)

Ingestion of toxic substances
  Elevated osmolar gap
    Methanol
    Ethylene glycol
  Normal osmolar gap
    Salicylate
    Paraldehyde
    Cyanide

TABLE 6-6   Causes of Normal Anion-Gap Metabolic Acidosis

With a tendency to hyperkalemia	With a tendency to hypokalemia
Subsiding diabetic ketoacidosis	Renal tubular acidosis, type I (classical distal acidosis)
Early uremic acidosis	Renal tubular acidosis, type II (proximal acidosis)
Early obstructive uropathy	Acetazolamide
Renal tubular acidosis, type IV	Acute diarrhea with losses of $[HCO_3^-]$ and $[K^+]$
Hypoaldosteronism (Addison's disease)	Ureterosigmoidostomy with increased resorption of $[H^+]$ and $[Cl^-]$ and losses of $[HCO_3^-]$ and $[K^+]$
Infusion or ingestion of HCl, NH_4Cl, lysine-HCl, or arginine-HCl	Obstruction of artificial ileal bladder
Potassium-sparing diuretics	Dilution acidosis

- Caution is necessary when serum ketone testing is performed, because the chemical reaction used to measure serum ketones has an important limitation: the nitroprusside reaction is positive only for acetoacetate. Patients presenting with clinically severe diabetic ketoacidosis or alcoholic ketoacidosis may have predominately β-hydroxybutyrate as the ketone species in their blood, and may therefore test negative or only weakly positive.
- An anion gap value less than 25 mEq/L has been found to be an insensitive indicator of elevated lactate levels in critically ill patients.[4]
- In trauma patients, the postresuscitation anion gap does not predict lactate levels.[5]
- A mnemonic to aid the recall the causes of increased anion-gap metabolic acidosis is: **a mud piles**: **a**lcohol, **m**ethanol, **u**remia, **D**KA, **p**araldehyde, **i**ron and isoniazid, **l**actic acidosis, **e**thylene glycol, **s**alicylates, and **s**tarvation.
- A mnemonic that can aid the recall the causes of normal anion-gap metabolic acidosis is: **used carp**: **u**reterostomy, **s**mall bowel fistulas, **e**xtra chloride, **d**iarrhea, **c**arbonic anhydrase inhibitors, **a**drenal insufficiency, **r**enal tubular acidosis, and **p**ancreatic fistula.

EMERGENCY DEPARTMENT CARE AND DISPOSITION

- Give supportive care by improving perfusion, administering fluids as needed, and improving oxygenation and ventilation.
- Correct the underlying problem. If the patient has ingested a toxin, give the appropriate treatment or antidote, as directed by the specific toxicology chapters in this book (see Chaps. 100 through 120). If septic, perform cultures and administer antibiotics, as directed by the appropriate chapters in this handbook. If in

shock, administer fluids and vasopressors as directed by the appropriate chapters (see Chaps. 7 through 11) of this book. If the patient is in DKA, treat as directed in Chap. 132, with IV fluids and insulin.
- Indications for bicarbonate therapy are listed in Table 6-7.
- When bicarbonate is used, Adrogue and Madias[6] recommend administering 0.5 mEq/kg bicarbonate for each mEq/dL desired rise in $[HCO_3^-]$. The goal is to restore adequate buffer capacity ($[HCO_3^-]$ >8 mEq/dL) or achieve clinical improvement in shock or dysrhythmias.
- Bicarbonate should be given as slowly as the clinical situation permits; 1.5 ampules of sodium bicarbonate in 500 mL D_5W produces a nearly isotonic solution for infusion.

METABOLIC ALKALOSIS

- The two most common causes of metabolic alkalosis are excessive diuresis (with loss of potassium, hydrogen ion, and chloride), and excessive loss of gastric secretions (with loss of hydrogen ion and chloride).
- Other causes of hypokalemia should also be considered.

CLINICAL FEATURES

- Symptoms of the underlying disorder (usually fluid loss) dominate the clinical presentation, but general symptoms of metabolic alkalosis include muscular irritability, tachydysrhythmias, and impaired oxygen delivery.
- The diagnosis of metabolic alkalosis is made from laboratory studies revealing a bicarbonate level above 26 mEq/L and a pH above 7.45.

TABLE 6-7   Indications for Bicarbonate Therapy in Metabolic Acidosis

INDICATION	RATIONALE
Severe hypobicarbonatemia (<4 mEq/L)	Insufficient buffer concentrations may lead to extreme increases in acidemia with small increases in acidosis
Severe acidemia (pH <7.20) with signs of shock or myocardial irritability that is not rapidly responsive to supportive measures	Therapy for the underlying cause of acidosis depends upon adequate organ perfusion
Severe hyperchloremic acidemia*	Lost bicarbonate must be regenerated by kidneys and liver, which may require days

*No specific threshold indication by pH exists. The presence of serious hemodynamic insufficiency despite supportive care should guide the use of bicarbonate therapy for this indication.

- In most cases, there is also an associated hypokalemia and hypochloremia.

DIAGNOSIS AND DIFFERENTIAL

- The differential diagnosis includes dehydration, loss of gastric acid, excessive diuresis, administration of mineralocorticoids, increased intake of citrate or lactate, hypercapnia, hypokalemia, and severe hypoproteinemia.

EMERGENCY DEPARTMENT CARE AND DISPOSITION

- Administer fluids in the form of normal saline in cases of dehydration.
- Administer potassium as KCl, no faster than 20 mEq/h, unless serum potassium is above 5.0 mEq/L.

RESPIRATORY ACIDOSIS

CLINICAL FEATURES

- Respiratory acidosis may be life threatening and a precursor to respiratory arrest. The clinical picture is often dominated by the underlying disorder.
- Typically, respiratory acidosis depresses the mental function, which may progressively slow the respiratory rate. Patients may be confused, somnolent, and eventually, unconscious.
- Although frequently hypoxic, in some disorders the fall in oxygen saturation may lag behind the elevation in P_{CO_2}. Pulse oximetry may be misleading, making arterial blood gases essential for the diagnosis.

DIAGNOSIS AND DIFFERENTIAL

- The differential diagnosis includes: chronic obstructive pulmonary disease (COPD), drug overdose, CNS disease, chest wall disease, pleural disease, and trauma.

EMERGENCY DEPARTMENT CARE AND DISPOSITION

- Increase ventilation. In many cases this requires intubation. The hallmark indication for intubation in respiratory acidosis is depressed mental status. Only in opiate intoxication is it acceptable to await treatment of the underlying disorder (rapid administration of naloxone) before reversal of the hypoventilation.
- Treat the underlying disorder. Remember that high-flow oxygen therapy may lead to exacerbation of CO_2

narcosis in patients with COPD and CO_2 retention. Monitor these patients closely when administering oxygen and intubate if necessary.

RESPIRATORY ALKALOSIS

CLINICAL FEATURES

- Hyperventilation syndrome is a problematic diagnosis for the emergency physician, as a number of life-threatening disorders present with tachypnea and anxiety: asthma, pulmonary embolism, diabetic ketoacidosis, and others.
- Symptoms of respiratory alkalosis often are dominated by the primary disorder promoting the hyperventilation.
- Hyperventilation by virtue of the reduction of P_{CO_2}, however, lowers both cerebral and peripheral blood flow, causing distinct symptoms.
- Patients complain of dizziness; painful flexion of the wrists, fingers, ankles, and toes; (carpopedal spasm); and frequently a chest pain described as tightness.

DIAGNOSIS AND DIFFERENTIAL

- The diagnosis of hyperventilation due to anxiety is a diagnosis of exclusion. Arterial blood gases can be used to rule out acidosis and hypoxia.
- Causes of respiratory alkalosis to consider include hypoxia, fever, hyperthyroidism, sympathomimetic therapy, aspirin overdose, progesterone therapy, liver disease, and anxiety.

EMERGENCY DEPARTMENT CARE AND DISPOSITION

- Treat the underlying cause. Only when more serious causes of hyperventilation are ruled out should you consider the treatment of anxiety. Anxiolytics may be helpful, such as lorazepam 1 to 2 mg, IV or PO.
- Rebreathing into a paper bag can cause hypoxia, and is not recommended.[7,8]

REFERENCES

1. Schrier RW: Treatment of hyponatremia. *N Engl J Med* 312: 1121, 1985.
2. Krause JA, Carlson RW: Rapid correction of hypokalemia using concentrated intravenous potassium chloride infusion. *Arch Intern Med* 150:613, 1990.

3. Graber ML, Quigg RJ, Stempsey WE, et al: Spurious hyperchloremia and decreased anion gap in hyperlipidemia. *Ann Intern Med* 98:607, 1983.
4. Levraut J, Bounatirou T, Ichai C, et al: Reliability of anion gap as an indicator of blood lactate in critically ill patients. *Intensive Care Med* 23:417, 1997.
5. Mikulaschek A, Henry SM, Donovan R, et al: Serum lactate is not predicted by anion gap or base excess after trauma resuscitation. *J Trauma* 40:218, 1996.
6. Adrogue HJ, Madias NE: Management of life-threatening acid-base disorders: Second of two parts. *N Engl J Med* 338:107, 1998.
7. Callaham M: Hypoxic hazards of traditional paper bag rebreathing in hyperventilating patients. *Ann Emerg Med* 18:622, 1989.
8. Callaham M: Panic disorders, hyperventilation, and the dreaded brown paper bag. *Ann Emerg Med* 30:838, 1997.

For further reading in *Emergency Medicine: A Comprehensive Study Guide,* 6th ed., see Chap. 25, "Acid-Base Disorders," by David D. Nicolaou and Gabor D. Kelen; Chap. 26, "Blood Gases: Pathophysiology and Interpretation," by Kelly L. Grogan and Peter Pronovost; and Chap. 27, "Fluid and Electrolytes," by Michael Londner, Darcie Hammer, and Gabor D. Kelen.

7 | **THERAPEUTIC APPROACH TO THE HYPOTENSIVE PATIENT**

John E. Gough

EPIDEMIOLOGY

- More than 1 million cases of shock present to emergency departments every year.
- Despite aggressive management, mortality remains high. One-month mortality for septic shock is 30 to 45%, and for cardiogenic shock it is 60 to 90%.[1,2]

PATHOPHYSIOLOGY

- Shock is defined as a circulatory insufficiency that creates an imbalance between tissue oxygen supply and demand.
- Shock is classified into four categories by etiology: (1) hypovolemic, (2) cardiogenic, (3) distributive (eg, neurogenic, anaphylaxis), and (4) obstructive (extracardiac obstruction to blood flow).
- Mean arterial pressure (MAP) is equal to the cardiac output (CO) times systemic vascular resistance (SVR). When oxygen demand exceeds delivery (DO_2), compensatory mechanisms attempt to maintain homeostasis. First, there is an increase in cardiac output. Next, the amount of oxygen extracted from hemoglobin increases. If the compensatory mechanisms are unable to meet oxygen demand, anaerobic metabolism occurs, resulting in the formation of lactic acid.

CLINICAL FEATURES

- The precipitating cause may be clinically obvious (eg, trauma, anaphylaxis), or occult (eg, adrenal insufficiency). The four main classes are hypovolemic, cardiogenic, distributive, and obstructive.
- A targeted history of the presenting symptoms and previously existing conditions including medication use may reveal the cause of the shock.
- Body temperature may be elevated, normal, or subnormal.
- Cardiovascular: Heart rate is usually elevated. Exceptions include paradoxical bradycardia in athletically conditioned individuals, intra-abdominal hemorrhage, hypoglycemia, cardiovascular drug (eg, β-blocker) use, and pre-existing cardiac disease. Blood pressure may initially be normal or elevated due to compensatory mechanisms, later falling when cardiovascular compensation fails. Neck veins may be distended or flattened, depending on the etiology of shock. Decreased coronary perfusion pressures can lead to ischemia, decreased ventricular compliance, and increased left ventricular diastolic pressure and pulmonary edema.
- Respiratory: Tachypnea, increased minute ventilation, and increased dead space are common. Bronchospasm, hypocapnia with progression to respiratory failure, and acute respiratory distress syndrome can be seen.
- Skin: Many skin findings are possible including pale, dusky, clammy skin with cyanosis, sweating, altered temperature, and decreased capillary refill.
- Gastrointestinal: The low-flow state found in shock can produce ileus, GI bleeding, pancreatitis, acalculous cholecystitis, and mesenteric ischemia.
- Renal: Oliguria may result from a reduced glomerular filtration rate; however, a paradoxical polyuria can occur in sepsis, which may be confused with adequate hydration status.
- Metabolic: Respiratory alkalosis is the first acid-base abnormality, progressing to metabolic acidosis as shock continues. Blood sugar may be increased or decreased. Hyperkalemia is a potentially life-threatening metabolic abnormality.

DIAGNOSIS AND DIFFERENTIAL

- The presumed etiology of shock will determine the specific diagnostic measures to be employed.
- Commonly performed laboratory studies include complete blood cell count (CBC), platelet count, electrolytes, blood urea nitrogen (BUN), creatinine, glucose, prothrombin and partial thromboplastin times, and urinalysis. Other laboratory tests frequently employed include arterial blood gases (ABG), lactic acid, fibrinogen, fibrin split products, D-dimer, cortisol levels, hepatic function tests, and cerebrospinal fluid studies.
- Cultures of blood, urine, cerebrospinal fluid, and wounds are ordered as necessary.
- Common diagnostic tests ordered include radiographs (chest and abdominal), electrocardiograms, ultrasound or CT scans (chest, head, abdomen, and pelvis) and echocardiograms.
- A pregnancy test should be performed in all females of childbearing age.
- Determination of the etiology of shock will guide therapy. Consider less common causes of shock when there is a lack of response to initial therapy. These include cardiac tamponade, tension pneumothorax, adrenal insufficiency, toxic or allergic reactions, and occult bleeding. Occult bleeding can occur from a ruptured ectopic pregnancy, or intra-abdominal or pelvic bleeding.

EMERGENCY DEPARTMENT CARE AND DISPOSITION

- The goal of the interventions is to restore adequate tissue perfusion and identify and treat the underlying etiology.
- Timely ED care can significantly decrease the predicted mortality of critically ill patients in as little as 6 hours of treatment.[3]
- Application of an algorithmic approach to optimize hemodynamic end points with early goal-directed therapy in the ED reduces mortality by 16% in patients with severe sepsis or septic shock.[4] The ABCDEs of shock resuscitation are establishing an **A**irway, controlling the work of **B**reathing, optimizing the **C**irculation, assuring adequate oxygen **D**elivery, and achieving **E**nd points of resuscitation.
- Airway control may be required, employing endotracheal intubation when necessary for respiratory distress or persistent shock. Remember that associated interventions such as sedative use and positive pressure ventilation may contribute to further hypotension and hemodynamic collapse.

- If mechanical ventilation is utilized, use of a neuromuscular blocking agent will decrease lactic acid production from respiratory muscle fatigue and increased oxygen consumption.
- Supplemental high-flow oxygen should be administered.
- Most external hemorrhage can be controlled by direct compression.
- Early surgical consultation for internal bleeding is essential. The need to rapidly correct internal bleeding is at the core of the "hypotensive resuscitation" controversy. Although a study of prehospital resuscitation found that delaying fluid resuscitation until surgical homeostasis improved survival,[5] these benefits could not be reproduced during hospital resuscitation.[6] Therefore the role for hypotensive resuscitation remains undefined.
- Large-bore peripheral intravenous catheters should be established and will usually allow adequate fluid resuscitation. Central venous access may be necessary for monitoring and employing some therapies, including pulmonary artery catheters, venous pacemakers, and long-term vasopressor therapy.
- Isotonic, intravenous crystalloid fluids (0.9% NaCl, Ringer's lactate) are preferred for the initial resuscitation phase.[7,8] The volume of crystalloids should be three times the estimated blood loss. Initial bolus volume is 20 to 40 mL/kg over 10 to 20 minutes. Blood is the ideal resuscitative fluid for hemorrhagic shock or in the presence of significant anemia. Fully cross-matched blood is preferred, but if more rapid intervention is required, type-specific or type O negative blood may be employed. The decision to use platelets or fresh frozen plasma (FFP) should be based on evidence of impaired hemostasis and frequent monitoring of coagulation parameters. Platelets are generally given if there is ongoing hemorrhage and the platelet count is 50,000 or less, and FFP is indicated if the prothrombin time is prolonged more than 1.5 times.
- Vasopressors should be used if there is persistent hypotension after adequate volume resuscitation.[9] American Heart Association recommendations based on blood pressure are dobutamine 2.0 to 20.0 μg/kg/min for systolic BP over 100 mm Hg, dopamine 5.0 to 20.0 μg/kg/min for systolic BP 70 to 100 mm Hg, and norepinephrine 0.5 to 30.0 μg/kg/min for systolic BP under 70 mm Hg.
- Acidosis should be treated with adequate ventilation and fluid resuscitation. Sodium bicarbonate (1 mEq/kg) use is controversial.[10] If it is used, it is given only in the setting of severe acidosis refractory to ventilation and fluid resuscitation.
- Early surgical or medical consultation for admission or transfer is done as indicated.

REFERENCES

1. Moscucci M, Bates ER: Cardiogenic shock. *Cardiol Clin* 13: 391, 1995.
2. Angus DC, Linde-Zwirble WT, Lidlicker J, et al: Epidemiology of severe sepsis in the United States: Analysis of incidence, outcome, and associated costs of care. *Crit Care Med* 29:1303, 2001.
3. Ngugen HB, Rivers EP, Havstad S, et al: Critical care in the emergency department: A physiologic assessment and outcome evaluation. *Acad Emerg Med* 7:1354, 2000.
4. Rivers EP, Nguyen HB, Havstad S, et al: Early goal-directed therapy in the treatment of severe sepsis and septic shock. *N Engl J Med* 345:1368, 2001.
5. Bickell WM, Wall MJ, Pepe PE, et al: Immediate versus delayed fluid resuscitation for hypotensive patients with penetrating torso injuries. *N Engl J Med* 331:1105, 1994.
6. Dutton RP, Mackenzie CF, Scalea TM: Hypotensive resuscitation during active hemorrhage: Impact on in-hospital mortality. *J Trauma* 52:1141, 2002.
7. Webb AR: The appropriate role of colloids in managing fluid imbalance: A critical review of the meta-analytic findings. *Crit Care Med* 4(Suppl 2):S26, 2000.
8. Alderson P, Schierhout G, Roberts I: Colloids versus crystalloids of fluid resuscitation in critically ill patients. *Cochrane Database Syst Rev* (2):CD00567, 2000.
9. Reinhart K, Sakka SG, Meier-Hellmann A: Haemodynamic management of a patient with septic shock. *Eur J Anaesthesiol* 17:6, 2000.
10. Arieff AI: Current concepts in acid-base balance: Use of bicarbonate in patients with metabolic acidosis. *Anaesth Crit Care* 7:182, 1996.

For further reading in *Emergency Medicine: A Comprehensive Study Guide,* 6th ed., see Chap. 30, "Approach to the Patient in Shock," by Emanuel P. Rivers, Ronny M. Otero, and H. Bryant Nguyen; and Chap. 31, "Fluid and Blood Resuscitation," by James E. Manning.

8 SEPTIC SHOCK

John E. Gough

EPIDEMIOLOGY

- Average mortality is 45%, ranging from 20 to 80%, depending on the patient's premorbid state.[1]
- Sepsis is more common in older adults, with a mean age of 55 to 60 years.[1]
- Factors that predispose to gram-negative bacteremia include diabetes mellitus, lymphoproliferative disorders, cirrhosis of the liver, burns, invasive procedures or devices, and chemotherapy.[1]
- Factors that predispose to gram-positive bacteremia include vascular[1] catheters, indwelling mechanical devices, burns, and IV drug use.
- Fungemia most often occurs in immunocompromised patients.[2]

PATHOPHYSIOLOGY

- Sepsis starts as a focus of infection that results in either bloodstream invasion or a proliferation of organisms at the infected site. These organisms release exogenous toxins that can include endotoxins and exotoxins.
- The host's reaction to these toxins results in the release of humoral defense mechanisms including cytokines (tumor necrosis factor, interleukins), platelet activating factor, complement, kinins, and coagulation factors. These factors can have deleterious effects including myocardial depression and vasodilation, resulting in refractory hypotension and multiple organ system failure.

CLINICAL FEATURES

- Hyperthermia or hypothermia may be seen in sepsis. Hypothermia is more often seen in patients at the extremes of age and in immunocompromised patients.
- Other vital sign abnormalities include tachycardia, wide pulse pressure, tachypnea, and hypotension.
- Mental status changes are commonly seen, ranging from mild disorientation to coma.
- Ophthalmic manifestations include retinal hemorrhages, cotton wool spots, and conjunctival petechiae.
- Cardiovascular manifestations initially include vasodilation resulting in warm extremities. Cardiac output is maintained or increased early in sepsis through a compensatory tachycardia. As sepsis progresses, hypotension may occur. Patients in septic shock may demonstrate a diminished response to volume replacement.
- Respiratory symptoms include tachypnea and hypoxemia. Sepsis remains the most common condition associated with acute respiratory distress syndrome (ARDS). ARDS may occur within minutes to hours from the onset of sepsis.
- Renal manifestations include acute renal failure (ARF) with azotemia, oliguria, and active urinary sediment.

- Liver dysfunction is common. The most frequent presentation is cholestatic jaundice. Increases in transaminases, alkaline phosphatase, and bilirubin are often seen. Severe or prolonged hypotension may induce acute hepatic injury or ischemic bowel necrosis. Painless mucosal erosions may occur in the stomach and duodenum and cause upper GI bleeds.
- Skin findings may be present in sepsis. Local infections can be present from direct invasion into cutaneous tissues. Examples include cellulitis, erysipelas, and fasciitis. Hypotension and disseminated intravascular coagulation (DIC) can also produce skin changes including acrocyanosis and necrosis of peripheral tissues. Infective endocarditis can produce microemboli that cause skin changes.
- Hematologic changes include neutropenia, neutrophilia, thrombocytopenia, and DIC. A leukocytosis with a left shift is common. Neutropenia occurs rarely but is associated with increased mortality. The hemoglobin and hematocrit are usually not affected unless the sepsis is prolonged or there is an associated GI bleed.
- Thrombocytopenia occurs in over 30% of patients with sepsis. DIC is more often associated with gram-negative sepsis. Decompensated DIC presents with clinical bleeding and thrombosis. Laboratory studies can show thrombocytopenia, prolonged PT and PTT, decreased fibrinogen level and antithrombin levels, and increased fibrin monomer, fibrin split values, and D-dimer values.
- Hyperglycemia may be seen even without a history of diabetes and is associated with an increased risk of adverse outcomes.[3] Hyperglycemia may result from increased catecholamines, cortisol, and glucagon. Increased insulin resistance, decreased insulin production, and impaired utilization of insulin may further contribute to hyperglycemia. Rarely, depletion of glucagon and inhibition of gluconeogenesis may lead to hypoglycemia.
- Arterial blood gas (ABG) studies in early sepsis may reveal hypoxemia and respiratory alkalosis. As perfusion worsens and glycolysis increases, a metabolic acidosis results.

DIAGNOSIS AND DIFFERENTIAL

- Septic shock should be suspected in any patient with a temperature of >38°C or <36°C, systolic blood pressure of <90 mm Hg, and evidence of inadequate organ perfusion. Hypotension may not reverse with volume replacement.
- Clinical features may include mental obtundation, hyperventilation, hot or flushed skin, and a wide pulse pressure.

- Immunocompromised patients and those at the extremes of age may have atypical presentations without fever or localized source of infection.
- Complete blood count (CBC), platelet count, DIC panel (prothrombin time, partial thromboplastin time, fibrinogen, D-dimer, and antithrombin concentration), electrolyte levels, liver function tests, renal function tests, ABG analysis, and urinalysis should be considered in a patient with suspected sepsis.
- Cultures of cerebrospinal fluid (CSF), sputum, blood, urine, and wounds should be obtained as indicated.
- Radiographs of suspected foci of infection (chest, abdomen, etc) should be obtained.
- Ultrasonography or CT scanning may help identify occult infections in the cranium, thorax, abdomen, and pelvis.
- Acute meningitis is the most common central nervous system infection associated with septic shock, and a lumbar puncture should be considered. If meningitis is a significant consideration, empiric antibiotics should be given as soon as possible.
- Differential diagnosis should include noninfectious causes of shock, including hypovolemic, cardiogenic, neurogenic, obstructive, endocrine, and anaphylactic.

EMERGENCY DEPARTMENT CARE AND DISPOSITION

- The first priority is aggressive airway management with high-flow oxygen (keeping oxygen saturations >90%). Endotracheal intubation may be necessary.
- Correction or stabilization of hypotension and inadequate perfusion is the second goal of resuscitation.[4] Rapid infusion of crystalloid IV fluid (Lactated Ringer's or normal saline) at 500 mL (20 mL/kg in children) every 5 to 10 minutes should be initiated; four to six liters (60 mL/kg in children) may be necessary. Crystalloids are preferred over colloids initially.[5] In addition to blood pressure, mental status, pulse, capillary refill, central venous pressure, pulmonary capillary wedge pressure, and urine output (>30 mL/h in adult, 1 mL/kg/h in children) can be monitored to evaluate therapy. If ongoing blood loss is suspected, blood replacement may be necessary.
- Dopamine 5 to 20 μg/kg/min titrated to response should be used if hypotension is refractory to IV fluid.[6]
- If the systolic blood pressure remains <70 mm Hg despite the preceding measures, a norepinephrine 8 to 12 μg/min loading dose and a 2 to 4 μg/min infusion to maintain mean arterial blood pressure of at least 60 mm Hg should be started.
- The source of infection must be removed if possible (remove indwelling catheters and incise and drain abscesses).

- Empiric antibiotic therapy: This measure is ideally begun after obtaining cultures, but administration should not be delayed. Dosages should be the maximum allowed and given intravenously. When the source is unknown, therapy should be effective against both gram-positive and gram-negative organisms. In adults a third-generation cephalosporin (ceftriaxone 1 g IV, cefotaxime 2 g IV, or ceftazidime 2 g IV) or an antipseudomonal β-lactamase-susceptible penicillin can also be used. Addition of an aminoglycoside (gentamycin 2 mg/kg IV or tobramycin 2 mg/kg IV) to this regimen is recommended. In immunocompromised adults ceftazidime 2 g IV, imipenem 750 mg IV, or meropenem 1 g IV alone is acceptable. If gram-positive infection is suspected (indwelling catheter or IV drug use) oxacillin 2 g IV or vancomycin 15 mg/kg IV should be added. If an anaerobic source is suspected (intra-abdominal, genital tract, odontogenic, and necrotizing soft tissue infection), metronidazole 7.5 mg/kg IV or clindamycin 900 mg IV should additionally be administered. If *Legionella* is a potential source, erythromycin 500 mg IV should be added.
- Acidosis is treated with oxygen, ventilation, and IV fluid replacement. If acidosis is severe, administration of sodium bicarbonate 1 mEq/kg IV is acceptable as directed by ABGs (see Chap. 6).
- DIC should be treated with fresh frozen plasma 15 to 20 mL/kg initially to keep PT at 1.5 to 2 times normal, and then treated with platelet infusion to maintain serum concentration of 50 to 100,000.
- If adrenal insufficiency is suspected, a glucocorticoid (hydrocortisone 100 mg IV) should be administered.
- Tight glucose control (between 80 and 100 mg/dL) with intensive insulin therapy has demonstrated decreased mortality from multiorgan failure.[3]
- Multiple innovative therapies are currently under investigation.

REFERENCES

1. Angus DC, Linde-Zwirble WT, Lidicker J, et al: Epidemiology of severe sepsis in the United States: analysis of incidence, outcome, and associated cost of care. *Crit Care Med* 29:1303, 2001.
2. Sands KE, Bates DW, Lanken PN: Epidemiology of sepsis syndrome in 8 academic medical centers. *JAMA* 278:234, 1997.
3. Van den Berghe G, Wouters P, Weekers F, et al: Intensive insulin therapy in the critically ill patients. *N Engl J Med* 345: 1359, 2001.
4. Task Force of the American College of Critical Care Medicine, Society of Critical Care Medicine: Practice parameters for hemodynamic support of sepsis in adult patients in sepsis. *Crit Care Med* 27:639, 1999.
5. Alderson P, Schierhout G, Roberts I: Colloids versus crystalloids of fluid resuscitation in critically ill patients. *Cochrane Database Syst Rev* (2):CD00567, 2000.
6. Reinhart K, Sakka SG, Meier-Hellmann A: Haemodynamic management of a patient with septic shock. *Eur J Anaesthesiol* 17:6, 2000.

For further reading in *Emergency Medicine: A Comprehensive Study Guide,* 6th ed., see Chap 32, "Septic Shock," by Jonathan Jui.

---

9 CARDIOGENIC SHOCK

Rawle A. Seupaul

EPIDEMIOLOGY

- Cardiogenic shock is the most common cause of in-hospital mortality from acute myocardial infarction (AMI), accounting for 50,000 to 70,000 deaths per year.
- Approximately 5 to 7% of patients with AMI will develop cardiogenic shock.
- Cardiogenic shock usually occurs early in the course of AMI, with a median time of 8 hours.
- Risk factors for developing cardiogenic shock after AMI are: advanced age, female gender, large MI, anterior wall MI, previous MI, previous congestive heart failure (CHF), multivessel disease, proximal left anterior descending artery occlusion, and diabetes mellitus.[1]
- With medical treatment alone, mortality from cardiogenic shock is high, 70 to 90%.

PATHOPHYSIOLOGY

- Cardiogenic shock most commonly occurs secondary to left ventricular (LV) infarction, involving approximately 40% of LV mass.
- Reduction in cardiac output leads to oliguria, hepatic failure, anaerobic metabolism, lactic acidosis, and hypoxia. These outcomes serve to further impair myocardial function.
- Multivessel disease, diastolic dysfunction, and arrhythmias hasten the development of cardiogenic shock. The presence of these factors may produce shock with less than 40% LV involvement.
- Compensatory mechanisms attempt to maximize cardiac output. Initially, sympathetic tone is increased,

resulting in increased myocardial contractility. This can be visualized as compensatory hyperkinesis by echocardiography.

- Sympathetic activity activates the renin-angiotensin system. This results in arterial and venous constriction, as well as increased blood volume. The latter is accomplished by sodium and water resorption mediated by aldosterone.
- Right ventricular (RV) infarction accounts for approximately 3 to 4% of cases of cardiogenic shock. However, this is usually associated with concomitant LV dysfunction.
- Cardiogenic shock occurs when there is insufficient pumping ability of the heart to support the metabolic needs of the tissues.

CLINICAL FEATURES

- Cardiogenic shock almost always presents with hypotension (systolic blood pressure <90 mm Hg). Systolic blood pressure may be >90 mm Hg if there is pre-existing hypertension or compensatory increases in systemic vascular resistance.
- Tachycardia or bradycardia may be present. If excessive, they should be treated appropriately.
- Patients may be cool, have clammy skin, and become oliguric.
- Diminished cerebral perfusion may lead to altered mentation.
- LV failure may result in tachypnea, rales, and frothy sputum.
- Valvular dysfunction and septal defects may be discernible by auscultating a murmur.
- Jugular venous distension and abdominal jugular reflex are usually present.

DIAGNOSIS AND DIFFERENTIAL

- The diagnosis of cardiogenic shock should be suspected from the initial history and physical exam. However, ancillary tests are essential to confirm the diagnosis. These include: (1) electrocardiogram (ECG) consistent with AMI (right-sided leads should be performed if posterior wall infarction is suspected); (2) chest radiograph for evidence of CHF, abnormal mediastinum, and evaluation of the cardiac silhouette; (3) two-dimensional transthoracic echocardiography done at the bedside can quickly evaluate regional hypokinesis, akinesis, or dyskinesis; and (4) lab studies including cardiac enzymes, coagulation parameters, serum lactate, and chemistries may also help establish the diagnosis.

- B-type natriuretic peptide (BNP) is an excellent predictor of the clinical development of heart failure after myocardial infarction.[2] Normal serum BNP levels are less than 100 pg/mL.
- Disease processes to be considered in the differential diagnosis include aortic dissection, pulmonary embolism, pericardial tamponade, acute valvular insufficiency, hemorrhage, and sepsis.

EMERGENCY DEPARTMENT CARE

- Medical therapy should be considered a temporizing measure while arranging for definitive treatment to re-establish coronary patency.[3]
- Stabilize the patient; perform endotracheal intubation if necessary, attain intravenous access, provide high-flow oxygen, place the patient on a monitor and pulse oximeter, and obtain an ECG and rhythm strip.
- Have the patient bite and chew 160 to 325 mg of aspirin unless contraindicated by allergy.[3]
- Identify rhythm disturbances, hypovolemia, hypoxemia, and electrolyte abnormalities early and treat accordingly.
- Intravenous nitroglycerin and/or morphine should be titrated for chest pain as well as hemodynamic parameters.
- If hypotension is present after adequate fluid resuscitation, consider dobutamine and/or dopamine (both dosed at 2 to 20 μg/kg/min IV) for inotropic and pressor support.[4,5]
- Norepinephrine (0.5 to 12 μg/min IV), a pure α-adrenergic agonist, may be used when there is an inadequate response to dopamine and/or dobutamine.
- Milrinone is a phosphodiesterase inhibitor that increases cyclic adenosine monophosphate, resulting in increased inotropism and cardiac output, and decreased peripheral vasoconstriction. Close hemodynamic monitoring is necessary with this agent as it may cause hypotension requiring pressor support.
- For preload and afterload reduction, the use of nitroglycerin (5 to 100 μg/min IV) or nitroprusside (0.5 to 10 μg/kg/min IV), respectively, may be indicated.
- Reperfusion modalities have been shown to significantly decrease mortality with the use of thrombolytics, intra-aortic balloon counterpulsation, and early revascularization.[3,6] If these modalities are not available, the patient should be transferred to an institution that can provide these services.
- Cardiology and/or thoracic surgery should be consulted early.
- Almost all patients with cardiogenic shock require admission to an intensive care unit.

REFERENCES

1. Peterson ED, Shaw LJ, Califf RM: Risk stratification after myocardial infarction. *Ann Intern Med* 126:561, 1997.
2. Sabatine MS, Morrow DA, de Lemos JA, et al: Multimarker approach to risk stratification in non-ST elevation acute coronary syndromes: Simultaneous assessment of troponin I, C-reactive protein, and B-type natriuretic peptide. *Circulation* 105:1760, 2002.
3. Menon V, Hochman JS: Management of cardiogenic shock complicating acute myocardial infarction. *Heart* 88:531, 2002.
4. Chernow B: New advances in the pharmacologic approach to circulatory shock. *J Clin Anesth* 8:67S, 1996.
5. McGhie AI, Goldstein RA: Pathogenesis and management of acute heart failure and cardiogenic shock: Role of inotropic therapy. *Chest* 102(Suppl 2):671S, 1992.
6. Sanborn TA, Sleeper LA, Bates ER, et al: Impact of thrombolysis, intra-aortic balloon pump counterpulsation, and their combination in cardiogenic shock complicating acute myocardial infarction: A report from the SHOCK trial registry. Should we emergently revascularize occluded coronaries for cardiogenic shock? *J Am Coll Cardiol* 36(Suppl A):1123, 2000.

For further reading in *Emergency Medicine: A Comprehensive Study Guide,* 6th ed., see Chap. 33, "Cardiogenic Shock," by W. Franklin Peacock IV and Jim Edward Weber.

10 ANAPHYLAXIS AND ACUTE ALLERGIC REACTIONS

Damian F. McHugh

EPIDEMIOLOGY

- The spectrum of allergic reactions ranges from mild cutaneous symptoms to life-threatening anaphylaxis.
- The prevalence of anaphylaxis ranges from as high as 5 per 1000 to as low as 2 per 10,000 emergency department visits.[1,2]
- Four fatalities per 10 million people are seen annually.[3]
- The faster the onset of symptoms, the more severe the reaction; half the fatalities occur within the first hour.[4]

PATHOPHYSIOLOGY

- The mechanism of allergic reactions is classically a type 1 hypersensitivity reaction, whereby allergen-induced IgE molecules cross-link on the surface of mast cells or basophils, causing degranulation and release of inflammatory mediators.
- Additional mechanisms have been described through complement activation[5,6] or by direct stimulation of the mast cell, or by unknown mechanisms—the so-called anaphylactoid reactions.[5,7]
- Common causes are penicillin, aspirin and other nonsteroidals, ACE inhibitors, trimethoprim-sulfamethoxazole, radiocontrast media, *Hymenoptera* stings, peanuts, shellfish, milk, eggs, monosodium glutamate, nitrites, and dyes.
- Idiopathic anaphylaxis is by definition of unknown cause.
- Anaphylaxis is not automatic on recurrent exposure; recurrence rates are 40 to 60% for insect stings, 20 to 40% for radiocontrast media, and 10 to 20% for penicillin.[7]
- Concurrent use of β-blockers is a risk for severe prolonged anaphylaxis.

CLINICAL FEATURES

- Urticaria (hives) is a cutaneous IgE-mediated reaction yielding itchy red wheals of varying sizes which promptly disappear. Angioedema is a similar reaction with edema in the dermis, usually of the face and neck. By definition, anaphylaxis includes either respiratory compromise or cardiovascular collapse.
- Reactions may occur in seconds, or may be delayed 1 hour or more after allergen exposure. Up to 20% of reactions are "biphasic," with further mediator release occurring up to 4 to 8 hours later.
- Pruritus and urticaria are the most common initial symptoms.
- Respiratory symptoms are stridor, dyspnea, and wheeze.
- GI features are nausea, cramps, diarrhea, and vomiting.

DIAGNOSIS AND DIFFERENTIAL

- Diagnosis is made clinically. A history of exposure to an agent, followed by symptoms and signs as described above make the diagnosis of acute allergic reaction.
- No tests are diagnostic. Work-up may focus on excluding other diagnoses, or stabilizing the cardiorespiratory systems.
- Differential diagnoses include vasovagal reaction, asthma, acute coronary ischemic syndromes or dysrhythmias, epiglottitis or foreign body, carcinoid, mastocytosis, or hereditary angioedema.

EMERGENCY DEPARTMENT CARE AND DISPOSITION

- **A:** *Airway*. Anticipate intubation earlier rather than later, especially in hoarse patients, or those with "a lump in my throat." Edema may necessitate an endotracheal tube one to two sizes smaller than expected. A cricothyrotomy kit should be open and ready before you start intubation.
- **B:** *Breathing*. Administer high flow oxygen as necessary. Treat bronchospasm with nebulized albuterol 0.5 mL of 5% solution in 3 mL saline.
- **C:** *Circulation*. Most patients, especially if hypotensive, need large volumes of crystalloid. If hypotension persists after 1 to 2 L of IV fluid is infused, IV epinephrine is needed.
- **D:** *Discontinue* the antigen exposure (eg, stop IV drug infusions or remove bee stingers).
- **E:** *Epinephrine*. If severe respiratory distress, laryngeal edema, or shock, IV epinephrine is indicated.[4] Put 0.1 mL of 1:1000 epinephrine in 10 mL saline and infuse over 5 to 10 minutes. If no response, start an epinephrine infusion with 1 mg (1 mL of 1:1000) in 500 mL saline at 0.5 to 2 mL/min (1 to 4 µg/min) and titrate to effect. For less severe signs, give intramuscular epinephrine 0.3 to 0.5 mL of 1:1000 every 5 to 10 minutes according to response. If repeated doses do not work, go to IV.
- **F:** *Further treatments*. Antihistamines, H_1 blockers such as diphenhydramine 25 to 50 mg IV are helpful and H_2 blockers such as ranitidine 50 mg can be helpful.[8] Steroids only help control persistent or delayed allergic reactions. Severe cases can be given methylprednisolone 125 mg IV; oral prednisone 60 mg can be used for less severe cases.
- **G:** *Glucagon*. In patients on β-blockers, glucagon 1 to 2 mg every 5 minutes may be helpful for hypotension refractory to epinephrine and fluids.
- Patients with symptomatic hereditary angioneurotic edema should be treated with C1 esterase inhibitor replacement in consultation with an appropriate specialist.[9]
- Observe patients with mild reactions for 1 hour, observe patients who receive epinephrine for 6 hours, and admit all patients with severe reactions to an ICU.
- Patients with angiotensin-converting enzyme inhibitor angioedema are often refractory to conventional therapy; patients with moderate to severe symptoms should be admitted for close observation.[10]
- Consider prescribing an Epi-Pen at discharge, and instruct patient in how and when to use it.
- Discharge patients with prescriptions for antihistamines and prednisone for 4 days.
- Referral of patients to an allergist for follow-up is prudent.

REFERENCES

1. Kemp SF, Lockey RF: Anaphylaxis: A review of causes and mechanisms. *J Allergy Clin Immunol* 110:341, 2002.
2. Stewart AG, Ewan PW: The incidence, aetiology and management of anaphylaxis presenting to an accident and emergency department. *QJ Med* 89:859, 1996.
3. Friday GA, Fireman P: Anaphylaxis. *Ear Nose Throat J* 75: 21, 1996.
4. Gavalas M, Sadana A, Metcalf S: Guidelines for the management of anaphylaxis in the emergency department. *J Accid Emerg Med* 15:96, 1998.
5. Atkinson TP, Kaliner MA: Anaphylaxis. *Med Clin North Am* 76:841, 1992.
6. Galli SJ: New concepts about the mast cell. *N Engl J Med* 328:257, 1993.
7. Bochner BS, Lichtenstein LM: Anaphylaxis. *N Engl J Med* 324:1785, 1991.
8. Winbery SL, Lieberman PL: Histamine and antihistamines in anaphylaxis. *Clin Allergy Immunol* 17:287, 2002.
9. Ebo DG, Stevens WF: Hereditary angioneurotic edema: A review of the literature. *Acta Clin Belg* 55:22, 2000.
10. Chiu AG, Newkirk KA, Davidson BJ, et al: Angiotensin-converting enzyme inhibitor-induced angioedema: A multicenter review and an algorithm for airway management. *Ann Otol Rhinol Larygol* 110:834, 2001.

For further reading in *Emergency Medicine, A Comprehensive Study Guide,* 6th ed., see Chap. 34, "Anaphylaxis and Acute Allergic Reactions," by Brian H. Rowe and Stuart Carr.

11 NEUROGENIC SHOCK

Rawle A. Seupaul

EPIDEMIOLOGY

- Approximately 10,000 spinal cord injuries occur in the U.S. each year.[1]
- The majority of cases are due to blunt trauma (motor vehicle crashes [MVC], falls, and sports-related), while penetrating trauma accounts for 10 to 15% of cases (gunshot and stab wounds).[2,3]

PATHOPHYSIOLOGY

- Neurogenic shock occurs when an acute spinal cord injury disrupts sympathetic flow, resulting in hypotension and bradycardia.[2]

- Spinal shock is a distinct entity that refers to transient loss of spinal reflexes below the level of a complete or partial cord injury.[4]
- Primary cord injury reflects the initial changes caused by the traumatic event (compression, laceration, or stretching of the spinal cord).
- Secondary injury ensues over several days to weeks and is caused mostly by continued cord ischemia.[4,5]

CLINICAL FEATURES

- Within the first 2 to 3 minutes, the initial cardiovascular response is hypertension, widened pulse pressure, and tachycardia.[2,6]
- As sympathetic tone is lost, the patient will be hypotensive with warm, dry skin.[7]
- The inability to redirect blood from the periphery to the core may result in hypothermia.[7]
- Most patients will be bradycardic secondary to overriding vagal tone.
- Any injury above T1 should disrupt the entire sympathetic chain. Injuries between T1 and L3 may result in partial sympathetic disruption.
- The symptoms of neurogenic shock may last from 1 to 3 weeks.[7]

DIAGNOSIS AND DIFFERENTIAL

- The diagnosis of neurogenic shock is always one of exclusion. Other potential causes of hypotension must be ruled out and treated aggressively.
- The diagnosis of neurogenic shock is clinical, and the diagnosis of spinal cord injury may be confirmed with magnetic resonance imaging.

EMERGENCY DEPARTMENT CARE AND DISPOSITION

- Once the ABCDs are addressed and the diagnosis of neurogenic shock is made, therapy is aimed at mitigating hypotension and bradycardia.
- Crystalloid should be infused with a goal mean arterial pressure above 70 mm Hg. If inotropic support is necessary, the use of dobutamine or dopamine (both dosed at 2 to 20 μg/kg/min) may be beneficial.[7]
- For symptomatic bradycardia, atropine should be used. In patients who develop heart block or asystole, a pacemaker may be necessary.[6]
- The use of steroids for spinal cord injury is discussed in Chap. 164.

REFERENCES

1. McDonald JW, Sadowsky C: Spinal-cord injury. *Lancet* 359: 417, 2002.
2. Zipnick RI, Scalea TM, Trooskin SZ, et al: Hemodynamic responses to penetrating spinal cord injuries. *J Trauma* 35:578, 1993.
3. Savitsky E, Votey S: Emergency department approach to acute thoracolumbar spine injury. *J Emerg Med* 15:49, 1997.
4. Bracken MB, Shepard MJ, Hellenbrand KG, et al: A randomized, controlled trial of methylprednisolone or naloxone in the treatment of acute spinal cord injury. *N Engl J Med* 322:1405, 1990.
5. Tator CH, Rowed DW: Current concepts in the immediate management of acute spinal cord injuries. *Can Med Assoc J* 121:1453, 1979.
6. Guha AB, Tator CH: Acute cardiovascular effects of experimental spinal cord injury. *J Trauma* 28:481, 1988.
7. Gilson GJ, Miller AC, Clevenger FW, Curet LB: Acute spinal cord injury and neurogenic shock in pregnancy. *Obstet Gynecol Surg* 50:556, 1995.

ANALGESIA, ANESTHESIA, AND SEDATION

12 ACUTE PAIN MANAGEMENT AND CONSCIOUS SEDATION

Diamond Vrocher

- Acute pain is present in 50 to 60% of patients presenting to the emergency department.
- Factors contributing to inadequate pain control, or oligoanalgesia, include a limited understanding of the related pharmacology, misunderstanding of the patient's perception of pain, and fear of serious side effects.
- Procedural sedation, formerly called conscious sedation, may be indicated for fracture manipulation or joint reduction, abscess drainage, laceration repair, tube thoracostomy, cardioversion, or a diagnostic study.

PATHOPHYSIOLOGY

- Noxious stimuli are first registered peripherally by nociceptors, C fibers, A-σ fibers, and free nerve endings, resulting in the release of glutamate, substance P, neurokinin A, and calcitonin gene-related peptide within the spinal cord.[1]
- Pain is modulated at the level of the dorsal root ganglion, inhibitory interneurons, and ascending pain tracts.
- Cognitive interpretation, localization, and identification of pain occur at the level of the hypothalamus, thalamus, limbus, and reticular activating system.

CLINICAL FEATURES

- The subjective interpretation of pain is variable. Therefore pain is best assessed using a validated, age-appropriate, objective pain scale.[2-3]

- Competent patients who are awake and cooperative can often reliably localize pain and determine its quality and severity.[4]
- Patients who have difficulty communicating with their caregivers due to cultural differences, extremes of age, language barriers, or mental illness may not be able to describe and localize pain.
- Physiologic responses to pain and anxiety are nonspecific, but include tachycardia, blood pressure elevation, tachypnea, diaphoresis, flushing or pallor, nausea, and muscle tension.
- Behavioral responses to pain and anxiety include facial expressions, posturing, crying, and vocalization.

EMERGENCY DEPARTMENT CARE AND DISPOSITION

- Nonpharmacologic treatment of pain may be used alone or adjunctively. Examples include application of heat or cold, immobilization or elevation of injured extremities, explanation and reassurance, relaxation, distraction, guided imagery, and biofeedback.
- Discussion and demonstration of a painful procedure with pediatric patients and their parent just prior to the intervention may minimize anxiety. Parents should be included in the interventional process to provide comfort.
- When pharmacologic intervention is necessary, the desired effect, the route of delivery, and the desired duration of effect should be considered in determining the ideal agent.

SYSTEMIC SEDATION AND ANALGESIA

- Sedation is a pharmacologically-induced decrease in environmental awareness. Analgesia is relief from the perception of pain.[5]

- Procedural sedation and analgesia (PSA) is divided into several classes. Minimal sedation is a sedated state characterized by normal responsiveness to voice. Moderate sedation and analgesia, or conscious sedation, is characterized by responsiveness to voice or light tactile stimulation while maintaining a patent airway and adequate ventilation. Deep sedation and analgesia is characterized by responsiveness only to repeated or painful stimuli, potential loss of a patent airway, and potentially inadequate ventilation.[6]
- PSA agents often have a narrow therapeutic index. Therefore these agents should be given in small incremental doses, allowing adequate time for the development and assessment of peak effect. Continuous reassessment is required.
- All patients undergoing PSA require continuous pulse oximetry, cardiac monitoring, immediate availability of suction and resuscitation equipment, and constant observation by a provider trained in airway management.
- Blood pressure, heart rate, respiratory rate, and level of consciousness should be assessed at baseline and every 5 to 10 minutes.
- Precalculated doses of "rescue" or reversal agents should be at the bedside: naloxone, 0.1 mg/kg every 2 to 3 minutes to reverse opiate-induced respiratory depression, and flumazenil, 0.01 to 0.02 mg/kg every 1 to 2 minutes to reverse benzodiazepine-induced respiratory depression during PSA.[7]
- Flumazenil should not be used on patients with a history of chronic benzodiazepine or tricyclic antidepressant use due to the risk of seizures.

ANALGESIA

NONOPIATES

- Nonopiate agents may be used alone for mild pain, or adjunctively with opiates for moderate to severe pain. Nonopiate analgesics cause no respiratory depression or sedation.
- Acetaminophen is an analgesic and anti-inflammatory agent with no anti-platelet effects that is safe in all age groups. Hepatotoxicity may occur in doses above 140 mg/kg/day.
- Nonsteroidal anti-inflammatory drugs (NSAIDs) include aspirin, naproxen, indomethacin, ibuprofen, and ketorolac. NSAIDs are analgesics and anti-inflammatory agents with opiate dose-sparing effects, but may cause platelet dysfunction, impaired coagulation, and gastrointestinal irritation, and bleeding.
- The safety and efficacy of ibuprofen has been established for children over 6 months of age.
- Aspirin use in children is discouraged because of the association with Reye's syndrome. Aspirin also may

induce bronchospasm and should be avoided in some asthmatic patients.

OPIATES

- Opiates have analgesic and sedative effects, but may cause respiratory depression, nausea and vomiting, constipation, urinary retention, pruritus, confusion, and muscle rigidity.
- Morphine is a naturally-occurring opiate with a 5- to 20-minute onset of effect, a 10- to 30-minute peak effect, and a 2- to 6-hour duration. The dose of morphine is 0.1 to 0.2 mg/kg and is commonly administered IV or IM. Morphine may cause hypotension due to histamine release.
- Fentanyl is a semisynthetic opiate with a 3- to 5-minute onset of effect and a 30- to 40-minute duration. The dose of fentanyl is 0.5 to 3 μg/kg IV, with additional 0.5 μg/kg doses until the desired effect is achieved. Fentanyl does not release histamine, and therefore rarely causes hypotension.[8] Chest wall rigidity may occur, especially at doses >5 μg/kg IV, and may not reverse with naloxone. In such cases, neuromuscular blockade and intubation may be required.
- Meperidine is a semisynthetic opiate whose use is discouraged in the ED due to the CNS toxicity of its metabolite normeperidine, significant histamine release,[8] and a higher risk of addiction than other opiates.
- Hydromorphone is a semisynthetic opiate with a 5- to 20-minute onset of effect, a 3- to 4-hour duration of effect, and less sedation and nausea than morphine. The dose of hydromorphone is 1 to 2 mg IV (0.015 mg/kg IV pediatric).
- The Demerol, Phenergan, Thorazine (DPT) cocktail is not recommended because of unreliable efficacy, the potential for respiratory depression, and an exceedingly long (7 hours) half-life.[9]

NITROUS OXIDE

- N_2O is an analgesic and sedative inhalation agent with a 3- to 5-minute onset of action and a 3- to 5-minute duration after withdrawal.
- N_2O is useful in adults and pediatrics for wound dressing and minor procedures.
- N_2O must be delivered with a minimum of 30% oxygen to avoid hypoxia, and a fail-safe scavenger system must be in place.
- Nitrous oxide may cause nausea and vomiting and is contraindicated in patients with altered mental status, head injury, suspected pneumothorax, chronic obstructive pulmonary disease (COPD), perforated viscus, or eye injuries, and in patients with balloon-tipped catheters.
- N_2O has opiate agonist properties, and therefore should be used with extreme caution if combined with

a sedative or opiate to avoid deep sedation or general anesthesia.[10]

KETAMINE

- Ketamine produces analgesia, amnesia, and dissociation with minimal respiratory depression. Ketamine has an onset of effect of 1 minute, and a duration of effect of 6 to 30 minutes. The dose of ketamine is 3 to 4 mg/kg PO, PR, or IM, with supplemental doses given at 2 mg/kg/dose. The IV dose is 0.5 to 2.0 mg/kg, with supplemental doses given at 0.25 mg/kg.
- Ketamine may cause bronchorrhea, bronchodilation, hypersalivation, laryngospasm, hallucinatory emergence reactions in older children and adults, and increased intracranial and intraocular pressure.[11]
- Ketamine is a direct myocardial depressant and vasodilator. However, its stimulation of CNS sympathetic outflow usually results in tachycardia and vasoconstriction.
- Atropine (0.01 mg/kg IV or IM) may be administered to control hypersalivation. Midazolam (0.025 to 0.05 mg/kg IV) may attenuate the emergence reaction, but caution must be taken to avoid respiratory depression.
- Contraindications include age ≤3 months, history of airway instability or tracheal stenosis, procedures involving stimulation of the posterior pharynx, cardiovascular disease (hypertension and congestive heart failure [CHF]), head injury, altered level of consciousness, CNS mass, hydrocephalus, poorly controlled seizure disorder, glaucoma, acute globe injury, or psychosis.

SEDATION

- Benzodiazepines (BNZ) are the sedative agents most commonly used for anxiolysis and PSA in the ED.
- BNZ potentiate the effects of CNS gamma-aminobutyric acid (GABA), resulting in chloride influx, which produces sedation, amnesia, anxiolysis, anticonvulsant effects, and respiratory depression.
- Midazolam, the most commonly used agent for PSA, has an onset of effect of 5 minutes and a duration of effect of 30 to 45 minutes. The adult dose of midazolam is 0.25 to 0.5 mg IV every 3 to 5 minutes titrated to desired effect. The pediatric dose is 0.05 to 0.1 mg/kg IV every 3 to 5 minutes with a maximum cumulative dose of 0.2 mg/kg. Lower doses should be considered in elderly or intoxicated patients because of the risk of cardiovascular and respiratory depression.
- Barbiturates are sedative agents used for PSA. Barbiturates may cause respiratory and CNS depression, especially when used with other sedatives or opiates.

- Methohexital is an ultra-short-acting barbiturate (0.5 to 2 mg/kg IV) with an onset of effect of 30 to 60 seconds and a duration of effect of 10 minutes. Methohexital may also be used rectally (20 to 25 mg/kg) for motionless sedation in children to facilitate imaging procedures.[12–13] Methohexital, unlike most barbiturates, may precipitate seizures and should therefore be avoided in patients with a seizure disorder.
- Chloral hydrate is a sedative agent (25 to 75 mg/kg PO or PR) used in children primarily for painless diagnostic procedures.[14] The onset of effect is 45 to 60 minutes and the duration of effect is 2 to 6 hours. Chloral hydrate is no longer recommended in the ED due to potential airway obstruction and the prolonged duration of action.
- Etomidate is an ultra-short-acting sedative agent increasingly used for PSA. Etomidate (0.1 to 0.2 mg/kg IV) has minimal hemodynamic effects and a low risk of apnea. Adverse effects may include vomiting, myoclonus, short-term adrenal suppression, and CNS depression.[15]

LOCAL AND REGIONAL ANESTHESIA

- Local anesthesia can be obtained by infiltrating directly into the area, infiltrating into the area of the peripheral nerves supplying the area, or infusing into the venous system supplying the area to be anesthetized.
- Local anesthetics are divided into two classes: amides and esters. Lidocaine is the prototype amide, and procaine the prototype ester. Bupivacaine is an amide anesthetic with a duration of action of 2 to 6 hours, and is preferred for prolonged procedures.
- The injection pain of local anesthetics can be minimized by slow injection of warm, bicarbonate-buffered solution through a 27- or 30-gauge needle.
- The addition of epinephrine to lidocaine extends the duration of anesthesia and slows systemic absorption. However, epinephrine may decrease local perfusion, and should not be used in the fingers, nose, toes, penis, or ears.
- Local anesthetic toxicity from excessive total dose or inadvertent IV injection can lead to cardiovascular depression, arrhythmias, seizures, and death. The maximum dose of lidocaine is 4.5 mg/kg without epinephrine, and 7 mg/kg with epinephrine.
- True allergic reactions to local anesthetics are rare and are usually due to the metabolite para-aminobenzoic acid in esters, and the preservative methylparaben in amides. If a true allergy is suspected, a preservative-free agent from the other class should be used. Diphenhydramine and benzyl alcohol are alternative local anesthetics.

- Regional anesthesia may have a delayed (up to 15 minutes) onset of effect. Prior to administering regional anesthesia, neurovascular status must be assessed.
- Before injection of regional anesthetic, aspiration should be performed to reduce the chance of intravascular injection.
- Topical anesthetics reduce the discomfort of painful procedures, decrease the need for local infiltration of anesthetics, and maintain wound edges. The most common topical anesthetics for ED use are tetracaine adrenaline cocaine (TAC), lidocaine epinephrine tetracaine (LET), and lidocaine prilocaine (EMLA). Neither TAC nor LET should be used on mucous membranes or in end-arterial fields. EMLA is reserved for use on intact skin.

REFERENCES

1. Grubb BD: Peripheral and central mechanisms of pain. *Br J Anaesthes* 81:8, 1998.
2. McCormack HM, Home DJ, Sheather S: Clinical applications of visual analog scales: A critical review. *Psychol Med* 10:1007, 1988.
3. Todd KH: Clinical versus statistical significance in the assessment of pain relief. *Ann Emerg Med* 27:439, 1996.
4. Acute Pain Management Guideline Panel: *Acute Pain Management: Operative or Medical Procedures and Trauma.* Guideline Report. AHCPR Pub. No. 92-002. Rockville MD: Agency for Health Care Policy and Research, Public Health Service, U.S. Department of Health and Human Services, 1993.
5. Sacchetti A, Schafermeyer R, Gerardi M, et al: Pediatric analgesia and sedation. *Ann Emerg Med* 23:237, 1994.
6. Joint Commission on Accreditation of Healthcare Organizations. 2001 Sedation and Anesthesia Care Standards. Available at: http://www.jcaho.org/accredited+organizations/behavioral+health+care/standards/revisions/2001/sedation+and+anesthesia.htm. Accessed June 28, 2002.
7. Chudnofsky CR: Group TEMCSS: Safety and efficacy of flumazenil in reversing conscious sedation in the emergency department. *Acad Emerg Med* 4:944, 1997.
8. Flacke JW, Flacke WE, Bloor BC, et al: Histamine release by four narcotics: A double-blind study in humans. *Anesth Analg* 66:723, 1987.
9. American Academy of Pediatrics: Reappraisal of the lytic cocktail/demerol, phenergan, and thorazine (DPT) for the sedation of children. *Pediatrics* 95:598, 1995.
10. Gillman MA: Analgesic (subanesthetic) nitrous oxide interacts with the endogenous opioid system: A review of the evidence. *Life Sci* 39:1209, 1986.
11. Green SM, Rothrock SG, Harris T, et al: Intramuscular ketamine for pediatric sedation in the emergency department: safety profile in 1,022 cases. *Ann Emerg Med* 31:688, 1998.
12. Pomeranz ES, Chudnofsky CR, Deegan TJ, et al: Rectal methohexital sedation for computed tomography imaging of stable pediatric emergency department patients. *Pediatrics* 105:1110, 2000.
13. Sedik H: Use of intravenous methohexital as a sedative in pediatric emergency departments. *Arch Pediatr Adolesc Med* 155:665, 2001.
14. Binder LS, Leake LA: Chloral hydrate for emergent pediatric procedural sedation: a new look at an old drug. *Am J Emerg Med* 9:530, 1991.
15. Vinson DR, Bradbury DR: Etomidate for procedural sedation in emergency medicine. *Ann Emerg Med* 39:592, 2002.

For further reading in *Emergency Medicine: A Comprehensive Study Guide,* 6th ed., see Chap. 36, "Acute Pain Management in the Adult Patient," by Gary D. Zimmer; Chap. 37, "Local and Regional Anesthesia," by Eric Higginbotham and Robert J. Vissers; Chap. 38, "Procedural Sedation and Analgesia," by David D. Nicolaou; and Chap. 134, "Acute Pain Management and Procedural Sedation in Children," by Michael N. Johnston and Erica Liebelt.

13 MANAGEMENT OF PATIENTS WITH CHRONIC PAIN
David M. Cline

- Chronic pain is defined as a painful condition that lasts longer than 3 months. Chronic pain can also be defined as pain that persists beyond the reasonable time for an injury to heal or a month beyond the usual course of an acute disease.

EPIDEMIOLOGY

- Chronic pain affects about a third of the population at least once during a patient's lifetime, at a cost of 80 to 90 billion dollars in health care payments and lawsuit settlements annually.
- Patients who attribute their chronic pain to a specific traumatic event experience more emotional distress, more life interference, and more severe pain than those with other causes.[1]
- Chronic pain may be caused by (1) a chronic pathologic process in the musculoskeletal or vascular system, (2) a chronic pathologic process in one of the organ systems, (3) a prolonged dysfunction in the peripheral or central nervous system, or (4) a psychological or environmental disorder.

PATHOPHYSIOLOGY

- The pathophysiology of chronic pain can be divided into three basic types. Nociceptive pain is associated with ongoing tissue damage. Neuropathic pain is associated with nervous system dysfunction in the absence of ongoing tissue damage. Finally, psychogenic pain has no identifiable cause.[2]

CLINICAL FEATURES

- Signs and symptoms of chronic pain syndromes are summarized in Table 13-1.
- "Transformed migraine" is a syndrome in which classic migraine headaches change over time and develop into a chronic pain syndrome. One cause of this change is frequent treatment with narcotics.
- Fibromyalgia is classified by the American College of Rheumatology as the presence of 11 of 18 specific tender points, nonrestorative sleep, muscle stiffness, and generalized aching pain, with symptoms present longer than 3 months (see www. rheumatology.org).
- Risk factors for chronic back pain following an acute episode include male gender, advanced age, evidence of nonorganic disease, leg pain, prolonged initial episode, and significant disability at onset.[3]
- Previous recommendations for bedrest in the treatment of back pain have proven counterproductive.[4]

Exercise programs have been found to be helpful in chronic low back pain.[5]

- Patients with complex regional pain type I, also known as reflex sympathetic dystrophy, and complex regional pain type II, also known as causalgia, may be seen in the ED as early as the second week after treatment of an acute injury.[6] These disorders cannot be differentiated from one another on the basis of signs and symptoms. Type I occurs because of prolonged immobilization or disuse, and type II occurs because of a peripheral nerve injury.

DIAGNOSIS AND DIFFERENTIAL

- The most important task of the emergency physician is to distinguish an exacerbation of chronic pain from a presentation that heralds a life- or limb-threatening condition. The history and physical examination should either confirm the chronic condition or point to the need for further evaluation when unexpected signs or symptoms are elicited.

EMERGENCY DEPARTMENT CARE AND DISPOSITION

- Before approximately 1990, the use of opioids for chronic pain was discouraged by pain specialists. Since that time, pain specialists have recommended

TABLE 13-1   Signs and Symptoms of Chronic Pain Syndromes

DISORDER	PAIN SYMPTOMS	SIGNS
Myofascial headache	Constant dull pain, occasionally shooting pain	Trigger points on scalp, muscle tenderness and tension
Transformed migraine	Initially migraine-like, becomes constant, dull, nausea, vomiting	Muscle tenderness and tension, normal neurologic examination
Fibromyalgia	Diffuse muscular pain, stiffness, fatigue, sleep disturbance	Diffuse muscle tenderness, >11 trigger points
Myofascial chest pain	Constant dull pain, occasionally shooting pain	Trigger points in area of pain
Myofascial back pain syndrome	Constant dull pain, occasionally shooting pain, pain does not follow nerve distribution	Trigger points in area of pain, usually no muscle atrophy, poor ROM in involved muscle
Articular back pain	Constant or sharp pain exacerbated by movement	Local muscle spasm
Neurogenic back pain	Constant or intermittent, burning or aching, shooting or electric shock-like, may follow dermatome; leg pain worse than back pain	Possible muscle atrophy in area of pain, possible reflex changes
Complex regional pain type I (RSD)	Burning persistent pain, allodynia, associated with immobilization or disuse	Early: edema, warmth, local sweating. Late: above alternates with cold; pale, cyanosis, eventually atrophic changes
Complex regional pain type II (causalgia)	Burning persistent pain, allodynia, associated with peripheral nerve injury	Early: edema, warmth, local sweating. Late: above alternates with cold; pale, cyanosis, eventually atrophic changes
Postherpetic neuralgia	Allodynia, shooting, lancinating pain	Sensory changes in the involved dermatome
Phantom limb pain	Variable: aching, cramping, burning, squeezing or tearing sensation	None

ABBREVIATIONS: ROM = range of motion; RSD = reflex sympathetic dystrophy.

opioids as an important option in a well-integrated treatment program.[7] However, treatment with opioids frequently contributes to the psychopathologic aspects of the disease.

• There are two essential points that affect the use of opioids in the ED on which there is agreement: (a) opioids should only be used in chronic pain if they enhance function at home and at work, and (b) a single practitioner should be the sole prescriber of narcotics or be aware of their administration by others.

• A previous narcotic addiction is a relative contraindication to the use of opioids in chronic pain, because when such patients are treated with opioids, addiction relapse rates approach 50%.[8]

• The management of chronic pain conditions is listed in Table 13-2.

• The need for long-standing treatment of chronic pain conditions may limit the safety of nonsteroidal anti-inflammatory drugs (NSAIDs).

• An evidence-based review found antidepressants to be effective in chronic low back pain, fibromyalgia, osteoarthritis, and neuropathic pain.[9] A separate meta-analysis found that tricyclic antidepressants were more effective in states in which symptoms were unexplained, such as fibromyalgia.[10]

• When antidepressants are prescribed in the ED, a follow-up plan should be in place. The most common drug and initial dose is amitriptyline, 10 to 25 mg, 2 hours prior to bedtime.

• Gabapentin, a structural analog of gamma-aminobutyric acid, has been shown to be effective in postherpetic neuralgia,[11] painful diabetic neuropathy,[12] and may have some benefit in complex regional pain syndromes. Gabapentin is started with an initial dose of 300 mg/day and is increased up to 1200 mg tid according to response.

• A meta-analysis has found calcitonin to be effective in the treatment of complex regional pain, type I (reflex sympathetic dystrophy).[13] Calcitonin can be given at a dose of 100 IU intranasal spray per day.

• Referral to the appropriate specialist is one of the most productive means to aid in the care of chronic pain patients who present to the ED. Chronic pain clinics have been successful at changing the lives of patients by eliminating opioid use, decreasing pain levels by one third, and increasing work hours twofold.

TABLE 13-2   Management of Selected Chronic Pain Syndromes

DISORDER	PRIMARY ED TREATMENT	SECONDARY TREATMENT*	POSSIBLE REFERRAL OUTCOME
Cancer pain	NSAIDs Opiates	Long-acting opiates	Optimization of medical therapy
Myofascial headache	NSAIDs Cyclobenzaprine	Antidepressants Phenothiazines	Trigger point injections Optimization of medical therapy
Transformed migraine	NSAIDs Cyclobenzaprine	Antidepressants	Optimization of medical therapy Narcotic withdrawal
Fibromyalgia	NSAIDs	Antidepressants Exercise program	Optimization of medical therapy Dedicated exercise program
Myofascial chest pain	NSAIDs	Antidepressants	Trigger point injections Optimization of medical therapy
Myofascial back pain syndrome	NSAIDs Stay active	Antidepressants	Trigger point injections Optimization of medical therapy
Articular back pain	NSAIDs		Surgery Physical therapy
Neurogenic back pain	Acute: tapered prednisolone or prednisone	NSAIDs Muscle relaxants	Epidural steroids Surgery Exercise program
Complex regional pain types I and II (RSD and causalgia)	Prednisone 60 mg per day x 4 days and then taper to include three weeks of therapy	Calcitonin Antidepressants Anticonvulsants	Spinal cord stimulation Intrathecal baclofen Sympathetic nerve blocks Spinal analgesia
Postherpetic neuralgia	Simple analgesics	Gabapentin Antidepressants	Regional nerve blockade
Phantom limb pain	Simple analgesics	Antidepressants Anticonvulsants	TENS Sympathectomy

*If started in the ED, consultation and/or follow-up with pain specialist or personal physician recommended.

ABBREVIATIONS: RSD = reflex sympathetic dystrophy, TENS = transcutaneous electrical nerve stimulation, NSAIDs = non-steroidal anti-inflammatory drugs.

MANAGEMENT OF PATIENTS WITH DRUG-SEEKING BEHAVIOR

EPIDEMIOLOGY

- The Drug Abuse Warning Network has tracked drug-related visits in a sampling of U.S. emergency departments and found that the incidence of visits to the ED involving abuse of narcotic-analgesic combinations rose 85% between 1994 and 2000.[14]
- A study conducted in Portland found that drug-seeking patients presented to the ED 12.6 times per year, visited 4.1 different hospitals, and used 2.2 different aliases. Patients who were refused narcotics at one facility were successful in obtaining narcotics at another facility 93% of the time and were later successful at obtaining narcotics from the same facility 71% of the time.[15]

CLINICAL FEATURES

- Because of the spectrum of drug-seeking patients, the history given may be factual or fraudulent.
- Drug seekers may be demanding, intimidating, or flattering.
- In one ED study, the most common complaints of patients who were seeking drugs were (in decreasing order): back pain, headache, extremity pain, and dental pain.[15]
- Many fraudulent techniques are used, including "lost" prescriptions, "impending" surgery, factitious hematuria with a complaint of kidney stones, self mutilation, and factitious injury.

DIAGNOSIS AND DIFFERENTIAL

- Drug-seeking behaviors can be divided into two groups: predictive and less predictive (Table 13-3). The behaviors listed under "predictive" are illegal in many states and form a solid basis to refuse narcotics to the patient.

EMERGENCY DEPARTMENT CARE AND DISPOSITION

- The treatment of drug-seeking behavior is to refuse the controlled substance, consider the need for alternative medication or treatment, and consider referral for drug counseling.

TABLE 13-3 Characteristics of Drug Seeking Behavior

BEHAVIORS PREDICTIVE OF DRUG SEEKING BEHAVIOR*

Sells prescription drugs
Forges/alters prescriptions
Factitious illness, requests narcotics
Uses aliases to receive narcotics
Admits to illicit drug addiction
Conceals multiple physicians prescribing narcotics
Conceals multiple ED visits receiving narcotics

LESS PREDICTIVE FOR DRUG SEEKING BEHAVIOR

Admits to multiple doctors prescribing narcotics
Admits to multiple prescriptions for narcotics
Abusive when refused
Multiple drug allergies
Uses excessive flattery
From out of town
Asks for drugs by name

*Behaviors in this category are unlawful in many states.

REFERENCES

1. Turk DC, Okifuji A: Perception of traumatic onset, compensation status, and physical findings: Impact on pain severity, emotional distress, and disability in chronic pain patients. *J Behav Med* 14:435, 1996.
2. Garcia J, Altman RD: Chronic pain states: Pathophysiology and medical therapy. *Semin Arthritis Rheum* 27:1, 1997.
3. Valat JP, Goupille P, Vedere V: Low back pain: Risk factors for chronicity. *Rev Rheum Engl Ed* 64.189, 1997.
4. Waddell G, Feder G, Lewis M: Systemic reviews of bed rest and advice to stay active for acute low back pain. *Br J Gen Pract* 47:647, 1997.
5. Faas A: Exercises: Which ones are worth trying, for which patients, and when. *Spine* 21:2874, 1996.
6. Cooney WP: Somatic versus sympathetic mediated chronic limb pain: Experiences and treatment options. *Hand Clin* 13: 355, 1997.
7. Khouzam RH: Chronic pain and its management in primary care. *South Med J* 93:946, 2000.
8. Dunbar SA, Katz NP: Chronic opioid therapy for nonmalignant pain in patients with a history of substance abuse. *J Pain Symptom Manage* 11:163, 1996.
9. Fishbain D: Evidence-based data on pain relief with antidepressants. *Ann Med* 32:305, 2000.
10. O'Malley PG, Jackson JL, Santoro J, et al: Antidepressant therapy for unexplained symptoms and symptom syndromes. *J Fam Prac* 48:980, 1999.
11. Rowbotham M, Harden N, Stacey B, et al: Gabapentin for the treatment of postherpetic neuralgia. *JAMA* 280:1837, 1998.
12. Backonja M, Beydoun A, Edwards KR, et al: Gabapentin for symptomatic treatment of painful diabetic neuropathy in patients with diabetes mellitus. *JAMA* 280:1831, 1998.
13. Perez RSGM, Kwakkel G, Zuurmond WWA, et al: Treatment of reflex sympathetic dystrophy (CRPS Type 1): A research

synthesis of 21 randomized controlled trials. *J Pain Symptom Manage* 21:511, 2001.

14. Anonymous: *Emergency Department Trends from the Drug Abuse Warning Network, Preliminary Estimates January–June 2001 with Revised Estimates 1994–2000.* Rockville, MD: National Clearinghouse for Alcohol and Drug Information, 2002.

15. Zechnich AD, Hedges JR: Community-wide emergency department visits by patients suspected of drug seeking behavior. *Acad Emerg Med* 3:312, 1996.

For further reading in *Emergency Medicine: A Comprehensive Study Guide,* 6th ed., see Chap. 39, "Management of Patients with Chronic Pain," by David M. Cline.

EMERGENCY WOUND MANAGEMENT

14 EVALUATING AND PREPARING WOUNDS

Timothy Reeder

EPIDEMIOLOGY

- Traumatic wounds account for more than 6% of all visits to emergency departments in the United States.[1]
- The most frequently involved body locations are the face, scalp, fingers, and hands.[2]
- Wounds in children are shorter, more frequently linear, located on the head, and more often caused by blunt trauma compared with wounds of adults.[3,4]

PATHOPHYSIOLOGY

- The mechanism of injury will help identify risk of foreign body, contamination, and wound complication.[5]
- A foreign body sensation increases the likelihood of a retained foreign object.
- The degree of contamination, the presence of foreign body, a laceration in an extremity, and a compromise in blood flow increase the incidence of wound infection.[6]
- Blunt forces compress the skin against underling bone, while sharp objects produce shear forces resulting in skin damage.
- Crush injuries are more likely to cause wound infection due to greater tissue damage.[7]
- Low-energy impact injuries may result in hematoma formation. These require aspiration or incision and drainage if they fail to resorb spontaneously.

CLINICAL FEATURES

- Document important medical conditions such as diabetes, renal disease, immunosuppression, malnutrition, and connective tissue disorders that impact wound healing.
- Self-inflicted injuries should prompt consideration of psychiatric evaluation.
- Most states have regulations requiring reporting of injuries that result from intentional acts.
- As the time from injury to wound closure increases, the bacterial inoculum increases, but a clear association with clinically relevant wound infection is less clear.[6,8] Therefore clinicians should consider time from injury to presentation, along with wound etiology, body location, degree of contamination, host risk factors, and the importance of cosmetic appearance in assessing the decision to close the wound.
- After 4 days of open wound management, the risk of infection after closure substantially decreases.

DIAGNOSIS AND DIFFERENTIAL

- A complete neurovascular examination should be documented prior to analgesia or anesthesia.
- A thorough visual inspection to the full depth and length of the wound will minimize missed foreign bodies and tendon and nerve injuries; such missed problems are a common cause of litigation.
- One should consider injecting a wound that extends over a joint to determine the integrity of the joint space.
- Consider imaging studies to help detect foreign bodies (see Chap. 19).

EMERGENCY DEPARTMENT CARE AND DISPOSITION

- Wound preparation is the most important step for adequate evaluation of the wound, prevention of infection, and optimal cosmetic outcome.
- Universal precautions and adherence to strict sterile technique remain the standard of care.
- Pain control with consideration of local or regional anesthesia should be provided before any wound manipulation.

HEMOSTASIS

- Control of bleeding is required for adequate wound evaluation. Direct pressure is the preferred method.
- Epinephrine-containing local anesthetics can be used except in distal anatomy such as fingers, nose, ear, and the penis.
- Other measures for control of bleeding include ligation of small vessels, electrocautery, absorbable gelatin foam (Gelfoam), oxidized cellulose (Oxycel), or collagen sponge (Actifoam).

IRRIGATION

- Use skin disinfectants only on the wound edges and outward as these substances may impair host defenses and promote bacterial growth in the wound.
- Wound irrigation with normal saline decreases bacterial counts and removes foreign bodies, thus reducing the infection rate. Use 60 mL of normal saline irrigation per centimeter of wound length, with a minimum of 200 mL.[8,9]
- Soaking wounds is not effective in cleaning contaminated wounds and may increase wound bacterial counts.[10]

DEBRIDEMENT AND HAIR REMOVAL

- Debridement of devitalized tissue by elliptical incision removes foreign matter and bacteria, resulting in a decreased infection risk. It also creates a clean wound edge, facilitating repair.
- Clip hair if necessary rather than shaving the skin, as shaving is associated with an increased infection rate. Do not remove hair from eyebrows due to the potential for abnormal or lack of regeneration.[8,9]

ANTIBIOTICS

- Although there is no clear evidence that antibiotic prophylaxis prevents wound infection in most ED patients, there may be a role in selected high-risk wounds and populations.
- If used, antibiotic prophylaxis should be (1) initiated before tissue manipulation, (2) effective against predicted pathogens, and (3) administered by routes that quickly achieve adequate blood levels.
- Reasonable coverage can be expected from penicillinase-resistant penicillin (eg, dicloxacillin 12 to 25 mg/kg per day PO divided qid for pediatric patients; 500 mg qid PO in adults), or a first-generation cephalosporin (eg, cephalexin 25 to 50 mg/kg per day PO divided qid in pediatric patients; 500 mg PO qid in adults). Clindamycin can be used in penicillin-allergic patients. Antibiotics should be given for 3 to 5 days.
- Patients with human and mammalian bites should receive penicillin or amoxicillin-clavulanate for *Pasteurella* and *Eikenella,* respectively (see Chap. 20 for discussion).
- Full-thickness oral lacerations should be treated for 3 to 5 days with penicillin (25 to 50 mg/kg per day PO divided qid for pediatric patients; 500 mg PO qid in adults).
- Wounds contaminated by freshwater and plantar puncture wounds through athletic shoes may require a fluoroquinolone (such as ciprofloxacin 500 mg PO bid in adults only) to cover *Pseudomonas* for 3 to 5 days.

TETANUS PROPHYLAXIS

- Guidelines for tetanus prophylaxis in wound management have been developed by several public and professional organizations.
- See Chap. 93 and Table 93-1 for the Centers for Disease Control and Prevention guidelines. Since the incubation period is from 7 to 21 days, it is acceptable to give the absorbed tetanus toxoid days after injury.
- Immunization and immunoglobulin administration are safe during pregnancy.

REFERENCES

1. McCaig LF, Burt CW: *National Hospital Ambulatory Medical Care Survey: 2001 Emergency Department Summary.* Adv Data 335:1, 2003.
2. Hollander JE, Singer AJ, Valentine S, Henry MC: Wound registry: Development and validation. *Ann Emerg Med* 25: 675, 1995.
3. Hollander JE, Singer AJ, Valentine SM: Comparison of wound care practices in pediatric and adult lacerations repaired in the emergency department. *Pediatr Emerg Care* 14: 15, 1998.
4. Baker MD, Lanuti M: The management and outcome of lacerations in urban children. *Ann Emerg Med* 19:1001, 1990.

5. Hollander JE: Patient and wound assessment: Basic concepts of the history and physical examination, in Singer AJ, Hollander JE (eds.): *Lacerations and Acute Wounds: An Evidence-Based Guide.* Philadelphia: FA Davis, 2002, p. 23.

6. Hollander JE, Singer AJ, Valentine SM, Shofer FS: Risk factors for infection in patients with traumatic lacerations. *Acad Emerg Med* 8:716, 2001.

7. Cardany CR, Rodeheaver G, Thacker J, Edgerton MT, Edlich RF: The crush injury: A high risk wound. *JACEP* 5:965, 1976.

8. Singer A, Hollander JE, Quinn JV: Evaluation and management of traumatic lacerations. *N Engl J Med* 337:1142, 1997.

9. Hollander JE, Singer AJ: Laceration management. *Ann Emerg Med* 34:356, 1999.

10. Lammers RL, Fourre M, Callaham ML, Boone T: Effect of povidone-iodine and saline soaking on bacterial counts in acute traumatic contaminated wounds. *Ann Emerg Med* 19:709, 1990.

For further reading in *Emergency Medicine: A Comprehensive Study Guide,* 6th ed., see Chap. 40, "Evaluation of Wounds," by Judd Hollander and Adam Singer; and Chap. 41, "Wound Preparation," by Susan C. Store and Wallace A. Carter.

15 METHODS FOR WOUND CLOSURE

David M. Cline

- Wounds can be closed primarily in the emergency department (ED) by the placement of sutures, surgical staples, skin-closure tapes, and adhesives.
- All wounds heal with some scarring; the goal is to use techniques that make the scar as small and invisible as possible.[1]
- In closing a laceration, it is important to match each layer of a wound edge to its counterpart. Care must be taken to avoid having one wound edge rolled inward. The rolled-in edge occludes the capillaries, promoting wound infection. The dermal side will not heal to the rolled epidermal side, causing wound dehiscence when the sutures are removed, resulting in an inferior scar appearance.
- The techniques described are an overview of basic wound closure, which should aid the practitioner in achieving acceptable results.

SUTURES

- Sutures are the strongest of all wound closure devices and allow the most accurate approximation of wound edges.[2]
- Sutures are divided into two general classes, nonabsorbable, and absorbable sutures, which lose all their tensile strength within 60 days.
- Monofilament synthetic sutures such as nylon or polypropylene have the lowest rates of infection and are the most commonly used suture materials in the ED.
- Synthetic monofilament absorbable sutures (eg, Monocryl) are preferred for closure of deep structures such as the dermis or fascia because of their strength and low tissue reactivity. Rapidly absorbing sutures (eg, Vicryl Rapide) can be used to close the superficial skin layers or mucous membranes, especially when the avoidance of removal is desired.[3]
- Sutures are sized according to their diameter. For general ED use, 6-0 suture is the smallest, and it is used for percutaneous closure on the face and other cosmetically important areas.
- Suture sizes 5-0 and 4-0 are progressively larger; 5.0 is commonly used for closure of hand and finger lacerations, and 4.0 is used to close lacerations on the trunk and proximal extremities.
- Very thick skin, such as that of the scalp and sole, may require closure with 3-0 sutures.

SUTURING TECHNIQUES

- Percutaneous sutures that pass through both the epidermal and dermal layers are the most common sutures used in the ED.
- Dermal, or subcuticular, sutures reapproximate the divided edges of the dermis without penetrating the epidermis. These two sutures may be used together in a layered closure as wound complexity demands. Sutures can be applied in a continuous fashion ("running" sutures) or as interrupted sutures.
- Improper tissue handling further traumatizes skin and results in an increased risk of infection and noticeable scarring.[4] Gentle pressure with fine forceps is recommended.

SIMPLE INTURRUPTED PERCUTANEOUS SUTURES

- Percutaneous sutures should be placed to achieve eversion of the wound edges. To accomplish this, the needle should enter the skin at a 90 degree angle. The needle point should also exit the opposite side at 90 degrees. The depth of the suture should be greater than the width. Sutures placed in this manner will encompass a portion of tissue that will evert when the knot is tied (Fig. 15-1).
- An adequate number of interrupted sutures should be placed so that the wound edges are closed without

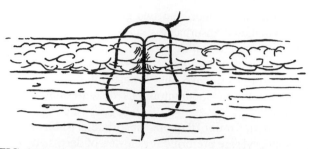

FIG. 15-1. A single interrupted percutaneous suture with everted edges.

gaping. Generally, the number of ties should correspond to the suture size (ie, 4 ties for 4-0 suture, 5 ties for 5-0 suture).

- Straight, shallow lacerations can be closed with percutaneous sutures only, sewing from one end toward the other and aligning edges with each individual suture bite. Deep, irregular wounds with uneven, misaligned, or gaping edges are more difficult to suture.

- Certain principles have been identified for these more difficult wounds:

  - Wounds with edges that cannot be brought together without excessive tension should have dermal sutures placed to partially close the gap.

  - When wound edges of different thickness are to be reunited, the needle should be passed through one side of the wound, and then drawn out before re-entry through the other side, to ensure that the needle is inserted at a comparable level.

  - Uneven edges can be aligned by first approximating the mid-portion of the wound with the initial suture. Subsequent sutures are then placed in the middle of each half until the wound edges are aligned and closed.

- Simple interrupted sutures are the most versatile and effective for realigning irregular wound edges and stellate lacerations (Fig. 15-2). An advantage of interrupted sutures is that only the involved sutures need to be removed in the case of wound infection.

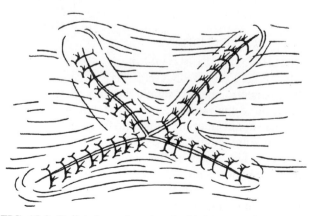

FIG. 15-2. Stellate laceration closed with interrupted sutures.

CONTINUOUS (RUNNING) PERCUTANEOUS SUTURES

- Continuous or running percutaneous sutures are best when repairing linear wounds. An advantage of the continuous suture is that it accommodates the developing edema of the wound edges during healing. However, a break in the suture may ruin the entire repair and may cause permanent marks if placed too tightly.

- Continuous suture closure of a laceration can be accomplished by two different patterns. In the first pattern, the needle pathway is at a 90 degree angle to the wound edges and results in a visible suture that crosses the wound edges at a 45 degree angle (Fig. 15-3A).

- In the other pattern, the needle pathway is at a 45 degree angle to the wound edges, so that the visible suture is at a 90 degree angle to the wound edges (Fig. 15-3B). In either case, the physician starts at the corner of the wound farthest away and sutures toward him- or herself.

DEEP DERMAL SUTURES

- The major role of these sutures is to reduce tension. They are also used to close dead spaces.

- However, their presence increases the risk of infection in contaminated wounds.[5]

- Sutures though adipose tissues do not hold tension, increase infection rates, and should be avoided.[6]

- With deep dermal sutures, the needle is inserted at the level of the mid-dermis on one side of the wound, and then exits more superficially below the dermal-

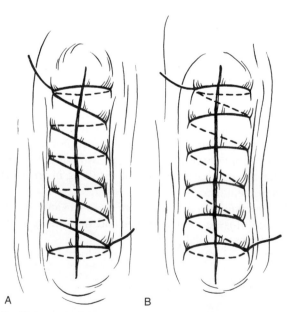

A   B

FIG. 15-3. A. Running suture crossing wound at 45 degrees. **B.** Running suture crossing wound at 90 degrees.

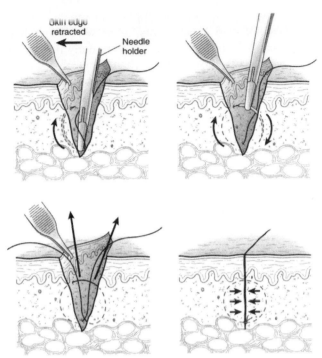

FIG. 15-4. Placement of a deep suture. The needle is inserted at the depth of the dermis and directed upward, exiting immediately beneath the dermal-epidermal junction. The needle is then inserted through the opposite side of the wound, starting at the dermal-epidermal junction and exiting at the depth of the dermis. (Reproduced with permission from Singer J, Hollander JE (eds.): *Lacerations and Acute Wounds: An Evidence-Based Guide.* Philadelphia: FA Davis, 2002, p. 121.)

epidermal junction (Fig. 15-4). The needle is then introduced below the dermal-epidermal junction on the opposite side of the wound and exits at the level of the mid-dermis. Thus the knot becomes buried in the tissue when tying of the suture is completed.
- The first suture is placed at the center of the laceration, while additional sutures then sequentially bisect the wound. The number of deep sutures should be minimized.

VERTICAL MATTRESS SUTURES

- Vertical mattress sutures (Fig. 15-5) and are also employed in certain situations.

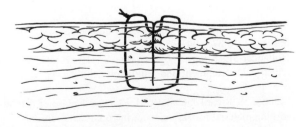

FIG. 15-5. Vertical mattress suture.

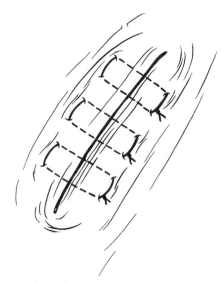

FIG. 15-6. Horizontal mattress suture.

- The vertical mattress suture is useful in areas of lax skin (eg, the elbow and the dorsum of the hand), where the wound edges tend to fold into the wound. It can act as an "all-in-one" suture, avoiding the need for a layered closure.

HORIZONTAL MATTRESS SUTURES

- Horizontal mattress sutures are faster and better at eversion than vertical mattress sutures.
- They are especially useful in areas of increased tension such as fascia, joints, and callus skin (Fig. 15-6). In order to avoid tissue strangulation, care must be taken not to tie the individual sutures too tightly.

DELAYED CLOSURE

- Delayed primary closure is an option for wounds suspected of contamination, or for wounds presenting beyond 12 hours after injury.
- With this method the wound is left open for a period of 3 to 5 days, after which it may be closed if no infection supervenes. A study conducted in 2002 randomized patients to delayed primary closure and secondary closure (ie, the wound is left open and allowed to close by secondary intention).[7] Healing times, appearance, and function were similar.

STAPLES

- Skin closure by metal staples is quick and economical, with the added advantage of low tissue reactivity.[8–10]

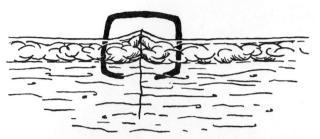

FIG. 15-7. A cutaneous staple properly placed will evert the skin edges and should not be in contact with the skin surface.

- However, the skin staple does not provide the same coaptation for lacerations with irregular skin edges that sutures can achieve, and staples should be reserved for lacerations where the healing scar is not readily apparent (eg, scalp).[9]
- When placing staples, the wound edges should be held together with tissue forceps. The device should be placed gently against the skin and the trigger squeezed slowly. A properly placed staple has the top portion somewhat above the skin surface (Fig. 15-7).

ADHESIVE TAPES

- Adhesive tapes are the least reactive of all wound closure devices.[11]
- Skin-closure tapes are used as an alternative to sutures and staples and for additional support after suture and staple removal.
- Tapes work best on flat, dry, immobile surfaces where the wound edges fit together without tension. Taped wounds are more resistant to infection than sutured wounds.[11]
- They can be used for skin flaps, where sutures may compromise perfusion, and for lacerations with thin, friable skin that will not hold sutures.
- Adhesion of tapes is enhanced by the application of benzoin to the skin surface 2 to 3 cm beyond the wound edges. Individual tapes are applied with some space between them, but not so much that there is a gap in the wound edges between the individual tapes. Tapes should stay in place about as long as an equivalent suture would, and will spontaneously detach as the underlying epithelium exfoliates.

CYANOACRYLATE TISSUE ADHESIVES

- Cyanoacrylate tissue adhesives close wounds by forming an adhesive layer on top of intact epithelium. Cyanoacrylate adhesives should never be applied within wounds due to their intense inflammatory reaction with subcutaneous tissue.

- Adhesives should not be applied to mucous membranes, infected areas, joints, areas with dense hair (eg, scalp), or on wounds exposed to body fluids.
- Adhesives are most useful when they are used on wounds that close spontaneously, have clean or sharp edges, and are located on clean, immobile areas.
- Compared to sutured wounds, wound closure with adhesives is faster, less painful, has comparable rates of infection and optimal cosmetic appearance, and when properly applied on selected wounds, has a similar dehiscence rate.[12–14]
- Wounds in which the edges are separated more than 5 mm are unlikely to stay closed with tissue adhesives alone. In this case, subcutaneous sutures can be inserted to relieve this tension.
- Tissue adhesives are equivalent in strength to 5-0 suture. Lacerations longer than 5 cm are prone to shear forces and unlikely to remain closed with tissue adhesives alone.
- The adhesive is carefully expressed through the tip of the applicator and gently brushed over the wound surface in a continuous, steady motion. The adhesive should cover the entire wound as well as an area covering 5 to 10 mm on either side of the wound edges. After allowing the first layer of the adhesive to polymerize for 30 to 45 seconds, two to three additional layers of the adhesive are similarly brushed onto the surface of the wound, waiting 5 to 10 seconds between successive layers.
- Care should be taken to position the patient parallel to the floor, cover the patient's eyes, and to gently squeeze the applicator to avoid problematic runoff.
- Once applied, cyanoacrylate should not be covered with ointment, bandages, or dressing. Patients should be instructed not to pick at the edges of the adhesive.
- After 24 hours, the area can be gently washed with plain water, but it should not be scrubbed, soaked, or exposed to moisture for any length of time.
- The adhesive will spontaneously slough off in 5 to 10 days. Should a wound open, the patient should immediately return for closure.

REFERENCES

1. Singer AJ, Clark RAF: Advances in cutaneous wound healing. *N Engl J Med* 341:738, 1999.
2. Hollander JE, Singer AJ, Valentine S, Henry MC: Wound registry: Development and validation. *Ann Emerg Med* 25: 675, 1995.
3. Canrelli JP, Ricard J, Collet LM, Marasse E: Use of fast absorbing material for skin closure in young children. *Int Surg* 73:151, 1988.

4. Singer AJ, Quinn JV, Thode CH, Hollander JE: Determination of poor outcome after laceration and incision repair. *Plast Reconstr Surg* 110:429, 2002.

5. Mehta PH, Dunn KA, Bradfield JF, Austin PE: Contaminated wounds: Infection rates with subcutaneous sutures. *Ann Emerg Med* 27:43, 1996.

6. Milewski PJ, Thomson H: Is a fat stitch necessary? *Br J Surg* 67:393, 1980.

7. Quinn J, Cummings S, Callaham M, Sellers K: Suturing versus conservative management of lacerations of the hand: Randomized controlled trial. *BMJ* 325:299, 2002.

8. Richie AJ, Rocke LG: Staples versus sutures in the closure of scalp wounds: A prospective, double blind, randomized trial. *Injury* 20:217, 1989.

9. Hollander JE, Giarrusso E, Cassara G, Valentine S, Singer AJ: Comparison of staples and sutures for closure of scalp lacerations (abstract). *Acad Emerg Med* 4:460, 1997.

10. George TK, Simpson DC: Skin wound closure with staples in the accident and emergency department. *Roy Coll Surg Edinburgh* 30:54, 1985.

11. Edlich RF, Rodeheaver G, Kuphal J, et al: Technique of closure: Contaminated wounds. *JACEP* 3:375, 1974.

12. Quinn J, Wells G, Sutcliffe T, et al: A randomized trial comparing octyl-cyanoacrylate tissue adhesive and sutures in the management of lacerations. *JAMA* 277:1527, 1997.

13. Singer AJ, Quinn JV, Hollander JE, Clark RE: Closure of lacerations and incisions with octyl-cyanoacrylate: A multicenter randomized clinical trial. *Surgery* 131:270, 2002.

14. Farion K, Osmand MH, Hartling L, et al: Tissue adhesives for traumatic lacerations in children and adults. *Cochrane Database Syst Rev* CD003326, 2002.

For further reading in *Emergency Medicine: A Comprehensive Study Guide,* 6th ed., see Chap. 42, "Methods for Wound Closure," by Adam J. Singer and Judd E. Hollander.

16   LACERATIONS TO THE FACE AND SCALP

Russell J. Karten

EPIDEMIOLOGY

- Lacerations to the face and scalp account for approximately 50% of the wounds treated in emergency departments (EDs) across the United States.[1] Cosmetically apparent facial wounds require meticulous repair for excellent results.
- Anyone with facial trauma should be questioned about the possibility of domestic violence; if this is suspected, notify the appropriate authorities. Prompt identification and intervention are critical in preventing future injury.[2]

PATHOPHYSIOLOGY

- Facial and scalp wounds are often caused by a combination of sharp and blunt mechanisms. It takes an average of ten times fewer bacteria to cause an infection in a blunt wound than in a wound caused by a sharp object.

SCALP AND FOREHEAD

ANATOMY

- The arterial supply to each side of the scalp involves three branches off the external carotid artery (occipital, superficial temporal, and posterior auricular arteries), and two branches from the internal carotid artery (supraorbital and supratrochlear arteries).[3]
- The scalp and forehead (which includes the eyebrows) are parts of the same anatomic structure (Fig. 16-1).

EVALUATION

- Wounds that fall along the lines of skin tension have better cosmetic results. Skin tension lines are always perpendicular to the underlying muscles.

WOUND PREPARATION

- Anesthesia can be provided by topical agents such as LET (lidocaine-epinephrine-tetracaine; effective in 50% of patients),[4] or local or regional infiltration (such as a supraorbital block). LET may also reduce the pain of lidocaine injection.[4]

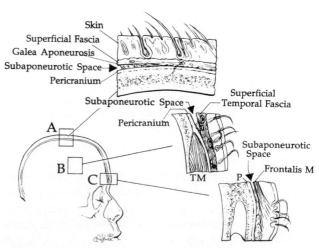

FIG. 16-1. The layers of the **A.** scalp, **B.** forehead, and **C.** eyebrow.

- All wounds are irrigated to reduce contamination and lessen the risk of infection.
- In nonbite, noncontaminated facial and scalp wounds presenting within 6 hours, routine irrigation does not alter the rate of infection or subsequent cosmetic appearance after suture repair.[5]
- Eyebrows should never be clipped or shaved because their delicate contour and form are valuable landmarks for the meticulous reapproximation of the wound edges.

REPAIR OF SCALP LACERATIONS

- It is not necessary to shave the scalp prior to closure; shaving actually increases the likelihood of a wound infection.
- When the edges of a laceration of either the eyebrow or the scalp are devitalized, debridement is mandatory. When debriding these sites, the scalpel should cut at an angle that is parallel to that of the hair follicles to reduce subsequent alopecia.
- Wound closure should be initiated with approximation of the galea aponeurotica with buried, interrupted absorbable 4-0 sutures.
- The divided edges of muscle and fascia must also be closed with buried, interrupted, absorbable 4-0 synthetic sutures to prevent the development of depressed scars.
- The skin can be closed by staples or by simple interrupted nylon sutures (consider using sutures that are a different color than the patient's hair). Some authors recommend single-layer closure with 3-0 nylon sutures.
- The use of staples saves money[6] and time, and is associated with similar outcomes to those of sutures.[7]

REPAIR OF FOREHEAD LACERATIONS

- The epidermal layer can be closed with 6-0 nonabsorbable nylon in a simple, interrupted fashion; with wound closure strips over tincture of benzoin; or with tissue adhesive.[8]
- The skin edges of anatomic landmarks on the forehead should be approximated first with key stitches, using interrupted, nonabsorbable monofilament 5-0 synthetic sutures.
- Accurate alignment of the eyebrow, transverse wrinkles of the forehead, and the hairline of the scalp is essential. It may be necessary to have younger patients raise their eyebrows to create wrinkles for accurate placement of the key stitches.

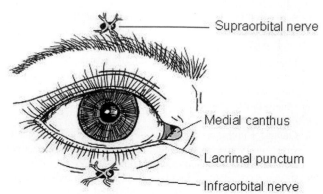

FIG. 16-2. External landmarks of eyelid anatomy.

EYELIDS

- A complete examination of the eye's structure and function is essential. Search for foreign bodies (see Chap. 152).
- The lid should be examined for involvement of the canthi, the lacrimal system, the supraorbital nerve, the infraorbital nerve, or penetration through the tarsal plate or lid margin (Fig. 16-2).
- The following wounds should be referred to an ophthalmologist: (1) those involving the inner surface of the lid, (2) those involving the lid margins, (3) those involving the lacrimal duct, (4) those associated with ptosis, and (5) those that extend into the tarsal plate.
- Failure to recognize and properly repair the lacrimal system can result in chronic tearing.
- Uncomplicated lid lacerations can be readily closed using nonabsorbable 6-0 suture which can be removed in 3–5 d. Tissue adhesive is contraindicated near the eye.

NOSE

- Lacerations of the nose may be limited to the skin or involve the deeper structures (sparse nasal musculature, cartilaginous framework, and nasal mucous membrane). They are repaired by accurate reapproximation of each tissue layer.
- Local anesthesia of the nose can be difficult because of the tightly adhering skin. Topical anesthesia may be successful with lidocaine, epinephrine, and tetracaine.
- When the laceration extends through all tissue layers, closure should begin with a marginal, nonabsorbable, monofilament 5-0 synthetic suture that aligns the skin surrounding the entrances of the nasal canals, to prevent malposition and notching of the alar rim.
- Traction on the long, untied ends of the marginal suture approximates the wound edges and aligns the anterior and posterior margins of the divided tissue layers.

- The mucous membrane should then be repaired with interrupted, braided, absorbable 5-0 synthetic sutures, with their knots buried in the tissue. The area is re-irrigated gently from the outside.
- The cartilage may rarely need to be approximated with a minimal number of 5-0 absorbable sutures. In sharply delineated linear lacerations, closure of the overlying skin is usually sufficient.
- The cut edges of the skin, with its adherent musculature, are closed with interrupted, nonabsorbable, monofilament 6-0 synthetic sutures. Removal of the external sutures may take place in 3 to 5 days.
- Following any nasal injury, the septum should be inspected for hematoma formation using a nasal speculum. The presence of bluish swelling in the septum confirms the diagnosis of septal hematoma. Treatment of the hematoma is evacuation of the blood clot.
- Drainage of a small septal hematoma can be accomplished by aspiration of the blood clot through an 18-gauge needle. A larger hematoma is drained through a horizontal incision at the base. Bilateral hematomas should be drained in the operating room by a specialist.
- Reaccumulation of blood can be prevented by nasal packing. Antibiotic treatment (penicillin) is recommended to prevent infection that may cause necrosis of cartilage.

LIPS

- Isolated intraoral lesions may not need to be sutured.
- Through-and-through lacerations that do not include the vermilion border can be closed in layers. Use 5-0 absorbable suture first for the mucosal surface. Re-irrigate, and close the orbicularis oris muscle with 5-0 absorbable suture. Close the skin with 6-0 nylon suture or tissue adhesive.
- Lacerations that cross the vermilion border are of utmost cosmetic importance. A repair with even 1 mm of step-off will be unappealing.
- Repair of a complex lip laceration requires a three-layered closure (Fig. 16-3). Using skin hooks, traction is applied to align the anterior and posterior borders of the laceration. Closure of the wound should start at the vermilion-skin junction with a nonabsorbable, monofilament 6-0 synthetic suture. The orbicularis oris muscle is then repaired with interrupted, braided, absorbable 4-0 synthetic sutures. The vermilion-mucous membrane junction is approximated with a braided, absorbable 5-0 synthetic suture. The suture ligature knot is buried in the subcutaneous tissue. The divided edges of the mucous membrane and vermilion are then closed using interrupted, braided, absorbable 5-0 synthetic sutures with a buried-knot construction.
- Skin edges of the laceration are usually jagged and irregular, but they can be fitted together as are the pieces of a jigsaw puzzle using interrupted, nonabsorbable, monofilament 6-0 synthetic sutures with their knots formed on the surface of the skin.
- Patients with sutured intraoral lacerations should receive prophylactic antibiotics.

CHEEKS AND FACE

- Facial lacerations are closed with 6-0 nonabsorbable suture. Simple interrupted sutures are used and are removed after 5 days. Tissue adhesive is an alternative.
- Attention to anatomic structures including the facial nerve and parotid gland is necessary (Fig. 16-4).

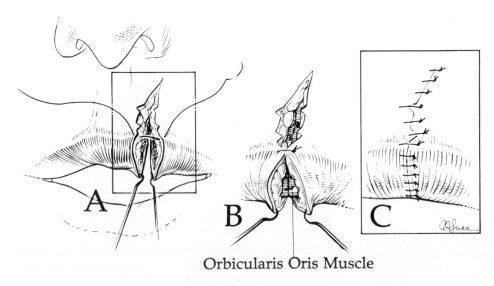

Orbicularis Oris Muscle

FIG. 16-3. Irregular-edged vertical laceration of the upper lip. **A.** Traction is applied to the lip and closure of the wound is begun first at the vermilion-skin junction. **B.** The orbicularis oris muscle is then repaired with interrupted, absorbable 4-0 synthetic sutures. **C.** The irregular edges of the skin are then approximated.

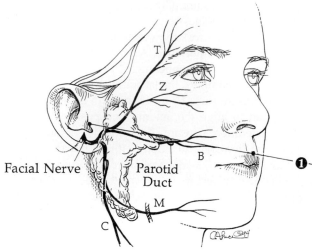

FIG. 16-4. Anatomic structures of the cheek. The course of the parotid duct is deep to a line drawn from the tragus of the ear to the midportion of the upper lip. Branches of the facial nerve: temporal (T), zygomatic (Z), buccal (B), mental (M), and cervical (C).

If these structures are involved, operative repair is indicated.

EAR

- Superficial lacerations of the ear can be closed with 6-0 nylon suture.
- Avoid epinephrine in lacerations involving the auricle.
- Exposed cartilage should be covered. Debridement of the skin is not advisable, since there is very little excess skin. In most through-and-through lacerations of the ear, the skin can be approximated and the underlying cartilage will be supported adequately (Fig. 16-5).

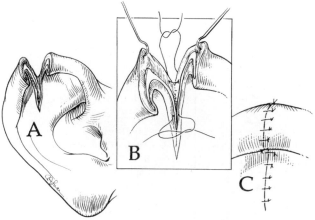

FIG. 16-5. A. Laceration through the auricle. **B.** One or two interrupted, 6-0 coated nylon sutures will approximate divided edges of cartilage. **C.** Interrupted nonabsorbable 6-0 synthetic sutures approximate the skin edges.

- Following repair of simple lacerations, a small piece of nonadherent gauze may be applied over the laceration only and a pressure dressing applied. Gauze squares are placed behind the ear to apply pressure and the head is wrapped circumferentially with gauze.
- Sutures should be removed in 5 days.
- An otolaryngologist or plastic surgeon should be consulted for more complex lacerations, ear avulsions, or auricular hematomas.

REFERENCES

1. Hollander JE, Singer AJ, Valentine S, et al: Wound registry: Development and validation. *Ann Emerg Med* 25:675, 1995.
2. Le BT, Dierks EJ, Ueek BA, et al: Maxillofacial injuries associated with domestic violence. *J Oral Maxillofacial Surg* 59: 1277, 2001.
3. Moore KL: *Clinically Oriented Anatomy,* 4th ed. Philadelphia: Williams & Wilkins, 1999.
4. Singer AJ, Stark MJ: LET versus EMLA for pretreating lacerations. A randomized trial. *Acad Emerg Med* 8:223, 2001.
5. Hollander JE, Richman PB, Werblud M, et al: Irrigation in facial and scalp lacerations: Does it alter outcome? *Ann Emerg Med* 31:73, 1998.
6. Orlinsky M, Goldberg RM, Chan L, et al: Cost analysis of stapling versus suturing for skin closure. *Am J Emerg Med* 13:77, 1995.
7. Hogg K, Carley S: Towards evidence based emergency medicine: Best BETs from the Manchester Royal Infirmary. Staples or sutures for repair of scalp laceration in adults. *Emerg Med J* 19:327, 2002.
8. Singer AJ, Quinn JV, Clark RE, et al: Closure of lacerations and incisions with octylcyanoacrylate: a multicenter randomized controlled trial. *Surgery* 131:270, 2002.

For further reading in *Emergency Medicine: A Comprehensive Study Guide,* 6th ed., see Chap. 43, "Lacerations to the Face and Scalp," by Wendy C. Coates.

17 INJURIES OF THE ARM, HAND, FINGERTIP, AND NAIL

David M. Cline

EPIDEMIOLOGY

- Soft tissue upper extremity injuries account for about 35% of the wounds and lacerations evaluated in the emergency department.[1]

PATHOPHYSIOLOGY

- Injuries may be classified as closed crush, simple lacerations, open crush with partial amputation, and complete amputation.[2]

CLINICAL FEATURES

- History should include occupation and hand dominance.
- Examination of arm and hand injuries includes inspection at rest, evaluation of motor nerve and tendon function, evaluation of sensory nerve function, and evaluation of perfusion.
- The wound should be examined for evidence of potential artery, nerve, tendon, and bone injury. Limited or painful movement suggests partial involvement of a tendon.[2]
- The wound should be evaluated for foreign bodies, debris, or bacterial contamination.
- Examining active motion and resistance to passive movement assesses motor function (Table 17-1).
- Sensation should be assessed in the median, ulnar, and radial nerve distribution (Table 17-2).

DIAGNOSIS AND DIFFERENTIAL

- For some injuries, a bloodless field may require a proximal tourniquet to temporarily halt arterial flow.
- A Penrose drain is commonly used for distal finger injuries and a manual blood pressure cuff is used for more proximal injures. Excessively high pressures and duration that can cause neurovascular damage may be avoided by limiting stretch of the drain to no more than 50% of the original length for 15- to 20-minute periods.[2,3]
- Once adequate visualization is obtained, the injury can be examined for foreign bodies and tendon and joint capsule injuries.
- It is essential to examine the hand and arm in the position of injury in order to avoid missing deep structure injuries that may have moved out of the field of view when examined in a neutral position.

TABLE 17-1   Motor Testing of the Peripheral Nerves of the Upper Extremity

NERVE	MOTOR EXAM
Radial	Dorsiflexion of wrist
Median	Thumb abduction away from the palm Thumb interphalangeal joint flexion
Ulnar	Adduction/abduction of digits

TABLE 17-2   Sensory Testing of Peripheral Nerves in the Upper Extremity

SENSORY NERVE	AREA OF TEST
Radial	First dorsal web space
Median	Volar tip of index finger
Ulnar	Volar tip of little finger

- For a forearm wound proximal to the wrist, an Allen's test should be performed. A Doppler probe is useful to detect a diminished pulse, detect flow in digital arteries, and to calculate an arterial pressure index (API; the ratio of the systolic blood pressure between the injured and uninjured side). In the absence of a diminished pulse or a ratio less than 1.0, the likelihood of a clinically significant occult arterial injury is exceedingly small.
- Injuries over joints should also be evaluated for possible penetration of the joint capsule. If this is a consideration, radiography may reveal air in the joint.
- An alternative approach to diagnose joint penetration is to inject sterile saline, with or without a few drops of sterile fluorescein, into the joint using a standard joint aspiration technique at a site separate from the laceration. Fluid dripping from the joint indicates an open joint capsule and requires specialty consultation.[4]
- Radiographic evaluation with anteroposterior (AP) and lateral films is indicated if bony injuries, retained radiopaque foreign bodies, or joint penetration are suspected.

EMERGENCY DEPARTMENT CARE AND DISPOSITION

- All wounds require scrupulous cleaning and irrigation after adequate anesthesia, which may require a regional or digital nerve block.
- Tetanus prophylaxis should be given as indicated (see Chap. 14).
- Consultation with a plastic or hand surgeon is required with complex or extensive injuries, injuries requiring skin grafting, or injuries requiring technically demanding skills. Consultation with a specialist is also recommended if the hand is vital to patient's career, for example a professional musician.
- Management of individual wound types should be directed by the sections that follow.

FOREARM AND WRIST LACERATIONS

- Injury over the wrist raises the possibility of a suicide attempt and the patient should be questioned about intent and a history of depression.

TABLE 17-3 Extensor Compartments in the Forearm

EXTENSORS IN THE FOREARM	FUNCTION
First compartment	
Abductor pollicis longus	Abducts and extends thumb
Extensor pollicis brevis	Extends thumb at MCP joint
Second compartment	
Extensor carpi radialis longus	Extends and radially deviates
Extensor carpi radialis brevis	wrist (both)
Third compartment	
Extensor pollicis longus	Extends thumb at IP joint
Fourth compartment	
Extensor digitorum communis	Splits into four tendons at level of the wrist.
	Extends index, long, ring, and little digits
Extensor indicis proprius	Extends index finger
Fifth compartment	
Extensor digiti minimi	Extends little finger at MCP joint
Sixth compartment	
Extensor carpi ulnaris	Extends and radially deviates wrist

ABBREVIATIONS: IP = interphalangeal; MCP = metacarpophalangeal.

- Tendons and distal nerves should be individually examined. The forearm has six extensor compartments located dorsally and innervated by the radial nerve (Table 17-3). Located on the volar surface of the forearm and crossing the wrist are the 12 flexor tendons innervated by the median and ulnar nerves (Table 17-4).
- Injuries that involve more than one parallel laceration, classic for suicide attempts, may require horizontal mattress sutures to cross all lacerations for closure to prevent compromising the vascular supply of the island of skin located between incisions (Fig. 17-1).

TABLE 17-4 Flexor Tendons in the Forearm

FLEXOR TENDON	FUNCTION
Flexor carpi radialis	Flexes and radially deviates wrist
Flexor carpi ulnaris	Flexes and ulnarly deviates wrist
Palmaris longus	Flexes wrist
Flexor pollicis longus	Flexes thumb at MCP and IP joint
At index, middle, ring, and little fingers:	
Flexor digitorum superficialis	Flexes digits at MCP and PIP joints
Flexor digitorum profundus	Flexes digits at MCP, PIP, and DIP joints

ABBREVIATIONS: DIP = distal interphalangeal; PIP = proximal interphalangeal; IP = interphalangeal; MCP = metacarpophalangeal.

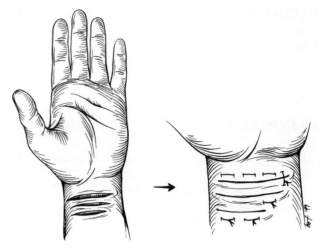

FIG. 17-1. Horizontal mattress sutures for multiple parallel lacerations.

HIGH PRESSURE INJECTION INJURIES

- These injuries often go unsuspected since they usually present with an initially benign appearance, most commonly an isolated puncture wound to the index finger of the nondominant hand.[5]
- These injuries should immediately be referred to a hand specialist for operative debridement.

PALM LACERATIONS

- Injuries to the palm may require a regional anesthetic, for example a median or ulnar nerve block.
- Very careful exploration is mandatory. If no deep injury is suspected, the wound is closed, paying particular attention to re-opposing the skin creases accurately.
- Care should be taken to avoid using deep "bites" with the needle, as this risks injury to the underlying tendons or tendon sheaths. Interrupted horizontal mattress sutures (see Chap. 15) with 5-0 monofilament suture are recommended to ensure that these sutures do not pull through.
- Deep injuries between the carpometacarpal joints and the distal creases of the wrist are difficult to manage and should be referred to a specialist for exploration and repair.

DORSAL HAND LACERATIONS

- On the dorsum of the hand, lacerations over the metacarpophalangeal joint suggest a closed fist injury and require special care (see Chap. 20).

- The pliable skin and extensive movements of the hand may hide tendon injuries, and therefore a careful examination of the wound and hand function is essential.
- Most dorsal hand lacerations can be repaired by emergency physicians using 5-0 nonabsorbable sutures.

EXTENSOR TENDON LACERATIONS

- Experienced emergency physicians may repair extensor tendon injuries over the dorsum of the hand, with the exception of the tendons to the thumb.
- The tendon injury should be discussed with a hand specialist for preferred technique and to arrange follow-up.
- Usually a figure-of-eight knot is used, with 4-0 nonabsorbable suture material (Fig. 17-2). The limb is then splinted.[2]
- Lacerations to the extensor tendons over the distal interphalangeal joint may produce a mallet deformity, while lacerations over the proximal interphalangeal joint may produce a boutonniere deformity. If the lacerations are open they are surgically repaired; if closed, they are splinted for up to 6 weeks.

FLEXOR TENDON LACERATIONS

- Injuries to flexor tendons should be referred to a specialist. Some hand surgeons prefer to repair these injuries within 12 to 24 hours.
- The repair can be delayed up to 7 days. In these cases the wound should be cleaned, the skin repaired, the limb splinted in a position of function, and arrangements made for follow-up within 2 to 3 days with a hand surgeon.

FINGER AND FINGERTIP INJURIES

- In general, finger lacerations are straightforward and can be repaired using 5-0 nonabsorbable suture materials.
- Digital nerve injuries should be suspected when static two-point discrimination is distinctively greater on one side of the volar pad than the other, or when it is greater than 10 mm. Digital nerve injuries can be repaired using microvascular techniques either acutely or days to weeks after the injury.
- Successful repair of fingertip injuries requires knowledge of anatomy (Fig. 17-3) and an understanding of techniques of reconstruction.
- Distal fingertip amputations with skin or pulp loss only are best managed conservatively, with serial dressing changes only, especially in children.

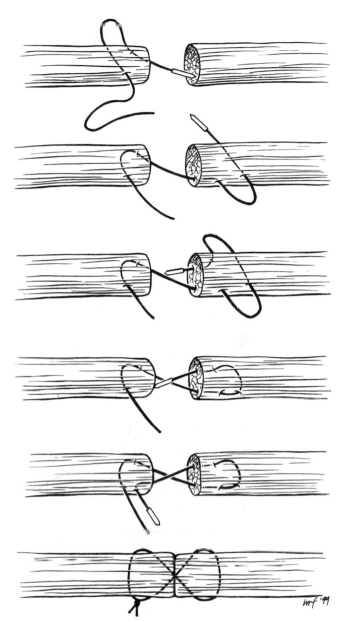

FIG. 17-2. Extensor tendon laceration repair with a figure-of-eight stitch.

- In cases with larger areas of skin loss (more than 1 cm²), a skin graft, either using the severed tip itself or skin harvested from the hypothenar eminence, may be required.
- Complications of the skin graft technique include decreased sensation of the fingertip, tenderness at the injury and graft site, poor cosmetic result, and hyperpigmentation in dark-skinned patients.
- Injuries with exposed bone are not amenable to skin grafting. Most of these injuries require specialist advice. If less than 0.5 mm of bone is exposed, and the wound defect is small, the bone may be trimmed back and the wound left to heal by secondary intention.

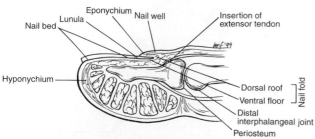

FIG. 17-3. Anatomy of the perionychium. (Reproduced with permission from Zook EG: The perionychium, in Green DP (ed.): *Operative Hand Surgery,* 2nd ed. New York: Churchill Livingstone, 1988, p. 1332.)

Injuries to the thumb or index finger with exposed bone nearly always require specialist attention.[6]

- Injuries to the nail bed require careful repair to reduce scar formation. They are associated with fractures of the distal phalanx in 50% of cases.
- Subungual hematomas require decompression by simple trephination of the nail plate. Use of a heated paper clip delays healing. Use of a nail drill, scalpel, or 18-gauge needle is recommended.
- Previously, it was recommended that if a subungual hematoma occupied more than 50% of the nail bed area, the nail should be removed to inspect and repair a likely nail bed laceration. Two prospective studies have shown that if other structures are intact, simple trephination produces an excellent result in patients with subungual hematoma regardless of size, injury mechanism, or presence of simple fracture.[7,8]
- Nail removal is needed if there is extensive crush injury, associated nail avulsion or surrounding nail fold disruption, or a displaced distal phalanx fracture on x-ray. The nail bed is inspected and repaired using 6-0 or 7-0 absorbable sutures. If the nail matrix is displaced from its anatomic position at the sulcus, the matrix should be carefully replaced and held in place with mattress sutures (Fig. 17-4).
- If there is extensive injury to the nail bed with avulsed tissue, specialist consultation is required.
- In children with fractures of the distal phalanx, the nail plate may come to lie upon the eponychium. After careful cleaning and adequate anesthesia, the nail plate should be replaced under the proximal nail fold.

RING TOURNIQUET SYNDROME

- Ring removal is required in all injured fingers. Swelling may require that the ring be cut off.
- If slower techniques are appropriate, simple lubrication may suffice.

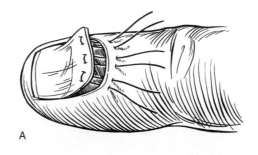
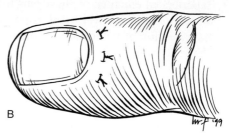

FIG. 17-4. Technique for repair of an avulsion of the germinal matrix using three horizontal mattress sutures. (Reproduced with permission from Chudnofsky CR, Sebastian S: Special wounds—Nail bed, plantar puncture, and cartilage. *Emerg Med Clin North Am* 10:808, 1992.)

- The string technique is an alternative method (Fig 17-5):
  1. String, umbilical tape, or 0-gauge silk may be used.
  2. The string is passed under the ring, and then wrapped firmly around the finger from proximal to distal.
  3. The proximal end of the string is then gently pulled and the ring advances down the finger.

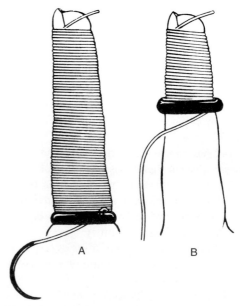

FIG. 17-5. String technique for ring removal. **A.** Completely wrapped. **B.** Unwrapping with ring advancing off with the string.

REFERENCES

1. Hollander JE, Singer AJ, Valentine S, Henry MC: Wound registry: Development and validation. *Ann Emerg Med* 25:675, 1995.
2. Harrison BP, Hilliard MW: Emergency department evaluation and treatment of hand injuries. *Emerg Med Clin North Am* 17: 793, 1999.
3. Shaw JA, DeMuth WW, Gillespy AW: Guidelines for the use of digital tourniquets based on physiologic pressure measurements. *J Bone Joint Surg Am* 67:1086, 1985.
4. Voit G, Irvine G, Beals RK: Saline load test for penetration of periarticular laceration. *J Bone Joint Surg [Br]* 78:732, 1996.
5. Vasilevski D, Noorbergen M, Depierreux M, et al: High-pressure injection injuries to the hand. *Am J Emerg Med* 18: 820, 2000.
6. Brown RE: Acute nail bed injuries. *Hand Clin* 18:561, 2000.
7. Seaberg DC, Angelos WF, Pans PM: Treatment of subungual hematomas with nail trephination: A prospective study. *Am J Emerg Med* 9:209, 1991.
8. Roser SE, Gellman H: Comparison of nail bed repair versus nail trephination for subungual hematomas in children. *J Hand Surg Am* 24:1166, 1999.

For further reading in *Emergency Medicine: A Comprehensive Study Guide,* 6th ed., see Chap. 44, "Injuries to the Arm, Hand, Fingertip, and Nail" by Fiona E. Gallahue and Wallace A. Carter.

18 LACERATIONS TO THE LEG AND FOOT

David M. Cline

EPIDEMIOLOGY

- Injuries to the leg and foot account for about 13% of traumatic wounds evaluated in the emergency department, distributed roughly into a third each for the foot, calf, and knee and thigh regions.[1]
- The foot is commonly injured in sports injuries.[2]
- Urban children can sustain foot lacerations while playing in water from fire hydrants, mostly due to stepping on broken glass.[3]
- Bicycle spoke injuries result in complex lacerations with marked surrounding abrasions and even tissue loss, usually occurring over the lateral malleolus and the base of the fifth metatarsal.[4]
- Lawn mower injuries are usually sustained from the blades of push mowers when being pulled back-

wards.[5] These wounds are heavily contaminated with multiple organisms.
- Metal lawn and garden edging is associated with plantar and knee injuries.[6]
- Hockey skates are associated with injury to the underlying tibialis anterior tendon, extensor hallucis tendon, and the dorsalis pedis artery and nerve.[7]

PATHOPHYSIOLOGY

- The mechanism of the injury determines the likelihood of disruption to underlying tissue, the risk of a retained foreign body, and the degree of potential contamination.
- The following circumstances are associated with specific pathogens: (1) farming accidents *(Clostridium perfringens),* (2) wading in a freshwater stream *(Aeromonas hydrophila),* and (3) high-pressure water systems used for cleaning surfaces *(Acinetobacter calcoaceticus).*
- Blunt force wounds often have irregular edges and are more likely to be associated with an underlying fracture. These characteristics increase the likelihood of wound infection compared to wounds caused by a sharp object.[8]

CLINICAL FEATURES

- Evaluation of wounds in general is discussed in Chap. 11. It is important to determine the position of the limb at the time of injury, which will help to uncover occult tendon injuries.
- Assessment for associated nerve, vessel, or tendon injury is mandatory.
- Prior to the use of anesthetic, the limb should be inspected for position at rest, and sensory neurologic function should be evaluated using light touch and two-point discrimination testing. One side can be compared to the other.

DIAGNOSIS AND DIFFERENTIAL

- Motor function may be better assessed after the wound is anesthetized (Tables 18-1 and 18-2). At this time, the wound can also be explored.

TABLE 18-1   Motor Function of Lower Extremity Peripheral Nerves

NERVE	MOTOR FUNCTION
Superficial peroneal	Foot eversion
Deep peroneal	Foot inversion Ankle dorsiflexion
Tibial	Ankle plantar flexion

TABLE 18-2   Tendon Function of the Lower Extremities

TENDON	MOTOR FUNCTION
Extensor hallucis longus	Great toe extension with ankle inversion
Tibialis anterior	Ankle dorsiflexion and inversion
Achilles tendon	Ankle plantar flexion and inversion

- The limb should be moved through its full range of motion in order to exclude tendon injury.
- Each tendon function should be tested individually, but the tendon should still be visibly inspected to rule out a partial laceration.
- Laboratory studies are usually not indicated.
- Radiology is required if there is a possibility of fracture or radiopaque foreign body. All injuries caused by glass should be x-rayed unless physical exam can reliably exclude a foreign body (see also Chap. 19).

EMERGENCY DEPARTMENT CARE AND DISPOSITION

GENERAL RECOMMENDATIONS

- See Chap. 14 for discussion of wound preparation; thorough irrigation of lower extremity wounds is essential.
- Wounds on the lower extremities are usually under greater tension than those on the upper limb. Consequently, a layered closure with 4-0 absorbable material to the fascia and interrupted 4-0 nonabsorbable sutures to the skin is preferred. The foot is an exception to this guideline.
- Deep sutures should be avoided in diabetics and patients with stasis changes, because of the increased risk of infection.[1]
- Tetanus immunization status should always be considered. The elderly are at particular risk for not being immunized.
- Cyanoacrylate glue is usually not used on the lower extremities because of greater wound tension.
- Lacerations involving the joint or tendons should be splinted in a position of function.

KNEE INJURIES

- Wounds over the knee, as for all wounds over joints, should be examined throughout the range of movement.
- Injuries over joints should also be evaluated for possible penetration of the joint capsule. Clinical evaluation alone is often incorrect.[9] If this is a consideration, radiography may reveal air in the joint.

- An alternative approach to diagnose joint penetration is to inject 60 mL of sterile saline, with or without a few drops of sterile fluorescein, into the joint using a standard joint aspiration technique at a site separate from the laceration. Leakage of the solution from the wound indicates joint capsule injury.[9]
- The popliteal artery, the popliteal nerve, and the tibial nerve are all at risk around the knee; their integrity should always be ascertained.
- After closure, the knee should be splinted to prevent excessive tension on the wound edges.

ANKLE INJURIES

- Lacerations to the ankle can easily damage underlying tendons. The joints should be moved through their full range with direct inspection of the wound to ensure there is no partial injury to the tendon. Particularly at risk are the Achilles tendon, the tibialis anterior, and the extensor hallucis longus.
- If any of these tendons are injured, they should be formally repaired.
- The Achilles tendon can rupture without a penetrating injury when a tensed gastrocnemius is suddenly contracted. This injury is most common in an athletic middle-aged male. Thompson's test can be utilized to assess the Achilles tendon. While kneeling on a chair, the patient's calf is gently squeezed at the midpoint. Absent plantar flexion of the foot indicates complete Achilles tendon laceration (a partial injury may still yield plantar flexion).

FOOT INJURIES

- Lacerations of the sole of the foot must be carefully explored to ensure not only the absence of tendon injury, but also the absence of foreign bodies. The patient lying prone with the foot supported on a pillow or overhanging the bed assists inspection.
- Regional anesthesia is often best for exploration and repair of lacerations in this area.
- Because of the high risk for infection, wounds older than 6 hours at presentation should probably not be repaired primarily.
- Large needles are required in order to adequately penetrate the thick dermis of the sole. Absorbable material is usually avoided in the foot. Nonabsorbable 3-0 or 4-0 material is used. Injuries to the dorsum of the foot can be repaired with 4-0 or 5-0 nonabsorbable sutures.
- Lacerations between the toes can be difficult to repair. The presence of an assistant can be a great help, holding the toes apart. An interrupted mattress suture is often required to ensure adequate skin apposition.

Crutches and a walking boot may be required after repair of any laceration on the foot.

- Other potentially serious injuries to the foot may be caused by lawn mowers and by bicycle spokes. Extensive soft tissue injury can occur, together with underlying fractures and tendon lacerations.[4,5] These severe injuries require the services of an orthopedic specialist.
- Infection occurs in 3 to 8% of lower extremity injuries, and up to 34% of foot lacerations.[3] However, there is no evidence that prophylactic antibiotics reduce the frequency of postrepair wound infections.[10] Therefore, the decision to use antibiotic prophylaxis is made using clinical judgment according to the degree of contamination, the presence of foreign debris, the presence of associated injuries, and host factors that predispose to infection.
- Wounds sustained while wading in fresh water are prone to infection with *Aeromonas hydrophila*.[11] In these cases a fluoroquinolone such as ciprofloxacin 500 mg bid is required. In children, trimethoprim-sulfamethoxazole, 5 mL of suspension per 10 kg up to 20 mL twice daily, is used. *Aeromonas hydrophila* should be considered in any rapidly progressive case of cellulitis in the foot after an injury.

HAIR-THREAD TOURNIQUET SYNDROME

- Hair-thread tourniquet syndrome is an unusual type of injury seen in infants. A strand or strands of hair wrap around one of the toes producing vascular compromise.[12,13]
- The hair must be completely cut to avoid compromising the neurovascular bundle to the toe.[13]
- This is best accomplished by making an incision on the extensor surface of the toe down to the extensor ligament.[13]

DISPOSITION

- Patients should be instructed to keep wounds clean and dry.
- Sutures should be removed in 10 to 14 days for the lower limb and in 14 days for lacerations over joints.
- Patients should receive routine wound care instructions. Elevation of the affected limb will reduce edema and aid healing.
- Wounds should be rechecked after 48 hours if they were heavily contaminated, or if a complex repair was required.
- Use crutches 7 to 10 days as needed to prevent additional tension on the wound.

REFERENCES

1. Hollander JE, Singer AJ, Valentine S, Henry MC: Wound registry: Development and validation. *Ann Emerg Med* 25: 675, 1995.
2. Nonfatal sports- and recreation-related injuries treated in the emergency departments—United States, July 2000–June 2001. *MMWR Morb Mortal Wkly Rep* 51:736, 2002.
3. Joffe M, Torry SB, Baker D: Fire hydrant play: Injuries and their prevention. *Pediatrics* 87:900, 1991.
4. Mine R, Fukui M, Nishimura G: Bicycle spoke injuries in the lower extremity. *Plast Reconstr Surg* 106:1501, 2000.
5. Anger DM, Ledbetter BR, Stasikelis PJ, Calhoun JH: Injuries of the foot related to the use of lawn mowers. *J Bone Joint Surg Am* 77:719, 1995.
6. Rittichier KK, Bassett KE: Metal lawn and garden edging: The hidden knife? *Pediatr Emerg Care* 17:28, 2001.
7. Simonet WT, Sim L: Boot-top tendon lacerations in ice hockey. *J Trauma* 38:30, 1995.
8. Singer AJ, Quinn JV, Thode HC, Hollander JE: Determinants of poor outcome after laceration and surgical incision repair. *Plast Reconstr Surg* 110:429, 2002.
9. Voit G, Irvine G, Beals RK: Saline load test for penetration of periarticular laceration. *J Bone Joint Surg [Br]* 78:732, 1996.
10. Stamou SC, Malterzou CH, Psaltipoulou T, et al: Wound infections after minor limb lacerations: Risk factors and the role of antimicrobial agents. *J Trauma* 46:1078, 1999.
11. Semel JD, Trenholme G: *Aeromonas hydrophila* water-associated traumatic wound infections: A review. *J Trauma* 30:324, 1990.
12. Liow RY, Budny P, Regan PJ: Hair thread tourniquet syndrome. *J Accid Emerg Med* 13:138, 1996.
13. Harris EJ: Acute digital ischemia in infants: The hair-thread tourniquet syndrome—a report of two cases. *J Foot Ankle Surg* 41:112, 2002.

For further reading in *Emergency Medicine: A Comprehensive Study Guide*, 6th ed., see Chap. 45, "Lacerations of the Leg and Foot," by Earl J. Reisdorff.

19 SOFT TISSUE FOREIGN BODIES
Rodney L. McCaskill

EPIDEMIOLOGY

- The potential exists for the presence of a foreign body in all wounds.
- Only a small proportion of wounds will contain a foreign body.[1,2]

PATHOPHYSIOLOGY

- Retained foreign bodies may lead to a severe local inflammatory response (eg, wood, thorns, spines), chronic local pain (eg, glass, metal, plastic), local toxic reactions (eg, sea urchin spines, catfish spines), systemic toxicity (eg, lead)[3], or infection.
- Infections are the most common complications of retained foreign bodies, and typically these infections are resistant to antibiotic therapy.[2]

CLINICAL FEATURES

- The mechanism of injury, composition and shape of the wounding object, and the shape and location of the resulting wound may increase the risk of a foreign body.[1,2]
- Lacerating objects that splinter, shatter, or break increase the risk of a foreign body.
- Since patients are often inaccurate in perceiving foreign bodies at the time of examination (sensitivity 43% and specificity 83%), wound evaluation is critical.[2]
- Careful exploration of the depths of all wounds increases the likelihood of finding a foreign body. Extending the edges of the wound is often necessary to thoroughly investigate for foreign bodies.
- Although puncture wounds and apparently superficial wounds can hold foreign bodies, wounds deeper than 5 mm and those whose depths cannot be investigated have a higher association with foreign bodies.[1]
- Blind probing with a hemostat is less effective, but may be utilized if the wound is narrow and deep and extending the wound is not desirable.
- Patients returning to the emergency department with retained foreign bodies may complain of sharp pain at the wound site with movement, a chronically irritated nonhealing wound, or a chronically infected wound.

DIAGNOSIS AND DIFFERENTIAL

- Imaging studies should be ordered if a foreign body is suspected.
- Most foreign bodies (80 to 90%) can be seen on plain radiographs.
- Metal, bone, teeth, pencil graphite, certain plastics, glass, gravel, sand, and aluminum are visible on plain film.[4–10]
- Wood, thorns, cactus spines, some fish bones, most plastics, and other organic matter cannot be seen on plain film, but because of its sensitivity in detecting different densities, CT scanning has been used successfully.[4,8,11]

- Ultrasound is probably less accurate than CT, but it reportedly has a 90% sensitivity for detecting foreign bodies larger than 4 to 5 mm in size.[12–16]
- MRI can detect radiolucent foreign bodies and is more accurate in identifying wood, plastic, spines, and thorns than the other modalities, but is less readily available for emergency use.[5]

EMERGENCY DEPARTMENT CARE AND DISPOSITION

- Not all foreign bodies need to be removed. Indications for foreign body removal include potential for infection, toxicity, functional problems, or potential for persistent pain.
- Vegetative material and heavily contaminated objects should always be removed.
- Radiopaque foreign bodies may be localized using skin markers and x-ray or fluoroscopy.
- Most busy emergency physicians will only be able to dedicate 15 to 30 minutes to removal procedures.
- Needles may be difficult to locate. If the needle is superficial and can be palpated, an incision can be made over one end and the needle removed. If the needle is deeper, then an incision can be made at the midpoint of the needle and the needle grasped with a hemostat and pushed back out through the entrance wound. If the needle is perpendicular to the skin, the entrance wound should be extended. Then pressure applied on the wound edges may reveal the needle so that it can be grasped and removed.
- Wooden splinters and organic spines are difficult to remove because of their tendency to break.
- Only splinters that are superficial should be removed by longitudinal traction. Otherwise the wound should be enlarged and the splinter lifted out of the wound intact. If the splinter is small and localization is difficult, then a block of tissue may be removed in an elliptical fashion and the remaining wound closed primarily. Since infection occurs frequently, subungual splinters should be removed with splinter forceps or by excising a portion of nail over the splinter and then removing the splinter intact.
- Cactus spines may be removed individually or with an adhesive such as facial gel, rubber cement, or household glue.[17]
- Several techniques have been established to remove fishhooks, including the string-pull method, the needle-cover technique, or the advance-and-cut technique. Alternatively, the wound may be enlarged down to the barb and the fishhook removed. When using any of these techniques, anesthesia should be injected around the fishhook entry site.
- After removal of a foreign body, the wound should be adequately cleaned and irrigated.

- If the potential for infection is low, the wound may be closed primarily.
- If there is a significant risk for infection, delayed primary closure is preferred.
- If a foreign body is suspected or identified radiographically but cannot be located even after thorough wound evaluation, or if the foreign body is located in an area that prohibits removal, then the patient should be informed and referred to a surgical specialist for delayed removal. If the foreign body is near a tendon or joint, the limb should be splinted. Prophylactic antibiotics are widely prescribed, but their efficacy has not been determined.

REFERENCES

1. Avner JR, Baker MD: Lacerations involving glass: The role of routine roentgenograms. *Am J Dis Child* 146:600, 1992.
2. Steele MT, Tran LV, Watson LA, Muelleman RL: Retained glass foreign bodies in wounds. Predictive value of wound characteristics, patient perception, and wound exploration. *Am J Emerg Med* 16:627, 1998.
3. Farrell SE, Vandevander P, Schoffstall JM, et al: Elevated serum lead levels in ED patients with retained lead foreign bodies. *Acad Emerg Med* 6:208, 1999.
4. Russell RC, Williamson DA, Sullivan JW, et al: Detention of foreign bodies in the hand. *J Hand Surg* 16A:2, 1991.
5. Courter BJ: Radiographic screening for glass foreign bodies: What does a "negative" foreign body series really mean? *Ann Emerg Med* 19:997, 1990.
6. Ellis G. Are aluminum foreign bodies detectable radiographically? *Am J Emerg Med* 11:12, 1993.
7. Roobottom CA, Weston MJ: The detection of foreign bodies in soft tissue: Comparison of conventional and digital radiography. *Clin Radiol* 49:330, 1994.
8. Reiner B, Siegel E, McLaurin T, et al: Evaluation of soft-tissue foreign bodies: Comparing conventional plain film radiography, computed radiography printed on film, and computed tomography displayed on a computer workstation. *AJR Am J Roentgenol* 167:141, 1996.
9. Chisholm CD, Wood CO, Chua G, et al: Radiographic detection of gravel in soft tissue. *Ann Emerg Med* 29:725, 1997.
10. Ell SR, Sprigg A, Parker AJ: A multi-observer study examining the radiographic visibility of fishbone foreign bodies. *J Roy Soc Med* 89:31, 1996.
11. Lue AJ, Fang WD, Manolidis S: Use of plain radiography and computed tomography to identify fish bone foreign bodies. *Otolaryngol Head Neck Surg* 123:435, 2000.
12. Jacobson JA, Powell A, Craig JG, et al: Wooden foreign bodies in soft tissue: Detection at ultrasound. *Radiology* 206:45, 1998.
13. Schlager D, Sanders AB, Wiggins D, et al: Ultrasound for the detection of foreign bodies. *Ann Emerg Med* 20:189, 1991.
14. Manthey DE, Storrow AB, Milbourn JM, et al: Ultrasound versus radiography in the detection of soft-tissue foreign bodies. *Ann Emerg Med* 28:7, 1996.
15. Graham DD: Ultrasound in the emergency department: Detection of wooden foreign bodies in the soft tissues. *J Emerg Med* 22:75, 2002.
16. Boyse TD, Fessell DP, Jacobsen JA, et al: US of soft-tissue foreign bodies and associated surgical complications with surgical correlation. *Radiographics* 21:1251, 2001.
17. Martinez TT, Jerome M, Barry RC, et al: Removal of cactus spines from the skin: A comparative evaluation of several methods. *Am J Dis Child* 141:1291, 1987.

For further reading in *Emergency Medicine: A Comprehensive Study Guide,* 6th ed., see Chap. 46, "Soft Tissue Foreign Bodies," by Richard L. Lammers.

20   PUNCTURE WOUNDS AND MAMMALIAN BITES

Chris Melton

PUNCTURE WOUNDS

PATHOPHYSIOLOGY

- The plantar surface of the foot is the most common site for puncture wounds.[1]
- Puncture wounds may injure underlying structures, introduce a foreign body, and plant inoculum for infection.
- Infection occurs in 6 to 11% of puncture wounds, with *Staphylococcus aureus* predominating.[2] *Pseudomonas aeruginosa* is the most frequent etiologic agent in post–puncture wound osteomyelitis, particularly when penetration occurs through the sole of an athletic shoe.[3]
- Post–puncture wound infections and failure of an infection to respond to antibiotics suggests the presence of a retained foreign body. Organized evaluation and management is necessary to minimize complications.

CLINICAL FEATURES

- Patients with a history of diabetes mellitus (DM), peripheral vascular disease (PVD), or immunosuppression (IS) are at increased risk of infection.[4]
- Wounds over 6 hours old with large and deep penetration and obvious visible contamination, which occurred outdoors with penetration through footwear and involving the forefoot carry the highest risk of infectious complications.[5]
- On physical examination, the likelihood of injury to structures beneath the skin must be determined.

Distal function of tendons, nerves, and vessels should be carefully assessed. The site should be inspected for location, condition of the surrounding skin, and the presence of foreign matter, debris, or devitalized tissue.

• Infection is suggested when there is evidence of pain, swelling, erythema, warmth, fluctuance, decreased range of motion, or evidence of drainage from the site.

DIAGNOSIS AND DIFFERENTIAL

• A high index of suspicion must be maintained for a retained foreign body. Patient perception of a foreign body is modestly useful in predicting one (sensitivity 43%, specificity 83%, positive likelihood ratio 2.49, and negative likelihood ratio 0.69).[6]

• Multiple view soft tissue plain-film radiographs should be obtained of all infected puncture wounds and of any wound suspicious for a retained foreign body. See Chap. 19 for recommendations on the diagnosis and management of retained foreign bodies.

EMERGENCY DEPARTMENT CARE AND DISPOSITION

• Many aspects of the treatment of puncture wounds remain controversial.[2]

• Uncomplicated, clean punctures treated <6 hours after injury require only low-pressure irrigation and tetanus prophylaxis as indicated. Soaking has no proven benefit. Healthy patients do not appear to require prophylactic antibiotics.

• Prophylactic antibiotics may benefit patients with PVD, DM, and IS. Plantar puncture wounds, especially those in high-risk patients, those located in the forefoot, or those through athletic shoes should be treated with prophylactic antibiotics.[7,8] Fluoroquinolones (such as ciprofloxacin 500 mg bid) are broad-spectrum antibiotics that rapidly achieve high blood levels following an oral dose and are acceptable alternatives to parenteral administration of both a cephalosporin and aminoglycoside. In general, prophylactic antibiotics should be continued for 5 to 7 days.

• Ciprofloxacin is not recommended for routine use for prophylaxis in children. Cephalexin 25 to 50 mg/kg/day divided qid up to 500 mg can be used with close follow-up.

• Wounds infected at presentation need to be differentiated into cellulitis, abscess, deeper spreading soft-tissue infections, and bone or cartilage involvement. Plain radiographs are indicated to detect the possibil-

ity of radiopaque foreign body, soft tissue gas, or osteomyelitis.

• Cellulitis is usually localized without significant drainage, developing within 1 to 4 days. There is no need for routine cultures, and antimicrobial coverage should be directed at gram-positive organisms, especially *S aureus*. Seven to ten days of a first-generation cephalosporin is usually effective.

• A local abscess may develop at the puncture site, especially if a foreign body remains. Treatment includes incision, drainage, and careful exploration for a retained foreign body. The wound should be rechecked in 48 hours. Serious, deep soft tissue infections require surgical exploration and débridement in the OR.

• Any patient who relapses or fails to improve after initial therapy should be suspected of having osteomyelitis or septic arthritis. Radiographs, white blood cell count (WBC), erythrocyte sedimentation rate (ESR), and orthopedic consultation should be obtained. Definitive management frequently necessitates operative intervention for debridement. Pending cultures, antibiotics are started that cover *Staphylococcus* and *Pseudomonas* species. A reasonable regimen would be parenteral nafcillin, 1 to 2 g IV every 4 hours, and ceftazidime, 1 to 2 g IV every 8 hours.

• Conditions for admission include wound infection in patients with DM, PVD, or other immunocompromised states;[9] wounds with progressive cellulitis and lymphangitic spread; osteomyelitis; septic arthritis; and deep foreign bodies necessitating operative removal.

• Tetanus prophylaxis should be provided according to guidelines (see Chap. 21). Outpatients should avoid weight bearing, should elevate and soak the wound in warm water, and have follow-up within 48 hours.

NEEDLESTICK INJURIES

• Needlestick injuries carry the risk of bacterial infection in addition to the risk of infection with hepatitis and human immunodeficiency virus (HIV).

• Each hospital should have a predesigned protocol developed by infectious disease specialists for the expeditious evaluation, testing, and treatment of needlestick injuries, because recommendations in this area are complex and changing.

HIGH-PRESSURE-INJECTION INJURIES

• High-pressure-injection injuries may present as a puncture wound, usually to the hand or foot. This equipment is designed to force liquids (usually paint or oil) through a small nozzle under high pressure.

- These injuries are severe owing to intense inflammation incited by the injected liquid spreading along fascial planes. Patients have pain and minimal swelling. Despite an innocuous appearance, serious damage can develop.
- Pain control should be achieved with parenteral analgesics; digital blocks are contraindicated so as to avoid increases in tissue pressure with resultant further compromise in perfusion.[10]
- An appropriate hand specialist should be consulted immediately and early surgical débridement implemented for an optimal outcome.

HUMAN BITES

- Human bites produce a crushing or tearing of tissue, with potential for injury to underlying structures and inoculation of tissues with normal human oral flora.
- Human bites are most often reported on the hands and upper extremities. Infection is the major serious sequela.

CLINICAL FEATURES

- Of particular concern is the clenched fist injury (CFI), which occurs in the metacarpophalangeal (MCP) region as the fist strikes the mouth and teeth of another individual.
- These hand injuries are at increased risk for serious infection and any questionable injury in the vicinity of the MCP joint should be considered a CFI until proven otherwise.
- The physical examination should include assessment of the direct injury and a careful evaluation of the underlying structures, including tendons, vessels, nerves, deep spaces, joints, and bone. Local anesthesia is usually required to perform a careful wound exploration.
- In a CFI, the wound must be examined through a full range of motion at the MCP joint to detect extensor tendon involvement, which may have retracted proximally in the unclenched hand.
- The exam must also assess a potential joint-space violation; see Chap. 18 for evaluation guidelines.
- Radiographs are recommended, particularly of the hand, to delineate foreign bodies and fractures.
- Human bites to the hand are frequently complicated by cellulitis, lymphangitis, abscess formation, tenosynovitis, septic arthritis, and osteomyelitis. Infections from human bites are polymicrobial, with staphylococcal and streptococcal species common isolates, as well as species-specific *Eikenella corrodens*.

DIAGNOSIS AND DIFFERENTIAL

- History and physical exam will usually reveal a straightforward diagnosis. There are times, however, when a patient may try to conceal or deny the true etiology of a human bite and a high degree of suspicion is warranted, particularly when the wound is on the hand.
- It is important to keep in mind that viral diseases can also be transmitted by human bites (eg, herpes simplex, herpetic whitlow, and hepatitis B). The potential risk of acquiring HIV through a human bite appears to be negligible due to low levels of HIV in saliva.

EMERGENCY DEPARTMENT CARE AND DISPOSITION

- Copious wound irrigation with normal saline solution and judicious limited débridement of devitalized tissue are critical to initial management.
- Human bites to the hand should initially be left open. Other sites can undergo primary closure unless there is a high degree of suspicion for infection.
- Prophylactic antibiotics should be considered in all but the most trivial of human bites. Amoxicillin-clavulanate 500 to 875 mg PO bid is the antibiotic of choice.[11]
- Uncomplicated fresh CFI wounds should be left open with an appropriate dressing. The hand should be immobilized and elevated for 24 hours, and prophylactic antibiotics should be administered. The patient should be re-evaluated in 1 to 2 days. If there is a laceration to either the extensor tendon or joint capsule, or radiographic findings, a hand specialist should be consulted for possible exploration in the operating room and admission for parenteral antibiotics.
- Wounds that are infected at presentation require systemic antibiotics after cultures are obtained. Local cellulitis in healthy and reliable patients may be managed on an outpatient basis with immobilization, antibiotics, and close follow-up. Moderate to severe infections require admission for surgical consultation and parenteral antibiotics. Appropriate coverage includes ampicillin-sulbactam, 3 g every 6 hours IV, or cefoxitin, 2.0 g every 8 hours IV. Penicillin-allergic patients may be treated with clindamycin plus ciprofloxacin.
- All patients should receive tetanus immunization according to guidelines.

DOG BITES

CLINICAL FEATURES

- Dog bites account for 80 to 90% of reported animal bites, with school-age children sustaining the majority of reported bites.

- Infection occurs in approximately 5% of cases and is more common in patients over 50 years old, those with hand wounds or deep puncture wounds, and those who delay seeking initial treatment for more than 24 hours.[11,12]
- A thorough history and exam as outlined in the section on human bites are required to assess the extent of the wound and the likelihood of infection.
- Infections from dog-bite wounds are often polymicrobial and include both aerobic and anaerobic bacteria.[12]

DIAGNOSIS AND DIFFERENTIAL

- Radiographs are recommended if there is evidence of infection, suspicion of a foreign body, bony involvement, or intracranial penetration bites to the heads of small children.

EMERGENCY DEPARTMENT CARE AND DISPOSITION

- All dog-bite wounds require appropriate local wound care with copious irrigation and débridement of devitalized tissue.
- Primary closure can be utilized in wounds to the scalp, face, torso, and extremities other than the feet and hands.[13,14] Lacerations of the feet and hands should be left open initially. Large, extensive lacerations, especially in small children, are best explored and repaired in the operating room.
- Puncture wounds, wounds to the hands and feet, and wounds in high-risk patients should receive 3 to 5 days of prophylactic antibiotics with amoxicillin-clavulanate 500 to 875 mg PO bid, or clindamycin plus ciprofloxacin. In children, clindamycin plus trimethoprim-sulfamethoxazole should be used.
- Penicillin (500 mg PO qid) is the drug of choice for *Capnocytophaga canimorsus,* and should be used prophylactically in high-risk immunocompromised patients (ie, those with asplenia, alcoholism, or chronic lung disease). Cephalosporins, tetracyclines, erythromycin, and clindamycin are reasonable alternatives.
- Wounds obviously infected at presentation need to be cultured and antibiotics initiated. Reliable, low-risk patients with only local cellulitis and no involvement of underlying structures can be managed as outpatients with close follow-up.
- Infection developing within 24 hours after injury suggests *Pasteurella multocida,* and treatment with penicillin, ciprofloxacin, or trimethoprim-sulfamethoxazole is recommended. Wound infection developing beyond 24 hours after the bite implicates *Staphylococcus* and *Streptococcus,* and these patients should receive dicloxacillin (12 to 25 mg/kg/day divided qid; 500 mg qid in adults), or a first-generation cephalosporin (eg, cephalexin, 25 to 50 mg/kg/day divided qid; 500 mg qid in adults).
- Significant wound infections require admission and parenteral antibiotics. Examples include infected wounds with evidence of lymphangitis, lymphadenitis, tenosynovitis, septic arthritis, osteomyelitis, systemic signs, and injury to underlying structures such as tendons, joints, or bones.
- Cultures should be obtained from deep structures, preferably during exploration in the operating room. Initial antibiotic therapy should begin with ampicillin-sulbactam 3 g IV every 6 hours, or clindamycin plus ciprofloxacin. If the Gram's stain reveals gram-negative bacilli, a third- or fourth-generation cephalosporin or aminoglycoside should be added.
- Tetanus prophylaxis should be provided according to standard guidelines.

CAT BITES

- Cat bites account for 5 to 18% of reported animal bites, with the majority resulting in puncture wounds on the arm, forearm, and hand.
- Up to 80% of cat bites become infected.[12]

CLINICAL FEATURES

- *P. multocida* is the major pathogen, isolated in 53 to 80% of infected cat bite wounds.
- *Pasteurella* causes a rapidly developing intense inflammatory response with prominent symptoms of pain and swelling. It may cause serious bone and joint infections and bacteremia.
- Many patients with septic arthritis due to *P. multocida* have altered host defenses due to glucocorticoids or alcoholism.

DIAGNOSIS AND DIFFERENTIAL

- Radiographs are recommended if there is evidence of infection, suspicion of a foreign body, or bony involvement.

EMERGENCY DEPARTMENT CARE AND DISPOSITION

- Treatment for cat-bite wounds is essentially the same as for dog-bite wounds.

- All cat-bite wounds require appropriate local wound care with copious irrigation and débridement of devitalized tissue.
- Primary wound closure is usually indicated, except in puncture wounds and lacerations smaller than 1 to 2 cm, as they cannot be adequately cleaned.[13,14] Delayed primary closure can also be employed in cosmetically important areas.
- Prophylactic antibiotics should be administered to high-risk patients, including those with punctures of the hand, immunocompromised patients, and patients with arthritis or prosthetic joints. The case can be made that all cat bites should receive prophylactic antibiotics because of the high risk of infection. Amoxicillin-clavulanate 500 to 875 mg PO bid (45 mg/kg/day divided bid in children), cefuroxime 500 mg PO bid (20 to 30 mg/kg/day divided bid in children), or doxycycline 100 mg PO bid, administered 3 to 5 days, are appropriate.
- For cat bites that develop infection, evaluation and treatment is similar to that of dog-bite infections. Penicillin is the drug of choice for *Pasteurella multocida* infections.
- Tetanus prophylaxis should be provided according to standard guidelines.

RODENTS, LIVESTOCK, AND EXOTIC AND WILD ANIMALS

- Rodent bites are typically trivial because they are not known to carry rabies and have a low risk for infection.
- Livestock and large game animals can cause serious injury. There is also a significant risk of infection and systemic illness caused by brucellosis, leptospirosis, and tularemia.
- Aggressive wound care and broad-spectrum antibiotics are recommended.

REFERENCES

1. Baldwin G, Colbourne M: Puncture wounds. *Pediatr Rev* 20:21, 1999.
2. Schwab RA, Powers RD: Conservative therapy of plantar puncture wounds. *J Emerg Med* 13:291, 1995.
3. Inaba AS, Zukin DD, Perro M: An update on the evaluation and management of plantar puncture wounds and *Pseudomonas* osteomyelitis. *Pediatr Emerg Care* 8:38, 1992.
4. Armstrong DG, Lavery LS, Quebedeaux TL, et al: Surgical morbidity and nondiabetic adults. *J Am Podiatr Med Assoc* 87:321, 1997.
5. Patzakis MJ, Wilkins J, Brien WW, et al: Wound site as a predictor of complications following deep nail punctures to the foot. *West J Med* 150:545, 1989.
6. Steele MT, Tran LV, Watson WA, Muelleman RT: Retained glass foreign bodies in wounds: Predicative value of wound characteristics, patient perception, and wound exploration. *Am J Emerg Med* 16:627, 1998.
7. Pennycook A, Makower R, O'Donnell A-M: Puncture wounds: Can infective complications be avoided? *J Roy Soc Med* 87:581, 1994.
8. Harrison M, Thomas M: Antibiotics after puncture wounds to the foot. *Emerg Med J* 19:49, 2002.
9. Lavery LS, Armstrong DG, Quebedeaux TL: Normal laboratory values in the face of severe infection in diabetics and nondiabetics. *Am J Med* 101:521, 1996.
10. Vasilevski K, Noorbergen M, Depierreux M, et al: High-pressure injection injuries to the hand. *Am J Emerg Med* 18:820, 2000.
11. Medeiros I, Saconato H: Antibiotic prophylaxis for mammalian bites. *Cochrane Database Syst Rev* 2:CD001738, 2001.
12. Talan DA, Citron DM, Abrahamian FM, et al: Bacteriologic analysis of infected dog and cat bites. *New Engl J Med* 340:85, 1999.
13. Fleisher G: The management of bite wounds. *New Engl J Med* 340:138, 1999.
14. Chen E, Hornig S, Shepherd SM, Hollander JE: Primary closure of mammalian bites. *Acad Emerg Med* 7:157, 2000.

For further reading in *Emergency Medicine: A Comprehensive Study Guide*, 6th ed., see Chap. 47, "Puncture Wounds and Mammalian Bites," by Robert A. Schwab and Robert D. Powers.

21 POSTREPAIR WOUND CARE

Eugenia B. Smith

DRESSINGS

- Dressings provide a moist environment, which speeds healing.[1]
- Semipermeable films such as Opsite are available in addition to conventional gauze dressings. They will not absorb large amounts of fluid.
- Topical antibiotics may be used as a dressing. They may be the only dressing needed on face and scalp wounds. Topical antibiotics may reduce the rate of wound infection and may also prevent scab formation.[2]
- Wounds closed with tissue adhesives should not be treated with topical antibiotic ointment, as it will loosen the adhesive.

PATIENT POSITIONING AFTER WOUND REPAIR

- The injured site should be elevated if possible.
- Splints are useful for extremity injuries.
- Pressure dressings are most useful for ear and scalp lacerations. A pressure dressing on the ear will reduce the likelihood of a cauliflower deformity.

PROPHYLACTIC ANTIBIOTICS

- There is no benefit to prophylactic antibiotics for routine laceration repair.[3]
- Prophylactic antibiotics should be used for human bites, dog or cat bites on the extremities, intraoral lacerations, open fractures, and wounds with exposed joints or tendons.[4,5]
- For most patients, an oral first-generation cephalosporin (eg, cephalexin 25 to 50 mg/kg/day divided four times per day, up to 500 mg per dose) or an antistaphylococcal penicillin (eg, dicloxacillin 25 to 50 mg/kg/day divided qid, up to 500 mg per dose) is reasonable.
- Oral penicillin (25 to 50 mg/kg/day divided qid, up to 500 mg per dose) should be used for intraoral wounds.
- Amoxicillin-clavulanate (20 to 40 mg/kg/day divided every 8 hours, up to 500 mg per dose) or a combination of penicillin and dicloxacillin are the preferred choices for high-risk mammalian bite wounds.
- For open fractures or joints, a parenteral antistaphylococcal agent and an aminoglycoside should be used (see Chaps. 17 and 18).
- A 3- to 5-day course is adequate for nonbite injuries and a 5- to 7-day course is adequate for bite wounds.

TETANUS PROPHYLAXIS

- Consider tetanus prophylaxis for every wounded patient.
- The only contraindication to tetanus toxoid is a history of neurologic or severe systemic reaction after a previous dose.
- Patients with clean minor wounds require tetanus prophylaxis if it has been greater than 10 years since the last dose.
- Tetanus prophylaxis (tetanus toxoid or diphtheria-tetanus toxoid, 0.5 mL IM) is indicated for all other wounded patients if it has been more than 5 years since the last dose.
- Tetanus immune globulin (250 units IM) should be administered to those without a history of a primary series of three tetanus immunizations. A second dose is required in 1 to 2 months and a third dose in 6 to 12 months.

WOUND DRAINS

- Gauze packing is the most common type of drain placed in the ED, usually used to pack an abscess cavity after incision and drainage. The packing should be replaced daily as long as the wound continues to drain.
- Open drainage using soft rubber tubing is used for infected or contaminated wounds that have been partially or completely closed. A safety pin placed through the tubing will prevent it from sliding into the wound.
- Closed drainage systems often have a self-inflating bulb that can be squeezed before attachment to the tubing to create a vacuum effect. Closed drains are generally removed after drainage slows to low levels (30 to 40 mL/day).

PAIN CONTROL

- Patients should be educated about the expected degree of pain and measures that might reduce pain.
- Medications may be needed, but narcotic analgesia is rarely necessary after the first 48 hours.

WOUND CARE INSTRUCTIONS AND FOLLOW-UP

- Standardized wound care instructions improve patient compliance and understanding.[5]
- Sutured or stapled lacerations should be gently washed and cleansed as early as 8 hours after closure.[6]
- Patients with dressings should remove their dressings after 24 to 48 hours to check the wound.
- All patients should be instructed to observe for redness, warmth, swelling, or drainage, and to initiate contact with their provider if any of these are seen.
- Facial sutures should be removed in 3 to 5 days.
- Most other sutures can be removed in 7 to 10 days, except for sutures in the hands or over joints, which should remain for 10 to 14 days.
- Tissue adhesives will slough off within 5 to 10 days of application.
- In the case of high-risk wounds, patients may be instructed to return for a wound check, usually in 48 hours.

PATIENT EDUCATION ABOUT LONG-TERM COSMETIC OUTCOME

- Instruct patients that all traumatic lacerations result in some scarring, and that short-term cosmetic appearance is not highly predictive of ultimate cosmetic outcome.[7]

- Instruct patients to avoid sun exposure while their wounds are healing, as it can cause permanent hyperpigmentation.[8] Patients should wear sunblock for at least 6 to 12 months after injury.

REFERENCES

1. Hinman CD, Maibach H: Effect of air exposure and occlusion on experimental human skin wounds. *Nature* 200:377, 1963.
2. Dire DJ, Coppola M, Dwyer DA, et al: A prospective evaluation of topical antibiotics for preventing infections in uncomplicated soft-tissue wounds repaired in the ED. *Acad Emerg Med* 2:4, 1995.
3. Cummings P, Del Beccaro MA: Antibiotics to prevent infection of simple wounds: A meta-analysis of randomized studies. *Am J Emerg Med* 13:396, 1995.
4. Singer AJ, Hollander JE, Quinn JV: Evaluation and management of traumatic lacerations. *N Engl J Med* 337:1142, 1997.
5. Hollander JE, Singer AJ: Laceration management. *Ann Emerg Med* 34:356, 1999.
6. Goldberg HM, Rosenthal SAE, Nemetz JC: Effect of washing closed head and neck wounds on wound healing and infection. *Am J Surg* 141:358, 1981.
7. Hollander JE, Blasko B, Singer AJ, et al: Poor correlation of short and long term appearance of repaired lacerations. *Acad Emerg Med* 2:983,1995.
8. Ship AG, Weiss PR: Pigmentation after dermabrasion: An avoidable complication. *Plast Reconstr Surg* 75:528, 1985.

For further reading in *Emergency Medicine: A Comprehensive Study Guide,* 6th ed., see Chap. 48, "Postrepair Wound Care," by Adam J. Singer and Judd E. Hollander.

22 APPROACH TO CHEST PAIN

Thomas Rebbecchi

EPIDEMIOLOGY

- Chest pain (CP) accounts for 5% of all ED visits (approximately 5 million visits/year).[1]

PATHOPHYSIOLOGY

- Chest pain can be visceral or somatic. Visceral pain originates from vessels or organs, enters the spinal cord at multiple levels, and is thus poorly described, using terms such as heaviness or aching. Somatic pain is dermatomal, from the parietal pleura or structures of the chest wall, and can be more precisely described.
- Ischemia is an imbalance of oxygen supply and demand.
- Coronary plaque formation occurs due to repetitive injury to the vessel wall. Plaque build-up leads to narrowing of the vessel.
- Angina pectoris is visceral pain due to lack of oxygen to myocytes. Anaerobic metabolism ensues; chemical mediators are released and pain results.
- Knowledge of coronary anatomy will help predict which coronary vessels are involved with an ischemic event (Fig. 22-1).

CLINICAL FEATURES

- Typical ischemic CP is felt as tightness, squeezing, crushing, or pressure in the retrosternal/epigastric area. Radiation of pain to the jaw or arm is associated

with a higher risk of ischemia.[2] Elderly patients may have less definitive symptoms.
- Symptoms lasting less than 2 minutes or longer than 24 hours are less likely to be ischemic. Atypical presentations (anginal equivalents) are the rule and are more common in women, diabetics, nonwhite minorities, and psychiatric patients.[3]
- Up to one third of acute myocardial infarctions (AMIs) may be silent.[1]
- The major cardiac risk factors are age over 40, male gender or postmenopausal woman, family history, cigarette use, hypertension, high cholesterol, truncal obesity, sedentary lifestyle, and diabetes mellitus (DM). Cocaine use should also be considered as a risk factor. These risk factors can only be used to predict coronary artery disease (CAD) in a given population and not in an individual.
- In the ED patient with chest pain, risk factors are not predictive in females, and DM and family history are only weakly predictive in males.[4]

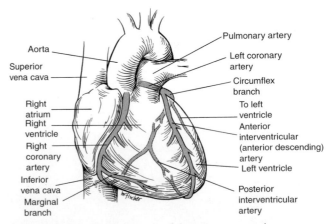

FIG. 22-1. Schematic diagram of the coronary arteries.

TABLE 22-1   Serious Causes of Chest Pain and Their Presentation

DIAGNOSIS	SYMPTOMS AT PRESENTATION
Pulmonary embolism (see Chap. 28)	Sudden onset, pleuritic pain, and dyspnea
Aortic dissection (see Chap. 30)	Tearing pain with radiation to back, possible neurologic symptoms
Pericarditis (see Chap. 27)	Positional ache, dyspnea
Pneumothorax (see Chap. 35)	Pleuritic pain and dyspnea
Acute coronary syndrome (see Chap. 23)	Vague, pressure-like pain, radiation to arm, neck, jaw
Esophageal rupture (see Chap. 40)	Constant retrosternal, epigastric pain, history of inciting event
Pneumonia (see Chap. 33)	Pleuritic pain, cough, dyspnea, chills

- A recent report looking at the presence of conventional risk factors in patients who were enrolled in controlled treatment trials for unstable angina or percutaneous coronary intervention found at least one risk factor (smoking, diabetes, hyperlipidemia, or hypertension) in 84.6% of women and 80.6% of men.[5]
- The character of the chest pain on presentation of the patient may aid in the differentiation of ischemic chest pain from other diagnostic possibilities (Table 22-1).
- Anginal pain is typically worsened with exertion and relieved with rest.
- Variant Prinzmetal angina is coronary vasospasm, usually at rest. The physical examination is often normal, but there is a higher incidence of abnormal heart sounds.

DIAGNOSIS AND DIFFERENTIAL

- Diagnosing angina is usually based on historical information.
- The electrocardiogram (ECG) is the most important single test and should be obtained within 10 minutes of arrival to the ED. Only 50% of patients will have a diagnostic ECG. Serial ECGs are imperative with continued CP.
- Serum cardiac markers are useful for ischemia and infarction. Creatine kinase (CK), specifically the MB fraction, measured over 24 hours is historically considered the gold standard for myocardial infarction.[6] Other conditions can elevate this blood level (Table 22-2).
- Troponin I is specific to cardiac muscle and has a high specificity and sensitivity for AMI.
- Myoglobin rises predictably in AMI, but there is a high false-positive rate due to its presence in all muscle tissue.
- The relationship between elevations of CK-MB, myoglobin, and troponin can be seen in Fig. 22-2.
- Echocardiography can diagnose impaired wall function, but cannot distinguish between ischemia and infarction.[7] Two-dimensional echocardiography may also aid in the diagnosis of other conditions that may mimic ischemic disease, such as pericarditis, aortic dissection, or hypertrophic cardiomyopathy.
- Stress-echo testing for low-risk patients has a negative predictive value of 97%.[7]
- Stress testing and nuclear imaging (sestamibi) can be used in the ED to risk stratify patients with CP.
- Chest x-ray can aid in the diagnosis of other noncardiac syndromes that may mimic ischemic CP (Table 22-3).

TABLE 22-2   Common Conditions Associated with Elevated CK-MB Levels

Unstable angina (intermediate coronary syndrome)

Acute coronary ischemia

Inflammatory heart diseases

Cardiomyopathies

Circulatory failure and shock

Cardiac surgery

Cardiac trauma

Skeletal muscle trauma (severe)

Dermatomyositis, polymyositis

Myopathic disorders

Muscular dystrophy, especially Duchenne

Vigorous exercise

Malignant hyperthermia

Reye's syndrome

Rhabdomyolysis of any cause

Delirium tremens

Ethanol poisoning (chronic)

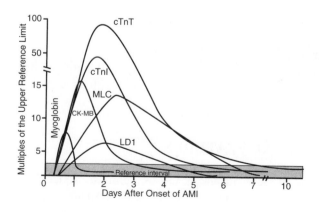

FIG. 22-2. Multiple marker curve.

TABLE 22-3   Important Causes of Acute Chest Pain

CHEST WALL PAIN	PLEURITIC PAIN	VISCERAL PAIN
Costosternal syndrome	Pulmonary embolism	Typical exertional angina
Costochrondritis (Tietze syndrome)	Pneumonia	Atypical (nonexertional) angina
Precordial catch syndrome	Spontaneous pneumothorax	Unstable angina
Slipping rib syndrome	Pericarditis	Acute myocardial infarction
Xiphodynia	Pleurisy	Aortic dissection
Radicular syndromes		Pericarditis
Intercostal nerve syndromes		Esophageal reflux or spasm
Fibromyalgia		Esophageal rupture
		Mitral valve prolapse

EMERGENCY DEPARTMENT CARE AND DISPOSITION

- Place the patient on a cardiac monitor, administer oxygen, and obtain IV access. Obtain an ECG.
- The patient should be treated aggressively if the clinical suspicion is high despite a nondiagnostic or normal ECG. Admit the patient to a high acuity setting in the presence of an acute coronary syndrome.
- The combination of ECG, clinical history, and cardiac markers can be used to risk stratify the patient for management and disposition (Table 22-4).
- Some patients can be observed in the ED and released after a series of normal cardiac markers and a provocative test.

TABLE 22-4   Prognosis-Based Classification System for ED Chest Pain Patients

I. **Acute myocardial infarction: immediate revascularization candidate**

II. **Probable acute ischemia: high risk for adverse events**
Any of the following:
   Evidence of clinical instability (ie, pulmonary edema, hypotension, arrhythmia)
   Ongoing pain thought to be ischemic
   Pain at rest associated with ischemic electrocardiographic changes
   One or more positive myocardial marker measurements
   Positive perfusion imaging study

III. **Possible acute ischemia: intermediate risk for adverse events**
History suggestive of ischemia with any of the following:
   Rest pain, now resolved
   New onset of pain
   Crescendo pattern of pain
   Ischemic pattern on electrocardiogram not associated with pain

IV.A. **Probably not ischemia: low risk for adverse events**
Requires all of the following:
   History not strongly suggestive of ischemia
   Electrocardiogram normal, unchanged from previous, or nonspecific changes
   Negative myocardial marker measurement

IV.B. **Stable angina pectoris: low risk for adverse events**
Requires all of the following:
   More than 2 weeks of unchanged symptom pattern or long-standing symptoms with only mild change
      in exertional pain threshold
   Electrocardiogram normal, unchanged from previous, or nonspecific changes
   Negative myocardial marker measurement

V. **Definitely not ischemia: very low risk for adverse events**
Requires all of the following:
   Clear objective evidence of nonischemic symptom etiology
   Electrocardiogram normal, unchanged from previous, or nonspecific changes
   Negative myocardial marker measurement

REFERENCES

1. Sigurdsson E, Thorgeirsson G, Sigvaldason H, et al: Unrecognized myocardial infarction: Epidemiology, clinical characteristics, and the prognostic role of angina pectoris: The Reykjavik Study. *Ann Intern Med* 122:96, 1995.
2. Panju AA, Hemmelgarn BR, Guyatt GH, Simel DL: Is this patient having a myocardial infarction? *JAMA* 280:1256, 1998.
3. Lee TH, Cook EF, Weisberg M, et al: Acute chest pain in the emergency room: Identification and examination of low-risk patients. *Arch Intern Med* 145:65, 1985.
4. Jayes RL, Beshansky JR, D'Agostino RB, Selker HP: Do patients' coronary risk factor reports predict acute cardiac ischemia in the emergency department? A multicenter study. *J Clin Epidemiol* 45:621, 1992.
5. Khot UN, Khot MB, Bajzer CT, et al: Prevalence of conventional risk factors in patients with coronary heart disease. *JAMA* 290:898, 2003.
6. Gibler WB, Lewis LM, Erb RE, et al: Early detection of acute myocardial infarction patients presenting with chest pain and nondiagnostic ECGs: Serial CK-MB sampling in the emergency department. *Ann Emerg Med* 19:1359, 1990.
7. Canto JG, Shilipak MG, Rogers WJ, et al: Prevalence, clinical characteristics and mortality among patients with myocardial infarction presenting without chest pain. *JAMA* 283:3227, 2002.

For further reading in *Emergency Medicine: A Comprehensive Study Guide,* 6th ed., see Chap 49, "Approach to Chest Pain," by Gary B. Green and Peter M. Hill.

23 ACUTE CORONARY SYNDROMES: MANAGEMENT OF MYOCARDIAL ISCHEMIA AND INFARCTION

Jim Edward Weber

EPIDEMIOLOGY

- Ischemic heart disease is the number one killer of adults in the United States.
- Acute coronary syndrome (ACS) is a spectrum of disease ranging from stable angina to acute myocardial infarction (AMI).[1]

PATHOPHYSIOLOGY

- Coronary plaque forms on coronary vessel walls after repetitive injury. With plaque rupture, thrombogenic substances are exposed to platelets.
- Platelet response involves adhesion, activation, and aggregation. Platelet adhesion molecules are strongly thrombogenic and bind to von Willebrand's factor (VWF). Thrombin, collagen, shearing forces, adenosine diphosphate (ADP), thromboxane A_2, and serotonin are potent platelet activators. Platelet glycoprotein IIB/IIIA receptors cross-link fibrinogen or VWF as the common pathway of aggregation.
- The severity of ACS depends upon the extent of O_2 deprivation by thrombus, with complete occlusion resulting in cell death.
- AMI results in injury to both the conduction system, leading to ectopy and dysrhythmia, and left ventricle (LV) pump function, leading to increased filling pressures.

CLINICAL FEATURES

- Cardiac risk factors are modestly predictive of CAD in asymptomatic patients, but poor emergency department (ED) predictors for AMI or other ACS.
- The physical examination of a patient with an ACS can range from normal to profound illness.
- Silent/atypical presentations of ischemia are common. Women and the elderly are more likely to present in this way.[2]
- Ischemic/anginal pain is similar to AMI pain. AMI pain usually resolves only with aggressive intervention, whereas anginal pain can resolve with rest or nitroglycerin (NTG).
- Extent and location of myocardial loss determines prognosis and predicts complications. A 25% loss of the LV leads to congestive heart failure (CHF). A 40% LV loss leads to shock. Right ventricle (RV) infarct leads to hypotension.
- Dysrhythmias occur in 72 to 100% of coronary care unit (CCU) patients with AMI. Premature ventricular contractions (PVCs) are common with AMI but not prognostic. Anterior injury leads to tachydysrhythmia. Inferior injury leads to increased vagal tone and first-degree and Mobitz 1 blocks. Mobitz 2 block is usually associated with anterior AMI and may lead to complete heart block. Anterior and/or inferior injury may lead to complete heart block.
- Fifteen to twenty percent of AMI patients have some degree of CHF.
- Free wall myocardial rupture accounts for 10% of AMI fatalities and occurs 1 to 5 days post-AMI.
- Interventricular wall rupture is signified by pain, shortness of breath (SOB), and a holosystolic murmur.
- Papillary muscle rupture occurs in 1% of all MIs 3 to 5 days into the event.
- Pericarditis is seen in up to 20% of all MIs 2 to 4 days after the event. Dressler's syndrome occurs 2 to 10 weeks post-AMI.

- Thirty percent of inferior AMIs involve the right ventricle, and are associated with increased mortality and complications.

DIAGNOSIS AND DIFFERENTIAL

- The history is usually suggestive, but the electrocardiogram (ECG) is the best single test available in the ED. In the setting of AMI, the ECG can range from normal (up to 5%) to distinct ST-segment elevation (Table 23-1).
- With a nondiagnostic ECG, serum markers may be helpful in determining myocardial necrosis and altering early intervention.
- Chest radiography may be useful in determining other causes of ischemic-like pain.

EMERGENCY DEPARTMENT CARE AND DISPOSITION

- The treatment of ACS and AMI require aggressive individualized treatment based on history, physical, and ECG findings (Table 23-2 and Fig. 23-1).
- The goal is to protect the myocardium by lowering oxygen demand and increasing oxygen delivery. Treatment strategies for AMI aim to achieve reperfusion and limit infarct size.
- Immediate management includes IV access, O₂, cardiac monitoring, and ECG.
- Patients with ST-elevation myocardial infarction (STEMI) should receive medical (fibrinolytic) or mechanical (angioplasty, stent, atherectomy) reperfusion. Patients with unstable angina or non-STEMI should be treated with antiplatelet and anticoagulant medications. Refractory non-STEMI patients who undergo percutaneous coronary intervention (PCI) benefit from glycoprotein IIb/IIIa inhibitors.
- Fibrinolytics resolve thrombus directly or indirectly by activating plasminogen.

TABLE 23-1 Localization of MI Based on ECG Findings

Anterior	V₂–V₄
Inferior	II, III, aVF, V₅, V₆
Anteroseptal	V₁–V₃
Lateral	I, aVL, V₄–V₆
Anterolateral	V₁–V₆
Right ventricular	V₄R–V₆R (often associated with inferior MI)
Posterior MI	large R >.04 mm, R/S >1, and ST depression in V₁ and V₂

ABBREVIATIONS: MI = myocardial infarction; ECG = electrocardiogram.

TABLE 23-2 Recommended Doses of Drugs Used in the Emergency Treatment of Acute Coronary Syndromes

Antiplatelet agents
Aspirin	160–325 mg PO
Clopidogrel	Loading dose of 300 mg PO followed by 75 mg/d

Antithrombins
Heparin	Bolus of 60–70 units/kg (maximum, 5000 units) followed by infusion of 12–15 units/kg per h (maximum, 1000 units/h) titrated to a PTT 1.5–2.5 times control
Enoxaparin (LMWH)	1 mg/kg SC q12h

Fibrinolytic agents
Streptokinase	1.5 million units over 60 min
Alteplase (tPA)	Body weight >67 kg: 15 mg initial IV bolus; 50 mg infused over next 30 min; 35 mg infused over next 60 min. Body weight <67 kg: 15 mg initial IV bolus; 0.75 mg/kg infused over next 30 min; 0.5 mg/kg over next 60 min
Reteplase (rPA)	10 mg IV bolus followed by 10 mg IV bolus 30 min later

Tenecteplase (TNKase)

Weight	Dose*
<60 kg	30 mg
≥60 but <70 kg	35 mg
≥70 but <80 kg	40 mg
≥80 but <90	45 mg
≥90	50 mg

*Total dose not to exceed 50 mg

Glycoprotein IIb/IIIa inhibitors
Abciximab	0.25 mg/kg bolus followed by infusion of 0.125 µg/kg per min (maximum, 10 µg/min) for 12–24 h
Eptifibatide	180 µg/kg bolus followed by infusion of 2.0 µg/kg per min for 72–96 h
Tirofiban	0.4 µg/kg per min for 30 min followed by infusion of 0.1 µg/kg per min for 48–96 h

Other anti-ischemic therapies
Nitroglycerin	SL: 0.4 mg q5 min × 3 prn pain. IV: start at 10 µg/min, titrate to 10% reduction in MAP if normotensive, 30% reduction in MAP if hypertensive
Morphine	2–5 mg IV q5–15 min prn pain
Metoprolol	5 mg IV over 2 min q5 min up to 15 mg, followed by 50 mg PO q6h 15 min after last IV dose
Atenolol	5 mg IV over 5 min, repeat once 10 min later, followed with 50 mg PO

ABBREVIATIONS: MAP = mean arterial pressure; PTT = partial thromboplastin time; SL = sublingual.

- Fibrinolytic treatment is indicated for patients with symptoms of AMI, onset to treatment of <12 hours, an ECG that has at least 1-mm ST-segment elevation in two or more contiguous limb leads or at least 2-mm ST-segment elevation in two or more contiguous chest leads, or a new left bundle-branch block (LBBB), in the absence of cardiogenic shock or contraindications[3] (Table 23-3).
- Streptokinase (SK) activates plasminogen, is antigenic, and is given as an infusion. Tissue plasminogen

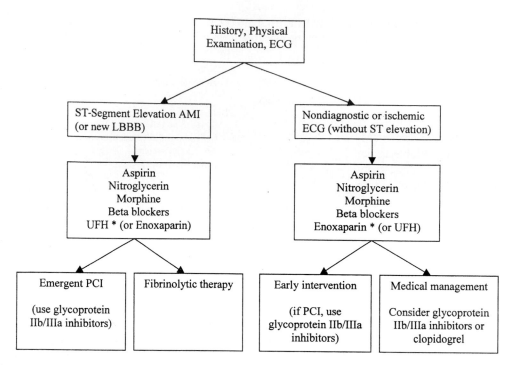

FIG. 23-1. Treatment considerations for patients with acute coronary syndrome. *Preferred antithrombin. AMI = acute myocardial infarction; ECG = electrocardiogram; LBBB = left bundle-branch block; PCI = percutaneous coronary intervention; UFH = unfractionated heparin.

Note: See text for discussion of individual treatment options, indications, and contraindications

activator (tPA) is fibrin specific. Front end (accelerated) loading is preferred and has been shown to be of greater benefit than SK.[4] Reteplase is a non–fibrin specific deletion mutant of tPA administered as a double bolus. Tenecteplase is a tPA substitution mutant with high fibrin specificity, given as a weight-based

TABLE 23-3 Contraindications to Fibrinolytic Therapy in Acute Myocardial Infarction

Absolute contraindications
Previous hemorrhagic stroke at any time
Bland CVA in past year
Known intracranial neoplasm
Active internal bleeding (excluding menses)
Suspected aortic dissection or pericarditis

Relative contraindications
Severe uncontrolled blood pressure (>180/100 mm Hg)
History of chronic severe hypertension
History of prior CVA of known intracranial pathology not covered in
  contraindications
Current use of anticoagulants with known INR >2–3
Known bleeding diathesis
Recent trauma (past 2 wk)
Prolonged CPR (>10 min)
Major surgery (<3 wk)
Noncompressible vascular punctures (including subclavian and
  internal jugular central lines)
Recent internal bleeding (2–4 wk)
Prior streptokinase should not receive streptokinase
Pregnancy
Active peptic ulcer disease
Other medical conditions likely to increase risk of bleeding

ABBREVIATIONS: CPR = cardiopulmonary resuscitation; CVA = cerebrovascular accident (stroke); INR = international normalized ratio.

bolus. Intracranial hemorrhage (ICH) is the most catastrophic risk of these drugs. Fresh frozen plasma (FFP) and cryoprecipitate are both needed to reverse the effects of fibrinbolytics.

• Primary (rescue) angioplasty can be used to open a vessel in place of fibrinolytics or if fibrinbolytics are not effective. There is a lower incidence of reinfarction, ischemia, and bleeding.[5] Complications include coronary artery dissection, platelet deposition, thrombus formation, and plaque hemorrhage.[6]

• Angioplasty reduces complications compared to fibrinolytics when performed in centers with significant expertise.[7] Similar results can be obtained in community settings after formalized training and program development.[8]

• Aspirin (ASA) alone reduces mortality by 23%, and should be given to patients with ACS.

• Clopidogrel + ASA is superior to ASA alone in reducing death, AMI, and stroke in patients with unstable angina/non-ST-elevation myocardial infarction (UA/NSTEMI).[9] It is recommended in patients with ASA allergy, and in UA/NSTEMI patients for whom noninvasive management or PCI is planned. Because of increased bleeding risk, it should be withheld 5 days prior to coronary artery bypass grafting (CABG).

• NTG will dilate coronary vessels to enhance oxygen delivery. The sublingual route (SL) is appropriate for patients with UA/NSTEMI. If not responsive after three SL doses 3 to 5 minutes apart, IV NTG can be titrated to blood pressure reduction rather than pain resolution. IV NTG is used for recurrent ischemia and AMI.

- Unfractionated heparin (UFH) is a potent anticoagulant that complexes with antithrombin III, inactivates thrombin, and prevents clot propagation. Dosing is based on weight, and efficacy is unpredictable. Heparin increases the risk of bleeding.
- Low molecular weight heparins have a reliable anticoagulant effect and can be given as a fixed dose. Enoxaparin is preferable to UFH for patients with UA/NSTEMI if CABG is not planned within 24 hours.
- β-Blockers lower myocardial O_2 demand and should be started in patients with UA/NSTEMI and within 12 hours of STEMI, when not contraindicated. Relative contraindications to the use of β-blockers are heart rate <60 bpm, systolic BP <100 mm Hg, moderate to severe CHF, signs of peripheral hypoperfusion, PR interval longer than 0.24 seconds, second- or third-degree atrioventricular block (AVB), severe chronic obstructive pulmonary disease (COPD), history of asthma, severe DM, and severe peripheral vascular disease. There is a sustained reduction in mortality with use of β-blockers compared with its absence.
- Glycoprotein IIb/IIIa inhibitors stop platelet aggregation and are effective for stabilization of ACS and in conjunction with PCI. In refractory angina and NSTEMI, glycoprotein IIb/IIIa inhibitors have been shown to reduce death, AMI, and refractory ischemia in the short term. The greatest benefit from glycoprotein IIb/IIIa inhibitors is for patients undergoing PCI.[10]
- Morphine reduces the pain of angina/MI as well as reducing preload.
- Calcium channel blockers have antianginal, vasodilatory, and antihypertensive properties, but have not been shown to reduce the mortality rate after MI.[3,11]
- All patients with ACS/AMI should be admitted to an intensive care setting and be evaluated by a cardiologist in an expeditious manner.

REFERENCES

1. Braunwald E, Mark DB, Jones RH, et al: Unstable Angina: Diagnosis and Management. Clinical Practice Guideline No. 10 (amended). AHCPR Publication No. 94-0602. Rockville, MD: Agency for Health Care Policy and Research and the National Heart, Lung, and Blood Institute, Public Health Service, U.S. Department of Health and Human Services, 1994.
2. Jayes RL, Beshansky JR, D'Agostino RB, Selker HP: Do patients' coronary risk factor reports predict acute cardiac ischemia in the emergency department? A multicenter study. *J Clin Epidemiology* 45:621, 1992.
3. Ryan TJ, Anderson JL, Antman EM, et al: ACC/AHA guidelines for the management of patients with acute myocardial infarction: A report of the American College of Cardiology/American Heart Association Task Force on Practice Guidelines (Committee on Management of Acute Myocardial Infarction). *J Am Coll Cardiol* 28:1328, 1996.
4. GUSTO Investigators: An international randomized trial comparing four thrombolytic strategies for acute myocardial infarction. *N Engl J Med* 329:673, 1993.
5. Grines CL, Browne KF, Marco J, et al: A comparison of immediate angioplasty with thrombolytic therapy for acute myocardial infarction. *N Engl J Med* 328:673, 1993.
6. Bittl JA: Advances in coronary angioplasty. *N Engl J Med* 335:1290, 1996.
7. Grines CL, Westerhausen Jr DR, Grines LL, et al: A randomized trial of transfer for primary angioplasty versus on-site thrombolysis in patients with high-risk myocardial infarction: The Air Primary Angioplasty in Myocardial Infarction study. *J Am Coll Cardiol* 39:1713, 2002.
8. Aversano T, Aversano LT, Passmani E, et al: Thrombolytic therapy vs primary percutaneous coronary intervention for myocardial infarction in patients presenting to hospitals without on-site cardiac surgery. *JAMA* 287:1943, 2002.
9. Yysyf S, Zhao F, Metha SR, et al: Effects of clopidogrel in addition to aspirin in patients with acute coronary syndromes without ST-segment elevation. *N Engl J Med* 345:494, 2001.
10. Platelet Receptor Inhibition in Ischemic Syndrome Management (PRISM) Study Investigators: A comparison of aspirin plus tirofiban with aspirin plus heparin for unstable angina. *N Engl J Med* 338:1498, 1998.
11. Hennekins CH, Albert CM, Godfried SL, et al: Adjunctive drug therapy of acute myocardial infarction: Evidence from clinical trials. *N Engl J Med* 335:1660, 1996.

For further reading in *Emergency Medicine: A Comprehensive Study Guide,* 6th ed., see Chap. 50, "Acute Coronary Syndromes: Acute Myocardial Ischemia and Unstable Angina," by Judd E. Hollander; and Chap. 51, "Intervention Strategies for Acute Coronary Syndromes," by Judd E. Hollander and Deborah B. Diercks.

24 SYNCOPE
Michael G. Mikhail

EPIDEMIOLOGY

- The elderly have the highest incidence of syncope, which accounts for 3% of ED visits each year.[1]
- Fifty percent of all patients will never have a definite etiology established.

PATHOPHYSIOLOGY

- The final common pathway of syncope is lack of vital nutrient delivery to the brainstem reticular activating system, leading to loss of consciousness and postural tone.

- The most common causes of syncope are vasovagal reflex, cardiac dysrhythmia, and orthostatic hypotension.[2,3]
- In the Framingham Heart Study 7814 patients were followed for 17 years and 822 reported syncope at one or more times (10.5%). The causes were vasovagal (21%), cardiac (10%), orthostatic (9%), and unknown (37%).[4]
- An inciting event causes a drop in cardiac output, which decreases oxygen and substrate delivery to the brain. The reclined posture and the response of autonomic autoregulation centers re-establish cerebral perfusion, leading to a spontaneous return of consciousness.
- In patients with reflex-mediated syncope, a stimulus produces an abnormal autonomic response, an increase in vagal tone. Hypotension with or without bradycardia ensues. Less commonly, the stimulus leads directly to vagal hyperactivity.

CLINICAL FEATURES

- The most common cause of syncope is reflex mediated, which leads to pronounced vagal tone with hypotension and/or bradycardia.
- The hallmark of vasovagal syncope is the prodrome of dizziness, nausea, diminished vision, pallor, and diaphoresis. This diagnosis requires an appropriate stimulus in combination with standing.
- Carotid sinus hypersensitivity, a form of reflex-mediated syncope that results in asystole greater than 3 seconds and/or hypotension, is more common in men, the elderly, and among those with ischemic heart disease. Only 25% of those patients who have some symptoms with carotid sinus stimulation actually have syncope.[2]
- Orthostatic syncope results from a sudden change in posture after prolonged recumbence, and the inability to mount an adequate increase in heart rate and/or peripheral vascular resistance.
- Cardiac syncope is due to dysrhythmia or structural heart disease. Syncope from dysrhythmia is usually sudden, with a brief prodrome of only seconds. Structural heart disease is usually unmasked as syncope during exertion or vasodilation. In the elderly this is most commonly due to aortic stenosis. In the young it is most commonly hypertrophic cardiomyopathy.
- A bradydysrhythmia is more likely to be an incidental finding on electrocardiogram (ECG) than an actual cause of syncope.
- Ten percent of patients with pulmonary embolism will present with syncope.[5]

- Hyperventilation has been used as a provocative maneuver in diagnosing panic disorders, and can lead to hypocarbia, cerebral vasoconstriction, and subsequent syncope.[6,7]
- In general, a patient with syncope and a psychiatric disorder is likely to be young, with repeated episodes of syncope, multiple prodromal symptoms, and generally a positive review of systems.[8]
- Less common causes of syncope include cerebrovascular disorders, subarachnoid hemorrhage, and subclavian steal syndrome.
- Multiple medications, such as β-blockers, calcium channel antagonists, and diuretics are frequent causes of syncope, especially in the elderly. The most commonly implicated medications include antihypertensives and antidepressants.[9]

DIAGNOSIS AND DIFFERENTIAL

- The most important tools in the work-up of syncope are a good history, physical examination, and ECG.
- The history is aimed at identifying any high-risk features, including age, history of structural heart disease, and prodromal events. Syncope without warning suggests a dysrhythmia; exertional syncope suggests outflow obstruction.
- The cardiac exam may uncover a murmur that would represent aortic stenosis or hypertrophic cardiomyopathy.
- An ECG may identify evidence of previous silent myocardial infarction, prolonged QT, or evidence of Wolff-Parkinson-White (WPW) syndrome.
- Selective laboratory testing of a hematocrit, pregnancy test, or electrolytes and glucose may reveal the etiology of syncope.
- Seizure is the most common disorder mistaken for syncope, which should be distinguished by the postictal phase.

EMERGENCY DEPARTMENT CARE AND DISPOSITION

- The main goal of ED care is to identify those patients at risk for further medical problems. With a thorough history, physical exam, and ECG, patients can be divided into three categories.
- If the diagnosis is established, then patients can be managed for the underlying cause. If the diagnosis is not established, then patients can be stratified as high-risk or non-high-risk. Features suggesting high risk for sudden cardiac death are age >45, abnormal ECG, history of ventricular arrhythmia, and conges-

tive heart failure.[10] Admission is directed at determining a possible structural or electrical cause of cardiac syncope.

- Non-high risk patients are unlikely to have a cardiac etiology and therefore are appropriate for outpatient follow-up.[11,12]
- Worrisome or recurrent cases may benefit from further outpatient work-up including 24-hour ambulatory or event monitoring and tilt testing.
- Patients should also be advised not to drive, work at heights, or place themselves in danger in the event of another syncopal episode.

REFERENCES

1. Kapoor WN: Syncope in older persons. *J Am Geriatr Soc* 42:426, 1994.
2. Sarasin FP, Louis-Simonet M, Carballo D, et al: Prospective evaluation of patients with syncope: A population based study. *Am J Med* 111:177, 2001.
3. Linzer M, Yang EH, Estes NA III, et al: Diagnosing syncope. Part 1: Value of history, physical examination and electrocardiography. The clinical efficacy assessment project of the American College of Physicians. *Ann Intern Med* 126:989, 1997.
4. Soteriades ES, Evans JC, Larson MG, et al: Incidence and prognosis of syncope. *N Engl J Med* 347:879, 2002.
5. Thames MD, Alpert JS, Dalen JE: Syncope in patients with pulmonary embolism. *JAMA* 238:2509, 1977.
6. Koenig D, Pontinen M, Divine GW: Syncope in young adults: evidence for a combined medical and psychiatric approach. *J Intern Med* 232:169, 1992.
7. Naschiz JE, Gattini L, Mazov I, et al: The capnography-tilt test for the diagnosis of hyperventilation syncope. *QJM* 90:139, 1997.
8. Kapoor WN, Fortunato M, Hanusa BH, et al : Psychiatric illness in patients with syncope. *Am J Med* 99:505, 1995.
9. Hanlon JH, Linzer M, MacMillan JP, et al: Syncope and presyncope associated with probable adverse drug reaction. *Arch Intern Med* 150:2309, 1990.
10. Martin TP, Hanusa BH, Kapoor WN: Risk stratification of patients with syncope. *Ann Emerg Med* 29:4, 1997.
11. Eagle KA, Black HR, Cook EF, et al: Evaluation of prognostic classifications for patients with syncope. *Am J Med* 79: 455, 1985.
12. Martin GJ, Adams SL, Martin HG, et al: Prospective evaluation of syncope. *Ann Emerg Med* 13:499, 1984.

For further reading in *Emergency Medicine: A Comprehensive Study Guide*, 6th ed., see Chap. 52, "Syncope," by Barbara K. Blok and Tina M. Newman.

25 CONGESTIVE HEART FAILURE AND ACUTE PULMONARY EDEMA

Chadwick Miller

EPIDEMIOLOGY

- Heart failure is the leading cause of hospitalization among those older than 65 years[1] and mortality rates are increasing. Only 50% of patients will survive 1 year after the development of pulmonary edema.

PATHOPHYSIOLOGY

- Three factors, preload, afterload, and contractility, determine ventricular stroke volume. Coupled with heart rate, stroke volume determines cardiac output.
- Low-output heart failure is due to an inherent problem in myocardial contraction.
- High-output heart failure occurs when functionally intact myocardium cannot meet excess systemic demands. The causes of high-output failure are relatively few and include anemia, thyrotoxicosis, large arteriovenous shunts, beriberi, and Paget's disease of the bone.
- Systolic dysfunction, defined as an ejection fraction of less than 40%, leads to afterload sensitivity and manifests as increased cardiac pressures with circulatory stress (eg, exercise).
- Diastolic dysfunction represents impaired ventricular relaxation with preserved ejection fraction and results in increased cardiac pressures with preload increases.
- The most common cause of right-sided failure is left-sided failure.
- Once heart failure has developed, several neurohormonal compensatory mechanisms occur. The reduction in cardiac output results in increased stimulation of the renin-angiotensin-aldosterone axis and secretion of antidiuretic hormone. The end result is enhanced sodium and water retention by the kidneys, which leads to fluid overload and the clinical manifestations of congestive heart failure (CHF). The increased adrenergic tone leads to arteriolar vasoconstriction, a significant rise in afterload, and finally, to increased cardiac work.
- See Table 25-1 for common causes of heart failure and pulmonary edema.
- Systolic dysfunction, defined as an ejection fraction less than 40%, is most commonly due to ischemic heart disease, but other causes may be considered. Mechanically, the ventricle has difficulty ejecting

TABLE 25-1   Common Causes of Heart Failure and Pulmonary Edema

Myocardial ischemia: Acute and chronic*

Valvular dysfunction
  Aortic valve disease
    Aortic stenosis
    Aortic insufficiency
      Aortic dissection
      Infectious endocarditis
  Mitral valve disease
    Mitral stenosis
    Mitral regurgitation
      Papillary muscle dysfunction or rupture
      Ruptured chordae tendineae
      Infectious endocarditis
    Prosthetic valve malfunction

Other causes of left ventricular outflow obstruction
  Supravalvular aortic stenosis
  Membranous subvalvular aortic stenosis

Cardiomyopathy*
  Hypertrophic cardiomyopathy
  Dilated†
  Restrictive

Acquired cardiomyopathy
  Toxic: Alcohol, cocaine, doxorubicin
  Metabolic: Thyrotoxicosis, myxedema

Myocarditis: Radiation, infection

Constrictive pericarditis

Cardiac tamponade

Systemic hypertension*

Miscellaneous
  Anemia
  Cardiac dysrhythmias*

*Seen in the ED with higher frequency.
†Includes idiopathic.

blood. Impaired contractility leads to increased intracardiac volumes and pressure and afterload sensitivity.

• In diastolic heart failure, contractile function is preserved and the ejection fraction is normal or elevated. The main pathology is impaired ventricular relaxation causing an abnormal relation between diastolic pressure and volume. This results in a left ventricle (LV) that has difficulty in receiving blood. Decreased LV compliance necessitates high atrial pressures to ensure adequate diastolic LV filling and results in preload sensitivity. Chronic hypertension and LV hypertrophy often lead to this condition.

CLINICAL FEATURES

• Acute pulmonary edema or congestion is the cardinal manifestation of left-sided heart failure, and patients usually present with severe respiratory distress, frothy pink or white sputum, moist pulmonary rales, and an S_3 or S_4. Patients frequently have tachycardia, cardiac dysrhythmias such as atrial fibrillation or premature ventricular contractions (PVCs), and are hypertensive.

• Symptoms of left-sided heart failure include dyspnea (especially with exertion), paroxysmal nocturnal dyspnea, orthopnea, nocturia, fatigue, and weakness.

• Patients with right-sided heart failure commonly have dependent edema of the extremities, and may have jugular venous distention, hepatic enlargement, and a hepatojugular reflex.

DIAGNOSIS AND DIFFERENTIAL

• The diagnosis of acute pulmonary edema is made with clinical findings and the chest x-ray.

• Chest x-ray may reveal vascular redistribution to the upper lung fields, cardiomegaly (cardiothoracic ratio grater than 0.6 on a posteroanterior [PA] film), Kerley B lines (short linear markings at the periphery of the lower lung fields), and pleural effusions.[2]

• The diagnosis of right-sided heart failure is made clinically, but if the cause is left-sided heart failure, the heart will be enlarged on chest x-ray.

• The ED diagnostic error rate is reported as 12%, equally divided between over- and underdiagnosis.[3] Errors occur because neither history nor physical examination are accurate for heart failure. Dyspnea has a sensitivity and specificity of about 50%, orthopnea has a specificity of 88% but with no better sensitivity, and rales have a predictive accuracy of only 70%. Edema is even worse as a heart failure indicator.

• Natriuretic peptides may help in the diagnosis of heart failure. B-type natriuretic peptide (BNP) levels <100 pg/mL yield a negative predictive value of 89 to 96%,[4,5] and suggest an alternative diagnosis; however, markedly elevated levels >250 pg/mL are strong evidence of heart failure. Intermediate values should prompt consideration of other confounding diagnoses and confirmatory testing.

• Differential diagnosis for acute pulmonary edema includes the common causes of acute respiratory distress: asthma, chronic obstructive pulmonary disease (COPD), pneumonia, pulmonary embolus, allergenic reactions, and other causes of respiratory failure.

EMERGENCY DEPARTMENT CARE AND DISPOSITION

• Administer 100% oxygen by face mask to achieve an oxygen saturation of 95% by pulse oximetry in cases of acute pulmonary edema.

• If hypoxia persists despite oxygen therapy, consider applying continuous positive airway pressure (CPAP) or biphasic positive airway pressure (BiPAP) via face mask.

- Immediate intubation is indicated for unconscious or visibly tiring patients.
- Administer nitroglycerin sublingually 0.4 mg (may be repeated up to every 1 to 5 minutes). If the patient does not respond, or the ECG shows ischemia, nitroglycerin may be given as an IV drip, 10 to 30 μg/min and titrate.
- Administer a potent intravenous diuretic such as furosemide 40 to 80 mg IV, or bumetanide, 0.5 to 1 mg IV. Electrolytes should be monitored, especially serum potassium.
- For patients with resistant hypertension, or those who are not responding well to nitroglycerin, nitroprusside may be used, starting at 2.5 μg/kg/min and titrated.
- Nesiritide antagonizes the renin-angiotensin-aldosterone axis and produces diuresis, preload reduction, afterload reduction, and coronary vasodilatation. This alternative to nitroglycerine is dosed with a 2 μg/kg bolus over 60 seconds and an IV drip of 0.01 μg/kg per minute, and may be used for acute decompensated heart failure without cardiogenic shock.
- For hypotensive patients or patients in need of additional inotropic support, begin dopamine at 5 to 10 μg/kg/min and titrate to a systolic BP of 90 to 100. Dobutamine can be given in combination with dopamine or as a single agent, provided the patient is not in severe circulatory shock. Start dobutamine at 2.5 μg/kg/min and titrate to the desired response.
- Consider thrombolytic agents for heart failure caused by myocardial infarction.
- Treat coexisting dysrhythmias (see Chap. 4) or electrolyte disturbances (see Chap. 6), avoiding those therapies that impair the inotropic state of the heart.
- Morphine can be given (2 to 5 mg IV) and repeated as needed. It may cause respiratory depression and adds little benefit beyond that of oxygen, diuretics, and nitrates; thus its use is controversial.
- Digoxin acts too slowly to be of benefit in acute situations.
- For anuric (dialysis) patients, sorbitol and phlebotomy may have some benefit, but dialysis is the treatment of choice in these patients who prove resistant to nitrates.
- Long-term treatment of congestive heart failure includes dietary salt reduction, preload reduction via chronic use of diuretics (eg, furosemide) and afterload reduction via β-blockers (eg, metoprolol), angiotensin-converting enzyme (ACE) inhibitors (eg, captopril), and digoxin.
- Most patients with heart failure require inpatient management. Candidates for outpatient management include those with mild symptoms due to a clearly correctable precipitant that have resolved. These patients must have a normal diagnostic evaluation and a strong social network.

REFERENCES

1. Masie BM, Shah NB: Evolving trends in epidemiologic factors of heart failure: Rationale for preventative strategies and comprehensive disease management. *Am Heart J* 133:703, 1997.
2. Chait A, Cohen HE, Meltzer LE, et al: The bedside chest radiograph in the evaluation of incipient heart failure. *Radiology* 105:563, 1972.
3. Remes J, Miettinen H, Reunanen A, et al: Validity of clinical diagnosis of heart failure in primary health care. *Eur Heart J* 12:15, 1991.
4. Peacock WF: The B-type natriuretic peptide assay: A rapid test for heart failure. *Cleve Clin J Med* 69:243, 2002.
5. Maisel AS, Krishnaswamy P, Nowak RM, et al: Rapid measurement of B-type natriuretic peptide in the emergency diagnosis of heart failure. *N Engl J Med* 347:161, 2002.

For further reading in *Emergency Medicine: A Comprehensive Study Guide,* 6th ed., see Chap. 53, "Congestive Heart Failure and Acute Pulmonary Edema," by W. Frank Peacock IV.

26 VALVULAR HEART DISEASE
David M. Cline

- Ninety percent of valvular disease is chronic, with decades between the onset of the structural abnormality and onset of symptoms.
- Through chronic adaptation by dilation and hypertrophy, cardiac function can be preserved for years, which may delay the diagnosis for 1 to 2 decades until a murmur is detected on auscultation.
- The four heart valves prevent retrograde flow of blood during the cardiac cycle, allowing efficient ejection of blood with each contraction of the ventricles. The mitral valve has two cusps, while the other three heart valves normally have three cusps. The right and left papillary muscles promote effective closure of the tricuspid and mitral valves, respectively.
- Compared to the general population, patients with hemodynamically significant valvular heart disease have a 2.5-fold increased rate of death and a 3.2-fold increased rate of stroke.[1]

MITRAL STENOSIS

EPIDEMIOLOGY

- Despite its declining frequency, rheumatic heart disease is still the most common cause of mitral valve stenosis.

PATHOPHYSIOLOGY

- The majority of patients eventually develop atrial fibrillation because of progressive dilation of the atria.
- Although the valvular obstruction is slowly progressive, acute symptoms are produced when the obstruction prevents an increase in cardiac output to meet an increased need, such as during exercise.

CLINICAL FEATURES

- As with all valvular diseases, exertional dyspnea is the most common presenting symptom (seen in 80% of patients with mitral stenosis).
- In the past, hemoptysis was the second most common presenting symptom, but is less common now with earlier recognition and treatment.
- Systemic emboli may occur and result in myocardial, kidney, central nervous system, or peripheral infarction.
- The classic murmur of mitral stenosis and associated signs are listed in Table 26-1.

DIAGNOSIS AND DIFFERENTIAL

- The electrocardiogram (ECG) may demonstrate notched or diphasic P waves and right axis deviation.
- On the chest radiograph, straightening of the left heart border, indicating left atrial enlargement, is a typical early radiographic finding. Eventually, findings of pulmonary congestion are noted: redistribution of flow to the upper lung fields, Kerley B lines, and an increase in vascular markings.
- The diagnosis of mitral stenosis should be confirmed with echocardiography and/or consultation with a cardiologist. The urgency for an accurate diagnosis and appropriate referral depends on the severity of symptoms.

EMERGENCY DEPARTMENT CARE AND DISPOSITION

- The medical management of mitral stenosis includes intermittent diuretics, such as furosemide 40 mg IV, to alleviate pulmonary congestion; the treatment of atrial fibrillation (see Chap. 4); and anticoagulation for patients at risk for arterial embolic events.
- Patients with mitral stenosis and paroxysmal or chronic atrial fibrillation or a history of an embolic event should be on long-term warfarin therapy with an international normalized ratio (INR) goal of 2 to 3.[2]
- Frank hemoptysis may occur in the setting of mitral stenosis and pulmonary hypertension.
- Bleeding may be severe enough to require blood transfusion, consultation with a thoracic surgeon, and emergency surgery.

MITRAL INCOMPETENCE

EPIDEMIOLOGY

- Infective endocarditis or myocardial infarction can cause acute rupture of the chordae tendineae or papillary muscles or cause perforation of the valve leaflets.

TABLE 26-1   Comparison of Heart Murmurs, Sounds, and Signs

VALVE DISORDER	MURMUR	HEART SOUNDS AND SIGNS
Mitral stenosis	Mid-diastolic rumble, crescendos into S_2	Loud snapping S_1, apical impulse is small and tapping due to underfilled ventricle
Mitral regurgitation	Acute: harsh apical systolic murmur that starts with S_1, and may end before S_2 Chronic: high-pitched apical holosystolic murmur that radiates into S_2	S_3 and S_4 may be heard
Mitral valve prolapse	Click may be followed by a late systolic murmur that crescendos into S_2	Mid-systolic click; S_2 may be diminished by the late systolic murmur
Aortic stenosis	Harsh systolic ejection murmur	Paradoxic splitting of S_2, S_3, and S_4 may be present, pulse of small amplitude; pulse has a slow rise and sustained peak
Aortic regurgitation	High-pitched blowing diastolic murmur immediately after S_2	S_3 may be present; wide pulse pressure

- Inferior myocardial infarction due to right coronary occlusion is the most common cause of ischemic mitral valve incompetence.
- Although an association between appetite suppressant drugs (fenfluramine and phentermine, or dexfenfluramine alone) and aortic regurgitation has generally been accepted,[3,4] the suspected association of mitral incompetence with the appetite suppressant drugs remains unclear.[5]

PATHOPHYSIOLOGY

- Acute regurgitation into a noncompliant left atrium quickly elevates pressures and causes pulmonary edema. In contrast, in the chronic state the left atrium dilates so that left atrial pressure increases little, even with a large regurgitant flow.

CLINICAL FEATURES

- Acute mitral incompetence presents with dyspnea, tachycardia, and pulmonary edema. Patients may quickly deteriorate to cardiogenic shock or cardiac arrest.
- Intermittent mitral incompetence usually presents with acute episodes of respiratory distress due to pulmonary edema and can be asymptomatic between attacks.
- Chronic mitral incompetence may be tolerated for years or even decades. The first symptom is usually exertional dyspnea, sometimes prompted by atrial fibrillation. If patients are not anticoagulated, systemic emboli occur in 20% and are often asymptomatic.
- The classic murmur and signs of mitral incompetence are listed in Table 26-1.

DIAGNOSIS AND DIFFERENTIAL

- In acute rupture, the ECG may show evidence of acute inferior wall infarction (more common than anterior wall infarction in this setting).
- On the chest radiograph, acute mitral incompetence from papillary muscle rupture may result in a minimally enlarged left atrium and pulmonary edema, with less cardiac enlargement than expected.
- In chronic disease, the ECG may demonstrate findings of left atrial and left ventricular hypertrophy (LVH). On chest radiography, chronic mitral incompetence produces left ventricular and atrial enlargement that is proportional to the severity of the regurgitant volume.
- Echocardiography is essential to make the diagnosis with certainty and bedside technique may be manda-

tory in the acutely ill patient. However, transthoracic echocardiography may underestimate lesion severity, and transesophageal technique should be undertaken as soon as the patient is adequately stable to leave the department. In stable patients, echocardiography can be scheduled electively.

EMERGENCY DEPARTMENT CARE AND DISPOSITION

- Pulmonary edema should be treated initially with oxygen, intubation for failing respiratory effort, diuretics, and nitrates as the patient tolerates.
- Nitroprusside increases forward output by increasing aortic flow and partially restoring mitral valve competence as left ventricular size diminishes. Start nitroprusside at 5 μg/kg/min IV unless the patient is hypotensive.
- There may be a subset of patients whose mitral regurgitation is worsened by nitroprusside (those patients who respond with dilation of the regurgitant orifice),[6] so careful monitoring is essential.
- Hypotensive patients should receive inotropic agents such as dobutamine 2.5 to 20 μg/kg/min in addition to nitroprusside.
- Aortic balloon counterpulsation increases forward flow and mean arterial pressure while diminishing regurgitant volume and left ventricular filling pressure, and can be used to stabilize a patient while awaiting surgery.
- Emergency surgery should be considered in cases of acute mitral valve rupture.

MITRAL VALVE PROLAPSE

EPIDEMIOLOGY

- Mitral valve prolapse (MVP) is the most common valvular heart disease in industrialized countries, affecting about 2.4% of the population.[7]
- Population studies comparing patients with mitral valve prolapse to those without the disorder have found no increased risk of atrial fibrillation, syncope, stroke, or sudden death.[7,8]

PATHOPHYSIOLOGY

- The etiology of MVP, or the click-murmur syndrome, is not known but may be congenital.
- Male sex, age over 45, and the presence of regurgitation, recognized clinically by a short systolic murmur, places the patient in a higher risk group for complications.[9]

CLINICAL FEATURES

- Most patients are asymptomatic. Symptoms include atypical chest pain, palpitations, and fatigue and dyspnea unrelated to exertion.
- The abnormal heart sounds are listed in Table 26-1.
- In patients with MVP without mitral regurgitation at rest, exercise provokes mitral regurgitation in 32% of patients, and predicts a higher risk for morbid events.[10]

DIAGNOSIS AND DIFFERENTIAL

- Echocardiography is recommended to confirm the clinical diagnosis of mitral valve prolapse and to identify any associated mitral regurgitation. Echocardiography and/or consultation with a cardiologist can be performed on an outpatient basis.

EMERGENCY DEPARTMENT CARE AND DISPOSITION

- Initiating treatment for mitral valve prolapse is rarely required for patients seen in the ED. Patients with palpitations, chest pain, or anxiety frequently respond to β-blockers, such as atenolol 25 mg qd. Avoiding alcohol, tobacco, and caffeine may also relieve symptoms.

AORTIC STENOSIS

EPIDEMIOLOGY

- Degenerative heart disease or calcific aortic stenosis, is the most common cause of aortic stenosis in adults residing in the United States.
- Congenital heart disease is the most common cause of aortic stenosis in young adults, with the presence of a bicuspid valve accounting for 50% of cases. Rheumatic heart disease is the third most common cause in the United States, but remains the most common cause worldwide.

PATHOPHYSIOLOGY

- Blood flow into the aorta is obstructed, producing progressive LVH and low cardiac output.

CLINICAL FEATURES

- The classic triad is dyspnea, chest pain, and syncope.
- Dyspnea is usually the first symptom, followed by paroxysmal nocturnal dyspnea, syncope on exertion, angina, and myocardial infarction.

- The classic murmur and associated signs of aortic stenosis are listed in Table 26-1.
- Blood pressure is normal or low, with a narrow pulse pressure.
- Brachioradial delay is an important finding in aortic stenosis.[11] The examiner simultaneously palpates the right brachial artery of the patient with the thumb and the right radial artery of the patient with the middle or index finger. Any palpable delay between the brachial artery and radial artery is considered abnormal.[11]

DIAGNOSIS AND DIFFERENTIAL

- The ECG usually demonstrates criteria for LVH and, in 10% of patients, left or right bundle-branch block.
- The chest radiograph is normal early, but eventually LVH and findings of congestive heart failure are evident if the patient does not have valve replacement.
- Echocardiography should be undertaken to confirm the suspected diagnosis of aortic stenosis in the hospital if the murmur is associated with syncope.

EMERGENCY DEPARTMENT CARE AND DISPOSITION

- Patients presenting with pulmonary edema can be treated with oxygen and diuretics, but nitrates should be used with caution as reducing preload may cause significant hypotension. Nitroprusside is not well tolerated in patients with aortic stenosis.
- New-onset atrial fibrillation may severely compromise cardiac output and therefore require anticoagulation with heparin and cardioversion.
- Patients with profound symptoms secondary to aortic stenosis such as syncope are usually admitted to the hospital.

AORTIC INCOMPETENCE

EPIDEMIOLOGY

- In 20% of patients, the cause of aortic incompetence is acute in nature. Infective endocarditis accounts for the majority of acute cases; aortic dissection at the aortic root causes the remainder. Calcific degeneration, congenital disease (most notably bicuspid valves), systemic hypertension, myxomatous proliferation, and rheumatic heart disease cause the majority of chronic cases.
- Marfan syndrome, syphilis, ankylosing spondylitis, Ehlers-Danlos syndrome, and Reiter syndrome are less frequent causes.

• An association between the appetite suppressant drugs (fenfluramine and phentermine or dexfenfluramine alone) has been found for aortic incompetence.[3–5]

PATHOPHYSIOLOGY

• In acute cases, a sudden increase in backflow of blood into the ventricle raises left ventricular end-diastolic pressure, which may cause acute heart failure.
• In chronic disease, the ventricle progressively dilates to accommodate the regurgitant blood volume. Wide pulse pressures result from the fall in diastolic pressure, and marked peripheral vasodilatation is seen.

CLINICAL FEATURES

• In acute disease, dyspnea is the most common presenting symptom, seen in 50% of patients. Many patients have acute pulmonary edema with pink frothy sputum. Patients may complain of fever and chills if endocarditis is the cause.
• Dissection of the ascending aorta typically produces a "tearing" chest pain that may radiate between the shoulder blades.
• The classic murmur and signs of aortic incompetence are listed in Table 26-1.
• In the chronic state, about one third of patients will have palpitations associated with a large stroke volume and/or premature ventricular contractions. Frequently these sensations are noticed in bed.
• In the chronic state, signs include a wide pulse pressure with a prominent ventricular impulse, which may be manifested as head bobbing.
• "Water hammer pulse" may be noted; this is a peripheral pulse that has a quick rise in upstroke followed by a peripheral collapse.
• Other classic findings may include accentuated precordial apical thrust, pulsus bisferiens, Duroziez sign (a to-and-fro femoral murmur), and Quincke pulse (capillary pulsations visible at the proximal nail bed, while pressure is applied at the tip).

DIAGNOSIS AND DIFFERENTIAL

• ECG changes may be seen with aortic dissection, including ischemia or findings of acute inferior myocardial infarction, suggesting involvement of the right coronary artery.
• In patients with acute regurgitation, the chest radiograph demonstrates acute pulmonary edema with less cardiac enlargement than expected.
• In chronic aortic incompetence, the ECG demonstrates LVH, and the chest radiograph shows LVH, aortic dilation, and possibly evidence of congestive heart failure.
• Echocardiography is essential for confirming the presence of and evaluating the severity of valvular regurgitation. Bedside transthoracic echocardiography should be undertaken in the unstable patient potentially in need of emergency surgery. Transesophageal echocardiography is recommended when aortic dissection is suspected, but may not be possible in acutely unstable patients.

EMERGENCY DEPARTMENT CARE AND DISPOSITION

• Pulmonary edema should be treated initially with oxygen and intubation for failing respiratory effort. Diuretics and nitrates can be used, but cannot be expected to be effective.
• Nitroprusside (start at 5 μg/kg/min) along with inotropic agents such as dobutamine (start at 2.5 μg/kg/min) or dopamine can be used to augment forward flow and reduce left ventricular end-diastolic pressure in an attempt to stabilize a patient prior to emergency surgery.
• Intra-aortic balloon counterpulsation is contraindicated.
• Although β-blockers are often used in treating aortic dissection, these drugs should be used with great caution, if at all, in the setting of acute aortic valve rupture because they will block the compensatory tachycardia.
• Emergency surgery may be life-saving.
• Chronic aortic regurgitation is typically treated with vasodilators such as angiotensin-converting enzyme (ACE) inhibitors or nifedipine (initiated by a patient's private physician).

PROSTHETIC VALVE DISEASE

EPIDEMIOLOGY

• Prosthetic valves are implanted in 40,000 patients per year in the United States. There are approximately 80 types of artificial valves, each with advantages and disadvantages. Patients who receive prosthetic valves are instructed to carry a descriptive card in their wallet.
• Patients with artificial valves develop endocarditis at a rate of 0.5% per year. Infections occur more frequently during the first 2 months after operation. The most common organisms during this period are *Staphylococcus epidermidis* and *S. aureus*. Gram-negative organisms and fungi are also frequent causes of endocarditis during this early period.
• Bleeding and systemic embolism originating from a thrombus on the prosthetic valve are the most important

complications of mechanical heart valves, occurring at a rate of 1.4% and 1% per year, respectively, for patients on warfarin.[12]

PATHOPHYSIOLOGY

- Prosthetic valves tend to be slightly stenotic, and a very small amount of regurgitation is common because of incomplete closure.
- Patients with mechanical valves require continuous anticoagulation. Some bioprostheses do not require long-term anticoagulation, unless atrial fibrillation is coexistent.
- Thrombi can form on a prosthetic valve and become large enough to obstruct flow or prevent closure. The dysfunction due to thrombi can be acute or slowly progressive.
- Bioprostheses may gradually degenerate, undergoing gradual thinning, stiffening, and possible tearing, which result in valvular incompetence.
- The sutures that secure the prosthetic valve may become disrupted, leading to paravalvular regurgitation as a fistula forms at the periphery of the valve.
- Mechanical models may suddenly fracture or fail. These failures usually bring sudden symptoms and often are fatal before corrective surgery can be accomplished.

CLINICAL FEATURES

- Many patients have persistent dyspnea and reduced effort tolerance after successful valve replacement. This is more common in the presence of pre-existing heart dysfunction or atrial fibrillation.
- Large paravalvular leaks usually present with congestive heart failure. Patients with new neurologic symptoms may have thromboembolism associated with the valve thrombi or endocarditis.
- Patients with prosthetic valves usually have abnormal cardiac sounds. Mechanical valves have loud, metallic closing sounds.
- Systolic murmurs are commonly present with mechanical models. Loud diastolic murmurs are generally not present with mechanical valves.
- Patients with bioprostheses usually have normal S_1 and S_2, with no abnormal opening sounds.
- The aortic bioprostheses are usually associated with short midsystolic murmur.

DIAGNOSIS AND DIFFERENTIAL

- New or progressive dyspnea of any form, new onset or worsening of congestive heart failure, decreased

exercise tolerance, or a change in chest pain compatible with ischemia all suggest valvular dysfunction.
- Persistent fever in patients with prosthetic valves should be evaluated for possible endocarditis with blood cultures.
- Blood studies that may be helpful include a blood count with red blood cell indices and coagulation studies if the patient is on warfarin.
- Emergency echocardiographic studies should be requested if there is any question about valve dysfunction. Ultimately, echocardiography and/or cardiac catheterization may be required for diagnosis.

EMERGENCY DEPARTMENT CARE AND DISPOSITION

- It is critical that patients suspected of having acute prosthetic valvular dysfunction have immediate referral to a cardiac surgeon for possible emergency surgery.
- The intensity of anticoagulation therapy varies with each type of mechanical valve, but ranges from an INR goal of 2 to 3.5.[13]
- Acute prosthetic valvular dysfunction due to thrombotic obstruction has been successfully treated with thrombolytic therapy,[2] but the diagnosis generally requires consultation with a cardiologist. Lesser degrees of obstruction should be treated with optimization of anticoagulation.
- Disposition of patients with worsening symptoms can be problematic, and consultation with the patient's regular physician may be needed prior to consideration for discharge.

PROPHYLAXIS FOR INFECTIVE ENDOCARDITIS

- See Chap. 92 for recommendations on prophylaxis prior to procedures performed in the emergency department.

REFERENCES

1. Petty GW, Khandheria BK, Whisnant JP, et al: Predictors of cerebrovascular events and death among patients with valvular heart disease: A population based study. *Stroke* 31:2628, 2000.
2. Bonow RO, Carabello B, de Leon AC Jr, et al: ACC/AHA guidelines for the management of patients with valvular heart disease: a report of the American College of Cardiology/American Heart Association Task Force on Practice Guidelines (Committee on Management of Patients with Valvular Heart Disease). *J Am Coll Cardiol* 32:1486, 1998.

3. Jollis JG, Landolfo CK, Kisslo J, et al: Fenfluramine and phentermine and cardiovascular findings: Effect of treatment duration and prevalence of valve abnormalities. *Circulation* 101:2071, 2000.
4. Gardin JM, Schumacher D, Constantine G, et al: Valvular abnormalities and cardiovascular status following exposure to dexfenfluramine or phentermine/fenfluramine. *JAMA* 283:1703, 2000.
5. Jick H: Heart valve disorders and appetite suppressant drugs. *JAMA* 283:1738, 2000.
6. Kizilbash AM, Willett DL, Brickner ME, et al: Effects of afterload reduction on vena contracta width in mitral regurgitation. *J Am Coll Cardiol* 32:427, 1998.
7. Freed LA, Levy D, Levine RA, et al: Prevalence and clinical outcome of mitral-valve prolapse. *N Engl J Med* 341:1, 1999.
8. Gilon D, Buonanno FS, Joffe MM, et al: Lack of evidence of an association between mitral-valve prolapse and stroke in young patients. *N Engl J Med* 341:8, 1999.
9. Zuppiroli A, Rinaldi M, Kramer-Fox R, et al: Natural history of mitral valve prolapse. *J Am Cardiol* 75:1028, 1995.
10. Stoddard MF, Prince CR, Dillon S, et al: Exercise-induced mitral regurgitation is a predictor of morbid events in subjects with mitral valve prolapse. *J Am Coll Cardiol* 25:693, 1995.
11. Leach RM, McBrian DJ: Brachioradial delay: A new clinical indicator of the severity of aortic stenosis. *Lancet* 335:1199, 1990.
12. Cannegieter SC, Rosendaal FR, Briet E: Thromboembolic and bleeding complications in patients with mechanical heart valves. *Circulation* 89:635, 1994.
13. Salem DN, Levine HJ, Pauker SG, et al: Antithrombotic therapy in valvular heart disease. *Chest* 114:590S, 1998.

For further reading in *Emergency Medicine: A Comprehensive Study Guide,* 6th ed., see Chap. 54, "Valvular Emergencies," by David M. Cline.

27 THE CARDIOMYOPATHIES, MYOCARDITIS, AND PERICARDIAL DISEASE

N. Stuart Harris

THE CARDIOMYOPATHIES

- Cardiomyopathies are the third most common form of heart disease in the United States and are the second most common cause of sudden death in the adolescent population.[1] It is a disease process that directly affects the cardiac structure and impairs myocardial function.
- Four types are currently recognized: (1) dilated cardiomyopathy (DCM), (2) hypertrophied cardiomyopathy (IICM), (3) restrictive cardiomyopathy, and (4) dysrhythmic right ventricular cardiomyopathy.[2]

DILATED CARDIOMYOPATHY

PATHOPHYSIOLOGY

- Dilation and compensatory hypertrophy of the myocardium result in depressed systolic function and pump failure leading to low cardiac output.[3]
- Eighty % of cases of DCM are not associated with specific cardiac or systemic disorders and are considered idiopathic. Idiopathic DCM is the primary indication for cardiac transplant in the United States.
- Blacks and males have a 2.5-fold increased risk compared to whites and females. The most common age at the time of diagnosis is 20 to 50 years.[3]

CLINICAL FEATURES

- Systolic pump failure leads to signs and symptoms of congestive heart failure (CHF) including dyspnea on exertion, orthopnea, and paroxysmal nocturnal dyspnea.
- Chest pain due to limited coronary vascular reserve may also be present.
- Mural thrombi can form from diminished ventricular contractile force, and there may be signs of peripheral embolization (eg, acute neurologic deficit, flank pain, hematuria, or a pulseless, cyanotic extremity).
- Holosystolic regurgitant murmur of the tricuspid and mitral valve may be heard along the lower left sternal border or at the apex. Other findings include a summation gallop, an enlarged and pulsatile liver, bibasilar rales, and dependent edema.

DIAGNOSIS AND DIFFERENTIAL

- Chest x-ray usually shows an enlarged cardiac silhouette, biventricular enlargement, and pulmonary vascular congestion ("cephalization" of flow and enlarged hila).
- The electrocardiogram (ECG) shows left ventricular hypertrophy, left atrial enlargement, Q or QS waves, and poor R wave progression across the precordium. Atrial fibrillation and ventricular ectopy are frequently present.
- Echocardiography confirms the diagnosis and demonstrates ventricular enlargement, increased systolic and diastolic volumes, and a decreased ejection fraction.
- Differential diagnosis includes acute myocardial infarction, restrictive pericarditis, acute valvular

disruption, sepsis, or any other condition that results in a low cardiac output state.

EMERGENCY DEPARTMENT CARE AND DISPOSITION

- Patients with newly diagnosed, symptomatic DCM require admission to a monitored bed or intensive care unit.
- Intravenous diuretics (eg, furosemide 40 mg intravenously) and digoxin (maximum dose 0.5 mg intravenously) can be administered. These drugs have symptomatic benefit, but have not been shown to increase survival.
- Angiotensin-converting enzyme (ACE) inhibitors (eg, enalaprilat 1.25 mg intravenously every 6 hours) and β-blockers (eg, carvedilol 3.125 mg orally) can be administered. These drugs have been shown to improve survival in DCM with CHF.[4,5]
- Amiodarone (loaded 150 mg intravenously over 10 minutes, then 1 mg/min for 6 hours) for complex ventricular ectopy can be administered.[6]
- Anticoagulation should be considered to reduce mural thrombus formation.

HYPERTROPHIC CARDIOMYOPATHY

PATHOPHYSIOLOGY

- This illness is characterized by left ventricular and/or right ventricular hypertrophy that is usually asymmetrical and involves primarily the intraventricular septum without ventricular dilation.[7]
- The result is abnormal compliance of the left ventricle leading to impaired diastolic relaxation and diastolic filling. Cardiac output is usually normal.
- Fifty percent of cases are hereditary. Molecular genetics demonstrate that HCM is a heterogeneous disease of the sarcomere with many mutations, most commonly involving the beta-myosin heavy chain.
- The prevalence is 1 in 500; the mortality rate is 1%, but 4 to 6% in childhood and adolescence.

CLINICAL FEATURES

- Symptom severity progresses with age.
- Dyspnea on exertion is the most common symptom, followed by angina-like chest pain, palpitations, and syncope.[8]
- Patients may be aware of forceful ventricular contractions and call these palpitations.

- Physical examination may reveal a fourth heart sound (S_4), hyperdynamic apical impulse, a precordial lift, and a systolic ejection murmur best heard at the lower left sternal border or apex.
- The murmur may be increased with Valsalva maneuver or standing after squatting. The murmur can be decreased by squatting, forceful hand gripping, or passive leg elevation with the patient supine (see Chap. 26 for contrasting murmurs).

DIAGNOSIS AND DIFFERENTIAL

- The ECG demonstrates left ventricular hypertrophy in 30% of patients and left atrial enlargement in 25 to 50%. Large septal Q waves (greater than 0.3 mV) are present in 25%. Another ECG finding is upright T waves in those leads with QS or QR complexes (T-wave inversion in those leads would suggest ischemia).
- Chest x-ray is usually normal. Echocardiography is the diagnostic study of choice, and will demonstrate disproportionate septal hypertrophy.

EMERGENCY DEPARTMENT CARE AND DISPOSITION

- Symptoms of HCM may mimic ischemic heart disease and treatment of those symptoms is covered in Chap. 23. Otherwise, general supportive care is indicated. Patients who present complaining of exercise intolerance or chest pain in whom the typical murmur of HCM is heard should be referred for echocardiographic evaluation. β-Blockers are the mainstay of treatment for patients with HCM and chest pain.[8]
- Patients should be discouraged from engaging in vigorous exercise.[9] Those with suspected HCM who have syncope should be hospitalized.

RESTRICTIVE CARDIOMYOPATHY

- This is one of the least common cardiomyopathies. In this form of the disease the ventricular volume and wall thickness is normal, but there is decreased diastolic volume of both ventricles.
- Most causes are idiopathic, but systemic disorders have been implicated, such as amyloidosis, sarcoidosis, hemochromatosis, scleroderma, carcinoid, hypereosinophilic syndrome, and endomyocardial fibrosis.[10] The idiopathic form is sometimes familial.

CLINICAL FEATURES

- Symptoms of CHF predominate, including dyspnea, orthopnea, and pedal edema. Chest pain is uncommon.
- Physical exam may reveal an S_3 or S_4 cardiac gallop, pulmonary rales, jugular venous distension, Kussmaul's sign (inspiratory jugular venous distension), hepatomegaly, pedal edema, and ascites.

DIAGNOSIS AND DIFFERENTIAL

- The chest x-ray may show signs of CHF without cardiomegaly.
- Nonspecific ECG changes are most likely. However, in cases of amyloidosis or sarcoidosis, conduction disturbances and low-voltage QRS complexes are common.
- Differential diagnosis includes constrictive pericarditis and diastolic left ventricular dysfunction (most commonly due to ischemic or hypertensive heart disease). Differentiating between restrictive cardiomyopathy and constrictive pericarditis is critical, because constrictive pericarditis can be cured surgically.

EMERGENCY DEPARTMENT CARE AND DISPOSITION

- Treatment is symptom-directed with the use of diuretics and ACE inhibitors.
- Corticosteroid therapy is indicated for sarcoidosis. Chelation is used for the treatment of hemochromatosis.
- Admission is determined by the severity of the symptoms and the availability of prompt subspecialty follow-up.

DYSRHYTHMOGENIC RIGHT VENTRICULAR CARDIOMYOPATHY

- This is the most rare form of cardiomyopathy and is characterized by progressive replacement of the right ventricular myocardium with fibrofatty tissue. The left ventricle and septum are usually spared.
- The typical presentation is that of sudden death or ventricular dysrhythmia in a young or middle-aged patient. All these patients require extensive work-up and hospitalization.
- Physical exam is normal. ECG may show right bundle-branch pattern. The echocardiogram has the highest sensitivity and positive predictive value for the diagnosis.[11]

MYOCARDITIS

PATHOPHYSIOLOGY

- Inflammation of the myocardium may be the result of a systemic disorder or an infectious agent.
- Viral etiologies include coxsackie B, echovirus, influenza, parainfluenza, Epstein-Barr, and HIV.
- Bacterial causes include *Corynebacterium diphtheriae, Neisseria meningitidis, Mycoplasma pneumoniae,* and beta-hemolytic streptococci.[12]
- Pericarditis frequently accompanies myocarditis.

CLINICAL FEATURES

- Systemic signs and symptoms predominate, including fever, tachycardia out of proportion to the fever, myalgias, headache, and rigors.
- Chest pain due to coexisting pericarditis is frequently present.
- A pericardial friction rub may be heard in patients with concomitant pericarditis.
- In severe cases, there may be symptoms of progressive heart failure (CHF, pulmonary rales, pedal edema, etc).

DIAGNOSIS AND DIFFERENTIAL

- Nonspecific ECG changes, atrioventricular block, prolonged QRS duration, or ST-segment elevation (in the setting of associated pericarditis) are seen. Chest x-ray is normal.
- Cardiac enzymes may be elevated.[13]
- Differential diagnosis includes cardiac ischemia or infarction, valvular disease, and sepsis.

EMERGENCY DEPARTMENT CARE AND DISPOSITION

- Supportive care is the mainstay of treatment. If a bacterial cause is suspected, antibiotics are appropriate. Many patients have progressive CHF, therefore hospitalization in a monitored environment is usually indicated (see Chap. 25 for management of CHF).

ACUTE PERICARDITIS

PATHOPHYSIOLOGY

- The pericardium consists of a loose fibrous membrane (visceral pericardium) overlying the epicardium, and a

dense collagenous sac (parietal pericardium) surrounding the heart. The space between these layers may contain up to 50 mL of fluid under normal conditions. Intrapericardial pressure is usually subatmospheric.
- Inflammation of the pericardium may be the result of viral infection (eg, coxsackie virus, echovirus, HIV), bacterial infection (eg, *Staphylococcus, Streptococcus pneumoniae,* beta-hemolytic *Streptococcus, Mycobacterium tuberculosis*), fungal infection (eg, *Histoplasma capsulatum*), malignancy (leukemia, lymphoma, melanoma, metastatic breast cancer), drugs (procainamide and hydralazine), radiation, connective tissue disease, uremia, myxedema, postmyocardial infarction (Dressler's syndrome), or may be idiopathic.[14]

CLINICAL FEATURES

- The most common symptom is sudden or gradual onset of sharp or stabbing chest pain that radiates to the back, neck, left shoulder, or arm. Radiation to the left trapezial ridge (due to inflammation of the adjoining diaphragmatic pleura) is particularly distinguishing.
- The pain may be aggravated by movement or inspiration. Typically, chest pain is made most severe by lying supine and is often relieved by sitting up and leaning forward.
- Associated symptoms include low-grade intermittent fever, dyspnea, and dysphagia.
- A transient, intermittent friction rub heard best at the lower left sternal border or apex is the most common physical finding. This rub is characteristically transient (eg, heard one hour and not the next).

DIAGNOSIS AND DIFFERENTIAL

- ECG changes of acute pericarditis and its convalescence have been divided into four stages. During stage 1, or the acute phase, there is ST-segment elevation in leads I, V_5, and V_6, with PR-segment depression in leads II, aVF, and V_4 through V_6. As the disease resolves (stage 2), the ST segment normalizes and T-wave amplitude decreases. In stage 3, inverted T waves appear in leads previously showing ST elevations. The final phase, stage 4, is characterized by the resolution of repolarization abnormalities and a return to a normal ECG.
- When sequential ECGs are not available, it can be difficult to distinguish pericarditis from the normal variant with "early repolarization." In these cases, a simple criterion offers considerable diagnostic utility: an ST segment:T-wave amplitude ratio greater than 0.25 in leads I, V_5, or V_6 is indicative of acute pericarditis.[15]
- Pericarditis without other underlying cardiac disease does not typically produce dysrhythmias.

- Chest x-ray is usually normal, but should be done to rule out other disease. Echocardiography is the best diagnostic test.
- Other tests that may be of value in establishing etiologic diagnosis include complete blood cell count with differential, blood urea nitrogen and creatinine levels (to rule out uremia), streptococcal serology, appropriate viral serology, other serology (eg, antinuclear and anti-DNA antibodies), thyroid function studies, erythrocyte sedimentation rate, and creatinine kinase levels with isoenzymes (to assess for myocarditis).

EMERGENCY DEPARTMENT CARE AND DISPOSITION

- Patients with idiopathic or presumed viral etiologies are treated as outpatients with nonsteroidal anti-inflammatory agents (eg, ibuprofen 400 to 600 mg orally four times daily) for 1 to 3 weeks.
- Patients should be treated for a specific cause if one is identified. Any patient with myocarditis or hemodynamic compromise should be admitted into a monitored environment. Any patient with enlarged cardiac silhouette on chest x-ray should be admitted for early Doppler echocardiography.

NONTRAUMATIC CARDIAC TAMPONADE

PATHOPHYSIOLOGY

- Tamponade occurs when the pressure in the pericardial sac exceeds the normal filling pressure of the right ventricle, resulting in restricted filling and decreased cardiac output.
- Causes include metastatic malignancy, uremia, hemorrhage (over-anticoagulation), idiopathic disorders, bacterial or tubercular disorders, chronic pericarditis, and others (eg, systemic lupus erythematosus, postradiation, myxedema).[16]

CLINICAL FEATURES

- The most common complaints are dyspnea and decreased exercise tolerance. Other nonspecific symptoms include weight loss, pedal edema, and ascites.
- Physical findings include tachycardia, low systolic blood pressure, and a narrow pulse pressure. Pulsus paradoxus (apparent dropped beats in the peripheral pulse during inspiration), neck vein distension, distant heart sounds, and right upper quadrant pain (due to hepatic congestion) may also be present. Pulmonary rales are usually absent.

DIAGNOSIS AND DIFFERENTIAL

- Low-voltage QRS complexes and ST-segment elevation with PR-segment depression may be present on the ECG. Electrical alternans (beat-to-beat variability in the amplitude of the P and R waves unrelated to inspiratory cycle) is a classic but uncommon finding (about 20% of cases). Chest x-ray may or may not reveal an enlarged cardiac silhouette. Echocardiography is the diagnostic test of choice.

EMERGENCY DEPARTMENT CARE AND DISPOSITION

- An intravenous fluid bolus of 500 to 1000 mL of normal saline will facilitate right heart filling and may temporarily improve the hemodynamics.
- Pericardiocentesis is both therapeutic and diagnostic. These patients require admission to an intensive care unit or monitored setting.

CONSTRICTIVE PERICARDITIS

PATHOPHYSIOLOGY

- Constriction occurs when fibrous thickening and loss of elasticity of the pericardium results in interference with diastolic filling. Cardiac trauma, pericardiotomy (open-heart surgery), intrapericardial hemorrhage, fungal or bacterial pericarditis, and uremic pericarditis are the most common causes.

CLINICAL FEATURES

- Symptoms develop gradually and mimic those of restrictive cardiomyopathy, including CHF, exertional dyspnea, and decreased exercise tolerance. Chest pain, orthopnea, and paroxysmal nocturnal dyspnea are uncommon.
- On physical examination patients may have pedal edema, hepatomegaly, ascites, jugular venous distension, and Kussmaul's sign. A pericardial "knock" (an early diastolic sound) may be heard at the apex. There is usually no friction rub.

DIAGNOSIS AND DIFFERENTIAL

- The ECG is not usually helpful, but may show low-voltage QRS complexes and inverted T waves.
- Pericardial calcification is seen in up to 50% of patients on the lateral chest x-ray, but is not diagnostic of constrictive pericarditis.
- Doppler echocardiography, cardiac computed tomography, and magnetic resonance imaging are diagnostic.
- Other diseases that should be considered include acute pericarditis or myocarditis, exacerbation of chronic ventricular dysfunction, or a systemic process resulting in decreased cardiac performance (eg, sepsis).

EMERGENCY DEPARTMENT CARE AND DISPOSITION

- General supportive care is the initial treatment. Symptomatic patients will require hospitalization and pericardiectomy.

REFERENCES

1. Liberthson RR: Sudden death from cardiac causes in children and young adults. *N Engl J Med* 334:1039, 1996.
2. Richardson P, McKenna W, Bristow M, et al: Report of the 1995 World Health Organization/International Society and Federation of Cardiology Task Force on the definition and classification of cardiomyopathies. *Circulation* 93:841, 1996.
3. Felker GM, Hu W, Hare JM, et al: The spectrum of dilated cardiomyopathy. The Johns Hopkins experience with 1278 patients. *Medicine* 78:270, 1999.
4. Hunt SA, Baker DW, Chin MH, et al: ACC/AHA guidelines for the evaluation and management of chronic heart failure in the adult: a report of the American College of Cardiology/American Heart Association Task Force on Practice Guidelines (Committee to Revise the 1995 Guidelines for the Evaluation and Management of Heart Failure). *J Am Coll Cardiol* 38:2101, 2001.
5. Foody JM, Farrell MH, Krumholz HM: Beta-blocker therapy in heart failure. A scientific review. *JAMA* 287:883, 2002.
6. Heidenreich PA, Keeffe B, McDonald KM, et al: Overview of randomized trials of antiarrhythmic drugs and devices for the prevention of sudden cardiac death. *Am Heart J* 144:422, 2002.
7. Maron BJ: Hypertrophic cardiomyopathy. A systematic review. *JAMA* 287:1308, 2002.
8. Spirito P, Seidman CE, McKenna WJ, et al: The management of hypertrophic cardiomyopathy. *N Engl J Med* 336:775, 1997.
9. Maron BJ, Thompson PD, Puffer JC, et al: Cardiovascular preparticipation screening of competitive athletes: A statement for health professionals from the Sudden Death Committee (Clinical Cardiology) and Congenital Cardiac Defects Committee (Cardiovascular Disease in the Young). American Heart Association. *Circulation* 94:850, 1996.
10. Kushwaha SS, Fallon JT, Fuster V: Restrictive cardiomyopathy. *N Engl J Med* 336:267, 1997.
11. Fontaine G, Fountaliran F, Frank R: Arrhythmogenic right ventricular cardiomyopathies: Clinical forms and main differential diagnoses. *Circulation* 97:1532, 1998.

12. Lieberman EB, Hutchins GM, Hershowitz A, et al: Clinico-pathologic description of myocarditis. *J Am Coll Cardiol* 18: 1617, 1991.
13. Parrillo JE: Inflammatory cardiomyopathy (myocarditis). Which patients should be treated with anti-inflammatory therapy? *Circulation* 104:4, 2001.
14. Oakley CM: Myocarditis, pericarditis, and other pericardial diseases. *Heart* 84:449, 2000.
15. Ginzton LE, Laks MM: The differential diagnosis of acute pericarditis from the normal variant: New electrocardiographic criteria. *Circulation* 65:1004, 1982.
16. Spodick DH: Pathophysiology of cardiac tamponade. *Chest* 113:1372, 1998.

For further reading in *Emergency Medicine: A Comprehensive Study Guide,* 6th ed., see Chap. 55, "The Cardiomyopathies, Myocarditis, and Pericardial Disease," by James T. Niemann.

28 PULMONARY EMBOLISM

Christopher Kabrhel

EPIDEMIOLOGY

- Pulmonary embolism (PE) accounts for 1/1000 ED visits and an estimated 200,000 to 500,000 cases occur each year in the U.S. It is the third most common cause of cardiovascular death.
- Up to two thirds of all ED patients with PE go undetected.[1]
- Risk factors can be categorized according to the points of Virchow's triad: (1) Hypercoagulable states include malignancy (the most common risk factor) like adenocarcinomas and brain cancers. Nonmalignant states include estrogen use (the most common nonmalignant risk factor), pregnancy, antiphospholipid antibody syndromes, genetic mutations such as factor V Leiden, the prothrombin mutation, and protein C or S deficiency.[2,3] (2) Venous stasis states include immobility secondary to recent trauma, surgery, paralysis, or debilitating illness. (3) Endothelial injury may be a result of trauma, surgery, vascular access, indwelling catheters, or prior deep venous thrombosis (DVT).

PATHOPHYSIOLOGY

- The pathophysiologic effects are the result of mechanical obstruction of right ventricular outflow and the release of inflammatory mediators from thrombus lodged in the pulmonary vasculature.

- The mechanism of the dyspnea and hypoxia is unclear. It is likely related to the V/Q mismatch caused by vasoactive mediators combined with the relative shunting of blood away from oxygenated alveoli.

CLINICAL FEATURES

- Common symptoms include dyspnea (the most common symptom, seen in 90% of PE patients), pleuritic chest pain (the second most common symptom, absent in one third of PE patients), nonpleuritic chest pain (epigastric or substernal and related to right ventricle [RV] subendocardial ischemia), anxiety, cough, and syncope.
- Common signs include hypoxemia (defined as SaO_2 <95% or PaO_2 <80% on room air), tachypnea, tachycardia (which may be absent in up to one half of PE patients), hemoptysis, diaphoresis, fever, and signs of DVT.
- Clinical signs of DVT occur in about 50% of patients, but it may be demonstrated venographically in up to 80% of patients with PE.[4]
- Massive PE can result in hypotension and severe hypoxia. Cardiac arrest occurs in about 2% of PE and usually presents as pulseless electrical activity from massive PE.[5]
- PE frequently presents atypically and may present without any symptoms or signs.

DIAGNOSIS AND DIFFERENTIAL

PRETEST PROBABILITY OF PULMONARY EMBOLISM

- The patient's pretest probability of PE guides the clinician's choice of diagnostic testing and helps determine when to terminate ancillary testing. The importance of determining the pretest probability should not be underestimated.
- Pretest probability can be subjectively determined by the clinician, though accuracy requires clinical experience.[6] Alternatively, clinical score systems and decision rules that incorporate symptoms, signs, and risk factors can categorize patients into large groups of low, intermediate, or high probability (Table 28-1).[7,8,9]

ANCILLARY TESTING

- Selective pulmonary angiography with cine angiofluoroscopy to evaluate for a filling defect in the pulmonary vasculature is the gold standard test for the diagnosis of PE. However, the test is invasive, has a

TABLE 28-1   Factors That Help Distinguish the Presence or Absence of an Outcome Diagnosis of PE in Outpatients Selected for Evaluation for PE*

	FACTORS ASSOCIATED WITH PE	FACTORS ASSOCIATED WITH ABSENCE OF PE	FACTORS CONTRIBUTING TO THE DECISION TO EVALUATE FOR PE BUT DO NOT DISTINGUISH PRESENCE OR ABSENCE OF PE
Symptoms	Unexplained dyspnea, hemoptysis	Substernal chest pain, nonspecific dizziness	Pleuritic chest pain, syncope, nonproductive cough, anxiety
Signs	Unilateral leg swelling, heart rate >100 beats/min, hypoxemia (room air pulse oximetry <95% with no history of lung disease)	Wheezing, temperature >102°F bilateral leg edema, pulse oximetry measured on room air consistently at 100%	Rales, temperature <102°F, respiratory distress, room air pulse oximetry reading of 95–99%
Risk factors	Age >50 y, recent surgery (requiring general anesthesia within past 4 wk), thrombophilia, adenocarcinoma (ovarian, pancreatic, prostate, and gastrointestinal) or brain cancer (especially glioblastoma multiforme), new-onset limb or body immobility >48 h	Age <30 y, COPD, asthma, smoking	Prior PE or DVT with a therapeutic INR and no thrombophilia, pregnancy, estrogen use, lung or breast cancer, postpartum status, congestive heart failure, or recent travel

*No individual criterion should be used as evidence to not test for PE.
ABBREVIATIONS: COPD = chronic obstructive pulmonary disease; DVT = deep venous thrombosis; INR = international normalized ratio; PE = pulmonary embolism.
SOURCE: Kline JA, Nelson RD, Jackson RE, Courtney DM: Criteria for the safe use of D-dimer testing in emergency department patients with suspected pulmonary embolism: A multicenter United States study. *Ann Emerg Med* 39:144, 2002; Wells PS, Anderson DR, Rodger M, et al: Derivation of a simple clinical model to categorize patients' probability of pulmonary embolism: Increasing the model's utility with the SimpliRED D-dimer. *Thromb Haemost* 83:416, 2000; and Wicki J, Perneger TV, Junod AE, et al: Assessing clinical probability of pulmonary embolism in the emergency ward: A simple score. *Arch Intern Med* 161:92, 2001.

morbidity and mortality rate of 1 to 5%, and about 1% of patients will be diagnosed with PE within a few months after a normal pulmonary angiogram. Recent practice has shifted away from this invasive and difficult procedure.

• D-dimer testing has become an important adjunct in the diagnosis or exclusion of PE. It is important to understand the type of D-dimer assay being used in the hospital laboratory. The sensitivity of qualitative D-dimers like the erythrocyte agglutination assay is about 85%. The sensitivity of quantitative D-dimers like enzyme-linked immunosorbent assay (ELISA) and the turbidimetric assay is about 95%. Most published research has restricted the use of D-dimer assays to patients with low pretest probability, though one recent study of a quantitative assay demonstrated excellent sensitivity (96%) regardless of pretest probability.[10] There are many conditions other than PE (eg, pregnancy, trauma, infection, malignancy, inflammatory conditions, recent surgery, advanced age) that can elevate the D-dimer. The specificity of all D-dimer assays is therefore low. Regardless of the assay used, a positive D-dimer must be followed by confirmatory testing for PE.

• Ventilation-perfusion scanning (V/Q) has traditionally been the first diagnostic imaging modality used in the diagnosis of PE. A normal V/Q scan implies a low enough risk of PE, even for patients with a high pretest probability, that the diagnosis is effectively excluded.[11] A high-probability V/Q scan effectively confirms the diagnosis of PE for patients with intermediate and high pretest probability.[11] However, only about 50% of patients with low pretest probability and a high-probability V/Q scan are subsequently found to have PE on pulmonary angiography. Therefore further testing should be performed to confirm the diagnosis in these patients. Unfortunately, up to 65% of patients in the ED will have low- or intermediate-probability V/Q scans, which should be considered indeterminate for PE. Strategies to evaluate PE for patients with indeterminate V/Q scans incorporate the use of quantitative D-dimer testing, serial venous ultrasound, computed tomography (CT) scanning, or pulmonary angiography.

• CT scanning has recently emerged in some centers as the imaging test of choice for the initial evaluation of PE. Images are obtained in 1.25- to 3.0-mm slices from the diaphragm to the apex of the lung. This may be followed by indirect venography to evaluate the lower extremity vasculature to increase the study's sensitvity.[12] Initial studies of CT for PE showed extremely high sensitivity, though further study has failed to reproduce these findings. Recent studies have shown sensitivity of between 70 and 90%.[13] Sensitivity is highest for large, central PE, and lowest for small, subsegmental PE, and can vary depending on the timing of the contrast bolus, movement of the patient, the addition of indirect venography, and the experience of the radiologist reading the study.[12] One advantage to CT scanning is its ability to identify alternative diagnoses that may explain the patient's symptoms.[14]

- Electrocardiography is neither sufficiently sensitive nor specific to evaluate PE. The classic findings of an S wave in lead I, a Q wave in lead III, and T-wave inversions in lead III are seen in a minority of PE patients.
- Arterial blood gas testing (ABG) cannot be used alone to either rule in or rule out PE. The overall sensitivity of a normal Pao_2 or A-a gradient is about 90%; however the specificity is only about 15%.[15]
- PE remains a common cause of pregnancy-related mortality and special consideration should be given to the evaluation of PE in these patients. For pregnant patients undergoing V/Q scanning, Foley catheter placement and IV hydration can reduce fetal exposure to ionizing radiation. In the case of a normal perfusion scan, the ventilation phase of the study can be avoided, thus limiting radiation exposure. For pregnant patients undergoing CT scanning, the abdomen should be shielded and indirect venography should be avoided. With these precautions in place, V/Q and CT probably expose the fetus to similarly low levels of ionizing radiation and should be considered safe techniques.

EMERGENCY DEPARTMENT CARE AND DISPOSITION

- As always, attention to airway stabilization and respiratory and circulatory support is paramount.
- The specific objectives in treating PE are to eliminate the clot burden and prevent recurrent thrombosis.
- Administer oxygen by nasal cannula or face mask as necessary.
- Crystalloid IV fluids should be given to augment preload and correct hypotension.
- Anticoagulation with a combination of heparin and warfarin is standard treatment for most cases of PE. Heparin therapy inhibits thrombin and prevents thrombus extension. Heparin has no intrinsic thrombolytic activity, but by allowing unopposed action of plasmin, it accelerates clot removal over 48 to 72 hours. Warfarin therapy is used for the long-term anticoagulation of patients with PE. However, because of a transient hypercoagulable state caused by a relative deficiency in protein C in the first days of warfarin therapy, treatment should always be preceded by heparin anticoagulation.

- Dosing of unfractionated heparin should be weight based, with 80 U/kg given as an initial bolus followed by 18 U/kg/h.
- Low molecular weight heparin has been shown to be safe and effective for the treatment of PE. Examples include enoxaparin 1 mg/kg subcutaneously as the initial dose in the ED.
- There are few absolute contraindications to anticoagulation with heparin for acute PE, though patients with recent intracranial hemorrhage or active gastrointestinal hemorrhage may have anticoagulation withheld.
- For patients with high pretest probability and no contraindications, heparin therapy should be initiated before diagnostic testing.
- Thrombolytic therapy should be considered for patients who require more aggressive treatment for PE. Currently, the only patients that have been shown to clearly benefit from thrombolytic therapy are those with hemodynamic instability.[16] Patients with echocardiographic evidence of right ventricular dysfunction may benefit from thrombolytic therapy, though evidence is conflicting as to whether the benefits outweigh the risks of hemorrhage in these patients.[17,18]
- The FDA has approved three regimens for treatment of PE: streptokinase, urokinase, and tissue plasminogen activator (tPA). Approved dosing is similar to that used in myocardial infarction. The most common regimen is 100 mg tPA infused over 2 hours, though it may be given as a bolus in the case of gross hemodynamic instability.
- Stable patients with PE can be admitted to a telemetry bed. Patients who exhibit signs of circulatory compromise and all patients who receive thrombolytic therapy should be admitted to an intensive care unit.

REFERENCES

1. Pineda LA, Hathwar VS, Grant BJB: Clinical suspicion of fatal pulmonary embolism. *Chest* 120:791, 2001.
2. Lane DA, Mannucci PM, Bauer KA, et al: Inherited thrombophilia: Part 1 [review]. *Thromb Haemost* 76:651, 1996.
3. Murin S, Marelich GP, Arroliga AC, Matthay RA: Hereditary thrombophilia and venous thromboembolism [review]. *Am J Resp Crit Care Med* 158:1369, 1998.
4. Hirsch J: Diagnosis of venous thrombosis and pulmonary embolism. *Am J Cardiol* 65:45C, 1990.
5. Courtney DM, Sasser H, Pincus B, Kline JA: Pulseless electrical activity with witnessed arrest as a predictor of sudden death from massive pulmonary embolism in outpatients. *Resuscitation* 49:265, 2001.

6. Rosen M, Sands D, Morris J, et al: Does a physician's ability to accurately assess the likelihood of pulmonary embolism increase with training? *Acad Med* 75:1199, 2000.

7. Kline JA, Nelson RD, Jackson RE, Courtney DM: Criteria for the safe use of D-dimer testing in emergency department patients with suspected pulmonary embolism: A multicenter United States study. *Ann Emerg Med* 39:144, 2002.

8. Wells PS, Anderson DR, Rodger M, et al: Excluding pulmonary embolism at the bedside without diagnostic imaging: management of patients with suspected pulmonary embolism presenting to the emergency department by using a simple clinical model and D-dimer. *Ann Intern Med* 135:98, 2001.

9. Chagnon I, Bounameaux H, Aujesky D, et al: Comparison of two clinical prediction rules and implicit assessment among patients with suspected pulmonary embolism. *Am J Med* 113:269, 2002.

10. Dunn KL, Wolf BS, Dorfman DM, et al: Normal D-dimer levels in emergency department patients suspected of acute pulmonary embolism. *J Am Coll Cardiol* 40:1475, 2002.

11. PIOPED Investigators: Value of the ventilation/perfusion scan in acute pulmonary embolism. Results of the Prospective Investigation of Pulmonary Embolism Diagnosis (PIOPED). *JAMA* 263:2753, 1990.

12. Richman PB, Wood J, Kasper DM, et al: Contribution of indirect computed tomography venography to computed tomography angiography of the chest for the diagnosis of thromboembolic disease in two United States emergency departments. *J Thromb Haemost* 1:652, 2003.

13. Perrier A, et al: Performance of helical computed tomography in unselected outpatients with suspected pulmonary embolism. *Ann Intern Med.* 135:88, 2001.

14. Richman PB, Courtney DM, Wood J, et al: Chest CT angiography (CTA) to rule out pulmonary embolism (PE) frequently reveals clinically significant ancillary findings—A multicenter study of 1025 emergency department patients. *Acad Emerg Med* 10:564, 2003.

15. Kline JA, Johns KL, Coluciello SA, Israel EG: New diagnostic tests for pulmonary embolism. *Ann Emerg Med* 35:168, 2000.

16. Dalen JE, Alpert JS, Hirsch J: Thrombolytic therapy for pulmonary embolism: Is it effective? Is it safe? When is it indicated? [review] *Arch Intern Med* 157:2550, 1997.

17. Grifoni S, Olivetto I, Cecchini P, et al: Short term clinical outcome of patients with acute pulmonary embolism, normal blood pressure, and echocardiographic right ventricular dysfunction. *Circulation* 101:2817, 2000.

18. Kasper W, Konstantinides S, Geibel A, et al: Management strategies and determinants of outcome in acute major pulmonary embolism: Results of a multicenter registry. *J Am Coll Cardiol* 30:1165, 1997.

For further reading in *Emergency Medicine: A Comprehensive Study Guide*, 6th ed., see Chap. 56, "Pulmonary Embolism," by Jeffrey A. Kline.

29 HYPERTENSIVE EMERGENCIES
Jonathan A. Maisel

EPIDEMIOLOGY

- Hypertension is the fourth most prevalent chronic medical condition in the United States, affecting up to 24% of the general adult population.[1,2]
- Thirty percent of patients presenting to emergency departments nationwide have a blood pressure equal to or greater than 140/90 mm Hg.[3]
- Seventy percent of those patients who have a blood pressure of 140/90 or greater at ED triage will have an elevated blood pressure at follow-up regardless of the presence of pain as the chief complaint. The higher the initial blood pressure, the more likely that blood pressure will be elevated at follow-up.[4]
- The risk of developing serious cardiovascular, renal, or cerebrovascular disease increases with poorly controlled blood pressure (BP).
- Nearly 75% of adult Americans with known hypertension (HTN) have inadequate control of their BP, and only half are compliant with prescribed medications.[1,2]
- The majority of patients require more than one mediation to control their blood pressure.[5]

PATHOPHYSIOLOGY

- At the cellular level, postsynaptic α_1 and α_2 receptors are stimulated by norepinephrine released from presynaptic sympathetic nerve endings, leading to the release of intracellular calcium. Free calcium activates actin and myosin, resulting in smooth muscle contraction, increased peripheral vascular resistance, and an increase in blood pressure. Presynaptic α_2 receptors help limit this response via a negative feedback loop.
- Hypertension develops: (1) as a result of alterations in the contractile properties of smooth muscle in arterial walls, or (2) as a response to failure of normal autoregulatory mechanisms within vascular beds of vital organs (ie, heart, kidney, brain).
- Long-standing, poorly controlled HTN may damage target organs by injuring vascular beds. Endothelial injury leads to deposition of fibrin within vessel walls and activation of mediators of coagulation and cell proliferation. A recurrent cycle of vascular reactivity develops, which leads to platelet aggregation and myointimal proliferation, and subsequent progressive narrowing of arterioles.

- Hypertension is associated with major cardiovascular risk factors such as smoking, hyperlipidemia, diabetes mellitus, age greater than 60, gender (men and post-menopausal women), obesity, and a family history of cardiovascular disease.[1] Although no single cause of HTN has been identified, a combination of factors such as these are believed to contribute to "essential" HTN. Several specific causes do exist, with intrinsic renal and renovascular disease being the most prevalent of the known causes.
- Hypertensive emergencies in childhood, defined as systolic or diastolic BP ≥95th percentile for age and sex, are most commonly caused by intrinsic renal or renovascular disease, or pheochromocytoma.

CLINICAL FEATURES

- Essential historical features include a prior history of HTN; noncompliance with antihypertensive medication; overall medication use, including over-the-counter and illicit drugs; and diet (especially products with sodium or tyramine).
- Any past medical history of cardiovascular, cerebrovascular, or renal disease; diabetes; hyperlipidemia; chronic obstructive pulmonary disease (COPD) or asthma; or a family history of HTN or premature heart disease should be elicited.[1]
- Precipitating causes such as pregnancy, illicit drug use (ie, cocaine and methamphetamine), and use of monoamine oxidase inhibitors or decongestants should be considered.
- Patients should be asked about central nervous system (CNS) symptoms (headache, visual changes, confusion, paresis, seizures), cardiovascular symptoms (chest pain, dyspnea, palpitations, pedal edema, tearing pain radiating to the back or abdomen), and renal symptoms (anuria, hematuria, edema).
- Blood pressure should be measured with an appropriately sized cuff (false elevations are seen with cuffs that are too small), at least twice if elevated, and in both arms and legs if substantially elevated.
- The physical exam should focus on target organ injury and its acuity, including mental status changes, focal neurologic deficits, funduscopic changes (hemorrhages, cotton-wool exudates, disk edema), and cardiovascular findings (carotid bruits, heart murmurs and gallops, asymmetric pulses [coarctation vs. dissection], pulmonary rales, and pulsatile abdominal masses).[1]
- In the pregnant or postpartum patient, assess for hyperreflexia and peripheral edema, suggesting pre-eclampsia.
- Children present with nonspecific complaints such as a throbbing frontal headache or blurred vision. Physical findings are similar to those seen in adults.

- Pheochromocytoma is another common etiology in childhood, presenting with nervousness, palpitations, sweating, blurry vision, and skin flushing.

DIAGNOSIS AND DIFFERENTIAL

- The diagnostic evaluation should be based on presenting symptoms and signs, or the existence of comorbidities.
- Renal impairment may present as hematuria, proteinuria, or red cell casts, or elevations in blood urea nitrogen (BUN), creatinine, and potassium levels.
- An electrocardiogram (ECG) may reveal ST-T wave changes consistent with coronary ischemia, electrolyte abnormalities, strain, or left ventricular hypertrophy.
- A chest x-ray may help identify congestive heart failure, aortic dissection, or coarctation.
- A urinalysis looking for protein may be the most cost effective test in the ED.[6]
- In patients with neurologic compromise or significant headache, computed tomography (CT) scan of the head may reveal ischemic changes, edema, or blood.
- A urine or serum drug screen may identify illicit drug use.
- A pregnancy test should be done on all hypertensive women of childbearing age.

EMERGENCY DEPARTMENT CARE AND DISPOSITION

- Although stage 1 HTN is defined as either a systolic BP >140 mm Hg or a diastolic BP >90 mm Hg,[5] management depends more on the patient's clinical condition than absolute systolic or diastolic values.
- Classification of HTN into four categories facilitates management:
  1. Hypertensive emergency: Elevated blood pressure associated with target organ (CNS, cardiac, renal) dysfunction. Requires immediate recognition and treatment.
  2. Hypertensive urgency: Elevated blood pressure associated with risk of imminent target organ dysfunction.
  3. Acute hypertensive episode: Systolic BP >180 and diastolic BP >110 without evolving or impending target organ dysfunction.
  4. Transient hypertension: Elevated blood pressure associated with another condition (eg, anxiety, alcohol withdrawal, "white-coat hypertension," and cocaine abuse). Patients usually become normotensive once the precipitating event resolves.
- Patients with hypertensive emergencies require O_2 supplementation, cardiac monitoring, and intravenous

access. After stabilizing the ABCs of resuscitation, the treatment goal is to reduce mean arterial pressure (diastolic BP + 1/3 [systolic BP − diastolic BP]) by 20 to 25% over 30 to 60 minutes.

- For hypertensive encephalopathy (characterized by severe headaches, nausea, vomiting, and altered mental status), use sodium nitroprusside, beginning at 0.3 μg/kg/min, titrating to a maximum of 10 μg/kg/min. Avoid rapid correction of BP to prevent cerebral ischemia secondary to hypoperfusion. Nitroprusside is a potent arteriolar and venous dilator, with an onset of action in seconds. An arterial line should be placed in order to closely monitor the BP, and the solution and tubing should be wrapped in aluminum foil to prevent degradation by light. Hypotension is the most common complication of nitroprusside infusions. Cyanide toxicity is seen rarely after prolonged infusions.

- Labetalol is useful as a second-line agent for hypertensive encephalopathy, providing a steady, consistent drop in BP without diminishing cerebral blood flow or producing a reflex tachycardia. It is a competitive, selective α_1-blocker, and a competitive, nonselective β-blocker, with the β-blocking action 4 to 8 times more potent than the α-blocking action. It has an onset of action of 5 to 10 minutes, and a duration of action of 8 hours. Its use should be avoided in patients with asthma, COPD, congestive heart failure (CHF), and heart block. The treatment should begin with incremental boluses of 20 to 40 mg IV, and repeated every 10 minutes, until the target blood pressure is achieved or a total dose of 300 mg is reached. Alternatively, after an initial bolus, a continuous infusion of 2 mg/min may be used, terminating the infusion when the target BP has been achieved. Labetalol is also ideal for use in syndromes associated with excessive catecholamine stimulation.

- Fenoldopam, a selective postsynaptic dopaminergic receptor agonist with potent vasodilatory and natriuretic properties, is a new agent which has been found to be as effective as nitroprusside for hypertensive emergencies, without affecting heart rate. The initial dose is 0.05 to 0.1 μg/kg/min, and can be increased by 0.1 μg/kg/min, up to 1.6 μg/kg/min.

- HTN associated with stroke is often a physiologic response to the stroke itself (to maintain adequate cerebral perfusion) and not its immediate cause. When the diastolic BP is >140 mm Hg, it may be slowly reduced by up to 20% using 5-mg increments of IV labetalol. In the case of subarachnoid hemorrhage, oral nimodipine 60 mg every 4 hours, or nicardipine 2 mg IV bolus, followed by a 4- to 15-mg/h infusion, may be used to reverse the vasospasm associated with blood in the subarachnoid space.

- For HTN associated with pulmonary edema, IV nitroglycerin or nitroprusside may be used. Nitroglycerin

is both an arteriolar and venous dilator, with greater effect on the venous system, and an onset of action within minutes. Initial infusion should be at a rate of 5 to 20 μg/min, with 5-μg/min incremental increases every 5 minutes until symptoms improve or side effects (headache, hypotension, tachycardia) ensue. Enalaprilat, the first FDA-approved IV angiotensin-converting enzyme (ACE) inhibitor, is also effective for hypertensive emergencies in the setting of congestive heart failure. It dilates the coronary vasculature, reduces pulmonary capillary wedge pressure (PCWP), and improves cardiac index and stroke volume. An initial IV bolus of 0.625 to 1.25 mg is effective within minutes, and can be repeated every 6 hours.

- For HTN associated with myocardial ischemia, IV nitroglycerin is first-line therapy. Because it is a better vasodilator of the coronary vessels than nitroprusside, it is the drug of choice for severe HTN complicating acute coronary ischemia or pulmonary edema.

- For HTN associated with aortic dissection, reducing the BP and ventricular ejection force may limit the extent of the dissection. Either labetalol alone or a combination of nitroprusside and a β-blocker can be used. Esmolol, an ultra-short-acting β_1-selective adrenergic blocker, is very effective, achieving 90% of β-blockade within 5 minutes of an IV bolus of 0.5 mg/kg, followed by an infusion of 0.05 to 0.3 mg/kg/min. Propranolol and metoprolol are alternatives. Esmolol, as well as other β-blockers, should be avoided in patients with asthma, COPD, and cocaine-induced cardiovascular complications (because of unopposed α-adrenergic effects).

- Worsening renal function in the setting of elevated BP, manifested by elevation of BUN and creatinine levels, proteinuria, or the presence of red blood cells or red cell casts in the urine, is considered a hypertensive emergency. Nitroprusside is the preferred agent. Dialysis-dependent patients presenting with volume overload may require emergent dialysis if they present with uncontrolled HTN and other evidence of end-organ dysfunction.

- For pregnancy-induced hypertension, including eclampsia, hydralazine can be given as a 10- to 20-mg IV dose or a 10- to 50-mg intramuscular (IM) dose, and can be repeated every 30 minutes.[7]

- The decision to treat a hypertensive emergency in a child is based on both the blood pressure and associated symptoms. Urgent treatment is required if the blood pressure exceeds prior measurements by 30%. The goal is to reduce the blood pressure by 25% within 1 hour. Nitroprusside (0.3 to 8.0 μg/kg/min) and labetalol (1 to 3 mg/kg/h) are the agents of choice.

- Treatment of pheochromocytoma requires surgical excision, and managing the elevated BP with an α-adrenergic blocker such as phentolamine.

- The treatment goal in hypertensive urgencies is the gradual reduction of BP within 24 to 48 hours by using oral antihypertensive agents. Useful agents include the following:
  - Labetalol 200 to 400 mg PO, repeated every 2 to 3 hours. Oral labetalol has an onset of action in 30 minutes, and a duration of action of 6 to 12 hours.
  - Captopril, an ACE inhibitor, has an onset of action in 15 to 30 minutes, a peak effect at 50 to 90 minutes, and a duration of effect of 4 to 6 hours. A 25-mg oral dose is effective in refractory CHF and renovascular HTN. Common side effects include rash, cough, and loss of taste, and rarely, life-threatening angioneurotic edema.
  - Sublingual nitroglycerin in the form of spray or 0.3- to 0.6-mg tablets, is the agent of choice for patients with angina or CHF. The hypotensive effect begins in minutes and can last several hours.
  - Clonidine is a centrally acting, α_2-adrenergic agonist that decreases central sympathomimetic activity, lowering plasma catecholamine levels. Its onset of action is 30 to 60 minutes, with peak effect in 2 to 4 hours. It is given as a dose of 0.1 mg hourly until the target BP is reached, or a total of 0.7 mg has been given. A patient treated with clonidine in the ED does not need to be discharged on this drug. Because an adequate response may take up to 6 hours, it is not a first-line agent.
  - Nifedipine, a dihydropyridine calcium channel antagonist, had been used commonly for hypertensive urgencies via the oral and sublingual routes. Serious adverse reactions such as acute coronary events and stroke preclude recommending it for the urgent treatment of HTN.[8]
  - Since a common cause of hypertensive urgency is noncompliance with medication, restarting a patient on a previously established regimen is an acceptable strategy.
- For nonemergent, nonurgent HTN, there is no evidence of a beneficial effect of acute BP reduction on long-term control or on the chronic effects of HTN. These patients do not require acute intervention, but should be referred for timely follow-up. Should an oral agent be started in the ED, the choice should be based on coexisting conditions, if any. Diuretics such as hydrochlorothiazide 25 mg/day are first-line agents in the elderly, as well as for patients with renal disease and CHF (consider potassium supplementation). β-Blockers such as metoprolol 50 mg bid are first-line agents for patients with angina or post–myocardial infarction. They are also useful in patients with a history of migraines, atrial fibrillation with a rapid ventricular response, and senile tremors. ACE inhibitors, such as captopril 25 mg bid to tid, can be used in patients with CHF or diabetes.

REFERENCES

1. Joint National Committee (JNC) on Prevention, Detection, Evaluation, and Treatment of High Blood Pressure: The Sixth Report of the Joint National Committee on Prevention, Detection, Evaluation, and Treatment of High Blood Pressure. *Arch Intern Med* 157:2413, 1997.
2. Burt VL, Whelton P, Roccella EJ, et al: Prevalence of hypertension in the U.S. adult population: Results from the Third Health and Nutrition Examination Survey, 1988–1991. *Hypertension* 25:305, 1995.
3. McCaig LF, Burt CW: National Hospital Ambulatory Medical Care Survey: 2001 emergency department summary. *Adv Data* 335:1, 2003.
4. Backer H, Decker L, Ackerson L: Reproducibility of increased blood pressure during an emergency department or urgent care visit. *Ann Emerg Med* 14:507, 2003.
5. Chobanian AV, Bakris GL, Black HR, et al: The Seventh Report of the Joint National Committee on Prevention, Detection, Evaluation, and Treatment of High Blood Pressure: The JNC 7 Report. *JAMA* 289:2560, 2003.
6. Karras DJ, Heilpern KL, Riley LJ, et al: Urine dipstick as a screening test for serum creatinine elevation in emergency department patients with severe hypertension. *Acad Emerg Med* 9:27, 2002.
7. Black HR, Lowe SA, Rubin PC: The pharmacologic management of hypertension in pregnancy. *J Hypertens* 10:201, 1992.
8. McCarthy M: US NIH issues warning on nifedipine. *Lancet* 346:689, 1995.

For further reading in *Emergency Medicine: A Comprehensive Study Guide,* 6th ed., see Chap. 57, "Hypertension," by Melissa M. Wu and Arjun Chanmugam.

30   AORTIC DISSECTION AND ANEURYSMS

David E. Manthey

ABDOMINAL AORTIC ANEURYSMS

EPIDEMIOLOGY

- The incidence of abdominal aortic aneurysm (AAA) increases with age; most patients are older than 60.
- Males are at increased risk.
- Eighteen percent of patients have a family history of aneurysm in a first-degree relative.
- Other risk factors include connective tissue disease, Marfan's syndrome, and atherosclerotic risk factors (smoking, hypertension, hyperlipidemia, and diabetes).

PATHOPHYSIOLOGY

- Destruction of the media of the aorta with a reduction in elastin and collagen is a prominent feature in aneurysm pathogenesis.
- Laplace's law [wall tension = (pressure × radius)/tensile force] dictates that as the aorta dilates, the force on the aortic wall increases, causing further aortic dilation.
- The rate of aneurysmal dilation is variable, with larger aneurysms expanding more quickly. An average rate may be .25 to .5 centimeter per year.[1]

CLINICAL FEATURES

- Three clinical scenarios exist: acute rupture, AAA as an incidental finding to aortoenteric fistula, and chronic contained rupture.
- Sudden death most commonly occurs with intraperitoneal rupture of the aneurysm.
- The classic presentation is an older male with severe back or abdominal pain who presents with syncope or hypotension.
- Pain, described as abrupt and severe at onset, is the most common presenting symptom; 50% describe this pain as "tearing."
- The presence of an AAA does not alter the femoral arterial pulsations.[2]
- Many patients present with a complaint of unilateral flank or groin pain, hip pain, or abdominal pain localized to a specific quadrant. An AAA is most commonly misdiagnosed as renal colic.[3]
- Lack of tenderness does not imply an intact aorta.
- There may be signs of retroperitoneal hemorrhage such as periumbilical (Cullen's sign) or flank ecchymosis (Grey-Turner's sign) or scrotal hematoma.
- Asymptomatic AAAs may be found on physical exam or during an unrelated radiologic evaluation. Those larger than 5 centimeters are at higher risk of rupture.
- Symptomatic aneurysms of any size should be considered emergent.
- Aortoenteric fistulas may present with a deceptively minor "sentinel" bleed or massive GI hemorrhage. This is classically seen after prior aortic grafting.[4]
- Chronic contained rupture is uncommon, but is seen when a AAA ruptures retroperitoneally with significant fibrosis that limits blood loss.[5]

DIAGNOSIS AND DIFFERENTIAL

- The differential for AAA depends on its presentation. The key is to keep AAA in your differential when evaluating patients for other symptoms such as back pain, syncope, and renal colic.
- Diagnostic studies should never unnecessarily delay the surgical repair of an AAA. They are only needed when the diagnosis of AAA is unclear.
- In the unstable patient, bedside abdominal ultrasound is approximately 100% sensitive for demonstrating the presence of an aneurysm and measuring its diameter.[6] It cannot reliably diagnose rupture.
- Computed tomographic (CT) scanning, approximately 100% accurate in determining the presence or absence of an AAA, is preferred in the stable patient as it better delineates the anatomic details of the aneurysm and any associated rupture.

EMERGENCY DEPARTMENT CARE AND DISPOSITION

- Stabilize the patient with volume resuscitation with isotonic fluids and/or blood transfusion via multiple large-bore IV lines.[7]
- Immediate surgical consultation is warranted for suspected rupturing AAA or aortoenteric fistula.
- Consult a vascular surgeon for urgent repair of chronically contained ruptured AAAs.
- For an incidentally discovered AAA, consultation with a vascular surgeon for admission or close outpatient follow-up based on the size of the aneurysm is appropriate.[8]

AORTIC DISSECTION

EPIDEMIOLOGY

- Aortic dissection has a bimodal distribution.
- Most patients are over the age of 50 years (mean age is 63).[9]
- Two thirds are male and 72% have hypertension.[9]
- Younger patients have identifiable risk factors such as congenital heart disease, connective tissue disease, and pregnancy.[10]
- Twenty-five to thirty percent of patients with Marfan's syndrome develop dissection.
- Dissection may also be iatrogenic from cardiac catheterization or surgery.

PATHOPHYSIOLOGY

- Aortic dissection occurs when the intima is violated, allowing blood to enter the media and dissect between the intimal and adventitial layers, developing a false lumen.

- Common sites for tearing include the ascending aorta and the region of the ligamentum arteriosum.
- The Stanford classification system categorizes a type A dissection as one with any involvement of the ascending aorta, and a type B dissection as one restricted to the descending aorta. The DeBakey system classifies type I dissections as those that involve the ascending aorta, the arch, and the descending aorta. Type II involves only the ascending aorta, and type III only the descending aorta.

CLINICAL FEATURES

- More than 85% of patients have abrupt onset of severe tearing chest or upper back pain.[9]
- Clinical presentation depends on the location of the dissection, with pain patterns that often change as the anatomic injury migrates.[10]
- Presentations include aortic valve insufficiency with or without pericardial tamponade, coronary artery occlusion with MI, stroke symptoms with carotid involvement, or paraplegia with occlusion of the vertebral blood supply. The dissection may progress distally, causing abdominal or flank pain or limb ischemia.
- Physical exam findings also depend on the location and progression of the dissection. A diastolic murmur or aortic insufficiency may be heard. Fifty percent of patients have decreased radial, femoral, or carotid pulses.[10]
- Hypertension and tachycardia are common, but hypotension may also be present.

DIAGNOSIS AND DIFFERENTIAL

- Ischemic end-organ manifestations associated with dissections may confuse the differential diagnosis, including myocardial infarction, pericardial disease, and spinal cord injuries.
- Rupture of the dissection back through the intima into the true lumen may cause a cessation of symptoms, leading to false reassurance.
- Ninety percent of patients with a thoracic dissection will have an abnormal chest x-ray. More common findings include a widening of the mediastinum, abnormal aortic contour, pleural effusion, apical capping, and depression of the left main stem bronchus.
- CT scanning may reliably diagnose dissection with a sensitivity of 83 to 100% and a specificity of 87 to 100%.
- Angiography, although still considered the gold standard, has a specificity of 94% and a sensitivity of 88%.[11,12] It can reliably show the complications of dissection.

- Transesophageal echocardiography has a sensitivity that ranges from 97 to 100% and a specificity of 97 to 99%.[11] It is highly operator dependent.

EMERGENCY DEPARTMENT CARE AND DISPOSITION

- Patients with suspected aortic dissection require prompt radiographic confirmation of the diagnosis and early consultation with the CT surgeon.
- Hypertension must be controlled with drugs that will not increase the shear force on the intimal flap. β-Blockers are the first-line choice, with nitroprusside added if the blood pressure remains elevated. Calcium channel blockers can be used if there is a contraindication to β-blockers.
- Dissection of the ascending aorta requires prompt surgical repair. Indications for repair of dissections involving only the descending aorta are controversial.[12]

REFERENCES

1. Faggioli GL, Stella A, Gargiulo M, et al: Morphology of small aneurysms: Definition and impact on risk of rupture. *Am J Surg* 168:131, 1994.
2. Satta J, Laara E, Immonen K, et al: The rupture type determines the outcome for ruptured abdominal aortic aneurysm patients. *Ann Chirurg Gynaecol* 86:24, 1997.
3. Henney AM, Adiseshiah M, et al: Abdominal aortic aneurysm: Report of a meeting of physicians and scientists, University College London Medical School. *Lancet* 341:215, 1993.
4. Batounis E, Georgopoulos S: The validity of current vascular imaging methods in the evaluation of aortic anastomotic aneurysms developing after abdominal aortic aneurysm repair. *Ann Vasc Surg* 10:537, 1996.
5. Jones CS, Reilly MK, Dalsing MC, Glover JL: Chronic contained rupture of abdominal aortic aneurysms. *Arch Surg* 121:542, 1986.
6. Kuhn M, Bonnin RLL, Davey MJ, et al: Emergency ultrasound scanning for abdominal aortic aneurysm: Accessible, accurate, and advantageous. *Ann Emerg Med* 36:219, 2000.
7. Crawford ED, Hess KR: Abdominal aortic aneurysm. *N Engl J Med* 321:1040, 1989.
8. Graham M, Chan A: Ultrasound screening for clinically occult abdominal aortic aneurysm. *Can Med Assoc* 138:627, 1988.
9. Hagan P, Nienaber C, Isselbacher EM, et al: The International Registry of Acute Aortic Dissection (IRAD): New insights into an old disease. *JAMA* 283:897, 2000.
10. Larson EW, Edwards WD: Risk factors for aortic dissection: A necropsy study of 161 cases. *Am J Cardiol* 53:849, 1984.

11. Erbel R, Bednarczyk I, Pop T, et al: Detection of dissection of the aortic intima and media after angioplasty of coarctation of the aorta. An angiographic, computed tomographic, and echocardiographic comparative study. *Circulation* 81: 805, 1990.

12. Cigarroa JE, Isselbacher EM, DeSanctis RW, et al: Medical progress: Diagnostic imaging in the evaluation of suspected aortic dissection—old standards and new directions. *N Engl J Med* 328:35, 1993.

For further reading in *Emergency Medicine: A Comprehensive Study Guide,* 6th ed., see Chap. 58, "Aortic Dissection and Aneurysms," by Louise A. Prince and Gary A. Johnson.

31 PERIPHERAL VASCULAR DISORDERS
Christopher Kabrhel

DEEP VENOUS THROMBOSIS AND THROMBOPHLEBITIS

EPIDEMIOLOGY

- Deep venous thrombosis (DVT) is a common condition with an estimated annual incidence of two million cases in the United States. DVT is part of the spectrum of venous thromboembolic disease that also includes pulmonary embolism (PE).
- The vast majority (90%) of DVT occur in the lower extremities, though thrombosis of the upper extremities can also occur, especially in the presence of an indwelling venous catheter.
- Acute arterial occlusion secondary to thrombosis or embolism is less common than venous occlusion, but is potentially life threatening and carries a mortality of 25%. In survivors of this condition, limb amputation is necessary in 20%.

PATHOPHYSIOLOGY

- Superficial thrombophlebitis is a common, self-limiting condition that presents with pain, redness, and tenderness along a superficial vein. The incidence of DVT from extension of superficial thrombophlebitis is about 3%.[1]
- DVT forms at sites of endothelial injury and venous stasis, and is augmented by hypercoagulable states. Thrombus is composed mostly of erythrocytes, fibrin, and platelets.

- The most significant risk factors for DVT are major surgery or trauma, prolonged immobilization, malignancy or other hypercoagulable state (factor V Leiden being the most common), and prior thromboembolic disease. Pregnancy, the immediate postpartum state, estrogen use, congestive heart failure, inflammatory conditions, and prolonged travel are also significant risk factors.
- DVT forms most commonly at the venous cusps of deep veins in the lower extremities, though it can also occur in the upper extremities, especially in the presence of indwelling catheters, pacemakers, or mechanical compression from tumor, cervical rib, or hypertrophied muscles.
- Thrombus may propagate, dissolve, or embolize, depending on the balance between thrombogenesis and thrombolysis. Proximal DVT is much more likely to cause PE than distal DVT, but 80% of symptomatic DVT will be located in or proximal to the popliteal vein. Furthermore, isolated calf DVT will extend proximally within 1 week in 20% of cases.[2]

CLINICAL FEATURES

- Unfortunately, the clinical examination is unreliable for DVT. The classic constellation of calf or leg pain, redness, swelling, tenderness, and warmth is present in fewer than 50% of patients with confirmed lower extremity DVT.[3]
- Homans' sign, pain in the calf with forced dorsiflexion of the ankle with the leg straight, is unreliable for DVT.
- Several decision instruments have been developed to categorize patients as having low, moderate, or high probability of DVT before diagnostic testing.[4]
- The scoring system developed by Wells and colleagues is presented in Table 31-1. The system is scored as follows: a score of ≥ 3 = high probability; a score of 1 to 2; = moderate probability; and a score of 0 = low probability.
- Uncommon but severe presentations of DVT include phlegmasia cerulea dolens and phlegmasia alba dolens. Phlegmasia cerulea dolens is a high-grade obstruction that elevates compartment pressures and can compromise limb perfusion.[5] It presents as a massively swollen, cyanotic limb. Phlegmasia alba dolens is usually associated with pregnancy and has a similar pathophysiology but presents as a pale limb secondary to arterial spasm.

DIAGNOSIS AND DIFFERENTIAL

- The history and physical examination is unreliable for DVT. Similar presentations can be seen with

TABLE 31-1 Predictors of Deep Vein Thrombosis

CLINICAL FEATURE	SCORE
Active cancer (treatment ongoing, palliative)	1
Paralysis, paresis, or recent plaster immobilization of lower extremities	1
Recently bedridden >3 d or major surgery within 4 wk	1
Localized tenderness along the distribution of the deep venous system	1
Entire leg swollen	1
Calf swelling >3 cm compared to the asymptomatic side (10 cm below tibial tuberosity)	1
Pitting edema confined to the symptomatic leg	1
Collateral superficial veins (nonvaricose)	1
Alternative diagnosis as likely or greater than that of deep vein thrombosis	−2

SOURCE: Used with permission from Wells et al.[4]

congestive heart failure, cellulitis, venous stasis without thrombosis, and musculoskeletal injuries. Therefore some type of objective testing for DVT is necessary.

- Assessing clinical probability using an objective and validated instrument can help guide the type and extent of objective testing necessary.
- A rapid enzyme-linked immunosorbent assay (ELISA) D-dimer has high sensitivity (97 to 99%) for DVT and can be used to exclude the diagnosis in low- to moderate-probability patients.[6] The use of latex D-dimer assays to exclude DVT is not recommended due to their low (80%) sensitivity.[4] Erythrocyte agglutination D-dimer assays have a sensitivity of 90 to 94% and the use of these tests to rule out DVT is controversial.[4,7]
- Duplex ultrasonography (real time B-mode imaging combined with Doppler flow imaging) is the test of choice for evaluating DVT in the ED. Duplex ultrasonography has high sensitivity (97%) and specificity (94%) for DVT.[2] Sensitivity is lower for pelvic and isolated calf DVT (73%). Some algorithms recommend serial ultrasonography for patients with high clinical probability of DVT and negative initial ultrasound. Two negative duplex scans 1 week apart carries less than 1% risk of symptomatic DVT or PE in 3 months.[2,4,7,8]
- For patients with suspected upper extremity DVT, duplex ultrasound has a sensitivity of 56 to 100%.[9] Venography or MRI may be necessary when there is high clinical suspicion and a negative duplex.
- Impedance plethysmography measures changes in electrical resistance in response to changes in calf volume secondary to venous obstruction. Sensitivity is 73 to 96% and specificity is 83 to 97%. However, due to its lower sensitivity this technique has been largely supplanted by duplex ultrasonography.[2,3]

- The traditional gold standard for DVT has been contrast venography. However, the technique is invasive and impractical, and so is rarely performed. Magnetic resonance imaging may represent a new gold standard for diagnosing DVT, but its application in the ED is unclear.

EMERGENCY DEPARTMENT CARE AND DISPOSITION

- Treatment of superficial thrombophlebitis is conservative. Mild cases can be treated with warm compresses, analgesia, and elevation. Antibiotics and anticoagulants are of no proven benefit in superficial thrombophlebitis, though it may be necessary to rule out associated DVT, especially in cases of proximal disease.
- Treatment of DVT centers on aggressive anticoagulation to prevent the extension of clot, allow for its lysis by the intrinsic fibrinolytic system, and prevent PE.
- Any patient with documented DVT on duplex ultrasonography should receive immediate anticoagulation with heparin and eventually warfarin. For patients with negative initial duplex ultrasound, several studies have demonstrated the safety of withholding anticoagulation pending repeat evaluation.[2,4,8]
- Low molecular weight heparins (LMWH) are safe and effective for the treatment of DVT.[9] The three most commonly used LMWHs are dalteparin (200 U/kg subcutaneously every 24 hours, maximum 18,000 U), enoxaparin (1.5 mg/kg subcutaneously every 24 hours, maximum 180 mg), and tinzaparin (175 U/kg subcutaneously every 24 hours, maximum 18,000 U). Low molecular weight heparins have a more predictable dose-response curve and fewer bleeding complications than unfractionated heparin, but should be avoided in patients with renal failure since they are renally cleared and levels are difficult to monitor.[10]
- When LMWH is unavailable or contraindicated, unfractionated heparin (UFH) therapy should be initiated. Dosing is weight based at 80 U/kg IV bolus followed by 18 U/kg/h infusion. The activated partial thromboplastin time (aPTT) should be maintained between 55 and 80 seconds (1.5 to 2.5 times normal). Traditional dosing using a 5000-U bolus and 1000 U/h infusion will underdose two thirds of patients.
- For patients with documented heparin-induced thrombocytopenia (HIT), a thrombin inhibitor such as lepirudin can be given as a 0.4-mg/kg IV slow bolus (up to 44 mg) followed by an infusion of 0.1 to 0.15 mg/kg/h.
- Oral anticoagulation with warfarin can be initiated simultaneously with heparin therapy. Usual initial

dosing is 5 mg/day with a target INR of 2 to 3. Anticoagulation should be continued for 3 months in patients with reversible risk factors, and 6 months or longer in other patients.[11]

- There is no evidence showing a survival benefit of thrombolytic therapy for DVT over heparin and warfarin.[12]
- An inferior vena cava filter can be placed to prevent PE when anticoagulation is contraindicated, a major complication occurs, or DVT continues to propagate despite adequate anticoagulation.
- Surgical thrombectomy is typically only considered for patients with DVT that have a persistently ischemic limb secondary to phlegmasia cerulea dolens.
- Many patients can be discharged from the ED following a dose of LMWH if appropriate follow-up is arranged and more invasive therapy is not required.

ACUTE ARTERIAL OCCLUSION

EPIDEMIOLOGY

- Peripheral arterial disease is noted in 11 to 27% of elderly patients.[13] Most of these patients have a history of smoking, though diabetes, hypertension, and hyperlipidemia are also significant risk factors. At least one half of these patients also have coronary or cerebrovascular disease.
- The most frequently involved arteries, in descending order, are the femoropopliteal, tibial, aortoiliac, and brachiocephalic.

PATHOPHYSIOLOGY

- Thrombotic arterial occlusion is more common than embolic arterial occlusion (20% of cases) in the lower extremities.[14]
- In the upper extremities, thrombosis also accounts for the largest proportion of arterial occlusion, but here, one third of cases are embolic and one quarter are secondary to arteritis.[15] Arteritis can be secondary to Takayasu's arteritis, Raynaud's disease, thromboangiitis obliterans (Buerger's disease), or collagen vascular disease such as rheumatoid arthritis, lupus, or polyarteritis nodosa. The embolus usually originates in the heart and atrial fibrillation is responsible for two thirds of these emboli. A mural thrombus after myocardial infarction is the second most common source of emboli. Noncardiac sources of emboli include tumor, vegetations, prosthetic devices, and thrombi from aneurysms or atheromatous plaques.
- The most common location for an embolus in the leg is the bifurcation of the common femoral artery, followed by the popliteal artery. The brachial artery is the most common site in the upper extremity. Thrombosis can occur at any site of vessel injury.

CLINICAL FEATURES

- Patients with acute arterial limb ischemia typically present with one of the "six P's": Pain, Pallor, Polar (coldness), Pulselessness, Paresthesias, and Paralysis.
- Pain is the earliest symptom and may increase with elevation of the limb. Changes in skin color and temperature are common.
- A decreased pulse distal to the obstruction is an unreliable finding for early ischemia, especially in patients with peripheral vascular disease and well developed collateral circulation.

DIAGNOSIS AND DIFFERENTIAL

- A history of an abruptly ischemic limb in a patient with atrial fibrillation or recent myocardial infarction is strongly suggestive of an embolus. A history of claudication suggests a thrombosis.
- A hand-held Doppler transducer can document flow or its absence over the dorsalis pedis, posterior tibial, popliteal, or femoral arteries in the lower extremity, and over the radial, ulnar, and brachial arteries in the upper extremity.
- The ankle-brachial index (ABI) is the ratio of the systolic blood pressure measured just above the malleoli to the brachial pressure in the arm. With arterial occlusion the ABI is usually markedly diminished (<0.5). A pressure difference of >30 mm Hg between any two adjacent levels can localize the site of obstruction.
- Duplex ultrasonography can detect an obstruction to flow with a sensitivity greater than 85%.
- The diagnostic gold standard is the arteriogram, which can define the anatomy of the obstruction and direct treatment.

EMERGENCY DEPARTMENT CARE AND DISPOSITION

- Patients with acute arterial occlusion should be treated with unfractionated heparin, though there is no equivocal evidence demonstrating the benefit of this practice (see DVT treatment section for dosing guidelines).
- Fluid resuscitation and treatment of heart failure may augment perfusion to the ischemic limb.
- Definitive treatment should be performed in consultation with a vascular surgeon. Catheter embolectomy

using a Fogarty balloon is the preferred method.[15] Other options include thrombolysis and standard surgery.

- All patients with an acute arterial occlusion should be admitted to a telemetry bed or to the ICU, depending on the stability of the patient and the planned course of therapy.

REFERENCES

1. Chengelis DL, Bendick PJ, Glover JL, et al: Progression of superficial venous thrombosis to deep vein thrombosis. *J Vasc Surg* 24:745, 1996.

2. Kearon C, Julian JA, Newman TE, et al: Noninvasive diagnosis of deep venous thrombosis. *Ann Intern Med* 128:663, 1998.

3. American Thoracic Society: The diagnostic approach to acute venous thromboembolism. *Am J Resp Crit Care Med* 160:1043, 1999.

4. Wells PS, Anderson DR, Ginsberg J: Assessment of deep vein thrombosis or pulmonary embolism by the combined use of clinical model and noninvasive diagnostic tests. *Semin Thromb Hemost* 26:643, 2000.

5. Garg SK: Developing venous gangrene in deep vein thrombosis: intraarterial low-dose burst therapy with urokinase: Case reports. *Angiology* 50:157, 1999.

6. Perrier A, Bounameaux H: Cost-effective diagnosis of deep vein thrombosis and pulmonary embolism. *Thromb Haemost* 86:475, 2001.

7. Anderson DR, Wells PS, Steill I, et al: Management of patients with suspected deep vein thrombosis in the emergency department: combining use of a clinical diagnosis model with D-dimer testing. *J Emerg Med* 19:225, 2000.

8. Birdwell BG, Raskob GE, Whitsett TL, et al: The clinical validity of normal compression ultrasonography in outpatients suspected of having deep venous thrombosis. *Ann Intern Med* 128:1, 1998.

9. Hirsh J, Warkentin TE, Shaughnessy SG, et al: Low-molecular-weight heparin. *Chest* 119:64S, 2001.

10. Gould MK, Dembitzer AD, Doyle RL, et al: Low-molecular-weight heparins compared with unfractionated heparin for the treatment of acute deep venous thrombosis: A meta-analysis of randomized controlled trials. *Ann Intern Med* 130:800, 1999.

11. Hirsh J, Dalen JE, Anderson DR, et al: Oral anticoagulants: mechanism of action, clinical effectiveness, and optimal therapeutic range. *Chest* 119:8S, 2001.

12. Wells PS, Forster AJ: Thrombolysis in deep vein thrombosis: Is there still an indication? *Thromb Haemost* 86:499, 2001.

13. Hiatt WR: Medical treatment of peripheral arterial disease and claudication. *N Engl J Med* 344:1608, 2001.

14. Sultan E, Evoy D, Eldin AS, et al: Atraumatic acute upper limb ischemia: A series of 64 patients in Middle East tertiary vascular center and literature review. *J Vasc Surg* 35:181, 2001.

15. Jackson MR, Clagett GP: Antithrombotic therapy in peripheral arterial occlusive disease. *Chest* 119:283S, 2001.

For further reading in *Emergency Medicine: A Comprehensive Study Guide,* 6th ed., see Chap. 59, "Thrombophlebitis and Occlusive Arterial Disease," by Anil Chopra.

32 RESPIRATORY DISTRESS

Matthew T. Keadey

DYSPNEA

PATHOPHYSIOLOGY

- Dyspnea is a subjective feeling of difficult, labored, or uncomfortable breathing. It is a complex sensation, without a defined neural pathway [1]
- Mechanical factors include a sense of skeletal muscle effort dependent on work of breathing and intraparenchymal stretch receptors.
- Chemoreceptors in the central medulla and carotid body respond to changes in CO_2 and O_2, respectively. Receptors in the atria and pulmonary arteries contribute, but in a poorly defined manner.
- Central and peripheral receptors send afferent neurons to the central nervous system (CNS), where the information is integrated in a complex manner.

CLINICAL FEATURES

- Patients may present with complaints of shortness of breath, air hunger, or dyspnea on exertion.
- Signs include tachypnea, tachycardia, difficulty speaking, use of accessory respiratory muscles, and/or stridor.
- The complaint of dyspnea must be rapidly evaluated with immediate identification of abnormal vital signs and abnormalities in the primary survey (airway, breathing, and circulation).[2] Airway obstruction, poor respiratory effort, and altered mental status mandate immediate intervention.
- Lesser degrees of dyspnea allow for a more thorough exam.

DIAGNOSIS AND DIFFERENTIAL

- A detailed history and physical exam will often lead to an accurate diagnosis of dyspnea.[2–4]
- Pulse oximetry provides an immediate assessment of oxygenation, but has poor sensitivity.[3]
- Arterial blood gas analysis (ABG) has improved sensitivity over pulse oximetry, but must be taken in the light of their work of breathing.
- Chest radiograph, electrocardiogram, peak flows, and hematocrit may prove helpful.[4]
- Elevated D-dimer and B-natriuretic peptide may lead to specific diagnoses.[5]
- Other ancillary tests include spirometry, cardiac and exercise stress testing, echocardiography, ventilation-perfusion scans, and lung biopsies.
- Table 32-1 lists common causes of dyspnea.

TABLE 32-1 Causes of Dyspnea

MOST COMMON CAUSES	MOST IMMEDIATELY LIFE-THREATENING
Obstructive airway disease: asthma, COPD	Upper airway obstruction: foreign body, angioedema, hemorrhage
Congestive heart failure/ cardiogenic pulmonary edema	Tension pneumothorax
Ischemic heart disease: unstable angina and myocardial infarction	Pulmonary embolism
Pneumonia	Neuromuscular weakness: myasthenia gravis, Guillain-Barré syndrome, botulism
Psychogenic	

ABBREVIATION: COPD = chronic obstructive pulmonary disease.

EMERGENCY DEPARTMENT CARE AND DISPOSITION

- Immediate priorities include maintaining the airway and supporting respiratory function. Supplemental oxygen is given to anyone in respiratory distress. Patients with chronic obstructive pulmonary disease (COPD) may tolerate lower Pa_{O_2} levels and must be treated symptomatically.[6]
- Noninvasive positive pressure ventilation including continuous positive airway pressure (CPAP) and biphasic positive airway pressure (BiPAP) ventilation may be initiated.
- Bag-valve-mask ventilation followed by endotracheal intubation with mechanical ventilation allow for long-term support.
- Definitive treatment depends on the etiology.
- All patients with an unclear cause of their dyspnea and hypoxia require admission to a monitored bed. Admission otherwise depends on the exact cause of their dyspnea.

HYPOXIA

PATHOPHYSIOLOGY

- Hypoxia is defined as the inadequate delivery of oxygen to the tissues and is caused by one of five mechanisms. Hypoxia is arbitrarily defined as a Pa_{O_2} < 60 mm Hg. Hypoxia is caused by:
  - **Hypoventilation:** rising Pa_{CO_2} displaces O_2 from the alveoli, decreasing the diffusion gradient across the pulmonary membrane.
  - **Right-to-left shunt:** unoxygenated blood enters the systemic circulation. Occurs with congenital heart abnormalities or perfusion of unoxygenated lung segments.
  - **Ventilation-perfusion mismatch:** results from abnormalities of ventilation or perfusion.
  - **Diffusion impairment:** caused by abnormalities of the alveolar-blood barrier.
  - **Low inspired O_2:** only a factor at high altitudes.

CLINICAL FEATURES

- Signs and symptoms are nonspecific, ranging from tachycardia and tachypnea to CNS manifestations such as lethargy, seizures, and coma.[7]
- At a Pa_{O_2} < 20 mm Hg, there is a paradoxical depression of the respiratory drive.
- Dyspnea does not occur sine qua non with hypoxia, and cyanosis is a poor indicator of oxygenation.

DIAGNOSIS AND DIFFERENTIAL

- Pulse oximetry is quick and frequently useful, but ABG analysis defines the diagnosis.
- Similar tests used to determine the cause of dyspnea might also elucidate the cause of hypoxia.

EMERGENCY DEPARTMENT CARE AND DISPOSITION

- Support, identify, and aggressively treat hypoxia, and try to maintain a Pa_{O_2} > 60 mm Hg. Lower Pa_{O_2} levels may be tolerated in COPD.
- All patients require admission until the underlying process is stabilized and or a definitive diagnosis made. Disposition is to a monitored bed.
- Frequent ABGs may require an arterial line for patient comfort.

HYPERCAPNIA

PATHOPHYSIOLOGY

- Hypercapnia is defined as a Pa_{CO_2} > 45 mm Hg and is caused by a decrease in minute ventilation. Minute ventilation is dependent on respiratory rate and tidal volume. Changes in either may lead to hypoventilation and hypercapnia.
- Hypercapnia is almost never due to increased CO_2 production.
- Alveolar ventilation is the product of tidal volume minus the dead space and respiratory rate. This is a more accurate measure of ventilation, but impractical to measure. Dead space is the volume that must be inhaled to reach the alveolus.
- Minute ventilation is controlled via a neural chemoreceptor in the medulla. Efferent outputs control the respiratory rate and tidal volume.

CLINICAL FEATURES

- Signs and symptoms of hypercapnia are not only dependent on the absolute value Pa_{CO_2}, but also the rate of increase.
- Acute elevations of Pa_{CO_2} cause an increase in intracranial pressure, leading to confusion, lethargy, seizures, and coma. Asterixis may be found on physical exam.
- Acute changes in Pa_{CO_2} > 100 mm Hg may lead to cardiovascular collapse.
- In acute hypercapnia, for every 10 mm Hg increase in CO_2, the pH will decrease .1 U.

TABLE 32-2 Causes of Hypercapnia

Depressed central respiratory drive
  Structural CNS disease: brainstem lesions
  Drug depression of respiratory center: opioids, sedatives, anesthetics
  Endogenous toxins: tetanus

Thoracic cage disorders
  Kyphoscoliosis
  Morbid obesity

Neuromuscular impairment
  Neuromuscular disease: myasthenia gravis, Guillain-Barré syndrome
  Neuromuscular toxin: organophosphate poisoning, botulism

Intrinsic lung disease associated with increased dead space
  Chronic obstructive pulmonary disease

Upper airway obstruction

- In chronic hypercapnia, patients may tolerate high levels of CO_2. For every 10 mm Hg increase in CO_2, the $[HCO_3^-]$ increases .35 mEq/L (see Chap. 6).

DIAGNOSIS AND DIFFERENTIAL

- The diagnosis is made by clinical suspicion and confirmed on ABG analysis. Pulse oximetry plays no role in the identification of hypercapnia. See Table 32-2 for further differential diagnoses.

EMERGENCY DEPARTMENT CARE AND DISPOSITION

- Aggressively support, treat, and identify causes of hypercapnia.
- Early identification of the etiology may make treatment options easier. For example, the patient with respiratory depression, pinpoint pupils, and altered mental status may have a heroin overdose that will respond to naloxone, while a patient with amyotrophic lateral sclerosis may only respond to assisted ventilation.
- Oxygen should be given to every patient with respiratory distress and not withheld over concern for decreasing the respiratory drive. Hypoxia will kill a patient, while only extreme hypercapnia will do the same.
- BiPAP or CPAP may be used to increase tidal volume and thus increase minute ventilation. However, if profound hypoxia or the inability to control the airway exists, endotracheal intubation and mechanical ventilation may be required.
- Disposition depends on the underlying cause and frequently requires admission to a monitored bed.

WHEEZES

PATHOPHYSIOLOGY

- Wheezes are high-pitched, musical, adventitious lung sounds produced by turbulent airflow through the central and distal airways.[8]
- Wheezes may occur in normal lungs in small children or during forced expiration. Wheezes are more pronounced in obstructed airways.
- Muscular hypertrophy, increased secretions, bronchospasm, and peribronchial inflammation can cause airway obstruction.

CLINICAL FEATURES

- Wheezes typically occur in asthma and other conditions with reactive airway disease, but "not all that wheezes is asthma." Clinicians must be savvy to recognize the subtle clues of alternate etiologies (Table 32-3).
- Not every patient with reactive airway disease will produce wheezes. Wheezing requires airflow and if airflow is minimal secondary to severe obstruction, no sounds may be heard at all.
- Lung sounds must be interpreted in the context of the clinical situation.

DIAGNOSIS AND DIFFERENTIAL

- Diagnosis is based on clinical suspicion and identification of wheezes upon auscultation of the lungs.
- Asthma and reactive airway disease is suspected in the proper clinical situation, while the patient's work of breathing, clinical exam, and peak expiratory flow

TABLE 32-3 Causes of Wheezing

Upper airway (more likely to be stridor, may have element of wheezing)
  Angioedema: allergic, ACE inhibitor, idiopathic
  Foreign body
  Infection: croup, epiglottis, tracheitis

Lower airway
  Asthma
  Transient airway hyperreactivity (usually caused by infection or irritation)
  Bronchiolitis
  Chronic obstructive pulmonary disease
  Foreign body

Cardiovascular
  Cardiogenic pulmonary edema ("cardiac asthma")
  Noncardiogenic pulmonary edema (ARDS)
  Pulmonary embolus (rare)

Psychogenic

ABBREVIATIONS: ACE = angiotensin-converting enzyme; ARDS = acute respiratory distress syndrome.

rate improves with treatment. Definitive diagnosis depends on spirometric testing, but is impractical in an acute setting.

- Other ancillary tests include a chest radiograph that is frequently helpful in a case of new-onset wheezing or suspicion of pulmonary infiltrates, and an electrocardiogram. In uncomplicated cases of asthma/COPD these tests may not be needed.
- Peak expiratory flow rates may be used to gauge response to treatment and as a measure of severity of airway obstruction. Its limitations include its dependence on effort and inability of children to use it effectively. Any peak flow greater than 80% of the predicted value is considered normal.

EMERGENCY DEPARTMENT DISPOSITION AND CARE

- Initially support, treat, and identify causes of wheezing. Supplemental oxygen is always administered and monitoring may be needed.
- Inhaled bronchodilators are the initial course of therapy (see Chap. 37). Steroids are also acutely used, but are of little help in the acute setting.
- Other agents of unproven significance include parenteral β-agonists, methylxanthines, and magnesium sulfate.
- Admission is required for those who have oxygen requirements or are capable of quick decompensation.

CYANOSIS

PATHOPHYSIOLOGY

- Cyanosis is a bluish color of the skin and mucous membranes resulting from an increased amount of deoxyhemoglobin.
- Typically 5 g/mL of deoxyhemoglobin must be present to produce cyanosis, but this is highly variable.
- Other factors that affect the ability to detect cyanosis include skin thickness and pigmentation, lighting, ambient temperature, and skin microcirculation.

CLINICAL FEATURES

- The presence of cyanosis usually indicates hypoxia, but this is not always the case. The tongue is very sensitive for identifying cyanosis. The earlobes, nail beds, and conjunctiva are less reliable.
- Cyanosis may be central or peripheral. Central cyanosis is usually the result of deoxyhemoglobin. Peripheral cyanosis is the result of poor peripheral cir-

TABLE 32-4   Causes of Cyanosis

CENTRAL CYANOSIS	PERIPHERAL CYANOSIS

Hypoxemia
    Decreased F_{IO_2}: high altitude
    Hypoventilation
    Ventilation-perfusion mismatch
    Right-to-left shunt: congenital heart disease, pulmonary arteriovenous fistulas, multiple intrapulmonary shunts
	Reduced cardiac output
	Cold extremities
	Maldistribution of blood flow: distributive forms of shock
	Arterial or venous obstruction

Hemoglobin abnormalities
    Methemoglobinemia: hereditary, acquired
    Sulfhemoglobinemia: acquired
    Carboxyhemoglobinemia (not true cyanosis)	

ABBREVIATION: F_{IO_2} = fraction of inspired oxygen.

culation, leading to increased oxygen extraction by the peripheral tissues.

DIAGNOSIS AND DIFFERENTIAL

- The presence of cyanosis must be taken in the context of the clinical situation (Table 32-4).
- ABG analysis will confirm the presence of hypoxia leading to cyanosis.
- Other useful tests include a hematocrit to detect anemia or polycythemia vera, a chest radiograph, and an electrocardiogram.
- Pseudocyanosis should be considered in any asymptomatic patient, but it should be a diagnosis of exclusion. Pseudocyanosis is caused by abnormal skin pigmentation, giving the skin a bluish or silver hue. Causative agents include heavy metals (iron, gold, lead, and silver) and certain drugs (phenothiazines, minocycline, amiodarone, and chloroquine).
- Methemoglobinemia, carboxyhemoglobin, and other acquired hemoglobinopathies, although rare, must be considered in certain clinical situations. Methemoglobinemia will turn blood a chocolate brown that will not turn red when exposed to air. Carboxyhemoglobin will cause an atypical cherry-pink cyanosis. It is important to identify these acquired hemoglobinopathies because they can be quickly and easily treated.

EMERGENCY DEPARTMENT CARE AND DISPOSITION

- Aggressive support, treatment, and identification of cyanosis are always indicated. Supplemental oxygen is an appropriate first-line treatment. If the patient is unresponsive to supplemental oxygen, poor perfusion, acquired hemoglobinopathies, or large right-to-left shunts may be present.

- Specific antidotes exist, including methylene blue (1 to 2 mg/kg IV) for methemoglobinemia, and supplemental oxygen possibly including hyperbaric treatments for carboxyhemoglobin poisoning.
- All patients with an unknown cause of cyanosis require admission until the condition is stabilized or definitively identified.

REFERENCES

1. Scano G, Ambrosion N: Pathophysiology of dyspnea. *Lung* 180:131, 2002.
2. Sharma OP: Symptoms and signs in pulmonary medicine: Old observations and new interpretations. *Dis Mon* 41:577, 1995.
3. American Thoracic Society: Dyspnea. Mechanism, assessment and management: A consensus statement. *Am J Respir Care Med* 159:321, 1999.
4. Morgan WC, Hodge HL: Diagnostic evaluation of dyspnea. *Am Fam Physician* 15:711, 1998.
5. McCullough PA, Nowak RM, McCord J, et al: B-type natriuretic peptide and clinical judgment in emergency diagnosis of heart failure: Analysis from Breathing Not Properly (BNP) Multinational Study. *Circulation* 106:416, 2002.
6. Thomas JR, von Gunten CF: Clinical management of dyspnea. *Lancet Oncol* 3:223, 2002.
7. Usen S, Webert M: Clinical signs of hypoxemia in children with acute lower respiratory infection: Indicators for oxygen therapy. *Int J Tuberc Lung Dis* 5:505, 2001.
8. Pasterknap H, Kraman SS, Wodicka GR: Respiratory sounds: Advances beyond the stethoscope. *Am J Respir Crit Care Med* 156:974, 1997.

For further reading in *Emergency Medicine: A Comprehensive Study Guide,* 6th ed., see Chap. 62, "Respiratory Distress," by J. Stephen Stapczynski.

33 BRONCHITIS, PNEUMONIA, AND SARS

David M. Cline

BRONCHITIS

EPIDEMIOLOGY

- Uncomplicated acute bronchitis (UAB) refers to an acute respiratory tract infection in which cough, occasionally with phlegm, is the predominant feature.[1]
- UAB usually lasts 1 to 3 weeks, but may last longer. Approximately 5% of adults in the United States report an episode of UAB each year, typically between October and March.[1]

PATHOPHYSIOLOGY

- UAB is an infection of the conducting airways of the lung. Respiratory viruses cause the vast majority of cases of UAB. Influenza B, influenza A, parainfluenza, and respiratory syncytial virus (RSV) are the most often implicated.[2]
- *Bordetella pertussis, Mycoplasma pneumoniae, Chlamydia pneumoniae,* and *Legionella* species are reported in 5 to 25% of cases of UAB.[1,3]
- Acute bronchitis in adults from *Bordetella pertussis* and parapertussis does not produce the characteristic whooping cough as these infections do in children.[3]
- *Bordetella pertussis, Mycoplasma pneumoniae,* and *Chlamydia pneumoniae* are recovered in 10 to 20% of adults with chronic or persistent cough lasting more than 2 to 3 weeks.[1]

CLINICAL FEATURES

- The cough of UAB is commonly productive and may last up to 2 months.[1]
- The presence of purulent sputum is unimportant in diagnosing or treating UAB unless other symptoms and signs suggest pneumonia. Fever >38°C (100.4°F), heart rate >100 bpm, respiratory rate >24 breaths/min, and chills suggest pneumonia; less than 10% of patients with UAB are febrile.
- The strongest independent predictors of UAB are cough and wheezing; nausea is the strongest negative predictor of UAB.[4]
- Approximately one third of patients presenting with symptoms of UAB may have asthma.[5]

DIAGNOSIS AND DIFFERENTIAL

- Clinical diagnosis of UAB is made with the following: (1) acute cough (less than 2 weeks), (2) no prior lung disease, and (3) no auscultatory abnormalities that suggest pneumonia.
- Pulse oximetry is indicated if the patient describes dyspnea or appears short of breath.
- Sputum Gram's stain and culture are not recommended for the routine diagnosis of UAB.[1]
- Bedside peak flow testing is indicated if wheezing is heard on examination.
- A chest radiograph is not required in patients who

appear nontoxic unless they have had symptoms for more than 3 weeks.

EMERGENCY DEPARTMENT CARE AND DISPOSITION

- Unless pertussis is a consideration, antibiotics do not improve the cough of UAB, but commonly produce side effects including nausea, vomiting, or vaginitis.[1,2]
- Patients with evidence of airflow obstruction should be treated with bronchodilators.[6] Albuterol by metered dose inhaler, 2 puffs q4h to q6h, is usually effective. Otherwise, supportive treatment is the rule.
- Cough suppression with a nonnarcotic or narcotic agent should be considered on an individual basis, taking into account comorbidities, sleep patterns, and potential side effects.

PNEUMONIA

EPIDEMIOLOGY

- Community-acquired pneumonia (CAP) is a common medical problem, accounting for about 4 million cases and 1 million hospitalizations per year in the United States.[7]
- Pneumonia is the sixth leading cause of death in the United States. Bacterial causes are the most common.

PATHOPHYSIOLOGY

- Pneumonia is an infection of the alveolar or gas exchange portions of the lung. Some forms of pneumonia produce an intense inflammatory response within the alveoli that leads to filling the air space with organisms, exudate, and white blood cells.
- Patients most at risk for pneumonia are those with a predisposition to aspiration, impaired mucociliary clearance, or risk of bacteremia.
- Pneumococcus is still the most common cause of bacterial pneumonia, with *Escherichia coli, Pseudomonas aeruginosa, Klebsiella pneumoniae, Staphylococcus aureus, Haemophilus influenzae,* and group A streptococci accounting for most of the rest.
- *Legionella* species and anaerobes are less frequent causes of bacterial pneumonia, with the latter primarily the result of aspiration.
- *Mycoplasma, Chlamydia,* and respiratory viruses account for the bulk of atypical pneumonia, which account for a third or more of all cases of pneumonia.
- Patients with chronic diseases, such as congestive heart failure, cancer, bronchiectasis, chronic obstruc-

tive pulmonary disease (COPD), diabetes, sickle-cell anemia, AIDS, and other immunodeficiencies, are at greater risk for pneumonia, as are smokers and postsplenectomy patients.
- Aspiration pneumonia occurs more frequently in alcoholics and patients with seizures, stroke, or other neuromuscular diseases.
- *Pneumocystis carinii* pneumonia is a common complication of HIV infection and is discussed in Chap. 91.

CLINICAL FEATURES

- Patients with bacterial pneumonia generally present with some combination of fever, dyspnea, cough, pleuritic chest pain, and sputum production.[7] Pneumococcal infection classically presents abruptly with fever, rigors, and rusty brown sputum. Pleural effusion occurs in 25% of patients.
- *Haemophilus influenzae* is more common in smokers and the elderly. *Staphylococcus aureus* frequently follows a viral respiratory illness, especially influenza and measles.
- Pneumonia due to *Legionella* is spread via airborne aerosolized water droplets rather than by person-to-person contact. This form of pneumonia presents as do *Mycoplasma, Chlamydia,* and viral pneumonia, with fever, chills, malaise, dyspnea, and a nonproductive cough. *Legionella* also commonly causes gastrointestinal symptoms of anorexia, nausea, vomiting, and diarrhea. Mental status changes may also be present.
- Physical findings of pneumonia vary with the offending organism and the type of pneumonia each causes, although most are associated with some degree of tachypnea and tachycardia.[8]
- Lobar pneumonias, such as those caused by pneumococcus and *Klebsiella,* exhibit signs of consolidation, including bronchial breath sounds, egophony, increased tactile and vocal fremitus, and dullness to percussion. A pleural friction rub and cyanosis may be present.
- Bronchopneumonias, such as those caused by *H. influenzae,* reveal rales and rhonchi on examination, without signs of consolidation. A parapneumonic pleural effusion may occur in either setting; empyemas are most common with *S. aureus, Klebsiella,* and anaerobic infections.
- *Legionella,* which begins with findings of patchy bronchopneumonia and progresses to signs of frank consolidation, has other common signs, including a relative bradycardia and confusion.
- Interstitial pneumonias, such as those caused by viruses, *Mycoplasma,* and *Chlamydia,* may exhibit fine rales, rhonchi, or normal breath sounds. Bullous

myringitis, when present in this setting, is pathogno
monic for *Mycoplasma* infection.

- Clinical features of aspiration pneumonitis depend on
the volume and pH of the aspirate, the presence of
particulate matter in the aspirate, and bacterial contamination. Although acid aspiration results in the rapid
onset of symptoms of tachypnea, tachycardia, and
cyanosis, and often progresses to frank pulmonary
failure, most other cases of aspiration pneumonia
progress more insidiously.
- Physical signs of aspiration pneumonia develop over
hours and include rales, rhonchi, wheezing, and copious frothy or bloody sputum. The right lower lobe is
most commonly involved due to the anatomy of the
tracheobronchial tree and to gravity.

DIAGNOSIS AND DIFFERENTIAL

- The diagnosis is suspected based on a constellation of
symptoms and signs, but individual symptoms and
clinical findings lack accuracy for precise diagnosis.[9]
- For an accurate diagnosis, a chest radiograph is
required.[9]
- Other tests include a white blood count with differential count, pulse oximetry analysis, blood cultures,
and pleural fluid examination. Arterial blood gas
analysis may be performed in ill-appearing patients.
- Sputum Gram's stain rarely changes therapy.[9]
- If *Legionella* is being considered, serum chemistry
studies and liver function tests should be performed,
as hyponatremia, hypophosphatemia, and elevated
liver enzymes are commonly found. Also, when appropriate, urine should be tested for *Legionella* antigen, and serologic testing for *Mycoplasma* can be performed, although these tests will have no impact on
the emergency management of the patient.
- Results of bedside cold agglutinin tests may be positive in cases of *Mycoplasma,* but are nonspecific.
- Most patients do not require identification of a specific organism.
- The differential diagnosis includes acute tracheobronchitis; pulmonary embolus or infarction; exacerbation
of COPD; pulmonary vasculitides, including Goodpasture's disease and Wegener's granulomatosis;
bronchiolitis obliterans; and endocarditis.

EMERGENCY DEPARTMENT CARE
AND DISPOSITION

- The emergency department treatment and disposition
of pneumonia depends primarily on the severity of the
clinical presentation and radiographic findings.[10]

- Oxygen should be administered as needed and antibiotic treatment should be initiated.
- Outpatient management is standard in otherwise
healthy patients who are nontoxic and without significant comorbid diseases.[7,10] Antibiotic choices include
azithromycin 500 mg on day 1 followed by 250 mg
daily for 4 additional days, clarithromycin 500 mg bid
for 10 days, cefpodoxime 200 mg bid for 10 days, or
amoxicillin-clavulanate 875 mg PO bid for 10 days.
Doxycycline 100 mg bid for 10 days is a low-cost
alternative.
- Oral fluoroquinolones, such as levofloxacin 500 mg
daily, moxifloxacin 400 mg daily, or gatifloxacin
400 mg daily for 10 to 14 days, are highly effective; however, because their overuse may promote
fluoroquinolone-resistant pneumonia, the CDC recommends reserving these agents for those who cannot tolerate or have failed other agents.
- For outpatient management of patients over 60 years old
or those with comorbid diseases, levofloxacin is a
good choice as a single agent. Otherwise, azithromycin
or clarithromycin in combination with either cefuroxime 500 mg orally daily for 10 days or amoxicillin-
clavulanate 875 mg PO twice a day for 10 days are excellent dual drug regimens.
- Close follow-up is necessary to monitor response to
therapy.
- Hospital admission should be reserved for patients at
the extremes of life, immunocompromised patients,
pregnant women, and those with clinical signs of toxicity (ie, respiratory rate >30 breaths/min, heart rate
over 125 bpm, systolic blood pressure <90 mm Hg,
hypoxemia, altered mental status, or volume depletion) or serious comorbid conditions (eg, neoplastic
disease, renal failure, diabetes, cardiac disease, or debilitated state).
- Patients requiring admission generally also receive empiric antibiotic therapy. Early antibiotic administration
in the ED may shorten the patient's hospital stay. Recommended treatments include ceftriaxone 1 to 2 g IV
daily, levofloxacin 500 mg IV daily, cefotaxime 1 to 2 g
IV every 8 hours, ampicillin-sulbactam 3 g IV every
6 hours, piperacillin-tazobactam 3.375 g every 6 hours,
or cefepime 1 to 2 g every 12 hours.
- Patients at high risk for gram-negative pneumonia or
Legionella (eg, alcoholics, diabetics, and institutionalized or intubated patients) should be treated with
either levofloxacin as monotherapy or with a combination of a macrolide such as erythromycin 1 g IV every
6 hours and either ampicillin-sulbactam 3 g IV every
6 hours or ceftriaxone 1 to 2 g IV daily.
- If *Pseudomonas* is suspected, double coverage with
an antipseudomonal penicillin (eg, ticarcillin) or
cephalosporin (eg, ceftazidime) plus either an antipseudomonal aminoglycoside (eg, tobramycin) or a
fluoroquinolone (eg, ciprofloxacin) is recommended.

- Local antibiotic sensitivities and resistance patterns, as well as local standards of care, should help determine final antibiotic selection.
- Aspiration pneumonitides require a different therapeutic approach. Witnessed aspirations should be treated with immediate tracheal suctioning, and the pH of the aspirate should be ascertained. Bronchoscopy is indicated for the removal of large particles and for further clearing of the airways. Patients requiring intubation should also be treated with positive end-expiratory pressure. Oxygen should be administered, but steroids and prophylactic antibiotics are of no value and should be withheld. For patients at risk of aspiration who present with signs and symptoms of infection, antibiotics are indicated. Levofloxacin 500 mg/day IV or PO, or ceftriaxone 1 to 2 g/day IV or IM, are sufficient for most cases of aspiration. In cases of severe periodontal disease, putrid sputum, or alcoholism, consider piperacillin-tazobactam 3.375 g every 6 hours or imipenem 500 mg every 8 hours or a fluoroquinolone plus clindamycin 600 mg every 8 hours.
- Failure of outpatient therapy generally requires hospital admission and broader-spectrum intravenous antibiotics. Patients with hypoxemia despite oxygen therapy or those with impending respiratory failure should be treated with endotracheal intubation and mechanical ventilation.

SEVERE ACUTE RESPIRATORY SYNDROME (SARS)

Up-to-date information regarding SARS can be found at the Centers for Disease Control and Prevention (CDC) web site: http://www.cdc.gov/ncidod/sars/, or by phone at 770-488-7100.

EPIDEMIOLOGY

- SARS came to worldwide attention in the winter of 2002–2003. Numerous deaths were reported in Asia, North America, and Europe.

PATHOPHYSIOLOGY

- The etiologic agent is a coronavirus, SARS-CoV.

CLINICAL FEATURES

- SARS should be considered in symptomatic individuals who have traveled to an area with current or previously documented or suspected community transmission of SARS. Currently those areas include China (mainland), Hong Kong, Hanoi, Singapore, Toronto, Taiwan, and Beijing.
- SARS also should be considered in symptomatic individuals with close contact within 10 days of symptom onset with a person known or suspected to have SARS.
- Moderate disease is defined as temperature >100.4°F (>38°C) and one or more findings of cough, shortness of breath, difficult breathing, or hypoxia.
- Severe respiratory illness is defined as criteria for moderate disease plus radiographic evidence of pneumonia, respiratory distress syndrome, or findings at autopsy.

DIAGNOSIS AND DIFFERENTIAL

- Initial diagnostic testing for suspected SARS patients should include chest radiograph, pulse oximetry, blood cultures, sputum Gram's stain and culture, and testing for viral respiratory pathogens, notably influenza A and B and RSV.
- Any patient who meets exposure and clinical criteria for SARS should be reported to local health agencies and have confirmatory testing.
- At this writing, the recommendation is for the testing of nasopharyngeal, oropharyngeal, and serum samples.
- Local health agencies and the CDC can provide additional information concerning testing and isolation procedures.

EMERGENCY DEPARTMENT CARE AND DISPOSITION

- No specific treatment recommendations can be made at this time.
- Clinicians evaluating suspected cases should use standard precautions (eg, hand hygiene) together with airborne (eg, N-95 respirator) and contact (eg, gowns and gloves) precautions. Consider eye protection.
- Empiric therapy should include coverage for organisms associated with any community-acquired pneumonia of unclear etiology, including agents with activity against both typical and atypical respiratory pathogens. Treatment choices may be influenced by severity of the illness. See section above.
- Infectious disease consultation is recommended.

REFERENCES

1. Gonzales R, Bartlett JG, Besser RE, et al: Principles of appropriate antibiotic use for treatment of uncomplicated acute bronchitis: Background. *Ann Intern Med* 134:521, 2001.

2. Macfarlane J, Holmes W, Gard P, et al: Prospective study of the incidence, etiology, and outcome of adult lower respiratory tract illness in the community. *Thorax* 56:109, 2001.

3. Bent S, Saint S, Vittinghoff E, Grady D: Antibiotics in acute bronchitis: A meta-analysis. *Am J Med* 107:62, 2001.

4. Hueston W, Mainous A, Dacus E, et al: Does acute bronchitis really exist? A reconceptualization of acute viral respiratory infections. *J Fam Pract* 49:401, 2000.

5. Thaidens H, Postma D, deBock G, et al: Asthma in adult patients presenting with symptoms of acute bronchitis in general practice. *Scand J Prim Health Care* 18:188, 2000.

6. Smucny J, Flynn C, Becher L, Glazier R: Are beta 2-agonists effective treatment for acute bronchitis or acute cough inpatients without underlying pulmonary disease? A systematic review. *J Fam Pract* 15:945, 2001

7. Halm EA, Teirstein AS: Management of community acquired pneumonia. *N Engl J Med* 347:2039, 2002.

8. Metlay JP, Kapoor WN, Fine MJ: Does this patient have community-acquired pneumonia? Diagnosing pneumonia by history and physical examination. *JAMA* 278:1440, 1997.

9. Theerthakarai R, El-Halees W, Ismail M, et al: Nonvalue of the initial microbiological studies in the management of non-severe community-acquired pneumonia. *Chest* 119:181, 2001.

10. Niederman MS, Mandell LA, Anqueto A, et al: Guidelines for the management of adults with community-acquired pneumonia. Diagnosis, assessment of severity, antimicrobial therapy, and prevention. *Am J Respir Crit Care Med* 163:1730, 2001.

For further reading in *Emergency Medicine: A Comprehensive Study Guide,* 6th ed., see Chap. 63, "Bronchitis, Pneumonia, and Pleural Empyema," by Donald A. Moffa, Jr. and Charles L. Emerman; and Chap. 64, "Aspiration Pneumonia and Lung Abscess," by Eric Anderson.

34 TUBERCULOSIS

Amy J. Behrman

EPIDEMIOLOGY

- Tuberculosis (TB) remains a major global problem. More than 30% of the world's population has latent or active TB which causes 2 million deaths yearly.[1]
- The incidence of TB in the United States rose sharply between 1984 and 1992, driven by factors including rising rates of incarceration, human immunodeficiency virus (HIV) infection, drug-resistant TB strains, and immigration from areas with endemic TB.[2]
- Stronger TB control programs targeting high-risk groups have reversed this trend; since 1993, U.S. TB case rates have fallen steadily..
- Rates remain disproportionately high in foreign-born persons, who account for nearly half of all U.S. cases.[3] Other populations with increased prevalence include HIV patients, the elderly and nursing home residents, alcoholics and illicit drug users, and residents and staff of prisons and homeless shelters.
- Patients with unrecognized TB frequently present to emergency departments (EDs) for evaluation and care, presenting challenges for diagnosis, treatment, and infection control.

PATHOPHYSIOLOGY

- *Mycobacterium tuberculosis* is a slow-growing aerobic rod with a unique, multilayered cell wall containing a variety of lipids that account for its acid-fast property.
- Transmission occurs through inhalation of droplet nuclei into the lungs. Persons with active tuberculosis who excrete stainable mycobacteria in saliva or sputum are the most infectious.[4]
- Hematogenous dissemination may occur. Survival of this organism is favored in areas of high oxygen content or blood flow, such as the apical and posterior segments of the upper lobe and the superior segment of the lower lobe of the lung, the renal cortex, the meninges, the epiphyses of long bones, and the vertebrae.[4]
- Latent tuberculosis infections (LTBI) are asymptomatic with positive tuberculin skin tests. LTBI will progress to active disease in 5% of cases within 2 years of primary infection; an additional 5% will reactivate over their lifetimes.[1] Reactivation rates are higher in the young, the elderly, persons with recent primary infection, those with immune deficiency (particularly HIV), and those with chronic diseases such as diabetes and renal failure.

CLINICAL FEATURES

- Primary TB infection is usually asymptomatic, presenting most frequently with only a new positive reaction to TB skin testing. Some patients may, however, present with active pneumonitis or extrapulmonary disease. Immunocompromised patients are much more likely to develop rapidly progressive primary infections.[1]
- Reactivation of LTBI accounts for most active cases. Patients with active TB usually present subacutely with fever, cough, weight loss, fatigue, and night sweats.

- Most patients with active TB have pulmonary involvement characterized by constitutional symptoms and (usually productive) cough. Hemoptysis, pleuritic chest pain, and dyspnea may develop.
- Rales and rhonchi may be found, but the pulmonary exam is usually nondiagnostic.[4]
- Extrapulmonary TB develops in up to 15% of cases.[4] Lymphadenitis, with painless enlargement and possible draining sinuses, is the most common example.
- Pleural effusion may occur when a peripheral parenchymal focus or local lymph node ruptures. Pericarditis with typical symptoms may develop by extension of infection from local lymph nodes or pleura.
- TB peritonitis usually presents insidiously after extension from local lymph nodes.
- TB meningitis may follow hematogenous spread, presenting with fever, headache, meningeal signs, and/or cranial nerve deficits.
- Miliary TB is a multisystem disease caused by massive hematogenous dissemination. It is most common in immunocompromised hosts and children. Symptoms and findings may include fever, cough, weight loss, adenopathy, hepatosplenomegaly, and cytopenias.
- Extrapulmonary TB may also involve bone, joints, skin, kidneys, and adrenals.
- Immunocompromised patients, and HIV patients in particular, are extremely susceptible to TB and far more likely to develop active infections with atypical presentations.[5] Disseminated extrapulmonary TB is also more common in HIV patients and should be considered in the evaluation of nonpulmonary complaints.[4,5]
- Prior partially treated TB is a risk factor for drug-resistant TB. It should be considered when TB is diagnosed, especially among those with suboptimal prior care, such as immigrants from endemic areas, prisoners, homeless persons, and drug users.
- Multidrug-resistant TB (MDR TB) is also more common in HIV patients than the general population and has a higher fatality rate in this group.[4,5]

DIAGNOSIS AND DIFFERENTIAL

- Consider the diagnosis of TB in any patient with respiratory or systemic complaints to facilitate early diagnosis, protect hospital staff, and make appropriate dispositions.
- Chest x-rays (CXRs) are the most useful diagnostic tool for active TB in the ED.[4] Active primary TB usually presents with parenchymal infiltrates in any lung area. Hilar and/or mediastinal adenopathy may occur with or without infiltrates. Lesions may calcify.

- Reactivation TB typically presents with lesions in the upper lobes or superior segments of the lower lobes. Cavitation, calcification, scarring, atelectasis, and effusions may be seen.[4] Cavitation is associated with increased infectivity.[4]
- Miliary TB may cause diffuse small (1- to 3-mm) nodular infiltrates.
- Patients coinfected with HIV and TB are particularly likely to present with atypical or even normal CXRs.[5]
- Acid-fast staining of sputum can detect mycobacteria in 60% of patients with pulmonary TB, although the yield is less in HIV patients. Atypical mycobacteria can yield false-positives. Many patients will have false-negatives on a single sputum sample. Microscopy of nonsputum samples (eg, pleural fluid, cerebrospinal fluid [CSF]) is even less sensitive.
- Definitive cultures generally take weeks, but new genetic tests employing DNA probes or polymerase chain reaction technology can confirm the diagnosis in hours.[4]
- Mantoux testing (intradermal tuberculin skin testing with purified protein derivative [PPD]) identifies most patients with latent, prior, or active TB infection. Results are read 48 to 72 hours after placement, limiting the usefulness of this test for ED patients. Persons with positive PPDs and no active TB disease should be evaluated for prophylactic treatment with INH to prevent reactivation TB.
- Patients with HIV or other immunosuppressive conditions and patients with disseminated TB may have false-negative skin tests even if not fully anergic.[6]

EMERGENCY DEPARTMENT CARE AND DISPOSITION

- Initial therapy should include at least four drugs until susceptibility profiles are available for the patient.[1,7] Beginning therapy usually includes isoniazid (INH), rifampin, pyrazinamide, and either streptomycin or ethambutol for 2 months. At least two drugs (usually INH and rifampin) are continued for four more months.
- Patients with immune compromise or MDR TB may require more drugs for longer periods.
- Table 34-1 summarizes usual initial daily drug doses and side effects.
- Patients with active TB who are discharged from the ED must have documented immediate referral to a public health department or qualified physician for long-term treatment and monitoring of drug toxicity. Patients should be educated about home isolation, follow-up, and screening of household contacts.
- Directly observed treatment (DOT) has improved

TABLE 34-1 Dosages and Common Side Effects of Some Drugs Used in Tuberculosis

DRUG	DAILY DOSE (MAX)	POTENTIAL SIDE EFFECTS
Isoniazid (INH)	Adult: 5 mg/kg (300 mg) Child: 10–20 mg/kg (300 mg) Route: PO	Hepatitis, neuritis, abdominal pain, acidosis, hypersensitivity, drug interactions
Rifampin	Adult: 10 mg/kg (600 mg) Child: 10–20 mg/kg (600 mg) Route: PO	Hepatitis, thrombocytopenia, GI disturbance, fever, drug interactions
Pyrazinamide	Adult: 15–30 mg/kg (2 g) Child: same Route: PO	Hepatitis, rash, arthralgia, GI disturbance, hyperuricemia
Ethambutol	Adult: 15–20 mg/kg (1.6 g) Child: same Route: PO	Optic neuritis, headache, peripheral neuropathy, GI disturbance
Ciprofloxacin	Adult: 750 mg bid Child: contraindicated Route: PO	Arthropathy, GI disturbance CNS disturbance
Streptomycin	Adult: 15 mg/kg (1 g) Child: 20–30 mg/kg (1 g) Route: IM	Eighth cranial neuropathy, rash, renal failure, proteinuria

ABBREVIATIONS: bid = twice daily, CNS = central nervous system, GI = gastrointestinal, IM = intramuscularly, PO = orally.

treatment outcomes for populations at high risk for noncompliance and the development of MDR TB.[8]

- Admission is indicated for clinical instability, diagnostic uncertainty, unreliable outpatient follow-up or compliance, and active known MDR TB. Physicians should know local laws regarding involuntary hospitalization and treatment.[9]
- Admission to respiratory or droplet isolation is mandatory for all cases of suspected TB.
- ED staff should be trained to identify patients at risk for active TB as early as possible in their ED and prehospital course. Patients with suspected TB should be masked or placed in respiratory isolation rooms.[10]
- Staff caring directly for patients with suspected TB should wear OSHA-approved respirator-masks.[10]
- ED staff should receive regular PPD skin testing to detect new primary infections, rule out active disease, and consider INH prophylaxis.[7,10]

REFERENCES

1. Small PM, Fujiwara PI: Management of tuberculosis in the United States. *N Engl J Med* 345:189, 2001.
2. Brudney K, Dobkin J: Resurgent tuberculosis in New York City. *Am Rev Respir Dis* 144:745, 1991.
3. Centers for Disease Control: Tuberculosis morbidity among US-born and foreign-born populations—United States, 2000. *Morb Mortal Wkly Rep* 51:101, 2000.
4. Rossman MD, MacGregor RR: *Tuberculosis*. New York: McGraw-Hill, 1995.
5. Havlir DV, Barnes PF: Tuberculosis in patients with human immunodeficiency virus infection. *N Engl J Med* 340:367, 1999.
6. Slovis BS, Plitman JD, Haas DW: The case against anergy testing as a routine adjunct to tuberculin skin testing. *JAMA* 283:2003, 2000.
7. American Thoracic Society: Targeted tuberculin testing and treatment of latent tuberculosis infection. *Am J Respir Crit Care Med* 157:729, 2000.
8. Nitta AT, Knowles KS, Kim J, et al: Limited transmission of multidrug-resistant tuberculosis despite a high proportion of infectious cases in Los Angeles County, California. *Am J Respir Crit Care Med* 165:812, 2002.
9. Gostin LO: Controlling the resurgent tuberculosis epidemic: A 50-state survey of TB statutes and proposals for reform. *JAMA* 269:255, 1993.
10. Behman AJ, Shofer FS: Tuberculosis exposure and control in an urban emergency department. *Ann Emerg Med* 31:370, 1998.

For further reading in *Emergency Medicine: A Comprehensive Study Guide,* 6th ed., see Chap. 65, "Tuberculosis," by Janet M Poponick.

35 PNEUMOTHORAX

Rodney L. McCaskill

EPIDEMIOLOGY

- Spontaneous pneumothorax occurs primarily in male smokers with a large height to weight ratio and probably results from bleb rupture.[1]
- Secondary pneumothorax occurs most often in patients with chronic obstructive pulmonary disease (COPD), but other underlying lung diseases such as asthma, cystic fibrosis, interstitial lung disease, cancer, and *Pneumocystis carinii* pneumonia have been implicated.[2]
- Iatrogenic pneumothorax occurs secondary to invasive procedures such as needle biopsy of the lung (50%), subclavian line placement (25%), nasogastric tube placement, or positive pressure ventilation, and should always be ruled out by a postprocedure chest x-ray.

PATHOPHYSIOLOGY

- Pneumothorax occurs when air enters the potential space between the parietal and visceral pleura leading to partial lung collapse.
- Tension pneumothorax is caused by positive pressure in the pleural space leading to decreased venous return, hypotension, and hypoxia.

CLINICAL FEATURES

- Symptoms resulting from a pneumothorax are directly related to the size, rate of development, and underlying lung disease.
- Acute onset pleuritic pain is found in 95%.[3]
- Dyspnea occurs in 80% and predicts a large pneumothorax.[3]
- Decreased breath sounds on the affected side are present 85% of the time.[3]
- Only 5% have tachypnea over 24 breaths per minute.[3]
- Electrocardiographic changes, including ST changes and T-wave inversion may be seen with pneumothorax.[4]

DIAGNOSIS AND DIFFERENTIAL

- The diagnosis of tension pneumothorax is based on clinical features including hypoxia, hypotension, distended neck veins, displaced trachea, and unilaterally decreased breath sounds. The gold standard for diagnosis is an upright posteroanterior chest x-ray, but it is only 83% sensitive.
- Expiratory films may slightly enhance visualization.[5]
- CT scan may be more sensitive.
- Recent studies have shown the sensitivity of ultrasound to be near 100%.[6]
- Differential diagnosis includes costochondritis, angina, myocardial infarction, pulmonary embolism, pericarditis, pleurisy, and pneumonia.

EMERGENCY DEPARTMENT CARE AND DISPOSITION

- Oxygen 2 to 4 L by nasal cannula helps increase resorption of pleural air.[7]
- In unstable patients (those with tension pneumothorax or pneumothorax with severe underlying lung disease), needle thoracostomy followed by tube thoracostomy should be performed before x-ray.
- Since pleural air is slowly resorbed, patients with small, spontaneous, asymptomatic pneumothoraces may be observed for 6 hours and discharged with surgical follow-up if there is no enlargement on x-ray; but 23 to 40% eventually will require tube thoracostomy.[7]
- Small asymptomatic pneumothoraces may be aspirated using a catheter and discharged with surgical follow-up at 6 hours if there is no recurrence.
- Tube thoracostomy is indicated for failed aspiration, recurrent pneumothorax, underlying lung disease, or abnormal vital signs.
- Helicopter transport, general anesthesia, or mechanical ventilation may also be indications for tube thoracostomy.

REFERENCES

1. Baumann MH, Strange C: The clinician's perspective on pneumothorax management. *Chest* 112:822, 1997.
2. Jantz MA, Pierson DJ: Pneumothorax and barotrauma. *Respir Emerg* 15:75, 1994.
3. Abolnik IZ, Lossos IS, Gillis D, Breuer R: Primary spontaneous pneumothorax in men. *Am J Med Sci* 305:297, 1993.
4. Kirby TJ, Ginsberg RJ: Management of the pneumothorax and barotrauma. *Clin Chest Med* 13:97, 1992.
5. Seow A, Kazerooni EA, Pernicano PG, Neary M: Comparison of upright inspiratory and expiratory chest radiographs for detecting pneumothoraces. *Am J Roentgenol* 166:313, 1996.
6. Rowan KR, Kirkpatrick AW, Lui D, et al: Traumatic pneumothorax detection with thoracic US: Correlation with chest radiography and CT—Initial experience. *Radiology* 225:210, 2002.

7. Baumann MH, Strange C: Treatment of spontaneous pneumothorax: A more aggressive approach? *Chest* 112:789, 1997.

For further reading in *Emergency Medicine: A Comprehensive Study Guide*, 6th ed., see Chap. 66, "Spontaneous and Iatrogenic Pneumothorax," by William Franklin Young, Jr. and Roger Loyd Humphries.

36 HEMOPTYSIS

James E. Winslow

EPIDEMIOLOGY

- Hemoptysis is defined as mild (less than 5 mL of blood seen in 24 hours), moderate, or massive (greater than 600 mL of blood seen in 24 hours).[1]
- The most common causes include infection (including tuberculosis), neoplasm, and cardiovascular disease. No cause is found in 28% of cases.[2]
- Hemoptysis is found in all age groups with a 60:40 male predominance.[3]

PATHOPHYSIOLOGY

- The lung has dual blood supply from the pulmonary and bronchial arteries. Bleeding may originate from either.
- Mechanism of bleeding is due to (1) increased intravascular pressure, (2) erosion by an inflammatory process into a blood vessel, or (3) complication of a bleeding diathesis.
- Hemoptysis due to increased intravascular pressure generally arises from a primary cardiac abnormality such as congestive heart failure (75% of cardiac cases), or less commonly, mitral stenosis.
- Erosion into bronchial vessels, which are under systemic pressure, can lead to severe hemoptysis. This is often due to tuberculosis or bronchiectasis.

CLINICAL FEATURES

- The acute onset of fever, cough, and bloody sputum suggests pneumonia or bronchitis. A more indolent productive cough may represent bronchitis or bronchiectasis.
- Dyspnea and pleuritic chest pain may be hallmarks of pulmonary embolism.

- Fever, night sweats, and weight loss often reflect TB or malignancy. Chronic dyspnea and minor hemoptysis may represent mitral stenosis or alveolar hemorrhage syndromes (often associated with renal disease).
- Smoking, male gender, and age greater than 40 years are the main risk factors for neoplasm.
- The physical examination is aimed at assessing the severity of hemoptysis and the underlying disease process, but is unreliable in localizing the site of bleeding.[4]
- Common signs include fever and tachypnea. Hypotension is rare except in massive hemoptysis. Cardiac examination may reveal mitral stenosis. Lung auscultation may reveal rales, wheezes, or focal consolidation. Adenopathy or muscle wasting may signify neoplasia.
- Careful inspection of the oral and nasal cavities is warranted to help exclude an extrapulmonary source of bleeding.

DIAGNOSIS AND DIFFERENTIAL

- The differential diagnosis of hemoptysis includes infection (bronchitis, pneumonia, TB, fungal pneumonia, and lung abscess), malignant lesions (primary lung neoplasms or metastatic tumors), cardiogenic causes (left ventricular failure or mitral stenosis), inflammatory causes (bronchiectasis or cystic fibrosis), trauma, foreign body aspiration, pulmonary embolism, primary pulmonary hypertension, vasculitis, and bleeding diathesis.
- Basic testing should include pulse oximetry and chest radiography, although 15 to 30% of patients presenting with hemoptysis will have a normal chest x-ray.[2,5] A chest computed tomography (CT) scan should be considered if there is hemoptysis with an abnormal chest radiograph.
- A hematocrit and type and cross-match should be obtained in major hemoptysis. Other testing should be ordered as indicated by the clinical situation.

EMERGENCY DEPARTMENT CARE AND DISPOSITION

- Initial management focuses on the ABCs. Cardiac and pulse oximetry monitoring along with noninvasive blood pressure machines should be utilized. Large-bore IV lines should be placed.
- Administer supplemental oxygen to maintain oxygenation.
- Administer normal saline or lactated Ringer's initially for hypotension. Packed red blood cells should be transfused as needed.

- Fresh frozen plasma should be given to those patients with coagulopathies; platelets should be administered to those with thrombocytopenia.
- Patients with ongoing massive hemoptysis should be placed in the decubitus position with the bleeding side down, which is thought to minimize spilling of blood into the contralateral lung.
- Cough suppression with codeine or opioids may prevent dislodgement of clots.
- Endotracheal intubation should be performed with a large tube (8.0 mm) for persistent hemoptysis and worsening respiratory status. This will optimize suctioning and permit bronchoscopy.
- Indications for ICU admission include massive to moderate hemoptysis or minor hemoptysis whose underlying cause carries a high risk of proximate massive bleeding. Some underlying conditions may warrant admission regardless of the degree of bleeding.
- All admissions should include consultation with a pulmonologist or a thoracic surgeon for help with decisions regarding bronchoscopy, CT scanning, or angiography for bronchial artery embolization.[6,7]
- Patients who are discharged should be treated for several days with cough suppressants, inhaled β-agonist bronchodilators, and if an infectious etiology is suspected, appropriate antibiotics. Close follow-up is important.

REFERENCES

1. Nelson JE, Forman M: Hemoptysis in HIV-infected patients. *Chest* 110:737, 1996.
2. Marshall TJ, Flower CDR, Jackson JE: Review: The role of radiology in the investigation and management of patients with hemoptysis. *Clin Radiol* 51:391, 1996.
3. Hirschberg B, Biran I, Glazer M, Kramer MR: Hemoptysis: Etiology, evaluation, and outcome in a tertiary referral hospital. *Chest* 112:440, 1997.
4. Haro Estarriol M, Vizcaya Sanchez M, Rubio Goday M, et al: Utility of the clinical history, physical examination and radiography in the localization of bleeding in patients with hemoptysis. *Ann Med Internat* 19:289, 2002.
5. Haponik EF, Chin R: Hemoptysis: Clinician's perspectives. *Chest* 97:469, 1990.
6. Haponik EF, Fein A, Chin R: Management of life-threatening hemoptysis: Has anything really changed? *Chest* 118:1431, 2000.
7. Karmy-Jones R, Cuschier J, Vallieres E: Role of bronchoscopy in massive hemoptysis. *Chest Surg Clin North Am* 11:873, 2001.

For further reading in *Emergency Medicine: A Comprehensive Study Guide,* 6th ed., see Chap. 67, "Hemoptysis," by William Franklin Young, Jr. and Michael W. Stava.

37 ASTHMA AND CHRONIC OBSTRUCTIVE PULMONARY DISEASE

Monika Ahluwalia

EPIDEMIOLOGY

- In the United States, asthma affects approximately 4 to 5% of the population.[1] The highest prevalence is at the extremes of age. Asthma affects 7 to 10% of the elderly population and is the most common chronic disease of childhood, with a prevalence of 5 to 10%.[2,3]
- Chronic obstructive pulmonary disease (COPD) is a worldwide respiratory health problem. It is the sixth leading cause of death in the world and the fourth most common cause of death in the United States.
- COPD is rarely seen in individuals younger than 40 years of age, but is very common among older individuals. In those aged 55 to 85 years, the prevalence of COPD is approximately 10%. The prevalence has doubled in the past few decades and is highest in countries with heavy cigarette use.
- In the United States, COPD is the third most common cause of hospitalization, the fourth most common cause of death, and the only leading cause of death with an increasing incidence.[3,4]
- Mortality from COPD ranges from 5 to 14% in hospitalized patients and increases to 24% in patients admitted to the intensive care unit.[3,5]

PATHOPHYSIOLOGY

- The pathophysiologic hallmark of asthma is the reduction in airway diameter caused by smooth muscle contraction, vascular congestion, bronchial wall edema, and thick secretions. The inflammatory reaction that triggers the decrease in airway diameter results in increasing work of breathing and has a significant effect on pulmonary function.
- Acute airway inflammation is triggered when antigens come into contact with mast cells, resulting in the release of inflammatory mediators like histamine, leukotrienes, chemokines, cytokines, and interleukins. These mediators result in bronchoconstriction, vascular congestion, edema formation, increased mucus production, and impaired mucociliary transport.[6]
- Antigens or precipitants of an acute attack include viral respiratory tract infections, environmental pollutants, medications, occupational exposures to industrial chemicals, exercise, and emotional stress.[7]
- COPD is characterized by airflow obstruction, espe-

cially in expiratory airflow secondary to airway secretions, mucosal edema, bronchospasm, and bronchoconstriction due to impaired lung elasticity.

- Physiologic consequences of airflow obstruction are demonstrated in increased airway resistance, decreased maximum expiratory flow rates, air trapping, increased airway pressures (with resultant barotrauma and adverse hemodynamic effects), ventilation-perfusion imbalance (causing hypoxemia/hypercarbia), and increased work of breathing causing respiratory muscle fatigue with ventilatory failure.
- An estimated 80 to 90% of the risk of developing COPD can be attributed to cigarette smoking. Other risk factors associated with COPD include environmental factors such as respiratory infections, occupational exposures, air pollution, passive smoke exposure, and diet. The only genetic risk factor is α_1 antitrypsin deficiency.[8]

CLINICAL FEATURES

- Classically, asthma and COPD exacerbations present with dyspnea, chest tightness, wheezing, and cough.
- Physical exam findings of a mild asthma attack include wheezing and a prolonged expiratory phase. Wheezing does not correlate with the degree of airflow obstruction, as a quiet chest may indicate severe airflow obstruction.
- A patient with a severe asthma exacerbation may present in a tripod position gasping for air with audible wheezing, diaphoresis, and using accessory muscles. Other signs of severe exacerbation include tachycardia, tachypnea, hypertension, and most importantly, hypoxia. Paradoxical respirations, alteration in mental status, lethargy, and quiet chest are all indicative of severe airflow obstruction and impending respiratory failure.
- The two dominant clinical forms of COPD are: (1) pulmonary emphysema and (2) chronic bronchitis. Emphysema is characterized by abnormal permanent enlargement and destruction of the air spaces distal to terminal bronchioles. By contrast, excess mucus secretion in the bronchial tree with a chronic productive cough occurring on most days for at least 3 months in the year for two consecutive years is characteristic of chronic bronchitis. Elements of both clinical forms are often present, although one may predominate.
- A pulsus paradoxus above 20 mm Hg is indicative of severe asthma and COPD exacerbation.
- Signs of hypercapnia include confusion, tremor, plethora, stupor, hypopnea, and apnea.
- Characteristics of patients who are at higher risk of respiratory failure with hypoxia and hypercarbia include patients with attacks lasting more than several days, steroid-dependent patients, and those with prior attacks requiring intubation.

DIAGNOSIS AND DIFFERENTIAL

- Diagnosis of asthma or COPD is made clinically, based on the history and physical examination, and the cause for the decompensation is investigated.
- Spirometry is commonly used to determine the severity of airflow obstruction and the effectiveness of therapy by measuring the forced expiratory volume in 1 second (FEV_1) and the peak expiratory flow rate (PEFR). Sequential measurements of FEV_1 and PEFR assess the response of treatment and can be used to predict need for hospitalization.[9,10]
- Pulse oximetry is a fast, easy, and noninvasive means for assessing and monitoring oxygen saturation during treatment, but does not aid in predicting clinical outcomes.[11] Pulse oximetry does not provide information about acid-base disturbances and hypercapnia.
- Arterial blood gases (ABG) may be used in asthma and COPD to assess for hypercapnia and respiratory acidosis. These are ominous findings and indicate extreme airway obstruction and fatigue with possible onset of acute respiratory failure.
- A chest radiograph should be obtained if there is clinical suspicion of pneumothorax, pneumomediastinum, pneumonia, or other medical concerns such as congestive heart failure (CHF), pleural effusions, or pulmonary neoplasia.
- Electrocardiograms are helpful in asthma and COPD to assess for cardiac ischemia, myocardial infarction, and arrhythmias such as multifocal atrial tachycardia. Electrocardiographic (ECG) findings in moderate to severe pulmonary disease may reveal right ventricular strain, abnormal P waves, or nonspecific ST-T wave abnormalities, which may resolve with treatment.
- The differential diagnosis of decompensated asthma and COPD includes CHF ("cardiac asthma"), upper airway obstruction, aspiration of a foreign body or gastric acid, pulmonary neoplasia, pleural effusions, interstitial lung diseases, pulmonary embolism, and exposure to asphyxiants.

EMERGENCY DEPARTMENT CARE AND DISPOSITION

- Although patients with COPD often have more underlying illness than do asthmatics, the therapy for acute bronchospasm and inflammation in each are similar.
- All patients should be placed on a cardiac monitor,

pulse oximeter, and noninvasive blood pressure monitor, and patients with moderate to severe attacks should have IV access.

- Oxygen should be administered. In COPD patients, the need for oxygen must be balanced against progressive hypercarbia and suppression of hypoxic ventilatory drive.[12] Arterial saturation should be corrected to above 90%.

- Adrenergic agonists that are specific for β_2 receptors are first-line agents used to treat acute bronchospasm in COPD and asthma attacks. β-Adrenergic agonists include albuterol, salmeterol, and formoterol. Binding of these drugs to β receptors triggers smooth muscle relaxation resulting in bronchodilation. Other effects of these agents include vasodilation and improved mucociliary clearance. Subcutaneous terbutaline sulfate (0.25 to 0.5 mL) or epinephrine 1:1000, 0.1 to 0.3 mL may also be administered in moderate to severe exacerbations provided the patient is not at risk for cardiac disease.[9,13]

- Anticholinergics are useful adjuvants when given with other therapies, and when used with β_2-agonists, their effects may be additive.[9,13] These agents competitively antagonize acetylcholine at the postganglionic junction and result in bronchodilation by blocking the vagal pathways. Ipratropium is the agent of choice (500 μg = 2.5 mL of the 0.02% inhalant solution), and is available as a nebulized solution or metered dose inhaler (MDI). A combined ipratropium and albuterol inhaler is also available. The effects of ipratropium peak in 1 to 2 hours and last 3 to 4 hours. Dosages may be repeated every 1 to 4 hours.[9,13]

- Systemic corticosteroids such as prednisone and methylprednisolone are commonly used to treat asthma and COPD. Although the complete mechanism of action of steroids is unknown, it is proposed that steroids increase responsiveness to β-adrenergic agents and reduce inflammation. Usually a short course of 3 to 10 days of prednisone 40 to 60 mg per day or its equivalent is prescribed.[9,13]

- Methylxanthines such as theophylline and aminophylline are not commonly used for acute asthma or COPD exacerbation.[9,13]

- Magnesium sulfate (1 to -2 g IV) may be used in severe asthma attack due to its bronchodilatory properties.[14]

- Heliox (80% helium and 20% oxygen) can be used in severe asthma exacerbations to lower airway resistance, provided the patient does not have an oxygen requirement.[15]

- In selected cooperative patients, noninvasive positive pressure ventilation (intermittent, continuous, or biphasic) may avert artificial ventilation when the patient begins to exhibit signs of acute ventilatory failure.[16]

- Mechanical ventilation is indicated for patients with hypoxia, severe hypercarbia, altered mental status, exhaustion, and worsening acidosis.

- In patients being discharged, continued treatment with β_2-agonists and oral steroids is important. In addition, patient education and close medical follow-up is essential.

REFERENCES

1. Centers for Disease Control and Prevention: Surveillance for asthma—United States, 1980–1999. *Morb Mortal Wkly Rep* 51:1, 1999.
2. Centers for Disease Control and Prevention: Asthma mortality rates and hospitalization among children and young adults: United States, 1980-1993. *Morb Mortal Wkly Rep* 45:350, 1966.
3. Cydulka RK, McFadden ER, Emerman CL, et al: Patterns of hospitalization in elderly patients with asthma and chronic obstructive pulmonary disease. *Am J Respir Crit Care Med* 156:1807, 1997.
4. Fiel SB: Chronic obstructive pulmonary disease mortality and mortality reduction. *Drugs* 52(Suppl 2):55, 1996.
5. Fuso L, Incalzi RA, Pistilli R, et al: Predicting mortality of patients hospitalized for acutely exacerbated chronic obstructive pulmonary disease. *Am J Med* 98:272, 1995.
6. Fabbri LM, Caramori G, Beghe B, et al: Physiologic consequences of long-term inflammation. *Am J Respir Crit Care Med* 157(Suppl 1):5195, 1998.
7. Busse WW, Gern JE: Viruses in asthma. *J Allergy Clin Immunol* 100:147, 1997.
8. American Thoracic Society: Standards for the diagnosis and care of patients with chronic obstructive pulmonary disease. *Am J Respir Crit Care Med* 152:578, 1995.
9. National Asthma Education and Prevention Expert Panel: Report 2: Guidelines for Diagnosis and Management of Asthma. Bethesda, MD: National Institutes of Health (NIH), 1997, NIH Pub. No. 97-4051.
10. Martin TG, Elenbaas RM, Pingleton SH: Use of peak expiratory flow rates to eliminate unnecessary arterial blood gases in acute asthma. *Ann Emerg Med* 11:70, 1982.
11. Harden R: Oxygen saturation in adults with acute asthma. *J Accid Emerg Med* 13:28, 1996.
12. Dunn WF, Nelson SB, Hubmayr RD: Oxygen induced hypercarbia in obstructive pulmonary disease. *Am Rev Respir Dis* 144:526, 1991.
13. Pauwels RA, Buist AS, Calverley PM, et al: Global strategy for the diagnosis, management, and prevention of chronic obstructive pulmonary disease. NHLBI/WHO Global Initiative for Chronic Obstructive Lung Disease (GOLD) Workshop Summary. *Am J Respir Crit Care Med* 163:1256, 2001.
14. Rowe BH, Bretzlaff JA, Bourdon C, et al: Magnesium sulfate

for treating exacerbations of acute asthma in the emergency department. *Cochrane Database Syst Rev* 2, 2000.

15. Carter ER: Heliox for acute severe asthma. *Chest* 117:1212, 2000.

16. Mehta S, Hill NS: Noninvasive ventilation. *Am J Respir Crit Care Med* 163:540, 2001.

For further reading in *Emergency Medicine. A Comprehensive Study Guide,* 6th ed., see Chap. 68, "Acute Asthma in Adults," by Rita K. Cydulka; and Chap. 69, "Chronic Obstructive Pulmonary Disease," by Rita K. Cydulka and Mohak Dave.

38 ACUTE ABDOMINAL PAIN

Peggy E. Goodman

EPIDEMIOLOGY

- Data from the United States National Center for Health Statistics indicate that abdominal pain was the single most frequently mentioned reason offered by patients for visiting the ED in 2000 (annual incidence of approximately 63/1000 adult ED visits).[1]
- Admission rates for abdominal pain vary markedly, ranging from 18 to 42%, with rates as high as 63% reported in patients over 65 years of age.

PATHOPHYSIOLOGY

- Visceral abdominal pain is usually caused by stretching of fibers innervating the walls or capsules of hollow or solid organs, respectively. Less commonly it is caused by early ischemia or inflammation.
- Foregut organs (stomach, duodenum, and biliary tract) produce pain in the epigastric region; midgut organs (most of the small bowel, and the appendix and cecum) cause periumbilical pain; and hindgut organs (most of the colon, including the sigmoid) as well as the intraperitoneal portions of the genitourinary system tend to cause pain initially in the suprapubic or hypogastric area.
- Visceral pain is usually felt at the midline.
- Parietal or somatic abdominal pain is caused by irritation of fibers that innervate the parietal peritoneum, usually the portion covering the anterior abdominal wall.
- In contrast to visceral pain, parietal pain can be localized to the dermatome directly above the site of the painful stimulus. As the underlying disease process evolves, the symptoms of visceral pain give way to the signs of parietal pain, with tenderness and guarding. As localized peritonitis develops further, rigidity and rebound appear.
- Referred pain is felt at a location distant from the diseased organ.

CLINICAL FEATURES

- The principal characteristics of abdominal pain include location, quality, severity, onset, duration, aggravating and alleviating factors, and change in any of these variables over time.
- Associated symptoms related to the gastrointestinal, genitourinary, gynecologic, and vascular systems should be sought.
- Contrary to conventional teaching, absent or diminished bowel sounds provide little clinically useful information. This is supported by the observation that in a series of 100 patients with operative confirmation of peritonitis due to perforation of peptic ulcer, about half were noted to have normal or increased bowel sounds.[2]
- The presence of hyperactive or obstructive bowel sounds is somewhat more helpful, as reflected by their presence in about half of 100 patients with small bowel obstruction (SBO), in contrast to only 5 to 10% of patients with 500 other surgical diagnoses. However, fully 25% of those with SBO had absent or diminished bowel sounds.[2]
- Rebound tenderness, often regarded as the main clinical criterion of peritonitis, has several important limitations. In patients with peritonitis, the combination of rigidity, referred tenderness, and especially "cough pain,"[3] usually provides sufficient diagnostic confirmation that little is gained by eliciting the unnecessary pain of rebound.[4]

- False-positive rebound tenderness occurs in about one patient in four without peritonitis,[4] perhaps because of a nonspecific startle response. Indeed, more recent work has led some authors to conclude that rebound tenderness, in contrast to cough pain, is of no predictive value.[5]
- There is little evidence that rectal tenderness in patients with right lower quadrant (RLQ) pain provides additional information beyond what has already been obtained by other, less uncomfortable components of the physical examination.[6]

DIAGNOSIS AND DIFFERENTIAL

- Based on three studies containing a total of over 1800 patients, a white blood cell (WBC) count exceeding the threshold value of 10,000 to 11,000/mm^3 only doubled the odds of appendicitis, while a WBC below this level cut the odds in half.[8,9,10]
- For acute cholecystitis, the likelihood ratios of the WBC count are virtually identical to those seen in appendicitis and are of equally limited clinical value.[7,8,9]
- In one large, well-conducted series of nonspecific abdominal pain (NSAP), 28% (95% CI 22 to 34%) of patients were reported to have WBC counts >10,500/mm^3.[10]
- Recent work has concluded that plain abdominal radiographs (PARs) continue to be markedly overutilized. One study concluded that restriction of the PAR to patients with suspected obstruction, perforation, ischemia, peritonitis, or renal colic would reduce imaging by 80%, with no impact on management.[11]
- Ultrasound can be helpful as a bedside screening test, but is operator dependent, and can be limited by patient factors such as bowel gas and obesity.
- Computed tomography (CT) is markedly superior for identifying virtually any abnormality that can be seen on plain films.[12,13,14]
- It is clear that diagnostic error in adults with abdominal pain increases in proportion to age, ranging from a low of 20% if only young adults are considered, to a high of 70% in the very elderly.[8,15]
- The most common causes of abdominal pain are listed in Table 38-1.

SPECIFIC DIAGNOSES

- Evaluation of specific diagnoses is discussed in the chapters that follow in this section. Exceptions include abdominal pain in the elderly, mesenteric ischemia, and abdominal wall pain.

TABLE 38-1 Most Common Causes of Abdominal Pain

FINAL DIAGNOSIS	PERCENTAGE OF >10,000 PATIENTS	
Nonspecific abdominal pain	34%	
Appendicitis	28%	
Biliary tract disease	10%	
Small bowel obstruction	4%	
Acute gynecologic disease	4%	
	Salpingitis	68%
	Ovarian cyst	21%
	Ectopic pregnancy	6%
	Incomplete abortion	5%
Pancreatitis	3%	
Renal colic	3%	
Perforated peptic ulcer	3%	
Cancer	2%	
Diverticular disease	2%	
Other	6%	

ABDOMINAL PAIN IN THE ELDERLY

- Over half of patients aged 65 or greater who present to the ED with abdominal pain require admission, 25 to 33% will require surgical intervention, and the combined mortality rate for abdominal pain in the elderly is 11 to 14%.
- Reliable history and physical examination are more difficult to elicit, due to decreased physiologic responses, comorbid illness, or effects of medications, and are more likely to result in inaccurate or delayed diagnosis; if elicited, the location of tenderness is generally reliable.
- Causes of abdominal pain stratified by age are listed in Table 38-2.

TABLE 38-2 Causes of Acute Abdominal Pain Stratified by Age

FINAL DIAGNOSIS	≥50 YEARS OLD (n = 2406)	<50 YEARS OLD (n = 6317)
Biliary tract disease	21%	6%
Nonspecific abdominal pain	16%	40%
Appendicitis	15%	32%
Bowel obstruction	12%	2%
Pancreatitis	7%	2%
Diverticular disease	6%	<0.1%
Cancer	4%	<0.1%
Hernia	3%	<0.1%
Vascular	2%	<0.1%
Gynecologic	<0.1%	4%
Other	13%	13%

MESENTERIC ISCHEMIA

- Mesenteric ischemia can be due to arterial or venous occlusion, and has a very high morbidity due to bowel vulnerability, delays in diagnosis, and patient comorbidities.
- The small bowel, which is supplied by the superior mesenteric artery, has a warm ischemia time of only 2 to 3 hours.
- The clinical picture of mesenteric ischemia is characterized initially by poorly localized visceral abdominal pain, without tenderness.
- Patients may become transiently better after a few hours of ischemia, at the time of onset of mucosal infarction, only to later develop peritoneal findings as full-thickness necrosis of the bowel wall becomes apparent.
- Timely diagnosis requires that an angiogram be obtained very early in the evolution of the pathologic process—so early in fact that it may seem clinically premature to order such an invasive test on an elderly patient who may not appear ill.[16]
- Persistently normal serial serum lactate levels markedly reduce the likelihood of mesenteric ischemia; elevated serum lactate is too nonspecific to reliably confirm the diagnosis.
- Contrast CT is 85 to 92% specific for mesenteric ischemia, but only 71 to 77% sensitive.[16,17,18]

ABDOMINAL WALL PAIN

- A useful and underutilized test to diagnose abdominal wall pain is the sit-up test, also known as Carnett's sign. Following identification of the site of maximum abdominal tenderness, the patient is asked to fold his or her arms across the chest and sit up halfway. The examiner maintains a finger on the tender area, and if palpation in the semisitting position produces the same or increased tenderness, the test is said to be positive for an abdominal wall syndrome.

EMERGENCY DEPARTMENT CARE AND DISPOSITION

- The management of abdominal emergencies is discussed in the diagnosis-specific chapters that follow.
- When required, judicious use of opioid pain medicine is recommended by the Agency for Healthcare Research and Quality.[19]
- If unable to determine the etiology of abdominal pain after detailed evaluation, the diagnosis of nonspecific abdominal pain is appropriate.

- The management of mesenteric ischemia is early identification and aggressive surgical intervention. Survival is 30% or less.

REFERENCES

1. McCaig LF, Nghi L: National Hospital Ambulatory Medical Care Survey: 2000 Emergency Department Summary. Advance data from vital and health statistics: no. 326. Hyattsville, MD: National Center for Health Statistics, 2002, p. 14.
2. Staniland JR, Ditchburn J, de Dombal FT: Clinical presentation of the acute abdomen: Study of 600 patients. *Br Med J* 3:393, 1972.
3. Jeddy TA, Vowles RH, Southam JA: Cough sign: A reliable test in the diagnosis of intra-abdominal inflammation. *Br J Surg* 81:279, 1994.
4. Bennett DH, Tambeur Luc J, Campbell WB: Use of coughing test to diagnose peritonitis. *Br Med J* 308:1336, 1994.
5. Liddington MI: Thomson WH: Rebound tenderness test. *Br J Surg* 78:795, 1991.
6. Dixon JM, Elton RA, Rainey JB, MacLeod DA: Rectal examination in patients with pain in the right lower quadrant of the abdomen. *Br Med J* 302:386, 1991.
7. de Dombal FT: The OMGE acute abdominal pain survey progress report, 1986. *Scand J Gastroenterol* 23(Suppl 144): 35, 1988.
8. de Dombal FT: Acute abdominal pain in the elderly. *J Clin Gastroenterol* 19:331, 1994.
9. Telfer S, Fonyo G, Holt, PR, de Dombal FT: Acute abdominal pain in patients over 50 years of age. *Scand J Gastroenterol* 144(Suppl):47, 1988.
10. Lukens TW, Emerman C, Effron D: The natural history and clinical findings of undifferentiated abdominal pain. *Ann Emerg Med* 22:690, 1993.
11. Anyanwu AC, Moalypour SM: Are abdominal radiographs still overutilized in the assessment of acute abdominal pain? A district general hospital audit. *J Roy Coll Surg Edinburgh* 43:267, 1998.
12. Rao PM, Rhea JT, Novelline RA, et al: Effect of computed tomography of the appendix on treatment of patients and the use of hospital resources. *N Engl J Med* 338:141, 1998.
13. Kircher MF, Rhea JT, Kihiczak D, et al: Frequency, sensitivity, and specificity of individual signs of diverticulitis on thin-section helical CT with colonic contrast material: Experience with 312 cases. *Am J Roentgenol* 178:1313, 2002.
14. Burkill GJ, Bell JR, Healy JC: The utility of computed tomography in small bowel obstruction. *Clin Radiol* 56:350, 2001.
15. Simmen HP, Decurtins M, Rotzer A, et al: Emergency room patients with abdominal pain unrelated to trauma: Analysis in a surgical university hospital. *Hepatogastroenterology* 38: 279, 1991.
16. Klein HM, Lensing R, Klosterhalfen B, Tons C, et al: Diagnostic imaging of mesenteric infarction. *Radiology* 197:79, 1995.

17. Taourel PG, Deneuville M, Pradel JA, et al: Acute mesenteric ischemia: Diagnosis with contrast-enhanced CT. *Radiology* 199:632, 1996.

18. Horton KM, Fishman EK: Volume-rendered 3D CT of the mesenteric vasculature: Normal anatomy, anatomic variants, and pathologic conditions. *Radiographics* 22:161, 2002.

19. Brownfield E: Pain management: Use of analgesics in the acute abdomen. Agency for Healthcare Research and Quality (AHRQ). http://www.AHRQ.GOV/CLINIC/PTSAFETY/CHAP37A.HTM 37.1. Accessed June 11, 2002.

For further reading in *Emergency Medicine: A Comprehensive Study Guide,* 6th ed., see Chap. 72, "Acute Abdominal Pain," by E. John Gallagher; and Chap. 73, "Abdominal Pain in the Elderly," by Robert McNamara.

39   GASTROINTESTINAL BLEEDING

Mitchell C. Sokolosky

EPIDEMIOLOGY

- Acute upper gastrointestinal (GI) bleeding has an annual incidence of 100 per 100,000.[1,2]
- Peptic ulcer disease accounts for 60% of all cases of upper GI bleeding followed by erosive gastritis and esophagitis, esophageal and gastric varices, and Mallory-Weiss syndrome.
- Lower GI bleeding has an annual incidence of 20 per 100,000.[3]
- The most common cause of apparent lower GI bleeding is upper GI bleeding. Hemorrhoids are the most common cause of actual lower GI bleeding, followed by diverticular disease, arteriovenous malformations, inflammatory disease, and polyps.[4]
- Both upper and lower GI bleeding are more common in males and the elderly.
- Factors associated with a high morbidity rate are hemodynamic instability, repeated hematemesis or hematochezia, failure to clear with gastric lavage, age over 60, and coexistent organ system disease.

PATHOPHYSIOLOGY

- Upper GI bleeding is defined as that originating proximal to the ligament of Treitz.
- Irritative factors such as alcohol, salicylates, and nonsteroidal anti-inflammatory agents are predisposing factors for peptic ulcer disease, gastritis, and esophagitis.

CLINICAL FEATURES

- Most patients will volunteer complaints of hematemesis, hematochezia, or melena.
- Some will have more subtle presentations of hypotension, tachycardia, angina, syncope, weakness, and confusion.
- Hematemesis or coffee-ground emesis suggests a source proximal to the right colon.
- Hematochezia indicates a more distal colorectal lesion.
- Weight loss and changes in bowel habits are classic symptoms of malignancy.
- Vomiting and retching followed by hematemesis is suggestive of a Mallory-Weiss tear.
- A history of aortic graft should suggest the possibility of an aortoenteric fistula.
- A history of medication or alcohol use should be sought. This history may suggest peptic ulcer disease, gastritis, or esophageal varices.
- Hypotension and tachycardia suggests severe bleeding. Cool clammy skin is an obvious sign of shock.
- Spider angiomata, palmar erythema, jaundice, and gynecomastia suggest underlying liver disease.
- Ingestion of iron or bismuth can simulate melena, and certain foods such as beets can simulate hematochezia; however, stool guaiac testing will be negative.
- Age >60 years, heart rate >100 bpm, systolic blood pressure <100 mm Hg, bright red blood in emesis or stool, or the presence of comorbidities all contribute to placing the patient in a higher-risk group for morbidity.[5]

DIAGNOSIS AND DIFFERENTIAL

- The diagnosis may be obvious with the finding of hematemesis, hematochezia, or melena.
- Nasogastric tube placement and aspiration may detect occult upper GI bleeding.
- A rectal exam is mandatory to detect the presence of blood, its appearance (bright red, maroon, or melanotic), and the presence of masses.
- A careful ear, nose, and throat (ENT) exam can exclude swallowed blood as a source.
- In patients with significant GI bleeding, the most important laboratory test is the type and cross-match of blood.
- Other important tests include a complete blood count, blood urea nitrogen (BUN), creatinine, electrolytes, glucose, coagulation studies, and liver function tests. The initial hematocrit level often will not reflect the actual amount of blood loss. Upper GI bleeding may elevate the BUN.
- Routine abdominal radiographs, including barium contrast studies, are of limited value in the emergency setting.

• Controversy in the literature remains as to whether scintigraphy, angiography, or colonoscopy, and in what order, should be the initial diagnostic procedure of choice in the evaluation of lower GI bleeding.[6–9]

EMERGENCY DEPARTMENT CARE AND DISPOSITION

• Emergency stabilization of the airway, breathing, and circulation is foremost.
• Oxygen, large-bore IVs, and monitors should be applied.
• Replace volume loss with crystalloids.
• The decision to start blood should be based on clinical factors (no improvement in perfusion after infusion of 2 L of crystalloids) rather than initial hematocrit.
• A nasogastric (NG) tube should be placed in all patients with significant bleeding, regardless of presumed source. Concerns that NG tube passage may provoke bleeding in patients with varices are unwarranted. Room temperature water is the preferred irrigant for gastric lavage.[10]
• Where available, early therapeutic endoscopy should be considered the treatment of choice for significant upper GI bleeding. Esophageal varices can be endoscopically treated by either band ligation or injection sclerotherapy. Endoscopic hemostasis (with injection sclerotherapy, electrocoagulation, heater probes, and lasers) has been used successfully in a variety of non-variceal etiologies of upper GI bleeding.
• Infusions of somatostatin and its synthetic longer-acting derivative octreotide have been shown to be effective in reducing bleeding from both varices and peptic ulcer disease. Octreotide (25 to 50 μg/h) has been shown to be as effective as sclerotherapy in acute variceal bleeding.[11] They should be considered useful adjuncts, either before endoscopy or when endoscopy is unsuccessful, contraindicated, or unavailable.
• Other treatment considerations may include the use of omeprazole and treatment of *Helicobacter pylori* infection with antibiotics.
• Balloon tamponade with the Sengstaken-Blakemore tube or its variants can control documented variceal hemorrhage in 40 to 80% of patients, but because of adverse reactions, it should be considered an adjunctive or temporizing measure only.
• In patients who do not respond to medical therapy, and in whom endoscopic hemostasis fails, emergency surgical intervention is indicated.
• Patients with GI hemorrhage will require hospital admission, and early referral to an endoscopist is advisable.

• Corley and colleagues[12] found five variables to be independent predictors of adverse outcomes in upper GI bleeding: initial hematocrit <30%, initial systolic BP <100 mm Hg, red blood in the nasogastric lavage, history of cirrhosis or ascites on examination, and a history of vomiting red blood.

REFERENCES

1. Rockall TA, Logan RF, Devlin HB, et al: Incidence of and mortality from acute upper gastrointestinal hemorrhage in the United Kingdom: Steering Committee and members of the National Audit of Acute Upper Gastrointestinal Hemorrhage. *BMJ* 311:222, 1995.
2. Longstreth GF: Epidemiology and outcome of patients hospitalized with acute lower gastrointestinal hemorrhage: A population-based study. *Am J Gastroenterol* 92:419, 1997.
3. Longstreth GF: Epidemiology of hospitalization for acute upper gastrointestinal hemorrhage: A population-based study. *Am J Gastroenterol* 90:206, 1995.
4. Machicado GA, Jensen DM: Acute and chronic management of lower gastrointestinal bleeding: Cost-effective approaches. *Gastroenterologist* 5:189, 1997.
5. Peter DJ, Dougherty JM: Evaluation of the patient with gastrointestinal bleeding: An evidence based approach. *Emerg Med Clin North Am* 17:239, 1999.
6. Suzman MS, Talmor M, Jennis R, et al: Accurate localization and surgical management of active lower gastrointestinal hemorrhage with technetium-labeled erythrocyte scintigraphy. *Ann Surg* 224:29, 1996.
7. Vernava AM, Moore BA, Longo WE, et al: Lower gastrointestinal bleeding. *Dis Colon Rectum* 40:846, 1997.
8. Richter JM, Christensen MR, Kaplan LM, et al: Effectiveness of current technology in the diagnosis and management of lower gastrointestinal hemorrhage. *Gastrointest Endosc* 41:93, 1995.
9. Ng DA, Opekla FG, Beck DE, et al: Predictive value of technetium Tc 99m-labelled red blood cell scintigraphy for positive angiogram in massive lower gastrointestinal hemorrhage. *Dis Colon Rectum* 40:471, 1997.
10. Leather RA, et al: Iced gastric lavage: A tradition without foundation. *Can Med Assoc J* 136:1245, 1987.
11. Jenkins SA, Shields R, Davies M, et al: A multicenter randomized trial comparing octreotide and injection sclerotherapy in the management and outcome of acute variceal hemorrhage. *Gut* 41:526, 1997.
12. Corley DA, Stefan AM, Wolf M, et al: Early indicators of prognosis in upper gastrointestinal hemorrhage. *Am J Gastroenterol* 93:336, 1998.

For further reading in *Emergency Medicine: A Comprehensive Study Guide,* 6th ed., see Chap. 74, "Gastrointestinal Bleeding," by David T. Overton.

40 ESOPHAGEAL EMERGENCIES

Mitchell C. Sokolosky

DYSPHAGIA

PATHOPHYSIOLOGY

- Dysphagia is defined as difficulty in swallowing.
- Most patients will have an identifiable, organic process causing their symptoms.
- Dysphagia can be grouped into two broad classification schemes: (1) transfer dysphagia (difficulty in initiating swallowing) and transport dysphagia[1] (feeling of food getting "stuck") and (2) obstructive disease (progressive symptoms, solids then liquids) and motor dysfunction (intermittent and variable symptoms).

CLINICAL FEATURES

- Historical information is the key to the diagnosis of dysphagia.
- Transport dysphagia that is present for solids only generally suggests a mechanical or obstructive process.
- Motility disorders typically cause transport dysphagia for solids and liquids.
- A poorly chewed meat bolus may obstruct the esophagus and be the presenting sign for a variety of underlying esophageal pathologies. These patients are often unable to swallow their own secretions on presentation.
- Physical examination of patients with dysphagia should focus on the head and neck and the neurologic exam. Unfortunately, the exam is often normal, despite the high-yield nature of this complaint.

DIAGNOSIS AND DIFFERENTIAL

- The diagnosis of the underlying pathology of dysphagia is most often made outside the emergency department (ED).
- Initial evaluation may include anteroposterior (AP) and lateral neck and chest x-rays.
- Barium swallow is usually the first test for patients with transport dysphagia.
- Direct laryngoscopy can be used to identify structural lesions.
- Oropharyngeal dysphagia is best worked up by videoesophagography.
- Structural or obstructive causes of dysphagia include neoplasms (squamous cell carcinoma is most common), esophageal strictures and webs, and diverticula.
- Motor lesions causing dysphagia include neuromuscular disorders (cerebrovascular accident [CVA] is most common), achalasia, and diffuse esophageal spasm.

EMERGENCY DEPARTMENT CARE AND DISPOSITION

- Protection of the airway and breathing is vital since aspiration is a major concern with most causes of dysphagia.
- Most causes of dysphagia can be further evaluated and managed in the outpatient setting.
- Many of the structural lesions will ultimately require dilatation as definitive therapy.

GASTROESOPHAGEAL REFLUX DISEASE (GERD)

PATHOPHYSIOLOGY

- GERD affects up to 25% of adults, possibly more among the elderly.[2]
- Transient relaxation of the lower esophageal sphincter (LES) complex (with normal tone in between periods of relaxation) is the primary mechanism causing reflux.
- Patients with moderate to severe reflux often have concomitant hiatal hernia.[3]
- Prolonged gastric emptying, agents that decrease LES pressure, and impaired esophageal motility predispose to reflux.

CLINICAL FEATURES

- Heartburn is the classic symptom of GERD.
- Chest discomfort may be the sole manifestation of the disease.
- The association of pain with meals, postural changes in pain, and relief of symptoms with antacids are more consistent with GERD.
- Less obvious presentations of GERD also occur such as pulmonary symptoms, especially asthma exacerbations, and multiple ear/nose/throat symptoms.
- GERD has also been implicated in the etiology of dental erosion, vocal cord ulcers and granulomas, laryngitis with hoarseness, chronic sinusitis, and chronic cough.[4,5]
- Over time, GERD can cause complications such as strictures, inflammatory esophagitis, and Barrett's esophagus (a premalignant condition).

DIAGNOSIS AND DIFFERENTIAL

- Diagnosis is often made by history and favorable response to antacid treatment.
- Unfortunately, like cardiac pain, GERD pain may be squeezing, pressure-like, and include a history of onset with exertion and rest. Both types of pain may be accompanied by diaphoresis, pallor, radiation, and nausea and vomiting.

EMERGENCY DEPARTMENT CARE AND DISPOSITION

- Comprehensive treatment of reflux disease involves decreasing acid production in the stomach, enhancing upper tract motility, and eliminating risk factors for the disease.
- Mild disease is often treated empirically with an H_2 blocker or proton pump inhibitor. A prokinetic drug may also greatly decrease symptoms.
- Patients should avoid agents that exacerbate GERD (ethanol, caffeine, nicotine, chocolate, fatty foods), sleep with the head of the bed elevated 30 degrees, and avoid eating within 3 hours of going to bed at night.

ESOPHAGEAL PERFORATION

PATHOPHYSIOLOGY

- Esophageal perforation represents a true emergency with a high mortality rate, regardless of the underlying cause.
- Iatrogenic injury (most common cause) accounts for 75% of all perforations.
- Boerhaave's syndrome, a well recognized clinical scenario of postemetic perforation, accounts for 10 to 15% of cases.

CLINICAL FEATURES

- Pain is classically described as acute, severe, unrelenting, and diffuse, and is reported in the chest, neck, and abdomen.
- Pain can radiate to the back and shoulders, or back pain may be the predominant symptom.
- Swallowing often exacerbates pain.
- Physical exam varies with the severity of the rupture and the elapsed time between the rupture and presentation.
- Abdominal rigidity with hypotension and fever often occur early.

- Tachycardia and tachypnea are common.
- Mediastinal emphysema takes time to develop. It is less commonly detected by examination or radiography in lower esophageal perforation, and its absence does not rule out perforation.[6]
- Hammon's crunch, caused by air in the mediastinum being moved by the beating heart, can sometimes be auscultated.
- Pleural effusions develop in half of patients with intrathoracic perforations and are uncommon in cervical perforations.

DIAGNOSIS AND DIFFERENTIAL

- Chest radiography and contrast esophagography with water-soluble contrast most often make the diagnosis.
- Endoscopy, computed topography (CT) of the chest, and thoracentesis can be useful adjuncts.
- Endoscopy is often done after negative esophagography in penetrating trauma with suspicion of esophageal perforation.
- Esophageal perforation is often ascribed to acute myocardial infarction (MI), pulmonary embolus, peptic ulcer disease, aortic catastrophe, or acute abdomen, resulting in critical delays in diagnosis, the most important factor in determining morbidity and mortality.

EMERGENCY DEPARTMENT CARE AND DISPOSITION

- Rapid, aggressive management is key to minimizing the morbidity and mortality associated with esophageal perforation.
- In the ED, resuscitation of shock (see Chaps. 7 and 8) and broad-spectrum parenteral antibiotics should be given to cover both aerobic and anaerobic organisms. Examples include single-drug coverage such as piperacillin-tazobactam 3.375 g IV, or double-drug coverage with cefotaxime 2 g IV or ceftriaxone 2 g IV plus clindamycin 600 mg IV or metronidazole 1 g IV.
- Emergent surgical consultation should be obtained as soon as the diagnosis is seriously entertained.
- All of these patients require admission to the hospital.

ESOPHAGEAL BLEEDING

PATHOPHYSIOLOGY

- Varices develop in patients with chronic liver disease in response to portal hypertension.
- Sixty percent of patients with chronic liver disease will develop varices.

- Of patients who develop varices, 25 to 30% experience hemorrhage.[7]
- Patients who develop varices from alcohol abuse have a higher risk of bleeding, especially if there is ongoing alcohol consumption.
- Mallory-Weiss tears (arterial bleeding from longitudinal mucosal lacerations of the distal esophagus/proximal stomach that usually following forceful vomiting) account for 5 to 15% of upper GI hemorrhages.

CLINICAL FEATURES

- Acute onset of upper GI bleeding is the usual presentation, though some patients can present with melena or hematochezia.
- The spectrum of severity of bleeding is broad.
- Less than half of patients with Mallory-Weiss tears will report a history of vomiting prior to hematemesis.

DIAGNOSIS AND DIFFERENTIAL

- Diagnosis is made by history and the presence of acute upper GI bleeding.
- Gastric aspiration may aid in the diagnosis.
- Endoscopy may be both diagnostic and therapeutic.
- Esophageal cancer often results in heme-positive stools, but is an uncommon cause of significant upper or lower GI bleeding.

EMERGENCY DEPARTMENT CARE AND DISPOSITION

- Resuscitation proceeds concurrently with the diagnostic effort of history, physical examination, and laboratory evaluation.
- Gastric lavage through a nasogastric tube is generally accepted, and early airway management should be considered.
- Prompt mobilization of resources including blood products, gastroenterology consult for endoscopy, and an appropriate inpatient level of care is important.
- About 60% of variceal bleeding will resolve with supportive care alone.
- The vast majority of Mallory-Weiss tears stop bleeding spontaneously, thus requiring only supportive care.
- With variceal bleeding, endoscopic therapy is often first-line therapy. Sclerotherapy and ligation are the main alternatives.
- Multiple pharmacotherapeutic agents (somatostatin analogues) have a role in controlling variceal bleeding. Consider infusing octreotide 25 to 50 µg/h IV.
- More recent review seems to support a trial of med-

ical therapy alone for variceal bleeding in cirrhotics, with results comparable to primary sclerotherapy.[8,9]
- Balloon tamponade is generally considered a last resort therapy.
- Surgical treatment can also be considered for patients who fail endoscopic and medical intervention.

REFERENCES

1. Trate DM, Parkman HP, Fisher RS: Dysphagia: Evaluation, diagnosis, and treatment. *Primary Care* 23:417, 1996.
2. Richter JE: Typical and atypical presentations of gastroesophageal reflux disease: The role of esophageal testing in diagnosis and management. *Gastroenterol Clin North Am* 25: 75, 1996.
3. Dent J: Patterns of lower esophageal sphincter function associated with gastroesophageal reflux. *Am J Med* 103:29S, 1997.
4. Hogan WJ: Spectrum of supraesophageal complications of gastroesophageal reflux disease. *Am J Med* 103:77S, 1997.
5. de Casestecker J: Medical therapy for supraesophageal complications of gastroesophageal reflux. *Am J Med* 103:138S, 1997.
6. Janjua KJ: Boerhaave's syndrome. *Postgrad Med J* 73:265, 1997.
7. Polio J, Groszmann RJ, Taylor MB: Acute management of portal hypertensive hemorrhage from the upper gastrointestinal tract, in Taylor MB (ed.): *Gastrointestinal Emergencies.* Baltimore: Williams & Wilkins, 1997.
8. Banares R, Alibillos A, Rincon D, et al: Endoscopic treatment versus endoscopic plus pharmacologic treatment for acute variceal bleeding: a mcta-analysis. *Hepatology* 3:609, 2002.
9. D'Amico G, Pietrosi G, Tarantino I, Pagliaro L: Emergency sclerotherapy versus medical interventions for bleeding oesophageal varices in cirrhotic patients (Cochrane Review), in *The Cochrane Library*, Issue 2. Oxford: Update Software, 2002.

For further reading in *Emergency Medicine: A Comprehensive Study Guide,* 6th ed., see Chap. 75, "Esophageal Emergencies," by Moss H. Mendelson.

41 SWALLOWED FOREIGN BODIES

Patricia Baines

EPIDEMIOLOGY

- Mortality from swallowed foreign bodies is approximately 1500 people per year.
- The pediatric population accounts for approximately 80% of all cases.

- Children most often ingest coins, toys, crayons, and ballpoint pen caps; adults are most likely to obstruct their esophagus with either meat or bones.[1]

PATHOPHYSIOLOGY

- Most objects pass spontaneously, 10 to 20% require some intervention, and only 1% requires surgical treatment.[2]
- There are five common areas where objects lodge: cricopharyngeal narrowing (C6 level), the most common site; thoracic inlet (T1 level); aortic arch (T4 level); tracheal bifurcation (T6 level); and hiatal narrowing (T10-T11 level).
- Once an object passes the pylorus, it usually continues and is passed in the stool.
- Objects lodged in the esophagus can result in airway obstruction, stricture, or perforation, with resulting mediastinitis, cardiac tamponade, paraesophageal abscess, or aortotracheoesophageal fistula.
- Perforation may be due to direct mechanical erosion or chemical corrosion.

CLINICAL FEATURES

- Common symptoms in adults are retching or vomiting, dysphagia, choking, coughing, or aspiration.
- Common symptoms in children include refusal to eat, vomiting, gagging, choking, stridor, neck or throat pain, inability to swallow, increased salivation, and foreign body sensation in the chest.

DIAGNOSIS AND DIFFERENTIAL

- The diagnosis can frequently be made clinically by examining the nasopharynx and oropharynx. Examine subcutaneous tissue for air secondary to perforation.
- Laryngoscopy is indicated (direct or indirect) when patients complain of foreign body sensation.
- In children, a red throat, dysphagia, palatal abrasion, temperature elevation, anxiety, distress, and peritoneal signs are all findings suggestive of foreign body ingestion.
- Radiographs of the neck, chest, or abdomen should be performed.
- Consultation and endoscopy is recommended before initiation of any contrast study.
- In cases of suspected perforation, use water-soluble contrast agent (Gastrografin).
- Barium should be used if aspiration is possible.
- Perform serial exams with repeated x-rays to monitor progress of the object.

The differential diagnosis includes dysphagia, esophageal carcinoma, and gastroesophageal reflux disease.[3]

EMERGENCY DEPARTMENT CARE AND DISPOSITION

FOOD IMPACTION

- Use conservative management if the patient can tolerate his or her own secretions. If the patient is unable to swallow fluids or if food does not pass within 12 hours, intervention is necessary.
- Administer glucagon 1 mg IV to relax esophageal smooth muscle.
- Nifedipine 10 mg sublingual is used to reduce lower esophageal sphincter pressure.[4] Sublingual nitroglycerin (0.4 mg) can be used, but may cause hypotension.
- Proteolytic enzymes such as papain (Adolph's meat tenderizer) are contraindicated due to risk of esophageal perforation.

COIN INGESTION

- Approximately 35% of children with coin ingestion will be asymptomatic.
- All children with suspected coin ingestion should have radiographs performed.
- Coins in the esophagus lie in the frontal plane with the flat side visible on the anteroposterior (AP) view. Coins in the trachea lie in the sagittal plane and are visible on end on the AP view.
- Lodged coins require endoscopic removal.
- Foley catheter removal of ingested coins may be used if less than 24 hours has passed since ingestion. Aspiration may be a complication. Airway equipment for airway control must be immediately available.

BUTTON BATTERY INGESTION

- A button battery ingestion is a true emergency because of the rapid action of the alkaline substance contained in the battery. Lithium cells are associated with more adverse outcome.
- Esophageal burns can occur within 4 hours and perforation can occur within 6 hours.
- Mercuric oxide cells contain heavy metals. Blood and urine mercury levels should be measured if a mercury cell opens within the GI tract.
- Emergent endoscopic removal of the button battery should occur after radiographic documentation. Ipecac is contraindicated.[5]
- Foley catheter technique may be used if the battery has been lodged for less than 2 hours.

- Button batteries that have passed the esophagus in an asymptomatic patient need not be retrieved. If the cell has not passed the pylorus within 48 hours, then retrieval is necessary.
- Most batteries pass through the GI tract within 48 to 72 hours.
- Early surgical consult is mandatory for symptomatic patients with acute abdomen, tarry or bloody stools, fever, or persistent vomiting.
- Assistance with cell identification may be obtained by calling the National Button Battery Ingestion Hotline (National Capital Poison Center, Washington, DC) at 202-625-3333.

INGESTION OF SHARP OBJECTS

- Objects longer than 5 cm and wider than 2 cm rarely pass the stomach.
- Open safety pins, razor blades, and other sharp pointed edges require removal before they pass from the stomach because 15 to 35% will cause intestinal perforation, generally at the ileocecal valve.
- Children who have swallowed sharp objects should have radiographs and an examination.[6] Asymptomatic children can be followed with serial exams and x-rays.
- Children who are symptomatic or have swallowed a sewing needle require surgical consultation.

COCAINE INGESTION

- A condom packet can hold up to 5 g of cocaine.
- Rupture of one packet may be fatal.
- Surgery is the safest method of retrieval, although spontaneous passage may occur.

FOREIGN BODY RETRIEVAL

- Endoscopy is the procedure of choice for foreign body removal, except for cocaine.[7]
- Consultation and possible admission is required with sharp or elongated objects, multiple foreign bodies, button batteries, evidence of perforation, a child with a nickel or quarter at the level of the cricopharyngeus muscle, airway compromise, or presence of a foreign body for more than 24 hours.

REFERENCES

1. Webb WA: Management of foreign bodies of the upper gastrointestinal tract: Update. *Gastrointest Endosc* 41:39, 1995.
2. American Society for Gastrointestinal Endoscopy: Guideline for the management of ingested foreign bodies. *Gastrointest Endosc* 41:622, 1995.
3. Klaus A, Swaim JM, Hinder RA: Laparoscopic antireflux surgery for supraesophageal complications of gastroesophageal reflux disease. *Am J Med* 111(Suppl 8A):2028, 2001.
4. Binder L, Anderson WA: Pediatric gastrointestinal foreign body ingestion. *Ann Emerg Med* 13:112, 1984.
5. Litovitz T, Schmitz BF: Ingestion of cylindrical and button batteries: An analysis of 2382 cases. *Pediatrics* 89:727, 1992.
6. Paul RI, Jaffe DM: Sharp object ingestions in children: Illustrative cases and literature review. *Pediatr Emerg Care* 4:245, 1988.
7. Mosca S, Manes G, Martino R, et al: Endoscopic management of foreign bodies in the upper gastrointestinal tract: Report on a series of 414 adult patients. *Endoscopy* 33:692, 2001.

For further reading in *Emergency Medicine: A Comprehensive Study Guide,* 6th ed., see Chap. 76, "Swallowed Foreign Bodies," by Wade R. Gaasch and Robert A. Barish.

42   PEPTIC ULCER DISEASE AND GASTRITIS

Mark R. Hess

EPIDEMIOLOGY

- The great majority of peptic ulcers are directly related to infection with *Helicobacter pylori* or nonsteroidal anti-inflammatory drug (NSAID) use.[1,2] For white Americans below the age of 35, the rate of *H. pylori* infection is 10% and this rate climbs to 80% by age 75. Black Americans have a higher infection rate of 45% below age 25.[3]
- One out of 10 Americans over age 17 will develop peptic ulcer disease (PUD) at some time.[4,5]

PATHOPHYSIOLOGY

- Hydrochloric acid and pepsin destroy gastric and duodenal mucosa and contribute to ulcer formation, usually after *H. pylori* has broken down the protective mucous gel. *H. pylori* infection is present in 80% of gastric ulcers and 95% of duodenal ulcers.[6]
- *Helicobacter pylori* infection generally causes a chronic active form of gastritis, but development of PUD occurs in only 10 to 20%.[3,7] Eradication of *H. pylori* reduces recurrence rates by about 65% in

duodenal ulcers and by about 40% in gastric ulcers.[6]
- NSAIDs inhibit prostaglandin synthesis. This contributes to ulcer formation by lowering mucus and bicarbonate production as well as blood flow to mucous membranes.[2]
- All ulcers generally respond to the traditional therapy of inhibiting acid production.
- Acute gastritis is generally caused by ischemia due to severe illness (burns, trauma, shock, etc), direct toxic effects (NSAIDs, alcohol, etc), or *H. pylori* infection.

CLINICAL FEATURES

- The most common symptom of PUD includes burning epigastric pain, usually after meals, that awakens the patient at night, and that is relieved with food, milk, or antacids. Acute gastritis may also present with nausea and vomiting, although the most common presentation is GI bleeding (microscopic to gross blood).
- The only physical sign of PUD may be epigastric tenderness unless a complication has occurred. Complications may present with rigid abdomen (perforation), abdominal distention and vomiting (gastric outlet obstruction), or GI bleeding. Gastric ulcers may perforate posteriorly, causing pancreatitis presenting with mid-back pain.

DIAGNOSIS AND DIFFERENTIAL

- The classic history with epigastric tenderness may suggest PUD, but definitive diagnosis cannot be made clinically.[8] Definitive diagnosis is made by upper GI series or endoscopy, with endoscopy having the highest yield.[1]
- The best ED test to detect *H. pylori* is a serologic study to detect IgG antibodies, which has a high sensitivity and specificity at a cost of $10 to $100 and a turnaround time less than 1 hour. However, antibodies do remain elevated for several years after eradication.
- Disorders to consider in the differential diagnosis of PUD include gastritis, gastroesophageal reflux disease (GERD), pancreatitis, hepatitis, cholelithiasis, cardiac ischemia, abdominal aortic aneurysm (AAA), gastroparesis, and gastric cancer.
- Ancillary tests to consider include complete blood cell count (CBC) to look for anemia in chronic GI blood loss, abdominal ultrasound for cholelithiasis and AAA, electrocardiogram and cardiac enzymes for cardiac ischemia, liver function tests for hepatitis and cholelithiasis, lipase for pancreatitis, and acute abdominal series for perforation.

EMERGENCY DEPARTMENT CARE AND DISPOSITION

- The acute treatment of PUD in the ED consists of antacids to neutralize gastric hydrochloric acid.[1] Often this is combined with viscous lidocaine.
- H_2-receptor antagonists (H2RAs) such as cimetidine, 300 mg IV or 800 mg orally at bedtime; ranitidine, 50 mg IV or 300 mg orally at bedtime; famotidine, 20 mg IV or 20 to 40 mg orally at bedtime; or nizatidine, 300 mg orally at bedtime are usually instituted for ongoing therapy to promote ulcer healing.[1,9] Proton pump inhibitors (PPIs, such as omeprazole, 20 mg daily, or lansoprazole, 15 mg daily) will heal ulcers faster and may have an inhibitory effect against *H. pylori*.[1,9]
- Finally if acute infection with *H. pylori* is found, antimicrobial and antisecretory therapy is instituted, with cure rates of 80 to 90%. Such a regimen might include lansoprazole, clarithromycin, and amoxicillin or metronidazole for 10 to 14 days.[10]
- All patients should receive discharge instructions, including avoidance of NSAIDs, alcohol, tobacco, caffeine, and non–enteric-coated aspirin. Early follow-up should be sought for patients at high risk for cancer, including those with anorexia, dysphagia, anemia, weight loss, or the elderly.

REFERENCES

1. Soll AH: Medical treatment of peptic ulcer disease: Practice guidelines. *JAMA* 275:622, 1996.
2. Sontag SJ: Guilty as charged: Bugs and drugs in gastric ulcer. *Am J Gastroenterol* 92:1255, 1997.
3. Damianos AJ, McGarrity TJ: Treatment strategies for *Helicobacter pylori* infection. *Am Fam Physician* 55:2765, 1997.
4. Sonnenberg A, Everhart JE: Health impact of peptic ulcer in the United States. *Am J Gastroenterol* 92:614, 1997.
5. NIH Consensus Development Panel: *Helicobacter pylori* in peptic ulcer disease. *JAMA* 272:65, 1994.
6. Forbes GM: Review: *Helicobacter pylori:* Current issues and new directions. *J Gastroenterol Hepatol* 12:419, 1997.
7. Falk GW: *H. pylori* 1997: Testing and treatment options. *Cleveland Clin J Med* 64:187, 1997.
8. Werdmuller BFM, Van der Putten ABMM, Loffeld RJLF: Review: The clinical presentation of peptic ulcer disease. *Neth J Med* 50:115, 1997.
9. Drugs for treatment of peptic ulcers. *Med Lett* 39:1, 1997.
10. Malfertheiner P, Megraud F, O'Morain C, et al: Current concepts in the management of *Heilicobacter pylori* infection –The Maastricht 2-2000 consensus report. *Aliment Pharmacol Ther* 16:167, 2002.

For further reading in *Emergency Medicine: A Comprehensive Study Guide*, 6th ed., see Chap. 77, "Peptic Ulcer Disease and Gastritis," by Matthew C. Gratton and Howard A. Werman.

43 APPENDICITIS

Peggy E. Goodman

EPIDEMIOLOGY

• The overall incidence of appendicitis is approximately 1 case per 1000 population per year. Six percent of the population will experience appendicitis at some point in their lifetime.[1] An estimated 1 million hospital days annually in the United States can be attributed to acute appendicitis.[1]

• Preoperative diagnosis of acute appendicitis is improving due to new imaging techniques,[2] but misdiagnosis remains an important cause of successful malpractice claims against emergency physicians.[3]

PATHOPHYSIOLOGY

• Acute appendicitis develops from obstruction of the appendiceal lumen. Increased luminal pressure leads to vascular compromise, bacterial invasion, inflammatory response, and resultant tissue necrosis.

• Classically, appendicitis is associated with the migration of pain from the periumbilical area to the right lower quadrant. However, there are many atypical presentations, often affected by variability of the anatomic location (eg, retrocecal, retroileal) of the appendix.[4]

CLINICAL FEATURES

• A summary of clinical examination operating characteristics for appendicitis is listed in Table 43-1.

• The most reliable symptom in acute appendicitis is abdominal pain.

• Right lower quadrant pain is 81% sensitive and 53% specific for the diagnosis of acute appendicitis. Migration of periumbilical pain to the right lower quadrant is 64% sensitive and 82% specific for the diagnosis of acute appendicitis.[5]

• After the onset of vague abdominal pain, the classic triad of symptoms in appendicitis includes anorexia, nausea, and vomiting. Sixty percent of patients with appendicitis will have some combination of these symptoms, but they are by themselves neither specific nor sensitive for appendicitis.[5]

• McBurney's point tenderness, Rovsing's sign, psoas sign, obturator sign, rectal exam tenderness, and rebound tenderness are all clinical exam findings that may be present.

TABLE 43-1 Summary of Clinical Examination Operating Characteristics for Appendicitis*

PROCEDURE	SENSITIVITY	SPECIFICITY	LR(+) [95% CI]	LR(−) [95% CI]
Right lower quadrant pain	0.81	0.53	7.31–8.46†	0–0.28†
Rigidity	0.27	0.83	3.76 (2.96–4.78)	0.82 (0.79–0.85)
Migration	0.64	0.82	3.18 (2.41–4.21)	0.50 (0.42–0.59)
Pain before vomiting‡	1.00	0.64	2.76 (1.94–3.94)	NA
Psoas sign	0.16	0.95	2.38 (1.21–4.67)	0.90 (0.83–0.98)
Fever	0.67	0.79	1.94 (1.63–2.32)	0.58 (0.51–0.67)
Rebound tenderness test	0.63	0.69	1.10–6.30†	0–0.86†
Guarding	0.74	0.57	1.65–1.78†	0–0.54†
No similar pain previously	0.81	0.41	1.50 (1.36–1.66)	0.323 (0.246–0.424)
Rectal tenderness	0.41	0.77	0.83–5.34†	0.36–1.15†
Anorexia	0.68	0.36	1.27 (1.16–1.38)	0.64 (0.54–0.75)
Nausea	0.58	0.37	0.69–1.20†	0.70–0.84†
Vomiting	0.51	0.45	0.92 (0.82–1.04)	1.12 (0.95–1.33)

*LR(+) indicates the positive likelihood ratio with its 95% CI; LR(−), the negative likelihood ratio with its 95% CI.
†In heterogeneous studies, the LRs are reported as ranges.
‡Only one study on this is included in the meta-analysis.
SOURCE: From Wagner et al.[5]

- Fever in appendicitis is a relatively late finding and rarely exceeds 39°C (102.2°F) unless rupture or other complications occur.

DIAGNOSIS AND DIFFERENTIAL

- The diagnosis of appendicitis is primarily clinical. Factors that increase the likelihood of appendicitis, listed in decreasing order of importance, are: right lower quadrant pain, rigidity, migration of pain to the right lower quadrant, pain before vomiting, positive psoas sign, rebound tenderness, and guarding.
- If the diagnosis is unclear, additional studies such as complete blood count, urinalysis, pregnancy test, and radiologic imaging should be considered.
- Elevation of the white blood cell count is sensitive, but has a very low specificity for appendicitis.[6] The positive and negative predictive values of an elevated WBC in acute appendicitis are 92% and 50%, respectively.[7]
- Obtaining a urinalysis is important to rule out other diagnoses, such as urolithiasis or urinary tract infection; however, pyuria and hematuria can occur when an inflamed appendix overlies a ureter.[8]
- Plain radiographs of the abdomen are often abnormal but are not specific.[6] Radiographic findings of possible acute appendicitis include appendiceal fecalith, appendiceal gas, localized paralytic ileus, blurred right psoas muscle, and free air.
- Ultrasonography has a high sensitivity but is limited in evaluating a ruptured appendix or an abnormally located (eg, retrocecal) appendix.[9,10]
- Computed tomography (CT) is more sensitive than ultrasound (98% vs. 87%), with comparable specificity (95% vs. 97%); debate exists whether focused appendiceal CT or traditional nonfocused abdominal CT is the better choice.[11] CT findings suggesting acute appendicitis include pericecal inflammation, abscess, and periappendiceal phlegmon or fluid collections.
- In order to avoid premature surgical intervention or discharge of the patient with an uncertain diagnosis, patients with atypical presentations may be observed with serial abdominal examination.[12]
- Patients under the age of 5 and the elderly have higher rates of misdiagnosis of appendicitis, leading to increased morbidity and mortality rates.[13,14]
- Appendicitis is the most common extrauterine surgical emergency in pregnancy, and occurs with an incidence equal to that of nonpregnant patients; if perforation and peritonitis occur, then fetal mortality rates are high.[15]
- Patients with AIDS have an increased risk of complications from appendicitis because of delays in diagnosis due to their frequently pre-existing gastrointestinal symptoms and immunocompromised state.[16]

EMERGENCY DEPARTMENT CARE AND DISPOSITION

- Prior to surgery, patients should have nothing by mouth, and should have IV access, analgesia, and antibiotic therapy started.
- Short-acting narcotic analgesics such as fentanyl (0.01 to 0.02 mg/kg) are preferred, since they can be reversed by naloxone if necessary.
- Antibiotics should cover anaerobes, enterococci, and gram-negative intestinal flora, such as monotherapy with tazobactam-piperacillin 3.375 g IV or ampicillin-sulbactam 3 g IV.[17]
- If no precise diagnosis is determined after evaluation and observation, the patient should be diagnosed as having nonspecific abdominal pain rather than be given a more specific diagnosis.
- Patients who have no contraindication to discharge should be given specific instructions to obtain close follow-up with their primary care physician, and to return if their condition worsens, or if they develop increased pain, fever, or nausea.

REFERENCES

1. Korner H, Soreide JA, Pederson EJ, et al: Stability of the incidence of acute appendicitis: A population based longitudinal study. *Dig Surg* 18:61, 2001.
2. Rao PM, Rhea JT, Rattner DW, Venus LG, Novelline RA: Introduction of appendiceal CT: impact on negative appendectomy and appendiceal perforation rates. *Ann Surg* 229:344, 1999.
3. Guss DA, Richards C: Comparison of men and women presenting to an ED with acute appendicitis. *Am J Emerg Med* 18:372, 2000.
4. Collins DC: 71,000 Human appendix specimens: A final report, summarizing forty years study. *Am J Proctol* 14:265, 1963.
5. Wagner J, McKinney WP, Carpenter JL: Does this patient have appendicitis? *JAMA* 276:1589, 1996.
6. Hoffman J, Rausmussen O: Aids in the diagnosis of acute appendicitis. *Br J Surg* 76:774, 1989.
7. Marchand A, Van Lente F, Galen RS: The assessment of laboratory tests in the diagnosis of acute appendicitis. *Am J Clin Pathol* 80:369, 1983.
8. Puskar D, Bedalov G, Fridrih S, et al: Urinalysis, ultrasound analysis, and renal dynamic scintigraphy in acute appendicitis. *Urology* 45:108, 1995.
9. Douglas CD, Macpherson NE, Davidson PM, Gani JS: Randomized controlled trial of ultrasonography in diagnosis of acute appendicitis, incorporating the Alvarado score. *BMJ* 321:919, 2000.
10. Jeffrey RB, Jain KA, Ngheim HV: Sonographic diagnosis of acute appendicitis: Interpretive pitfalls. *AJR Am J Roentgenol* 162:55, 1994.

11. Jacobs JE, Birnbaum BA, Macari M, et al: Acute appendicitis: comparison of helical CT diagnosis focused technique with oral contrast material versus nonfocused technique with oral and intravenous contrast material. *Radiology* 220:683, 2001.

12. Paulson EK, Kalady MF, Papas TN: Suspected appendicitis. *N Engl J Med* 348:236, 2003.

13. Cappendijk VC, Hazebroek FW: The impact of diagnostic delay on the course of acute appendicitis. *Arch Dis Child* 83: 64, 2000.

14. Franz M, Norman J, Fabri PJ: Increased mortality of appendicitis with advancing age. *Am Surg* 61:40, 1995.

15. Mahmoodian S: Appendicitis complicating pregnancy. *South Med J* 85:19, 1992.

16. Flum DR, Steinberg SD, Sarkis AY, et al: Appendicitis in patients with acquired immunodeficiency syndrome. *J Am Coll Surg* 184:481, 1997.

17. Anderson BR, Kallehave FL, Anderson HK: Antibiotics versus placebo for prevention of post-operative infection after appendectomy. *Cochrane Review* 1, 2003. Oxford Update Software.

For further reading in *Emergency Medicine: A Comprehensive Study Guide,* 6th ed., see Chap. 78, "Acute Appendicitis," by Denis J. FitzGerald and Arthur M. Pancioli.

44 INTESTINAL OBSTRUCTION

Roy L. Alson

EPIDEMIOLOGY

- Small bowel obstruction (SBO) is more common than large bowel obstruction (LBO).
- Intestinal obstruction is due to mechanical obstruction or functional (adynamic or paralytic ileus) obstruction, with ileus being more common. Mechanical obstruction may be due to either intrinsic or extrinsic mechanisms.
- Adhesions following surgery are the most common cause of SBO.[1] Incarcerated inguinal hernias are the second most common cause of SBO. Other causes of bowel obstruction are listed in Table 44-1.
- Large bowel obstruction is most commonly due to neoplasm.[2] Fecal impaction is common in elderly and debilitated patients.
- Complications and mortality rises in those over 60 years of age.[1] Mortality also increases dramatically if corrective surgery is delayed beyond 24 hours.[4]
- Ileus may be due to injury, infection, medications, or electrolyte abnormalities.

TABLE 44-1   Common Causes of Bowel Obstruction

DUODENUM	SMALL BOWEL	COLON
Stensois	Adhesions	Carcinoma
Foreign body/bezoar	Hernia	Fecal impaction
Stricture	Intussusception	Ulcerative colitis
Superior mesenteric artery syndrome	Lymphoma	Volvulus
	Stricture	Diverticulitis (strictures or abscess)
		Intussusception
		Pseudo-obstruction

PATHOPHYSIOLOGY

- Blockage prevents passage of luminal contents and results in dilatation due to accumulation of gastric, biliary, and pancreatic secretions.
- With distention, intraluminal pressure rises, decreasing bowel wall blood flow. When pressure exceeds capillary pressure, absorption ceases and leakage of fluids (third-spacing) may occur. Microvascular changes may allow entry of gut flora into the circulation, resulting in bacteremia and sepsis. Necrosis and bowel perforation may follow.
- With obstruction, oral fluid intake stops and vomiting occurs. This fluid loss, coupled with the third space losses mentioned above, leads to hypovolemia and shock.[2]
- Closed loop obstruction has a more rapid progression.

CLINICAL FEATURES

- Classic history includes vomiting, abdominal distention, and pain, with a past history of abdominal surgery or hernia.
- Abdominal pain is crampy and intermittent. SBO results in primarily periumbilical pain versus hypogastric pain for LBO.[1,3] Pain with ileus may be constant.
- Emesis is often bilious early and may be feculent with late SBO or with LBO.
- Early in the disease course, bowel sounds have high-pitched rushes, but this finding diminishes with time.
- The patient may have surgical scars, hernias, or intra-abdominal masses.
- Peritoneal signs suggest perforation.
- Clinical signs of dehydration and/or shock may be present (tachycardia, hypotension).
- Rectal exam may reveal impaction, occult blood, or carcinoma. Passage of stool does not rule out obstruction.
- Women may have palpable gynecologic neoplasms on pelvic exam.

DIAGNOSIS AND DIFFERENTIAL

- Radiographs help localize small versus large bowel obstruction. Plicae circulares are linear densities that traverse the small bowel lumen. Haustrae in the large bowel do not extend fully across the lumen.
- Dilated loops of bowel on supine film with stepladder air-fluid levels on upright film are diagnostic (Fig. 44-1). Look on upright or decubitus film for free air suggesting perforation, and for pneumonia or pleural effusions on the chest film.
- Laboratory tests include complete blood count (CBC), blood urea nitrogen (BUN), serum electrolytes, serum amylase, and urinalysis. Liver function tests as well as cross-match and coagulation studies may also be needed.
- Leukocytosis with a left shift may suggest peritonitis, gangrene of the bowel, or an abscess.[2] Serum lactate may be useful in assessing the presence of mesenteric vascular occlusion.
- As dehydration and shock develop, elevated urine specific gravity and metabolic acidosis may be seen along with hemoconcentration.
- Sigmoidoscopy or barium enema may be useful in localizing the site of LBO.
- Contrast-enhanced abdominal CT has been advocated to identify partial versus complete bowel obstruction.[5,7]
- Pseudo-obstruction (Ogilvie's syndrome) is most commonly seen in the low colonic region.[6] Intestinal motility is depressed (often due to tricyclic antidepressants or anticholinergic agents), resulting in large volumes of retained gas. Air-fluid levels are rarely seen on x-ray. Pseudo-obstruction is treated by colonoscopy.

EMERGENCY DEPARTMENT CARE AND DISPOSITION

- With mechanical bowel obstruction, prompt surgical consultation is required.
- A nasogastric tube is used to decompress the bowel. Use of long intestinal tubes in the ED is not indicated.
- Fluid resuscitation should be started using crystalloid. Monitor vital signs and urine output to measure response to fluids.
- Appropriate antibiotic therapy (such as piperacillin-tazobactam 3.375 g, or ampicillin-sulbactam 3.0 g IV) should be started if perforation is suspected or surgery is anticipated.
- For adynamic ileus, conservative treatment including nasogastric decompression, fluid replacement, and observation are usually effective.

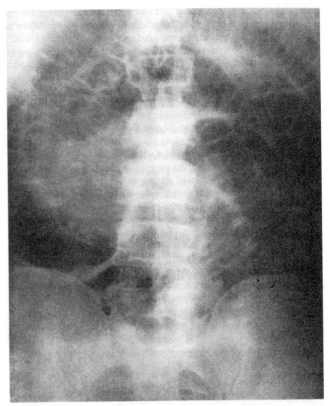

A

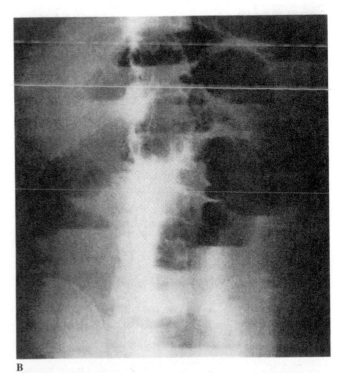

B

FIG. 44-1. A. Flat-plate abdominal film illustrates distended loops of small bowel. **B.** Upright film demonstrates multiple air-fluid levels and stepladder appearance. (Reproduced with permission from Harris JH, Harris WH: *The Radiology of Emergency Medicine*, 3rd ed. Baltimore: Williams & Wilkins, 1993, p. 843.)

REFERENCES

1. Becker WF: Intestinal obstruction: An analysis of 1007 cases. *South Med J* 48:41, 1955.
2. Cheadle WC, Garr FE, Richardson JD: The importance of early diagnosis of small bowel obstruction. *Am Surg* 54:565, 1988.
3. Shatila AH, Chamberlain BE, Webb WR: Current status of diagnosis and management of strangulation obstruction of the small bowel. *Am J Surg* 132:299, 1976.
4. Brolin RE, Krasna MJ, Mast BA: Use of tubes and radiographs in bowel obstruction. *Ann Surg* 206:126, 1987.
5. Frager D, Baer JW, et al: Detection of intestinal ischemia in patients with acute small bowel obstruction due to adhesions or hernia: Efficacy of CT. *AJR Am J Roentgenol* 167:1451, 1996.
6. Doudi S, Berry AR, Kettlewell MS: Acute colonic pseudo obstruction. *Br J Surg* 79:99, 1992.
7. Daneshmand S, Hedley CG, Stain SC: The utility and reliability of computed tomography scan in the diagnosis of small bowel obstruction. *Am Surg* 65:922, 1999.

For further reading in *Emergency Medicine, A Comprehensive Study Guide,* 6th ed., see Chap. 79, "Intestinal Obstruction," by Salvator J. Vicario and Timothy G. Price.

---

45 HERNIA IN ADULTS AND CHILDREN

N. Heramba Prasad

- A hernia is an external or internal protrusion of a body part from its natural location.

EPIDEMIOLOGY

- Abdominal wall hernias occur in six locations: inguinal, femoral, umbilical, anterior abdominal, pelvic, or lumbar (Fig. 45-1).
- Incidence of abdominal wall hernia is 10 to 20 per 1000 births and is greater in premature infants.[1]
- Predisposing factors include prematurity, family history, genitourinary abnormalities, ascites, peritoneal dialysis, ventriculoperitoneal shunt, cystic fibrosis, chronic obstructive pulmonary disease, pregnancy, or wounds.
- Groin hernias occur more frequently in males. Indirect inguinal hernias in males are more common on the right side due to later passage of the right testis, and have a bimodal incidence, with peaks in infants and in adults older than 40 years. Umbilical and femoral hernias are more common in females. Anterior abdominal wall hernias have a similar incidence in both genders.

PATHOPHYSIOLOGY

- Hernias occur in structural areas with inherent weakness, including penetration sites for extraperitoneal structures, areas lacking strong multilayer support, and wound sites (either surgical or traumatic).
- Specific hernia types: (1) an indirect inguinal hernia passes through the inguinal canal, which is an internal ring defect lateral to the inferior epigastric vessels; (2) a direct inguinal hernia occurs primarily in adults and is an acquired defect through the external ring medial to the inferior epigastric vessels; (3) a femoral hernia protrudes below the inguinal ligament in the femoral canal; (4) the umbilical hernia occurs in infants; (5) the epigastric hernia passes through the linea alba of the rectus sheath above the umbilicus; (6) the spigelian hernia occurs at the site of the semilunar or arcuate line, just lateral to the rectus muscle; (7) pelvic hernias are rare and pass through sciatic foramen; (8) lumbar hernias are extremely rare; (9) incisional hernias occur through incision sites and are more likely with infection and obesity.

CLINICAL FEATURES

- Symptoms may include pain, nausea and vomiting, or possibly even clinical toxicity. Infants may exhibit irritability.
- Most hernias are detected during routine physical examination.
- Complications include: (1) inclusion of a viscus (a sliding hernia); (2) incarceration or irreducibility; (3) vascular compromise of the incarcerated contents (strangulation); (4) bowel obstruction due to incarceration and local edema; (5) bowel perforation due to strangulation; (6) gangrene, abscess formation, peritonitis, and sepsis due to ischemic bowel.

DIAGNOSIS AND DIFFERENTIAL

- Most of the above-described hernias are palpable on exam; however, the spigelian hernia is frequently intraperitoneal, and may not be detectable on physical exam.
- Chest x-ray and multiple views of the abdomen are useful to exclude bowel obstruction or perforation.
- A groin hernia must be differentiated from a lymph node, vascular aneurysm, scrotal hydrocele, epi-

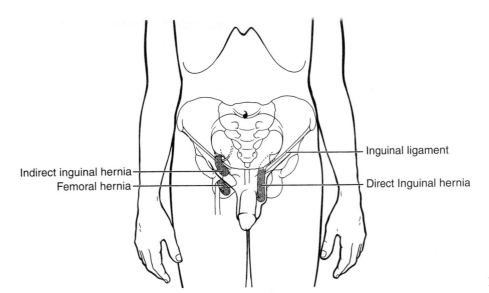

FIG. 45-1. Groin hernias.

didymitis, testicular torsion, undescended testis, groin abscess, cellulitis, or tumor.

- Suspicion of spigelian or pelvic hernias often necessitates the use of ultrasonography or computed tomography.[2]

EMERGENCY DEPARTMENT CARE AND DISPOSITION

- Recently incarcerated hernias may be gently reduced in the ED. The patient may be discharged with outpatient surgical referral.
- Infants with inguinal hernias have a high risk of incarceration and should be referred for surgical repair within the next few days.[3] In contrast, umbilical hernias rarely incarcerate.
- The need for repair of all groin hernias has recently been questioned.[4]
- For cases suspected of strangulation and ischemic bowel, treatment should include broad-spectrum antibiotics (such as piperacillin-tazobactam 3.375 g IV, or double drug coverage with cefotaxime 2 g IV or ceftriaxone 2 g IV plus clindamycin 600 mg IV or metronidazole 1 g IV), IV fluids, nasogastric decompression, and an immediate surgical consultation.

REFERENCES

1. Mensching DJ, Musielewicz AJ: Abdominal wall hernias. *Emerg Med Clin North Am* 14:739, 1996.
2. Hojer AM, Rygaard H, Jess P: CT in the diagnosis of abdominal wall hernias: A preliminary study. *Eur Radiology* 7:1416, 1997.
3. Gahukamble DE, Khamage AS: Early versus delayed repair of reduced incarcerated inguinal hernias in the pediatric population. *J Pediatr Surg* 31:1218, 1996.
4. Crawford DL, Phillips EH: laparoscopic repair and groin hernia surgery. *Surg Clin North Am* 78:1047, 1998.

For further reading in *Emergency Medicine: A Comprehensive Study Guide,* 6th ed., see Chap. 80, "Hernia in Adults and Children," by Frank W. Lavoie and Mary Harkins Becker.

46 ILEITIS, COLITIS, AND DIVERTICULITIS

Jonathan A. Maisel

CROHN'S DISEASE

- Crohn's disease—also described as regional enteritis, terminal ileitis, and granulomatous ileocolitis—is an idiopathic gastrointestinal (GI) tract disease. Segmental involvement of any part of the GI tract, from the mouth to the anus, by a nonspecific granulomatous inflammatory process characterizes the disease.

EPIDEMIOLOGY

- The peak incidence of Crohn's disease occurs in patients between 15 and 22 years of age with a secondary peak at age 55 to 60 years.
- Crohn's disease is seen worldwide, but is more common in people of European descent.

- There is a 20 to 30% increased risk of Crohn's disease among women as compared to men. It is four times more common among Jews than non-Jews, and is more common in whites than blacks, Asians, or Native Americans.
- A family history of inflammatory bowel disease is present in 10 to 15% of patients.

PATHOPHYSIOLOGY

- The cause is still unknown.
- The most important pathologic feature of Crohn's disease is the involvement of all the layers of the bowel and extension into mesenteric lymph nodes. This may lead to the development of fissures, fistulas, and abscesses. In addition, the disease is discontinuous, with normal areas alternating with diseased areas.

CLINICAL FEATURES

- Abdominal pain, anorexia, diarrhea, and weight loss are present in up to 80% of cases, although the clinical course is variable and unpredictable.
- Patients commonly report a history of recurring fever, abdominal pain, and diarrhea over several years, without a definitive diagnosis.
- One third of patients develop perianal fissures or fistulas, abscesses, or rectal prolapse. Fistulas occur between the ileum and sigmoid colon, the cecum, another ileal segment, or the skin. Abscesses are characterized as intraperitoneal, retroperitoneal, interloop, or intramesenteric.
- Growth retardation can be seen in children.[1]
- Obstruction, hemorrhage, and toxic megacolon also occur. Obstruction is caused by edema of the bowel wall, and stricture formation secondary to the inflammatory process. Half of all cases of toxic megacolon occur in patients with Crohn's disease, frequently associated with massive GI bleeding.[2]
- Up to 30% of patients develop extraintestinal manifestations including arthritis, uveitis, and skin disease (eg, erythema nodosum and pyoderma gangrenosum).
- Hepatobiliary disease, including gallstones, pericholangitis, and chronic active hepatitis, is commonly seen, as is pancreatitis.
- Hyperoxaluria, caused by increased colonic absorption of dietary oxalate, leads to the development of nephrolithiasis in up to 25% of patients.
- Some patients develop thromboembolic disease as a result of a hypercoagulable state; they have a 25% mortality rate.
- Malabsorption, malnutrition, and chronic anemia develop in long-standing disease, and the incidence of GI tract malignant neoplasm is triple that of the general population.
- The recurrence rate for patients with Crohn's disease is 25 to 50% when treated medically, and higher for patients treated surgically.

DIAGNOSIS AND DIFFERENTIAL

- The definitive diagnosis of Crohn's disease is usually established months or years after the onset of symptoms. Common misdiagnoses are appendicitis and pelvic inflammatory disease.
- A careful and detailed history for previous bowel symptoms that preceded acute presentation may provide clues for correct diagnosis. The absence of true guarding or rebound is noted.
- Peritonitis and leukocytosis can be masked in patients taking glucocorticoids.
- The differential diagnosis of Crohn's disease includes lymphoma, ileocecal amebiasis, sarcoidosis, tuberculosis, Kaposi's sarcoma, *Campylobacter* enteritis, and *Yersinia* ileocolitis. Most of these are uncommon, and the latter two can be differentiated by stool cultures.
- Laboratory evaluation should include a complete blood count (CBC), chemistries, and type and crossmatch when indicated.
- Plain abdominal radiography may identify perforation, obstruction, and toxic megacolon, which may appear as a long, continuous segment of air-filled colon greater than 6 cm in diameter.
- Computed tomography of the abdomen is the most useful test to identify both intra- and extraintestinal manifestations of Crohn's disease.
- A definitive diagnosis is confirmed by an upper GI series, an air contrast barium enema, and colonoscopy.

EMERGENCY DEPARTMENT CARE AND DISPOSITION

- Initial treatment requires restoration of fluid loss and correction of electrolyte abnormalities.[2,3]
- Sulfasalazine 3 to 4 g/day is effective for mild to moderate active Crohn's disease, but has multiple toxic side effects, including GI and hypersensitivity reactions. Mesalamine, up to 4 g/day, is equally effective with fewer side effects.[2,3]
- Glucocorticoids (prednisone) 40 to 60 mg/day are reserved for severe small intestine disease and ileocolitis.
- Immunosuppressive drugs, 6-mercaptopurine (1 to 1.5 mg/kg/day), or azathioprine (1 to 2.5 mg/kg/day), are used as steroid-sparing agents, in healing fistulas, and in patients with serious surgical contraindications.[2,3]

- Metronidazole 10 to 20 mg/kg/day or ciprofloxacin 500 to 750 mg twice daily is useful in patients with perianal complications and fistulous disease.[4]
- Patients with medically resistant moderate to severe Crohn's disease may benefit from the anti–tumor necrosis factor antibody infliximab, given 5 mg/kg IV.[5] Patients must be screened for tuberculosis prior to treatment.[5]
- Diarrhea can be controlled by loperamide 4 to 16 mg/day, diphenoxylate 5 to 20 mg/day, and cholestyramine 4 g 1 to 6 times per day.
- Patients who should be admitted include those who demonstrate signs of fulminant colitis, peritonitis, obstruction, significant hemorrhage, severe dehydration, electrolyte imbalance, or those with less severe disease who fail outpatient management.
- Surgical intervention is indicated in patients with intestinal obstruction or hemorrhage, perforation, abscess or fistula formation, toxic megacolon, perianal disease, and sometimes in those who fail medical therapy.
- The recurrence rate after surgery is nearly 100%.

ULCERATIVE COLITIS

- Ulcerative colitis is an idiopathic chronic inflammatory and ulcerative disease of the colon and rectum, characterized most often clinically by bloody diarrhea.

EPIDEMIOLOGY

- Ulcerative colitis is more prevalent in the United States and northern Europe.
- Peak incidence occurs in the second and third decades of life.
- First-degree relatives have a 15-fold increased risk of developing ulcerative colitis and a 3.5-fold increased risk of developing Crohn's disease.
- There is a slight predominance in men.

PATHOPHYSIOLOGY

- Ulcerative colitis involves primarily the mucosa and submucosa, with sparing of the outer layers of the bowel wall.
- Microscopically, the disease is characterized by mucosal inflammation with formation of crypt abscesses, epithelial necrosis, and mucosal ulceration.
- The rectosigmoid colon is involved in 95% of cases.

CLINICAL FEATURES

- Ulcerative colitis is commonly characterized by intermittent attacks of acute disease with complete remission between bouts.
- Patients with mild disease (60%) have fewer than four bowel movements per day, no systemic symptoms, and few extraintestinal manifestations. Disease is limited to the rectum in 80%.
- Severe disease (15%) is associated with frequent daily bowel movements, weight loss, fever, tachycardia, anemia, and more frequent extraintestinal manifestations, including peripheral arthritis, ankylosing spondylitis, episcleritis, uveitis, pyoderma gangrenosum, and erythema nodosum.
- Ninety percent of the mortality from ulcerative colitis is in patients with severe disease.
- The most serious complication is toxic megacolon. This occurs when the disease extends through all layers of the colon, resulting in a loss of muscular tone, dilatation, and potential perforation and peritonitis.
- Mortality from perforation is 50%, but is reduced to 10% if surgery is undertaken prior to perforation.
- Abscess and fistula formation, which is much more common in patients with Crohn's disease, occurs in 20% of patients with ulcerative colitis.[6] GI hemorrhage (most common), obstruction secondary to stricture formation, and acute perforation are other complications.
- There is a 10- to 30-fold increased risk of developing colon carcinoma.

DIAGNOSIS AND DIFFERENTIAL

- The diagnosis of ulcerative colitis may be considered with a history of abdominal cramps, diarrhea, and mucoid stools. Laboratory findings are nonspecific and may include leukocytosis, anemia, thrombocytosis, decreased serum albumin, abnormal liver function tests, and negative stool studies for ova, parasites, and enteric pathogens.
- Barium enema can confirm the diagnosis and defines the extent of colonic involvement, but colonoscopy is the most sensitive method. Rectal biopsy can exclude amebiasis and metaplasia.
- The differential diagnosis includes infectious, ischemic, irradiation, antineoplastic agent–induced, pseudomembranous, and Crohn's colitis. When the disease is limited to the rectum, consider sexually acquired diseases such as rectal syphilis, gonococcal proctitis, lymphogranuloma venereum, and inflammation caused by herpes simplex virus, *Entamoeba histolytica*, *Shigella*, and *Campylobacter*.

EMERGENCY DEPARTMENT CARE AND DISPOSITION

- Patients with severe ulcerative colitis should be treated with fluid replacement and correction of electrolyte abnormalities.
- Patients on steroids should receive hydrocortisone 300 mg/day, methylprednisolone 48 mg/day, or prednisone 60 mg/day.[7]
- Cyclosporine 4 mg/kg/day has been advocated for cases of fulminant colitis that have failed treatment with intravenous steroids.[8]
- Intravenous antibiotics active against coliforms and anaerobes, such as ampicillin (2 g every 6 hours), gentamicin (1.5 mg/kg every 8 hours), and clindamycin (300 to 600 mg every 6 hours) or metronidazole (500 mg every 8 hours) should be initiated.
- Patients with significant gastrointestinal hemorrhage, toxic megacolon, and bowel perforation should be admitted with consultation with both a gastroenterologist and a surgeon.
- The majority of patients with mild and moderate disease can be treated as outpatients. Therapy listed below should be discussed with a gastroenterologist, and close follow-up must be ensured.
  1. Prednisone 40 to 60 mg/day is usually sufficient and can be adjusted depending on the severity of the disease. Once clinical remission is achieved, steroids should be slowly tapered and discontinued, as there is no evidence that maintenance dosages of steroids reduce the incidence of relapses.
  2. Sulfasalazine 1.5 to 2 g/day is inferior to steroids in treating acute attacks and is most useful as maintenance therapy by reducing the recurrence rate. Newer 5-aminosalicylic derivatives such as mesalamine are quite effective in inducing and maintaining remission, with fewer side effects.
  3. In patients with active proctitis, 5-aminosalicylic enemas and topical steroid preparations such as beclomethasone and hydrocortisone can be used acutely and to maintain remission with fewer side effects.
  4. In refractory cases, a combination of glucocorticoids and immunomodulators, such as 6-mercaptopurine 1 to 1.5 mg/kg/day or azathioprine 1 to 2 mg/kg/day, should be considered.
  5. Supportive measures include replenishment of iron stores, dietary elimination of lactose, and addition of bulking agents such as psyllium. Antidiarrheal agents can precipitate toxic megacolon and should be avoided.

PSEUDOMEMBRANOUS COLITIS

- Pseudomembranous colitis is an inflammatory bowel disorder in which membrane-like yellowish plaques of exudate overlie and replace necrotic intestinal mucosa.

EPIDEMIOLOGY

- *Clostridium difficile* is a spore-forming obligate anaerobic bacillus that causes pseudomembranous colitis.
- Risk factors for this disease include recent antibiotic use, GI surgery or manipulation, severe underlying medical illness, and advanced age.
- Three different syndromes have been described: neonatal pseudomembranous enterocolitis, postoperative pseudomembranous enterocolitis, and antibiotic-associated pseudomembranous colitis.
- *C. difficile* is the most common enteric pathogen associated with nosocomial diarrhea.[9]

PATHOPHYSIOLOGY

- Hospitalized patients are colonized with *C. difficile* in 10 to 25% of cases.
- Broad-spectrum antibiotics—most notably clindamycin, cephalosporins, and ampicillin/amoxicillin—alter the gut flora in such a way that toxin-producing *C. difficile* can flourish within the colon, producing clinical manifestations of pseudomembranous colitis.
- Chemotherapeutic agents[10] and antiviral agents[11] have been implicated as well.

CLINICAL FEATURES

- Clinical manifestations can vary from frequent, watery, mucoid stools, to a toxic picture including profuse diarrhea, crampy abdominal pain, fever, leukocytosis, and dehydration.
- Examination of the stool may reveal fecal leukocytes. Toxic megacolon, colonic perforation, and extraintestinal complications occur rarely.

DIAGNOSIS AND DIFFERENTIAL

- The disease typically begins 7 to 10 days after the institution of antibiotics, but the range is between a few days up to 8 weeks.
- The diagnosis is confirmed by the demonstration of *C. difficile* in the stool and by the detection of toxin in

stool filtrates. Colonoscopy is not routinely needed to confirm the diagnosis.

EMERGENCY DEPARTMENT CARE AND DISPOSITION

- The treatment of pseudomembranous colitis includes discontinuing antibiotic therapy, initiating intravenous fluid replacement, and correcting electrolyte abnormalities. This is effective without additional treatment in 25% of patients.
- Metronidazole 250 mg PO four times daily is the treatment of choice in patients with mild to moderate disease that do not respond to supportive measures. Vancomycin 125 to 250 mg PO four times daily should be reserved for cases in which the patient has not responded to or is intolerant of metronidazole, as well as for children and pregnant patients.[12,13]
- Patients with severe diarrhea, those with a systemic response (fever, leukocytosis, severe abdominal pain), and those whose symptoms persist despite appropriate outpatient management must be hospitalized and should receive vancomycin 125 to 250 mg 4 times daily for 10 days. The symptoms usually resolve within a few days.
- Antidiarrheal agents may prolong or worsen symptoms and should be avoided.
- Relapses occur in 10 to 20% of patients.

DIVERTICULITIS

- Diverticulitis is caused by bacterial proliferation within an existing colonic diverticulum, leading to microperforation and inflammation of pericolonic tissue.

EPIDEMIOLOGY

- Clinical diverticulitis occurs in 10 to 25% of patients with diverticulosis. One third of the population will have acquired the disease by age 50, and two thirds by age 85.[14]
- Only 2 to 4% of patients with diverticulitis are under the age of 40, but the younger age group tends to have a more virulent form of the disease, with frequent complications requiring earlier surgical intervention.[15]

PATHOPHYSIOLOGY

- It remains unresolved whether diverticular disease is a disorder of colonic motility, a colonic muscle abnormality, a connective tissue disorder, or a normal concomitant of aging. A low-residue diet has been implicated as a major factor in the pathogenesis of diverticular disease.
- Most commonly, clinical diverticulitis results from high colonic pressures, resulting in erosion and microperforation of the diverticular wall, leading to inflammation of pericolonic tissue.

CLINICAL FEATURES

- The most common symptom is a steady, deep discomfort in the left lower quadrant of the abdomen. Other symptoms include tenesmus and changes in bowel habits such as diarrhea or increasing constipation.
- The involved diverticulum can irritate the urinary tract and cause frequency, dysuria, or pyuria.
- If a fistula develops between the colon and the bladder, the patient may present with recurrent urinary tract infections or pneumaturia.
- Paralytic ileus with abdominal distension, nausea, and vomiting may develop secondary to intra-abdominal irritation and peritonitis. Small bowel obstruction and perforation can also occur.
- Right lower quadrant pain, which may be indistinguishable from acute appendicitis, can occur with ascending colonic diverticular involvement and in patients with a redundant right-sided sigmoid colon.
- Physical examination frequently demonstrates a low-grade fever, but the temperature may be higher in patients with generalized peritonitis and in those with an abscess.
- The abdominal exam reveals localized tenderness, often with voluntary guarding and rebound tenderness. A fullness or mass may be appreciated over the affected area of colon.
- Occult blood may be present in the stool.

DIAGNOSIS AND DIFFERENTIAL

- The differential diagnosis includes appendicitis, peptic ulcer disease, pelvic inflammatory disease, endometriosis, ischemic colitis, aortic aneurysm, renal calculus, irritable bowel syndrome, lactate intolerance, colon carcinoma, intestinal lymphoma, Kaposi's sarcoma, sarcoidosis, collagen vascular disease, irradiation colitis or proctosigmoiditis, fecal impaction, foreign body granuloma, and any bacterial, parasitic, or viral infectious cause.
- Laboratory studies should include routine screening blood tests, urinalysis, and an abdominal radiographic series.
- Leukocytosis is present in only 36% of patients with diverticulitis.

- The abdominal series may be normal or may demonstrate an associated ileus, partial small bowel obstruction, colonic obstruction, free air indicating bowel perforation, or extraluminal collections of air, suggesting a walled-off abscess.
- Computed tomography of the abdomen is the diagnostic procedure of choice and may demonstrate presence of diverticulae, inflammation of pericolic fat, bowel wall thickening, or peridiverticular abscess.[16,17]

EMERGENCY DEPARTMENT CARE AND DISPOSITION

- If a patient has systemic signs and symptoms of infection, has failed outpatient management, or demonstrates signs of peritonitis, hospitalization and surgical consultation is necessary.
- Inpatient treatment includes IV antibiotics, usually an aminoglycoside such as gentamicin or tobramycin (1.5 mg/kg every 8 hours), and either metronidazole (500 mg every 8 hours) or clindamycin (300 to 600 mg every 6 hours), for aerobic and anaerobic organism coverage. Ticarcillin-clavulanic acid or imipenem have been used as alternate agents.
- The patient is placed on bowel rest, nothing by mouth is given, and IV fluids are administered. Nasogastric suction may be indicated in patients with bowel obstruction or adynamic ileus.[18]
- Outpatient management is acceptable for patients with localized pain without signs and symptoms of local peritonitis or systemic infection. Treatment consists of bowel rest and broad-spectrum oral antibiotic therapy. Common agents effective against aerobic organisms include ampicillin (500 mg every 6 hours), trimethoprim-sulfamethoxazole (2 tablets every 12 hours), ciprofloxacin (500 mg every 12 hours), or cephalexin (500 mg every 6 hours). One of these medications is taken in combination with an agent effective against anaerobic organisms, such as metronidazole (500 mg every 8 hours) or clindamycin (300 mg every 6 hours). Patients should limit activity and maintain a liquid diet for 48 hours. If symptoms improve, low-residue foods are added to the diet. Patients should seek medical care if they develop increasing abdominal pain, fever, or are unable to tolerate oral intake.

REFERENCES

1. Walker-Smith JA, Savage MO: Effects of inflammatory bowel disease on growth: Growth matters. *Kabi Pharmacia* 12:10, 1993.
2. Robert JR, Sachar DB, Greenstein AJ: Severe gastrointestinal hemorrhage in Crohn's disease. *Ann Surg* 213:207, 1991.
3. Hanauer SB, Sandborn W: The practice Parameters Committee of the American College of Gastroenterology: Management of Crohn's disease in adults. *Am J Gastroenterol* 96: 635, 2001.
4. Podolsky DK: Inflammatory bowel disease. *N Engl J Med* 347:417, 2002.
5. Targan SR, Hanauer SB, Ven Deventer SJH, et al: A short-term study of chimeric monoclonal antibody CA2 to tumor necrosis factor α for Crohn's disease. *N Engl J Med* 337: 1029, 1997.
6. Farraye FA, Peppercorn MA: Inflammatory bowel disease: Advances in the management of ulcerative colitis and Crohn's disease. *Consultant* 28:39, 46, 1988.
7. Meyers S, Sachar DB, Goldberg JD, et al: Corticotropin versus hydrocortisone in the intravenous treatment of ulcerative colitis. *Gastroenterology* 85:351, 1983.
8. Lichtiger S, Present DH, Kornbluth A, et al: Cyclosporine in severe ulcerative colitis refractory to steroid therapy. *N Engl J Med* 330:1841, 1994.
9. Viscidi R, Willey S, Bartlett JG: Isolation rates and toxigenic potential for *Clostridium difficile* isolates from various patient populations. *Gastroenterology* 81:5, 1981.
10. Silva J, Fekety R, Werk C, et al: Inciting and etiologic agents of colitis. *Rev Infect Dis* 6(Suppl 1):S214, 1984.
11. Colarian J: *Clostridium difficile* colitis following antiviral therapy in the acquired immunodeficiency syndrome. *Am J Med* 84:1081, 1988.
12. Demaio J, Bartlett JG: Update on diagnosis of *Clostridium difficile*–associated diarrhea. *Curr Clin Top Infect Dis* 15:97, 1995.
13. Fekety R, Silva J, Kauffman C, Buggy B, Deery G: Treatment of antibiotic associated *Clostridium difficile* colitis with oral vancomycin: Comparison of two dosage regimens. *Am J Med* 86:15, 1989.
14. Parks TC: Natural history of diverticular disease of the colon. *Clin Gastroenterol* 4:53, 1975.
15. Freischlag J, Bennion RS, Thompson JE: Complications of diverticular disease of the colon in young people. *Dis Col Rectum* 29:639, 1986.
16. Ferzoco LB, Raptopoulos V, Sileu W: Acute diverticulitis. *N Engl J Med* 338:1521, 1998.
17. Johnson CD, Baker ME, Rice RP: Diagnosis of acute colonic diverticulitis: Comparison of barium enema and CT. *Am J Radiol* 148:541, 1987.
18. Hackford AW, Schoetz DJ, Coller JA, et al: Surgical management of complicated diverticulitis. *Dis Colon Rectum* 28:317, 1985.

For further reading in *Emergency Medicine: A Comprehensive Study Guide,* 6th ed., see Chap. 81, "Ileitis, Colitis, and Diverticulitis," by Howard A. Werman, Hagop S. Mekhjian, and Douglas A. Rund.

47 ANORECTAL DISORDERS

N. Heramba Prasad

HEMORRHOIDS

EPIDEMIOLOGY

- Hemorrhoids are associated with constipation and straining at stool, pregnancy, obesity, chronic liver disease, portal hypertension, and rarely, tumors of the rectum and sigmoid colon.

PATHOPHYSIOLOGY

- Internal hemorrhoidal veins are located above the dentate line and drain into the portal venous system (Fig. 47-1).
- External hemorrhoidal veins are located below the dentate line and drain through the pudendal and iliac venous systems.

CLINICAL FEATURES

- Internal hemorrhoids are only visible through an anoscope and cause painless, bright-red rectal bleeding with defecation. Constant locations are at the 2, 5, and 9 o'clock positions in a prone patient.

- External hemorrhoids may be visualized on external exam and commonly cause pain and discomfort, most severe at the time of defecation.
- Thrombosis of external hemorrhoids is the usual cause of pain.
- Prolapse may occur with larger hemorrhoids, spontaneously reducing or requiring periodic manual reduction. Failure to reduce may lead to incarceration and even gangrene, requiring surgical intervention. Prolapse may cause mucous discharge and pruritus ani.
- The common complications of hemorrhoids are strangulation, thrombosis, and severe bleeding.

DIAGNOSIS AND DIFFERENTIAL

- Clinical signs cannot differentiate colonic lesions from hemorrhoids.[1]
- Other causes of rectal pain include malignancy, abscess, cryptitis, anal fissure, trauma, foreign bodies, rectal prolapse, and venereal proctitis.

EMERGENCY DEPARTMENT CARE AND DISPOSITION

- For most patients, treatment is nonsurgical and includes hot sitz baths and good hygiene, with the addition of bulk laxatives (psyllium seed compounds or gentle stool softeners) after the acute phase has

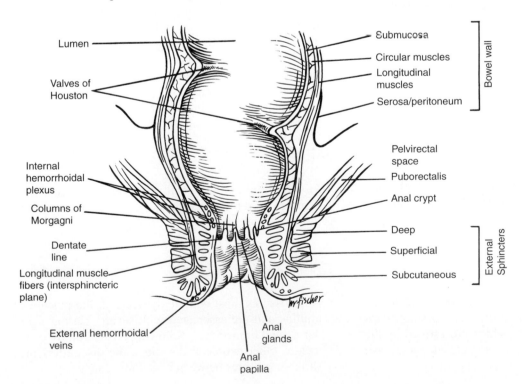

Lumen

Valves of Houston

Internal hemorrhoidal plexus

Columns of Morgagni

Dentate line

Longitudinal muscle fibers (intersphincteric plane)

External hemorrhoidal veins

Anal papilla

Anal glands

Submucosa

Circular muscles

Longitudinal muscles

Serosa/peritoneum

Bowel wall

Pelvirectal space

Puborectalis

Anal crypt

Deep

Superficial

Subcutaneous

External Sphincters

FIG. 47-1. Coronal section of the anorectum.

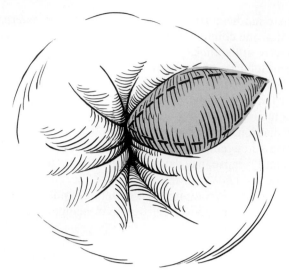

FIG. 47-2. Elliptical excision of thrombosed external hemorrhoid. (Reproduced with permission from Goldberg SM, et al: *Essentials of Anorectal Surgery*. Philadelphia: Lippincott, 1980.)

subsided. Topical analgesics or steroids may provide temporary relief.[2]
- Thrombosed external hemorrhoids require excision of the clots for relief. The thrombosed vein should be unroofed by an elliptical incision that allows evacuation of the multiloculated clots. Initial conservative treatment may be tried for less severe cases present for less than 48 hours (Fig. 47-2).
- Surgical referral and intervention is indicated for continued bleeding, intractable pain, incarceration, or strangulation. Rare complications of surgical repair include acute thrombosis, and for immunocompromised patients, potential pelvic sepsis.

CRYPTITIS

EPIDEMIOLOGY

- Cryptitis is associated with repetitive sphincter trauma, either secondary to spasm, recurrent diarrhea, or passage of large, hard stools.

PATHOPHYSIOLOGY

- The pleated columns of Morgagni, proximal to the dentate line, are connected at the base by small flaps of mucosa, the anal crypts, which are formed by the puckering action of the sphincter muscles and have the potential to become infected (cryptitis).

CLINICAL FEATURES

- Anal pain, spasm, and itching, with or without bleeding, are the usual symptoms.
- The posterior crypts are most commonly involved and are tender, swollen, and nodular.

DIAGNOSIS AND DIFFERENTIAL

- Diagnosis is confirmed by palpation or visualization by anoscopy.
- See hemorrhoid section for differential of anal pain. Cryptitis may coexist and lead to the development of fissures, fistulae, and abscess formation.

EMERGENCY DEPARTMENT CARE AND DISPOSITION

- Bulk laxatives, dietary fiber, hot sitz baths, and warm rectal irrigations will enhance healing. Surgical excision may be necessary in refractory cases.

FISSURE IN ANO

EPIDEMIOLOGY

- Anal fissures are the most common cause of painful rectal bleeding.
- In most cases, anal fissures occur in the midline posteriorly.
- An atypical anal fissure not located in the midline should alert the physician to other potentially life-threatening causes, including Crohn's disease, ulcerative colitis, carcinomas, lymphomas, syphilis, other sexually transmitted diseases (STDs), and tuberculosis.

PATHOPHYSIOLOGY

- Fissure in ano is the result of a linear tear from the dentate line through the sensitive anodermal tissue of the anal canal.

CLINICAL FEATURES

- Anal fissures most commonly occur in the posterior midline and are associated with severe, tearing pain during and immediately following defecation. In contrast to other anorectal disorders, the discomfort invariably subsides between bowel movements.

- Rectal examination may be limited secondary to severe pain; however, a characteristic sentinel pile, the result of swollen and hypertrophied papillae, may be visualized externally.

DIAGNOSIS AND DIFFERENTIAL

- See hemorrhoid section for differential of anal pain. Abscess and stricture formation may result from prolonged and severe fissure in ano.

EMERGENCY DEPARTMENT CARE AND DISPOSITION

- Hot sitz baths, a diet rich in bran, and local analgesic and/or hydrocortisone-containing ointments will provide symptomatic relief and alleviate sphincter spasm.

ANORECTAL ABSCESSES

EPIDEMIOLOGY

- Abscess may develop from prolonged or severe fissure in ano. Specific diseases associated with development of fistulous abscesses include gonococcal proctitis, carcinomas, Hodgkin's lymphoma, Crohn's disease, radiation fibrosis, trauma, immunocompromised states, and tuberculosis.
- The most common abscess is the perianal abscess.

PATHOPHYSIOLOGY

- Abscesses originate in the anal crypts with gland obstruction and spread to involve the perianal, intersphincteric, ischiorectal, deep perianal, or supralevator (pelvirectal) spaces.

CLINICAL FEATURES

- The perianal abscess occurs in the midline posteriorly and may be palpated as a superficial, tender mass with or without fluctuance.
- A dull, aching, throbbing pain persists between bowel movements, but also increases with defecation. Fever and leukocytosis may be present.

DIAGNOSIS AND DIFFERENTIAL

- See hemorrhoid section for differential of anal pain. Deeper perirectal abscesses may be difficult to detect on physical exam only. Endorectal ultrasonography[3] may be useful to confirm diagnosis.

EMERGENCY DEPARTMENT CARE AND DISPOSITION

- Most abscesses must be drained in the operating room by a surgeon, including all perirectal abscesses. Only simple perianal abscesses may be drained in the ED; however, caution is still advised.
- Once a simple abscess has been adequately drained, antibiotics need to be considered only for patients whose immune system may be compromised.

PILONIDAL SINUS

EPIDEMIOLOGY

- Most commonly occurs before the fourth decade of life.
- Carcinoma is a rare complication of recurrent pilonidal sinus disease occurring more frequently in men.

PATHOPHYSIOLOGY

- A pilonidal sinus or cyst is formed by a classically chronic and recurring foreign-body granuloma reaction to an ingrown hair.

CLINICAL FEATURES

- A pilonidal sinus or cyst will occur in the midline, upper part of the natal cleft overlying the lower sacrum and coccyx, causing pain, redness, and swelling.
- It is usually a chronic and recurring disease.

EMERGENCY DEPARTMENT CARE AND DISPOSITION

- Acute abscesses should be incised, drained, and packed in the ED.
- Once a simple abscess without complicating cellulitis has been adequately drained, antibiotics only need to be considered for patients whose immune system may be compromised.
- In order to prevent recurrence, definitive surgical excision of the entire pilonidal sinus system must be performed at least 6 weeks after all evidence of infection has resolved.

FISTULA IN ANO

EPIDEMIOLOGY

- A fistula most commonly results as a complication of a perianal or ischiorectal abscess; however, fistulae may be seen in association with ulcerative colitis, Crohn's disease, trauma, STDs, or tuberculosis.

PATHOPHYSIOLOGY

- A fistula is an abnormal tract connecting the anal canal with the skin.
- The Goodsall rule purports that anterior-opening fistulae follow a direct course to the anal canal; however, posterior-opening fistulae may course through a more unpredictable and circuitous path.

CLINICAL FEATURES

- Malodorous and bloody discharge persists as long as the fistula remains open. Most cases involve recurrent blockages of the path, resulting in chronic repetitive abscess formation and subsequent spontaneous drainage.

DIAGNOSIS AND DIFFERENTIAL

- Abscess may be the presenting sign for fistula in ano.
- A 7-MHz endoprobe ultrasonograph may be used for diagnosis.[3]

EMERGENCY DEPARTMENT CARE AND DISPOSITION

- Surgical excision is the definitive treatment.

RECTAL PROLAPSE/PROCIDENTIA

EPIDEMIOLOGY

- Prolapse of the rectal mucosa only is most commonly seen in children under the age of 2 years; however, it is also associated with third- and fourth-degree hemorrhoids in adults.
- Complete rectal prolapse (procidentia) occurs at the extremes of age and is most common in elderly women, with a higher incidence noted among women who have undergone hysterectomy.

PATHOPHYSIOLOGY

- The three classes of rectal prolapse are based upon anatomic differences: (1) prolapse of the rectal mucosa only; (2) prolapse of all three layers of the rectum; and (3) intussusception or telescoping of the upper rectum through the lower rectum.
- The second and third classes of prolapse are due to both a laxity in the pelvic floor and a weakening of the sphincter musculature.

CLINICAL FEATURES

- Clinical features include the detection of a protruding mass, blood-stained mucus anal discharge, and fecal incontinence.

DIAGNOSIS AND DIFFERENTIAL

- The prolapsed rectum may be mistaken for hemorrhoids. A rectal tumor must be ruled out in adults.

EMERGENCY DEPARTMENT CARE AND DISPOSITION

- Reduction may be accomplished after appropriate analgesia and sedation. If the tissue is ischemic, there is high risk of perforation and sepsis.
- Surgical correction is indicated; however, the patient may be discharged on stool softeners and referred for outpatient proctosigmoidoscopy after successful reduction in the ED.

ANORECTAL TUMORS

EPIDEMIOLOGY

- The most common (80%) and most aggressive anorectal tumor is the anal canal tumor, located proximal to the dentate line and including the transitional zone of epithelium. Neoplasms that occur in this group include adenocarcinoma, malignant melanoma, and Kaposi's sarcoma.

CLINICAL FEATURES

- Patients present with nonspecific symptoms including sensation of a mass, pruritus, pain, and blood in the stool. Constipation, anorexia and weight loss, narrowing of the stool caliber, and tenesmus eventually develop.

- An anal margin neoplasm will frequently present as an ulcer that fails to heal in a timely manner.

DIAGNOSIS AND DIFFERENTIAL

- Tumors may be misdiagnosed as hemorrhoids. Complications of anorectal tumors include rectal prolapse, prolonged blood loss, and perirectal abscesses or fistulas.

EMERGENCY DEPARTMENT CARE AND DISPOSITION

- Referral for proctoscopic or sigmoidoscopic examination and biopsy is mandatory.

RECTAL FOREIGN BODIES

CLINICAL FEATURES

- The most common location for a rectal foreign body is in the ampulla.
- The most common complication of rectal foreign body is perforation, which can result in overwhelming sepsis.

DIAGNOSIS AND DIFFERENTIAL

- A radiograph must be obtained to review the position, shape, and number of foreign bodies, and to exclude the presence of free air due to rectal perforation.

EMERGENCY DEPARTMENT CARE AND DISPOSITION

- Most foreign bodies are low in the rectum and may be removed in the ED after local anesthesia to obtain sphincter relaxation and administration of IV sedation.
- A surgeon or gastroenterologist should be consulted in cases with high risk of perforation or anticipated difficulty of removal. A broad-spectrum antibiotic should be administered.

PRURITUS ANI

EPIDEMIOLOGY

- Pruritus most commonly occurs during the fifth and sixth decades of life, affecting men primarily.

- Secondary pruritus ani may be due to anorectal disease, infection, diet, irritants, dermatologic conditions, or systemic diseases.

CLINICAL FEATURES

- Chronic pruritus ani may result in a thickened, depigmented appearance of the perianal skin.

EMERGENCY DEPARTMENT CARE AND DISPOSITION

- Referral to a proctologist and/or dermatologist is usually necessary.
- Symptomatic treatments include sitz baths, zinc oxide ointment, and 1% hydrocortisone cream.

REFERENCES

1. Segal WN, Greenberg PD, Rochay DC, et al: The outpatient evaluation of hematochezia. *Am J Gastroenterol* 93:179, 1998.
2. Maltz C, Black A: Anorectal disorders. *Emerg Med* 33:11, 2001.
3. Cataldo PA, Scenagore AJ, Luchtfeld MA: Intrarectal ultrasound in the evaluation of perirectal abscesses. *Dis Colon Rectum* 36:554, 1993.

For further reading in *Emergency Medicine; A Comprehensive Study Guide*, 6th ed., see Chap. 82, "Anorectal Disorders," by Brian E. Burgess and James K. Bouzoukis.

48 VOMITING, DIARRHEA, AND CONSTIPATION

Jonathan A. Maisel

VOMITING AND DIARRHEA

EPIDEMIOLOGY

- In the 1990s diarrhea accounted for less than 0.5% of all deaths in the United States.[1] Most diarrheal deaths occur in the elderly and the young.[1,2]
- Diarrhea is the second most common reason for work absenteeism and is estimated to cost $608 million in lost productivity per year.[3,4]

- Food-borne diseases are estimated to cause approximately 76 million illnesses, 325,000 hospitalizations, and 5000 deaths in the United States each year. The majority of these illnesses are caused by unknown or unidentified pathogens.[5] Most food-borne diseases go undiagnosed or unreported.
- Three pathogens, *Salmonella, Listeria,* and *Toxoplasma,* cause 1500 deaths each year, more than 75% of all deaths caused by known pathogens.[5] Newly recognized pathogens include *Campylobacter jejuni, Escherichia coli* O157:H7, *Listeria monocytogenes,* and *Cyclospora cayetanensis.*[5]
- A growing number of foods previously thought to be safe have been identified as new vehicles for transmission. *E. coli* O157:H7, generally associated with undercooked beef or unpasteurized dairy products, is now linked with items such as fruits, salad vegetables, yogurt, water, and acidic foods.
- Imported fresh fruits and vegetables, international travel, a trend towards eating meals outside the home, routine use of antibiotics to promote growth in farm animals, and increasing numbers of persons with compromised immunity, all contribute to the increasing incidence of food-borne disease.[6,7]
- Viral gastroenteritis, caused by Norwalk viruses, astroviruses, rotaviruses, and enteric adenoviruses are the most common form of food-borne disease with an estimated annual incidence in the United States of 23 million illnesses.[5,7] Simultaneous infection with more than one viral pathogen is common. Food-borne viruses are usually transmitted person to person by the fecal-oral route, and are infectious in very low doses.
- The most common causes of bacterial food-borne illnesses in the United States are *Campylobacter, Salmonella, Shigella,* and *E. coli.*[8]

PATHOPHYSIOLOGY

- Vomiting is a complex, highly coordinated activity involving the gastrointestinal tract, the central nervous system, and the vestibular system.
- Three stages of vomiting have been described: nausea, retching, and emesis.[9] With nausea comes hypersalivation and tachycardia. Retching occurs when the pylorus contracts and the fundus relaxes, thereby moving food to the gastric cardia. Finally, emesis occurs when the powerful abdominal muscles contract simultaneously and thus eject food or gastric secretions from the stomach.
- There are four basic mechanisms of diarrhea: increased intestinal secretion, decreased intestinal absorption, increased osmotic load, and abnormal intestinal motility.

- At a cellular level, intestinal absorption occurs through the villi, while secretion occurs though the crypts. In diarrheal states, enterotoxins, inflammation, or ischemia often damage the intestinal villi preferentially. As a result, diarrhea occurs because of diminished absorption by the intestinal villi and unopposed crypt secretion (crypts are more resilient after injury).[10]
- Normal physiologic defense mechanisms designed to prevent food-borne disease include gastric acid, normal GI flora, intestinal motility, and intestinal mucous glycoproteins.
- Direct invasion of the mucosal epithelial cells occurs with many food-borne pathogens, such as *Shigella, Salmonella,* enteroinvasive *E. coli, Campylobacter,* and *Vibrio parahaemolyticus.* Intracellular multiplication of these organisms is followed by epithelial cell death.
- Cytotoxins such as the Shiga toxin of *Shigella dysenteriae* or Shiga-like toxins produced by enterohemorrhagic *E. coli* O157:H7, enteropathogenic *E. coli,* and *Vibrio parahaemolyticus,* also cause cellular membrane disruption and cell lysis.
- *Vibrio cholerae* and enterotoxic *E. coli* produce protein toxins that alter fluid and electrolyte transfer across epithelial cell membranes and produce large volumes of fluid that exceed the absorptive capacity of the colon. The resultant excessive diarrhea can lead to rapid dehydration.

CLINICAL FEATURES

- Vomiting with blood can represent gastritis, peptic ulcer disease, or carcinoma. However, aggressive nonbloody vomiting followed by hematemesis is more consistent with a Mallory-Weiss tear.
- The presence of bile rules out gastric outlet obstruction, as from pyloric stenosis or strictures.
- An associated symptom such as fever would direct one to an infectious or inflammatory cause.
- Vomiting with chest pain suggests myocardial infarction or pneumonia.
- Vomiting with back pain can be seen with aortic aneurysm or dissection, pancreatitis, pyelonephritis, or renal colic.
- Headache with vomiting suggests increased intracranial pressure, such as with subarachnoid hemorrhage or head injury.
- Vomiting in a pregnant patient is consistent with hyperemesis gravidarum in the first trimester; but in the third trimester it could represent pre-eclampsia if accompanied by hypertension.
- Associated medical conditions are also useful in discerning the cause of vomiting: diabetes mellitus sug-

gests ketoacidosis, peripheral vascular disease suggests mesenteric ischemia, previous abdominal surgery suggests intestinal obstruction, and medication use (eg, lithium or digoxin) suggests toxicity.

- The physical examination in a vomiting patient includes a careful assessment of the gastrointestinal, pelvic, and genitourinary systems. In addition, assessment of hydration status is important.

- Other clues to specific causes for vomiting may come from the dermal exam (eg, hyperpigmentation with Addison's disease) or pulmonary examination (eg, signs of consolidation, suggesting pneumonia).

- By definition, diarrhea represents a daily stool output of >200 g, but generally refers to any increase in frequency or liquidity.[11] Other important historical factors include duration of illness and presence of blood.

- Acute diarrhea of less than 2 to 3 weeks' duration is more likely to represent a serious cause, such as infection, ischemia, intoxication, or inflammation.

- Associated factors such as fever, pain, presence of blood, or type of food ingested may suggest the diagnosis of infectious gastroenteritis or diverticulitis.

- Neurologic symptoms can be seen in certain diarrheal illnesses, such as seizure with shigellosis or theophylline toxicity, or paresthesias with ciguatoxin.

- Details about the host can also better define the diagnosis. Malabsorption from pancreatic insufficiency or HIV-related bowel disorders need not be considered in a healthy host.

- Dietary practices—including frequent restaurant meals, exposure to day care centers, consumption of street vendor food or raw seafood, overseas travel, and camping with the ingestion of lake or stream water—may isolate the vector and narrow the differential diagnosis for infectious diarrhea (eg, oysters suggest *Vibrio;* rice suggests *Bacillus cereus;* eggs suggest *Salmonella;* and meat suggests *Campylobacter, Staphylococcus, Yersinia, E. coli,* or *Clostridium*).

- Certain medications, particularly antibiotics, colchicine, lithium, and laxatives, can all contribute to diarrhea.

- Travel may predispose the patient to enterotoxigenic *E. coli* or *Giardia.* Social history—such as sexual preference, drug use, and occupation—may suggest such diagnoses as HIV-related illness or organophosphate poisoning.

- The physical examination should initially focus on assessment of hydration status.

- Abdominal examination can narrow the differential diagnosis, as well as reveal the need for surgical intervention. Even appendicitis can present with diarrhea in up to 20% of cases.

- Rectal examination can rule out impaction or presence of blood, the latter suggesting inflammation, infection, or mesenteric ischemia.

DIAGNOSIS AND DIFFERENTIAL

- A mnemonic to prompt the physician's recall of disease groupings causing vomiting and diarrhea is GASTROENTERITIS: **g**astrointestinal disease, **a**ppendicitis or aorta, **s**pecific disease (eg, glaucoma), **t**rauma, medications (**R**x), **o**bstetric-gynecologic disorders, **e**ndocrine disorders, **n**eurologic disease, **t**oxicology, **e**nvironmental disorders, **r**enal disease, **i**nfection, **t**umors, **i**schemia, and **s**upratentorial.

- In a presumed food-borne illness, determining the exact time of exposure may suggest a particular causative agent (Table 48-1).[12]

TABLE 48-1 Etiologic Agents for Food-Borne Diseases and Usual Incubation Periods

1–6 h
  Norwalk viruses
  Astrovirus, calicivirus
  Staphylococcus aureus
  Bacillus cereus vomiting toxin
  Ciguatoxin
  Scombroid toxins
  Paralytic or neurotoxic shellfish poisoning
  Puffer fish, tetrodotoxin
  Heavy metals
  Monosodium glutamates
  Short-acting mushroom toxins

6–24 h
  Bacillus cereus diarrheal toxin
  Clostridium perfringens
  Vibrio parahaemolyticus
  Long-acting mushroom toxins

24–48 h
  Nontyphoidal *Salmonella*
  Enterotoxigenic *E. coli* (ETEC)
  Clostridium botulinum
  Trichinella spp. intestinal phase

2–6 days
  Shigella
  Campylobacter
  Escherichia coli O157:H7
  Vibrio cholerae
  Streptococcus group A
  Yersinia enterocolitica

6–14 days
  Cryptosporidium parvum
  Salmonella typhi
  Cyclospora
  Giardia lamblia

>14 days
  Hepatitis A
  Brucella
  Listeria monocytogenes invasive disease
  Trichinella spp. systemic phase

SOURCE: From Centers for Disease Control and Prevention (CDC): Surveillance summaries: Surveillance for foodborne-disease outbreaks: United States, 1988–1992. *MMWR Morb Mortal Wkly Rep* 45:SS-5:1, 1996.

- All women of childbearing age warrant a pregnancy test.
- In vomiting associated with abdominal pain, liver function tests, urinalysis, and lipase or amylase determinations may be useful.
- Electrolyte determinations and renal function tests are usually of benefit only in patients with severe dehydration or prolonged vomiting. In addition, they may confirm addisonian crisis with hyperkalemia and hyponatremia.
- The electrocardiogram and chest radiograph can be reserved for patients with suspected ischemia or pulmonary infection.
- An acute abdominal series can be used to confirm the presence of obstruction.
- The most specific tests in diarrheal illness all involve examination of the stool in the laboratory. Wright's stain for fecal leukocytes has an 82% sensitivity and 83% specificity for the presence of invasive bacterial pathogens.[13] Current therapeutic strategies, however, suggest this test is no longer useful.
- Stool culture is expensive and labor intensive. To limit cost and increase yield, testing should be limited to severely dehydrated or toxic patients, children, immunocompromised patients, and those with diarrhea lasting longer than 3 days. In addition, it may be useful for patients involved in public health–sensitive occupations.
- In patients with chronic persistent diarrhea, an examination for ova and parasites may be useful to rule out *Giardia* or *Cryptosporidium.*
- Assay for *Clostridium difficile* toxin may be useful in ill patients with antibiotic-associated diarrhea.
- Because of the low sensitivity and delay in results, laboratory testing in routine diarrheal cases is not indicated.
- In extremely dehydrated or toxic patients, electrolyte determinations and renal function tests may be useful.
- If toxicity is suspected, tests for levels for theophylline, lithium, or heavy metals will aid in the diagnosis.
- Radiographs are reserved for ruling out intestinal obstruction or pneumonia, particularly *Legionella.*
- Hemolytic-uremic syndrome (HUS), characterized by acute renal failure, thrombocytopenia, and hemolytic anemia, may complicate *E. coli* O157:H7 infections in children and the elderly.

EMERGENCY DEPARTMENT CARE AND DISPOSITION

- Replacement of fluids can be intravenous (bolus 500 mL IV in adults, 10 to 20 mL/kg in children), with normal saline solution in seriously ill patients. Mildly dehydrated patients may tolerate an oral rehydrating solution containing sodium (at least 45 mEq/L in children) as well as glucose to enhance fluid absorption. The World Health Organization advocates a mixture of 1 cup orange juice, 4 teaspoons sugar, 1 teaspoon baking powder, and 3/4 teaspoon salt in 1 L of boiled water.[10] The goal is to infuse 50 to 100 mL/kg over the first 4 hours.
- Nutritional supplementation should be started as soon as nausea and vomiting subside. Patients can quickly advance from clear liquids to solids, such as rice and bread. Patients may benefit from avoiding raw fruit, caffeine, and lactose- and sorbitol-containing products.
- Antibiotics are recommended for adult patients with severe or prolonged diarrhea.[14–16] In addition, they are indicated for travelers from tropical or Third World countries. Although single-dose fluoroquinolones show some effectiveness, ciprofloxacin 500 mg orally bid for 3 days is recommended. Although inferior, trimethoprim-sulfamethoxazole (TMP-SMX), TMP 10 mg/SMX 50 mg/kg/day (maximum dose TMP 160 mg and SMX 800 mg) for 3 days is indicated for children or nursing mothers, if antibiotics are truly necessary. It should be noted that antibiotics are of questionable value in infectious diarrhea from *E. coli* O157:H7.
- Metronidazole 250 to 750 mg PO tid for 5 to 14 days is indicated for *C. difficile, Giardia,* or *Entamoeba* infection. Antibiotics are especially indicated in patients or workers in the food industry or institutional settings, such as day care centers and nursing homes.
- Antidiarrheal agents, especially in combination with antibiotics, have been shown to shorten the course of diarrhea.[15,16] Loperamide is given 4 mg PO initially and then 2 mg PO after each diarrheal stool, maximum of 16 mg/day (for children over 2 years, 1 to 2 mg bid to tid on day 1, then 0.1 mg/kg after each loose stool). Diphenoxylate and atropine 1 to 2 tablets PO every 6 hours for 2 days or less may be helpful for more severe diarrhea.
- Antiemetic agents are useful in actively vomiting patients with dehydration. Promethazine 25 mg (0.25 to 1 mg/kg in children over 2 years) intramuscularly (IM), or rectally (PR) every 6 hours is prescribed. Prochlorperazine 5 to 10 mg IV or IM, or 25 mg PR every 6 to 8 hours is effective. Metoclopramide 5 to 10 mg IV (children 0.1 to 0.2 mg/kg) IV/IM every 6 to 8 hours is useful and can be given in pregnancy (category B). For severe or refractory cases, ondansetron 4 to 8 mg (children 0.15 mg/kg) IV may be used.[17]
- Admission is dependent on toxic appearance and response to therapy, as well as concomitant and preexistent medical conditions.

CONSTIPATION

EPIDEMIOLOGY

- Constipation is the most common digestive complaint in the United States and accounts for 2.5 million physician visits per year.[18]
- There is an age-related increase in the incidence of constipation, with 30 to 40% of adults over age 65 citing constipation as a problem.[19,20]

PATHOPHYSIOLOGY

- Fluid intake, fiber intake, exercise, medications, and medical condition affect gut motility.

CLINICAL FEATURES

- Constipation is demonstrated by the presence of hard stools that are difficult to pass.
- Acute onset implies obstruction until proven otherwise. Chronic constipation is less ominous and can be managed on an outpatient basis.
- Associated symptoms, such as vomiting and inability to pass flatus, confirm obstruction.
- Associated illnesses can help disclose the underlying diagnosis: cold intolerance (hypothyroidism), diverticulitis (inflammatory stricture), or nephrolithiasis (hyperparathyroidism).
- Physical examination should focus on detection of hernias or abdominal masses.
- Rectal examination will detect masses, such as fecal impaction, anal fissures, or fecal blood. The latter, accompanied by weight loss or decreasing stool caliber, may confirm colon carcinoma.
- Fecal impaction itself can cause rectal bleeding from stercoral ulcers.
- The presence of ascites in postmenopausal women raises suspicion of ovarian or uterine carcinoma.

DIAGNOSIS AND DIFFERENTIAL

- Directed testing in acute constipation, based on suspicion, can include a complete blood count (to rule out anemia), a thyroid panel (to rule out hypothyroidism), and electrolyte determinations (to rule out hypokalemia or hypercalcemia).
- Flat and erect abdominal films may be useful in confirming obstruction or assessing stool burden.
- The differential diagnosis of constipation is listed in Table 48-2.

TABLE 48-2   Differential Diagnosis of Constipation

ACUTE OR SUBACUTE
Gastrointestinal: obstructing cancer, volvulus, stricture, hernia, adhesion, pelvic or abdominal masses
Medicinal: addition of new medicine (eg, antipsychotic, anticholinergic, narcotic analgesic, antacids)
Environmental: change in defecation regimen (eg, forced to use bedpan)
Exercise and diet: decrease in level of exercise, fiber intake, fluid intake

CHRONIC
Gastrointestinal: slowly growing tumor, colonic dysmotility, anal pathology
Medicinal: chronic laxative abuse, antipsychotics, anticholinergics, narcotic analgesics
Neurologic: neuropathy, Parkinson's disease, paraplegia, cerebral palsy
Endocrine: diabetes, hypothyroidism, hyperparathyroidism
Rheumatologic: scleroderma
Toxicologic: lead poisoning

- Chronic constipation is a functional disorder that can be worked up on an outpatient basis. Nevertheless, complications of chronic constipation, such as fecal impaction and intestinal pseudo-obstruction, will require either manual, colonoscopic, or surgical intervention.

EMERGENCY DEPARTMENT CARE AND DISPOSITION

- The most important prescription for functional constipation is a dietary and exercise regimen that includes fluids (1.5 L/day), fiber (10 g/day), and exercise. Fiber in the form of bran (1 cup/day) or psyllium (1 teaspoon tid) increases stool volume and gut motility.
- Medications can provide temporary relief for this chronic problem. Stimulants can be either given PO, as with anthraquinones (eg, Peri-Colace 1 to 2 tablets PO at bedtime), or PR, as with bisacodyl (10 mg PR tid in adults or children). In the absence of renal failure, saline laxatives such as milk of magnesia 15 to 30 mL PO daily to bid or magnesium citrate 200 mL PO once, are useful. Hyperosmolar agents such as lactulose or sorbitol 15 to 30 mL PO bid may also be helpful. In children, glycerine rectal suppositories or mineral oil (age 5 to 11 years: 5 to 15 mL PO daily; age >12: 15 to 45 mL PO daily) have been advocated.
- Enemas of soap suds (1500 mL PR) or phosphate (eg, Fleet 1 unit PR, 1 oz/10 kg in children) are generally reserved for severe cases or after fecal disimpaction. Use care to avoid rectal perforation.
- Fecal impaction should be removed manually using local anesthetic lubricant. In female patients, transvaginal pressure with the other hand may be helpful.

An enema or suppositories to complete evacuation can follow.

- Early follow-up is indicated in patients with recent severe constipation or systemic symptoms, such as weight loss, anemia, or change in stool caliber. Patients with organic constipation from obstruction require hospitalization and surgical evaluation.
- Intestinal pseudo-obstruction and sigmoid volvulus can sometimes be corrected colonoscopically.

REFERENCES

1. Lew JF, Glass RI, Gangarosa RE, et al: Diarrheal deaths in the United States, 1979 through 1987. *JAMA* 265:3280, 1991.
2. Bennett RJ, Greenough WB: Approach to acute diarrhea in the elderly. *Gastroenterol Clin North Am* 22:517, 1993.
3. Siegel D, Cohen PT, Neighbor M, et al: Predictive value of stool examination in acute diarrhea. *Arch Pathol Lab Med* 111:715, 1987.
4. Brownlee HJ: Introduction: Management of acute nonspecific diarrhea. *Am J Med* 88(Suppl 6A):1S, 1990.
5. Mead PS, Slutsker L, Deitz V, et al: Food-related illness and death in the United States. *Emerg Infect Dis* 5:607, 1999.
6. Altekruse S, Cohen M, Swerdlow D: Perspective: Emerging foodborne disease. *Emerg Infect Dis* 3:285, 1997.
7. Altekruse S, Swerdlow D: The changing epidemiology of foodborne disease. *Am J Med Sci* 311:23, 1996.
8. Preliminary FoodNet data on the incidence of foodborne illnesses—selected sites, United States, 2000. *MMWR Morb Mortal Wkly Rep* 50:13, 2001.
9. Lumsden K, Holden WS: The act of vomiting in man. *Gut* 10:173, 1969.
10. Park SI, Giannella RA: Approach to the adult patient with acute diarrhea. *Gastroenterol Clin North Am* 22:483, 1993.
11. Kroser JA, Metz DC: Evaluation of the adult patient with diarrhea. *Primary Care* 23:629, 1996.
12. Centers for Disease Control and Prevention: Diagnosis and management of foodborne illness: a primer for physicians. *MMWR Morb Mortal Wkly Rep* 50(No. RR-2):1, 2001.
13. DuBois D, Binder L, Nelson B: Usefulness of the stool Wright's stain in the emergency department. *J Emerg Med* 6:483, 1988.
14. Goodman LJ, Trenholme GM, Kaplan RL, et al: Empiric antimicrobial therapy of domestically acquired acute diarrhea in urban adults. *Arch Intern Med* 150:541, 1990.
15. Ericsson CD, DuPont HL, Mathewson JJ, et al: Treatment of traveler's diarrhea with sulfamethoxazole and trimethoprim and loperamide. *JAMA* 263:257, 1990.
16. Murphy GS, Bodhidatta L, Echeverria P, et al: Ciprofloxacin and loperamide in the treatment of bacillary dysentery. *Ann Intern Med* 118:582, 1993.
17. Reeves JJ, Shannon MV, Fleisher GR: Ondansetron in the treatment of nausea and vomiting associated with gastroenteritis: A randomized controlled trial. *Pediatrics* 109:62, 2002.
18. Sonnenberg A, Koch TR: Physician visits in the United States for constipation: 1958 to 1986. *Dig Dis Sci* 34:606, 1989.
19. Romero Y, Evans JM, Fleming KC, et al: Constipation and fecal incontinence in the elderly population. *Mayo Clin Proc* 71:81, 1996.
20. Abyad A, Mourad F: Constipation: Common sense care of the older patient. *Geriatrics* 51:28, 1996.

For further reading in *Emergency Medicine: A Comprehensive Study Guide,* 6th ed., see Chap. 83, "Vomiting, Diarrhea, and Constipation," by Annie T. Sadosty and Jennifer J. Hess; and Chap. 150, "Foodborne and Water-Borne Diseases," by William T. Anderson.

49 JAUNDICE, HEPATIC DISORDERS, AND HEPATIC FAILURE

Gregory S. Hall

JAUNDICE

PATHOPHYSIOLOGY

- Jaundice, a yellowish discoloration of the skin, sclerae, and mucous membranes, is a symptom that results from hyperbilirubinemia (excessive serum levels of hemoglobin breakdown products) and thus the deposition of bile pigments.[1]
- It has many etiologies (Table 49-1).
- Hyperbilirubinemia can be divided into two types. The unconjugated form results from increased bilirubin production (eg, hemolysis) or a liver defect in its uptake or conjugation. The conjugated form occurs in the setting of intra- or extrahepatic cholestasis, resulting in decreased excretion of conjugated bilirubin via the intestinal tract. Intrahepatic cholestasis may result from hepatocellular damage or damaged biliary endothelium. Extrahepatic cholestasis results from bile duct obstruction by mass, gallstones, inflammation, stricture, or congenital defect.
- The total serum bilirubin should be elevated in a jaundiced patient. Clinically, jaundice usually becomes noticeable at a serum bilirubin level of 2.0 to 2.5 mg/dL and is often first seen in the sclera.
- An indirect fraction of serum bilirubin of 85% or higher is consistent with the unconjugated type, whereas a direct fraction of 30% or above indicates the conjugated form.

TABLE 49-1   Causes of Jaundice

Disorders of bilirubin metabolism
   Neonatal jaundice
   Hemolysis
   Hemoglobinopathy
   Transfusion reaction
   Inborn errors of metabolism

Hepatocellular causes
   Infections
      Viral hepatitis
      Leptospirosis
      Infectious mononucleosis
   Drugs and toxins
      Ethanol
      Acetaminophen
      Amanita toxin
      Carbon tetrachloride
      Anabolic steroids
      Chlorpromazine
      Isoniazid
   Metabolic
      Wilson disease
      Reye's syndrome
      Hemochromatosis
   Granulomatous
      Wegener's granulomatosis
      Sarcoidosis
      Lymphoma
      Mycobacterial
   Miscellaneous
      Fatty liver of pregnancy
      Ischemia
      Primary biliary cirrhosis
      Benign recurrent intrahepatic cholestasis
      Postoperative cholestasis
      Amyloidosis

Bile duct obstruction
   Gallstones
   Cholangiopathy due to acquired immunodeficiency syndrome
   Primary sclerosing cholangitis
   Bile duct stricture
   Pancreatic tumors or cysts
   Pancreatitis
   Cholangiocarcinoma

- Conjugated bilirubin is water soluble and is detectable in the urine even with low serum levels.

CLINICAL FEATURES

- Jaundice is a symptom with a myriad of possible underlying causes.[2]
- Sudden onset of jaundice in a previously healthy young person, together with a prodrome of fever, malaise, myalgias, and a tender enlarged liver, points to hepatitis (probably viral) as a likely cause.
- Heavy ethanol use suggests alcoholic hepatitis. In the setting of alcoholic liver disease and cirrhosis, jaundice usually develops gradually (discussed later).
- A family history of jaundice or a history of recurrent mild jaundice that spontaneously resolves usually ac-

companies inherited causes of jaundice such as Gilbert's syndrome.
- Cholecystitis in itself may not cause jaundice unless there is acute biliary obstruction present such as with a retained common bile duct gallstone.
- Painless jaundice in an older patient classically suggests pancreatic or hepatobiliary malignancy.
- Patients with a known prior malignancy and a hard, nodular liver accompanied by jaundice may be found to have liver metastases.
- Biliary tract scarring or strictures must always be suspected as a cause of jaundice in patients with a prior history of biliary tract surgery, pancreatitis, cholangitis, or inflammatory bowel disease.
- Hepatomegaly with jaundice, accompanied by pedal edema, jugular venous distention, and a gallop rhythm, suggest chronic heart failure.

DIAGNOSIS AND DIFFERENTIAL

- Initial laboratory testing that should be obtained in the work-up of a jaundiced patient includes serum bilirubin level (both total and direct fraction—the indirect fraction can be deduced by simple subtraction), serum aminotransferases and alkaline phosphatase levels, urinalysis to check for bilirubin and urobilinogen, and a complete blood count (CBC).
- Additional laboratory tests may be indicated based on the clinical setting (serum amylase and lipase levels, prothrombin time [PT], electrolytes and glucose levels, blood urea nitrogen [BUN] and creatinine levels, viral hepatitis panels, drug levels, and pregnancy test).
- Prothrombin time (PT) is the most sensitive measure of hepatic synthetic function, and if elevated, suggests significant hepatocellular dysfunction or necrosis.
- With normal liver enzyme levels, the jaundice is more likely to be caused by sepsis or systemic infection, inborn errors of metabolism, or pregnancy, rather than by primary hepatic disease.
- With abnormally elevated liver enzymes, the pattern of abnormalities may suggest the etiology. Aminotransferase elevation, if predominant, suggests hepatocellular diseases such as viral or toxic hepatitis or cirrhosis, whereas markedly elevated alkaline phosphatase levels (two to three times normal) and GGT (gamma-glutamyl transferase) points to intra- or extrahepatic obstruction (gallstones, stricture, or malignancy).
- A Coombs test and hemoglobin electrophoresis may be useful if anemia is present, along with normal liver aminotransferase levels (to look for hemolysis and hemoglobinopathy).
- If clinical features and initial laboratory results reveal conjugated hyperbilirubinemia, ultrasound studies of the biliary tract, liver, and pancreas should be

performed to rule out gallstones, dilated extrahepatic biliary ducts, or mass/tumor in the liver, pancreas, and portal region.

- A computed tomography (CT) scan may also be considered, but is more costly and is not as sensitive as ultrasound for detection of gallstones in the gallbladder.

EMERGENCY DEPARTMENT CARE AND DISPOSITION

- Jaundice by itself is not an adequate justification for hospital admission. In some situations, discharge from the emergency department pending further outpatient work-up may be appropriate, if a patient is hemodynamically stable with new-onset jaundice, has no evidence of liver failure or acute biliary obstruction, if appropriate laboratory studies have been ordered, if the patient has timely follow-up readily available and is reliable and has adequate social support.
- Patients suffering significant drug- or toxin-induced hepatitis or alcoholic hepatitis are best managed by admission for supportive care and in the case of alcoholics, treatment for potential withdrawal symptoms.
- If extrahepatic biliary obstruction is suspected, surgical consultation should be obtained in the emergency department. See further advice on admissions with regard to hepatitis and cirrhosis later in this chapter.

HEPATITIS

EPIDEMIOLOGY

- As of the year 2000, chronic liver disease was the twelfth leading cause of death overall and the tenth leading cause of death among young men in the United States, accounting for 17,214 deaths (1.5%). Many cases of end-stage liver disease (ESLD) (approximately 50%) are related to alcohol abuse. However, in recent decades, an increasing number of cases can be attributed to chronic viral hepatitis.[3-5]
- Currently, hepatitis C virus (HCV) infection is the most common of all blood-borne infections in the United States, with approximately 28,000 to 180,000 new cases yearly. An estimated 3.9 million (1.8%) Americans have been infected.
- HCV infection is often subclinical, with symptoms of chronic liver disease and cirrhosis delayed one to two decades. It is anticipated that the number of cases of chronic liver disease related to HCV will increase sharply in the next 10 to 20 years.[6,7]
- Effective vaccination against hepatitis B virus (HBV) has lead to a decline in the prevalence of related disease in the general population. Still, there are an esti-

mated 140,000 to 320,000 cases of HBV infection yearly, with 140 to 320 deaths due to acute infections.[8]
- Hepatitis A virus (HAV) is commonly encountered by Americans, with 33% of the population having acquired immunity secondary to exposure.[4,9]

PATHOPHYSIOLOGY

- Common to essentially all causes of chronic liver disease is ongoing hepatocellular injury and death with the progressive disruption of the functional microanatomy of the liver. Eventually, the metabolic function of the liver becomes both compromised and isolated, resulting in nutritional deficiencies, bleeding diatheses, and the accumulation of toxic metabolic wastes.
- Risk factors for viral hepatitis include male homosexuality, hemodialysis, intravenous drug abuse, raw seafood ingestion, blood product transfusion, tattoos or body piercing, needle punctures, foreign travel, or close contact with an infected source patient.

CLINICAL FEATURES

- Viral hepatitis may range in severity from asymptomatic infection to fulminant hepatic failure to chronic cirrhosis.
- Symptomatic patients usually report sudden or insidious onset of prodrome of anorexia, nausea, emesis, fatigue, malaise, and altered taste.
- Low-grade fever, accompanied by pharyngitis, coryza, and headache, may confuse the picture and lead to an initial misdiagnosis of upper respiratory infection or flu-like illness.
- A few days of generalized pruritus, clay-colored stools, and dark urine may precede the onset of gastrointestinal (GI) symptoms and jaundice. Malaise usually persists while the other prodromal symptoms resolve. Right upper quadrant pain with an enlarged tender liver and splenomegaly may be found. Many patients do not become clinically jaundiced, and most will recover gradually over the ensuing 3 to 4 months.
- Rarely, fulminant hepatic failure develops with a clinical picture of encephalopathy, coagulopathy, and rapidly worsening jaundice.
- Chronic persistent infection (usually with hepatitis B or C) can lead to the development of cirrhosis with gradual jaundice, ascites, peripheral edema, and liver failure over a period of 10 to 20 years.
- Hepatitis A (HAV) is transmitted predominantly by the fecal-oral route and is commonly seen in Americans. Children and adolescents are more commonly

affected, but often subclinically, whereas most adults are symptomatic with a longer, more severe course. Symptom onset is often more abrupt than with other viruses. Epidemic outbreaks have been seen in children at day care centers, institutionalized patients, and in patients exposed to a common source case via contaminated food or water.

- Hepatitis B (HBV) is acquired primarily via a percutaneous exposure to infected blood or body fluids. Most cases are subclinical without jaundice. Often symptom onset is insidious, and in 5 to 10% of cases is preceded by a serum sickness–like syndrome with polyarthritis, proteinuria, and angioneurotic edema. Symptomatic patients usually have a more severe and protracted course than those with HAV.
- Chronic HBV infection occurs in 6 to 10% of patients, who may go on to develop cirrhosis, ESLD, and hepatocellular carcinoma.
- Hepatitis C (HCV) is the most common of all bloodborne infections in the United States, and may be contracted via parenteral, sexual, and perinatal contact. Most patients remain asymptomatic or have milder symptoms than those with HBV or HAV. Unfortunately, chronic HCV infection occurs in 85% of patients, the majority of whom remain subclinically infected. Up to 70% of chronic HCV cases progress to the development of chronic liver disease (cirrhosis and ESLD) and are at increased risk for hepatocellular carcinoma.

DIAGNOSIS AND DIFFERENTIAL

- Establishment of a diagnosis of viral hepatitis depends primarily on liver function abnormalities, coupled with the clinical picture. Serum transaminases, GGT, aspartate aminotransferase (AST), and alanine aminotransferase (ALT) should be checked because elevations are suggestive of hepatitis.[10,11]
- Values in the hundreds of units per liter are consistent with mild viral inflammation, but elevations into the thousands suggest extensive acute hepatocellular necrosis and more fulminant disease.
- In acute and chronic viral hepatitis, the ratio of AST:ALT is usually <1 (whereas a ratio >2 is more suggestive of alcoholic hepatitis—alcohol stimulates AST production).
- The serum alkaline phosphatase level should also be determined—mild to moderate elevations are seen in virtually all hepatobiliary disease, but if elevated greater than four times normal, cholestasis should be suspected (a concurrently elevated GGT supports this).
- Isolated significant elevation of alkaline phosphatase (AP) without marked hyperbilirubinemia (AP:bilirubin ratio of 1000:1) suggests an infiltrative or granulomatous disease such as lymphoma, tuberculosis, sarcoidosis, or fungal infection.
- Total serum bilirubin along with its direct fraction (the indirect fraction can be deduced by simple subtraction) may also be useful since a conjugated (direct) fraction of 30% or higher is consistent with viral hepatitis.
- The magnitude of transaminase elevation is, however, not a reliable marker of disease severity, but a persistent total bilirubin level >20 mg/dL or a PT prolonged by more than a few seconds indicates a poor prognosis (hence, the PT should be checked).
- Serum electrolytes, BUN, and creatinine should be checked if there is clinical suspicion of volume depletion or electrolyte abnormalities.
- Abnormal mental status should prompt an immediate determination of serum glucose level, which may be low due to poor oral intake or hepatic failure. (Other causes of abnormal mental status such as hypoxia, sepsis, intoxication, structural intracranial process, or encephalopathy must also be considered.)
- A CBC may be useful, as an early transient neutropenia followed by a relative lymphocytosis with atypical forms is often seen with viral hepatitis. Anemia, if present, may be more suggestive of alcoholic hepatitis, decompensated cirrhosis, GI bleeding, or a hemolytic process.
- Serologic studies to determine the specific viral agent responsible may be ordered in the emergency department to facilitate the final diagnosis, but these results are rarely immediately available and thus play no significant role in emergency department management.
- Important differential diagnoses include alcohol- or toxin-induced hepatitis, infectious mononucleosis, cholecystitis, ascending cholangitis, sarcoidosis, lymphoma, liver metastases, and pancreatic or biliary tumors.

EMERGENCY DEPARTMENT CARE AND DISPOSITION

- Most patients can be successfully managed as outpatients with emphasis on rest, adequate oral intake, strict personal hygiene, and avoidance of hepatotoxins (ethanol and drugs). Close follow-up arrangements should be made.
- Patients with any of the following should be admitted to the hospital: encephalopathy, PT prolonged by more than a few seconds, intractable vomiting, hypoglycemia, bilirubin >20 mg/dL, age >45 years, immunosuppression, or suspected toxin-induced hepatitis.
- Volume depletion and electrolyte imbalances should be corrected with intravenous crystalloid. Hypoglycemia

should be initially treated with 1 amp of 50% dextrose in water intravenously followed by the addition of dextrose to intravenous fluids and careful monitoring.

- Fulminant hepatic failure should warrant admission to the intensive care unit with aggressive support of circulation and respiration, monitoring and treatment of increased intracranial pressure if present (consider hyperventilation and mannitol), correction of hypoglycemia and coagulopathy, administration of oral lactulose or neomycin, and a protein-restricted diet.[12,13] See following section on treatment of cirrhosis. Consultation with a hepatologist and liver transplant service are indicated.
- Glucocorticoid therapy has no value in acute viral hepatitis, even with fulminant hepatic failure, and should be avoided.

ALCOHOLIC LIVER DISEASE AND CIRRHOSIS

PATHOPHYSIOLOGY

- Three clinical syndromes best describe liver injury secondary to alcohol: hepatic steatosis (fatty liver), alcoholic hepatitis, and alcoholic cirrhosis. An enlarged, non- or mildly tender liver from steatosis is usually seen in a relatively asymptomatic alcoholic patient.[14]
- The cirrhotic liver becomes increasingly resistant to blood flow. Portal hypertension results in splenomegaly and the development of gastroesophageal varices. Splenomegaly contributes to anemia and thrombocytopenia. Ascites develops secondary to portal hypertension and abnormalities in renal sodium and water excretion caused by diminished glomerular filtration rate (GFR) and elevations in both aldosterone and antidiuretic hormone.

CLINICAL FEATURES

- Alcoholic hepatitis is typically found in the chronic alcoholic who presents with a gradual onset of anorexia, nausea, fever, dark urine, jaundice, weight loss, abdominal pain, and generalized weakness.
- Physical exam reveals a tender, enlarged liver, low-grade fever, and icteric mucous membranes, sclera, or skin.
- Patients suffering from cirrhosis generally report a gradual deterioration in their health with anorexia, muscle loss (often masked by edema or ascites), fatigue, nausea, emesis, diarrhea, and increasing abdominal girth (ascites). Low-grade intermittent or continuous fever may also be present, while hypothermia may be seen at end-stage disease.[3]

- Abdominal palpation may reveal a small firm liver and possibly splenomegaly. Jaundice, pedal edema, ascites, palmar erythema, testicular atrophy, gynecomastia, and spider angiomata are also common.
- Hepatic encephalopathy, characterized by a fluctuating level of consciousness and confusion, and possibly hyperreflexia, spasticity, and generalized seizures may also be present.
- Asterixis ("liver flap") is characteristic, but not specific for encephalopathy due to liver failure.
- Patients with cirrhosis often come to the emergency department because of worsening ascites or edema, complications such as GI or variceal bleeding (see Chap. 39, "Gastrointestinal Bleeding"), encephalopathy, spontaneous bacterial peritonitis (abdominal pain), and various concurrent infections (urinary tract infection, pneumonia, etc).

DIAGNOSIS AND DIFFERENTIAL

- Alcoholic hepatitis and cirrhosis may be diagnosed by their clinical features and laboratory findings. Laboratory studies that should be checked include levels of serum transaminases (GGT, ALT, AST), serum alkaline phosphatase, total bilirubin (and its fractions), serum albumin, serum glucose and electrolytes, BUN, and creatinine, CBC, and PT.
- In the setting of alcoholic hepatitis, serum transaminase levels are usually elevated to a range of two to ten times that of normal with AST:ALT ratio of >1.5 to 2.0 (AST production is stimulated by ethanol). With cirrhosis, transaminase levels are often only mildly elevated. Alkaline phosphatase and bilirubin levels are usually only mildly elevated with both alcoholic hepatitis and cirrhosis.
- Anemia, leukopenia, and thrombocytopenia are commonly seen in chronic ethanol abusers. If concurrent pancreatitis is suspected, serum lipase and amylase levels should be checked.
- Fever with or without leukocytosis in a chronic alcoholic warrants a chest x-ray to rule out pneumonia; cultures of blood, urine, and ascitic fluid (if present); and a thorough search for other sources of sepsis (meningitis, cholecystitis, cellulitis, perirectal abscess, etc).[15]
- Elevated serum ammonia level unfortunately does not correlate well with acute deterioration of liver function due to cirrhosis, and while it may be checked as a marker of encephalopathy, it cannot be used as an index of its severity or response to treatment.
- **Spontaneous bacterial peritonitis** (SBP), the most common complication of cirrhotic ascites, should be suspected in any cirrhotic patient with fever, abdominal pain or tenderness, worsening ascites, subacute

functional decline, or encephalopathy.[16] Other subtle clues to SBP include deteriorating renal function, hypothermia, and diarrhea.

- SBP may be confirmed through sampling of ascitic fluid by paracentesis, ideally under ultrasound guidance to minimize the risk of bowel puncture. Ascitic fluid should be tested for total protein and glucose levels, lactic (acid) dehydrogenase (LDH), Gram's stain, and white blood cell count (WBC) with differential. A total WBC count >1000 per cubic millimeter or neutrophil (PMN) count >250 per cubic millimeter is diagnostic for SBP. Some authorities suggest that a WBC count of >250 per cubic millimeter in a symptomatic patient should be treated until cultures return.

- Gram's stain and culture results from ascitic fluid are often negative (30 to 40%), but placing 10 mL of ascitic fluid in a blood culture bottle may have an improved yield. Gram-negative Enterobacteriaceae (*E. coli, Klebsiella,* etc) account for 63% of SBP, followed by the pneumococcus (15%) and the enterococcus (6 to 10%). Empirical therapy with antimicrobial agents to cover typical enteric flora should be instituted as soon as SBP is suspected from ascitic fluid analysis.

- Hepatorenal syndrome, a refractory form of acute renal failure that occurs in cirrhotic patients, may develop in the setting of sepsis, acute dehydration, overzealous diuresis, or high-volume paracentesis. The differential diagnosis includes other forms of hepatitis (drugs, toxins, etc), as well as other causes of upper abdominal pain (cholecystitis, biliary colic, gastritis or peptic ulcer disease, pancreatitis, etc).[17]

- Gastroesophageal varices form as a result of intrahepatic fibrosis and scarring, leading to portal vein resistance and hypertension, with resulting collateral flow through veins at the gastroesophageal junction. Bleeding may take the form of frank hematemesis, "coffee grounds" emesis, with melena, or with massive hemorrhage, hematochezia. Symptoms may be more insidious with light-headedness, generalized weakness, fatigue, or increased confusion being the presenting features.

- Cirrhosis is often caused by ethanol or chronic viral hepatitis; uncommon causes include drugs or toxins, hemochromatosis, Wilson's disease, and primary (idiopathic) biliary cirrhosis.

EMERGENCY DEPARTMENT CARE AND DISPOSITION

ALCOHOLIC HEPATITIS

- Hospital admission is generally required except for mild cases of alcoholic hepatitis.

- Fluid therapy with dextrose-containing intravenous fluids should be given with the goal of maintaining adequate intravascular volume while avoiding fluid overload in the edematous or ascitic patient.

- Thiamine (100 mg) should always be given with initial intravenous fluids and dextrose. Vitamin supplements should also be given to any malnourished alcoholic.

- Correction of electrolyte abnormalities should be initiated (many alcoholic patients will require supplemental magnesium and potassium).

- Alcohol-dependent patients must be monitored closely for symptoms of withdrawal (ie, tremors, confusion, agitation, hallucination, seizures, etc), and judicious use of benzodiazepines (eg, lorazepam) should be given as prophylaxis and therapy for withdrawal symptoms.

- Large-volume paracentesis is sometimes required for symptomatic ascites (shortness of breath or abdominal pain). When more than 4 L are removed, the patient may experience significant fluid shifts and hypotension.

- Identified bacterial coinfection should be promptly treated with appropriate parenteral antibiotics and broad-spectrum coverage should be initiated in any alcoholic with suspected sepsis, pending culture results.[18]

CIRRHOSIS AND LIVER FAILURE

- Abstinence from alcohol and other hepatotoxins (drugs, etc) is essential for outpatient management. Adjunctive measures may include salt and water restriction, cautious diuretic use (spironolactone), protein-restricted diet, and therapeutic paracentesis for relief of abdominal distention.

- Emergency management often includes changing diuretic dosage, correction of fluid or electrolyte abnormalities, and blood transfusion for symptomatic anemia.

- New-onset or worsening encephalopathy warrants hospital admission. Management includes supplemental oxygen, support of perfusion and respiration as needed, and supplemental dextrose in intravenous fluids. Precipitating factors such as a coexisting infection, GI bleeding, or renal failure must be carefully investigated and aggressively treated.[19] Lactulose may be given orally, by nasogastric tube, or by enema, up to three times a day until one to two soft stools per day are produced. The oral dose is 20 g in a glass of water or fruit juice; for enemas 300 mL of lactulose syrup is diluted with 700 mL of water or normal saline, and the enema should be retained for 30 minutes.[19]

- Cefotaxime 2 g intravenously followed by 1 to 2 g intravenously every 4 to 8 hours is an acceptable antibiotic regimen for spontaneous bacterial peritonitis (alternatives include ticarcillin-clavulanate 3.1 g IV every 6 hours, piperacillin-tazobactam 3.375 g IV every 6 hours, ampicillin-sulbactam 3 g IV every 6 hours, or the quinolones IV).[18] Patients with prior history of SBP due to resistant *E. coli* or *Klebsiella* should have a fluoroquinolone, imipenem, or meropenem added to the above therapy pending culture results.
- Addition of intravenous albumin (1.5 g/kg at diagnosis of SBP, and 1 g/kg on day 3) to antimicrobial therapy may reduce the incidence of renal failure and hospital mortality in patients with SBP.[20]
- Acute liver failure from any cause (with prolonged PT, hypoglycemia, coagulopathy, encephalopathy, marked jaundice, etc) should warrant admission to the intensive care unit, aggressive treatment, and consultation with a hepatologist and transplant team if available.[12,13]
- Any cirrhotic patient whose clinical stability is in doubt should always be considered for admission. All patients with clearly decompensated cirrhosis, fever, or hypothermia, or complications such as concurrent infection, SBP, GI bleeding, encephalopathy, and acute or worsening renal function should be admitted.
- Gastroesophageal varices and hemorrhage should be suspected in any bleeding patient with liver disease. See Chap. 39 for management.
- A recent Cochrane Review found that empirical antimicrobial therapy against enteric organisms reduced all-cause mortality from variceal bleeding by 27% and infections by 60% with minimal side effects.[21]

REFERENCES

1. Sherlock S, Dooley J: *Diseases of the Liver and Biliary System,* 10th ed. London: Blackwell Science Ltd., 1997, p. 201.
2. Lewis JH, Zimmerman HJ: Drug- and chemical-induced cholestasis. *Clin Liver Dis* 3:433, 1999.
3. Williams EJ, Iredale JP: Liver cirrhosis. *Postgrad Med J* 74:193, 1998.
4. Centers for Disease Control and Prevention: Hepatitis home page: www.cdc.gov/ncidod/diseases/hepatitis/index.htm.
5. Anderson RN: Deaths: Leading causes for 2000. *Natl Vital Stat Rep* 50:1, 2002.
6. Alter MJ, Margolis H: Recommendations for prevention and control of hepatitis C virus (HCV) infection and HCV-related chronic disease. *MMWR Recomm Rep* 47:1, 1998.
7. Gross JB Jr: Clinician's guide to hepatitis C. *Mayo Clin Proc* 73:355, 1998.
8. Lee WM: Medical progress: Hepatitis B virus infection. *N Engl J Med* 337:1733, 1997.
9. Koff R: Hepatitis A. *Lancet* 351:1643, 1998.
10. Kamath PS: Clinical approach to the patient with abnormal liver test results. *Mayo Clin Proc* 71:1089, 1996.
11. Aranda-Michel J, Sherman KE: Tests of the liver: Use and misuse. *Gastroenterologist* 6:34, 1998.
12. Lee WM: Medical progress: Acute liver failure. *N Engl J Med* 329:1862, 1993.
13. Caraceni P, Van Thiel DH: Acute liver failure. *Lancet* 345: 163, 1995.
14. Friedman S: Seminars in medicine of the Beth Israel Hospital, Boston: The cellular basis of hepatic fibrosis. Mechanisms and treatment strategies. *N Engl J Med* 328:1828, 1993.
15. King PD, Rumbaut R, Sanchez C: Pulmonary manifestations of chronic liver disease. *Dig Dis* 14:73, 1996.
16. Guarner C, Soriano G: Spontaneous bacterial peritonitis. *Semin Liver Dis* 17:203, 1997.
17. Roberts R, Kamath PS: Ascites and hepatorenal syndrome: Pathophysiology and management. *Mayo Clin Proc* 71:874, 1996.
18. Soares-Weiser K, Brezis M, Leibovici L: Antibiotics for spontaneous bacterial peritonitis in cirrhotics (Cochrane Review), in *The Cochrane Library,* Issue 4. Oxford: Update Software, 2002.
19. Riordan SM, Williams R: Current concepts: Treatment of hepatic encephalopathy. *N Engl J Med* 337:473, 1997.
20. Sort P, Navasa M, Arroyo V, et al: Effect of intravenous albumin on renal impairment and mortality in patients with cirrhosis and spontaneous bacterial peritonitis. *N Engl J Med* 341:403, 1999.
21. Soares-Weiser K, Brezis M, Tur-Kaspa R, Leibovici L: Antibiotic prophylaxis for cirrhotic patients with gastrointestinal bleeding (Cochrane Review), in *The Cochrane Library,* Issue 4. Oxford: Update Software, 2002.

For further reading in *Emergency Medicine: A Comprehensive Study Guide,* 6th ed., see Chap. 84, "Jaundice," by Richard O. Shields, Jr.; and Chap. 86, "Hepatic Disorders and Hepatic Failure," by Joshua S. Broder and Rawden Evans.

50 CHOLECYSTITIS AND BILIARY COLIC

Gregory S. Hall

EPIDEMIOLOGY

- Symptomatic gallstone disease, though classically noted to afflict the obese female patient between 20 and 40 years old, may in fact be found in all age groups, especially diabetics and the elderly.[1,2]
- Gallstones cause four major biliary tract emergencies: biliary colic (symptomatic cholelithiasis), cholecystitis, gallstone pancreatitis, and ascending cholangitis.

- Risk factors associated with gallstone formation and its complications include increased age, female sex and parity, pregnancy, obesity, marked weight loss or prolonged fasting, familial tendency, oral contraceptives, clofibrate, ceftriaxone, Asian descent, chronic liver disease, and hemolytic disorders (eg, sickle cell disease).[2–4]

PATHOPHYSIOLOGY

- Gallstones form into three major types: 70% are cholesterol stones (usually radiolucent), 20% are pigment stones (often radiopaque), and 10% are mixed.
- Symptomatic cholelithiasis or biliary colic occurs when a gallstone is forced from the gallbladder into the cystic or common bile duct, producing obstruction, subsequent rise in intraluminal pressure, and gallbladder distention, which leads to visceral ischemia and a chemical inflammatory response. Pain, nausea, and vomiting follow; persistent obstruction may result in bacterial contamination and hence acute cholecystitis or ascending cholangitis and possibly pancreatitis.
- Bacterial pathogens are present in 50 to 80% of patients with acute cholecystitis, and include Enterobacteriaceae (70%, usually *Escherichia coli* and *Klebsiella* species), enterococci (15%), *Bacteroides* (10%), *Clostridium* species (10%), and group D *Streptococcus* and *Staphylococcus* species.

CLINICAL FEATURES

- Common symptoms of acute biliary colic in decreasing order of frequency include right upper quadrant pain or epigastric pain (one study suggests epigastric pain as the predominant symptom in over 60%),[5] nausea and vomiting, pain referred to the right shoulder or left upper back, and pain that is typically persistent and not colicky, lasting for 2 to 6 hours; pain episodes may be associated with meals, though it is not in up to one third of patients.[5,6]
- Clinical studies have not demonstrated a correlation with fatty food intolerance that is different from its association with other upper GI disorders.[5–7]
- Symptoms of acute biliary colic tend to occur between 9 am and 4 am, with a peak between midnight and 1 am, and repeat attacks tend to recur at the same time.[6]
- Signs of acute biliary colic include epigastric or right upper quadrant (RUQ) tenderness without peritoneal irritation or rebound, and at times volume depletion due to emesis.
- Because of similar symptoms and/or signs, biliary colic is easily mistaken for dyspepsia, peptic ulcer disease, gastritis, or gastroesophageal reflux disease.
- Symptoms of acute cholecystitis include right upper quadrant or epigastric pain that persists beyond 6 hours, or changes from dull and poorly localized (visceral) to sharp and localized to RUQ (parietal); and fever and chills, nausea, emesis, and anorexia.
- Signs of acute cholelithiasis include well-localized RUQ tenderness; Murphy's sign (increased pain or inspiratory arrest during deep subcostal palpation of the right upper quadrant with inspiration) 97% sensitive for acute cholecystitis,[7] but only 48% sensitive in the elderly[8]; toxic appearance; fever; volume depletion; abdominal distension; and hypoactive bowel sounds.
- Gallstones are the cause of 30 to 70% of cases of acute pancreatitis (depending on patient population), and of all patients with gallstones, 15 to 20% will develop pancreatitis due to biliary calculi; presentation is similar to that of ethanol-induced pancreatitis, with epigastric or diffuse abdominal pain that radiates into the back, nausea, and emesis (symptoms and findings of acute cholecystitis may be concurrent).
- Ascending cholangitis is a life-threatening illness (mortality approaches 100% if untreated), usually resulting from obstruction of the common bile duct (most commonly from a gallstone, and not stricture or tumor) and subsequent reflux of bacteria into lymphatics and hepatic veins. Presenting symptoms include fever, jaundice, and RUQ pain (known as Charcot's triad, but all three symptoms are found in only 25%), along with mental confusion and shock.

DIAGNOSIS AND DIFFERENTIAL

- Laboratory studies that may aid diagnosis include white blood cell count (WBC) (leukocytosis with a left shift suggests cholecystitis, but its absence does not exclude it), serum bilirubin and alkaline phosphatase (normal or mild elevation), amylase and/or lipase (to exclude pancreatitis), urinalysis, electrolytes, glucose, blood urea nitrogen (BUN), creatinine, and pregnancy test (serum or urine) in females with childbearing potential (to exclude an obstetric emergency).
- No single laboratory test or combination of tests has a sufficiently high sensitivity to determine a diagnosis of cholecystitis[9]; patients with biliary colic often have normal labs.
- Radiographic studies that are helpful include plain abdominal films (but show gallstones only 10 to 20% of the time), chest x-rays to rule out pneumonia, and an electrocardiogram should always be performed in older patients to detect myocardial ischemia/infarction as a potential cause of nausea and upper abdominal pain.
- Hepatobiliary ultrasound is the initial diagnostic

study of choice to detect gallstone disease (sensitivity of 94% and specificity of 78% for acute cholecystitis).[10] Studies of bedside hepatobiliary ultrasound by emergency physicians have demonstrated similar sensitivity and specificity for detection of gallstones or a sonographic Murphy's sign compared to radiologists,[11] but decreased accuracy in determination of pericholecystic fluid, wall thickening, gallbladder air, and ductal dilation.[12] Thus, emergency physicians with limited experience should interpret scans showing possible cholecystitis with caution, and a confirmatory study should be done by a radiologist before cholecystectomy is advised.[13]

- On occasion, the gallbladder may not be visualized well on ultrasound and consideration should be given to a radioisotope cholescintigraphy scan using technetium iminodiacetic acid analogues (HIDA scan), which has a sensitivity of 97% and a specificity of 90% (a normal patient will have a clearly outlined gallbladder and cystic duct within 1 hour; if not, cystic duct obstruction is very likely). If the serum bilirubin level is elevated above 5 mg/dL, an alternative radioisotope is used, a diisopropyl iminodiacetic acid (DISIDA) scan.
- Computed tomographic (CT) scanning has a sensitivity of only 50% for cholecystitis, though it may be useful to detect other intra-abdominal conditions in the differential.
- Differential diagnosis includes gastritis, peptic ulcer disease, hepatitis, pancreatitis, gastroesophageal reflux, renal colic, pyelonephritis, appendicitis, pneumonia, acute myocardial infarction, pelvic inflammatory disease, perihepatitis, and ectopic pregnancy.

EMERGENCY DEPARTMENT CARE AND DISPOSITION

- Uncomplicated biliary colic will resolve spontaneously, while cholecystitis, pancreatitis, and cholangitis need hospital admission.
- Administer isotonic crystalloid IV fluids to correct volume deficits and electrolyte abnormalities. In some cases (eg, septic shock) IV pressor support may be required to support perfusion.
- Antiemetics (promethazine 12.5 to 25 mg IV) or antispasmodics (glycopyrrolate 0.1 mg IV) should be given for vomiting.
- Meperidine (0.5 to 1.0 mg/kg IV or IM) has traditionally been the preferred drug for analgesia because it causes less spasm of the sphincter of Oddi. Morphine 0.1 mg/kg is an acceptable alternative. Ketorolac (15 to 30 mg IV or 30 to 60 mg IM) may help relieve the pain of uncomplicated biliary colic, but is less likely to be effective with bacterial cholecystitis.
- Antibiotics should be given to any patient suspected

of having cholecystitis or cholangitis. For nonseptic patients a third-generation cephalosporin is often adequate (cefotaxime or ceftazidime 1 to 2 g IV every 8 hours or ceftizoxime 1 to 2 g IV every 8 to 12 hours or ceftriaxone 1 to 2 g IV every 12 to 24 hours). Triple therapy with ampicillin (0.5 to 1.0 g IV every 6 hours), gentamicin (3 mg/kg/day IV every 8 hours), and clindamycin (1200 to 2700 mg/day divided into two, three, or four equal doses) should be given to patients who appear septic.

- Patients diagnosed with acute cholecystitis, gallstone pancreatitis, or cholangitis require immediate surgical consultation and hospital admission.
- Patients with uncomplicated biliary colic who are asymptomatic or improved with supportive treatment after 4 to 6 hours and are able to maintain oral hydration can be discharged. Oral narcotic-acetaminophen analgesics may be prescribed for 24 to 48 hours. Timely outpatient follow-up should be arranged. The patient should be carefully instructed to return to the ED for fever, worsening abdominal pain, intractable vomiting, or another significant attack.

REFERENCES

1. Ikard RW: Gallstones, cholecystitis, and diabetes. *Surg Gynecol Obstet* 171:528, 1990.
2. Ross SO, Forsmark CE: Pancreatic and biliary disorders in the elderly. *Gastroenterology Clin* 30:531, 2001.
3. Landers D, Carmona R, Cromblehome W: Acute cholecystitis in pregnancy *Obstet Gynecol* 69:131, 1987.
4. Burghart LJ: Cholangitis in viral disease. *Mayo Clin Proc* 73:479, 1998.
5. Diehl AK, Sugarek NJ, Todd K: Clinical evaluation for gallstone disease: Usefulness of symptoms and signs in diagnosis. *Am J Med* 89:29, 1990.
6. Rigas B, Torosis J, McDougall C, et al: The circadian rhythm of biliary colic. *J Clin Gastroenterol* 12:409, 1990.
7. Jorgenson T: Abdominal symptoms and gallstone disease: An epidemiological investigation. *Hepatology* 8:856, 1989.
8. Adedji OA, McAdam A: Murphy's sign, acute cholecystitis, and elderly people. *J Roy Coll Surg Edinburgh* 41:88, 1996.
9. Singer AJ, McCracken G, Henry MC: Correlation among clinical, laboratory, and hepatobiliary scanning findings in patients with suspected acute cholecystitis. *Ann Emerg Med* 28:267, 1996.
10. Shea JA, Berlin JA, Escarce JJ, et al: Revised estimates of diagnostic test sensitivity and specificity in suspected biliary tract disease. *Arch Intern Med* 154:2573, 1994.
11. Kendall JL, Shimp RJ: Performance and interpretation of focused right upper quadrant ultrasound by emergency physicians. *J Emerg Med* 19:32, 2001.
12. Lanoix R, Leak LV, Gaeta T, Gernsheimer JR: A preliminary evaluation of emergency ultrasound in the setting of an emer-

gency medicine training program. *Am J Emerg Med* 18:11, 2000.

13. Rosen CL, Brown DFM, Chang Y, et al: Ultrasonography by emergency physicians in patients with suspected cholecystitis. *Am J Emerg Med* 19:32, 2001.

For further reading in *Emergency Medicine: A Comprehensive Study Guide*, 6th ed., see Chap. 85, "Cholecystitis and Biliary Colic," by William J. Brady, Tom P. Aufderheide, and Judith E. Tintinalli.

---

51 PANCREATITIS

Robert J. Vissers

EPIDEMIOLOGY

- In the United States cholelithiasis or alcohol abuse account for 90% of all cases of acute pancreatitis (AP).[1]
- The list of other factors associated with AP is extensive (Table 51-1).
- The overall prevalence is estimated to be 0.5%.[1]
- About 5 to 10% of patients with acute pancreatitis develop complications or death.

PATHOPHYSIOLOGY

- The central cause is believed to be the intracellular activation of digestive enzymes and autodigestion of the pancreas.[2]
- Pancreatic digestion from activated proteolytic enzymes leads to edema, interstitial hemorrhage, vascular damage, coagulation, and cellular necrosis.
- AP can also cause a generalized systemic inflammatory response that may lead to shock, acute respiratory distress syndrome (ARDS), and multisystem organ failure.[2]

CLINICAL FEATURES

- The patient typically presents with moderate distress, a boring epigastric pain that radiates to the back, tachycardia, nausea and vomiting, and abdominal distension.[1]
- Cullen's sign, a bluish discoloration around the umbilicus, and Grey Turner's sign, a bluish discoloration in the left flank, are characteristic but rare signs of hemorrhagic pancreatitis.

TABLE 51-1   Common Etiologic or Contributing Factors in Acute Pancreatitis

Ethanol ingestion

Biliary tract disease

Trauma, penetrating or blunt

Penetrating peptic ulcer

Following endoscopic procedures

Obstruction secondary to neoplasms, diverticula, and polyps

Metabolic disturbances
   Hyperlipemia (Frederickson types I, IV, V)
   Hypercalcemia
   Diabetes mellitus, diabetic ketoacidosis
   Uremia

Viral infections
   Viral hepatitis
   Infectious mononucleosis
   Coxsackie group B
   HIV

Pregnancy—any trimester, postpartum

Collagen vascular disease

Liver disease

Generalized infections

Drugs
   Oral contraceptives
   Azathioprine
   Glucocorticoids
   Tetracyclines
   Isoniazid
   Indomethacin
   Thiazides
   Salicylates
   Calcium
   Warfarin

- Complications may be life-threatening (Table 51-2).
- Blood loss, refractory hypotension, and respiratory failure may accompany more severe forms.[3]

DIAGNOSIS AND DIFFERENTIAL

- Diagnosis is made by a suggestive history and physical exam, associated with elevated pancreatic enzymes.[3,4]
- Amylase is primarily found in the pancreas and salivary glands; however, low levels can also be found in the fallopian tubes, ovaries, testes, adipose tissue, small bowel, lung, thyroid, skeletal muscle, and certain neoplasms, making this a relatively nonspecific test.[5] Amylase greater than three times the upper limit of normal has a specificity of 75% and a sensitivity of 80 to 90% for AP.[4]
- Lipase is more specific than amylase for AP and is the preferred test. At a cutoff of two times the upper limit of normal, lipase is 90% sensitive and specific. There is no benefit to ordering both amylase and lipase.[6]

TABLE 51-2   Complications of Acute Pancreatitis

Pulmonary
    Pleural effusions, usually left-sided
    Atelectasis
    Hypoxemia
    Acute respiratory distress syndrome (>50% mortality)
Cardiovascular
    Myocardial depression
    Hemorrhage, hypovolemia, and myocardial depressant factor
Metabolic
    Hypocalcemia
    Hyperglycemia
    Hyperlipidemia
    Coagulopathy, disseminated intravascular coagulopathy
Other
    Hemorrhage
    Colonic perforation
    Renal failure
    Erythemia-nodosum dermatitis
    Arthritis
    Pseudocyst
    Abscess

- Leukocytosis may be present, and an elevated alkaline phosphatase suggests biliary disease.
- Hypotension, tachycardia >130 beats per minute, P_{O_2} <60 mm Hg, oliguria, increasing blood urea nitrogen (BUN) or creatinine, or hypocalcemia are indicators of a potentially complicated course.[7]
- Plain radiographs of the abdomen are usually not helpful. Calcification is suggestive of chronic pancreatitis, and a sentinel loop or a colon cut-off sign suggesting ileus may be present, but are not diagnostic.[1]
- Ultrasonography is helpful in the identification of gallstones or dilatation of the biliary tree.
- Computed tomography (CT) is the study of choice for visualizing the pancreas, confirmation of inflammation, and the identification of phlegmons, abscesses, or pseudocysts. It cannot be used to rule out AP.[8] CT scanning gives an estimation of severity of illness.[9]
- Endoscopic retrograde cholangiopancreatography (ERCP) is rarely used in the ED, but can be useful when the etiology remains unclear after initial evaluation. The utility of magnetic resonance imaging (MRI) in AP is unclear.
- Differential diagnosis of AP includes left lower lobe pneumonia, rupture of a pseudocyst, gallbladder disease, peritonitis, peptic ulcer disease, small bowel obstruction, renal colic, dissecting aortic aneurysm, diabetic ketoacidosis, and gastroenteritis.[3]

EMERGENCY DEPARTMENT CARE AND DISPOSITION

- Treatment of AP primarily involves pancreatic rest (nothing or only clear fluids by mouth), fluid resuscitation, pain control, and prevention of vomiting.[1,3]
- The mainstay of treatment for AP is fluid resuscitation with normal saline to maintain blood pressure and adequate urine output.[1]
- Pressors such as dopamine 2 to 20 μg/kg/min are indicated in patients with persistent hypotension despite adequate fluid resuscitation.
- Oxygen should be administered to maintain a pulse oximetry of greater than 95%.
- A nasogastric tube may be used if the patient is distended with persistent vomiting; however, no studies have demonstrated that its presence alters the course of the illness.
- Parenteral analgesia should be given as necessary for patient comfort. Intravenous narcotics such as morphine 0.1 mg/kg are often required.
- Antiemetics, such as promethazine 12.5 to 25 mg IV, may be helpful to reduce vomiting (see Chap. 48).[1]
- Urgent decompression by endoscopic sphincterotomy of the ampulla of Vater is indicated in persistent biliary obstruction.[3]
- Patients with mild pancreatitis, no evidence of systemic complications, and a low likelihood of biliary tract disease may be managed as outpatients if they are able to tolerate oral fluids and their pain is well controlled.
- Patients with significant systemic complications, shock, or extensive pancreatic necrosis will necessitate an intensive care setting.[10]

REFERENCES

1. Mergener K, Baillic J: Fortnightly review: acute pancreatitis. *BMJ* 316:44, 1998.
2. Karne S, Baillic J: Etiopathogenesis of acute pancreatitis. *Surg Clin North Am* 79:699, 1999.
3. Moscati RM: Pancreatitis. *Emerg Med Clin North Am* 14: 719, 1996.
4. Vissers RJ, Abu-Laban RB, McHugh DF: Amylase and lipase in the emergency department evaluation of acute pancreatitis. *J Emerg Med* 17:1027, 1999.
5. Rosenblum J: Serum lipase is increased in disease states other than acute pancreatitis: amylase revisited. *Clin Chem* 37:315, 1991.
6. Vissers RJ, Dagnone J, Abu-Laban R, Walls RM: Serum amylase offers no additional benefit to serum lipase in the ED diagnosis of acute pancreatitis. *Acad Emerg Med* 4:396, 1998.
7. De Bernadinis M, Violi V, Roncuroni L, et al: Discriminant power and information content of Ranson's prognostic signs in acute pancreatitis: a meta-analytic study. *Crit Care Med* 27:2272, 1999.
8. Balthazar EM: CT diagnosis and staging of acute pancreatitis. *Radiol Clin North Am* 27:19, 1989.
9. Balthazar EM: Acute pancreatitis: Assessment of severity with clinical CT evaluation. *Radiology* 223:603, 2002.

10. Pitchumoni S, Agarwal N, Jain NK: Systemic complications of acute pancreatitis. *Am J Gastroenterol* 83:597, 1988.

For further reading in *Emergency Medicine: A Comprehensive Study Guide,* 6th ed., see Chap. 87, "Acute and Chronic Pancreatitis," by Robert J. Vissers and Riyad B. Abu-Laban.

52 COMPLICATIONS OF GENERAL SURGICAL PROCEDURES

N. Heramba Prasad

- Fever, respiratory complications, genitourinary complaints, wound infections, vascular problems, and complications of drug therapy are some common postoperative disorders seen in the emergency department (ED). Most of these are discussed elsewhere in this book; certain specific problems will be mentioned here.
- The causes of postoperative fever are listed as the five Ws: **W**ind (respiratory), **W**ater (urinary tract infection [UTI]), **W**ound, **W**alking (deep venous thrombosis [DVT]), and **W**onder drugs (pseudomembranous colitis [PMC]).[1]

CLINICAL FEATURES

- Fever in the first 24 hours is usually due to atelectasis, necrotizing fasciitis, or clostridial infections.
- In the 24 to 72 hours postsurgery, pneumonia, atelectasis, intravenous-catheter-related thrombophlebitis, and infections are the major causes of complications.
- UTIs are seen 3 to 5 days postoperatively.
- DVT typically occurs 5 days after the procedure, and wound infections generally manifest 7 to 10 days after surgery.
- Antibiotic-induced PMC is seen 6 weeks after surgery.

RESPIRATORY COMPLICATIONS

- Postoperative pain and inadequate clearance of secretions contribute to the development of atelectasis. Fever, tachypnea, tachycardia, and mild hypoxia are usually seen. Pneumonia may develop 24 to 96 hours later.
- Hypoxia, tachycardia, a widened A-a gradient, and respiratory distress should point to the diagnosis of pulmonary embolism (see Chap. 28 for diagnosis and management).

GENITOURINARY COMPLICATIONS

- UTIs are more common after instrumentation of the urinary tract. Urinary retention occurs in 4% of all surgical patients[2] and in 60% of patients after urethral surgery. It is more common in elderly males, especially after excessive fluid administration and after spinal anesthesia. Lower abdominal pain, urgency, and inability to void should alert the clinician to suspect urinary retention.[2,3]
- Oliguria or anuria commonly results from volume depletion. Intrinsic factors such as acute tubular necrosis (ATN), drug nephrotoxicity, and postrenal obstructive uropathy also may lead to acute renal failure.

WOUND COMPLICATIONS

- Hematomas result from inadequate hemostasis. Careful evaluation to rule out infections must be undertaken.
- Seromas are collections of clear fluid under the wound. Extremes of age, diabetes, poor nutrition, necrotic tissue, poor perfusion, foreign bodies, and wound hematomas contribute to the development of wound infections.
- Necrotizing fasciitis is characterized by extremely painful, erythematous, swollen, and warm areas without sharp margins. This staphylococcal infection spreads rapidly. Patients will exhibit marked systemic toxicity, and crepitance and bullae may be present.[4]
- Wound dehiscence can occur due to diabetes, poor nutrition, chronic steroid use, and inadequate or improper closure of the wound. Dehiscence of abdominal wounds may result in evisceration of abdominal organs.

VASCULAR COMPLICATIONS

- Superficial thrombophlebitis usually occurs in the upper extremities after intravenous catheter insertion, or in the lower extremities because of stasis and varicosity of veins.
- DVT commonly occurs in the lower extremities. Swelling and pain of the calf are commonly encountered (see Chap. 31 for diagnosis and management).

DRUG THERAPY COMPLICATIONS

- Many drugs are known to cause fever and antibiotic-induced diarrhea.[5]
- PMC, a dreaded complication, is caused by *Clostridium difficile* toxin. Bloody, watery diarrhea, fever, and crampy abdominal pain are the usual complaints.

DIAGNOSIS AND DIFFERENTIAL

- Patients with suspected respiratory complications should have chest x-rays. They may reveal plate-like or discoid atelectases, pneumonia, or pneumothorax. Pneumothorax occurs early after certain surgical procedures or catheter insertion, and a chest x-ray will help confirm the diagnosis.
- Patients with oliguria or anuria should be evaluated for signs of hypovolemia or urinary retention.
- Diagnosis of PMC is established by demonstrating *C. difficile* cytotoxin in the stool. In 27% of the cases, however, the assay can be negative.

EMERGENCY DEPARTMENT CARE AND DISPOSITION

- Always discuss patients and proposed treatments with the surgeon who initially cared for the patients.
- Although debilitated patients may need hospitalization, many patients with atelectasis can be treated as outpatients.
- Postoperative pneumonia is polymicrobial, and an antipseudomonal antibiotic with an aminoglycoside is usually recommended. Most patients with UTI can be managed as outpatients with oral antibiotic therapy (see Chap. 55).
- Insertion of a Foley catheter and prompt drainage will alleviate urinary retention. There is no need for clamping the catheter periodically. Prophylactic antibiotics are reserved for patients who have had urinary tract instrumentation, those with prolonged retention, and those at risk for infection.
- Wound hematomas may require removal of some sutures and evacuation. Surgical consultation before treatment is appropriate. Seromas can be treated with needle aspiration and wound cultures. Admission may not always be necessary.
- Most wound infections can be treated with oral antibiotics (usually the surgeon's choice), unless the patients manifest systemic symptoms and signs. Perineal infections usually require admission and parenteral antibiotics. As surgical debridement and parenteral antibiotics are indicated for necrotizing fasciitis, physicians should start clindamycin 900 mg and penicillin G, 6 million units IV.[6]
- Most patients with superficial thrombophlebitis can be treated with local heat and elevation of the affected area if there is no evidence of cellulitis or lymphangitis. Patients with suppurative thrombophlebitis, characterized by erythema, lymphangitis, fever, and severe pain, should be hospitalized and treated with excision of the affected vein.
- Fluid resuscitation, oral vancomycin, and metronida-

zole, orally or intravenously, are currently available treatment modalities for drug-induced PMC (see Chap. 46).

SPECIFIC CONSIDERATIONS

COMPLICATIONS OF BREAST SURGERY

- Wound infections, hematomas, pneumothorax, necrosis of the skin flaps, and lymphedema of the arms after mastectomy are common problems seen after breast surgery.
- Lymphedema of the arm occurs in 5 to 10% of patients. Elevation and minor activity restriction will help reduce swelling.

COMPLICATIONS OF GI SURGERY

INTESTINAL OBSTRUCTION
- Neuronal dysfunction following any surgery in which the peritoneum is entered may cause paralytic ileus. Following gastrointestinal (GI) surgery, small bowel tone returns to normal within 24 hours, gastric function within 2 days, and colonic function within 3 days.
- Prolonged ileus should alert the clinician to peritonitis, abscesses, hemoperitoneum, pneumonia, sepsis, and electrolyte imbalance. Clinical features include nausea, vomiting, obstipation, constipation, abdominal distension, and pain.
- Abdominal x-rays, complete blood count, electrolytes, blood urea nitrogen and creatinine levels, and urinalysis should be obtained.
- Treatment of adynamic ileus consists of nasogastric suction, bowel rest, and hydration. Mechanical obstruction is usually due to adhesions and may require surgical intervention.
- Differentiation between mechanical versus paralytic ileus may be difficult in the ED.

NONOBSTRUCTIVE COMPLICATIONS
- Intra-abdominal abscesses are caused by preoperative contamination or postoperative anastomotic leaks. Diagnosis can be confirmed by computed tomography (CT) scan or ultrasonography. Percutaneous drainage or surgical exploration, evacuation, and parenteral antibiotics will be required.
- Pancreatitis occurs, especially after direct manipulation of the pancreatic duct. Patients typically have nausea, vomiting, abdominal pain, and leukocytosis. Lumbar pain, left pleural effusion, Turner's sign (discoloration of the flank), and Cullen's sign (periumbilical ecchymosis) may be present. Serum amylase and lipase levels are usually elevated.

- Serum amylase levels may also be elevated in cholecystitis, bowel obstruction, and mesenteric ischemia.
- Cholecystitis and biliary colic have been reported as postoperative complications. Elderly patients are more prone to develop acalculous cholecystitis.
- Fistulas, either internal or external, may result from direct bowel injury and require surgical consultation and hospitalization.
- Anastomotic leaks are especially devastating after esophageal or colon surgery. Esophageal leaks occur 10 days after the procedure. Dramatic presentation with shock, pneumothorax, and pleural effusion is usually seen.
- Dumping syndrome is noticed in gastric bypass procedures. It is due to the sudden influx of hyperosmolar chyle into the small intestine, resulting in fluid sequestration and hypovolemia. Patients experience nausea, vomiting, epigastric discomfort, palpitations, dizziness, and sometimes syncope.
- Alkaline reflux gastritis is caused by the reflux of bile into the stomach. Endoscopic evaluation will establish the diagnosis. Postvagotomy diarrhea and afferent loop syndrome are seen in some patients.
- Colonoscopy may cause hemorrhage, perforation, retroperitoneal abscesses, pneumoscrotum, pneumothorax, volvulus, and infection.
- Rectal surgery complications include urinary retention, constipation, prolapse, bleeding, and infections.
- Finally, tetanus has been known to occur following surgical wounds.[7,8]
- Complications of percutaneous endoscopic gastrostomy (PEG) tubes include infections, hemorrhage, peritonitis, aspiration, wound dehiscence, sepsis, and obstruction of the tube.

Replacement of PEG and J-Tubes (Jejunostomy)
- Prevention is the best form of treatment for gastrostomy tube (G-tube) obstruction. If the tube cannot be unclogged, replacement will be necessary.
- A tube placed by surgery or endoscopy that has not since been replaced may have a bolster device preventing removal. The bolster must be removed endoscopically, or the tube may be cut off and the bolster allowed to pass through GI tract. This latter technique is not recommended for children.
- If the G-tube was placed radiologically or has been previously replaced, it will have an inflated balloon.

The balloon should be deflated or cut off to remove the tube.
- Tracts that are 7 to 10 days old probably will remain open long enough for replacement of the tube.
- If the size and the type of tube (jejunostomy [J-tube] versus gastrostomy) cannot be determined, it is reasonable to use a 16F G-tube or Foley catheter. Tube placement should be confirmed by a Gastrografin study. Jejunostomy tubes are replaced with smaller size Foley catheters and the balloon is not inflated, as the jejunal lumen may be obstructed by the balloon.
- Complications arising from stomas are due to technical errors or from underlying disease such as Crohn's disease and cancer. Ischemia, necrosis, bleeding, hernia, and prolapse are sometimes seen.

REFERENCES

1. O'Grady NP, Barie PS, Bartlett J, et al: Practice parameters for evaluating fever in critically ill adult patients. *Crit Care Med* 26:392, 1998.
2. Tammela T, Kontturi M, Lukkarinen O: Postoperative urinary retention: I. Incidence and predisposing factors. *Scand J Urol Nephrol* 20:197, 1986.
3. Nyman MA, Schwenk NM, Silverstein MD: Management of urinary retention: Rapid versus gradual decompression and risk of complications. *Mayo Clin Proc* 72:951, 1997.
4. Wysoki MG, Santora TA, Shah RM, Friedman AC: Necrotizing fasciitis: CT characteristics. *Radiology* 203:859, 1997.
5. Johnaon DH, Cunha BA: Drug fever. *Infect Dis Clin North Am* 10:85, 1996.
6. Gilbert DN, Moellering RC, Sande MA: *The Sanford Guide to Antimicrobial Therapy*, 28th ed. Dallas: Antimicrobial Therapy Inc., 1998.
7. Meyer KA, Spector BK: Incidence of tetanus bacilli in stools and on regional skins of one hundred urban herniotomy cases. *Surg Gynecol Obstet* 54:785, 1932.
8. LaForce FM, Young LS, Bennett JV: Tetanus in the United States: 1965-1969. *N Engl J Med* 280:569, 1969.

For further reading in *Emergency Medicine: A Comprehensive Study Guide*, 6th ed., see Chap. 88, "Complications of General Surgical Procedures," by Edmond A. Hooker.

RENAL AND GENITOURINARY DISORDERS

53 ACUTE RENAL FAILURE

Marc D. Squillante

- Renal dysfunction and acute renal failure (ARF) present with a wide variety of manifestations, depending on the underlying etiology.
- The demographics of ARF show it evolving not as a result of specific primary renal diseases, but as a complication of multiorgan disease processes.
- Risk factors include cardiac disease, hypovolemia from any cause, vascular or thrombotic disorders, glomerular diseases, diseases affecting the renal tubules, use of nephrotoxic drugs, and a variety of anatomic problems of the genitourinary tract.

EPIDEMIOLOGY

- The distinction between community- and hospital-acquired ARF is important in diagnosis, treatment, and outcome. Hospital-acquired ARF is more common, is usually multifactorial, with an aging population at increased risk of ARF and many nephrotoxic exposures, and has a higher mortality.
- The majority of community-acquired ARF is due to volume depletion, and up to 90% of ED cases have a potentially reversible cause.[1]
- Most adult ARF deaths are due to sepsis and cardiac and pulmonary failure.
- Pediatric ARF has a different set of etiologies and mortality averages 25%.[2]

PATHOPHYSIOLOGY

- Regardless of the cause of ARF, reductions in renal blood flow (RBF) represent a common pathologic pathway for decreasing glomerular filtration rate (GFR).[3] This relationship is most clear in prerenal failure, defined by conditions with normal tubular and glomerular function, where GFR is depressed by compromised renal perfusion.
- Intrinsic renal failure occurs with diseases of the glomerulus, interstitium, or tubule, associated with the release of renal vasoconstrictors.[4]
- Postobstructive renal failure initially produces an increase in tubular pressure decreasing the filtration driving force. This pressure gradient soon equalizes, and the maintenance of depressed GFR depends on vasoconstrictors.[5] During periods of decreased RBF, the kidneys are especially vulnerable to further insults. Recovery from ARF is first dependent on restoration of RBF.
- **Prerenal failure** is produced by conditions that decrease renal perfusion (Table 53-1), and is the most common cause of community-acquired ARF (40 to 80% of cases).[6] It is a common precursor to ischemic and nephrotoxic causes of intrinsic renal failure as well.[7] For adults in a community hospital, prerenal failure accounted for 70% of ARF cases as compared with only 11% from intrinsic renal etiologies.[8]
- The etiologies of intrinsic renal failure are subdivided anatomically into diseases of the tubules, interstitium, glomeruli, and vessels (see Table 53-1). Intrinsic renal failure accounts for approximately 11 to 45% of all cases, depending on the population studied. ARF has a different spectrum in the pediatric population: a higher incidence of intrinsic renal causes for ARF (45%) secondary to diseases such as glomerulonephritis and hemolytic-uremic syndrome (HUS).[9]
- Acute tubular necrosis (ATN) secondary to renal ischemia accounts for the majority of cases of intrinsic renal failure. Nephrotoxins are the second most common cause of ATN, accounting for approximately 25%.
- **Postrenal failure** accounts for 5 to 17% of all cases of community-acquired ARF, but has a significantly higher incidence in selected populations (such as elderly men).

TABLE 53-1   Common Causes of Acute Renal Failure

PRERENAL	RENAL	POSTRENAL

Decreased cardiac output
  Myocardial ischemia/infarction
  Valvular heart disease
  Cardiomyopathy
  Pericardial tamponade
  High-output failure
 	
Hypovolemia
  Blood loss/hemorrhagic shock
  Vomiting/diarrhea
  Diuretics
  Postobstructive diuresis
  Fluid sequestration
    Cirrhosis
    Pancreatitis
    Burns
    General anesthesia
    Septic shock
	Vascular/ischemia
	  Renal vasculature thrombosis, TTP, DIC,
	    NSAIDs, severe hypertension, hemolytic-uremic
	    syndrome
	Glomerular
	  Primary glomerular diseases (acute glomerulonephritis)
	    or systemic disease with glomerular involvement
	    (SLE, vasculitis, HSP, endocarditis)
	Tubulointerstitial
	  Ischemic ATN, rhabdomyolysis, toxin-induced tubular
	    damage (aminoglycosides, radiocontrast, solvents,
	    heavy metals, ethylene glycol, myoglobin/
	    hemoglobin), acute interstitial nephritis, infiltrative
	    and autoimmune diseases, infectious agents
		Penile lesions
		  Phimosis
		  Meatal stenosis
		  Urethral stricutre
		
		Prostatic enlargement—BPH, cancer
		
		Upper urinary tract/ureteral diseases (usually
		  requires bilateral involvement/obstruction)
		    Calculi, tumors, blood clots
		    Papillary necrosis
		    Vesicoureteral reflux
		    Stricture
		    AAA
		    Retroperitoneal

ABBREVIATIONS: DIC = disseminated intravascular coagulation; NSAIDs = nonsteroidal anti-inflammatory agents; ATN = acute tubular necrosis; TTP = thrombotic thrombocytopenic purpura; SLE = systemic lupus erythematosus; HSP = Henoch-Schönlein purpura; BPH = benign prostatic hypertrophy; AAA = abdominal aortic aneurysm.

CLINICAL FEATURES

- Reported mortality rates from ARF have remained fairly constant, even with the advent of dialysis, at 40 to 90%.[10,11]
- Patients usually have signs and symptoms of their underlying causative disorder, but eventually develop stigmata of renal failure. Volume overload, hypertension, pulmonary edema, mental status changes or neurologic symptoms, nausea and vomiting, bone and joint problems, anemia, and increased susceptibility to infection (a leading cause of death) can occur, as patients develop more chronic uremia.
- Deterioration in renal function leads to excessive accumulation of nitrogenous waste products in the serum.
- ARF can be classified as oliguric (<400 mL urine per 24 hours) and nonoliguric (>400 mL urine per 24 hours). Oliguric renal failure has a higher mortality rate.[12]
- Approximately 20 to 60% of patients experiencing ARF will require dialysis,[13] but the majority will recover, with only 25% requiring long-term dialysis.[14]

DIAGNOSIS AND DIFFERENTIAL

- The history and physical exam, directed towards discovery of underlying illnesses, should assess vital signs, volume status, establish urinary tract patency and output, and search for signs of chemical intoxication, drug use, muscle damage, associated systemic diseases, or infection.

- Diagnostic studies include urinalysis, blood urea nitrogen (BUN) and creatinine levels, serum electrolytes, urinary sodium and creatinine levels, and urinary osmolality. Creatinine provides the most accurate and consistent estimation of GFR. Analysis of these tests allows most patients to be placed in either the prerenal, renal, or postrenal group (Table 53-2).
- Fractional excretion of sodium and renal failure index can be calculated to help in this categorization[15] (see Table 53-2).
- Normal urinary sediment may be seen in prerenal and postrenal failure, HUS, and thrombotic thrombocytopenic purpura.
- Granular casts are seen in ATN. Albumin and red blood cell (RBC) casts are found in both glomerulonephritis and malignant hypertension. White blood cell casts are seen in interstitial nephritis and pyelonephritis.
- Crystals can be present with renal calculi and certain drugs (sulfas, ethylene glycol, and radiocontrast agents).
- Ultrasonography is the radiologic procedure of choice in most patients with acute renal failure when hydronephrosis and upper urinary tract obstruction is suspected.

EMERGENCY DEPARTMENT CARE AND DISPOSITION

- Initial care of patients with ARF focuses on treating the underlying cause and correcting fluid and electrolyte derangement. Resuscitation is the first priority. Efforts should be made to prevent further renal damage and provide supportive care until renal function

TABLE 53-2   Laboratory Studies Aiding in the Differential Diagnosis of Acute Renal Failure

TEST EMPLOYED	PRERENAL	RENAL*	POSTRENAL†
Urine sodium (mEq/L)	<20	>40	>40
FE_{Na} (%)‡	<1	>1	>1
Renal failure index (RFI)‡	<1	>1	>1
Urine osmolality (mOsm/L)	>500	<350	<350
Urine/serum creatinine ratio	>40:1	<20:1	<20:1
Serum urea nitrogen/creatinine ratio	>20:1	=10:1	>10:1

*FE_{Na} may be <1 in intrinsic renal failure patients with glomerulonephritis, hepatorenal syndrome, radiocontrast acute tubular necrosis, myoglobinuric and hemoglobinuric acute renal failure, renal allograft rejection, and with certain drugs (captopril and nonsteroidal anti-inflammatory agents).

†Can see indices similar to prerenal early in course of obstruction. With continued obstruction, tubular function is impaired and indices mimic those of renal causes.

‡Fractional excretion of sodium (%) $= \dfrac{\text{Urine sodium/serum sodium}}{\text{Urine creatinine/serum creatinine}} \times 100$

§RFI $= \dfrac{\text{Serum sodium}}{\text{Urine creatinine/serum creatinine}} \times 100$

has recovered (see Chap. 6 for treatment of electrolyte and acid-base disorders).

PRERENAL FAILURE

- Effective intravascular volume should be restored with isotonic fluids (normal saline or lactated Ringer's) at a rapid rate in appropriate patients.[16]
- If cardiac failure is causing prerenal azotemia, cardiac output should be optimized to improve renal perfusion, and reduction in intravascular volume (ie, with diuretics) may be appropriate.

POSTRENAL FAILURE

- Appropriate urinary drainage should be established; the exact procedure depends on the level of obstruction.
- A Foley catheter should be placed to relieve obstruction caused by prostatic hypertrophy. There is no support for the practice of intermittent catheter clamping to prevent hypotension and hematuria; urine should be completely and rapidly drained. Percutaneous nephrostomy may be required for ureteral occlusion until definitive surgery to correct the obstruction can take place once the patient is stabilized.
- For the acutely anuric patient, obstruction is the major consideration. If no urine is obtained on initial bladder catheterization, emergency urologic consultation should be considered.
- With chronic urinary retention, postobstructive diuresis may occur due to osmotic diuresis or tubular dysfunction. Patients may become suddenly hypovolemic and hypotensive. Urine output must be closely monitored, with appropriate fluid replacement.

RENAL FAILURE

- Adequate circulating volume must be restored first; hypovolemia potentiates and exacerbates all forms of ARF.
- Nephrotoxic agents (drugs, intravenous contrast) should be avoided. Patients with nonoliguric ARF have improved mortality and renal function recovery. However, the use of diuretics to "convert" oliguric to nonoliguric ARF is not beneficial.[17] Diuretics are useful in the management of volume-overloaded patients.
- Low-dose dopamine (1 to 5 μg/kg/min) may improve renal blood flow and urine output, but does not lower mortality rates or improve recovery.[18] It is probably best used in ARF patients with congestive heart failure.
- Mannitol may be protective against myoglobinuric ARF in early rhabdomyolysis. Large-volume crystalloid infusions are the primary treatment here. Urinary alkalinization with sodium bicarbonate is also recommended.
- Renally-excreted drugs (digoxin, magnesium, sedatives, and narcotics) should be used with caution since therapeutic doses may accumulate to excess and cause serious side effects. Fluid restriction may be required.
- Interventions useful in the prevention of radiocontrast nephropathy include acetylcysteine,[19] fenoldopam,[20] and crystalloid infusions.

DIALYSIS

- If treatment of the underlying cause fails to improve renal function, hemodialysis or peritoneal dialysis should be considered. Decisions about dialysis are usually made by the nephrology consultant.

- Dialysis is often initiated when the BUN level is >100 mg/dL or the serum creatinine level is >10 mg/dL.
- Patients with complications of ARF such as cardiac instability (due to metabolic acidosis and hyperkalemia), intractable volume overload, hyperkalemia, and uremia (ie, encephalopathy, pericarditis, and bleeding diathesis) not easily corrected by other measures should be considered for emergency dialysis.

DISPOSITION

- Patients with new-onset ARF usually require hospital admission, often to an intensive care unit.
- Transferring patients to another institution should be considered if nephrology consultation and dialysis facilities are not available.

REFERENCES

1. Kaufman J, Dhakai M, Bulabhai P, Hamburger R: Community-acquired acute renal failure. *Am J Kidney Dis* 17:191, 1991.
2. Moghal NE, Brocklebank JT, Meadow SR: A review of acute renal failure in children: Incidence, etiology, and outcome. *Clin Nephrol* 49:91, 1998.
3. Brezis M, Rosen S: Hypoxia of the renal medulla: Its implications for disease. *N Engl J Med* 332:647, 1995.
4. Thurau K, Boylan JW: Acute renal success: The unexpected logic of oliguria in acute renal failure. *Am J Med* 61:308, 1976.
5. Vaughn ED Jr, Sorenson EJ, Gillenwater JY: The renal hemodynamic response to chronic unilateral complete ureteral occlusion. *Invest Urol* 8:78, 1970.
6. Hou SH, et al: Hospital-acquired renal insufficiency: A prospective study. *Am J Med* 74:243, 1983.
7. Shusterman N, Strom BL, Murray TG, et al: Risk factors and outcome of hospital-acquired acute renal failure: Clinical epidemiologic study. *Am J Med* 83:65, 1987.
8. Kaufman J, Dhakal M, Patel B, et al: Community-acquired acute renal failure. *Am J Kidney Dis* 17:191, 1991.
9. Moghal NE, Brocklebank JT, Meadow SR: A review of acute renal failure in children: Incidence, etiology and outcome. *Clin Nephrol* 49:91, 1998.
10. Alkhunaizi AM, Schrier RW: Management of acute renal failure: New perspectives. *Am J Kidney Dis* 28:315, 1996.
11. Druml W: Prognosis of acute renal failure 1975–1995 [editorial]. *Nephron* 73:8, 1996.
12. Corwin HL, Teplick RS, Schreiber MJ, et al: Prediction of outcome in acute renal failure. *Am J Nephrol* 7:8, 1987.
13. Liano F, Junco E, Pascual J, et al: The spectrum of acute renal failure in the intensive care unit compared with that seen in other settings: The Madrid Acute Renal Failure Study Group. *Kidney Int* 66(Suppl):S16, 1998.
14. Spurney RF, Fulkerson JW, Schwab SJ: Acute renal failure in critically ill patients: Prognosis for recovery of kidney function after prolonged dialysis support [see comments]. *Crit Care Med* 19:8, 1991.
15. Miller TR, Anderson RJ, Linas SL, et al: Urinary diagnostic indices in acute renal failure: A prospective study. *Ann Intern Med* 89:47, 1978.
16. Conger JD: Interventions in clinical acute renal failure: What are the data? *Am J Kidney Dis* 26:565, 1995.
17. Shilliday IR, Quinn KJ, Allison ME: Loop diuretics in the management of acute renal failure: A prospective, double-blind, placebo-controlled, randomized study. *Nephrol Dial Transplant* 12:2592, 1997.
18. Denton M, Chertow GM, Brady HR: "Renal-dose" dopamine for the treatment of acute renal failure: Scientific rationale, experimental studies and clinical trials. *Kidney Int* 50:4, 1996.
19. Tepel M, Van Der Geit M, Schwarzfeld C, et al: Prevention of radiographic-contrast-agent-induced reductions in renal function by acetylcysteine. *N Engl J Med* 343:180, 2000.
20. Tumlin JA, Wang A, Murray PT, Mathur VS: Fenoldopam mesylate blocks reductions in renal plasma flow after radio-contrast dye infusion: A pilot trial in the prevention of contrast nephropathy. *Am Heart J* 143:894, 2002.

For further reading in *Emergency Medicine: A Comprehensive Study Guide,* 6th ed., see Chap. 92, "Acute Renal Failure," by Richard Sinert and Peter R. Peacock, Jr.

54 EMERGENCIES IN RENAL FAILURE AND DIALYSIS PATIENTS

Jonathan A. Maisel

- Patients with end-stage renal disease (ESRD) may sustain multiple complications of their disease process and treatment. (See the appropriate chapters for discussion on the management of hypertension, heart failure, bleeding disorders, and electrolyte disorders.)

EPIDEMIOLOGY

- The 2001 annual data report of the United States Renal Data System (USRDS) noted there were 89,252 new cases of ESRD, with 424,179 patients being treated for ESRD during that year.[1]
- ESRD is primarily a disease of the elderly, with patients over 65 years of age comprising 47.9% of new cases, and 37.2% of all living individuals with the disease.

- Diabetes mellitus is the most common disease causing ESRD, accounting for 42.8% of patients, followed by hypertension (25.9%), glomerulonephritis (9%), and cystic kidney disease (2.3%).[1]
- Cardiac causes account for approximately 50% of all cases of ESRD death. Infectious etiologies account for 10 to 25% of deaths.

PATHOPHYSIOLOGY

- The pathophysiology of renal failure can be categorized by three mechanisms: (1) excretory failure (ie, inability to excrete over 70 chemicals known to accumulate in renal failure, most notably urea); (2) biosynthetic failure (ie, the loss of renal hormones vitamin D and erythropoietin); and (3) regulatory failure (ie, the disruption of normal feedback mechanisms, leading to the oversecretion of hormones that exacerbate uremia).
- The diagnosis of uremia is a clinical one, based on a constellation of symptoms. Though a correlation exists between the symptoms of uremia and a low glomerular filtration rate (8 to 10 mL/min), routine laboratory tests are inaccurate markers of the syndrome. The decision to institute renal replacement therapy (RRT) is a clinical one.

CARDIOVASCULAR COMPLICATIONS

- Cardiovascular disease is more prevalent in ESRD patients than in the general population. The etiology is multifactorial, including pre-existing conditions (eg, hypertension, diabetes), uremia, and complications of dialysis.
- Creatine protein kinase (and the MB fraction), troponin I, and troponin T are not significantly elevated in ESRD patients, and have been shown to be specific markers of myocardial ischemia in these patients.
- Hypertension occurs in 80 to 90% of patients starting dialysis, largely due to increases in total peripheral resistance. Management includes control of blood volume, followed by use of adrenergic-blocking drugs, angiotensin-converting enzyme inhibitors, or vasodilating agents.
- Congestive heart failure (CHF) may be caused by hypertension, coronary ischemia, and valvular disease, as well as uremic cardiomyopathy, fluid overload, and arteriovenous (AV) fistulas (high-output failure). Treatment is similar to that in non-ESRD patients. Diuretics (eg, furosemide 60 to 100 mg) are useful, even in oliguric patients, as they cause pulmonary vessel vasodilatation. Preload can be reduced by inducing diarrhea with sorbitol and with phlebotomy (minimum 150 mL). Hemodialysis (HD) is the definitive treatment.
- Pericarditis in ESRD patients is usually due to uremia, and is seen when other symptoms of uremia are most severe. Because inflammatory cells do not penetrate the myocardium, electrocardiographic (ECG) changes typical of acute pericarditis are not seen. Pericardial friction rubs are louder than in most other forms of pericarditis, often palpable, and frequently persist after the metabolic abnormalities have been corrected. Uremic pericarditis is treated with intensive dialysis therapy.
- Cardiac tamponade is the most serious complication of uremic pericarditis. It rarely presents with the classic signs of Beck's triad, but rather with changes in mental status, hypotension, or dyspnea. An enlarged heart on chest x-ray may suggest the diagnosis, which can be confirmed with echocardiography. Hemodynamically significant pericardial effusions require pericardiocentesis under fluoroscopic or ultrasonographic guidance.

NEUROLOGIC COMPLICATIONS

- Uremic encephalopathy presents with cognitive defects, memory loss, slurred speech, and asterixis. The progressive neurologic symptoms of uremia are the most common indications for initiating HD. However, it should remain a diagnosis of exclusion until structural, vascular, infectious, toxic, and metabolic causes of neurologic dysfunction have been ruled out.
- Peripheral neuropathy, manifested by impaired vibration sense and stocking-glove pain or anesthesia, occurs in more than 50% of patients with ESRD.
- Autonomic dysfunction, characterized by impotence, postural dizziness, gastric fullness, bowel dysfunction, and reduced sweating, is common in ESRD patients, but is not responsible for intradialytic hypotension.[2]
- Subdural hematoma is seen in 3.5% of HD patients, presumably related to trauma, anticoagulation, excessive ultrafiltration, or hypertension. It should be considered in any ESRD patient presenting with a change in mental status.
- Dialysis disequilibrium, generally occurring at the end of dialysis, is characterized by nausea, vomiting, and hypertension, which can progress to seizures, coma, and death. Treatment consists of terminating dialysis and administering mannitol intravenously to increase serum osmolarity. This syndrome should be distinguished from other neurologic disorders, such as subdural hematoma, stroke, hypertensive crisis, hypoxia, and seizures.

GASTROINTESTINAL COMPLICATIONS

- Anorexia, nausea, and vomiting are common symptoms of uremia, and are used as an indication to initiate dialysis and assess its efficacy.

HEMATOLOGIC COMPLICATIONS

- Abnormal hemostasis in ESRD is multifactorial in origin, resulting in an increased risk of gastrointestinal (GI) tract bleeding, subcapsular liver hematomas, subdural hematomas, and intraocular bleeding.
- Immunologic compromise, caused by impaired leukocyte chemotaxis and phagocytosis, leads to high mortality rates from infection. Dialysis therapy does not appear to improve immune system function.

COMPLICATIONS OF HEMODIALYSIS

- Hypotension is the most frequent complication of HD. Excessive ultrafiltration from underestimation of the patient's ideal blood volume (dry weight) is the most common cause of intradialytic hypotension.
- Cardiac compensation for fluid loss may be compromised by diastolic dysfunction common in ESRD patients.
- Other causes of intradialytic hypotension include myocardial dysfunction from ischemia, hypoxia, arrhythmias, and pericardial tamponade; abnormalities of vascular tone secondary to sepsis, overproduction of nitric oxide, and antihypertensive medications; and volume loss from vomiting, diarrhea, GI bleeding, or blood tubing or filter leaks.
- Treatment consists of Trendelenburg positioning, oral salt solution, or infusion of parenteral normal saline solution.

COMPLICATIONS OF VASCULAR ACCESS

- Complications of vascular access account for more inpatient hospital days than any other complication of HD.
- Thrombosis or stenosis are the most common complications, presenting with loss of the bruit and thrill over the access. These need to be treated within 24 hours with angiographic clot removal or angioplasty.
- Vascular access infections often present with signs of systemic sepsis, including fever, hypotension, and an elevated white blood cell (WBC) count. Classic signs of pain, erythema, swelling, and discharge are often missing. *Staphylococcus aureus* is the most common infecting organism, followed by gram-negative bacteria. Patients usually require hospitalization, and treatment with vancomycin (1 g IV), and an aminoglycoside (eg, gentamicin 100 mg IV initially, and after each dialysis).
- Potential life-threatening hemorrhage from a vascular access may result from a ruptured aneurysm or anastomosis, or overanticoagulation. Bleeding can often be controlled with 5 to 10 minutes of pressure at the puncture site. Life-threatening hemorrhage may require placement of a tourniquet proximal to the access, and vascular surgery consultation. If the etiology is excessive anticoagulation, the effects of heparin can be reversed with protamine 0.01 mg/IU heparin dispensed during dialysis (10 to 20 mg protamine if the heparin dose is unknown). If a newly inserted vascular access continues to bleed, desmopressin acetate (0.3 μg/kg IV) can be given as an adjunct to direct pressure.

COMPLICATIONS OF PERITONEAL DIALYSIS

- Peritonitis is the most common complication of peritoneal dialysis (PD). Signs and symptoms are similar to those seen in other patients with peritonitis, and include fever, abdominal pain, and rebound tenderness. A cloudy effluent supports the diagnosis.
- Laboratory evaluation should include complete blood cell count and analysis of peritoneal fluid for cell count, Gram's stain, culture, and sensitivity. In the setting of peritonitis, cell counts usually reveal more than 100 leukocytes, with more than 50% neutrophils. Gram's stain is positive in only 10 to 40% of culture-proven peritonitis. Organisms isolated include *Staphylococcus epidermidis, S. aureus, Streptococcus* species, gram-negative bacteria, anaerobes, and fungi.
- Empiric therapy begins with a few rapid exchanges of dialysate to decrease the number of inflammatory cells within the peritoneum. The addition of heparin (500 to 1000 IU/L dialysate) decreases fibrin clot formation. Next, empiric antibiotics, covering gram-positive organisms (eg, cephalothin or vancomycin 500 mg/L dialysate) and gram-negative organisms (eg, gentamycin 100 mg/L dialysate) are added to the dialysate.
- Inpatient versus outpatient treatment of PD-related peritonitis should be based on clinical presentation.

REFERENCES

1. U.S. Renal Data System: *USRDS 2001 Annual Data Report: Atlas of End-Stage Renal Disease in the United States.*

Bethesda, MD: National Institutes of Health, National Institute of Diabetes and Digestive and Kidney Diseases, 2001.

2. Straver B, DeVries PM, ten Voorde BJ, et al: Intradialytic hypotension in relation to pre-existent autonomic dysfunction in hemodialysis patients. *Int J Artif Organs* 21:794, 1998.

For further reading in *Emergency Medicine: A Comprehensive Study Guide,* 6th ed., see Chap. 93, "Emergencies in Renal Failure and Dialysis Patients," by Richard Sinert and Mark Spektor.

55 URINARY TRACT INFECTIONS AND HEMATURIA

Kama Guluma

URINARY TRACT INFECTIONS

EPIDEMIOLOGY

- There are four groups of patients at risk for urinary tract infection (UTI): neonates, girls, young women, and older men.
- In neonates, UTI occurs with a male:female (M:F) incidence ratio of 1.5:1, often as part of a gram-negative sepsis syndrome.
- In preschool, the M:F ratio inverts, with girls being affected 10 times as often as boys. By school age, the incidence increases to 5%, and is almost exclusively in girls.
- In young adult women, the incidence of UTI rises with commencement of sexual activity. Bacteriuria in men under age 50, on the other hand, is rare, and is typically associated with a sexually transmitted infection of the urethra or prostate.
- The incidence of UTI in postmenopausal women increases with age as, under the influence of decreased estrogen, *Escherichia coli* replaces vaginal lactobacilli. In males over the age of 50, the incidence of UTI approaches and eventually exceeds that of females, due to the increasing prevalence of prostate hypertrophy and related instrumentation.
- Asymptomatic bacteriuria (ABU), defined as two successive urine cultures with more than 10^5/mL of a single bacterial species in an asymptomatic patient, occurs in up 5% of women aged 18 to 40 years,[1] in up to 40% of female nursing home residents, and commonly in patients with indwelling urinary catheters.

PATHOPHYSIOLOGY

- A thin film of urine remains in the functionally intact bladder after each void. Urinary pathogens, adhering to the uroepithelium with adhesins, fibrae or pili, are removed from the film by mucosal production of organic acids. Incomplete bladder emptying renders this mechanism ineffective, and is responsible for the increased frequency of UTI in patients with structural or neurogenic bladder outflow abnormalities.
- Ureteral valves restrict the majority of uncomplicated UTIs to the bladder. If ascending infection of the urinary tract occurs, renal defense mechanisms including local antibody secretion and complement activation are induced.
- In uncomplicated UTIs, the most common urinary pathogen is *E. coli* (Table 55-1). Up to one half of women with symptomatic UTI may have low-grade or early infection, usually with 10^2 to 10^4 colony-forming units (CFU) per milliliter of *E. coli, Staphylococcus saprophyticus,* or *Chlamydia trachomatis.* In complicated UTIs (ie, in those occurring in patients with underlying urologic or neurologic dysfunction), *Pseudomonas* spp. and enterococci are likely pathogens.
- In young women, the risk of UTI is independently associated with recent sexual intercourse, recent use of a diaphragm with spermicide, and a history of UTI.[1,2] A "milking action" of the female urethra during intercourse can increase the concentration of bacteria in the bladder by up to a factor of ten.[3] The use of a spermicide enhances vaginal colonization with *E. coli.*[3]

TABLE 55-1   Etiologic Agents in Uncomplicated Urinary Tract Infection

ORGANISM	INCIDENCE
Escherichia coli	>80%
Klebsiella spp.	5–20%
Proteus spp.	5–20%
Enterobacter spp.	5–20%
Pseudomonas spp.	5–20%
Group D streptococci	<5%
*Chlamydia trachomatis**	<5%
*Staphylococcus saprophyticus**	<5%

*Much more common in the "dysuria pyuria" syndrome in which sterile or low-colony-count culture results are obtained. *Staphylococcus saprophyticus* may account for up to 15% of acute lower tract infections in young, sexually active females, but rarely progresses to involve the upper tract.

CLINICAL FEATURES

- UTIs presenting to the emergency department are categorized into two major clinical syndromes: acute cystitis and acute pyelonephritis.
- Patients with acute cystitis, in which infection is localized to the bladder, will typically present with internal dysuria (as opposed to external dysuria from pain as urine passes over inflamed urethral tissue), frequency, and suprapubic discomfort. In the young male, however, dysuria is likely to represent urethritis or prostatitis.[4]
- Patients with acute pyelonephritis, in which infection has spread to the kidney, typically present with localized kidney pain, fever, chills, nausea, vomiting, malaise, and costovertebral angle tenderness, in addition to the preceding symptoms of cystitis.
- Subclinical pyelonephritis, a syndrome in which infection has spread to the kidneys without overt symptoms and signs beyond those of cystitis, is clinically indistinguishable from acute cystitis without the use of specialized diagnostic techniques, and is estimated to be present in about 25 to 30% of patients diagnosed with acute cystitis. Epidemiologic risk factors include lower socioeconomic status, pregnancy, structural urinary tract abnormality, history of UTI relapse after treatment, prior history of acute pyelonephritis, frequent UTIs, symptoms for more than 7 days, or diabetes or immunosuppressing infections.[5,6]

DIAGNOSIS AND DIFFERENTIAL

- The differential diagnosis of UTI includes vulvovaginitis, cervicitis, mechanical or chemical urethritis, and urolithiasis. Factors that are independent predictors of a UTI in a patient with dysuria are advanced age, history of UTI, back pain, pyuria, hematuria, and bacteriuria.[6]
- A midstream urine specimen, or a sample from urethral catheterization if necessary, should be analyzed for nitrite and leukocyte esterase reactions, and pyuria, bacteriuria, and hematuria.
- The urine nitrite reaction has a >90% specificity for UTI, but a low sensitivity (50%); a negative result does not rule out the diagnosis.[7,8]
- A positive urine leukocyte esterase reaction from pyuria has a sensitivity of 48% as an indicator of UTI in emergency department patients in general,[7] but approaches 88% in symptomatic women with high levels of pyuria.
- Abnormal pyuria in women is defined as two to five leukocytes (WBC) per high-power field (hpf, or 400× magnification) from a centrifuged specimen. In men, more than 1 to 2 WBC/hpf in the presence of bacteriuria is significant.[4,5] False-negatives can occur with large, dilute urine volumes, partially treated UTI, renal obstruction, or systemic leukopenia.
- Bacteriuria may be absent in women with low-grade, non-coliform or chlamydial UTIs, but is a specific marker for detection of UTI. More than 1 bacteria per oil-power field (1000× magnification) in an uncentrifuged specimen, or more than 15 per oil-power field in a centrifuged specimen, is significant and highly correlates with a culture result of >10^5 CFU/mL. False-positives can occur with vaginal or fecal contamination.
- In a male with dysuria, a Gram's stain of urethral discharge may reveal evidence suggestive of a gonococcal or chlamydial urethritis, or another sexually transmitted infection.
- Urine cultures should be sent in the following settings of UTI: acute pyelonephritis, patients needing to be hospitalized, patients with chronic indwelling urinary catheters, pregnant women, children, and adult males.[4,6,9,10]
- Elderly, diabetic, or severely ill patients with acute pyelonephritis that has been poorly responsive to therapy should undergo imaging with renal ultrasound or other modalities to evaluate for obstruction. Profoundly ill diabetic patients may have a rare gas-forming (emphysematous) pyelonephritis, the diagnosis of which can be facilitated by renal computed tomography.[11]

EMERGENCY DEPARTMENT CARE AND DISPOSITION

- For adult females with a clinical diagnosis of simple cystitis, and few prior episodes of UTI, brief duration of symptoms, no risk factors for subclinical pyelonephritis, and good available follow-up, a 3-day course of oral antibiotic therapy will suffice.[5,12,13] Options include a fluoroquinolone such as ciprofloxacin 250 to 500 mg bid, ofloxacin 200 to 400 mg bid, or levofloxacin 250 mg daily; or trimethoprim-sulfamethoxazole, 1 double-strength tablet twice daily. Amoxicillin-clavulanate 250/125 mg twice daily, or nitrofurantoin macrocrystals 100 mg four times daily can be used, especially in pregnant patients (who can also be treated with cephalexin 500 qid for 7 days or amoxicillin 250 mg three times daily for 7 days), but may require 5 to 7 days of treatment. Emerging resistance to these routinely used antibiotics, with the exception of the quinolones, has made quinolone therapy a first-line choice.
- Adult females with risk factors for subclinical pyelonephritis and a low likelihood of compliance with follow-up should receive a 10- to 14-day course of one of the

above-mentioned antibiotics, as they are likely to respond poorly to a shorter course of therapy.[14]

- Adult males with lower UTI should also receive a 10-day course of antibiotics, once urethritis and prostatitis are ruled out, and referred to a urologist for evaluation of a suspected underlying anatomic abnormality.
- Asymptomatic bacteriuria should be treated if two or more sequential cultures are positive. It poses a special problem in pregnancy; if untreated, it has a likelihood of progression to symptomatic UTI or pyelonephritis that is three- to fourfold the progression rate in nonpregnant patients, leading to subsequent complications including miscarriage. Treatment of ABU in pregnancy, with a 7-day course, is therefore unequivocally indicated.[10]
- Patients with acute pyelonephritis are distinguished from those with cystitis by the clinical symptoms and signs described above. The decision to admit the patient with acute pyelonephritis is based on age, host factors, comorbidity, and response to initial emergency department interventions.
  - Administer adequate intravenous fluid to dehydrated or vomiting patients.
  - Send cultures and administer a dose of an oral or intravenous antibiotic. Intravenous options include a fluoroquinolone such as ciprofloxacin 400 mg every 12 hours or levofloxacin 250 mg every 24 hours, ampicillin 1 g every 6 hours plus gentamicin 2 mg/kg every 8 hours, a third generation cephalosporin such as ceftriaxone 1 g every 12 hours, or an extended-spectrum penicillin plus a beta-lactamase inhibitor.[13]
  - Eighty to ninety percent of young patients who are able to take oral antibiotics respond to outpatient oral antibiotic therapy.[15,16] These patients can be discharged on a 10- to 14-day course of a fluoroquinolone, now considered first-line therapy, or one of the oral regimens described above if available culture sensitivities suggest susceptibility.[13]
  - Patients with intractable nausea and vomiting, unremitting fever, and loss of vasomotor tone should be admitted.
  - Additional indications for admission involve factors associated with an unfavorable prognosis, such as old age, debility, renal calculi or obstruction, a history of recent hospitalization or instrumentation, diabetes mellitus, chronic nephropathy, sickle cell anemia, underlying carcinoma, or intercurrent cancer chemotherapy. In these cases antimicrobial coverage should be broadened and an antipseudomonal agent added. Patients with emphysematous pyelonephritis may require nephrectomy.
- A relapse of UTI less than 1 month after treatment usually represents a treatment failure. A cluster of more than three recurrences in 1 year suggests rein-

fection and should prompt a referral for a search for structural urologic abnormalities or underlying systemic disease.

HEMATURIA

EPIDEMIOLOGY

- At least one episode of painless, atraumatic hematuria is reported by approximately 3% of the general population.[17]
- The incidence is higher in women (because of UTI) and older patients (because of malignancy, and in men, benign prostatic hypertrophy).

PATHOPHYSIOLOGY

- Hematuria can result from infection, inflammation, trauma, or uroepithelial breakdown in any part of the genitourinary tract, from kidneys to urethra.
- Causes include UTI, nephrolithiasis, autoimmune or immune-mediated disease (such as Henoch-Schönlein purpura, IgA nephropathy, and poststreptococcal glomerulonephritis), schistosomiasis, renal vein thrombosis, malignant hypertension, sickle cell anemia, strenuous exercise (a common benign cause in younger patients),[18] and urogenital malignancy (typically in older patients).[17,19] Coagulopathy and anticoagulant use are other causes.

CLINICAL FEATURES

- Hematuria may present as either microscopic or gross hematuria.
- Microscopic hematuria, which is primarily a laboratory entity, suggests, though not exclusively, a renal source. Gross (visible) hematuria, which presents in a spectrum from discoloration of the urine to passage of frank blood and clots, suggests a lower tract source.
- The time of occurrence of gross hematuria during micturition may be indicative of the source of bleeding. Blood at the beginning of urination that then clears suggests a urethral source; blood throughout urination suggests a kidney, ureter, or bladder source; and blood at the termination of an initially clear urination suggests a bladder neck or prostatic source.

DIAGNOSIS AND DIFFERENTIAL

- The differential diagnosis of apparent gross hematuria includes myoglobinuria, hemoglobinuria, bilirubinuria, porphyrinuria, pigmenturia from various foods, and medication metabolite excretion.

- In the analysis of a clean-catch urine sample, free hemoglobin, myoglobin, porphyrins, or povidone iodine in urine may lead to a false-positive urine test strip reaction for blood, so confirmatory microscopic analysis is helpful.
- Microscopic hematuria is defined as greater than 5 RBCs/hpf in centrifuged urine. Abnormal RBC morphology, RBC casts, and proteinuria suggest glomerular disease.[19,20]
- Other diagnostic studies with pertinence to individual etiologies can be ordered as guided by the history and physical exam. Patients taking anticoagulants should have the appropriate coagulation studies checked. Analysis of serum chemistries, including blood urea nitrogen and creatinine when indicated, will give a preliminary assessment of renal function.

EMERGENCY DEPARTMENT CARE AND DISPOSITION

- Treatment of hematuria should be directed at the underlying cause, if known and amenable. The crux of subsequent ED management is the minimization of complications and appropriate referral or admission for additional evaluation.
- In patients with gross hematuria likely to lead to bladder outlet obstruction by coagulated blood, insertion of a triple lumen urinary catheter and bladder irrigation with saline until clearing will facilitate drainage.
- Patients with bladder outlet obstruction, pregnancy, or new diagnosis of glomerulonephritis (especially with evidence of pulmonary edema, volume overload, or renal dysfunction) warrant admission.
- Patients younger than 40 years with painless hematuria, which is usually benign and transient, may be referred to a primary care provider for a repeat urine analysis. In those older than 40 years, especially with risk factors for urogenital malignancy, referral to a urologist for a timely outpatient evaluation is indicated.
- All patients with hematuria and significant proteinuria (which implies glomerular disease) require a referral for an expeditious outpatient work-up.[20]

REFERENCES

1. Hooton TM, Scholes D, Stapleton AE, et al: A prospective study of asymptomatic bacteriuria in sexually active young women. *N Engl J Med* 343:992, 2000.
2. Scholes D, Hooton TM, Roberts PL, et al: Risk factors for re-
current urinary tract infection in young women. *J Infect Dis* 182:1177, 2000.
3. Strom BL, Collins M, West SL, et al: Sexual activity, contraceptive use, and other risk factors for symptomatic and asymptomatic bacteriuria: A case control study. *Ann Intern Med* 107:816, 1987.
4. Lipsky BA: Prostatitis and urinary tract infection in men: What's new; what's true? *Am J Med* 106:327, 1999.
5. Krieger JN: Urinary tract infections: What's new? *J Urol* 168:2531, 2002.
6. Bent S, Nallmothu BK, Simel DL, et al: Does this woman have an acute uncomplicated urinary tract infection? *JAMA* 287:2701, 2002.
7. Propp DA, Weber D, Ciesla M: Reliability of a urine dipstick in emergency department patients. *Ann Emerg Med* 18:560, 1989.
8. Holloway J, Joshi N, O'Bryan T: Positive urine nitrite test: An accurate predictor of absence of pure enterococcal bacteriuria. *South Med J* 93:681, 2000.
9. Foxman B: Epidemiology of urinary tract infections: Incidence, morbidity, and economic costs. *Am J Med* 113(Suppl): 5S, 2002.
10. Connolly A, Thorp JM Jr: Urinary tract infections in pregnancy. *Urol Clin North Am* 26:779, 1999.
11. Stapleton A: Urinary tract infections in patients with diabetes. *Am J Med* 113(Suppl):80S, 2002.
12. Abramowicz M: The choice of antibacterial drugs. *Med Lett Drug Ther* 40:33, 1998.
13. Warren JW, Abrutyn E, Hebel JR, et al: Guidelines for antimicrobial treatment of uncomplicated acute bacterial cystitis and acute pyelonephritis in women. *Clin Infect Dis* 29: 745, 1999.
14. Stamm WE, Hooton TM: Management of urinary tract infections in adults. *N Engl J Med* 329:1328, 1993.
15. Pinson AG, Philbrick JT, Lindbeck GH, Schorling JB: Oral antibiotic therapy for acute pyelonephritis: A methodologic review of the literature. *J Gen Intern Med* 7:544, 1992.
16. Pinson AG, Philbrick JT, Lindbeck GH, et al: Emergency department management of acute pyelonephritis in women: A cohort study. *Am J Emerg Med* 12:271, 1994.
17. Sutton MJ: Evaluation of hematuria in adults. *JAMA* 263: 2475, 1990.
18. Jones GR, Newhouse I: Sport-related hematuria: A review. *Clin J Sport Med* 7:119, 1997.
19. Summerton N, Mann S, Rigby AS, et al: Patients with new onset haematuria: Assessing the discriminant value of clinical information in relation to urologic malignancies. *Br J Gen Pract* 52:284, 2002.
20. Tomson C, Porter T: Asymptomatic microscopic or dipstick haematuria in adults: Which investigations for which patients? A review of the evidence. *BJU Int* 90:185, 2002.

For further reading in *Emergency Medicine: A Comprehensive Study Guide,* 6th ed., see Chap. 94, "Urinary Tract Infections" and Chap. 97, "Hematuria and Hematospermia," by David S. Howes and Mark P. Bogner.

56 MALE GENITAL PROBLEMS

Stephen H. Thomas

TESTICULAR TORSION

CLINICAL FEATURES

- Due to potential for infarction and infertility, testicular torsion must be the primary consideration in any male complaining of testicular pain.[1]
- Though torsion is most common in the peripubertal period (when hormonal stimulation is maximal), this organ-threatening emergency may occur at any age.
- Pain usually occurs suddenly, is severe, and is felt in either the lower abdominal quadrant, the inguinal canal, or the testis
- Though pain may follow strenuous activity such as athletics, torsion also occurs during sleep (when unilateral cremasteric contraction is the cause). The pain may be constant or intermittent but is not positional, since torsion is primarily an ischemic event.

DIAGNOSIS AND DIFFERENTIAL

- When the diagnosis is obvious, urologic consultation is indicated for exploration, since imaging tests can be too time consuming. The often-quoted 4-hour warm ischemia time for 90% chance of testicular preservation is based on sparse evidence, and thus the emergency physician should move as expeditiously as possible in cases of suspected torsion.
- In indeterminate cases, color-flow duplex ultrasound, and less commonly radionuclide imaging, may be helpful. Both techniques are subject to limitations associated with need for timely test availability and image interpretation.
- Compared to radionuclide imaging, ultrasound offers the advantage of providing additional information about scrotal anatomy and differential diagnoses, but is more likely to yield indeterminant results.[2,3]
- Torsion of the appendages is more common than testicular torsion but is not dangerous, since the appendix testis and appendix epididymis have no known function. If the patient is seen early, diagnosis can be supported by the following: pain is most intense near the head of the epididymis or testis; there is an isolated tender nodule; or the pathognomonic blue-dot appearance of a cyanotic appendage is illuminated through thin prepubertal scrotal skin.
- The differential for testicular torsion also includes epididymitis, inguinal hernia, hydrocele, and scrotal hematoma.

EMERGENCY DEPARTMENT CARE AND DISPOSITION

- The ED physician can attempt manual detorsion.[4] Most testes twist in a lateral-to-medial direction, so detorsion is performed in a medial-to-lateral direction, similar to the opening of a book. The end point for successful detorsion is pain relief; worsening of pain with detorsion may indicate the need for attempts at detorsion by lateral-to-medial rotation.
- Regardless of whether detorsion appears successful, urologic referral is indicated.
- If normal intratesticular blood flow can be demonstrated with color Doppler, immediate surgery is not necessary for torsion of the appendages, since most appendages calcify or degenerate over 10 to 14 days and cause no harm.
- If the diagnosis cannot be assured, urologic exploration is needed to rule out testicular torsion.[?]

EPIDIDYMITIS AND ORCHITIS

CLINICAL FEATURES

- Epididymitis, an inflammatory process, is characterized by gradual onset of pain.
- Bacterial infection is the most common, with infecting agents dependent on the patient's age. In patients younger than 40 years old, epididymitis is primarily due to sexually transmitted diseases (STDs); culture or DNA probe analysis for gonococci and *Chlamydia* is indicated in patients <40 years old, even in the absence of urethral discharge. In older men (>40 years), common urinary pathogens predominate.
- Epididymitis causes lower abdominal, inguinal canal, scrotal, or testicular pain, alone or in combination. Due to the inflammatory nature of the pain, patients with epididymitis may note transient pain relief when elevating the scrotal contents while recumbent (positive Prehn's sign).

DIAGNOSIS AND DIFFERENTIAL

- Initially, tenderness is well localized to the epididymis, but progression of inflammation and swelling-mediated obliteration of the sulcus between the epididymis and testis results in the physical examination finding of a single, large testicular mass (epididymo-orchitis).
- Orchitis in isolation is rare; it usually occurs with viral or syphilitic disease and is treated with disease-specific therapy, symptomatic support, and urologic follow-up.

- Testicular malignancy should be suspected in patients presenting with asymptomatic testicular mass, firmness, or induration. Ten percent of tumors present with pain due to hemorrhage within the tumor. Urgent urologic follow-up is indicated.

EMERGENCY DEPARTMENT CARE AND DISPOSITION

- If the patient appears toxic, admission for intravenous antibiotics (eg, ceftriaxone 1 to 2 g every 12 hours or trimethoprim-sulfamethoxazole 5 mg/kg of the trimethoprim component every 6 hours) is indicated.
- Outpatient treatment is the norm in patients who do not appear toxic; urologic follow-up within a week is indicated. Oral antibiotic regimens should include 10 days of therapy with one of the following: doxycycline 100 mg bid or ofloxacin 300 mg bid for patients under 40; for patients age 40 or older, trimethoprim-sulfamethoxazole, one double-strength tablet bid, or a quinolone such as levofloxacin 250 mg daily are indicated.
- Additionally, scrotal elevation, ice application, non-steroidal anti-inflammatory drugs (NSAIDs), opioids for analgesia, and stool softeners are indicated.
- Orchitis is treated with disease-specific therapy, symptomatic support, and urologic follow-up. Patients at risk for syphilitic disease should be treated as directed in Chap. 88.

SCROTUM

- Scrotal abscesses may be localized to the scrotal wall or may arise from extensions of infections of scrotal contents (ie, testis, epididymis, and bulbous urethra). A simple hair follicle scrotal wall abscess can be managed by incision and drainage; no antibiotics are required in immunocompetent patients.
- When a scrotal wall abscess is suspected of coming from an intrascrotal infection, ultrasound and retrograde urethrography may demonstrate pathology in the testis and/or epididymis and urethra, respectively. Definitive care of any complex abscess calls for a urology consultation.
- **Fournier's gangrene** is a polymicrobial infection of the perineal subcutaneous tissues. Immunocompromised males, particularly diabetics, are at highest risk. Prompt diagnosis is essential to prevent extensive tissue loss. Early surgical consultation is recommended for at-risk patients who present with scrotal, rectal, or genital pain. Treatment is with aggressive fluid resuscitation (with normal saline); broad-spectrum antibiotics to cover gram-positive, gram-negative, and anaerobic organisms, such as ampicillin-sulbactam 3 g IV; surgical débridement; and hyperbaric oxygen.[5]

PENIS

- **Balanoposthitis** is inflammation of the glans (balanitis) and foreskin (posthitis). Upon foreskin retraction, the glans and prepuce appear purulent, excoriated, malodorous, and tender. Treatment consists of cleansing with mild soap, assuring adequate dryness, application of antifungal creams (nystatin qid or clotrimazole bid) and an oral azole (such as fluconazole), and urologic referral for follow-up and possible circumcision. An oral cephalosporin (eg, cephalexin 500 mg qid) should be prescribed in cases of secondary bacterial infection.
- **Phimosis** is the inability to retract the foreskin proximally. Hemostatic dilation of the preputial ostium relieves the urinary retention until definitive dorsal slit or circumcision can be performed. Circumcision can often be averted by application of topical steroids (eg, triamcinolone 0.025% bid for 4 to 6 weeks).[6]
- **Paraphimosis** is the inability to reduce the proximal edematous foreskin distally over the glans. Paraphimosis is a true urologic emergency because resulting glans edema and venous engorgement can progress to arterial compromise and gangrene. If surrounding tissue edema can be successfully compressed, as by wrapping the glans with 2 × 2-inch elastic bandages for 5 minutes, the foreskin may be reduced. Making several puncture wounds with a small (22- to 25-gauge) needle may help with expression of glans edema fluid. Local anesthetic block of the penis is helpful if patients cannot tolerate the discomfort associated with edema compression and removal. If arterial compromise is suspected or has occurred, local infiltration of the constricting band with 1% plain lidocaine followed by superficial vertical incision of the band will decompress the glans and allow foreskin reduction.
- **Penile entrapment injuries** occur when various objects are wrapped around the penis. Such objects should be removed, and urethral integrity (retrograde urethrogram) and distal penile arterial blood supply (Doppler studies) should be confirmed when indicated.
- **Penile fracture** occurs when there is an acute tear of the penile tunica albuginea. The penis is acutely swollen, discolored, and tender in a patient with history of intercourse-related trauma accompanied by a snapping sound.[7] Urologic consultation is indicated.
- **Peyronie's disease** presents with patients noting sudden or gradual onset of dorsal penile curvature with erections. Examination reveals a thickened plaque

on the dorsal penile shaft. Assurance and urologic follow-up are indicated.

- **Priapism** is a painful pathologic erection, which may be associated with urinary retention. Infection and impotence are other complications. In most cases, the initial therapy for priapism is terbutaline 0.25 to 0.5 mg (repeated in 20 minutes if needed) injected subcutaneously in the deltoid area. If patients present early (within 4 hours), oral pseudoephedrine (60 to 120 mg) may be effective. Patients with priapism from sickle-cell disease are usually treated with simple or exchange transfusion. Corporal aspiration and irrigation with either normal saline solution or an α-adrenergic antagonist is the next step and may need to be performed by the emergency physician when urologic consultation is not available. Even when emergency physicians provide stabilizing care, urologic consultation is indicated in all cases.

URETHRA

URETHRAL STRICTURE

- Urethral stricture is becoming more common due to the rising incidence of sexually transmitted diseases. If a patient's bladder cannot be cannulated with a 14F or 16F Foley or Coudé catheter, the differential diagnosis includes urethral stricture, voluntary external sphincter spasm, bladder neck contracture, or benign prostatic hypertrophy.
- Retrograde urethrography can be performed to delineate the location and extent of urethral stricture. Endoscopy is necessary to confirm bladder neck contracture or define the extent of an obstructing prostate gland.
- Suspected voluntary external sphincter spasm can be overcome by holding the patient's penis upright and encouraging him to relax his perineum and breathe slowly during the procedure.
- After no more than three gentle attempts to pass a 12F Coudé catheter into a urethra prepared with anesthetic lubricant, urology consultation should be obtained.
- In an emergency situation, suprapubic cystotomy can be performed. The infraumbilical and suprapubic area is prepped with povidone iodine solution. A 25- to 27-gauge spinal needle is used to locate the bladder (ED ultrasound can facilitate this), followed by placement of the cystotomy using the Seldinger technique.
- Urologic follow-up should occur within 2 to 3 days.

URETHRAL FOREIGN BODIES

- Urethral foreign bodies are associated with bloody urine and slow, painful urination.

- X ray of the bladder and urethral areas may disclose a foreign body.
- Removal of the foreign body may be achieved with a gentle milking action; retrograde urethrography or endoscopy is required in such cases to confirm an intact urethra.
- Often, urologic consultation for endoscopy or open cystotomy is required for foreign-body removal.

URINARY RETENTION

CLINICAL FEATURES

- Urinary retention syndromes can range from overt retention to insidious overflow incontinence that can fool the unsuspecting physician.[8]
- A detailed history, including use of over-the-counter cold and diet aids, may reveal the cause of urinary retention.
- Men do not void as completely when sitting down, and infrequent ejaculation may lead to secondary prostatic congestion and symptoms of outlet obstruction.
- An intact sensory examination, anal sphincter examination, and bulbocavernosus reflex test differentiate chronic outlet obstruction from the sensory or motor neurogenic bladder and spinal cord compression.

DIAGNOSIS AND DIFFERENTIAL

- Physical examination should include a search for meatal stenosis, palpation of urethral length for masses or fistulae consistent with urethral stricture disease or abscess formation, lower abdominal examination for palpation of suprapubic mass, and rectal examination to evaluate anal sphincter tone and prostate size and consistency.

EMERGENCY DEPARTMENT CARE AND DISPOSITION

- Most patients with bladder outlet obstruction are in distress, and passage of a urethral catheter alleviates their pain and their urinary retention. Copious intraurethral lubrication including a topical anesthetic (eg, using a urethral injector device and lidocaine gel) should be used, and a 16F Coudé catheter is recommended if straight catheters fail. Be certain to pass the catheter to its fullest extent, obtaining free urine flow, before inflating the balloon.
- The catheter should be left indwelling and connected to a leg drainage bag.
- Belladonna and opium suppositories (one every 4 to 6 hours) can be prescribed to alleviate the constant urge to void secondary to bladder spasm, which frequently accompanies an indwelling catheter.
- In patients whose bladder catheter will be left in longer than 5 to 7 days, prophylactic antibiotics (eg, trimethoprim, 100 mg/day) should be instituted.

Otherwise, antibiotics are indicated only if urinalysis is consistent with urinary tract infection.

- If urinary retention has been chronic, postobstructive diuresis may occur even in the presence of normal blood urea nitrogen and creatinine levels. In such patients, close monitoring of urinary output is indicated, and they should be observed for 4 to 6 hours after catheterization.
- In all cases of urinary retention, urologic follow-up is indicated for a complete genitourinary evaluation.

REFERENCES

1. Cuckow PM, Frank JD: Torsion of the testis. *BJU Int* 86:349, 2000.
2. Marcozzi D, Suner S: The nontraumatic, acute scrotum. *Emerg Med Clin North Am* 19:547, 2001.
3. Blaivas M, Sierzenski P, Lambert M: Emergency evaluation of patients presenting with acute scrotum using bedside ultrasonography. *Acad Emerg Med* 8:90, 2001.
4. Garel L, Dubois J, Azzie G, et al: Preoperative detorsion of the spermatic cord with Doppler ultrasound monitoring in patients with intravaginal acute testicular torsion. *Pediatr Radiol* 30:41, 2000.
5. Dahm P, Roland FH, Vaslef SN, et al: Outcome analysis in patients with primary necrotizing fasciitis of the male genitalia. *Urology* 56:31, 2000.
6. Webster TM, Leonard MP: Topical steroid therapy for phimosis. *Can J Urol* 9:1492, 2002.
7. Eke N: Fracture of the penis. *Br J Surg* 89:555, 2002.
8. Curtis LA, Dolan TS, Cespedes RD: Acute urinary retention and urinary incontinence. *Emerg Med Clin North Am* 91:591, 2001.

For further reading in *Emergency Medicine: A Comprehensive Study Guide,* 6th ed., see Chap. 95, "Male Genital Problems," by Robert E. Schneider.

57 UROLOGIC STONE DISEASE
Geetika Gupta

The acute phenomenon of renal stones migrating down the ureter is referred to as renal colic.

EPIDEMIOLOGY

- Stones are three times more common in males and usually occur in the third to fifth decades.[1]
- Children under 16 years of age constitute approximately 7% of all cases of renal stones with a 1:1 sex distribution.[2]
- Overall incidence is around 12%.[1]
- There is an increased incidence from genetic predisposition and hereditary diseases (eg, renal tubular acidosis, hyperparathyroidism, cystinuria).
- Lifestyle factors augment stone growth. Increasing water intake results in a decreased incidence of calculi. Patients in mountainous, desert, or tropical regions, and those in sedentary jobs suffer a higher frequency of stone disease.
- Medications such as protease inhibitors and diuretics have also shown an increase in prevalence.[1]
- Approximately one third of the patients suffer recurrences within 1 year and 50% in 5 years.[1]

PATHOPHYSIOLOGY

- The precise cause of urinary stone formation is unknown. It requires three elements: supersaturation, lack of inhibitors, and stasis.[1,3]
- Approximately 75% of calculi are composed of calcium, occurring in conjunction with oxalate, phosphate, or a combination of both. Calcium excretion is elevated in conditions such as high dietary calcium intake, immobilization syndrome, or hyperparathyroidism. Oxalate excretion is enhanced in patients with inflammatory bowel disease and as a result of small bowel bypass surgery.
- Ten percent of stones are magnesium-ammonium-phosphate (struvite). These are associated with infection by urea-splitting bacteria and are the most common cause of staghorn calculi.[1] Antibiotic penetration into these calculi is low and makes patients with stones prone to urosepsis.
- Uric acid causes 10% of uroliths, with cystine and other uncommon stones making up the remainder.
- The majority (90%) of urinary calculi are radiopaque. Calcium phosphate and calcium oxalate stones have a density similar to bone.
- Common areas of impaction include the renal calyx, ureteropelvic junctions, and the ureterovesical junction (UVJ). The UVJ has the smallest diameter of the urinary tract and is the most common location for impacted stones.
- Common etiologies in pediatrics are metabolic abnormality (50%), urologic anomalies (20%), infection (15%), and immobilization syndrome (5%).

CLINICAL FEATURES

- Patients are usually asymptomatic until there is at least partial obstruction.

- Patients complain of the acute onset of severe pain which can be associated with diaphoresis, nausea, and emesis. During extreme presentations, the patient is anxious, pacing or writhing, and may be unable to hold still or converse.
- Typically pain originates in either flank, radiating ipsilaterally and anteroinferiorly around the abdomen and toward the ipsilateral testicle or labium majus. The radiating pattern is the result of autonomic nerve fibers serving both the kidney and respective gonad. Anterior abdominal pain may radiate back toward the flank and is associated with midureteral stones. Stones near the bladder may cause urinary frequency and urgency.
- Extracorporeal shock wave lithotripsy (ESWL) fractures stones into small particles using focused sound waves. The resulting sludge is passed in the urine. When there are large fragments, an acute episode of renal colic occurs. The presentation is identical to de novo episodes of renal colic.

DIAGNOSIS AND DIFFERENTIAL

- All patients with suspected renal colic require a urinalysis. In 11 to 14% of the cases, urinary blood is absent.[4] In addition, 20 to 30% of pediatric cases may have painless hematuria. Pyuria indicates the need for a thorough investigation to exclude infection.
- The kidney-ureter-bladder (KUB) radiograph's greatest utility is in the exclusion of other pathologies.
- Intravenous pyelogram (IVP) yields information regarding renal function as well as anatomy. The first and most reliable indication of the presence of obstruction is a delay in the appearance of the nephrogram. Adjuncts to diagnosis include distension of the renal pelvis, calyceal distortion, dye extravasation, hydronephrosis, and visualization of the entire ureter.[5]
- The sensitivity of an IVP is 64 to 90% and the specificity is 94 to 100%. A falsely negative IVP infrequently occurs when there is a radiolucent, partially obstructing stone.[6,7]
- Advantages of the IVP is that it provides information on renal function and the degree of obstruction. The major disadvantages are time to perform the exam, contrast allergy, and the risk of nephrotoxicity.
- Noncontrast helical computed tomography (CT) is the diagnostic procedure of choice in the emergency department (ED).[1,6] The sensitivity is 95 to 97% and the specificity is 96 to 98%.[8] Advantages of CT include its speed and that it avoids the risk of contrast allergy.[8] The disadvantage is that it doesn't evaluate for renal function or define the degree of obstruction.
- Positive findings of CT include ureteral caliber changes, suspicious calcifications, stranding of perinephric fat, and dilation of the collecting system.

- Ultrasound (US) is reserved for patients unable to undergo an IVP or CT.[7,9] US is not a functional test and provides anatomic information only. It is useful in the detection of hydronephrosis and larger stones (>5 mm) in the proximal and distal ureter.[7]
- Differential diagnosis includes a symptomatic abdominal aortic aneurysm, incarcerated hernia, epididymitis, testicular torsion, ectopic pregnancy, salpingitis, pyelonephritis, papillary necrosis (due to sickle cell disease, diabetes, nonsteroidal analgesic abuse, or infection), renal infarction, appendicitis, herpes zoster, drug-seeking behavior, and musculoskeletal strain. A right ureteral stone can resemble cholecystitis.

EMERGENCY DEPARTMENT CARE AND DISPOSITION

- Pain medication including narcotics and nonsteroidal anti-inflammatory drugs should not be delayed pending test results.
- In cases complicated by urinary tract infection (UTI), routine cultures of urine and blood are indicated and renal obstruction must be excluded. Antibiotics should be started promptly while the patient is in the emergency department.
- Hospitalization is required if the patient has an infection with concurrent obstruction, solitary kidney and complete obstruction, uncontrolled pain, or intractable emesis. Disposition should be discussed with a urologist in patients with a stone >6 mm, renal insufficiency, severe underlying disease, IVP with extravasation or complete obstruction, or failed outpatient management.[1]
- Stones with diameters less than 4 mm will pass in 90% of cases. Stones 4 to 6 mm pass about 50% of the time, and only 10% of stones exceeding 6 mm pass spontaneously. Irregularly shaped stones with spicules and sharp edges will have a lower passage rate.[1]
- Rates of passage for stones found in the proximal, middle, and distal ureter are approximately 20, 50, and 70%, respectively, regardless of stone size.
- Discharge is appropriate in patients with rounded stones <4 to −5 mm, in the absence of infection, and when pain is controlled by oral analgesics.
- Patients need to be counseled to return promptly for fever, vomiting, or uncontrolled pain, and they should receive a prescription for oral narcotics.
- Follow-up with a urologist is recommended within 7 days.[10]
- All urine should be collected and strained for the identification of any passed stones. Patients whose stones pass in the emergency department require no further treatment.

REFERENCES

1. Manthey DE, Teicheman J: Nephrolithiasis. *Emerg Med Clin North Am* 19:633, 2001.
2. Minevich E: Pediatric urolithiasis. *Pediatr Clin North Am* 48:1571, 2001.
3. Shokeir AA: Renal colic: new concepts related to pathophysiology, diagnosis, and treatment. *Curr Opin Urol* 12:263, 2002.
4. Bove P, Kaplan D, Darlyample N, et al: Reexamining the value of hematuria testing in patients with acute flank pain. *J Urol* 162(Pt 1):685, 1999.
5. Rivers K, Shetty S, Menon M: When and how to evaluate a patient with nephrolithiasis. *Urol Clin North Am* 27:203, 2000.
6. Worster A, Preyra I, Weaver B, Haines T: The accuracy of noncontrast helical computed tomography versus intravenous pyelography in the diagnosis of suspected acute urolithiasis; A meta-analysis. *Ann Emerg Med* 40:780, 1997.
7. Svedstrom E, Alanen A, Nurmi M: Radiologic evaluation of renal colic: The role of plain films, excretory urography, and sonography. *Eur J Radiol* 11:180, 1990.
8. Smith RC, Verga M, McCarthy S, Rosenfield AT: Diagnosis of acute flank pain: Value of unenhanced helical CT. *Am J Roentgenol* 166:97, 1996.
9. Fowler KA, Locken JA, Duchesne JH, Williamson MR: US for detecting renal calculi with nonenhanced CT as a reference standard. *Radiology* 222:109, 2002.
10. Singal RK, Denstedt JD: Contemporary management of ureteral stones. *Urol Clin North Am* 24:59, 1997.

For further reading in *Emergency Medicine: A Comprehensive Study Guide,* 6th ed., see Chap. 96, "Urologic Stone Disease," by Rakesh Engineer and W. Frank Peacock IV.

58 COMPLICATIONS OF UROLOGIC DEVICES
David M. Cline

COMPLICATIONS OF URINARY CATHETERS

- Infection is the most common complication of urinary catheters (10 to 30%)[1] and management is discussed in Chap. 55.
- Minor traumatic complications of urinary catheters may require no therapy, while major complications (such as bladder perforation) require consultation with a urologist.

NONDRAINING CATHETER

- Obstruction is suggested if the catheter does not flush easily or if there is no return of the irrigant. Obstruction of the catheter by blood clots often creates a situation in which the catheter is easily flushed, but little or no irrigant is returned. If this occurs, the catheter can be replaced with a triple-lumen catheter so the bladder can be easily irrigated. If after clearing the bladder of all clots evidence of continued bleeding is present, urologic consultation is recommended for possible cystoscopy.
- Some physicians advocate the use of single-lumen catheters to lavage the bladder, as its larger lumen may aid in the evacuation of larger clots.

NONDEFLATING RETENTION BALLOON

- If the obstruction is distal, the result of a crush or defective valve, the catheter can be cut proximal to the defect. If this does not deflate the balloon, a lubricated guidewire can be introduced into the cut inflation channel in an attempt to clear the obstruction.
- The balloon can be ruptured within the bladder. However, consider urologic consultation prior to rupturing the balloon, as overinflation (using sterile water) often requires 10 to 20 times the normal balloon volume.
- Urologic consultation may be required if simple measures are not successful.

COMPLICATIONS OF PERCUTANEOUS NEPHROSTOMY TUBES

- Percutaneous nephrostomy is a urinary drainage procedure used for supravesical or ureteral obstruction secondary to malignancy, pyonephrosis, genitourinary stones, or ureteral strictures.
- Bleeding may occur, and most episodes can be managed with irrigation to clear the nephrostomy tube of clots. In resistant cases check complete blood count (CBC), renal function, and coagulation studies (as indicated by comorbidities).
- Treat the patient for hemodynamic instability and consult urology.
- Infectious complications of nephrostomy tubes range from simple bacteriuria and pyelonephritis to renal abscess, bacteremia, and urosepsis. Culture any wound drainage, start an antibiotic such as ciprofloxacin 400 mg IV, and consult urology.[2]
- Mechanical complications, such as catheter dislodgement and tube blockage, can occur with these devices. The urologist has several techniques available to reestablish access to an obstructed nephrostomy tube.

COMPLICATIONS OF URETERAL STENTS

- Dysuria, urinary urgency, and frequency, as well as abdominal and flank discomfort, are common complaints in patients with ureteral stents.[3,4] The baseline discomfort in a functioning, well-positioned stent can range anywhere from minimal to debilitating. However, an abrupt change in the character, location, or intensity of the pain requires further evaluation for stent malposition or malfunction.
- Ureteral stents may remain in place for weeks to months and often function with no complications during the entire period. However, stents can often become encrusted with mineral deposits and may obstruct. Complete obstruction of urine flow is possible, although this tends to occur more often in patients with stents in place for long-term use. These patients may require urologic consultation, and in some cases may require stent replacement.

URINARY TRACT INFECTION VERSUS STENT MIGRATION OR MALFUNCTION

- Changing abdominal or flank pain or bladder discomfort may be indicative of stent migration. X-ray examination is indicated with comparison to a previous film to evaluate stent position, and urologic consultation with further studies to evaluate stent position may eventually be necessary.

- When a urinary tract infection occurs in the presence of a stent, stent removal is not mandatory, because most infections can be managed with outpatient antibiotics. However, if pyelonephritis or systemic infection is evident, then further evaluation and emergent intervention are indicated. Plain x-ray examination to check for stent migration, and urologic consultation for evaluation of stent migration and malfunction are indicated, as well as initiation of antibiotic therapy.

REFERENCES

1. Cancio LC, Sabanegh ES, Thompson IM: Managing the Foley catheter. *Am Fam Physician* 48:829, 1993.
2. Millward SF: Percutaneous nephrostomy: A practical approach. *J Intervasc Radiat* 11:955, 2000.
3. Richter S, Ringel A, Shaley M, Nissenkorn I: The indwelling ureteric stent: A "friendly" procedure with unfriendly high morbidity. *BJU Int* 85:408, 2000.
4. Adams J: Renal stents. *Emerg Med Clin North Am* 12:750, 1994.

For further reading in *Emergency Medicine: A Comprehensive Study Guide,* 6th ed., see Chap. 98, "Complications of Urologic Procedures and Devices," by Elaine B. Josephson and Jatinder Singh.

59 VAGINAL BLEEDING AND PELVIC PAIN IN THE NONPREGNANT PATIENT

Cherri D. Hobgood

ABNORMAL VAGINAL BLEEDING

EPIDEMIOLOGY

- Five percent of women between the ages of 30 and 49 will consult a physician for treatment of menorrhagia.[1]

PATHOPHYSIOLOGY

- The normal menstrual cycle is 28 days and has four phases: follicular, ovulation, luteal or secretory, and menses (see Fig. 59-1).[2]
- Menopause is the result of ovarian burnout and occurs at the average age of 51.[1] The perimenopausal period is characterized by marked variation in the intermenstrual period and very high serum levels of follicle-stimulating hormone (FSH) and luteinizing hormone (LH) as well as low levels of serum estrogen.
- Anovulatory cycles result from an imbalance of follicle degeneration and stimulation. In the presence of an estrogen steady state, the endometrium enters a prolonged proliferative phase and becomes hyperplastic. When the estrogen steady state is insufficient to meet the needs of the hyperplastic endometrium, a relative estrogen insufficiency occurs and the thickened endometrium sloughs. This hormonal pattern produces prolonged periods of amenorrhea with intermittent menorrhagia, which is char-

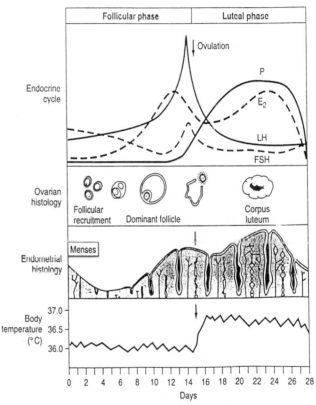

FIG. 59-1. The hormonal, ovarian, endometrial, and basal body temperature changes and relationships throughout the normal menstrual cycle. (Reproduced with permission from Carr BR, Wilson JD: Disorders of the ovary and female reproductive tract, in Isselbacher KJ, Braunwald E, Wilson JD, et al (eds): *Harrison's Principles of Internal Medicine,* 13th ed. New York, McGraw-Hill, 1998, p 2101.)

acteristic of anovulatory cycles. These cycles are typically painless due to the lack of progesterone-mediated myometrial contractions, and are most common in the perimenarchal and perimenopausal age groups.

CLINICAL FEATURES

- Abnormal vaginal bleeding is defined as vaginal bleeding occurring outside the normal menstrual cycle.
- Menorrhagia is defined as menses >7 days, menstruation >60 mL, or <21-day recurrence due to any cause.
- Metrorrhagia is defined as irregular vaginal bleeding outside the normal cycle.
- Menometrorrhagia is defined as excessive irregular vaginal bleeding.
- Dysfunctional uterine bleeding is defined as abnormal vaginal bleeding due to anovulation.
- Postcoital bleeding is defined as vaginal bleeding after intercourse, suggestive of cervical pathology.

DIAGNOSIS AND DIFFERENTIAL

- A thorough physical examination may reveal structural or traumatic causes of bleeding; this should include a complete abdominal and pelvic examination. Once the bleeding site is identified, a ranked differential may be formulated.
- Ultrasound is the most useful diagnostic imaging modality in the patient presenting with vaginal bleeding, adnexal or uterine masses, and pain.
- In all women of childbearing age, pregnancy must be excluded as a potential diagnosis.
- In adolescents, bleeding may be due to anovulation, exogenous hormone use, or coagulopathy.
- In premenopausal women, bleeding may be due to cervicitis, endometrial or cervical polyps, cervical or endometrial cancer, submucosal fibroids, exogenous hormone use, anovulation, thyroid dysfunction, local trauma, or retained foreign body.
- In postmenopausal women, the most common causes of vaginal bleeding are exogenous estrogens, atrophic vaginitis, and endometrial lesions including cancer, with each accounting for approximately 30% of cases. Other tumors such as vulvar, vaginal, and cervical compose approximately 10% of cases.
- Anovulatory dysfunctional uterine bleeding is likely if the pelvic exam is normal. This is most common in perimenarcheal girls and perimenopausal women who present with prolonged menses, irregular cycles, and/or intermenstrual bleeding.
- Primary coagulation disorders such as von Willebrand's disease, myeloproliferative disorders, and immunothrombocytopenia are present in 19% of teens presenting with menorrhagia. Petechiae or other signs are frequently absent.
- Ovarian hyperstimulation syndrome, characterized by ovarian enlargement and fluid loss, occurs in up to 10%

of in-vitro fertilization (IVF) patients. Mild forms present with weight gain, thirst, and abdominal pain. Severe forms present with hypovolemia, hypotension, and acute respiratory distress. Physical manifestations may include pericardial effusion, ascites, hydrothorax, hepatorenal failure, and thromboembolism.

EMERGENCY DEPARTMENT CARE AND DISPOSITION

- If pregnancy is ruled out, the only diagnoses that must be identified acutely are trauma (including sexual assault), bleeding dyscrasias, infections, and foreign bodies.
- Most patients require no immediate intervention.
- Hemodynamically unstable patients will require resuscitation and gynecologic consult for possible dilation and curettage (D&C). Uterine packing should be avoided due to increased risk of infection.
- Life-threatening hemorrhage may be treated with conjugated estrogens.
- Hemodynamically stable patients with anovulatory dysfunctional uterine bleeding can be managed with either of the following hormonal therapies.
  - IV conjugated estrogen 25 mg every 2 to 4 hours for 24 hours or oral conjugated estrogen 2.5 mg PO four times daily (10 mg total per day). After bleeding subsides, add medroxyprogesterone 10 mg every day. Both medications should be continued for 7 to 10 days and then discontinued for a synchronized withdrawal bleed.
  - Oral contraceptive pills: ethinyl estradiol 35 μg and norethindrone 1 mg, 4 tabs for 7 days; or slow taper (ethinyl estradiol 35 μg and norethindrone 1 mg), 4 tabs for 2 days, then 3 tabs for 2 days, then 2 tabs for 2 days, then 1 tab for 3 days.
  - Progesterone therapy with medroxyprogesterone acetate 10 mg/day for 10 days.
- Older patients in whom there is a concern for malignancy should not be started on hormonal therapy, but must be promptly referred to a gynecologist for possible endometrial biopsy.
- Teens presenting with menorrhagia should be evaluated with a complete blood count (CBC), coagulation studies, and a bleeding time.
- For patients identified as having a blood dyscrasia, treatment options include antifibrinolytics such as tranexamic acid. Desmopressin acetate (DDAVP) may also be effective; however, patients with von Willebrand's disease must be typed prior to DDAVP therapy due to the risk of severe thrombocytopenia.
- In most cases nonsteroidal anti-inflammatory drugs (NSAIDs) are useful as adjunctive therapy and serve to decrease bleeding and painful cramping. Important

exceptions are patients with blood dyscrasias in whom NSAIDs may increase bleeding,[1] and patients with fibroids who will achieve little additional therapeutic advantage from NSAID therapy.[3]

- HIV-positive women are subject to higher rates of vaginal and pelvic infections and cervical dysplasia, but the diagnostic and therapeutic approach to management is unchanged.
- Patients with ovarian hyperstimulation syndrome all should be evaluated with liver and renal function tests, coagulation screens, and chest x-ray (CXR). Treatment consists of IV fluids, avoidance of diuretic therapy, and heparin where indicated.

PELVIC PAIN

EPIDEMIOLOGY

- Up to 15% of all women have some degree of endometriosis. After dysmenorrhea it is the most common etiology for cyclic pain in women of reproductive age.
- Leiomyomas or fibroids are the most common pelvic tumor. By the age of 40, 20% of all women will develop fibroids. They are more common, have an increased rate of growth, and are frequently multiple in black women.

PATHOPHYSIOLOGY

- Pelvic pain may arise from either gynecologic or nongynecologic conditions, and may be referred to the back, buttocks, perineum, or legs.
- Visceral pain is colicky and caused by distention of a hollow viscus or stretching of a ligament. Pain of this type is produced by distention of the fallopian tube in ectopic pregnancy, uterine contractions in dysmenorrhea, and stretch of the round ligament with adhesions or in pregnancy.
- Peritoneal or somatic pain is sharp and localized to the region of inflamed tissue. This type of pain is seen in salpingitis, appendicitis, and endometritis. Generalized peritonitis may be seen with large degrees of inflammation (ie, spillage of blood, pus, or gastrointestinal contents into the peritoneal cavity).

CLINICAL FEATURES

- Ovarian cysts are the most common noninfectious cause of acute pelvic pain. Ovarian cyst enlargement may be asymptomatic or produce poorly localized visceral pain mimicking ectopic pregnancy. When cyst leakage or rupture occurs, acute pain develops secondary to peritoneal irritation. Associated hemorrhage may be significant.
- Ovarian/adnexal torsion is a surgical emergency. The ovary or tubule elements twist on their pedicle, compromising the blood supply and producing ischemic pain and subsequent necrosis. Patients with ovarian masses and pelvic adhesions are at increased risk of torsion.
- Mittelschmerz is physiologic midcycle pain at ovulation. It occurs at day 14 to 16 of the menstrual cycle. Pain is typically unilateral, mild to moderate, and may last a day or less. Vaginal spotting may occur.
- Dysmenorrhea is the most common cause of midcycle pain.
  - Primary dysmenorrhea occurs most often in young girls just after menarche. Pain is crampy and may be associated with nausea, backache, and headache.
  - Secondary dysmenorrhea occurs later in life, and is associated with other gynecologic problems such as infection, fibroids, endometriosis, and adhesions.
- Endometriosis produces symptoms of pelvic pain, usually at menses, as well as dyspareunia and dysmenorrhea. Primary diagnosis is rarely established during an ED visit.
- Leiomyomas or fibroids rarely produce acute pain, but if severe pain is present, torsion of a pedunculated fibroid or degeneration should be considered. Degeneration is particularly common during pregnancy, when rapid fibroid growth results in outstripping of the blood supply, resulting in degeneration.

DIAGNOSIS AND DIFFERENTIAL

- The differential diagnosis of pelvic pain is extensive (Table 59-1).[4]
- A thorough history and physical examination should be performed, including a complete set of vital signs and an abdominal and gynecologic examination. The location and type of pain, its severity, onset, exacerbating and alleviating factors, and reproducibility on examination, as well as the presence or absence of masses or abnormalities in the organs of reproduction will guide the formulation of the differential diagnosis.
- Laboratory evaluation should include pregnancy testing in all women of childbearing age. If indicated by the history and physical exam, consideration should be given to a complete blood count, urinalysis, coagulation studies, sexually transmitted disease (STD) testing, and/or specific endocrine evaluations.
- Ultrasound is the test of choice for determining adnexal pathology, detecting free fluid in the pelvis, and evaluation of the thickness of the endometrium. Leiomyomas, ovarian cysts, hydrosalpinx, pelvic

TABLE 59-1   Differential Diagnosis of Acute Pelvic Pain

Acute pain
1. Complication of pregnancy
   a. Ruptured ectopic pregnancy
   b. Abortion, threatened or incomplete
   c. Degeneration of a leiomyoma
2. Acute infections
   a. Endometritis
   b. Pelvic inflammatory disease (acute PID)
   c. Tubo-ovarian abscess
3. Acute infections
   a. Hemorrhagic functional ovarian cyst
   b. Torsion of adnexa
   c. Twisted parovarian cyst
   d. Rupture of functional or neoplastic ovarian cyst

Recurrent pelvic pain
1. Mittelschmerz (midcycle pain)
2. Primary dysmenorrhea
3. Secondary dysmenorrhea

Gastrointestinal
1. Gastroenteritis
2. Appendicitis
3. Bowel obstruction
4. Diverticulitis
5. Inflammatory bowel disease
6. Irritable bowel syndrome

Genitourinary
1. Cystitis
2. Pyelonephritis
3. Ureteral lithiasis

Musculoskeletal
1. Abdominal wall hematoma
2. Hernia

Other
1. Acute porphyria
2. Pelvic thrombophlebitis
3. Aneurysm
4. Abdominal angina

SOURCE: From Rapkin et al,[4] with permission.

adhesions, tubo-ovarian abscesses, endometriosis, and ovarian carcinoma may all be visualized by this method.[5]

- Computed tomography may also be used in this setting and has a high sensitivity when differentiating between acute appendicitis and gynecologic conditions.[6]
- In a 15-year review of ovarian torsion, only 25% had a history of ovarian cyst, pain characteristics were variable, and objective findings on pelvic examination were uncommon.[7]
- Laparoscopy and/or laparotomy may be required in pelvic pain if the etiology is uncertain or direct visualization of an ambiguous adnexal mass is required. It is the gold standard for the diagnosis of pelvic inflammatory disease. It may also be required to make the final diagnosis in ovarian torsion and endometriosis.[8]
- The diagnosis of mittelschmerz is clinical; more serious etiologies should be ruled out by physical exami-

nation and a pregnancy test, and extensive evaluation is unwarranted.

EMERGENCY DEPARTMENT CARE AND DISPOSITION

- The ED treatment for the majority of patients with pelvic pain is analgesia and gynecologic follow-up. Leiomyomas, endometriosis, mittelschmerz, secondary dysmenorrhea, and chronic pelvic pain may all be treated in this manner.
- Ovarian cysts are treated primarily with analgesia and follow-up if unruptured. If the cyst has ruptured and the patient is hemodynamically stable, the same treatment protocol may be used. If cyst rupture produces hemoperitoneum, surgical intervention may be required.
- Ovarian torsion requires surgical intervention for adnexal detorsion or removal of the ischemic ovary and fallopian tube elements.

PREPUBERTAL CHILDREN

EPIDEMIOLOGY

- Of prepubertal children presenting with vaginal bleeding, 21% are associated with precocious puberty, 54% are associated with other etiologies, and 24% are idiopathic.
- Ten years of age is the lower limit for menarche; the mean age in North America is 12.5 years. The average time required to establish ovulatory cycles is 2 years after menarche.
- Genital trauma represents 0.2% of all injuries in children younger than 15. The most common mechanisms of injury are bicycle accidents, straddle injuries, and falls. The labia majora was most commonly injured. The majority of injuries were superficial, with only 5% of children requiring surgical repair.
- Urethral prolapse occurs most frequently between the ages of 2 and 10 years; it is most common in black children.
- Labial adhesions or labial agglutination are a common, recurring condition of girls from 1 to 6 years of age. They are the result of minor labial trauma or irritation and are typically asymptomatic.

PATHOPHYSIOLOGY

- In newborn females, the placental transfer of maternal hormones estradiol and gonadotropin are responsible for minor breast development and blood-tinged vaginal discharge. Normal neonates may experience uterine bleeding in the first 6 weeks of life secondary to maternal estrogen withdrawal.

- Secondary sex characteristics develop on average 2 years prior to menarche, and any variation of this is pathologic and a specific etiology must be sought.

CLINICAL FEATURES

- Vaginitis is the most common cause of pelvic pain and bleeding in prepubertal children. Flora is generally mixed and may include respiratory, enteric, and fungal pathogens. *Candida* is uncommon and may herald early diabetes.
- Trauma to the perineum can produce ecchymoses and lacerations that may be associated with injury to the vagina, urethra, rectum, and intra-abdominal organs. The hypoestrogenic skin of the vagina tears easily, and there is a significant risk of wall perforation with any penetrating injury to the vagina and rectum.
- Vaginal foreign bodies generally present with foul-smelling vaginal discharge, which may be bloody. Toilet paper is the most common foreign body.
- Congenital vaginal obstruction may be due to transverse vaginal septum or imperforate hymen. These typically present as abdominal or perineal masses or complaints of difficulty urinating. More severe cases may present with constipation, hydronephrosis, respiratory compromise, and lower extremity edema.
- Urethral prolapse presents as a soft, spongy mass 1 to 2 cm in diameter with a central dimple at the urethral meatus. Vaginal bleeding, urinary frequency, dysuria, and hematuria are the most common complaints.
- Seborrhea and psoriasis may present with bleeding, pruritus, fissuring, and pain. Lichen sclerosus appears as an hourglass-shaped depigmented area on the vulva and perineal and adjacent skin. The skin is atrophic and thin with tiny ivory papules that coalesce. The patches are frequently dry and itchy.

DIAGNOSIS AND DIFFERENTIAL

- Prepubertal children presenting with vaginal bleeding require a thorough history as to the circumstances of bleeding, times of occurrence, associated symptoms (including pain), and possible exposure to diethylstilbestrol (DES) or sexual abuse.
- The physical exam in prepubertal children should include a careful assessment of subtle signs of disease, injury, and/or abuse; the Tanner stage of sexual development should also be noted. Speculum exam and vaginoabdominal exam should not be performed unless vaginal trauma or bleeding is present. If performed, anesthesia should be utilized. If a pelvic mass

or foreign body is suspected, rectoabdominal examination with the child in the frog-leg position should be performed.
- Diagnoses of congenital vaginal malformations are made by careful examination of the perineum. The diagnosis may be unsuspected until the patient develops difficulty with urination, or an abdominal or a perineal mass develops and prompts evaluation.
- Urethral prolapse may be differentiated from vaginal masses by observing the child urinate in a bedpan.

EMERGENCY DEPARTMENT CARE AND DISPOSITION

- Care of traumatic injuries to the perineum should be based on the extent of injury. Hematomas can spread liberally and should be observed until expansion has stopped. All penetrating injuries require a careful vaginal and rectal examination. Any traumatic bleeding should be referred to a pediatric gynecologist for examination under anesthesia.
- Removal of vaginal foreign bodies may be attempted by irrigation of the vaginal vault with warm water, or by milking hard objects from the vagina via the rectum. Failure to remove the object should prompt gynecologic consultation for removal under anesthesia.
- Congenital vaginal obstruction is treated surgically. The urgency of referral depends upon presenting symptoms. Urologic, fecal, or vascular compromise should prompt emergent referral.
- Urethral prolapse is best treated with sitz baths and estrogen creams. If the mucosa is red or necrotic, surgical intervention may be required.
- Symptomatic labial adhesions may be treated with estrogen cream for 2 to 4 weeks, followed by a 2-week course of emollients such as petroleum jelly.
- Mild forms of lichen sclerosus may be treated with sitz baths and short courses of 1% hydrocortisone cream. Longer periods of steroid treatment lead to atrophy and should be avoided.

REFERENCES

1. Jones JS, Montgomery M: Gynecologic disorders in the older patient. *Acad Emerg Med* 1:580, 1994.
2. Carr B, Wilson J: Disorders of the ovary and female reproductive tract, in Isselbacher K, Braunwald E, Fauci AS, et al (eds.): *Harrison's Principles of Internal Medicine,* 13th ed. New York: McGraw-Hill, 1998, p. 2101.
3. Duncan KM, Hart LL: Nonsteroidal anti-inflammatory drugs in menorrhagia. *Ann Pharmacother* 27:1353, 1993.

4. Rapkin A: Pelvic pain and dysmenorrhea, in Berek JS, Adashi EY, Hilliard PA (eds.): *Novak's Gynecology,* 12th ed. Baltimore: Williams & Wilkins, 1998, p. 400.
5. Clinical policy: Critical issues for the initial evaluation and management of patients presenting with a chief complaint of nontraumatic acute abdominal pain. *Ann Emerg Med* 36:406, 2000.
6. Rao PM, Feltmate CM, Rhea JT, Schulick AH, Novelline RA: Helical computed tomography in differentiating appendicitis and acute gynecologic conditions. *Obstet Gynecol* 93:417, 1999.
7. Houry D, Abbott JT: Ovarian torsion: A fifteen-year review. *Ann Emerg Med* 38:156, 2001.
8. Porpora MG, Gomel V: The role of laparoscopy in the management of pelvic pain in women of reproductive age. *Fertil Steril* 68:765, 1997.

For further reading in *Emergency Medicine: A Comprehensive Study Guide,* 6th ed., see Chap. 101, "Vaginal Bleeding in the Nonpregnant Patient," by Laurie J. Morrison and Julie M. Spence; and Chap. 102, "Abdominal and Pelvic Pain in the Nonpregnant Patient," by Reb Close.

60 ECTOPIC PREGNANCY

David M. Cline

EPIDEMIOLOGY

- Ectopic pregnancy (EP) occurs in 2% of all pregnancies and is the leading cause of maternal death in the first trimester.[1]
- Twenty percent of EPs are ruptured at the time of presentation.[1]
- Major risk factors include: history of pelvic inflammatory disease; surgical procedures on the fallopian tubes, including tubal ligation; previous EP; diethylstilbestrol exposure; intrauterine device use; and assisted reproduction techniques.[2]
- This diagnosis must be considered in every woman of childbearing age presenting with abdominal pain.

PATHOPHYSIOLOGY

- EP is postulated to be caused by: (1) mechanical or anatomic alterations in the tubal transport mechanism, or (2) functional/hormonal factors that alter the fertilized ovum.

- Tubal rupture is thought to be spontaneous, but trauma associated with coitus or a bimanual examination may precipitate tubal rupture. Tubal rupture may occur in the early weeks of an EP or as late as 16 weeks' estimated gestational age.

CLINICAL FEATURES

- The classic triad of abdominal pain, vaginal bleeding, and amenorrhea used to describe EP may be present, but many cases occur with more subtle findings.
- Presenting signs and symptoms may be different in ruptured versus nonruptured EP. Only 90% of women with EP complain of abdominal pain; 80% have vaginal bleeding; and only 70% give a history of amenorrhea.[3]
- The pain described may be sudden, lateralized, extreme, or it may be relatively minor and diffuse.[3]
- The presence of hemoperitoneum causing diaphragmatic irritation may cause pain to be referred to the shoulder or upper abdomen.
- Vaginal bleeding is usually light; heavy bleeding is more commonly seen with threatened abortion or other complications of pregnancy.
- Presenting vital signs may be entirely normal even with a ruptured ectopic pregnancy, or may indicate advanced hemorrhagic shock.
- There is poor correlation with the volume of hemoperitoneum and vital signs in ectopic pregnancy. Relative bradycardia may be present even in cases with rupture and intraperitoneal hemorrhage.[4]
- Physical examination findings are highly variable. The abdominal examination may show signs of localizing or diffuse tenderness with or without peritoneal signs.[5]
- The pelvic examination findings may be normal, but more often reveals cervical motion tenderness, adnexal tenderness with or without a mass, and possibly an enlarged uterus.
- Fetal heart tones are only rarely audible.[5]

DIAGNOSIS AND DIFFERENTIAL

- Urine pregnancy testing (for urinary beta-human chorionic gonadotropin [β-hCG]) should be performed immediately.
- Dilute urine may result in a false-negative result; serum testing will give a more definitive result in such situations.
- Transvaginal ultrasound is the test of choice to identify EP. If an intrauterine pregnancy is identified, the

chance of a coexisting EP is extremely small in most patients. However, if a patient has been on fertility drugs, has had in vitro fertilization, or has multiple risk factors for EP, further evaluation for EP is warranted.[6]

- A progesterone level of ≤5 ng/mL with an empty uterus or nonspecific fluid collection in the uterus determined by ultrasound is highly suggestive of EP, but a progesterone level cannot be used to exclude EP.[7]
- Sonographic findings of an empty uterus with adnexal mass (other than a simple cyst) with or without free fluid in the abdomen are highly suggestive of EP.
- Sonographic findings of empty uterus without an adnexal mass or free fluid in a woman with a positive pregnancy test result is considered indeterminate. In such situations, the findings must be evaluated in context with the patient's quantitative β-hCG level. A high β-hCG level (greater than 6000 mIU/mL) with an empty uterus is suggestive of EP.
- If the β-hCG is low (less than 1000 mIU/mL), then the pregnancy may indeed be intrauterine or ectopic but too small to be visualized on ultrasound. In this situation, repeat quantitative β-hCG testing in 2 days must be performed.[8]
- A normal intrauterine pregnancy should show at least a 66% increase in the β-hCG level in that period of time; EP would show a slower rate of increase.
- Levels between 1000 and 6000 mIU/mL may warrant dilation and curettage (D&C) or laparoscopy to diagnose EP following evaluation by an obstetric-gynecologic consultant.
- Individual hospitals may vary in the expertise of the sonographers available, and levels other than 1000 and 6000 mIU/mL may be reasonable guidelines in certain institutions.
- Differential diagnosis in the patient presenting with abdominal pain, vaginal bleeding, and early pregnancy includes threatened, incomplete, or missed abortion; recent elective abortion; or endometritis.

EMERGENCY DEPARTMENT CARE AND DISPOSITION

- Treatment of patients with suspected EP is dependent on the patient's vital signs, physical signs, and symptoms. Close communication with the obstetric-gynecologic consultant is essential.[8]
- For unstable patients, start two large-bore intravenous lines for rapid infusion of crystalloid and/or packed red blood cells to maintain blood pressure.
- Perform a bedside urine pregnancy test.
- Notify an obstetric-gynecologic consultant immediately for the unstable patient, even before laboratory and diagnostic tests are complete.
- Draw blood for complete blood count, blood typing, and Rh (rhesus factor) determination (or cross-matching for the unstable patients), quantitative β-hCG determination (if indicated), and serum electrolyte determination as required.
- If the patient is stable, proceed with diagnostic work-up, including transvaginal ultrasound. In reliable patients with indeterminate ultrasound results and a β-hCG level below 1000 mIU/mL, discharge with ectopic precautions and arranged follow-up in 2 days for repeat β-hCG determination and obstetric-gynecologic re-evaluation is appropriate.
- Definitive treatment, as determined by the obstetric-gynecologic consultant, may involve laparoscopy, D&C, or medical management with methotrexate.[8]

REFERENCES

1. Leads from the Morbidity and Mortality Weekly Report: Ectopic pregnancy—United States. 1990-1992. *JAMA* 273:533, 1995.
2. Ankum WM, Mol BWJ, Van der Veen F, et al: Risk factors for ectopic pregnancy: A meta-analysis. *Fertil Steril* 65:1093, 1996.
3. Stovall TG, Kellerman AL, Ling FW, et al: Emergency department diagnosis of ectopic pregnancy. *Ann Emerg Med* 19: 1098, 1990.
4. Hick JL, Rodgerson JD, Heegard WG, et al: Vital signs fail to correlate with hemoperitoneum from ruptured ectopic pregnancy. *Am J Emerg Med* 19:488, 2001.
5. Kaplan BC, Dart RG, Moskos M, et al: Ectopic pregnancy: Prospective study with improved diagnostic accuracy. *Ann Emerg Med* 28:10, 1996.
6. Tal J, Haddad S, Gordon N, Timor Tritsch I: Heterotopic pregnancy after ovulation induction and assisted reproductive technologies: A literature review from 1971 to 1993. *Fertil Steril* 66:1, 1996.
7. Dart R, Ramanujum P, Dart L: Progesterone as a predictor of ectopic pregnancy when the ultrasound is indeterminate. *Am J Emerg Med* 20:575, 2002.
8. American College of Emergency Physicians: Clinical policy: Critical issues in the initial evauation and management of patients presenting to the emergency department in early pregnancy. *Ann Emerg Med* 41:123, 2003.

For further reading in *Emergency Medicine: A Comprehensive Study Guide,* 6th ed., see Chap. 103, "Ectopic Pregnancy," by Richard S. Krause and David M. Janicke.

61 COMORBID DISEASES IN PREGNANCY

Sally S. Fuller

- For information on hypertension in pregnancy, see Chap. 62. For information on pulmonary embolism, see Chap. 28.

MEDICATION USE DURING PREGNANCY

- Table 61-1 lists recommendations for drug use during pregnancy.

DIABETES

- Diabetics are at increased risk for hypertensive diseases, preterm labor, spontaneous abortion, pyelonephritis, fetal demise, hypoglycemia, and diabetic ketoacidosis (DKA).
- Oral hypoglycemic agents are contraindicated. Insulin requirements increase throughout the pregnancy from 0.7 U/kg/day to 1.0 U/kg/day at term.
- DKA may develop at lower glucose levels than in the nonpregnant patient.
- DKA and hypoglycemia are treated the same as in the nonpregnant patient.

HYPERTHYROIDISM

- Hyperthyroidism in pregnancy increases the risk of preeclampsia and neonatal morbidity. Clinical features may be subtle, and may include hyperemesis gravidarum. Propylthiouracil (PTU) is the treatment of choice.
- Thyroid storm presents with fever, volume depletion, and cardiac decompensation, and has a high mortality rate. PTU, sodium iodide, and propranolol (unless cardiac failure is present) can control symptoms.
- For further information, see Chap. 134.

DYSRHYTHMIAS

- Dysrhythmias, rare in pregnancy, are treated with lidocaine, digoxin, procainamide, and verapamil in the usual doses.
- β-Blockers may be used acutely for control, but not for long-term use.[1]

- Cardioversion has not been shown to be harmful to the fetus.[2]
- For anticoagulation, unfractionated or low molecular weight heparin is used.

THROMBOEMBOLISM

- Thromboembolic disease is 5 to 20 times more likely to develop in the postpartum period[3] (see Chaps. 28 and 31).
- The incidence of deep venous thrombosis (DVT) ranges between 0.5 and 0.7%.[4]
- Factors associated with increased risk include advanced maternal age, increasing parity, multiple gestation, operative delivery (13- to 16-fold increase compared to vaginal delivery), bedrest, obesity, and hypercoagulable states.[4]
- Diagnosis may be made by duplex Doppler studies, impedance plethysmography, or technetium-99m radionuclide venography. For pulmonary embolism (PE), ventilation and perfusion scanning or pulmonary angiography can be performed. Iodine-125 fibrinogen scanning should not be used. Spiral computed tomographic (CT) scanning for PE has not been studied in pregnancy.
- Treatment of DVT and PE is with heparin or enoxaparin; warfarin is contraindicated (see Chaps. 28 and 31).

ASTHMA

- Clinical features, diagnosis, and management are similar in pregnant and nonpregnant patients. Clinical presentation includes cough, wheezing, and dyspnea.
- Peak expiratory flow rates are unchanged in pregnancy.[5] However, the normal P_{CO_2} on the arterial blood gas (ABG) test is 27 to 32 with a normal pH of 7.40 to 7.45.
- Acute therapy includes β_2-agonists such as albuterol via nebulizer. Intravenous methylprednisolone and oral prednisone can be used in pregnancy. Epinephrine 0.3 mL (1:1000 dilution) can be given subcutaneously. Oxygen should be administered to maintain a P_{O_2} of >65 mm Hg. Fetal monitoring should be done after 20 weeks.
- Criteria for intubation or admission are similar in pregnant and nonpregnant patients; standard agents for rapid sequence intubation are used.

URINARY TRACT INFECTIONS

- Urinary tract infection is the most common bacterial infection in pregnancy.
- Simple cystitis may be treated for 3 days with slow-

TABLE 61 1   Drug Use in Pregnancy

DRUG	CATEGORY*	COMMENT
Antibiotics		
Cephalosporins	B	May use
Penicillins	B	May use
Erythromycin	B	Estolate salt contraindicated due to hepatotoxicity; otherwise may use
Azithromycin	B	May use
Nitrofurantoin	B	May use
Clindamycin	B	May use
Metronidazole	B	Should be avoided during first trimester
Isoniazid	C	May use when necessary
Ethambutol	B	May use
Antivirals		
Acyclovir	C	May use in life-threatening maternal illness
Antihypertensive agents		
Alpha-methyldopa	B	May use
β-blockers	B, C	May use when necessary
Calcium channel blockers	C	May use when necessary
Prazosin	C	May use when necessary
Hydralazine	C	Widely used
Anticonvulsants		
All	C, D	Congenital malformations reported with all anticonvulsants, but benefits may outweigh risks; use of folic acid (1 mg/day) may help prevent teratogenesis; valproic acid has especially high risk of neural tube defects
Corticosteroids	C	May be used in pregnancy for serious maternal conditions; gestational diabetes may develop
Anticoagulants		
Heparin	C	Drug of choice for pregnant women requiring anticoagulation
Analgesics		
Acetaminophen	A	May use
Propoxyphene	C	Caution advised when used close to term; neonatal withdrawal may occur
Opiates	C	Caution advised when used close to term; neonatal withdrawal may occur; avoid aspirin combinations
Nonsteroidal anti-inflammatory drugs	D, C, D	May be used for short duration (48–72 h) and not at all after 32 weeks; ibuprofen widely used
Antiemetics		
Meclizine	B	May use
Dimenhydrinate	B	May use
Diphenhydramine	B	Avoid first trimester
Trimethobenzamide	C	Used widely
Phenothiazines	C	Used widely
Over-the-counter cold medications		
Pseudoephedrine	C	Topical sprays preferable
Phenylpropanolamine	C	Topical nasal sprays preferable
Vaccines		
Live vaccines (measles-mumps-rubella)	X	Contraindicated
Inactivated viral vaccines (rabies, hepatitis B, influenza)	C	May be given
Pneumococcal vaccine	C	May be given
Tetanus and diphtheria	C	May be given

*Categories: A = safe, human studies; B = presumed safe, animal studies; C = uncertain safety, animal studies show an adverse effect; D = unsafe, use may be justifiable in certain circumstances; X = contraindicated.

release nitrofurantoin 100 mg PO, amoxicillin 500 mg PO tid, or cephalexin 500 mg PO qid.
- Patients with pyelonephritis should be admitted for IV antibiotics because of increased risk of preterm labor and sepsis. IV hydration and antibiotics should be used: cefazolin 1 to 2 g IV, or ampicillin 1 g IV plus gentamicin 1 mg/kg IV.
- Quinolones are contraindicated during pregnancy. Sulfonamides should be avoided close to term. Trimethoprim may be used after the first trimester.

INFLAMMATORY BOWEL DISEASE

- The general treatment of the pregnant patient with inflammatory bowel disease is the same as that of the nonpregnant patient. Antidiarrheal drugs including codeine and Lomotil may be safely used. Sulfasalazine, in combination with folic acid supplements, may also be used.

SICKLE CELL DISEASE

- Women with sickle cell disease are at higher risk for miscarriage, preterm labor, and vaso-occlusive crises.
- Clinical features, evaluation, and treatment are similar in pregnant and nonpregnant patients. Management includes aggressive hydration and analgesic therapy. Narcotics should be used; nonsteroidal anti-inflammatory agents should be avoided after 32 weeks' gestation. Hydroxyurea should be discontinued in pregnancy.
- Aplastic crises occur rarely, and are associated with parvovirus infection (fifth disease) and hydrops fetalis.

MIGRAINE

- Treatment includes acetaminophen and narcotics.
- Ergot alkaloids and triptans should not be used.

SEIZURE DISORDERS

- Management of a pregnant patient with a known seizure disorder is similar to that of a nonpregnant patient. Valproic acid is avoided because of an association with neural tube defects.
- Status epilepticus with prolonged maternal hypoxia and acidosis has a high mortality rate for the mother and infant and should be treated aggressively with early intubation and ventilation. Place the patient in the left lateral decubitus position to maximize placental oxygenation.

HIV INFECTION

- All pregnant HIV-infected women beyond 14 weeks' gestation should be on zidovudine therapy to reduce the risk of transmission to the fetus.[6]
- Patients with CD4 counts <200 should be on prophylaxis for *Pneumocystis carinii* pneumonia. Treatment of opportunistic infections is unchanged in pregnancy.

SUBSTANCE ABUSE

- Cocaine use is associated with increased incidence of fetal death in utero, placental abruption, preterm labor, premature rupture of membranes, spontaneous abortion, intrauterine growth restriction, and fetal cerebral infarcts. Treatment of toxicity is unchanged in pregnancy.
- Opiate withdrawal in pregnant women is treated with methadone or clonidine (0.1 to 0.2 mg every hour until signs of withdrawal resolve, up to 0.8 mg total).
- Alcohol use contributes to increased rates of spontaneous abortion, low birth weight infants, preterm deliveries, and fetal alcohol syndrome. Acute withdrawal is treated with short-acting barbiturates and benzodiazepines are avoided in early pregnancy.

DOMESTIC VIOLENCE

- Approximately 15% of pregnant women are victims of domestic violence.[7] They are at risk for placental abruption, uterine rupture, preterm labor, and fetal fractures. Rh immune globulin (Rhogam 300 μg IM) should be considered following blunt abdominal trauma in Rh-negative patients.

DIAGNOSTIC IMAGING IN PREGNANCY

- The risk of radiation exposure varies with gestational age. The second to the eighth week postconception is the period of organogenesis, the most vulnerable period for birth defects. Mental retardation and other problems may occur with significant x-ray exposure between weeks eight and twenty-five.
- A cumulative dose of 10 rads is the threshold for human teratogenesis, and the fetus is most vulnerable at 8 to 15 weeks' gestation.
- Ultrasound, ventilation-perfusion scanning, and magnetic resonance imaging have not shown any teratogenic effects.

REFERENCES

1. Frishman WH, Chesner M: Beta-adrenergic blockers in pregnancy. *Am Heart J* 115:147, 1988.
2. Schroeder JS, Harrison DC: Repeated cardioversion during pregnancy. *Am J Cardiol* 27:445, 1971.
3. Bonnar J: Epidemiology of venous thromboembolism in pregnancy and the puerperium, in Greer I, Turpie A, Forbes C (eds.): *Haemostasis and Thrombosis*. London: Chapman and Hall Medical, 1992, p. 260.

4. McColl MD, Ramsay JE, Tait RC, et al: Risk factors for pregnancy related venous thromboembolism. *Thromb Haemost* 78:1183, 1997.
5. Brancazio LR, Laifer SA, Schwartz T: Peak expiratory flow rate in normal pregnancy. *Obstet Gynecol* 89:383, 1997.
6. Recommendations of the USPHS task force on the use of zidovudine to reduce the perinatal transmission of HIV. *Morb Mortal Wkly Rep* 43:1, 1994.
7. Mayer L, Liebschutz J: Domestic violence in the pregnant patient: Obstetric and behavioral interventions. *Obstet Gynecol Surv* 53:627, 1998.

For further reading in *Emergency Medicine: A Comprehensive Study Guide*, 6th ed., see Chap. 105, "Comorbid Diseases in Pregnancy," by Jessica L. Bienstock and Harold E. Fox.

62 EMERGENCIES DURING PREGNANCY AND THE POSTPARTUM PERIOD

Sally S. Fuller

- The leading causes of maternal death are pulmonary embolus (see Chap. 28), ectopic pregnancy (see Chap. 60), hypertensive disorders of pregnancy, hemorrhage, and infection.[1]
- Risk increases with increased maternal age, increased birth order, lack of prenatal care, unmarried status, and minority race.[1]

EMERGENCIES IN THE FIRST 20 WEEKS

THREATENED ABORTION AND ABORTION

EPIDEMIOLOGY
- Twenty to forty percent of pregnancies abort spontaneously.

PATHOPHYSIOLOGY
- Chromosomal abnormalities account for most fetal wastage. Risk increases with increasing maternal age and concurrent medical disorders, previous abortion, infections, and anatomic abnormalities.

CLINICAL FEATURES
- Threatened abortion is vaginal bleeding with a closed cervical os and benign physical examination.

- Inevitable abortion will occur with vaginal bleeding and dilatation of the cervix.
- Incomplete abortion is defined as partial passage of the conceptus and is more likely between 6 and 14 weeks of pregnancy.
- Complete abortion is passage of all fetal tissue before 20 weeks' gestation.
- Missed abortion is fetal death at less than 20 weeks' gestation without passage of fetal tissue.
- Septic abortion implies evidence of infection during any stage of abortion, such as pelvic pain, fever, cervical motion or uterine tenderness, and purulent or foul-smelling discharge.

DIAGNOSIS AND DIFFERENTIAL
- The differential diagnosis includes ectopic pregnancy (see Chap. 60), and gestational trophoblastic disease (GTD). GTD is a neoplastic disease of trophoblastic tissue, and is distinguished from threatened abortion by ultrasound. It may be noninvasive (hydatidiform mole) or invasive (choriocarcinoma).[3]

EMERGENCY DEPARTMENT CARE AND DISPOSITION
- Manage hemodynamic instability. Consult a gynecologist emergently in the unstable patient. Perform a pelvic exam, and obtain a complete blood count (CBC), blood typing and Rh factor determination, quantitative β-hCG, and urinalysis. Rh-negative women should receive Rh (D) immune globulin 300 μg IM.
- Vaginal ultrasound should reveal a gestational sac in a normal pregnancy with a β-hCG >1000 mIU/mL.[2] Absence of a gestational sac with a β-hCG >1000 mIU/mL suggests complete abortion or ectopic pregnancy.
- Incomplete abortion or GTD requires dilatation and curettage. GTD patients must receive close follow-up until quantitative β-hCG has returned to zero. Failure of the β-hCG to return to normal could indicate choriocarcinoma.
- Septic abortion requires gynecologic consultation and broad-spectrum antibiotics such as ampicillin-sulbactam 3.0 g IV or clindamycin 600 mg plus gentamycin 1 to 2 mg/kg IV.
- Threatened abortion or complete abortion patients may be discharged with close follow-up arranged. Discharge instructions include pelvic rest (no intercourse or tampons) and instructions to return for heavy bleeding, fever, or pain.

NAUSEA AND VOMITING OF PREGNANCY

- Hyperemesis gravidarum (intractable nausea and vomiting without significant abdominal pain) can cause hypokalemia or ketonemia and may result in a low birth weight infant. The pathophysiology is unknown.

- Diagnostic work-up should include a CBC, electrolyte panel, and urinalysis.
- Treatment consists of rehydration with IV fluid (5% dextrose in normal saline [D_5NS] or 5% dextrose in lactated Ringer's [D_5LR]), along with antiemetics,[4] until ketonuria clears. Antiemetics that are frequently used are metoclopramide 10 mg IV, promethazine 25 mg IV (pregnancy class C, but widely used), or ondansetron 4 mg IV.

EMERGENCIES DURING THE SECOND HALF OF PREGNANCY

VAGINAL BLEEDING

- Abruptio placentae, placenta previa, and preterm labor are the most common causes.
- Speculum and digital pelvic exam is contraindicated until ultrasound has been obtained to rule out placenta previa.
- Manage hemodynamic instability with IV NS and/or packed RBCs.
- Obtain emergent obstetric consultation, CBC, type and cross-matching, disseminated intravascular coagulation (DIC) profile, and electrolyte studies on all patients. Rh (D) immune globulin 300 μg should be given to Rh-negative patients.

ABRUPTIO PLACENTAE

- Abruptio placentae is the premature separation of the placenta from the uterine wall.
- Risk factors include hypertension, advanced maternal age, multiparity, smoking, cocaine use, previous abruption, and abdominal trauma.
- Clinical features include vaginal bleeding, abdominal pain, uterine tenderness, or fetal distress; in severe cases, DIC and fetal and/or maternal death.
- Emergency delivery may be needed to save the life of the fetus and/or mother.

PLACENTA PREVIA

- Placenta previa is the implantation of the placenta over the cervical os.
- Risk factors include multiparity and prior cesarean section.
- Clinical features are painless bright red vaginal bleeding. Diagnosis is made by transabdominal pelvic ultrasound, and pelvic exams are contraindicated.[5]

PREMATURE RUPTURE OF MEMBRANES (PROM)

- Premature rupture of membranes (PROM) is rupture of membranes prior to the onset of labor.
- Clinical presentation is a rush of fluid or continuous leakage of fluid from the vagina.
- Diagnosis is confirmed by finding a pool of fluid with pH greater than 6.5 (dark blue on nitrazine paper) in the posterior fornix, and ferning pattern on smear. Sterile speculum exam may be done; however, if possible, digital pelvic exam should be deferred or done with sterile gloves.
- Tests for chlamydia, gonorrhea, bacterial vaginosis, and group B streptococci should be performed.
- Patients with suspected PROM should be admitted.

PRETERM LABOR

- Preterm labor is defined as labor prior to 37 weeks' gestation.[6] It occurs in 10% of deliveries and is the leading cause of neonatal deaths.
- Risk factors include PROM, abruptio placentae, drug abuse, multiple gestation, polyhydramnios, incompetent cervix, and infection.
- Clinical features include regular uterine contractions with effacement of the cervix. The diagnosis is made by observation, with external fetal monitoring and serial sterile speculum examinations.
- Consult an obstetrician for admission and decision regarding tocolytics. If tocolytics are initiated, the mother should receive glucocorticoids to hasten fetal lung maturity.[7] Do not use tocolytics if abruptio placentae is suspected.
- Gestational age less than 34 weeks is associated with poorer outcomes; consider transfer to a tertiary care center with a high-risk intensive care unit if possible.

HYPERTENSION, PRE-ECLAMPSIA, AND RELATED DISORDERS

- Diagnostic criteria are listed in Table 62-1.
- Hypertension with pregnancy is associated with pre-eclampsia, eclampsia, HELLP (**h**emolytic anemia, **el**evated **l**iver enzymes, and **l**ow **p**latelets) syndrome, abruptio placentae, preterm birth, and low birth weight infants.
- Hypertension in pregnancy is defined as a blood pressure greater than 140/90 mm Hg, a 20–mm Hg rise in systolic blood pressure, or a 10–mm Hg rise in diastolic blood pressure above the prepregnancy level.

TABLE 62-1   Criteria for Hypertension, Pre-eclampsia, and Eclampsia

Hypertension	BP >140/90 measured twice at least 6 h apart
Transient hypertension	BP >140/90 without other signs of pre-eclampsia or eclampsia
Pre-eclampsia	BP >140/90, or >20 mm Hg rise in systolic, or >10 mm Hg rise in diastolic BP Proteinuria (300 mg/24 h or 1 g/mL) Generalized or pedal edema or weight gain of at least 5 lb over 1 week
Eclampsia	Above findings plus generalized seizure

PRE-ECLAMPSIA

- Pre-eclampsia complicates 5 to 10% of pregnancies. Risk factors include obesity, chronic hypertension, renal disease, insulin-resistant diabetes, prior pre-eclampsia, twin gestation, and primagravida. The cause is unknown; however, uteroplacental blood flow is known to be decreased.[8]
- Clinical presentation is hypertension, proteinuria, and edema in patients of 20 or more weeks' gestation through the postpartum period. Patients may present with headache, visual disturbances, edema, or abdominal pain. Eclampsia is pre-eclampsia with seizures.
- HELLP syndrome, a variant of pre-eclampsia, usually presents with abdominal pain, and hypertension may not be present initially. HELLP syndrome should be considered in the evaluation of all pregnant women (at greater than 20 weeks' gestation) with abdominal pain. Diagnosis is made by lab tests: schistocytes on peripheral smear, platelet count less than 150,000/mL, elevated AST (aspartate aminotransferase) and ALT (alanine aminotransferase) levels, and abnormal coagulation profile.
- Consult an obstetrician and obtain CBC, urinalysis, electrolyte panel, liver panel, and coagulation profile. Severe pre-eclampsia or eclampsia is treated with magnesium sulfate loading dose 4 to 6 g in 100 mL of fluid over 20 minutes, followed by maintenance infusion of 1 to 2 g/h to prevent seizure. Treat hypertension with hydralazine 2.5 mg initially, followed by 5 to 10 mg every 10 minutes IV, or labetalol 20 mg IV initial bolus, with repeat boluses of 40 to 80 mg if needed to a maximum of 300 mg for blood pressure control.9 Definitive treatment requires delivery of the fetus.

EMERGENCIES DURING THE POSTPARTUM PERIOD

- Hemorrhage and infection are the most common postpartum complications presenting to the ED.

- Postpartum pre-eclampsia or eclampsia, amniotic fluid embolism, and postpartum cardiomyopathy are rare but life-threatening complications.
- Thromboembolic disease is common in the postpartum period.

POSTPARTUM HEMORRHAGE

- The differential diagnosis of hemorrhage includes uterine atony (most common), uterine rupture, laceration of the lower genital tract, retained placental tissue, uterine inversion, and coagulopathy.
- Diagnose by physical examination. The uterus is enlarged and "doughy" with uterine atony; a vaginal mass is suggestive of an inverted uterus. Bleeding in spite of good uterine tone and size may indicate retained products of conception.
- Manage hemorrhage with crystalloid IV fluids and/or packed red blood cells if needed. Obtain CBC, clotting studies, and type and cross-match. Uterine atony is treated with oxytocin 20 U in 1 L of IV fluid at 200 mL/h. Minor lacerations may be repaired using local anesthetic. Extensive lacerations, retained products of conception, uterine inversion, or uterine rupture require emergency operative treatment by the obstetrician.

INFECTION

- Postpartum endometritis is usually polymicrobial. Risk factors include cesarean delivery, prolonged ruptured membranes or labor, younger maternal age, and internal fetal monitoring.
- Clinical features include fever, lower abdominal pain, and foul-smelling lochia.
- Diagnosis is made by physical examination revealing uterine or cervical motion tenderness and discharge. Discharge may be minimal in group B *Streptococcus* infections. CBC, urinalysis, and cervical cultures should be obtained.
- Admit for broad-spectrum antibiotic treatment, such as cefoxitin 1 to 2 g IV every 6 hours, or combination therapy with ampicillin 1 g IV every 6 hours and gentamicin 1.5 mg/kg IV every 8 hours.

AMNIOTIC FLUID EMBOLISM

- Amniotic fluid embolism is a sudden, catastrophic illness with mortality rates of 60 to 80%. Clinical features include sudden cardiovascular collapse with hypoxemia, seizures, and DIC. Care is supportive.[6]

MASTITIS

- Mastitis is cellulitis of the periglandular breast tissue. Treatment is with cephalexin or dicloxacillin 500 mg qid. Patients should continue nursing on the affected breast.

REFERENCES

1. Berg CJ, Atrash HK, Koonin LM, et al: Pregnancy-related mortality in the United States, 1987-1990. *Obstet Gynecol* 88: 161, 1996.
2. Cacciatore B, Tiitenen A, Stenman U, et al: Normal early pregnancy: Serum hCG levels and vaginal ultrasonography findings. *Br J Obstet Gynaecol* 97:899, 1990.
3. Shapter AP, McLellan R: Gestational trophoblastic disease. *Obstet Gynecol Clin North Am* 28:805, 2001.
4. Pearlman M, Tintinalli JE (eds.): *Emergency Care of the Woman.* New York: McGraw-Hill, 1998.
5. Hertzberg BS, Bowie JD, Carroll BA, et al: Diagnosis of placenta previa during the third trimester: Role of transperineal sonography. *Am J Roentgenol* 159:83, 1992.
6. American College of Obstetricians and Gynecologists: Preterm labor. ACOG Technical Bulletin No. 206, June 1995.
7. National Institutes of Health: NIH consensus development statement: Effect of corticosteroids for fetal maturation on perinatal outcomes. Washington: NIH Consensus Development Conference, 1994.
8. Sibai B, Ramadan M: Preeclampsia and eclampsia, in Sciarra J (ed.): *Gynecology and Obstetrics.* Philadelphia: Lippincott Williams & Wilkins, 1995, p. 1.
9. Sibai BM: Treatment of hypertension in pregnant women. *N Engl J Med* 335:257, 1996.

For further reading in *Emergency Medicine: A Comprehensive Study Guide,* 6th ed., see Chap. 106, "Emergencies During Pregnancy and the Postpartum Period," by Gloria J. Kuhn.

63 EMERGENCY DELIVERY

David M. Cline

EPIDEMIOLOGY

- The incidence of out-of-hospital delivery has fallen to less than 1% of deliveries.[1]
- In a study in Washington State of 7000 planned home deliveries, 500 were rushed emergently to the hospital for delivery.[2]

CLINICAL FEATURES

- Every patient presenting with signs of active labor should receive immediate monitoring of maternal vital signs and fetal heart rate. Maternal blood pressure should be monitored, and Doppler heart tones are helpful to confirm normal fetal heart rate (120 to 160 beats per minute).
- A persistently slow fetal heart rate (less than 100 beats per minute) is an indicator of fetal distress, and emergent obstetric consultation is necessary.
- False labor is characterized by irregular, brief contractions usually confined to the lower abdomen. These contractions, commonly called Braxton-Hicks contractions, are irregular in both intensity and duration. True labor is characterized by painful, regular contractions of steadily increasing intensity and duration, leading to progressive cervical dilatation. True labor typically begins in the fundal region and upper abdomen and radiates into the pelvis and lower back.

DIAGNOSIS AND DIFFERENTIAL

- Patients without vaginal bleeding should be examined both bimanually and with a sterile speculum.
- Patients presenting with vaginal bleeding should initially be evaluated with ultrasound prior to any speculum or bimanual examination to rule out placenta previa.[3]
- If spontaneous rupture of membranes (SROM) is suspected, examination with a sterile speculum should be performed and digital exam avoided, as studies have shown an increased risk of infection after a single digital examination.[4]
- Determining whether membranes have ruptured is an important predictor of the likelihood of imminent labor as well as the potential for complications such as infection or cord prolapse.[5]
- SROM occurs during the course of active labor in most patients, although it may occur prior to the onset of labor in 10% of third-trimester patients. SROM typically occurs with a gush of clear or blood-tinged fluid. It can be confirmed by using nitrazine paper to test residual fluid in the fornix or vaginal vault while a sterile speculum examination is performed. Amniotic fluid has a pH of 7.0 to 7.4 and will turn nitrazine paper dark blue. Vaginal fluid typically has a pH of 4.5 to 5.5 and will make the nitrazine strip remain yellow.

PLACENTA PREVIA

- Placenta previa occurs when the placenta partially or completely overlies the internal cervical os. The presence of placenta previa should be suspected in any third-trimester patient presenting with painless vaginal bleeding, particularly bright red blood per vagina.
- If previa is suspected, an emergent ultrasound prior to speculum or bimanual examination is required.[6] If previa is present on ultrasound and the patient is actively laboring, no further examination should be performed and arrangements should be made for immediate transport to labor and delivery for cesarean section.

PLACENTAL ABRUPTION

- Abruptio placentae (or placental abruption) is the separation of the placenta from its implantation site prior to delivery.
- Placental abruption is classically characterized by the vaginal bleeding, a "rock-hard" painful uterus, and fetal distress (decrease in fetal heart rate to <100 beats per minute).[7]
- Risk factors for abruption include maternal hypertension, smoking, cocaine use, and trauma.

EMERGENCY DEPARTMENT CARE AND DISPOSITION

EMERGENCY DELIVERY

- The use of routine episiotomy for a normal spontaneous vaginal delivery has been discouraged in recent years and increases the incidence of third- and fourth-degree lacerations at the time of delivery.[8,9]
- If an episiotomy is necessary, it may be performed as follows.
  1. A solution of 5 to 10 mL of 1% lidocaine is injected with a small-gauge needle into the posterior fourchette and perineum.
  2. While protecting the infant's head, a 2- to 3-cm cut is made with scissors to extend the vaginal opening.
  3. The incision must be supported with manual pressure from below, taking care not to allow the incision to extend into the rectum.
- Control of the delivery of the neonate is the major challenge. As the infant's head emerges from the introitus, the physician should support the perineum with a sterile towel placed along the inferior portion of the perineum with one hand while supporting the fetal head with the other. Mild counterpressure is exerted to prevent the rapid expulsion of the fetal head, which may lead to third- or fourth-degree perineal tears.

- As the infant's head presents, the left hand may be used to control the fetal chin while the right remains on the crown of the head, supporting the delivery. This controlled extension of the fetal head will aid in the atraumatic delivery.
- The mother is then asked to breathe through contractions rather than bearing down and attempting to push the baby out rapidly.
- Immediately following delivery of the infant's head, the infant's nose and mouth should be suctioned. This is particularly important in infants presenting with meconium in order to prevent aspiration. A simple bulb will assist in the routine clearing of the infant's nose and mouth.
- After suctioning, the neck should be palpated for the presence of a nuchal cord. This is a common condition, found in 25% of all cephalad-presenting deliveries. If the cord is loose, it should be reduced over the infant's head; the delivery may then proceed as usual. If the cord is tightly wound, it may have to be clamped in the most accessible area by two clamps in close proximity and cut to allow delivery of the infant.
- After delivery of the head, the head will restitute, or turn to one side or the other. As the head rotates, the physician's hands are placed on either side of it, providing gentle downward traction to deliver the anterior shoulder. The physician's hand then gently guides the fetus upward, delivering the posterior shoulder and allowing the remainder of the infant to be delivered.
- It is useful to prepare for the delivery by placing the posterior (left) hand underneath the infant's axilla prior to delivering the rest of the body. The anterior hand may then be used to grasp the infant's ankles and ensure a firm grip.
- The infant is then loosely wrapped in a towel and stimulated as it is dried. The umbilical cord is double clamped and cut with sterile scissors.
- The infant is then further dried and warmed in an incubator, where postnatal care may be provided and Apgar scores calculated at 1 and 5 minutes after delivery.
- Scoring includes general color, tone, heart rate, respiratory effort, and reflexes.

CORD PROLAPSE

- In the event that the bimanual examination reveals a palpable, pulsating cord, the examiner's hand should not be removed, but rather should be used to elevate the presenting fetal part to reduce compression of the cord.[10]

- Immediate obstetric assistance is then necessary, as a cesarean section is indicated.
- The examiner's hand should remain in the vagina while the patient is transported and prepped for surgery in order to prevent further compression of the cord by the fetal head.[11]

SHOULDER DYSTOCIA

- Shoulder dystocia is first recognized after the delivery of the fetal head, when routine downward traction is insufficient to deliver the anterior shoulder.
- After delivery of the infant's head, the head retracts tightly against the perineum (the "turtle sign").[12]
- Upon recognizing shoulder dystocia, the physician should suction the infant's nose and mouth and call for assistance to position the mother in the extreme lithotomy position, with legs sharply flexed up to the abdomen (the McRoberts maneuver) with the legs held by the mother or an assistant.
- The bladder should be drained if this has not already been done.
- A generous episiotomy may also facilitate delivery.
- Next, an assistant should apply suprapubic pressure to disimpact the anterior shoulder from the pubic symphysis.
- It is important to remember never to apply fundal pressure, as this will further force the shoulder against the pelvic rim.[13]

BREECH PRESENTATION

- Breech presentations may be classified as frank, complete, incomplete, or footling.
- The frank breech and the complete breech presentation serve as a dilating wedge nearly as well as the fetal head, and delivery may proceed in an uncomplicated fashion.
- The main point in a frank or complete breech presentation is to allow the delivery to progress spontaneously. This lets the presenting portion of the fetus dilate the cervix maximally prior to the presentation of the fetal head. It is recommended that the examiner refrain from touching the fetus until the scapulae are visualized.
- Footling and incomplete breech positions are not considered safe for vaginal delivery because of the possibility of cord prolapse or incomplete dilatation of the cervix. In any breech delivery, immediate obstetric consultation should be requested.

POSTPARTUM CARE

- The placenta should be allowed to separate spontaneously, assisted with gentle traction. Aggressive traction on the cord risks uterine inversion, tearing of the cord, or disruption of the placenta, which can result in severe vaginal bleeding.[14]
- After the removal of the placenta, the uterus should be gently massaged to promote contraction. Oxytocin (20 U in 1 L of 0.9 normal saline) is infused at a moderate rate to maintain uterine contraction.
- Episiotomy or laceration repair may be delayed until an experienced obstetrician is able to close the laceration and inspect the patient for fourth-degree (rectovaginal) tears.[15]

REFERENCES

1. Curtin SC: Trends in the attendant, place, and timing of births, and in the use of obstetric interventions: United States, 1989-1997. *Nat Vital Stat Rep* 47:1, 1999.
2. Pang JW, Heffelfinger JD, Huang GJ, et al: Outcomes of planned home births in Washington State: 1989-1996. *Obstet Gynecol* 100:253, 2002.
3. Leerentveld RA, Gilberts EC, Arnold MJ, Wladimiroff JW: Accuracy and safety of transvaginal sonographic placental localization. *Obstet Gynecol* 76:759, 1990.
4. Johnston MM, Sanchez-Ramos L, Vaughn AJ, et al: Antibiotic therapy in preterm, premature rupture of membranes: A randomized prospective double blind trial. *Am J Obstet Gynecol* 163:743, 1990.
5. Mercer BM, Lewis R: Preterm labor and premature rupture of membranes: Diagnosis and management. *Infect Dis Clin North Am* 11:177, 1997.
6. Iyasu S, Saftlas AK, Rowley DL, et al: The epidemiology of placenta previa in the United States. *Am J Obstet Gynecol* 168:1424, 1987.
7. Lowe TW, Cunningham FG: Abruptio placentae. *Clin Obstet Gynecol* 33:406, 1990.
8. Borgatta L, Picning SJ, Cohen WR: Association of episiotomy and delivery position with deep perineal laceration during spontaneous delivery in nulliparous women. *Am J Obstet Gynecol* 160:294, 1989.
9. Shino P, Klebanoff MA, Corey JC: Midline episiotomies: More harm than good? *Obstet Gynecol* 75:765, 1990.
10. Barnett WM: Umbilical cord prolapse: A true obstetrical emergency. *J Emerg Med* 7:149, 1989.
11. Critchlow CW, Leef TL, Benedetti TJ, et al: Risk factors and infant outcomes associated with umbilical cord prolapse: A population based case-control study among births in Washington state. *Am J Obstet Gynecol* 170:613, 1994.
12. Naef RW, Martin JN: Emergency management of shoulder dystocia. *Obstet Gynecol Clin North Am* 22:247, 1995.

13. Nocon JJ, McKenzie DK, Thomas LJ, et al: Shoulder dystocia: An analysis of risks and obstetric maneuvers. *Am J Obstet Gynecol* 168:1732, 1993.
14. Combs CA, Murphey EL, Laros RK: Factors associated with postpartum hemorrhage with vaginal birth. *Obstet Gynecol* 77:69, 1991.
15. Zahn CM, Yoemans ER: Postpartum hemorrhage, placenta accreta, uterine inversion, and puerperal hematomas. *Clin Obstet Gynecol* 33:422, 1990.

For further reading in *Emergency Medicine: A Comprehensive Study Guide,* 6th ed., see Chap. 107, "Emergency Delivery," by Michael J. VanRooyen and Kimberly B. Fortner.

64 VULVOVAGINITIS

David A. Krueger

EPIDEMIOLOGY

- Vulvovaginitis accounts for 10 million physician visits per year in the United States, and is the most common gynecologic complaint in prepubertal girls.[1]
- Bacterial vaginosis (BV) is the most common cause of malodorous discharge and is seen almost exclusively in women who have been sexually active. BV is associated with preterm labor and premature rupture of membranes (PROM).[2]
- *Candida* vaginitis will affect 75% of women at least once during their childbearing years.[3] Factors associated with increased rates of colonization include pregnancy, oral contraceptives, uncontrolled diabetes mellitus, and frequent visits to STD clinics. It is rare in premenarcheal girls and decreases in incidence after menopause unless hormone replacement therapy is used.
- *Trichomonas vaginalis* causes an STD that affects 2 to 3 million women annually. The prevalence correlates with overall sexual activity. It is associated with preterm delivery and PROM.[4] Seventy percent of men and eighty-five percent of women who have intercourse with an infected partner develop *Trichomonas* infection. There is a high prevalence of gonorrhea in women with *Trichomonas.*
- Genital herpes is sexually transmitted and is the most frequent cause of painful lesions of the lower genital tract in American women.

PATHOPHYSIOLOGY

- The pathophysiology of vulvovaginitis is related to inflammation of the vulva and vaginal tissues. Causes include infection, irritants and allergens, foreign bodies, and atrophy.
- In females of childbearing age, estrogen causes the development of a thick vaginal epithelium with glycogen stores that support the normal flora. The glycogen is converted by lactobacilli and acidogenic corynebacteria to lactic acid and acetic acid that forms the acidic environment (pH 3.5 to 4.1) that discourages the growth of pathogenic bacteria.
- Causes of infectious vulvovaginitis include: trichomoniasis, caused by *Trichomonas vaginalis;* bacterial vaginosis, caused by replacement of normal flora by overgrowth of both anaerobes and *Gardnerella vaginalis;* and candidiasis, usually caused by *Candida albicans.*
- Contact dermatitis results from exposure of vulvar epithelium and vaginal mucosa to chemical irritants or allergens. Secondary infections can occur.
- Foreign bodies left in place longer than 48 hours can cause severe localized infections from *Escherichia coli,* anaerobes, or overgrowth of other vaginal flora.
- Atrophic vaginitis during menarche, pregnancy, lactation, and after menopause results from the lack of estrogen stimulation on the vaginal mucosa, resulting in loss of normal rugae, atrophy of squamous epithelium, and increase in vaginal pH.

CLINICAL FEATURES

- Bacterial vaginosis causes vaginal discharge and pruritus. Examination findings range from mild vaginal redness to a frothy gray-white discharge.
- *Candida* vaginitis causes vaginal discharge, severe pruritus, dysuria, and dyspareunia. Examination reveals vulvar and vaginal erythema and edema, and thick "cottage cheese" discharge.
- *Trichomonas vaginalis* causes vaginal discharge, perineal irritation, dysuria, spotting, and pelvic pain. Examination reveals vaginal erythema and a frothy, malodorous discharge.
- Genital herpes causes painful, fluid-filled vesicles that progress to shallow-based ulcers. Local symptoms include dysuria and pelvic pain. Systemic symptoms such as fever, malaise, headache, and myalgias are common.
- Contact vulvovaginitis causes pruritus and a burning sensation. Examination reveals an edematous, erythematous vulvovaginal area.
- Vaginal foreign bodies can cause a bloody or foul-smelling discharge. Examination generally reveals the foreign body.

- Atrophic vaginitis causes vaginal soreness, dyspareunia, and occasional spotting or discharge. Examination reveals a thin, inflamed, and even ulcerated vaginal mucosa.

DIAGNOSIS AND DIFFERENTIAL

- A detailed gynecologic history should be obtained and a gynecologic exam should be performed.
- Microscopic evaluation of vaginal secretions using normal saline (demonstrating clue cells for BV and motile *T. vaginalis* for trichomoniasis) and 10% potassium hydroxide (KOH) (demonstrating yeast or pseudohyphae for candidiasis and fishy odor for BV) will frequently provide the diagnosis.
- Secretions should be tested for pH using nitrazine paper. A pH greater than 4.5 is typical of BV or trichomoniasis. A pH less than 4.5 is typical of physiologic discharge or a fungal infection.
- Bacterial vaginosis is diagnosed according to the Centers for Disease Control (CDC) by three of the following (1) discharge, (2) pH >4.5, (3) fishy odor when 10% KOH is added to the discharge (positive amine test result), and (4) clue cells, which are epithelial cells with clusters of bacilli stuck to the surface, seen on saline wet prep.[5]
- *Candida* vaginitis is diagnosed microscopically by the presence of yeast buds and pseudohyphae. Using a 10% KOH solution will dissolve the epithelial cells, making the findings easier to see. Sensitivity is 80%.
- Trichomoniasis is diagnosed microscopically by the presence of motile, pear-shaped, flagellated trichomonads that are slightly larger than leukocytes. Sensitivity is 40 to 80%.
- Genital herpes is diagnosed based on clinical suspicion, and is confirmed by either culture or polymerase chain reaction of fluid obtained from the ulcer or vesicle.
- Contact vulvovaginitis is diagnosed by ruling out an infectious cause and identifying the offending agent.
- On wet preparation, atrophic vaginitis will show erythrocytes and increased polymorphonuclear leukocytes (PMNs) associated with small, round epithelial cells, which are immature squamous cells that have not been exposed to sufficient estrogen.

EMERGENCY DEPARTMENT CARE AND DISPOSITION

- Bacterial vaginosis is treated with metronidazole 500 mg PO bid for 7 days or clindamycin 300 mg PO bid for 7 days. All symptomatic patients should be treated regardless of pregnancy status. All pregnant women, particularly those at high risk for preterm labor, should be treated because of the negative impact this infection has on pregnancy.[5] No treatment is necessary for male partners or asymptomatic women. If the patient is in the first trimester of pregnancy, treat with metronidazole 0.75%, one applicatorful intravaginally bid for 5 days.
- For trichomoniasis, metronidazole 2 g orally in a single dose is the treatment of choice (or alternatively 500 mg orally bid for 7 days). Metronidazole gel is much less effective, achieving cure in less than 50%.
- Oral metronidazole is still considered to be a class C agent in pregnancy by many authorities, and many clinicians avoid treatment during the first trimester. However, the CDC points out that multiple studies of metronidazole use in pregnancy have not demonstrated a consistent association with teratogenic or mutagenic effects. The CDC guidelines state that pregnant women may be treated with a single 2-gram oral dose of metronidazole.
- *Candida* vaginitis is treated with the topical imidazoles (butoconazole, clotrimazole, or miconazole cream applied topically for 3 to 7 days). Alternative treatment in the nonpregnant patient is fluconazole 150 mg PO.[5] Treatment of sexual partners is not necessary unless candidal balanitis is present.
- Genital herpes is treated by antiviral agents within 1 day of onset of symptoms to help control the symptoms and to accelerate healing of the lesions. Treatment is not curative and does not affect the frequency or severity of recurrences. Patients with severe disease may require hospitalization for IV therapy. Systemic analgesics may also be needed.
- Contact vulvovaginitis is treated by removal of the offending agent. Cool sitz baths and wet compresses of dilute boric acid or Burow's solution may provide some relief. Topical corticosteroids can also be used to relieve symptoms and promote healing.
- Vaginal foreign bodies require removal of the object. No other therapy is necessary.
- Atrophic vaginitis is treated with topical vaginal estrogen cream or tablets. Nightly use for 1 to 2 weeks should alleviate symptoms. Estrogen should not be used if there is a history of cancer of any of the reproductive organs or postmenopausal bleeding. Referral should be made to a gynecologist.

REFERENCES

1. Jaquiery A, Stylianopoulos A, Hogg G, et al: Vulvovaginitis: Clinical features, aetiology, and microbiology of the genital tract. *Arch Dis Child* 81:64, 1999.

2. French JI, McGregor JA, Draper D, et al: Gestational bleeding, bacterial vaginosis, and common reproductive tract infections: risk for preterm birth and benefit of treatment. *Obstet Gynecol* 93:715, 1999.
3. Sobel JD: Vaginitis. *N Engl J Med* 337:1896, 1997.
4. Fiscella K: Racial disparities in preterm births: The role of urogenital infections. *Public Health Rep* 111:104, 1996.
5. Centers for Disease Control and Prevention: 2002 guidelines for treatment of sexually transmitted diseases: Recommendations and reports. *Morb Mortal Wkly Rep* 51:1, 2002.

For further reading in *Emergency Medicine: A Comprehensive Study Guide,* 6th ed., see Chap. 108, "Vulvovaginitis," by Gloria J. Kuhn.

65 PELVIC INFLAMMATORY DISEASE AND TUBO-OVARIAN ABSCESS

Robert W. Shaffer

EPIDEMIOLOGY

- Pelvic inflammatory disease (PID) occurs at an annual rate of 10 to 20 cases per 1000 women of reproductive age.[1]
- Up to 25% of patients develop long-term sequelae which include infertility, ectopic pregnancy, and chronic pain.
- Ten to twenty percent of untreated gonococcal or chlamydial cervicitis may progress to PID.
- Risk factors include multiple sexual partners, sexual abuse, young age, HIV-1 infection, bacterial vaginosis, history of other STDs, frequent vaginal douching, and use of intrauterine devices (IUDs).[2–6]
- Risk is reduced with use of barrier contraception and pregnancy; however, PID can occur during the first trimester and may cause fetal loss.
- Bilateral tubal ligation does not confer protection from PID, but disease severity may be less.[7]

PATHOPHYSIOLOGY

- PID represents an ascending infection from the lower genital tract. The spectrum of disease includes salpingitis, endometritis, tubo-ovarian abscess (TOA), and peritonitis.
- *Neisseria gonorrhoeae* and/or *Chlamydia trachomatis* are isolated from almost all cases.
- At least 30 to 40% of infections are polymicrobial and include anaerobes, *Gardnerella vaginalis,* enteric gram-negative rods, *Haemophilus influenzae, Streptococcus agalactiae, Mycoplasma hominis,* and *Ureaplasma urealyticum.*[8,9] PID may result from *Mycoplasma tuberculosis* infection in endemic areas.[10]
- *N. gonorrhoeae* and *C. trachomatis* may be instrumental in the initial infection of the upper genital tract, whereas other bacterial species are isolated increasingly as inflammation increases and abscesses form.
- Infection may extend beyond the pelvis via direct or lymphatic spread to involve the hepatic capsule, resulting in perihepatitis and focal peritonitis (Fitz-Hugh–Curtis syndrome).

CLINICAL FEATURES

- Lower abdominal pain is the most common presenting complaint.
- Other common symptoms include abnormal vaginal discharge, vaginal bleeding, postcoital bleeding, dyspareunia, irritative voiding symptoms, fever, malaise, nausea, and vomiting. However, PID may produce minimal or no symptoms.[11]
- Physical exam findings include lower abdominal tenderness, mucopurulent cervicitis, cervical motion tenderness, and uterine and/or adnexal tenderness. Peritoneal signs may be present.
- Unilateral adnexal tenderness and palpable fullness or mass may indicate TOA.
- Right upper quadrant tenderness, especially with jaundice, suggests Fitz-Hugh–Curtis syndrome.

DIAGNOSIS AND DIFFERENTIAL

- PID is a clinical diagnosis (Table 65-1).
- Laboratory evaluation should include a pregnancy test, wet prep, and endocervical swabs for gonorrhea and chlamydia. Elevations in white blood cell count, erythrocyte sedimentation rate, and C-reactive protein help support the diagnosis of PID.
- Transvaginal pelvic ultrasound is used to detect TOA, which appears as a complex adnexal mass with multiple internal echoes.
- Procedures such as endometrial biopsy, culdocentesis, and laparoscopy may facilitate or confirm the diagnosis; however, their utility in the emergency department setting is limited.
- The differential diagnosis includes cervicitis, ectopic pregnancy, endometriosis, ovarian cyst, ovarian torsion, spontaneous abortion, septic abortion, cholecystitis, gastroenteritis, appendicitis, diverticulitis, pyelonephritis, and renal colic.

TABLE 65-1   Treatment Guidelines for PID Based on Diagnostic Criteria

Group 1: Minimum criteria
Empirical treatment indicated if no other etiology to explain findings
Uterine or adnexal tenderness
Cervical motion tenderness

Group 2: Additional criteria improving diagnostic specificity
Oral temperature >101°F (38.3°C)
Abnormal cervical or vaginal mucopurulent secretions
Elevated erythrocyte sedimentation rate
Elevated C-reactive protein
Laboratory evidence of cervical infection with *N. gonorrhoeae* or *C. trachomatis* (ie, culture or DNA probe techniques)

Group 3: Specific criteria for PID based on procedures that may be appropriate for some patients
Laparoscopic confirmation
Transvaginal ultrasound (or MRI) showing thickened, fluid-filled tubes with/without free pelvic fluid or tubo-ovarian complex
Endometrial biopsy showing endometritis

SOURCE: Adapted from CDC.[11]

EMERGENCY DEPARTMENT CARE AND DISPOSITION

- Analgesia and IV hydration should be given as needed.
- Immediate initiation of broad-spectrum antibiotics improves long-term outcomes.[11] See Tables 65-2 and 65-3 for treatment options as recommended by the Centers for Disease Control and Prevention.
- Any IUD must be removed after antibiotics are started.
- Sixty to eighty percent of TOAs resolve with antibiotics alone. The remainder require drainage.
- The decision for hospitalization should be made based on severity of illness, inability to tolerate PO medications/fluids, likelihood of anaerobic infection (IUD use, suspected abscess, recent instrumentation), uncertainty of diagnosis, immunosuppression, pregnancy, patient age, fertility issues, or concerns for compliance.[12]

TABLE 65-2   Parenteral Treatment Regimens for PID

1. Cefotetan 2 g IV q12h *or* cefoxitin 2 g IV q6h
   +
   Doxycycline 100 mg IV/PO q12h
2. Clindamycin 900 mg IV q8h
   +
   Gentamicin 2 mg/kg IV loading dose followed by 1.5 mg/kg q8h
3. Ofloxacin 400 mg IV q12h *or* levofloxacin 500 mg IV q24h
   +
   Doxycycline 100 mg PO or IV q12h
   ±
   Metronidazole 500 mg IV q8h *or* ampicillin-sulbactam 3 g IV q6h

SOURCE: Adapted from the CDC.[11]

TABLE 65-3   Oral/Outpatient Treatment Regimens for PID

1. Ofloxacin 400 mg PO bid for 14 days *or* levofloxacin 500 mg PO qd for 14 days
   ±
   Metronidazole 500 mg PO bid for 14 days
2. Ceftriaxone 250 mg IM × 1 *or* cefoxitin 2 g IM × 1 *and* probenecid 1 g PO × 1
   +
   Doxycycline 100 mg PO bid for 14 days
   ±
   Metronidazole 500 mg PO bid for 14 days

SOURCE: Adapted from the CDC.[11]

- Patients started on IV antibiotics may be switched to oral treatment 24 hours after clinical improvement. With outpatient treatment, patients should be followed-up within 72 hours to assess substantial response to antibiotic therapy and compliance.
- Patients should be educated regarding prevention, compliance, and the need to have all sexual partners treated. Appropriate referrals for further STD testing including HIV and syphilis should be provided.

REFERENCES

1. Rein DB, Kassler WJ, Irwin KL, et al: Direct medical cost of pelvic inflammatory disease and its sequelae: Decreasing but still substantial. *Obstet Gynecol* 95:397, 2000.
2. Marks C, Tideman RL, Estcourt CS, et al: Assessment of risk for pelvic inflammatory disease in an urban sexual health population. *Sex Transm Infect* 76:470, 2000.
3. Ness RB, Soper DE, Holley RL, et al: Douching and endometritis: Results from the PID Evaluation and Clinical Health (PEACH) study. *Sex Transm Dis* 28:240, 2001.
4. Champion JD, Piper J, Shain R, et al: Minority women with sexually transmitted diseases, sexual abuse and risk for pelvic inflammatory disease. *Res Nurs Health* 24:38, 2001.
5. Dayal M, Barnhart RT: Noncontraceptive benefits and therapeutic uses of the oral contraceptive pill. *Semin Reprod Med* 19:295, 2001.
6. Shelton, JD: Risk of clinical pelvic inflammatory disease attributable to an intrauterine device. *Lancet* 357:443, 2001.
7. Levgur M, Duvivier R: Pelvic inflammatory disease after tubal sterilization: A review. *Obstet Gynecol Surv* 55:41, 2001.
8. Mcneeley SG, Hendrix SL, Mezzoni MM, et al: Medically sound, cost-effective treatment for pelvic inflammatory disease and tuboovarian abscess. *Am J Obstet Gynecol* 178: 1272, 1998.
9. Peipert JF, Montagno AB, Cooper AS, Sung CJ: Bacterial vaginosis as a risk factor for upper genital infection. *Am J Obstet Gynecol* 177:1184, 1997.
10. Avan BI, Fatmi Z, Rashid S: Comparison of the clinical and laparoscopic features of infertile women suffering from genital tuberculosis (TB) or pelvic inflammatory disease or endometriosis. *J Pakistan Med Assoc* 51:393, 2001.

11. Centers for Disease Control and Prevention: 2002 Guidelines for treatment of sexually transmitted diseases. *Morb Mortal Wkly Rep* 51(RR-6):1, 2002.
12. Peipert JF, Ness RB, Blume J, et al: Clinical predictors of endometritis in women without symptoms and signs of pelvic inflammatory disease. *Am J Obstet Gynecol* 184:856, 2001.

For further reading in *Emergency Medicine: A Comprehensive Study Guide,* 6th ed., see Chap. 109, "Pelvic Inflammatory Disease," by Amy J. Behrman, William H. Shoff, and Suzanne M. Shepherd.

66 COMPLICATIONS OF GYNECOLOGIC PROCEDURES

Debra Houry

- The most common reasons for emergency department visits during the postoperative period following gynecologic procedures are pain, fever, and vaginal bleeding. A focused but thorough evaluation should be performed including cervical cultures and bimanual examination. (Complications common to gynecologic and general surgery are covered in Chap. 52.)

COMMON COMPLICATIONS OF ENDOSCOPIC PROCEDURES

LAPAROSCOPY

- The incidence of major complications of laparoscopy in the United States is low, with visceral injuries occurring 2.5% of the time in gynecologic procedures and major vascular injuries 0.15% of the time (20% of these vascular injuries are fatal).[1]
- The overall incidence of complications in major operative laparoscopy is 10.4%.[2]
- The major complications associated with the use of the laparoscope are the following: (1) thermal injuries to the bowel; (2) bleeding at the site of tubal interruption or sharp dissection; (3) incisional hernia; and (4) rarely, ureteral or bladder injury, large bowel injury, and pelvic hematoma or abscess.
- Of these complications, the most serious and dreaded is that of thermal injury to the bowel. These patients generally appear 3 to 7 days postoperatively, depending upon the degree of necrosis, with signs and symptoms of peritonitis, including bilateral lower abdominal pain, fever, elevated white blood cell (WBC)

count, and direct and rebound tenderness. Although gas has been used to insufflate the abdomen, it should be absorbed totally within 3 postoperative days.
- Patients who have increasing pain after laparoscopy, either early or late, have a bowel injury until proved otherwise. If thermal injury is a serious consideration and cannot be distinguished from other causes of peritonitis, it is best to err on the side of early laparotomy.

HYSTEROSCOPY

- Complications of hysteroscopy occur in approximately 2% of cases including the following: (1) reaction to the distending media, (2) uterine perforation, (3) cervical laceration, (4) anesthesia reaction, (5) intra-abdominal organ injury, (6) infection, and (7) postoperative bleeding.[3]
- Postoperative bleeding will be the most likely cause of hospital revisit. After hemodynamic stabilization of the patient, the gynecologist can insert a pediatric Foley or balloon catheter to tamponade the bleeding.

MISCELLANEOUS COMPLICATIONS OF MAJOR GYNECOLOGIC PROCEDURES

CUFF CELLULITIS

- **Cuff cellulitis** refers to infections of the contiguous retroperitoneal space immediately above the vaginal apex and including the surrounding soft tissue. It is a common complication following both abdominal and vaginal hysterectomy.
- It usually produces a fever between postoperative days 3 and 5. These patients complain of fever, pelvic pain, and abnormal vaginal discharge. Pelvic tenderness and induration are prominent during the bimanual examination. A vaginal cuff abscess may be palpable.
- The treatment of choice is readmission, drainage, and intravenous antibiotics as determined by the gynecologist.

PELVIC ABSCESS

- Patients who present with fever and abdominal or pelvic pain shortly after hospital discharge for pelvic surgery may have a pelvic (usually ovarian) abscess.
- Sudden increase in pain may indicate ruptured abscess, a surgical emergency.
- The treatment of choice is readmission, drainage, and intravenous antibiotics as determined by the gynecologist.

POSTCONIZATION BLEEDING

- The most common complication associated with LEEP (loop electrical excision procedure) or cold-knife conization of the cervix is bleeding. If delayed hemorrhage occurs, it usually occurs 7 days postoperatively. Bleeding following this procedure can be rapid and excessive. Visualization of the cervix is the key to controlling such bleeding.
- Application of Monsel's solution is a reasonable first step if it is easily available; otherwise cauterization with silver nitrate may be attempted.
- Usually suturing of the bleeding arteriole is necessary. Quite often the patient must be taken to the operating room for repair secondary to poor visualization.

INDUCED ABORTION

- Causes for bleeding and pain within 24 hours of an abortion are retained products of conception, uterine perforation, and cervical lacerations; delayed complications (up to 4 weeks) are due to retained products of conception and endometritis.[4]
- Cervical lacerations can be treated with direct pressure and application of Monsel's solution or silver nitrate.
- Patients with a firm, boggy uterus should have a sonogram to look for retained products. IV antibiotics and repeat D&C are usually necessary if retained products are suspected.
- If the patient has pain, bleeding, or both—but unaccompanied by fever—missed ectopic pregnancy must be ruled out.

VESICOVAGINAL FISTULAS

- Vesicovaginal fistulas may occur after total vaginal hysterectomy. Patients return 10 to 14 days after surgery with watery vaginal discharge. Gynecologic consultation is necessary.

ASSISTED REPRODUCTIVE TECHNOLOGY

- Complications related to ultrasound-guided retrieval of oocytes are rare and include ovarian hyperstimulation syndrome, pelvic infections, intraperitoneal bleeding, and adnexal torsions.[5,6]

- Ovarian hyperstimulation syndrome can be a life-threatening complication of induction of ovulation. The incidence of the moderate-to-severe form is 1 to 2%.
- Symptoms include abdominal distention, ovarian enlargement, and weight gain in the mildest form. In the most severe form, patients have massive third-spacing of fluids into the abdominal cavity, which can lead to ascites, electrolyte imbalances, pleural effusions, and hypovolemia.
- Abdominal and pelvic examinations are contraindicated due to extremely fragile ovaries that are at high risk of rupture or hemorrhage.
- Electrolyte studies, renal function tests, a complete blood count, coagulation studies, and blood for type and cross-match should be obtained. An electrocardiogram to evaluate potential hyperkalemic changes should also be obtained.
- The gynecologist should be consulted for admission.

REFERENCES

1. Rein H: Complications and litigation in gynecologic endoscopy. *Curr Opin Obstet Gynecol* 13:425, 2001.
2. Saidi MH, Vancaillie TG, White AJ, et al: Complications of major operative laparoscopy: A review of 452 cases. *J Reprod Med* 41:471, 1996.
3. Hulka JF, Peterson JB, Phillips JM, Surrey MW: Operative hysteroscopy: American Association of Gynecologic Laparoscopists 1991 membership survey. *J Reprod Med* 38:572, 1993.
4. Hakim-Elahi E, Tovell HMM, Burnhhill MS: Complications of first trimester abortion: A report of 170,000 cases. *Obstet Gynecol* 76:129, 1990.
5. Dicker D, Ashkenazi J, Feldberg D, et al: Severe abdominal complications after transvaginal ultrasonographically guided retrieval of oocytes for in vitro fertilization and embryo transfer. *Fertil Steril* 59:1313, 1993.
6. Govaerts I, Devreker F, Delbaere A, et al: Short-term medical complications of 1500 oocyte retrievals for in-vitro fertilization and embryo transfer. *Eur J Obstet Gynecol Reprod Biol* 77:239, 1998.

For further reading in *Emergency Medicine: A Comprehensive Study Guide,* 6th ed., see Chap. 112, "Complications of Gynecologic Procedures," by Michael A. Silverman and Karen M. Hardart.

67 FEVER

Douglas K. Holtzman

EPIDEMIOLOGY

- In the pediatric population, fever is the most common chief complaint presenting to an emergency department and accounts for 30% of outpatient visits each year.

PATHOPHYSIOLOGY

- Fever is the result of the body's thermostat being reset by exogenous pyrogens, such as bacteria, bacterial endotoxins, antigen-antibody complexes, and viruses, which stimulate the production of endogenous pyrogens.
- The thermostat is thought to be located in the preoptic region of the anterior hypothalamus located near the floor of the third ventricle.
- Once reset, the body attempts to adjust to the higher setting by undergoing peripheral vasoconstriction, shivering, central pooling, and (if able) behavioral activity such as putting on more clothing or seeking a warmer environment.[1]

CLINICAL FEATURES

- It has long been argued that "fever is good" and should be allowed to persist. Most children, however, feel uncomfortable and certain children are at risk for febrile seizures, thus fever is generally treated.
- Present pediatric guidelines consider any rectal temperature $\geq 38°C$ (100.4°F) to be a fever and warrants an evaluation.[2]

- In general, higher temperatures are associated with a higher incidence of bacteremia.[3]

DIAGNOSIS AND DIFFERENTIAL

INFANTS UP TO 3 MONTHS OLD

- Early studies suggested that infants under the age of 3 months were at high risk of a serious bacterial infection (SBI). Today, practice guidelines use 0 to 8 weeks of age, with some using an upper limit of 6 weeks.[4,5]
- Febrile infants less than 1 month old are at the greatest risk, with an average risk of 13% for bacteremia. During their second month, the risk of bacteremia is about 10%.[6]
- Young infants are especially problematic in assessing severity of illness based on clinical exam because of lack of development of social skills and inability to communicate with the examiner.
- The birth history is important to obtain as some of the etiologies of infection may be related to that time.
- Poor feeding, irritability, lethargy, or temperature instability suggest a potentially serious bacterial illness.[7]
- Infants lack reliable exam findings of meningitis such as nuchal rigidity, and often present with inconsolable crying or irritability.
- A history of cough, tachypnea, or hypoxia should alert the examiner to a possible lower respiratory tract infection and indicate the need for a chest x-ray.
- The general recommendations for laboratory evaluation to detect a SBI include a complete blood count (CBC) with differential, blood culture, catheterized urinalysis with culture, and lumbar puncture. A chest x-ray and stool culture are performed when dictated by history or physical exam.[8]
- Accurately identifying the high-risk infant is difficult in this age group, but certain criteria when collectively

assessed have been shown to help identify those at low risk.

- These criteria include: well-appearing without a history of prematurity, white blood cell count (WBC) between 5000 and 15,000/mm^3, absolute neutrophil count (ANC) less than 10000/μL, urinalysis with less than 10 WBC per high powered field (hpf),[9] and stool with less than 5 WBC/hpf in infants with diarrhea.[10,11]
- Management of infants at low risk remains a subject of significant debate. It is generally considered appropriate to treat and hospitalize all infants less than 1 month old. Ceftriaxone (50 mg/kg) pending culture results is typically recommended, with cefotaxime (50 mg/kg) used in infants less than 1 week old.
- Low-risk infants 4 to 8 weeks old may be managed with hospitalization and ceftriaxone (50 mg/kg) pending culture results, hospitalization alone, ceftriaxone (50 mg/kg) and discharged home, or discharged home with no antibiotics. Discharged patients must be able to follow-up in 24 hours.[12]

INFANTS 3 TO 24 MONTHS OLD

- Physical exam findings appear to be more reliable in this age group. The willingness to make eye contact, alertness, response to noxious stimuli, ability to be consoled, and playfulness are important findings in the examination.
- Viral illnesses including pneumonia account for the majority of febrile illnesses in this age group.
- Of the bacterial etiologies, *Streptococcus pneumoniae* is the most common, with *Haemophilus influenzae* now an uncommon organism since the institution of the HIB vaccine.[13]
- Otitis media is typically caused by *Streptococcus pneumoniae* or nontypeable *H. influenzae*.
- Although pneumonia is commonly caused by viral etiologies, it is considered appropriate to institute antibiotic coverage (primarily for *S. pneumoniae*; see Chap. 73).
- The typical meningitic symptoms of nuchal rigidity and Kernig's or Brudzinski's signs may not be apparent in children less than 2 years old. Seizure activity, inconsolability, bulging fontanelle, or irritability may be the only signs.
- The most common organism causing occult bacteremia is *Streptococcus pneumoniae*. Of those children ages 3 to 36 months with *S. pneumoniae* bacteremia, only 0.019% develop meningitis.[14]

OLDER FEBRILE CHILDREN

- The risk for bacteremia in children over 3 years of age is significantly low.

- Other etiologies to consider include streptococcal pharyngitis (particularly between the ages of 5 and 10 years old), mononucleosis, or pneumonia which may be caused by *S. pneumoniae* or *Mycoplasma pneumoniae*. See Chap. 73 for treatment recommendations.

EMERGENCY DEPARTMENT CARE AND DISPOSITION

- Current recommendations for treating suspected occult bacteremia include ceftriaxone (50 mg/kg) or amoxicillin (45 mg/kg twice daily) with a 24-hour follow-up regardless of the therapy chosen.
- **Note:** Ceftriaxone should never be initiated without appropriate antecedent or coincident diagnostic studies.[15]
- Fever may be reduced by use of acetaminophen 10 to 15 mg/kg given every 4 hours (maximum of 5 doses in 24 hours). Some clinicians advocate the use of 40 to 45 mg/kg as an initial loading dose when using it rectally.
- Alternatively, ibuprofen may be given at 5 to 10 mg/kg every 6 hours (maximum of 40 mg/kg/24 hours).
- Slowly sponging the child with tepid water will reduce fever by evaporation.
- Aspirin should be avoided in children due to the possible link between it and Reye's syndrome.
- All children with positive blood cultures should be recalled for a repeat evaluation. If the patient is afebrile and clinically well, they should complete a 10-day course of antibiotic therapy.
- If the child with a positive blood culture remains febrile or is ill-appearing, a full septic evaluation (complete blood count [CBC], blood culture, lumbar puncture, urine culture, and chest x-ray) should be performed. The patient should be hospitalized and receive parenteral antibiotics.[16]

REFERENCES

1. Kluger MJ: Fever revisited. *Pediatrics* 90:846, 1992.
2. Baraff LJ, Bass JW, Fleisher GR, et al: Practice guidelines for the management of infants and children 0-36 months of age with fever without source. *Ann Emerg Med* 22:1198, 1993.
3. McCarthy PL, Jekel JF, Dolan TF: Temperature less than or equal to 40°C in children less than 24 months of age: A prospective study. *Pediatrics* 59:663, 1977.
4. Roberts KB: Fever in the first eight weeks of life. *Johns Hopkins Med J* 141:9, 1977.
5. McCarthy PL, Dolan TF: Hyperpyrexia in children. *Am J Dis Child* 130:849, 1976.
6. Baker MD, Bell LM, Avner JR: Outpatient management without antibiotics of fever in selected infants. *N Engl J Med* 324:1437, 1993.

7. Krober MS, Bass JW, Powell JM, et al: Bacterial and viral pathogens causing fever in infants less than 3 months old. *Am J Dis Child* 139:889, 1985.

8. Berkowitz CD, Uchiyama N, Tully SB, et al: Fever in infants less than two months of age: Spectrum of disease and predictors of outcome. *Pediatr Emerg Care* 1:128, 1985.

9. Hoberman A, Wald ER: Urinary tract infections in young febrile children. *Pediatr Infect Dis J* 16:11, 1997.

10. Dagan R, Powell KR, Hall CD, et al: Identification of infants unlikely to have serious bacterial infection although hospitalized for suspected sepsis. *J Pediatr* 107:855, 1985.

11. Dagan R, Sofer S, Phillip M, Shachak E: Ambulatory care of febrile infants younger than 2 months of age classified as being at low risk for having bacterial infections. *J Pediatr* 112:355, 1987.

12. Lieu TA, Baskin MN, Schwartz S, Fleisher GR: Clinical and cost-effectiveness of outpatient strategies for management of febrile infants. *Pediatrics* 89:1135, 1992.

13. Giebink GS: The prevention of pneumococcal disease in children. *N Engl J Med* 345:1177, 2001.

14. Baker MD, Bell LM, Avner JR: The efficacy of routine outpatient management of fever without antibiotics in selected infants. *Pediatrics* 92:524, 1999.

15. Fleisher GR, Rosenberg N, Vinci R, et al: Intramuscular versus oral antibiotic therapy for the prevention of meningitis and other bacterial sequelae in young febrile children at risk for occult bacteremia. *J Pediatr* 124:504, 1994.

16. McCarthy PL, Dolan TF: The serious implications of high fever in infants during their first three months. *Clin Pediatr* 15:794, 1976.

For further reading in *Emergency Medicine: A Comprehensive Study Guide*, 6th ed., see Chap. 115, "Fever," by Carol D. Berkowitz.

68 BACTEREMIA, SEPSIS, AND MENINGITIS IN CHILDREN
Milan D. Nadkarni

BACTEREMIA

- The identification of bacteremia and the management of infants and young children with fever and no identifiable source of infection on initial presentation is currently an area of great controversy.

EPIDEMIOLOGY

- The risk of bacteremia in well-appearing children aged 3 to 36 months with temperatures of 39°C (102.2°F) or higher is 1.6%.[1] This rate has fallen significantly since the advent of the *Haemophilus influenzae* type b (Hib) immunization.
- Neonates with a temperature of 38°C or higher have a 5% risk of bacteremia and a 15% risk of a serious bacterial infection.[2]
- Children aged 3 to 36 months with fever and a recognizable viral syndrome (including croup, varicella, bronchiolitis, and stomatitis) were found to have an even lower risk of bacteremia (0 to 1.1%).[3]

PATHOPHYSIOLOGY

- Bacteremia is present when pathogenic bacteria are present in the blood.
- The term **occult bacteremia** is used when a patient presents without a clinically identifiable source of infection at initial presentation, but the blood culture is subsequently positive.
- Infants and young children are thought to be at increased risk for bacteremia due to their immature reticuloendothelial system. The likelihood of various organisms is age dependent.
- Neonates are at risk for bacteremia and resultant sepsis from organisms acquired around the time of birth. These include group B *Streptococcus, Escherichia coli, Listeria monocytogenes,* and enterococcus species. Risk factors include premature delivery, ruptured amniotic membranes more than 24 hours prior to delivery, and maternal amnionitis.
- In older infants and children, *Streptococcus pneumoniae* accounts for more than 90% of occult bacteremia with *Neisseria meningitidis,* group A *Streptococcus,* and *Salmonella* responsible for the remainder. *Haemophilus influenzae* type b was a significant cause of bacteremia, but has been nearly eliminated since vaccination against this organism began in the early 1990s.[4]

CLINICAL FEATURES

- By definition, occult bacteremia has only fever and a well appearance.
- The presence of croup, bronchiolitis, and uncomplicated varicella makes bacteremia very unlikely.[3]
- The presence of otitis media does not appear to change the risk of bacteremia.[5]

DIAGNOSIS AND DIFFERENTIAL

- The diagnosis of bacteremia is made by blood culture, the results of which are not available during the initial emergency department visit.

- Other tests such as the complete blood count (CBC), erythrocyte sedimentation rate, and C-reactive protein are neither sensitive nor specific.[6-8]
- A greater elevation in temperature does correlate with a higher risk of bacteremia, but even with temperatures of 41°C or higher, most well-appearing children are not bacteremic.[9]

EMERGENCY DEPARTMENT CARE AND DISPOSITION

- All febrile infants under 6 weeks of age should undergo a septic work-up, be given intravenous (IV) antibiotics (Table 68-1), and be admitted to the hospital.
- Febrile infants 6 to 12 weeks of age may not require a full septic evaluation if they have no risk factors, have reliable caretakers, and follow up can be arranged within 12 hours. Acceptable options are:
  - Perform a CBC, blood culture, catheter urinalysis, culture and sensitivities (C&S), but give no antibiotics and follow up within 12 hours.
  - Perform a complete septic work-up including lumbar puncture, give ceftriaxone 50 mg/kg intramuscularly (IM), and follow up in 12 hours.
  - Perform a complete septic work-up including lumbar puncture, give no antibiotics, and follow up in 12 hours.
  - Perform a complete septic work-up including lumbar puncture, admit to the hospital, and give IV antibiotics.
- Indications for empiric antibiotic treatment for occult bacteremia include: temperature >39°C (102.2°F) in children between 3 months and 36 months of age, WBC >15,000/μL or <5000/μL, absolute neutrophil count >10,000/μL (regardless of the total white count), and >10% band count (regardless of the total white count).

TABLE 68-1   Initial Intravenous Antibiotic Therapy for Sepsis and Meningitis

AGE	SEPSIS*	MENINGITIS
<60 days	Ampicillin 100 mg/kg plus Cefotaxime 50 mg/kg consider acyclovir 20–30 mg/kg†	Ampicillin 100 mg/kg plus Cefotaxime 50 mg/kg consider acyclovir 20–30 mg/kg
2 months and older	Cefotaxime 50 mg/kg or Ceftriaxone 50 mg/kg plus consider vancomycin 15 mg/kg‡	Cefotaxime 100 mg/kg or Ceftriaxone 100 mg/kg plus vancomycin 15 mg/kg

*Use meningitis doses if the patient is considered too unstable for lumbar puncture.
†Consider acyclovir for patients with CSF pleocytosis or neonatal seizures.
‡Consider addition of vancomycin in sepsis with critical illness.

- There is considerable debate about the choice of empiric antibiotic treatment of occult bacteremia.[10] Options include:
  - Ceftriaxone 50 mg/kg IV/IM 3 1, which effectively covers the patient until culture results are available. There is good evidence that this action prevents sequelae.
  - Ceftriaxone as above plus amoxicillin (80 mg/kg/day divided tid) for 7 days. This action provides presumptive treatment, as cultures can sometimes be negative even if bacteremia is present.
  - Oral amoxicillin only (80 mg/kg/day divided bid or tid). There is debate about whether this prevents meningitis and other sequelae.
- All children who are presumptively treated for occult bacteremia should have a follow-up at 24 and 48 hours.
- If the child is toxic appearing at follow-up, perform a lumbar puncture, repeat blood cultures, and admit for IV antibiotics.
- If the child appears nontoxic but febrile at follow-up, give a second dose of ceftriaxone with another follow-up appointment in 24 hours.
- If the child appears nontoxic and afebrile, no further treatment may be required, or a second dose of ceftriaxone may be administered while awaiting cultures.

SEPSIS

EPIDEMIOLOGY

- Sepsis is an infectious inflammatory syndrome with clinical evidence of infection that may include focal infections and meningitis. Multiorgan failure and death may rapidly develop. The clinical situations in which sepsis may develop or be suspected are quite varied and therefore the true incidence is not well described.

PATHOPHYSIOLOGY

- The progression from bacteremia to sepsis is related to colonization with a bacterial pathogen (usually nasopharyngeal), invasion of the blood by encapsulated organisms, the release of inflammatory mediators, and failure of host defenses.
- Risk factors include impaired splenic function, congenital metabolic disease, humoral or cellular immunodeficiency states, presence of an indwelling foreign body (eg, central venous catheter), and obstruction to drainage of a body cavity.
- The likelihood of various pathogens as the etiologic agent for sepsis is age dependent (Table 68-2).

TABLE 68-2   Common Organisms Causing Sepsis and Meningitis

AGE	ORGANISMS
0–2 months	Group B *Streptococcus* *Escherichia coli* *Listeria monocytogenes*
2 months to 5 years	*Streptococcus pneumoniae* *Neisseria meningitidis* β-Hemolytic *Streptococcus* *Haemophilus influenzae* b* *Rickettsia rickettsii*† *Salmonella* spp. (gastroenteritis) *Escherichia coli* (pyelonephritis)

*Marked decline in cases since introduction of Hib vaccine; consider in those who are unimmunized.

†Etiologic agent for Rocky Mountain spotted fever, seen in endemic areas following tick bites with sumer/fall predominance.

CLINICAL FEATURES

- Sepsis is a clinical diagnosis. The clinical findings of advanced sepsis are related to alteration in functioning of end organs, including the brain, heart, blood vessels, lungs, kidneys, and skin.
- Sepsis may present early and more subtly or obvious and late. Clinical deterioration may be very rapid.
- Neurologic symptoms include altered mental status with irritability, confusion, or lethargy. A history of poor feeding, a lack of spontaneous motor activity, and hypotonia are common.
- Fever is typical. Infants younger than 3 months of age may be hypothermic, a grave prognostic finding.
- Tachypnea and respiratory distress with retractions may develop due to hypoxia or metabolic acidosis.
- In early septic shock, the cardiovascular system responds with resting tachycardia, warm distal extremities, and brisk capillary refill. In later stages of septic shock, circulatory collapse ensues with weak distal pulses, delayed capillary refill, and cool extremities. Hypotension is a very late, very ominous sign in young children.
- Skin findings may include petechiae that may progress to coalescent purpura, particularly in meningococcal disease.
- Poor renal perfusion typically leads to oliguria and then anuria.

DIAGNOSIS AND DIFFERENTIAL

- The diagnosis of sepsis is based on clinical appearance. A positive blood culture is generally expected, but not necessary for this clinical diagnosis.
- A child with a toxic appearance should be considered septic and appropriately treated with antibiotics promptly. However, in addition to infectious etiologies, the differential diagnosis of the septic appearing infant and child includes toxicologic ingestion, cardiac disease (eg, myocarditis), trauma (eg, shaken-baby syndrome), and metabolic etiologies (eg, previously unrecognized inborn errors of metabolism).
- The peripheral white blood cell count is typically elevated but may be normal.

EMERGENCY DEPARTMENT CARE AND DISPOSITION

- Treatment of shock takes precedence over the diagnostic work-up.
- The administration of high-flow oxygen, the initiation of cardiac monitoring, and the placement of intravenous or intraosseous access are important first steps.
- Endotracheal intubation may be required for respiratory failure.
- Fluid resuscitation with 20-mL/kg boluses of normal saline should be administered.
- Dopamine may be necessary to support perfusion after three to four fluid boluses.
- Hypoglycemia should be identified and treated.
- Broad-spectrum antibiotics should be administered as soon as access is available (and after the blood culture if possible). The administration of antibiotics should not be delayed awaiting lab test results or lumbar puncture.
- Antibiotic selection is empiric and age based (see Table 68-1).

MENINGITIS

EPIDEMIOLOGY

- Since the advent of the *Haemophilus influenzae* type b (Hib) vaccine, the epidemiology of meningitis in the United States has changed dramatically. In 1986 the median age for all patients with meningitis was 15 months. In 1995 the median age was 25 years.[11] Meningitis has shifted from being predominantly a disease of infants and young children to a disease predominantly of adults.

PATHOPHYSIOLOGY

- Typically, meningitis is a complication of primary bacteremia. It is thought that the products of bacterial multiplication alter the permeability of the blood-brain barrier and extend the infection to the brain and surrounding cerebrospinal fluid spaces.

- Less commonly, meningitis may result from hematogenous spread from a distant primary focal infection, direct extension from adjacent infection, or following cribriform plate or sinus fracture.
- The neurologic damage that sometimes follows meningitis is thought to result from direct inflammatory effects, brain edema, increased intracranial pressure, decreased cerebral blood flow, and vascular thrombosis.
- Impaired splenic function and immunosuppression or immunodeficiency is associated with a relatively higher risk of meningitis.
- The bacterial agents responsible for meningitis vary with age. Group B streptococci, *Escherichia coli,* and *Listeria monocytogenes* predominate in neonates. *Streptococcus pneumoniae* and *Neisseria meningitidis* are most common in older infants and children.

CLINICAL FEATURES

- The presentation of meningitis is age dependent.
- Neonates often present with nonspecific signs and symptoms. Symptoms may include decreased responsiveness, poor feeding, vomiting, fever (or normothermia or hypothermia), a bulging fontanelle, or apparent respiratory distress. Paradoxical irritability is present when the infant prefers to be lying still (resting the meninges) rather than held or rocked.
- In infants outside of the neonatal age range, generalized lethargy and a toxic appearance is typical. Nuchal rigidity is not generally appreciable until the patient reaches the toddler age group.
- Older children present more like adults with headache, photophobia, neck stiffness, nausea, vomiting, and fever.
- *Neisseria meningitidis* meningitis may lead to a fulminant, rapid progression to shock and death over a period of hours.
- Seizures may present in as many as 25% of patients with bacterial meningitis, and although usually generalized, may be focal.[12]
- Pretreatment with oral antibiotics may mute the presenting symptoms and lead to a longer duration of symptoms before diagnosis.

DIAGNOSIS AND DIFFERENTIAL

- The diagnosis of meningitis is made by analysis of cerebrospinal fluid (CSF) obtained from a lumbar puncture. A CSF leukocytosis with a preponderance of polymorphonucleocytes, a CSF protein greater than 100 mg/mL, and a CSF glucose level less than 50% of the blood glucose level are suggestive of a bacterial source of meningitis. A Gram's stain is considered 70% sensitive for identifying a causative bacterial agent.
- Other conditions that may present similarly to bacterial meningitis include sepsis without meningitis, intracranial mass lesions, aseptic meningitis, trauma, cardiac or respiratory failure, toxic ingestion, and metabolic abnormalities.
- If there is a CSF leukocytosis and the patient has previously been on antibiotics, bacterial antigen testing of the CSF may be helpful in making an accurate diagnosis of partially treated meningitis.[13]
- Unusual organisms have a higher likelihood of causing meningitis in immunocompromised patients.

EMERGENCY DEPARTMENT CARE AND DISPOSITION

- Critically ill children should be treated as indicated in the section on sepsis above.
- Rapid administration of antibiotics is critical to maximize the likelihood of a good neurologic outcome for the patient. In critically ill or toxic-appearing infants and children, antibiotic administration should not be delayed for computed tomographic (CT) scan of the head or lumbar puncture.
- The empiric antibiotic selection is based on the likely organism, that is in turn based on age. Doses are generally higher when meningitis is suspected to enhance drug penetration across the blood-brain barrier. Neonates should be given intravenous ampicillin and cefotaxime. Ceftriaxone should be avoided in neonates because it is known to cause kernicterus. Consider acyclovir for the treatment of all neonates who present with seizures, are ill-appearing, or have CSF pleocytosis. Infants and children should be given intravenous cefotaxime or ceftriaxone. Vancomycin should be added to all critically-ill-appearing infants or if the CSF is suspicious for meningitis.
- The use of steroids (dexamethasone) has been controversial and its use has decreased markedly because of the decreased incidence of *Haemophilus influenzae* type b. Steroids have been implicated in a worse neurologic outcome in patients with pneumococcal or meningococcal meningitis.[12]

REFERENCES

1. Lee GM, Harper MB: Risk of bacteremia for febrile young children in the post-*Haemophilus influenzae* type b era. *Arch Pediatr Adolesc Med* 152:624, 1998.

2. Bonadio WA, Webster H, Wolfe A, et al: Correlating infectious outcome with clinical parameters of 1130 consecutive febrile infants aged zero to eight weeks. *Pediatr Emerg Care* 9:84, 1993.
3. Greenes DS, Harper MB: Low risk of bacteremia in febrile children with recognizable viral syndromes. *Pediatr Infect Dis J* 18:258, 1999.
4. Talan DA, Morgan GJ, Pinner RW: Progress toward eliminating *Haemophilus influenzae* type b disease among infants and children-United States, 1987-1997. *Ann Emerg Med* 34:109, 1999.
5. Schutzman SA, Petrycki S, Gleisher GR: Bacteremia with otitis media. *Pediatrics* 87:48, 1991.
6. Bennish M, Beem MO, Orniste V: C reactive protein and zeta sedimentation ratio as indicators of bacteremia in pediatric patients. *J Pediatr* 104:729, 1984.
7. McCarthy PL, Jekel JF, Dolan TF: Comparison of acute-phase reactants in pediatric patients with fever. *Pediatrics* 62:716, 1978.
8. Rothrock SG: Occult bacteremia: Overcoming controversy and confusion in the management of infants and children. *Pediatr Emerg Med Rep* 1:21, 1999.
9. Harper MG, Fleisher GR: Occult bacteremia in the 3-month-old to 3-year-old age group. *Pediatr Ann* 22:484, 1993.
10. Green SM, Rothrock SG: Evaluation styles for well-appearing febrile children: Are you a "risk-minimizer" or a "test-minimizer"? *Ann Emerg Med* 33:211, 1999.
11. Schuchat A, Robinson K, Wenger JD, et al: Bacterial meningitis in the United States in 1995. *N Engl J Med* 337:970, 1997.
12. Arditi M, Mason EO, Bradley JS, et al: Three-year multicenter surveillance of pneumococcal meningitis in children: Clinical characteristics and outcome related to penicillin susceptibility and dexamethasone use. *Pediatrics* 99:289, 1998.
13. Bhisitkul DM, Hogan AE, Tanz RR: The role of bacterial antigen detection tests in the diagnosis of bacterial meningitis. *Pediatr Emerg Care* 10:67, 1994.

For further reading in *Emergency Medicine: A Comprehensive Study Guide,* 6th ed., see Chap. 116, "Bacteremia, Sepsis, and Meningitis in Children," by Peter Mellis.

69 COMMON NEONATAL PROBLEMS

Lance Brown

- In general, the signs and symptoms of illness are vague and nonspecific in neonates (ie, infants in the first month of life), making the identification of specific diagnoses very challenging (Table 69-1).

TABLE 69-1   Nonspecific Signs and Symptoms of Neonatal Illness

Fever or hypothermia
Abnormal tone (limp or stiff)
Weak suck
Poor feeding
Jaundice
Grunting respirations
Cyanosis or mottling
Vomiting

- Parents of these infants are often very fatigued from the erratic sleep patterns of their neonate and may be quite inexperienced at parenting if this is their first baby. Worry and fatigue may combine to prompt an emergency department visit.
- The survival of premature infants has produced a population of children whose corrected gestational age (chronological age since birth in weeks minus number of weeks of prematurity) makes them similar to neonates. Some of these children have multiple medical problems and may become frequent visitors to the emergency department.
- Neonates present to the emergency department with a wide range of conditions, from normal to critical.

NORMAL VEGETATIVE FUNCTIONS

- Bottle-fed infants will generally take six to nine feedings per 24-hour period, with a relatively stable pattern developing by the end of the first month of life. Breast-fed infants will generally prefer feedings every 2 to 4 hours.
- Infants typically lose 5 to 10% of their birth weight during the first 3 to 7 days of life. After this time, infants are expected to gain about 1 ounce per day (20 to 30 g) during the first 3 months of life.
- The number, color, and consistency of stool varies in the same infant from day to day, and certainly among infants. Normal breast-fed infants may go 5 to 7 days without stooling or have 6 to 7 stools per day. Color has no significance unless blood is present.
- Respiratory rates in newborns can vary, with normal ranges from 30 to 60 breaths per minute. Periodic breathing with brief (less than 5 to 10 seconds) pauses in respiration may be normal.
- Normal newborns awaken at variable intervals that can range from about 20 minutes to 6 hours. Neonates and young infants tend to have no day-night differentiation until about 3 months of age.

TABLE 69-2 Conditions Associated with Acute, Unexplained, Excessive Crying in Neonates

Corneal abrasion

Hair tourniquet (toe, penis)

Stomatitis

Subdural hematoma (nonaccidental trauma)

Fracture (nonaccidental trauma)

Dehydration

Inborn error of metabolism

Acute infections (sepsis, urinary tract infection, meningitis)

Congenital heart disease (including supraventricular tachycardia)

Encephalitis (herpes)

ACUTE, UNEXPLAINED, EXCESSIVE CRYING (INCONSOLABILITY)

- There are multiple causes of prolonged crying in infants (Table 69-2). These causes range from the relatively benign to the life-threatening. True inconsolability represents a serious condition in the majority of infants.[1,2]

INTESTINAL COLIC

- Intestinal colic is the most common cause of excessive (but not inconsolable) crying. The cause is unknown. The incidence is about 13% of all neonates. The formal definition includes crying for 3 hours per day or more for 3 days per week or more over a 3-week period. Intestinal colic seldom lasts beyond 3 months of age.

NONACCIDENTAL TRAUMA (CHILD ABUSE)

- A battered child may present with unexplained bruises at varying ages, skull fractures, intracranial injuries identifiable on computed tomographic (CT) scan of the head, extremity fractures, cigarette burns, retinal hemorrhages, and unexplained irritability, lethargy, or coma.

FEVER AND SEPSIS

- Fever in the neonate (28 days of age or younger) is defined as the history of or presence of a rectal temperature of 38°C (100.4°F) or more. Fever in the neonate must be taken seriously, and proper management includes a septic work-up (complete blood count [CBC], urinalysis, blood culture, urine culture, lumbar puncture and analysis of cerebrospinal fluid, cerebrospinal fluid culture, chest x-ray if respiratory symptoms are present, and stool culture if diarrhea is present), the administration of parenteral antibiotics (ampicillin gentamicin or ampicillin 1 cefotaxime), and admission. Well appearance on clinical exam and initial tests with results available in the emergency department cannot reliably rule out serious bacterial infection in the neonate.[3]

- Neonates with fever have about twice the risk of having a serious bacterial infection when compared to infants in the second month of life.

- Sepsis in neonates is typically grouped into early-onset disease, occurring in the first 5 days of life, and late-onset disease, occurring after the first week of life. Risk factors for early-onset sepsis include maternal fever, prolonged rupture of membranes, and fetal distress. Late-onset sepsis typically develops somewhat more gradually and is more commonly associated with meningitis. The signs and symptoms of neonatal sepsis are typically nonspecific (see Table 69-1).

- Bacteria associated with neonatal sepsis include group B streptococci, enteric organisms such as *Escherichia coli* and *Klebsiella, Haemophilus influenzae,* and *Listeria monocytogenes.*

GASTROINTESTINAL SYMPTOMS

SURGICAL LESIONS

- Surgically correctable abdominal emergencies in neonates are uncommon, may present with nonspecific symptomatology, and when suspected require prompt consultation with an experienced pediatric surgeon.

- The most common signs and symptoms are nonspecific and include irritability and crying, poor feeding, vomiting, constipation, and abdominal distention. Bilious vomiting is suggestive of malrotation with midgut volvulus and requires emergent surgical consultation. A groin mass may represent an incarcerated hernia, although inguinal hernias are usually seen in older infants.

FEEDING DIFFICULTIES

- An emergency department visit may arise when there is a parental perception that an infant's food intake is inadequate. If the patient's weight gain is adequate (see above) and the infant appears satisfied after feeding, parental reassurance is appropriate. A successful trial of feeding in the emergency department can reassure parents, emergency department nurses, and physicians alike.

- When there is an underlying anatomic abnormality interfering with feeding or swallowing (eg, esophageal stenosis, esophageal stricture, laryngeal clefts, compression of the esophagus or trachea by a double aortic arch), the infant typically has had trouble feeding since birth and usually presents with malnourishment and dehydration.
- Infants with a recent and true decrease in intake usually have an acute disease, most commonly an infection.[4]

REGURGITATION

- Regurgitation is due to reduced lower esophageal sphincter pressure and relatively increased intragastric pressure in neonates.
- Regurgitation is typically a self-limited condition, and if an infant is thriving and gaining weight appropriately, reassurance alone is appropriate.

VOMITING

- Vomiting is differentiated from regurgitation by forceful contraction of the diaphragm and abdominal muscles. Vomiting has a variety of causes and is rarely an isolated symptom.
- Vomiting from birth is usually due to an anatomic anomaly and usually inhibits an infant from being discharged from the newborn nursery.
- Vomiting is a nonspecific but serious symptom in neonates. Etiologies are diverse and include increased intracranial pressure (eg, shaken-baby syndrome), infections (eg, urinary tract infections, sepsis, gastroenteritis), hepatobiliary disease (usually accompanied by jaundice), and inborn errors of metabolism (usually accompanied by hypoglycemia and metabolic acidosis).
- Bilious vomiting in a neonate should be considered a surgical emergency (presumed malrotation until proven otherwise).

DIARRHEA

- Although bacterial diarrhea is a cause of bloody diarrhea, it is rare in neonates. The most common causes of blood in the stool in infants less than 6 months of age are cow's milk intolerance and anal fissures. Breast-fed infants may have heme-positive stool from swallowed maternal blood due to bleeding nipples.
- Necrotizing enterocolitis may present as bloody diarrhea and usually presents with other signs of sepsis (eg, jaundice, lethargy, fever, poor feeding, abdominal

distention). Abdominal radiography may demonstrate pneumatosis intestinalis or free air.
- Dehydrated neonates (and neonates with impending dehydration from rotavirus) should be admitted for rehydration.

ABDOMINAL DISTENTION

- Abdominal distention can be normal in the neonate and is usually due to lax abdominal muscles and relatively large intra-abdominal organs. In general, if the neonate appears comfortable, is feeding well, and the abdomen is soft, there is no need for concern.

CONSTIPATION

- Infrequent bowel movements in neonates do not necessarily mean that the infant is constipated. Stool patterns can be quite variable, and breast-fed infants may go a week without passing stool and then pass a normal stool.
- If an infant has never passed stool, the differential diagnosis includes intestinal stenosis or atresias, Hirschsprung's disease, and meconium ileus or plug.
- Constipation that develops later in the first month of life suggests Hirschsprung's disease, hypothyroidism, or anal stenosis.

CARDIORESPIRATORY SYMPTOMS

NOISY BREATHING AND STRIDOR

- Noisy breathing in a neonate is usually benign. Infectious causes of stridor seen commonly in older infants and young children (eg, croup) are rare in neonates.
- Stridor in a neonate is often due to a congenital anomaly, laryngomalacia being the most common. Other causes include webs, cysts, atresias, stenoses, clefts, and hemangiomas.
- Nasal congestion from a mild upper respiratory tract infection may cause significant problems in a neonate. Neonates are obligate nasal breathers and feed for relatively prolonged times breathing only through their noses (having the bottle or breast occlude the mouth). The use of saline drops and suctioning is typically effective.

APNEA AND PERIODIC BREATHING

- Periodic breathing may be normal in neonates.
- Apnea is formally defined as a cessation of respiration for greater than 10 to 20 seconds with or without

bradycardia and cyanosis. Apnea generally signifies a critical illness and prompt investigation (especially for sepsis) and admission for monitoring and therapy (including empiric antibiotics) should be initiated.
- Apnea may be the first sign of bronchiolitis with respiratory syncytial virus in neonates and occurs before wheezing.

CYANOSIS AND BLUE SPELLS

- Many disorders may present with cyanosis, and differentiating them may present quite a diagnostic challenge. However, some symptom patterns may help differentiate various causes and assist in suggesting the correct diagnosis and course of action.
- Rapid, unlabored respirations and cyanosis suggest cyanotic heart disease with right-to-left shunting.
- Irregular, shallow breathing and cyanosis suggests sepsis, meningitis, cerebral edema, or intracranial hemorrhage.
- Labored breathing with grunting and retractions is suggestive of pulmonary disease such as pneumonia or bronchiolitis.
- All cyanotic neonates should be admitted to the hospital for monitoring, therapy, and further investigation.[5,6]

BRONCHOPULMONARY DYSPLASIA

- Premature infants who have survived the neonatal intensive care unit (NICU) may have residual lung injury and bronchopulmonary dysplasia (BPD). Young infants with BPD may be on home oxygen, diuretics, bronchodilators, or steroids.
- Infants with BPD may have respiratory deterioration due to acute illnesses including bronchiolitis, pneumonia, dehydration, sepsis, gastroesophageal reflux and aspiration, and congestive heart failure.
- The most common cause of acute respiratory deterioration in an infant with BPD is a lower respiratory tract infection. Respiratory syncytial virus (RSV) infections are particularly common and may be quite severe.
- Basic treatment for BPD exacerbations includes oxygenation and bronchodilators. Antibiotics, admission, and mechanical ventilation may be required based on the clinical presentation.

JAUNDICE

- There are multiple causes of jaundice, and the likelihood of these causes is based on the age at which the patient has the onset of jaundice.

- Jaundice that occurs within the first 24 hours of life tends to be serious in nature and is usually addressed while the patient is in the newborn nursery.
- Jaundice which develops during the second or third day of life is usually physiologic, and if the neonate is gaining weight, feeding well, is not anemic, and does not have a bilirubin approaching 20 mg/dL, reassurance and close follow-up is appropriate.
- Jaundice that develops after the third day of life is generally serious. Causes include sepsis, congenital infections, congenital hemolytic anemias, breast-milk jaundice, and hypothyroidism. Work-up of these infants usually includes a septic work-up, including a lumbar puncture, a peripheral blood smear, direct and total bilirubin levels, reticulocyte count, and a Coombs test. Empiric antibiotics (see Chaps. 67 and 68) are generally administered when sepsis is suspected.

ORAL THRUSH

- Intraoral lesions due to *Candida* are typically white and pasty, covering the tongue, lips, gingiva, and mucous membranes.
- The presence of oral thrush may prompt a visit to the emergency department because the parent notices something white in the mouth or because the discomfort of extensive lesions interferes with feeding.
- Treatment consists of the topical application of oral nystatin suspension.

APPARENT LIFE-THREATENING EVENTS (ALTE)

- An apparent life-threatening event (ALTE) is defined as an episode that is frightening to the observer and involves a period of apnea, transient color change (pale or cyanotic), a transient change in tone (limp or stiff), and a period of choking or gagging.[7,8] By the conventional use of the term "ALTE," these children appear well on presentation to the emergency department and all abnormal behaviors have stopped.
- The presentation of a child with ALTE is nonspecific. Once it is determined that an ALTE has occurred, the work-up typically includes pulse oximetry, CBC, glucose, electrolytes, calcium, phosphorus, magnesium, ammonia levels, chest x-ray, electrocardiogram, and a septic work-up including blood, urine, and cerebrospinal fluid. Currently these patients are typically admitted to the hospital for further work-up and apnea monitoring. The utility of apnea monitoring (particularly in the home) has been questioned recently.[9]

- At the conclusion of hospitalization, diagnoses of infants with ALTE may remain elusive. When identified, diagnoses may include inborn errors of metabolism, seizure, gastroesophageal reflux, lower respiratory tract infection, pertussis, gastroenteritis, asthma, head injury, feeding difficulties, and urinary tract infections.[10]
- There appears to be a relationship between ALTEs and sudden infant death syndrome (SIDS), but the nature of this relationship is not clear.

REFERENCES

1. Poole SR: The infant with acute, unexplained, excessive crying. *Pediatrics* 88:450, 1991.
2. Brown L, Hicks M: Subclinical mastitis presenting as acute, unexplained, excessive crying in an afebrile 31-day-old female. *Pediatr Emerg Care* 17:189, 2001.
3. Baker MD, Bell LM: Unpredictability of serious bacterial illness in febrile infants from birth to 1 month of age. *Arch Pediatr Adolesc Med* 153:508, 1999.
4. Schmitt BD: The first week at home with your new baby. *Contemp Pediatr* 10:77, 1993.
5. Carroll JL, Marcus CL, Loughlin GM: Disordered control of breathing in infants and children. *Pediatr Rev* 14:51, 1993.
6. Korones SB, Bada-Ellzey HS (eds.): Cyanosis, in *Neonatal Decision Making*. St. Louis: Mosby, 1993, p. 62.
7. National Institutes of Health Consensus Development Conference on Infantile Apnea and Home Monitoring, Sept. 29 to Oct. 1, 1986. Consensus statement. *Pediatrics* 79:292, 1987.
8. Perkin RM, Swift JD, Baron H, et al: Apparent life-threatening events: Recognition, differentiation, and management. *Pediatr Emerg Med Reports* 3:99, 1998.
9. Ramanathan R, Corwin MJ, Hunt CE, et al: Cardiorespiratory events recorded on home monitors: Comparison of healthy infants with those at increased risk for SIDS. *JAMA* 285:2199, 2001.
10. Gray C, Davies F, Molyneux E: Apparent life-threatening events presenting to a pediatric emergency department. *Pediatr Emerg Care* 15:195, 1999.

For further reading in *Emergency Medicine: A Comprehensive Study Guide*, 6th ed., see Chap. 117, "Common Neonatal Problems" by Tonia J. Brousseau and Niranjan Kissoon; Chap. 118, "The NICU Graduate," by Daniel G. Batton; and Chap. 119, "Sudden Infant Death Syndrome and Apparent Life-Threatening Event," by Carol D. Berkowitz.

70 PEDIATRIC HEART DISEASE

David M. Cline

- This chapter will cover three main presentations of pediatric heart disease as they present to the emergency department: cyanosis and shock, congestive heart failure, and complications of known congenital heart disease. Other cardiovascular topics such as dysrhythmias (Chap. 4), syncope (Chap. 81), pediatric hypertension (Chap. 29), and myocarditis and pericarditis (Chap. 27) are covered in other chapters and will not be discussed here.
- There are six common clinical presentations of pediatric heart disease: cyanosis, congestive heart failure (CHF), pathologic murmur in an asymptomatic patient, abnormal pulses, hypertension, and syncope. Table 70-1 lists the most common lesions in each category.
- Pediatric heart disease is frequently misdiagnosed as a viral upper respiratory tract illness or feeding intolerance. In fact, feeding intolerance may be the first symptom of congenital heart disease.
- Evaluation of an asymptomatic murmur is an elective diagnostic work-up that can be done on an outpatient basis. The Still murmur, which is the most common innocent murmur, is early systolic in timing, located at the apex or the left sternal border, and does not radiate.[1] Common pathologic murmurs in children are holosystolic, continuous or diastolic in timing, and usually radiate.[2]

TABLE 70-1 Clinical Presentation of Pediatric Heart Disease

Cyanosis	TGA, TOF, TA, Tat, TAVR
Congestive heart failure	See Table 70-2
Murmur/symptomatic patient	Shunts: VSD, PDA, ASD Obstructions Valvular incompetence
Abnormal pulses	
Bounding	PDA, AI, AVM
Decreased with prolonged amplitude	Coarctation, HPLV
Hypertension	Coarctation
Syncope	
Cyanotic	TOF
Acyanotic	Critical AS

ABBREVIATIONS: AI = aortic insufficiency; AS = aortic stenosis; ASD = atrial septal defect; AVM = arteriovenous malformation; HPLV = hypoplastic left ventricle; PDA = patent ductus arteriosus; TA = truncus arteriosus; Tat = tricuspid atresia; TAVR = total anomalous venous return; TGA = transposition of the great arteries; TOF = tetralogy of Fallot; VSD = ventricular septal defect.

EPIDEMIOLOGY

- Pediatric cardiac conditions are relatively rare. Congenital heart disease is a broad term encompassing a multitude of anatomic abnormalities. Congenital heart disease is the most common form of pediatric heart disease and is present in only 8 cases per 1000 live births in all forms.[3]
- Acquired heart disease is less common and includes complications secondary to rheumatic fever (now quite uncommon), Kawasaki's disease, severe chronic anemias, myocarditis, pericarditis, and endocarditis.

CYANOSIS AND SHOCK

PATHOPHYSIOLOGY

- Five main conditions present with cyanosis: transposition of the great arteries, tetralogy of Fallot, truncus arteriosus, tricuspid atresia, and total anomalous venous return (all five start with "T").
- The anatomy of each of these conditions is different, but a few simple principles are common among them. Cyanosis is present and is generally due to an anatomic shunt with mixing of oxygenated and deoxygenated blood.

CLINICAL FEATURES

- An accurate set of vital signs including pulse oximetry and blood pressure is essential. Cyanosis associated with a heart murmur strongly suggests congenital heart disease, but the absence of a murmur does not exclude a structural heart lesion.
- Early signs of inadequate cardiac output in the neonate may be suggested by slow feeding or tachypnea, diaphoresis, or staccato cough with feeding.
- Shock with or without cyanosis, especially during the first 2 weeks of life, should alert the clinician to the possibility of congenital heart disease associated with closure of a patent ductus arteriosus. Neonates with shunt-dependent lesions will experience profound symptoms with closure of the ductus.
- Shock in the neonate is recognized by inspection of the patient's skin for pallor, cyanosis, and skin mottling, and assessment of the mental status appropriate for age. Mental status changes may be fluctuating signs of apathy, irritability, or failure to respond to pain or parents.
- Tachycardia and tachypnea are commonly present as the initial signs. Tachypnea associated with congenital heart disease is typically effortless, without accessory muscle use commonly seen with respiratory disease.

- Distal pulses should be assessed for quality, amplitude, and duration (see Table 70-1).

DIAGNOSIS AND DIFFERENTIAL

- Determining the cause of cyanosis and respiratory distress in the critically ill neonate is difficult. The clinician should consider congenital heart disease, respiratory disorders, central nervous system disease, and sepsis.
- The hyperoxic test helps to differentiate respiratory disease from cyanotic congenital heart disease (although imperfectly). The infant should be placed on 100% oxygen. Persistence of hypoxemia suggests the presence of a shunt from congenital heart disease.
- The work-up for congenital heart disease begins with chest x-ray and electrocardiogram (ECG) with pediatric analysis. Chest x-ray should be assessed for heart size, shape, and pulmonary blood flow.
- An abnormal right position of the aortic arch may be a clue to the diagnosis of congenital cardiac lesion. Increased pulmonary vascularity may be seen with significant left-to-right shunting or left-sided failure.
- Echocardiography is generally required to define the diagnosis.
- The differential diagnosis for cyanosis or shock due to congenital heart disease includes typically cyanotic lesions: transposition of the great vessels, tetralogy of Fallot, and other forms of right ventricular outflow tract obstruction or abnormalities of right heart formation.
- Typically acyanotic lesions that can present with shock include severe coarctation of the aorta, critical aortic stenosis, and hypoplastic left ventricle. It should be noted that cyanosis may accompany shock of any cause.
- **Tetralogy of Fallot** produces the following features: a holosystolic murmur of a ventricular septal defect (VSD), a diamond-shaped murmur of pulmonary stenosis, and cyanosis. The toddler may relieve symptoms by squatting. Chest x-ray may reveal a boot-shaped heart with decreased pulmonary vascular markings or a right-sided aortic arch. The ECG may reveal right ventricular hypertrophy and right axis deviation.
- **Hypercyanotic episodes,** or **"tet spells,"** may bring children with tetralogy of Fallot to the ED with dramatic presentations. Symptoms include paroxysmal dyspnea, labored respiration, increased cyanosis, and possibly syncope. If the condition is accompanied by polycythemia, the patient may suffer seizures, cerebrovascular accidents, or death. These episodes frequently follow exertion due to feeding, crying, or straining at stool, and last from minutes to hours.[4]
- **Transposition of the great vessels** represents the most common cyanotic defect presenting with symp-

toms during the first week of life. This entity is easily missed due to the absence of cardiomegaly or murmur. Symptoms (prior to shock) include dusky lips, increased respiratory rate, and/or feeding difficulty. ECG may show right-sided-force dominance.[5]

- **Left ventricular outflow obstruction syndromes** may present with shock, with or without cyanosis. Several congenital lesions fall into this category, but in all these disorders, systemic blood flow is dependent on a large contribution of shunted blood from a patent ductus arteriosus.[6] When the ductus closes, these infants present with decreased or absent perfusion, hypotension, and severe acidosis.

EMERGENCY DEPARTMENT CARE AND DISPOSITION

- Cyanosis and respiratory distress are first managed with high-flow oxygen, cardiac and oxygen monitoring, and a stable IV line.
- Noncardiac causes of symptoms should be considered and treated appropriately, including a fluid challenge of 20 mL/kg of normal saline solution as indicated.
- Immediate consultation should be obtained with a pediatric cardiologist, and if the patient is in shock, a pediatric intensivist.
- Management of hypercyanotic spells consists of positioning the patient in knee-chest position and administration of morphine sulfate subcutaneously or intramuscularly 0.2 mg/kg. Resistant cases should prompt immediate consultation with a pediatric cardiologist for consideration of phenylephrine for hypotension or propranolol for tachycardia.
- For severe shock in infants suspected of having shunt-dependent lesions, prostaglandin E_1 can be given in an attempt to reopen the ductus.[7] Start 0.05 to 0.1 μg/kg/min initially; this may be increased to 0.2 μg/kg/min if there is no improvement. Side effects include fever, skin flushing, diarrhea, and periodic apnea. Intubation and ventilation are often required.
- Epinephrine is the initial drug of choice for hypotension. Start an infusion at 0.05 to 0.5 μg/kg per minute, and titrate to desired blood pressure.
- By definition, these children are critically ill and require admission, usually to the pediatric intensive care unit.

CONGESTIVE HEART FAILURE

PATHOPHYSIOLOGY

- Multiple causes of congestive heart failure are seen and the likely etiology is based on the age of the patient at the time of presentation (Table 70-2).

TABLE 70-2   Differential Diagnosis of Congestive Heart Failure Based on Age of Presentation

AGE	SPECTRUM	
1 minute	Noncardiac origin: anemia, acidosis, hypoxia, hypoglycemia, hypocalcemia, sepsis	Acquired
1 hour		
1 day	PDA in premature infants	Congenital
1 week	HPLV	
2 weeks	Coarctation	
1 month	Ventricular septal defect	
3 months	Supraventricular tachycardia	Acquired
1 year	Myocarditis	
	Cardiomyopathy	
	Severe anemia	
10 years	Rheumatic fever	

ABBREVIATIONS: HPLV = hypoplastic left ventricle; PDA = patent ductus arteriosus.

- The most common general cause of congestive heart failure in infants is afterload increase due to an anatomic abnormality. Less commonly, increases in preload or general volume overload are responsible for the heart failure. Older infants and children may have acquired causes of poor contractility (eg, myocarditis) leading to heart failure.

CLINICAL FEATURES

- The distinction between pneumonia and CHF in infants requires a high index of clinical suspicion and is a difficult one to make.
- Pneumonia can cause a previously stable cardiac condition to decompensate; thus both problems can present simultaneously.
- The predominant symptoms include poor feeding, diaphoresis, irritability or lethargy with feeding, weak cry, and in severe cases, grunting and nasal flaring.
- Note that the tachypnea associated with congestive heart failure in infants is typically "effortless" and is the first manifestation of decompensation, followed by rales on exam.

DIAGNOSIS AND DIFFERENTIAL

- Cardiomegaly evident on chest x-ray is universally present except in constrictive pericarditis. A cardiothoracic index greater than 0.6 is abnormal.
- The primary radiographic signs of cardiomegaly on the lateral chest x-ray are an abnormal cardiothoracic index and lack of retrosternal air space due to the direct abutment of the heart against the sternum.

- Once CHF is recognized, age-related categories simplify further differential diagnosis (see Table 70-2).
- In contrast to the gradual onset of failure with a VSD, coarctation of the aorta can present with abrupt onset of congested heart failure precipitated by a delayed closure of the ductus arteriosus during the second week of life.
- Onset of CHF after 3 months of age usually signifies acquired heart disease. The exception is when pneumonia, endocarditis, or other complications cause a congenital lesion to decompensate.
- Myocarditis is often preceded by a viral respiratory illness and needs to be differentiated from pneumonia. As with pneumonia, the infant usually presents in distress with fever, tachypnea, and tachycardia.
- ECG may reveal diffuse ST changes, dysrhythmias, or ectopy, signaling increased risk of sudden death.
- Chest x-ray shows cloudy lung fields either from inflammation or pulmonary edema. However, cardiomegaly with poor distal pulses and prolonged capillary refill distinguish it from common pneumonia.
- Once cardiomegaly is discovered, hospital admission and an echocardiogram are indicated.
- Usually pericarditis presents as cardiomegaly discovered on a chest x-ray. Clinical signs such as chest pain, muffled heart sounds, and a rub may be present. An echocardiogram is performed urgently to distinguish a pericardial effusion from dilated or hypertrophic cardiomyopathy, as well as to determine the need for pericardiocentesis.
- If an infant presents in pure right-sided CHF, the primary problem is most likely to be pulmonary, such as cor pulmonale.
- In early stages, lid edema is often the first noticeable sign. This may progress to hepatomegaly, jugular venous distention, peripheral edema, and anasarca.

EMERGENCY DEPARTMENT CARE AND DISPOSITION

- The infant who presents with mild tachypnea, hepatomegaly, and cardiomegaly should be seated upright in a comfortable position, oxygen should be given, and the child should be kept in a neutral thermal environment to avoid metabolic stresses imposed by either hypothermia or hyperthermia.
- If the work of breathing is increased or CHF is apparent on chest x-ray, 1 to 2 mg/kg of furosemide parenterally is indicated.
- Hypoxemia can usually be corrected by fluid restriction, diuresis, and an increased F_{IO_2}, although continuous positive airway pressure is sometimes necessary.

- Stabilization and improvement of left ventricular function can often first be accomplished with inotropic agents. Digoxin is used in milder forms of CHF. The appropriate first digitalizing dose to be given in the ED would be 0.02 mg/kg.
- At some point, CHF progresses to cardiogenic shock, in which distal pulses are absent and end-organ perfusion is threatened. In such situations, continuous infusions of inotropic agents, such as dopamine or dobutamine, are indicated instead of digoxin. The initial starting range is 2 to 10 μg/kg/min.
- Aggressive management is often necessary for secondary derangements, including respiratory insufficiency, acute renal failure, lactic acidosis, disseminated intravascular coagulation, hypoglycemia, and hypocalcemia.
- For definitive diagnosis and treatment of congenital lesions presenting in CHF, cardiac catheterization followed by surgical intervention is often necessary. See the previous section for recommendations regarding administration of prostaglandin E_1 as a temporizing measure prior to surgery.

REFERENCES

1. Rosenthal A: How to distinguish between innocent and pathological murmurs in childhood. *Pediatr Clin North Am* 31:511, 1984.
2. McNamara DG: Value and limitation of auscultation in the management of congenital heart disease. *Pediatr Clin North Am* 37:93, 1990.
3. Grabitz RG, Joffres MR: Congenital heart disease incidence in the first year of life: The Alberta Pediatric Cardiology Program. *Am J Epidemiol* 128:318, 1988.
4. Van Roenkens CN, Zuckerman AL: Emergency management of hypercyanotic crises in tetralogy of Fallot. *Ann Emerg Med* 25:256, 1995.
5. Kirklin JW, Colvin EV, McConnell ME, et al: Complete transposition of the great arteries: Treatment in the current era. *Pediatr Clin North Am* 37:171, 1990.
6. Starnes VA, Griffin ML, Pitlick PT, et al: Current approach to hypoplastic left heart syndrome: Palliation, transplantation or both? *J Thorac Cardiovasc Surg* 104:189, 1992.
7. Perkin RM, Levin DL: Shock in the pediatric patient: II, Therapy. *J Pediatr* 101:319, 1982.

For further reading in *Emergency Medicine: A Comprehensive Study Guide,* 6th ed., see Chap. 120, "Pediatric Heart Disease," by C. James Corrall.

71 OTITIS AND PHARYNGITIS

David M. Cline

OTITIS MEDIA

- Acute otitis media (AOM), an infection of the middle ear, commonly affects infants and young children because of relative immaturity of the upper respiratory tract, especially the eustachian tube.

EPIDEMIOLOGY

- Each year there are 25 to 30 million office visits for otitis media, over 3.7 million emergency department visits, and indirect costs of $5.7 billion a year.[1,2]
- The incidence is higher in males, children who attend day care, children exposed to smoke, and those with a family history of otitis media.[1,2]
- Bacteria are the most important cause of AOM and can be isolated in pure culture from the middle ear exudate in 60 to 75% of cases.
- *Streptococcus pneumoniae* is the most prevalent and most virulent cause, accounting for approximately 40% of infections.[3] *Haemophilus influenzae* NT (nontypable) and *Moraxella catarrhalis* account for another 40% and have a high rate of spontaneous resolution.[4] *Chlamydia pneumoniae* is more common in those less than 6 months of age, and *Staphylococcus aureus* is more common in those less than 6 weeks of age.[5,6]

PATHOPHYSIOLOGY

- Abnormal function of the eustachian tube appears to be the dominant factor in the pathogenesis of middle ear disease. Both obstruction and abnormal patency play a role in eustachian tube dysfunction.

CLINICAL FEATURES

- The peak age is 6 to 18 months.[1] Symptoms include fever, poor feeding, irritability, vomiting, earache, and otorrhea.[1]
- Signs include a dull, bulging, immobile tympanic membrane (TM), loss of visualization of bony landmarks within the middle ear, air-fluid levels or bubbles within the middle ear, and bullae on the TM.[6] The light reflex is of no diagnostic value.

DIAGNOSIS AND DIFFERENTIAL

- Diagnosis is based on presenting symptoms and changes of the TM and middle ear. A red TM alone does not indicate the presence of an ear infection. Fever, prolonged crying, and viral infections can cause hyperemia of the TM.[6]
- Pneumatic otoscopy can be a helpful diagnostic tool; however, a retracted drum for whatever reason will demonstrate decreased mobility.[7]

EMERGENCY DEPARTMENT CARE AND DISPOSITION

- Amoxicillin 45 to 60 mg/kg/day PO divided twice to three times daily remains the first drug of choice despite the increasing incidence of penicillin-resistant *Streptococcus pneumoniae* and the predominance of β-lactamase–producing *H. influenzae* NT and *M. catarrhalis*.[1,6]
- Risk factors for drug-resistant *Streptococcus pneumoniae* (DRSP) include age <2 years, day care attendance, antibiotics in the last 3 months, and immunoincompetence. High-dose amoxicillin (80 to 90 mg/kg/day PO divided twice daily) is considered the first-line treatment for those at risk for DRSP.[8]
- Other antibiotics appropriate for DRSP include amoxicillin-clavulanate 45 mg/kg/day PO divided twice daily (a higher dose can be considered, 80 to 90 mg/kg/day divided twice daily, but do not exceed 10 mg/kg/day of the clavulanate component). Further choices include cefuroxime axetil 30 mg/kg/day PO divided twice daily, cefdinir 14 mg/kg/day PO divided once to twice daily, and ceftriaxone 50 mg/kg/day IM for three doses.[8] For patients allergic to the previously mentioned antibiotics, azithromycin 10 mg/kg PO the first day followed by 5 mg/kg PO for four more days can be used.
- Infants less than 30 days of age with AOM are at risk for infection with group B *Streptococcus, Staphylococcus aureus,* and gram-negative bacilli and should undergo evaluation and treatment for presumed sepsis (see Chap. 68).
- Recurrent AOM is characterized as three or more episodes within 6 months or four or more within 12 months.
- Persistent AOM occurs when the signs and symptoms of AOM do not improve with appropriate antibiotic therapy.
- High-dose amoxicillin therapy or other antibiotics suitable for DRSP coverage should be considered for both recurrent and persistent AOM.[8]

- In uncomplicated AOM, symptoms resolve within 48 to 72 hours; however, the middle ear effusion may persist as long as 8 to 12 weeks. Routine follow-up is not necessary unless the symptoms persist or worsen.

OTITIS MEDIA WITH EFFUSION (OME)

- OME is fluid within the middle ear without the associated signs and symptoms of an acute infection.[9] Chronic OME (duration >3 months) can result in significant hearing loss and language delay.

CLINICAL FEATURES

- OME is characterized by a middle ear effusion, distortion of bony landmarks, and decreased mobility of the TM.[6]
- Absent are symptoms of acute infection such as fever, irritability, and otalgia.[6]

DIAGNOSIS AND DIFFERENTIAL

- The diagnosis is based upon the appearance of the TM in the absence of systemic symptoms. Audiometry is of limited value for diagnosis, but is crucial to the evaluation of hearing deficit.

EMERGENCY DEPARTMENT CARE AND DISPOSITION

- Treatment of OME includes careful observation for resolution (standard treatment of choice),[9] or ear, nose, and throat (ENT) referral and hearing evaluation for chronic OME. There is no indication for antihistamines, decongestants, or steroids.[9]
- Antibiotics achieve resolution in only 14% of cases.[9]
- Bilateral myringotomy tubes may be required if effusion does not resolve.

OTITIS EXTERNA

EPIDEMIOLOGY

- Otitis externa (OE) is an inflammatory process involving the auricle, external auditory canal (EAC), and surface of the TM. It is commonly caused by gram-negative enteric organisms, *Staphylococcus aureus, Pseudomonas aeruginosa,* or fungi.[10]

PATHOPHYSIOLOGY

- Any compromise of the normal shape of the canal or normal process of cerumen production can lead to OE due to colonization and tissue invasion of pathogenic organisms.[14]

CLINICAL FEATURES

- Peak seasons for OE are spring and summer, and the peak age is 9 to 19 years. Symptoms include earache, itching, and fever.[14]
- Signs include erythema, edema of the EAC, white exudate on the EAC and TM, pain with motion of tragus or auricle, and periauricular or cervical adenopathy.[14]

DIAGNOSIS AND DIFFERENTIAL

- Diagnosis of OE is based on clinical signs and symptoms. A foreign body within the external canal should be excluded by carefully removing any debris that may be present.

EMERGENCY DEPARTMENT CARE AND DISPOSITION

- Cleaning the ear canal with a small tuft of cotton attached to a wire applicator is the first step. The clinician should place a wick in the canal if significant edema obstructs the EAC.
- Mild OE can be treated with acidifying agents alone, such as Otic Domeboro.
- Fluoroquinolone otic drops are now considered the preferred agents over neomycin-containing drops. Ciprofloxacin with hydrocortisone 0.2%/1% suspension (Cipro HC) 3 drops twice daily or ofloxacin 0.3% solution 10 drops twice daily can be used.[10] Ofloxacin is used when TM rupture is found or suspected.[10]
- Oral antibiotics are indicated if auricular cellulitis is present.
- Follow-up should be advised if improvement does not occur within 48 hours; otherwise re-evaluation at the end of treatment is sufficient.

PHARYNGITIS

EPIDEMIOLOGY

- It is estimated that $300 million are spent annually on the diagnosis and treatment of pharyngitis.[11]

PATHOPHYSIOLOGY

- Etiologies include multiple viruses and bacteria, but only Group A β-hemolytic *Streptococcus* (GABHS), Epstein-Barr virus, and *Neisseria gonorrhoeae* require accurate diagnosis.[11]
- The identification and treatment of GABHS pharyngitis is important in order to prevent the suppurative complications and the sequelae of acute rheumatic fever.

CLINICAL FEATURES

- Peak seasons for GABHS are late winter or early spring, and the peak age is 4 to 11 years. Symptoms (sudden onset) include sore throat, fever, headache, abdominal pain, enlarged anterior cervical nodes, palatal petechiae, and tonsillar hypertrophy.[11]
- With GABHS there is absence of cough, coryza, laryngitis, stridor, conjunctivitis, and diarrhea.[11]
- A scarlatiniform rash associated with pharyngitis is almost always GABHS and is commonly referred to as scarlet fever. Diagnosis based on clinical findings alone results in only 50 to 70% accuracy at best.
- Epstein-Barr virus (EBV) is a herpes virus and often presents much like streptococcal pharyngitis.[11] Common symptoms are fever, sore throat, and malaise. Cervical adenopathy may be prominent and often is posterior as well as anterior. Hepatosplenomegaly may be present.
- EBV should be suspected in the child with pharyngitis nonresponsive to antibiotics, in the presence of a negative throat culture.
- Gonococcal (CG) pharyngitis in children and non–sexually active adolescents should alert one to the possibility of child abuse. GC pharyngitis tends to have a more benign clinical presentation than GABHS pharyngitis.

DIAGNOSIS AND DIFFERENTIAL

- Definitive diagnosis of GABHS is made with the throat culture; however, this may not always be practical in the ED, because of the time involved and potential problems with follow-up.[12]
- Rapid antigen-detection tests, if properly performed, achieve sensitivity and specificity close to that of the throat culture.[13,14]
- A negative rapid strep test does not exclude GABHS and should be verified with a throat culture. Other etiologies of pharyngitis to recognize are Epstein-Barr virus (infectious mononucleosis) and *N. gonorrhoeae*.
- With EBV, the white blood cell count will typically show a lymphocytosis with a preponderance of atypical lymphocytes. Diagnosis is confirmed with a positive heterophil antibody (mono spot).
- Diagnosis of GC pharyngitis is made by culture on Thayer-Martin medium.[15] Vaginal, cervical, and rectal cultures should also be obtained if GC pharyngitis is suspected.[15]

EMERGENCY DEPARTMENT CARE AND DISPOSITION

- Antibiotic choices[11] for GABHS include benzathine penicillin 1.2 million U IM (600,000 U IM for patients less than 27 kg), penicillin V 1 g PO twice daily for 10 days (500 mg PO twice daily for patients less than 27 kg), amoxicillin 60 mg/kg/day PO divided three times daily for 10 days, erythromycin ethylsuccinate 40 to 50 mg/kg/day PO divided three times daily for 10 days, cefprozil 30 mg/kg/day PO divided twice daily for 10 days, cefuroxime 30 mg/kg/day divided twice daily for 10 days, and azithromycin 12 mg/kg daily for 5 days.
- Antibiotic choices for GC pharyngitis include ceftriaxone 125 mg plus azithromycin 12 mg/kg daily for 5 days or spectinomycin 40 mg/kg IM for 7 days plus doxycycline 100 mg twice daily for 7 days.[15]
- Antipyretics and sometimes analgesics will be necessary during the first 48 to 72 hours of treatment. Appropriate follow up should be encouraged for treatment failure and symptomatic contacts. Follow-up for suspected GC pharyngitis should include child sexual abuse and social service investigations.[15]
- An increase in the number of treatment failures with penicillin has been reported. The evidence does not support the abandonment of penicillin as a mainstay of treatment.[11]
- EBV is usually self-limited and requires only supportive treatment of antipyretics, fluids, and bedrest. Occasionally EBV is complicated by airway obstruction and can be effectively treated with prednisone, 2.5 mg/kg/day tapered over 5 days, or dexamethasone, 0.5 mg/kg to a maximum of 10 mg daily tapered over 5 days.
- Steroids may also be helpful in other forms of pharyngitis with moderate to severe swelling.

REFERENCES

1. McCracken GH Jr: Diagnosis and management of acute otitis media in the urgent care setting. *Ann Emerg Med* 39:413, 2002.

2. Weiss HB, Mathers LJ, Forjuoh SH, et al: *Child and Adolescent Emergency Department Visit Databook.* Pittsburgh: Center for Violence and Injury Prevention, Allegheny University of the Health Sciences, 1997.

3. Maxon S, Yamauchi T: Acute otitis media. *Pediatr Rev* 17:191, 1996.

4. Steele RW: Management of otitis media. *Infect Med* 15:174, 1998.

5. Block SL: Causative pathogens, antibiotic resistance and therapeutic considerations in acute otitis media. *Pediatr Infect Dis* 16:449, 1997.

6. Bluestone CD, Klein JO: *Otitis Media in Infants and Children,* 3rd ed. Philadelphia: Saunders, 2000.

7. Hobberman A, Paradise JL: Acute otitis media: Diagnosis and management in the year 2000. *Pediatr Ann* 29:609, 2000.

8. Dowell SF, Butler JC, Giebink GS, et al: Acute otitis media: Management and surveillance in an era of pneumococcal resistance—A report from the Drug-Resistant *Streptococcus pneumoniae* Therapeutic Working Group. *Pediatr Infect Dis J* 18:1, 1999.

9. Stool SE, Berg AO: *Clinical Practice Guideline: Otitis Media with Effusion in Young Children.* Rockville, MD: Agency for Health Care Policy and Research, 1994, Pub. No. 94-0622.

10. Hughes E, Lee JH: Otitis externa. *Pediatr Rev* 22:191, 2001.

11. Bisno AL, Acute pharyngitis. *N Engl J Med* 344:205, 2001.

12. Dajani A, Taubert K, Ferrieri P, et al: Treatment of acute streptococcal pharyngitis and prevention of rheumatic fever: A statement for health professionals. *Pediatrics* 96:758, 1995.

13. Gerber MA, Tanz RR, Kabat W, et al: Optical immunoassay test for group A beta-hemolytic streptococcal pharyngitis: An office-based, multicenter investigation. *JAMA* 277:899, 1997.

14. Bisno AL, Gerber MA, Gwaltney JM, et al: Diagnosis and management of group A streptococcal pharyngitis: A practice guideline. *Clin Infect Dis* 25:574, 1997.

15. Peter G (ed.): *American Academy of Pediatrics: 2000 Red Book: Report of the Committee on Infectious Diseases,* 25th ed. Elk Grove Village, IL: American Academy of Pediatrics, 2000.

For further reading in *Emergency Medicine: A Comprehensive Study Guide,* 6th ed., see Chap. 121, "Otitis and Pharyngitis in Children," by Kimberly S. Quayle, Susan Fuchs, and David M. Jaffe.

72 SKIN AND SOFT TISSUE INFECTIONS

David M. Cline

- This chapter discusses several common skin and soft-tissue infections of childhood. Impetigo is discussed in Chap. 84.

CONJUNCTIVITIS

EPIDEMIOLOGY

- Conjunctivitis is the most common ocular infection of childhood and is usually a sporadic illness, but may occur with epidemic periodicity with viral pathogens in summer months.
- Although *Chlamydia trachomatis* is more common, *Neisseria gonorrhoeae* poses the greatest threat to the integrity of the eye in the neonate.
- Later in childhood, viruses, such as adenovirus, and the respiratory tract pathogens predominate, particularly untypable *Haemophilus* species.

PATHOPHYSIOLOGY

- Pathogens introduced into the conjunctival sac may proliferate and produce hyperemia and an inflammatory exudate. This exudate may be purulent, fibrinous, or serosanguineous. With certain organisms, corneal involvement (keratitis) also may occur.

CLINICAL FEATURES

- Older children with conjunctivitis may complain of photophobia, ocular pain, or the sensation of a foreign body in the eye, which is associated with crusting of the eyelids or conjunctival injection.
- Erythema and increased secretions characterize conjunctivitis, with intense redness and purulence being more common with infectious rather than allergic causes.
- Allergic conjunctivitis is typically recurrent, seasonal, and accompanied by pruritus and sneezing.
- Fever and other systemic manifestations do not occur with isolated conjunctivitis.
- The duration of symptoms with infectious causes is often 2 to 4 days.

DIAGNOSIS AND DIFFERENTIAL

- The diagnosis of infectious conjunctivitis depends on the clinical examination.
- A Gram stain should be performed in infants less than 1 month old or in confusing cases. It will show more than five white blood cells (WBCs) per field, and in many cases, bacteria. The finding of gram-negative intracellular diplococci identifies *N. gonorrhoeae.*
- Conjunctival scrapings or cultures may be performed to diagnose *Chlamydia trachomatis* or other viral or bacterial pathogens.

- Fluorescein staining helps to identify the dendrites of herpes simplex.
- Conjunctivitis may be a manifestation of a systemic disorder, such as measles or Kawasaki's disease.
- Differential diagnosis of the red eye includes conjunctivitis, orbital and periorbital infection, retained foreign body, corneal abrasion, uveitis, and glaucoma.

EMERGENCY DEPARTMENT CARE AND DISPOSITION

- Treatment is directed at the most common causes of conjunctivitis based on the patient's age and examination findings as well as slitlamp exam, fluorescein staining pattern, and Gram staining, if indicated.
- Infants less than 1 month of age with exceptionally purulent conjunctivitis or gram-positive results for *N. gonorrhoeae* should receive ceftriaxone, 125 mg IM.[1] Close follow-up the next day should be arranged. Infants appearing toxic should be admitted. Public health reporting and investigation are mandatory.
- For infants under 3 months of age, treatment with erythromycin 50 mg/kg/day divided four times a day for 14 days plus erythromycin ointment 0.5% four times daily is instituted to treat *C. trachomatis* and to prevent later development of the associated vertically transmitted pneumonia syndrome.
- Older children require only topical antibiotic instillation into the conjunctival sac, such as tobramycin, or gentamicin 1 to 2 drops every 4 hours while awake.
- For herpes simplex infections, urgent consultation with an ophthalmologist is required. Topical and oral antiviral therapy is indicated. Examples include trifluridine, 1 drop 9 times daily and acyclovir 10 to 20 mg/kg PO four times daily.
- The administration of diphenhydramine (5 mg/kg/day divided every 6 hours PO) or hydroxyzine (2 mg/kg/day divided every 6 hours PO) may be useful for allergic conjunctivitis along with eradication of exposure to offending agents. In older children, olopatadine 0.1%, 1 to 2 drops bid can be used.
- All children with conjunctivitis should have re-evaluation within 48 hours of treatment if there is no improvement, and no child should be treated for longer than 5 days with topical therapy without improvement. Failure to improve indicates further investigation and ophthalmologic consultation.

SINUSITIS

- Sinusitis is an inflammation of the paranasal sinuses that may be secondary to infection and allergy, and may be acute, subacute, or chronic in time course.

EPIDEMIOLOGY

- The major pathogens in acute bacterial sinusitis in childhood are *Streptococcus pneumoniae, Moraxella catarrhalis,* and nontypable *Haemophilus influenzae.*[2]
- The incidence of *H. influenzae* sinusitis in children would be expected to decline with Hib vaccination.

PATHOPHYSIOLOGY

- The ethmoid and maxillary sinuses are present at birth, but the frontal and sphenoid sinuses do not become aerated until 6 or 7 years of age.
- The sinuses are lined primarily by ciliated columnar epithelium and connect with the nasopharynx via narrow ostia.
- Resistance to infection depends on the patency of the ostia, the function of the ciliary mechanism, and the quality of the secretions.
- Obstruction of the ostia results either from mucosal swelling, or less commonly, mechanical obstruction. By far the most frequent offenders are viral upper respiratory infection and allergic inflammation.

CLINICAL FEATURES

- Two major types of sinusitis may be differentiated on clinical grounds: acute severe sinusitis and mild subacute sinusitis.
- Acute severe sinusitis is associated with elevated temperature, headaches, and localized swelling and tenderness or erythema in the facial area corresponding to the sinuses. Such localized findings are most often seen in older adolescents and adults.
- Mild subacute sinusitis is manifest in childhood as a protracted upper respiratory infection (URI) with a predominance of purulent nasal discharge and the absence of swelling. Rather than improve in 3 to 7 days, these children have persistent symptoms in excess of 2 weeks. Fever is infrequent. This latter type of sinusitis may be confused with congestion of brief duration found with some URIs.

DIAGNOSIS AND DIFFERENTIAL

- The diagnosis is made on clinical grounds without laboratory or radiographic studies. Transillumination of the maxillary or frontal sinuses is seldom helpful in children.

- Standard radiographs should be obtained for patients with uncertain clinical diagnosis and in cases of severe sinusitis. The most diagnostic finding is an air-fluid level or complete opacification of the sinus.
- Computed tomography (CT) is a more accurate and expensive tool for cases that fail to respond to standard therapy.
- Few other conditions masquerade as sinusitis, and the differential is limited, particularly in children.
- Appropriate indications for aspiration of the maxillary sinus by an otolaryngologist include: (1) life-threatening complications, (2) immunosuppressive conditions, (3) clinical unresponsiveness, and (4) unusually severe disease. The presence of organisms on Gram's stain and a count of at least 104 colony-forming units point to bacterial infection.[3]

EMERGENCY DEPARTMENT CARE AND DISPOSITION

- For acute severe disease, intravenous therapy is recommended: ceftriaxone (75 mg/kg/day) or ampicillin-sulbactam (200 mg/kg/day of ampicillin component divided every 8 hours).
- Persistent disease demands ear, nose, and throat referral for surgical drainage.
- Mild subacute disease can be treated with amoxicillin (80 mg/kg/day orally divided three times a day).
- Persistent subacute disease can be treated with cefprozil, 30 mg/kg/day PO divided bid, or cefdinir 14 mg/kg/day PO divided twice daily or qd.
- For patients failing prior antibiotics, give amoxicillin-clavulanate 40 to 45 mg/kg/day PO divided twice daily or cefpodoxime 10 mg/kg/day PO divided twice daily.

CELLULITIS

- Cellulitis is an infection of the skin and subcutaneous tissues that extends below the dermis, differentiating it from impetigo.

EPIDEMIOLOGY

- It is a frequent infection in warm weather.
- Under normal circumstances, *Staphylococcus aureus*, *Streptococcus pyogenes* and *H. influenzae* are the most commonly isolated organisms.
- Since the advent of effective conjugated vaccines against *H. influenzae*, such infections are rare in childhood, but now more common in infants under the age of 6 months.

PATHOPHYSIOLOGY

- Cellulitis may occur either when a pathogen is directly inoculated into the subcutaneous tissue or following an episode of bacteremia. The majority of infections involve local invasion after a breach in the integument.
- The organisms responsible are usually *S. aureus* and *S. pyogenes*. In contradistinction, *H. influenzae* disseminates hematogenously.

CLINICAL FEATURES

- Cellulitis manifests a local inflammatory response at the site of infection, with erythema, warmth, and tenderness.
- Fever is unusual, except in severe cases including those caused by *H. influenzae*.

DIAGNOSIS AND DIFFERENTIAL

- The diagnosis of cellulitis is made by inspection. Cellulitis must be differentiated from other causes of erythema and edema, including trauma, allergic reaction, and cold-induced lesions.
- Laboratory studies, including WBC concentration, blood culture, and rarely aspirate culture, are obtained in specific circumstances, including immunocompromise, fever, severe local infection, facial involvement, and failure to respond to standard therapy.
- A WBC count over 15,000 is more common in *H. influenzae* infections.

EMERGENCY DEPARTMENT CARE AND DISPOSITION

- For toxic patients with fever and leukocytosis, intravenous therapy should be used. Antibiotic choices include: nafcillin 25 to 37 mg/kg IV given every 6 hours, oxacillin 25 to 37 mg/kg IV given every 6 hours, or ampicillin-sulbactam (200 mg/kg/day of ampicillin divided every 8 hours). Alternatives include cefazolin 20 mg/kg given every 6 hours plus gentamicin 5 to 7.5 mg/kg/day divided every 8 hours.

- For nontoxic patients, dicloxacillin (50 to 100 mg/kg/day divided four times daily), amoxicillin-clavulanate 45 mg/kg/day PO divided bid, or cephalexin (50 to 100 mg/kg/day divided four times daily) can be used.
- For patients allergic to previously mentioned antibiotics, azithromycin 10 mg/kg PO the first day followed by 5 mg/kg PO for four more days, or erythromycin ethylsuccinate 40 to 50 mg/kg/day PO divided three times daily can be used, but may be less effective.
- Patients who fail to respond to reasonable outpatient antibiotic therapy must be further evaluated and considered for admission and intravenous antibiotic therapy. Other underlying conditions, such as diabetes or underlying immune compromise, must be sought.

PERIORBITAL/ORBITAL CELLULITIS

- Periorbital cellulitis is an inflammatory process of the tissues anterior to the orbital septum or within the orbit (orbital cellulitis).

EPIDEMIOLOGY

- *Staphylococcus aureus* and *Streptococcus pneumoniae* are the principal etiologic agents.[4] *H. influenzae* is declining in frequency.[4]
- Orbital infections are most often due to *S. aureus*, particularly when puncture wounds are involved.[5]
- Children under 3 years old are more likely to be bacteremic, thus experiencing the highest incidence of periorbital cellulitis.
- Orbital cellulitis can occur at any age, but is usually seen in children less than 6 years old.

PATHOPHYSIOLOGY

- Organisms reach the periorbital area either hematogenously or by direct extension from the ethmoid sinus. In the case of orbital disease, contiguous spread is most common.

CLINICAL FEATURES

- Orbital and periorbital cellulitis causes the periorbital area to appear red and swollen. Periorbital edema is usually more pronounced with preseptal infections.
- Proptosis or limitation of extraocular muscle function indicates orbital involvement.
- The eye is usually painful to touch but is nonpruritic.

DIAGNOSIS AND DIFFERENTIAL

- Allergic and traumatic causes for edema must be considered.
- Tumors and metabolic disease may cause swelling and discoloration, particularly thyrotoxicosis in adolescents and neuroblastoma in the young child.
- Leukocytosis occurs frequently with cellulitis and more often with bacteremic preseptal infections. Blood cultures in patients with leukocytosis are often positive.
- CT is performed when orbital involvement is suspected and may easily demonstrate an inflammatory mass or tumor.

EMERGENCY DEPARTMENT CARE AND DISPOSITION

- Admission and treatment with intravenous antibiotics is the usual course to prevent complications of meningitis and subperiosteal abscess.
- Antibiotic choices include: nafcillin 25 to 37 mg/kg IV given every 6 hours, oxacillin 25 to 37 mg/kg IV given every 6 hours, or ampicillin-sulbactam (200 mg/kg/day of the ampicillin component divided every 8 hours). Alternatives include cefazolin 20 mg/kg given every 6 hours plus gentamicin 5 to 7.5 mg/kg/day divided every 8 hours.
- Surgical drainage may be necessary with abscess formation.

REFERENCES

1. Laga M, Naamara W, Brunham RC, et al: Single-dose therapy of gonococcal ophthalmia neonatorum with ceftriaxone. *N Engl J Med* 315:1382, 1986.
2. Nash D, Wald E:Sinusitis *Pediatr Rev* 22:11, 2001.
3. American Academy of Pediatrics, Subcommittee on Management of Sinusitis and Committee on Quality Improvement. *Pediatrics* 108:798, 2001.
4. Schwartz GR, Wright SW: The changing bacteriology of periorbital cellulitis. *Ann Emerg Med* 28:617, 1996.
5. Starkey CR, Steele RW: Medical management of orbital cellulitis. *Pediatr Infect Dis J* 20:1002, 2001.

For further reading in *Emergency Medicine: A Comprehensive Study Guide*, 6th ed., see Chap. 122, "Skin and Soft Tissue Infections," by Richard Malley.

73   PNEUMONIA IN CHILDREN

Lance Brown

EPIDEMIOLOGY

- Pneumonia is more common in early childhood than at any other age. The incidence of pneumonia decreases as a function of age (eg, 40 per 1000 in preschool children, 9 per 1000 in 10 year olds in North America).[1,2]
- Etiologic agents tend to have a seasonal variation. Parainfluenza virus tends to occur in the fall. Respiratory syncytial virus (RSV) and bacteria in the winter, and influenza in the spring.
- Risk factors that increase the incidence or severity of pneumonia include prematurity, malnutrition, low socioeconomic status, passive exposure to smoke, and day care attendance.
- Although the mortality rate is less than 1% in industrialized nations, 5 million children younger than 5 years of age in developing countries die each year from pneumonia.

PATHOPHYSIOLOGY

- Most cases of pneumonia develop after the aspiration of infective viruses or bacteria into the lower respiratory tract.
- Protective mechanisms against the development of pneumonia include nasal entrapment of aerosolized particles, mucus and ciliary movement in the upper respiratory tract, laryngeal reflexes and coughing, alveolar macrophages, the activation of complement and antibodies, and lymphatic drainage. Any derangement of these protective mechanisms leads to an increased risk for pneumonia.
- Children who are at a higher risk for pneumonia include those with anatomic abnormalities of the airways, immune deficiencies, neuromuscular weakness, and abnormal mucus production.
- Even with extensive laboratory testing, the specific etiologic agent often remains elusive. The best predictor of the etiologic agent is the age of the patient (Table 73-1).

CLINICAL FEATURES

- Clinical features of pneumonia are quite variable and are most dependent on the age of the patient. Other factors include the specific respiratory pathogen, the severity of the disease, and any underlying illnesses.
- Neonates and young infants with pneumonia typically present with a sepsis syndrome.[3] The signs and symptoms are nonspecific and include fever or hypothermia, apnea, tachypnea, poor feeding, vomiting, diarrhea, lethargy, grunting, bradycardia, and shock.
- Tachypnea is the most commonly seen physical sign in children with pneumonia. In an otherwise well-appearing child, the absence of tachypnea suggests another diagnosis.[4]
- In older children, signs and symptoms of pneumonia include fever, abnormal lung examination, cough, and pleuritic chest pain. Associated signs and symptoms may include headache, malaise, wheezing, rhinitis,

TABLE 73-1   Likely Etiologic Agents for Pneumonias in Infants and Children

AGE	TYPICAL ETIOLOGIC AGENTS	COMMENT
Neonates (<28 days)	Group B *Streptococcus* *Escherichia coli* *Klebsiella* species	Neonates are the only age group for whom typical bacterial infections are more common than viral infections. Pneumonia is thought to develop after aspiration of maternal genital organisms during birth.
1–24 months	Respiratory syncytial virus Parainfluenza virus Influenza virus Adenovirus *Streptococcus pneumoniae* *Streptococcus pyogenes* *Staphylococcus aureus* *Haemophilus influenzae* (nontypeable)	Viruses are the most common etiologic agents in this age group. Infants 1–3 months of age may also develop afebrile pneumonitis due to *Chlamydia trachomatis* and present with a staccato cough, relatively well appearance, and rales on lung examination.
2–5 years	Influenza A and B Adenovirus *S. pneumoniae* *H. influenzae* (nontypeable)	Historically, *H. influenzae* type b was a relatively common cause of pneumonia in this age group. Immunizations have decreased the incidence of *H. influenzae* dramatically. The impact of immunization against *S. pneumoniae* as an etiologic agent for pneumonia has not yet been fully described.
6–18 years	*Mycoplasma pneumoniae* *S. pneumoniae* *Chlamydia pneumoniae* *S. aureus* Adenovirus	*M. pneumoniae* is most commonly seen in children 10–15 years of age and is the most common etiologic agent for all school-aged children.

conjunctivitis, pharyngitis, and rash. The clinical manifestations of bacterial and viral pneumonias significantly overlap, making the clinical distinction between them problematic.[5]

- Lower lobe pneumonias may cause significant abdominal pain and distention.[6] This presentation may mislead the unsuspecting physician into pursuing an intra-abdominal diagnosis and inappropriately consulting a surgeon.

DIAGNOSIS AND DIFFERENTIAL

- Several conditions may present similarly to pneumonia, and these include congestive heart failure, atelectasis, tumors, congenital pulmonary anomalies, aspiration pneumonitis, poor inspiration or technical difficulties with the chest x-ray, allergic alveolitis, and chronic pulmonary diseases.
- Chest x-rays are commonly used to make the diagnosis of pneumonia. Consolidation on chest x-ray is considered a reliable sign of pneumonia.[7] Viral pneumonias tend to have diffuse interstitial infiltrates with hyperinflation, peribronchial thickening or cuffing, and areas of atelectasis. Bacterial pneumonias tend to have lobar or segmental infiltrates. However, there is overlap, and identifying the etiologic agent by chest x-ray is only somewhat reliable (42 to 80% sensitive and 42 to 100% specific).[4]

- Blood cultures are positive less than 10% of the time in children with proven bacterial pneumonia.[8]
- Sputum cultures may be diagnostic, but are difficult to obtain in young children who are not intubated or do not have a tracheostomy.
- Nasopharyngeal or throat cultures may reveal the causative agent when chlamydia, pertussis, mycoplasma, or a viral pathogen is isolated. Rapid viral antigen tests are available for RSV and influenza. These tests have no role in identifying bacterial etiologies for pneumonia.
- Leukocytosis with a left shift is typical for bacterial pneumonia.[9]
- Most children with radiographically evident pneumonia have normal pulse oximetry readings.[10]

EMERGENCY DEPARTMENT CARE AND DISPOSITION

- General care of the pediatric patient with pneumonia includes assessing for and treating hypoxia, dehydration, and fever. With significant bronchospasm and wheezing, bronchodilators are suggested.
- Empiric antibiotic selection is based on the likely etiologic agents (based on age) and whether the patient is

TABLE 73-2   Empiric Treatment of Pediatric Pneumonias

PATIENT CHARACTERISTICS	TREATMENT RECOMMENDATIONS
Neonates (<28 days)	Inpatient treatment with intravenous: Ampicillin (50 mg/kg per dose) plus Cefotaxime (50 mg/kg per dose) or Ampicillin (50 mg/kg per dose) plus Gentamicin (2.5 mg/kg per dose)
1–3 months old Afebrile, staccato cough, rales, relatively well appearance; 50% have had prior conjunctivitis	Inpatient treatment with intravenous: Erythromycin (10 mg/kg per dose)
1 month–5 years	Inpatient treatment with intravenous: Cefuroxime (50 mg/kg per dose) or Ampicillin (50 mg/kg per dose) Outpatient treatment with oral: Amoxicillin (45 mg/kg per dose twice daily) or Erythromycin (15 mg/kg per dose 3 times per day)
6 years–18 years	Inpatient treatment with intravenous: Erythromycin (10 mg/kg per dose) Outpatient treatment with oral: Erythromycin (15 mg/kg per dose 3 times per day) May substitute another macrolide
Critically ill-appearing child and/or resistant *Streptococcus pneumoniae* suspected	To standard therapy, add intravenous: Vancomycin (20 mg/kg per dose)
Technology- or ventilator-dependent child with multiple hospitalizations (suspect *Pseudomonas aeruginosa*)	Inpatient treatment with intravenous: Ceftazidime (50 mg/kg per dose)

admitted to the hospital or discharged home (Table 73-2). Most children with pneumonia are treated as outpatients.

- The exact pulse oximetry threshold at which an otherwise well-appearing young child with pneumonia should be admitted to the hospital is unknown.[11]
- Indications for admission include age less than 3 months, a history of apneic episodes or cyanosis, toxic appearance, respiratory distress, oxygen requirement, dehydration, vomiting, failed outpatient therapy, immunocompromised state, associated pleural effusion or pneumatocele, or an unreliable caretaker. Pediatric intensive care unit admission should be considered in children with severe respiratory distress or impending respiratory failure.

REFERENCES

1. Murphy TF, Henderson FW, Clyde WA Jr, et al: Pneumonia: An eleven-year study in a pediatric practice. *Am J Epidemiol* 113:12, 1981.
2. Wright AL, Taussig LM, Ray CG, et al: The Tucson Children's Respiratory Study: II. Lower respiratory tract illness in the first year of life. *Am J Epidemiol* 129:1232, 1989.
3. Bohin S, Field DJ: The epidemiology of neonatal respiratory distress. *Early Hum Dev* 37:73, 1994.
4. Margolis P, Gadomoski A: Does this infant have pneumonia? *JAMA* 279:308, 1998.
5. Fang GD, Fine M, Orloff J, et al: New and emerging etiologies for community-acquired pneumonia with implications for therapy. *Medicine* 69:307, 1990.
6. Kanegaye JT, Harley JR: Pneumonia in unexpected locations: An occult cause of pediatric abdominal pain. *J Emerg Med* 13:773, 1995.
7. Davies HD, Wang EE, Manson D, et al: Reliability of the chest radiograph in the diagnosis of lower respiratory infections in young children. *Pediatr Infect Dis J* 15:600, 1996.
8. Turner RB, Lande AE, Chase D, et al: Pneumonia in pediatric outpatients: Cause and clinical manifestations. *J Pediatr* 111:194, 1987.
9. Triga MG, Syrogiannopoulos GA, Thoma KD, et al: Correlation of leukocyte count and erythrocyte sedimentation rate with the day of illness in presumed bacterial pneumonia. *J Infect* 36:63, 1998.
10. Tanen DA, Trocinski DR: The use of pulse oximetry to exclude pneumonia in children. *Am J Emerg Med* 20:521, 2002.
11. Brown L, Dannenberg B. Pulse oximetry in discharge decision-making: a survey of emergency physicians. *Can J Emerg Med* 4:388, 2002.

For further reading in *Emergency Medicine: A Comprehensive Study Guide,* 6th ed., see Chap. 123, "Viral and Bacterial Pneumonia in Children" by Kathleen Brown and Willie Gilford, Jr.

74   ASTHMA AND BRONCHIOLITIS

Douglas R. Trocinski

ASTHMA

EPIDEMIOLOGY

- Asthma affects approximately 4.8 million U.S. children[1] and accounts for 570,000 emergency department visits in patients under the age of 14.[2,3]
- The percentage of patients with adverse outcomes (intubation, need for cardiopulmonary resuscitation, and death) tripled between 1986 and 1993.[4]
- Risk factors associated with development of asthma in children include low birth weight, family history of asthma, urban household, low-income household, and race (children of African-American, Asian, and Hispanic descent).[6,7]
- Risk factors that may contribute to asthma deaths include: socioeconomic background, limited access to health care, improper medication administration, unrecognized severity or extreme lability of disease, nocturnal asthma and history of prior respiratory failure and intubation.

PATHOPHYSIOLOGY

- Asthma is classified as extrinsic (IgE mediated), intrinsic (infection induced), and mixed (both IgE and infection induced).
- The most common triggers for children older than 2 years are allergens and irritants, while viral respiratory infections are thought to predominate in those below age 2.
- Asthma is a two-stage process: (1) bronchoconstriction due to histamine and leukotriene release (early stage) and (2) airway mucosal edema with mucous plugging (late stage).
- Bronchospasm, mucosal edema, and mucous plugging cause variable and reversible airflow obstruction and air trapping, which may impair oxygen exchange and lead to ventilation-perfusion mismatches in areas of atelectasis, resulting in hypoxia.
- Compensatory hyperventilation may cause a fall in Pa_{CO_2} and respiratory alkalosis. More severe obstruction and inadequate alveolar ventilation ultimately result in marked CO_2 retention, respiratory acidosis, and respiratory failure. Pseudonormalization of Pa_{CO_2} is therefore ominous.
- Cessation of symptoms depends largely on resolution of mucosal inflammation and may take days to weeks.

- Age-specific anatomic differences in children increase their risk of respiratory failure. These include increased compliance of rib cage and diaphragm immaturity, a predisposition to atelectases secondary to a lack of lung tissue elastic recoil, and thicker airway walls that result in proportionally greater narrowing with bronchoconstriction. These factors result in an increased work of breathing and a predisposition to respiratory muscle fatigue.[4]

CLINICAL FEATURES

- Wheezing is the most common symptom of asthma.
- In cases of severe bronchospasm, the "silent wheezer" may reveal only diminished breath sounds and decreased air movement on auscultation.
- Persistent nonproductive cough or exercise-induced cough may be the result of bronchospasm.
- The amount of air movement, retractions, nasal flaring, degree of accessory muscle use and/or a tripod position usually reflect the severity of the asthma attack.
- Cyanosis, altered mental status, and somnolence may indicate respiratory failure. Bradycardia and shock herald impending cardiac arrest.

DIAGNOSIS AND DIFFERENTIAL

- Chest x-ray usually reveals hyperinflation and flattening of the diaphragm, but is generally not useful for a recurrent, typical exacerbation.
- Indications for chest x-ray in asthma include a first episode of wheezing, unilateral wheezing or rales, and fever.
- Measuring a peak expiratory flow rate (PEFR) may be useful in children over 4 years of age. PEFR less than 50% of the predicted value indicates more severe obstruction.
- Hypercarbia on arterial blood gas measurement may be the initial sign of respiratory failure.
- Other causes of wheezing include viral infection, bronchopulmonary dysplasia, congestive heart failure, gastroesophageal reflux, vascular rings, bronchial stenosis, mediastinal cysts, cystic fibrosis, pneumonia, and aspiration of foreign body.

EMERGENCY DEPARTMENT CARE

- Albuterol, the mainstay of acute therapy, can be administered as episodic treatments at 0.15 mg/kg/dose (2.5 to 5 mg) every 20 minutes, or as a continuous nebulization up to 0.5 mg/kg/hour (10 to 15 mg per hour).

- Oxygen should be administered if oxygen saturation is below 94%. Of note, transient decrease in oxygen saturation may accompany effective therapy secondary to ventilation-perfusion mismatch.
- Steroids are indicated for nearly all acute exacerbations to decrease mucosal inflammation, thereby preventing progression of an attack, decreasing incidence of emergency department visits and hospitalization, and reducing morbidity. Prednisone or prednisolone, 2 mg/kg/day, should be administered early in presentation and continued for 5 days safely with no need for a taper.[5,6]
- Ipratropium should be considered for most exacerbations in a dose of 125 to 250 μg if less than age 14, and 500 μg if the patient is 14 years of age or older.[7,8]
- Magnesium sulfate 25 to 50 mg/kg (maximum dose 2 g) IV over 20 minutes may benefit a subset of children with severe exacerbation.[9,10]
- Helium-oxygen (Heliox) may benefit children with severe exacerbations by decreasing airway resistance and work of breathing, but should not be used for children with an oxygen requirement greater than the delivered oxygen.[11]
- IV fluids may be required in patients with status asthmaticus because of increased insensible water loss and decreased oral intake.
- If mechanical ventilation is required, low inflating pressures and long expiratory times may reduce the risk of barotrauma.
- Ketamine (1 to 2 mg/kg IV) is a useful induction agent for intubation due to its bronchodilating effects.
- Subcutaneous epinephrine (0.01 mL/kg of 1:1000 solution, maximum 0.3 mL) should be given if the patient is unresponsive to therapy or respiratory distress increases while IV access is obtained.
- The intravenous β_2-agonist terbutaline may be given to refractory patients at a dose of 0.5 to 1.0 μg/kg/min. These patients require continuous cardiac monitoring in an ICU setting to protect from myocardial ischemia and tachyarrhythmias. Terbutaline may also be administered subcutaneously prior to IV access (0.01 mL/kg of a 1-mg/mL solution, maximum 0.25 mL).
- Chronic therapies may include levalbuterol, the R-isomer of albuterol, inhaled glucocorticoids, leukotriene-receptor inhibitors, cromolyn sodium, nedocromil, and theophylline.

DISPOSITION

- Admission is warranted for persistent oxygen requirement, refractory respiratory distress, or dyspnea on exertion despite intensive therapy over 2 to 4 hours.

Level of inpatient care is dependent on severity of exacerbation and degree of response to therapy.

- Children who respond to conventional therapy should be discharged with detailed instructions, β_2-agonist therapy (generally an MDI with a spacer), a prescription for oral steroids, and confirmed follow-up with the primary care provider.

BRONCHIOLITIS

EPIDEMIOLOGY

- Bronchiolitis occurs typically from October to May.
- Infants less than 2 years old are most commonly affected. The peak incidence in urban populations is at 2 months of age.
- Young infants (under 2 months of age) and those with history of prematurity, bronchopulmonary dysplasia, congenital heart disease, or immunosuppression are at increased risk of complicated courses of the disease.
- The infectious agent is highly contagious and is transmitted by direct contact with secretions and self-inoculation by contaminated hands via the eyes and nose.

PATHOPHYSIOLOGY

- Respiratory syncytial virus (RSV) causes 50 to 70% of clinically significant bronchiolitis.[12]
- Non-RSV bronchiolitis is caused by influenza virus, parainfluenza virus, echovirus, rhinovirus, *Mycoplasma pneumoniae,* and *Chlamydia trachomatis.*
- Mucous plugging results from necrosis of the respiratory epithelium and destruction of ciliated epithelial cells. This and submucosal edema lead to peripheral airway narrowing and variable obstruction.
- Increased airway resistance and decreased compliance result in increased work of breathing.

CLINICAL FEATURES

- Bronchiolitis, or inflammation of the bronchioles, often begins with nasal discharge, pharyngitis, cough, and fever. The predominant symptom, wheezing and respiratory distress, generally follow upper respiratory infection symptoms.
- Tachypnea, retractions, nasal flaring, and grunting may be present.
- Decreased breath sounds or absence of breath sounds signifies severe bronchoconstriction. Cyanosis and altered mental status are ominous signs of respiratory failure.

- Symptoms peak in 3 to 5 days and usually resolve within 2 weeks.
- Immunity is variable and reinfection may occur.

DIAGNOSIS AND DIFFERENTIAL

- Chest x-ray is recommended in all children with an initial episode of wheezing. The chest x-ray may show hyperinflation and peribronchial cuffing.
- Pulmonary consolidation on the chest x-ray may reflect primary pneumonia or superinfection.
- Identification of RSV can be made from nasal washings using fluorescent monoclonal antibody testing, but may be unnecessary except for children with underlying conditions that predispose to a complicated course, or as required locally for bed placement and isolation determination.
- Initial pulse oximetry is recommended in all children with respiratory distress, with continuous monitoring maintained for initial readings less than 93%.
- Complete blood count and blood culture are generally not helpful.

EMERGENCY DEPARTMENT CARE AND DISPOSITION

- Children with bronchiolitis and a history of reactive airway disease may respond to an inhaled β-agonist (albuterol 0.15 mg/kg/dose). If improvement occurs, treatments may be repeated as needed.
- Nebulized epinephrine (1:1000) 0.5 mL in 2.5 mL normal saline may be beneficial if albuterol fails. Epinephrine may be repeated every 2 hours.[13]
- Helium-oxygen (heliox) should be considered for children with severe symptoms, unless the child's oxygen requirement makes its use unsafe.[14]
- Dehydration from increased insensible water loss may require IV fluid therapy.
- Corticosteroids are not indicated in bronchiolitis unless there is a history of underlying reactive airway disease.[15]
- Indications for hospitalization include (1) apnea, (2) respiratory distress unresponsive to treatment, (3) hypoxia, (4) vomiting and/or dehydration, and (5) persistent tachypnea greater than 60 breaths/min.
- Admission should be considered for children with underlying conditions that predispose to a complicated course of therapy (bronchopulmonary disease, congenital heart disease, immune compromise).
- All children discharged from the emergency department require confirmed 24-hour follow-up with their primary care provider.

REFERENCES

1. Calmes D, Leake BD, Carlisle DM: Adverse outcomes among children hospitalized with asthma in California. *Pediatrics* 101:845, 1998.
2. Surveillance for Asthma—United States 1960-1995. *MMWR* 47:6, 1998.
3. Goodman DC, Stukel TA, Chang CH: Trends in pediatric asthma hospitalization rates: Regional and socioeconomic differences. *Pediatrics* 101:208, 1998.
4. Wohl M: Developmental physiology of the respiratory system, in Sherlock V, Boat T (eds.): *Kendig's Disorders of the Respiratory Tract in Children,* 6th ed., Philadelphia: Saunders, 1998, p. 19.
5. Tal A, Levy N, Bearman JE: Methylprednisolone therapy for acute asthma in infants and toddlers: A controlled clinical trial. *Pediatrics* 86:350, 1990.
6. Scarfone RJ, Fuchs SM, Nager AL, Shane SA, et al: Controlled clinical trial of oral prednisone in emergency department treatment of children with acute asthma. *Pediatrics* 92: 513, 1993.
7. Schuh S, Johnson DW, Callahan S, Canny G, et al: Efficacy of frequent nebulized ipratropium bromide added to frequent high dose albuterol therapy in severe childhood asthma. *J Pediatrics* 126:639, 1995.
8. Qureshi F, Pestian J, Davis P, Zaritsky A: Effect of nebulized ipratropium on the hospitalization rates of children with asthma. *N Engl J Med* 339:1030, 1998.
9. Ciarallo L, Sauer AH, Shannon MW: IV magnesium therapy for moderate to severe pediatric asthma: Results of a randomized, placebo-controlled trial. *J Pediatrics* 129:809, 1996.
10. Devi PR, Kumar L, Singhi SC, Prasad R, et al: IV MgSO$_4$ in acute severe asthma not responding to conventional therapy. *Indian Pediatrics* 34:389, 1997.
11. Kudukis TM, Manthous CA, Schmidt GA, Hall JB, et al: Inhaled heliox revisited: Effect of inhaled helium oxygen mixture during treatment of status asthmaticus in children. *J Pediatrics* 130:217, 1997.
12. Wohl ME: Bronchiolitis, in Chernick V, Boat T (eds.): *Kendig's Disorders of the Respiratory Tract in Children,* 6th ed. Philadelphia: Saunders, 1998, p. 473.
13. Menon K, Sutcliffe T, Klassen TP: A randomized trial comparing the efficacy of epinephrine with salbutamol in the treatment of acute bronchiolitis. *J Pediatrics* 126:1004, 1995.
14. Hollman G, Shen G, Zeng L, Yngsdal-Krenz R, et al: Helium-oxygen improves clinical asthma scores in children with acute bronchiolitis. *Crit Care Med* 26:1731, 1998.
15. Klassen TP, Sutcliffe T, Watters LK, et al: Dexamethasone in salbutamol treated inpatients with acute bronchiolitis: a randomized controlled trial. *J Pediatrics* 130:191, 1997.

For further reading in *Emergency Medicine: A Comprehensive Study Guide,* 6th ed., see Chap. 124, "Pediatric Asthma and Bronchiolitis," by Maybelle Kou and Thom Mayer.

75 SEIZURES AND STATUS EPILEPTICUS IN CHILDREN
Michael C. Plewa

- Both the causes and the manifestations of seizure activity are numerous, ranging from benign to life-threatening.
- Although idiopathic seizures (eg, epilepsy) comprise the largest category of seizures, several risk factors include encephalitis, disorders of amino acid metabolism, structural abnormalities (eg, neoplasm, hydrocephalus, shunt malfunction, microcephaly, or arteriovenous malformations), systemic disorders (eg, sickle cell anemia, systemic lupus erythematosus), congenital infections, or neurocutaneous syndromes (eg, tuberous sclerosis, neurofibromatosis, Sturge-Weber syndrome).
- Precipitants of seizures can include fever, sepsis, hypoglycemia, hypocalcemia, hypoxemia, hyper- or hyponatremia, hypotension, toxin or medication exposure, and head injury.

EPIDEMIOLOGY

- Approximately 1 to 2% of the United States population has epilepsy, although the lifetime likelihood of at least one seizure is nearly 9%.
- In children aged 0 to 9 years, the prevalence is 4.4 cases per 1000, and in those 10 to 19 years old, the prevalence is 6.6 cases per 1000.
- Simple febrile convulsions constitute a separate category, with an incidence of 3 to 4% in children.

PATHOPHYSIOLOGY

- A seizure is an abnormal, sudden, and excessive electric discharge of neurons (gray matter) that propagates down the neuronal processes (white matter) to affect end organs in a clinically measurable fashion.
- Neuronal depolarizations may be precipitated by a deficiency of inhibitory neurotransmitter (eg, gamma-aminobutyric acid [GABA]), excess of excitatory neurotransmitter (eg, glutamate), or dysfunction of these receptors.

CLINICAL FEATURES

- Symptoms of seizure may include any of the following: loss of or alteration in consciousness, including behavioral changes, and auditory, sensory, or olfactory hallucinations; involuntary motor activity, including vocalizations, tonic or clonic contractions, spasms, automatisms (staring, blinking, lip-smacking, chewing, pedaling) or choreoathetoid movements; atony (loss of tone resulting in fall); and incontinence.

- Signs could include alteration in consciousness or motor activity; autonomic dysfunction, such as mydriasis, diaphoresis, hypertension, tachypnea or apnea, tachycardia, and salivation; and postictal somnolence.
- Neonatal seizures may have subtle manifestations, sometimes only autonomic changes such as mydriasis, apnea, or cardiac irregularity.

DIAGNOSIS AND DIFFERENTIAL

- The diagnosis of seizure disorder is based primarily on history and physical examination, with laboratory studies (other than a bedside assay for glucose) obtained in a problem-focused manner.[1]
- Serum drug level determinations are useful for phenobarbital, phenytoin, valproic acid, carbamazepine, and ethosuximide in patients with breakthrough seizures or status epilepticus, whereas levels of the newer agents may not be immediately available or useful in guiding therapy.
- Serum chemistry studies (ie, electrolytes, magnesium, calcium, creatinine, and blood urea nitrogen levels) are usually not indicated except in neonatal seizures, infantile spasms, febrile seizures that are complex in nature (with duration over 15 minutes, focal involvement, or several recurrences in 24 hours), status epilepticus, or suspected metabolic or gastrointestinal disorders.[2]
- Serum ammonia, TORCH (**t**oxoplasmosis, **r**ubella, **c**ytomegalovirus, and **h**erpes) titers, and urine and serum amino acid screening may be useful in neonatal seizures.
- Blood gas analysis is indicated in neonatal seizures and status epilepticus.
- Cardiac monitoring is useful to assess the PR and QT intervals and the possibility of cardiac dysrhythmia as the precipitant of seizure.
- Toxicology screening may be useful in adolescents suspected of recreational drug use (eg, cocaine).
- Magnetic resonance imaging is the preferred neuroimaging procedure for most cases of new-onset seizures,[3] whereas cerebral ultrasound is useful in neonates and immediate noncontrast computed tomography is indicated in cases of head trauma, nonfebrile status epilepticus, and focal seizures or focal neurologic signs.[2]
- Lumbar puncture should be performed in patients with neonatal seizure, infantile spasms, and complex febrile seizures under 18 months of age, meningeal signs, or persistent alteration in consciousness.

- Emergent electroencephalographic (EEG) monitoring is indicated for neonatal seizures, nonconvulsive status epilepticus, and refractory status epilepticus, especially when a paralytic agent is used.
- It is important to differentiate true seizure activity from one of several nonepileptic paroxysmal disorders, such as neonatal jitteriness (precipitated by stimulation), shuddering, hyperexplexia (startle disease), near-miss sudden death syndrome, breath-holding spells (of cyanotic or pallid types), hyperventilation, syncope, migraine, pseudoseizures, narcolepsy, Tourette's syndrome, or chorea, which are characterized by normal EEGs and are unresponsive to antiepileptic drugs.

EMERGENCY DEPARTMENT CARE AND DISPOSITION

- Initial management should include: (1) airway maintenance (supplemental oxygen, suctioning, airway opening, or intubation when necessary), (2) seizure termination, (3) correction of reversible causes, (4) initiation of appropriate diagnostic studies, and (5) arrangement of follow-up or admission, as appropriate.
- Termination of seizure activity is important to prevent irreversible pathologic changes and risk of persistent seizure disorder, especially in the setting of status epilepticus, defined as one seizure greater than 30 minutes in duration.[4] For this reason, seizures lasting greater than 10 minutes are treated as status epilepticus.[4]
- Intravenous (IV) access is essential in cases of neonatal seizures, status epilepticus, and recurrent seizures.
- Admission is essential for neonatal seizures and status epilepticus, and should be considered for complex febrile seizures (especially if sepsis or meningitis is suspected), recurrent breakthrough seizures (especially with therapeutic or toxic drug levels), first seizure with focal involvement, persistent abnormal neurologic exam, or suspected neurologic or systemic disease.

FIRST SEIZURE

- Only patients with prolonged or repetitive witnessed seizures, especially with concomitant neurologic deficit, are started on antiepileptic drugs. The choice of antiepileptic drug is based on seizure type, side effect profile, and ease of administration, and should usually be discussed with the primary physician or neurologist.
- Generalized tonic-clonic seizures are commonly treated with valproate 20 to 60 mg/kg/day, or topiramate 1 to

10 mg/kg/day, or lamotrigine 2 to 15 mg/kg/day (with lower doses when used with valproate). Other drugs are also effective.

- Partial seizures are primarily treated with carbamazepine 10 to 40 mg/kg/day. Other first-line agents include phenytoin 4 to 8 mg/kg/day, phenobarbital 3 to 8 mg/kg/day, and primidone 5 to 20 mg/kg/day.
- Complex partial seizures are commonly treated with felbamate 45 mg/kg/day or gabapentin 20 to 30 mg/kg/day.
- Absence seizures are primarily treated (after confirmatory EEG) with ethosuximide 20 to 30 mg/kg/day, and with valproate, lamotrigine, or topiramate if present with other seizure types.
- Myoclonic as well as tonic/atonic seizures are commonly treated with valproate, lamotrigine, topiramate, or felbamate.
- IV loading can be achieved with the IV form of valproate Depacon 10 to 30 mg/kg over 15 minutes, or fosphenytoin 15 to 20 mg phenytoin equivalents (PE)/kg at 3 PE/kg/min, a phenytoin prodrug without infusion-related complications.

FEBRILE SEIZURE

- Febrile seizures occur in children aged 3 months to 5 years.
- Identification and treatment of the cause of fever is the primary goal of therapy for febrile seizures.[5,6] Fever can be controlled by acetaminophen or ibuprofen and tepid water baths.
- Antiepileptic drug therapy with oral phenobarbital or valproate are only used in those with an underlying neurologic deficit (eg, cerebral palsy), complex (prolonged or focal) febrile seizure, repeated seizures in the same febrile illness, onset under 6 months of age, or more than three febrile seizures in 6 months.[7,8]

NEONATAL SEIZURES

- The cause of neonatal seizures should be thoroughly investigated and treated aggressively in an intensive care setting.
- Persistent or uncertain cause of seizures should be treated with empiric IV pyridoxine 100 mg/day; hypoglycemia with 10% dextrose solution 5 mL/kg IV; hypocalcemia with calcium gluconate (10% solution) 200 to 500 mg/kg/day IV (in four daily doses) and magnesium sulfate 25 to 50 mg/kg IV or IM; and biotinidase deficiency with biotin 10 mg/day.
- The first-line agent is IV phenobarbital 20 mg/kg at 1 mg/kg/min followed by 3 to 4 mg/kg/day.[9]

- Second-line agents include IV fosphenytoin 20 mg PE/kg at 3 mg PE/kg/min and then 4 to 8 mg PE/kg/day, midazolam 0.2 mg/kg over 2 minutes, or lorazepam 0.1 mg/kg IV over 2 minutes.
- Refractory seizures are treated with continuous IV infusion of midazolam 0.04 to 0.5 mg/kg/hour or pentobarbital 0.5 to 3.0 mg/kg/hour.
- Diazepam might exacerbate hyperbilirubinemia.

INFANTILE SPASMS

- Therapy with adrenocorticotropic hormone (ACTH) or with topiramate, clonazepam, vigabatrin, or valproate is often started in the inpatient setting after specialty consultation. Glucose transporter defect syndrome (diagnosed by lumbar puncture [LP]) is treated with a ketogenic diet.

HEAD TRAUMA AND SEIZURES

- Immediate seizures following head trauma may require short-term treatment with fosphenytoin, especially following severe head injury.[10] Early and late posttraumatic seizures may require long-term antiepileptic therapy if recurrent.[11]

BREAKTHROUGH SEIZURES IN THE KNOWN EPILEPTIC

- Precipitants of breakthrough seizures include low anticonvulsant levels (from noncompliance, infection, altered metabolism, or drug interaction), toxic anticonvulsant levels (eg, phenytoin, carbamazepine), altered sleep patterns, stress, alcohol or recreational drug use (especially stimulants), or medication use (eg, lindane, theophylline, cyclosporine, isoniazid, meperidine, or tricyclic antidepressants).
- Those with recurrent or frequent tonic, tonic-clonic, or clonic seizures and low antiepileptic drug levels should receive rapid loading of antiepileptic drug IV (phenobarbital, fosphenytoin, or Depacon) or rectally (liquid valproate, phenobarbital, phenytoin, primidone, or carbamazepine). Lamotrigine should not be loaded because of risk of rash.
- A second antiepileptic agent should be considered (after consultation with the neurologist) if levels are in the high therapeutic range, such as phenobarbital, phenytoin, or valproate for focal or partial seizures, and lamotrigine, ethosuximide, valproate, clonazepam, or acetazolamide for absence seizures.

STATUS EPILEPTICUS

- Airway maintenance is of primary importance in status epilepticus because all therapeutic agents can result in respiratory depression.
- With IV access, lorazepam 0.1 mg/kg to a total of 8 mg, diazepam 0.2 to 0.5 mg/kg to a total of 2.6 mg/kg, or midazolam 0.1 to 0.2 mg/kg are the primary agents of choice.[12–14] Lorazepam may be preferred because of its longer effective half-life in the brain. Midazolam usually requires continuous infusion.
- Without IV access, alternatives include rectal, nasal, or IM midazolam 0.1 to 0.2 mg/kg; rectal diazepam 0.5 mg/kg; rectal valproic acid 60 mg/kg; or intraosseous (IO) infusion of lorazepam, diazepam, or midazolam (in similar dosages as IV).[15,16]
- Fosphenytoin 20 mg PE/kg IV or IO should be started immediately after the primary agent, followed by phenobarbital 20 to 30 mg/kg IV or IO repeated 10 mg/kg every 20 minutes to levels of 60 mg/mL, or Depacon 10 to 30 mg/kg IV (over 15 minutes) if fosphenytoin is ineffective.
- If seizures still persist, consider continuous midazolam IV infusion 0.04 to 0.05 mg/kg/h, propofol 1 mg/kg IV bolus followed by 2 mg/kg/h infusion, or general anesthesia (along with continuous EEG monitoring) with pentobarbital 2 mg/kg bolus followed by 1 to 2 mg/kg/h IV infusion or inhalational agents, or IV lidocaine 2 mg/kg bolus followed by infusion at 5 to 10 mg/kg/h.[12]
- Consider treatable causes such as hypoglycemia (treated with 10% dextrose 5 mL kg IV or IO), hyponatremia, toxin exposure (eg, iron, lead, carbon monoxide, salicylates, stimulants, etc.), or infections (eg. meningoencephalitis or brain abscess). Specific toxicologic therapy (eg, activated charcoal, hyperbaric oxygen, or chelation therapy) should be used where appropriate for suspected toxin exposure.

COMPLICATIONS OF ANTIEPILEPTIC THERAPY

- Carbamazepine use can result in hyponatremia and movement disorder.
- Clonazepam use can result in sedation and bladder dysfunction.
- Ethosuximide can cause movement disorder.
- Gabapentin use can result in myoclonic seizures, hepatic injury, and dizziness.
- Lamotrigine can cause rash (eg, Stevens-Johnson syndrome, toxic epidermal necrolysis) and drug interactions.
- Oxcarbazepine interacts with oral contraceptives.

- Phenobarbital use can result in sedation, hepatic dysfunction, or weakness.
- Phenytoin use can result in gingival hyperplasia, neuropathy, osteomalacia, macrocytic anemia, weakness, rash, hepatic injury, ataxia, and nausea. Extravasation can cause the "purple glove syndrome."
- Tiagabine can cause sedation, myoclonic seizures, and interactions with other antiepileptic agents.
- Topiramate can cause memory loss, sedation, and renal stones.
- Valproate use can result in hepatic injury, hyperammonemia, pancreatitis, and thrombocytopenia.
- Zonisamide can cause oligohidrosis and hyperthermia.
- Ketogenic diet can result in pancreatitis and renal calculi. Avoid glucose infusions that reverse the ketogenic state.
- Vagus nerve stimulators can occasionally cause hoarseness; these can be temporarily deactivated with a magnet.

REFERENCES

1. Nypuaver MM, Reynolds SL, Tanz RR, Davis AT: Emergency department laboratory evaluation of children with seizures: dogma or dilemma? *Pediatr Emerg Care* 8:13, 1992.
2. Pellock JH: Management of acute seizure episodes. *Epilepsia* 39:S28, 1998.
3. Pellegrino TR: An emergency department approach to first-time seizures. *Emerg Med Clin North Am* 12:925, 1994.
4. Lowenstein DH, Bleck T, Macdonald RL: It's time to revise the definition of status epilepticus. *Epilepsia* 40:120, 1999.
5. Millichap JG, Colliver JA: Management of febrile seizures: Survey of current practice and phenobarbital usage. *Pediatr Neurol* 7:243, 1991.
6. Consensus Development Conference on Febrile Seizures. Proceedings. *Epilepsia* 2:377, 1981.
7. Berg AT, Shinnar S, Hauser WA, et al: A prospective study of recurrent febrile seizures [see comments]. *N Engl J Med* 327: 1161, 1992.
8. Farwell JR, Lee YJ, Hertz DG, et al: Phenobarbital for febrile seizures: Effects on intelligence and on seizure recurrence. *N Engl J Med* 322:364, 1990.
9. Maytal J, Novak GP, King KC: Lorazepam in the treatment of refractory neonatal seizures. *J Child Neurol* 6:319, 1991.
10. Boeve BF, Wijdicks FM, Benarrock EE, Schidt KD: Paroxysmal sympathetic storms ("diencephalic seizures") after severe diffuse axonal head injury. *Mayo Clin Proc* 73:148, 1998.
11. Rosman NP, Herskowitz J, Carter AP, O'Connor JF: Acute head trauma in infancy and childhood. *Pediatr Clin North Am* 26:707, 1979.
12. Lowenstein DH, Alldredge BK: Status epilepticus. *N Engl J Med* 338:970, 1998.

13. Leppik IE, Derivan AT, Homan RW, et al: A double blind study of lorazepam and diazepam in status epilepticus. *JAMA* 249:1452, 1983.

14. Rivera R, Segnini M, Baltodano A, Perez V: Midazolam in the treatment of status epilepticus in children [see comments]. *Crit Care Med* 21:955, 1993.

15. Chamberlain JM, Altieri MA, Futterman C, et al: A prospective, randomized study comparing intramuscular midazolam with intravenous diazepam for the treatment of seizures in children. *Pediatr Emerg Care* 13:92, 1997.

16. Treiman DM, Meyers PD, Walton NY, et al: A comparison of four treatments for generalized convulsive status epilepticus. *N Engl J Med* 339:792, 1998.

For further reading in *Emergency Medicine: A Comprehensive Study Guide,* 6th ed., see Chap. 125, "Seizures and Status Epilepticus in Children," by Michael A. Nigro.

76 VOMITING AND DIARRHEA IN CHILDREN

Debra G. Perina

EPIDEMIOLOGY

- In the United States, children younger than 3 years of age have 1.3 to 2.3 episodes of diarrhea each year. The most common cause of diarrhea in children is infectious. The prevalence is higher in children attending day care centers.
- Up to one fifth of all acute care outpatient visits to hospitals are by families with infants or children with acute gastroenteritis, and 9% of all hospitalizations of children younger than 5 years of age are for diarrhea.[1]
- Most enteric infections are self-limited, but excessive water and electrolyte loss resulting in clinical dehydration may occur in 10% and is life threatening in 1%.[2]
- Pathogenic viruses, bacteria, or parasites may be isolated from nearly 50% of children with diarrhea. Viral infection is the most common, but bacterial pathogens may be isolated in 1 to 4% of cases.
- Rotaviruses, Norwalk viruses, and the enteric adenoviruses are the most recognized viral pathogens that affect children, with rotavirus being the most common.
- The major bacterial enteropathogens in the United States are *Campylobacter jejuni, Shigella* species, *Salmonella* species, *Yersinia enterocolitica, Clostridium difficile,* and *Escherichia coli. Escherichia coli* has three pathogenic varieties, with the enterohemor-

rhagic (serotype O157:H7) being the most aggressive, releasing a cytotoxin that has been responsible for several deaths.
- *Giardia lamblia* is a parasitic infection and a common cause of diarrhea in infants and young children in day care centers.

PATHOPHYSIOLOGY

- Viral, parasitic, and bacterial pathogens cause disease by tissue invasion and alteration of intestinal absorption of water and electrolytes.
- Some bacterial pathogens such as *Escherichia coli, Vibrio cholerae,* and *Shigella* cause diarrhea by the production of enterotoxins and cytotoxins and invasion of the mucosal absorptive surface.
- The small bowel absorbs the vast majority of water in the gastrointestinal tract. Pathogens that interfere with water absorption in this area tend to produce voluminous diarrhea. By contrast, disease processes that affect the colonic region, such as dysentery, produce frequent, small volume, often bloody stools. Table 76-1 lists common causative agents, clinical features, and treatment for diarrhea in children.

CLINICAL FEATURES

- Evaluation of a child's state of hydration is most important. If possible, it is best to determine the degree of fluid loss by comparing the child's current weight to a recent previous weight.
- When objective measurements are not available, the state of hydration can be assessed by physical examination. Combinations of physical signs, including ill general appearance, capillary refill of greater than 3 seconds, dry mucous membranes, and absent tears are good predictors. The presence of two or more signs predicts 5% or greater dehydration, whereas three or more signs predict 10% or greater dehydration.[3]
- Severe dehydration accompanied by lethargy, hypotension, and delayed capillary refill requires immediate administration of parenteral fluids. Although capillary refill may be affected by conditions other than dehydration, it should be considered a sign of significant dehydration until proven otherwise.[4]

DIAGNOSIS AND DIFFERENTIAL

- The most important aspect of diagnosis is a thorough history and physical examination. Selective laboratory testing may be useful if enteric pathogens are suspected.

TABLE 76-1   Common Agents, Clinical Features, and Treatment of Diarrhea

AGENT	CLINICAL FEATURES	TREATMENT
Viral		
Rotavirus	Watery diarrhea, winter, most common agent	Rehydration
Enteric adenovirus	Watery diarrhea, concurrent respiratory symptoms	Rehydration
Norwalk	Watery diarrhea, epidemic, fever, headache, myalgias	Rehydration
Bacterial		
Campylobacter jejuni	Fever, abdominal pain, watery or bloody diarrhea; may mimic appendicitis, animal reservoir	Rehydration, erythromycin
Shigella	Fever, abdominal pain, headache, mucoid diarrhea	Rehydration, TMP-SMX or ampicillin
Salmonella	Fever, bloody diarrhea, animal reservoir; antibiotics prolong the carrier state	Rehydration, TMP-SMX if complicated
Escherichia coli		
Enterotoxigenic	Watery diarrhea	Rehydration, TMP-SMX
Enterohemorrhagic	Dysentery, associated with HUS	Rehydration, check CBC, BUN, creatinine
Enteroinvasive	Dysentery, *Shigella*-like	Rehydration, TMP-SMX
Vibrio cholerae	Rice-water diarrhea	Rehydration, TMP-SMX
Yersinia enterocolitica	Fever-vomiting, diarrhea, abdominal pain; may mimic appendicitis	Rehydration, Ceftriaxone (controversial)
Clostridium difficile	Recent antibiotic use	Rehydration, metronidazole
Staphylococcus aureus	Food poisoning	Rehydration
Parasitic		
Giardia lamblia	Diarrhea, flatulence; exposure to day care centers, mountain streams	Rehydration, metronidazole
Entamoeba histolytica	Bloody, mucoid stools; hepatic abscess	Rehydration, metronidazole

DOSES: ampicillin 50 mg/kg/d divided qid; ceftriaxone 50 mg/kg/d; erythromycin 40 mg/kg/d divided qid; metronidazole 30 mg/kg/d divided bid; TMP-SMX based on 8 to 12 mg/kg/d of the TMP component divided bid.
ABBREVIATIONS: bid = twice a day; BUN = blood urea nitrogen; CBC = complete blood count; qid = four times a day; HUS = hemolytic-uremic syndrome; TMP-SMX = trimethoprim-sulfamethoxazole.

- Dehydration caused by diarrhea is usually isotonic, and serum electrolyte determinations are not necessary unless signs of severe dehydration are present.
- Protracted vomiting and/or diarrhea in infants and toddlers may cause hypoglycemia. Blood glucose determinations are useful in this setting.
- The fecal leukocyte test, sometimes used as a screening tool, has poor sensitivity and guaiac testing has poor specificity.[5]
- A febrile child with abrupt onset of diarrhea occurring more than four times per day or with blood in the stool is more likely to have an illness caused by a bacterial pathogen and stool cultures are indicated.[6]
- Vomiting and diarrhea may be a nonspecific presentation for other disease processes, such as otitis media, urinary tract infection, sepsis, malrotation, increased intracranial pressure, metabolic acidosis, intussusception, and drug or toxin ingestion.
- Infants under 1 year of age are at particularly high risk for rapid dehydration and hypoglycemia.

- Special attention should be given to those children who have chronically debilitating illnesses, high-risk social situations, or malnutrition, since they are at particular risk for rapid decompensation.

EMERGENCY DEPARTMENT CARE AND DISPOSITION

If vomiting is the prominent symptom:
- Since most cases are self-limited, oral rehydration is generally all that is necessary.[7,8] Vomiting is not a contraindication to oral rehydration with glucose-electrolyte solutions. The key is to give small amounts of the solution frequently.
- If oral rehydration is not possible or not tolerated by the patient, intravenous (IV) rehydration with normal saline may be necessary.
- Antiemetics are controversial and generally not recommended.[8] If they are used, the physician should be

aware of potential adverse side effects associated with these drugs, such as dystonic reactions.

If diarrhea is the prominent symptom:

- Children with mild diarrhea who are not dehydrated may continue routine feedings.[9]
- Children with moderate to severe dehydration should first receive adequate rehydration before resuming routine feedings. Food should be reinstated after the rehydration phase is completed and never delayed more than 24 hours. There is no need to dilute formula, since over 80% of children with acute diarrhea can tolerate full-strength milk safely.[9]
- Dietary recommendations include a diet high in complex carbohydrates, lean meats, vegetables, fruits, and yogurt. Fatty foods and foods high in simple sugars should be avoided. The bananas, rice, applesauce, and toast (BRAT) diet is discouraged, since it does not provide adequate energy sources.
- Antimotility drugs are not helpful and should not be used to treat acute diarrhea in children.[8–11]
- Antibiotics are considered if the diarrhea has persisted longer than 10 to 14 days or the patient has a significant fever, systemic symptoms, or blood or pus in the stool.[11] See Table 76-1 for antibiotic recommendations.
- All infants and children who appear toxic or have high-risk social situations, significant dehydration, intractable vomiting, 10% dehydration, altered mental status, an inability to drink, bloody diarrhea, or laboratory evidence of hemolytic anemia, thrombocytopenia, or elevated creatinine levels should be admitted.
- If the patient is discharged, the family should be given instructions to return or seek care with their primary physician if the child has increased emesis, bilious vomiting, decreased activity level, or decreased urination.

REFERENCES

1. Cicrello HG, Glass RI: Current concepts of the epidemiology of diarrheal diseases. *Pediatr Infect Dis* 5:163, 1994.
2. Glass RJ, Lew JF, Gangorosa RE, et al: Estimate of morbidity and mortality rates for diarrheal diseases in American children. *J Pediatr* 118(Suppl):527, 1991.
3. Gorelick MH, Shaw KN, Murphy KO: Validity and reliability of clinical signs in the diagnosis of dehydration in children. *Pediatrics* 99:e6, 1997.
4. Gorelick MH, Shaw KN, Murphy KO, Baker D: Effect of fever on capillary refill time. *Pediatr Emerg Care* 13:305, 1997.
5. Hiricho L, Campos M, Rivera J, Guerrant RL: Fecal screening tests in the approach to acute infectious diarrhea; a scientific overview. *Pediatr Infect Dis J* 15:486, 1996.
6. DeWitt TC, Humphrey KF, McCarthy P: Clinical predictors of acute bacterial diarrhea in young children. *Pediatrics* 76: 551, 1985.
7. Santosham M, Daum RS, Dillman L, et al: Oral rehydration therapy of infantile diarrhea: A controlled study of well-nourished children hospitalized in the United States and Panama. *N Engl J Med* 306:1070, 1982.
8. American Academy of Pediatrics, Provisional Committee on Quality Improvement, Subcommittee on Acute Gastroenteritis Practice Parameter: The management of acute gastroenteritis in young children. *Pediatrics* 97:424, 1996.
9. Brown KH, Peerson JM, Fontaine O: Use of nonhuman milks in the dietary management of young children with acute diarrhea: A meta-analysis of clinical trials. *Pediatrics* 93:17, 1994.
10. World Health Organization. *The Rational Use of Drugs in the Management of Acute Diarrhea in Children.* Geneva: World Health Organization, 1990.
11. Richards L, Claeson M, Pierce N: Management of acute diarrhea in children: Lessons learned. *Pediatr Infect Dis J* 12:5, 1993.

For further reading in *Emergency Medicine: A Comprehensive Study Guide,* 6th ed., see Chap. 126, "Vomiting and Diarrhea in Children," by Christopher M. Holmes and Summer A. Smith.

77   PEDIATRIC ABDOMINAL EMERGENCIES
Debra G. Perina

EPIDEMIOLOGY

- The causes of abdominal pain vary with age. See Table 77-1 for a listing of causes stratified by age.

PATHOPHYSIOLOGY

- Differentiation between two types of abdominal pain, peritoneal and obstructive, can aid in diagnosis.
- Peritoneal pain is exacerbated by motion, while obstructive pain is spasmodic with restlessness. See Chap. 38 for further discussion of the pathophysiology of abdominal pain.

CLINICAL FEATURES

- Presenting signs and symptoms will vary with the child's age. The key gastrointestinal signs and symptoms are pain, vomiting, diarrhea, constipation,

TABLE 77-1   Etiology of Abdominal Pain

UNDER 2 YEARS	6–11 YEARS
Appendicitis*	Appendicitis*
Colic (first 4 months)	Diabetic ketoacidosis
Congenital abnormalities*	Functional
Gastroenteritis	Gastroenteritis
Incarcerated hernia*	Henoch-Schönlein purpura
Intussusception*	Incarcerated hernia*
Malabsorption	Inflammatory bowel disease
Malrotation	Obstruction
Metabolic acidosis*	Peptic ulcer disease*
Obstruction	Pneumonia*
Sickle cell pain crisis	Renal stones
Toxins*	Sickle cell syndrome
Urinary tract infection	Streptococcal pharyngitis
Volvulus*	Torsion of ovary or testicle
	Toxins*
	Trauma*
	Urinary tract infection

2–5 YEARS	OVER 11 YEARS
Appendicitis*	Appendicitis*
Diabetic ketoacidosis	Cholecystitis
Gastroenteritis	Diabetic ketoacidosis*
Hemolytic-uremic syndrome*	Dysmenorrhea
Henoch-Schönlein purpura	Ectopic pregnancy*
Incarcerated hernia*	Functional
Intussusception*	Gastroenteritis
Malabsorption	Incarcerated hernia*
Metabolic acidosis*	Inflammatory bowel disease
Obstruction	Obstruction
Pneumonia*	Pancreatitis
Sickle cell pain crisis	Peptic ulcer disease*
Toxins*	Pneumonia*
Trauma*	Pregnancy
Urinary tract infection	Renal stones
Volvulus*	Sickle cell syndrome
	Torsion of ovary or testicle
	Toxins*
	Trauma*
	Urinary tract infection

*Life-threatening causes of abdominal pain.

bleeding, jaundice, and masses. These symptoms can be the result of a benign process or may indicate a life-threatening illness.
- The origin of abdominal pain may be extra-abdominal, such as with pneumonia or pharyngitis.[1,2]
- Pain in children less than 2 years of age usually manifests as fussiness, irritability, or lethargy.
- Pain of gastrointestinal (GI) origin is usually referred to the periumbilical area in children 2 to 6 years old.
- Associated symptoms or the presence of illness in other family members may be useful in arriving at a diagnosis.
- Vomiting and diarrhea are common in children. These symptoms may be the result of a benign process or indicate the presence of a life-threatening process (see Chap. 76). Bilious vomiting is frequently indicative of a serious process.
- Constipation may be functional or pathologic. The

shape and girth of the abdomen, presence of bowel sounds or masses, and abnormalities in the anal area should be noted.
- GI bleeding can be from upper or lower sources.[3] Upper sources are vascular malformation, swallowed maternal blood, bleeding diathesis, foreign body, peptic ulcer disease, and Mallory-Weiss tear. Lower GI bleeding can be from fissures, intussusception, hemolytic-uremic syndrome, swallowed maternal blood, vascular malformations, polyps, inflammatory bowel disease, or diverticulum. The cause of minimal to moderate amounts of blood in the stool is frequently never identified.
- Bleeding in the neonate may be a sign of necrotizing enterocolitis, GI duplication, infection, milk allergy, or anal fissure.
- Jaundice outside of infancy is usually an ominous sign.

DIAGNOSIS AND DIFFERENTIAL

- Table 77-1 lists common causes of abdominal pain seen in various age groups and identifies those that are potentially life-threatening.
- It is clinically useful to differentiate the most serious causes of GI emergencies in children in the first year of life from those of older children. Common emergencies in the first year of life include malrotation of the gut, incarcerated hernia, intestinal obstruction, pyloric stenosis, and intussusception.
- Malrotation of the gut, although rare, can present with a volvulus, which can be life-threatening.[4] Presenting symptoms are usually bilious vomiting, abdominal distention, and streaks of blood in the stool. The vast majority of cases present within the first month of life. Distended loops of bowel overriding the liver on abdominal radiographs are suggestive of this diagnosis.
- The symptoms of incarcerated hernia include irritability, poor feeding, vomiting, and an inguinal or scrotal mass. The mass will not be detected unless the infant is totally undressed. The incidence of incarcerated hernia is highest in the first year of life. It is possible to manually reduce the hernia on examination in most cases (see Chap. 45).
- Intestinal obstruction may be caused by atresia, stenosis, meconium ileus, malrotation, intussusception, volvulus, incarcerated hernia, imperforate anus, and Hirschsprung's disease. Presentation includes irritability, vomiting, and abdominal distention, followed by absence of bowel sounds. Flat and upright films of the abdomen are diagnostic of obstruction, but a barium enema can help to differentiate the etiology.
- Pyloric stenosis usually presents with nonbilious projectile vomiting occurring just after feeding, most

commonly seen in the second or third week of life. It is familial and male predominant, with first-born males being particularly affected. Palpation of the pyloric mass, or "olive," in the left upper quadrant is diagnostic. Ultrasound may also aid in the diagnosis if the mass is not palpated.

- Intussusception occurs when one portion of the gut telescopes into another. GI bleeding and edema give rise to bloody mucus-containing stools, producing "currant-jelly" stool.[5] The greatest incidence is between 3 months and 6 years of age and it is more common in males. The classic presentation is sudden epigastric pain along with pain-free intervals during which the examination can reveal the classic sausage-shaped mass in the right side of the abdomen. Lethargy or mental status changes may be the only symptom.[6,7] This mass is palpated in up to two thirds of patients. A barium enema or insufflation can be both diagnostic and therapeutic, since the intussusception is reduced while doing the procedure in 80% of cases.[8]
- GI emergencies in children 2 years of age and older include appendicitis, bleeding, Meckel's diverticulum, colonic polyps, foreign bodies, and Henoch-Schönlein purpura and hemolytic-uremic syndrome.
- Classic symptoms of appendicitis are pain, fever, and anorexia. However, the presentation may be extremely varied, making the diagnosis challenging.[9]
- Appendicitis does occur in children under 2 years of age, but the presentation is usually as sepsis or peritonitis since symptoms at this age are so nonspecific that the appendix has usually perforated by the time of definitive diagnosis. Early in the course of the illness the symptoms are often attributed to gastroenteritis.
- Over age 2, appendicitis becomes an important part of the differential diagnosis. Again, the clinician may be misled by the absence of classic symptoms. Guarding and rebound may not be present, the temperature may be normal, the white blood cell count may be normal, and the child may be asking for food. Associated gastroenteritis is fairly common.[10]
- Computed tomography (CT) has better sensitivity and specificity than ultrasound in detecting appendicitis in atypical or indeterminate cases; however, CT may be less accurate in younger children due to the relative lack of body fat, which makes it more difficult to differentiate surrounding tissue from an inflamed appendix.[11,12]
- Meckel's diverticulum can cause bleeding, a volvulus, or intestinal obstruction. Acute inflammation may mimic appendicitis or act as a nidus for intussusception.
- GI bleeding in children over age 2 can be caused by several sources. Upper GI bleeding usually results from peptic ulcer disease, gastritis, or varices. Lower GI bleeding can be due to GI polyps, internal hemorrhoids, severe gastroenteritis or infectious colitis, inflammatory bowel disease, coagulopathies, anal fissures, hemolytic-uremic syndrome, and Henoch-Schönlein purpura. A small amount of blood in the diaper is most likely related to anal fissure or ingested foodstuffs.
- Henoch-Schönlein purpura (HSP) and hemolytic-uremic syndrome (HUS) can cause abdominal pain and bleeding. Associated symptoms in HSP include joint pain and a petechial or purpuric rash on buttocks and lower extremities. Low-grade fever, hematuria, pallor, lethargy, or altered mental status are seen in HUS. A history of gastroenteritis, sometimes with bloody diarrhea, is present up to 2 weeks before the onset of HUS. Hypertension occurs in up to 50% and seizures in up to 40% of cases of HUS.
- Colonic polyps may cause painless hematochezia and can be single (juvenile) or multiple. The parent may discover a prolapsed polyp as a mass protruding from the rectum. Multiple polyps may suggest familial polyposis, which is a rare and often premalignant syndrome.
- Pancreatitis is not common in childhood. The most common causes are abdominal trauma, post-viral complications, drugs and toxin exposure, systemic diseases such as cystic fibrosis, and idiopathic.
- Intra-abdominal masses generally grow silently until causing obstruction. For this reason a careful abdominal exam should be done on all children. Common abdominal tumors include Wilms' tumor (an intrarenal tumor), neuroblastomas (arising from the adrenal glands or sympathetic chain), and rhabdomyosarcoma (from striated muscle, most commonly in the pelvis).
- Portal hypertension, although rare, is one of the common causes of major upper GI bleeding. Ascites is the most common presenting sign in infants, while massive hematemesis and hematochezia are the usual presenting symptoms in children. Etiologies include congenital liver disease, hepatitis, inborn errors of metabolism, extrahepatic biliary thrombosis, and biliary atresia.

EMERGENCY DEPARTMENT CARE AND DISPOSITION

- If the child is critically ill, resuscitation efforts should begin immediately as the examination is done concurrently.
- Remove all clothing prior to examination. The examination should always include a good abdominal exam and rectal examination with testing of stool for occult blood.
- The most important laboratory studies are complete blood count with differential, urinalysis, and guaiac test for occult blood. Other tests should be guided by how ill-appearing the child is. Determinations of electrolyte and amylase, hepatic, or lipase levels or pregnancy test may be indicated.

- Chest and abdominal radiographs can be useful to diagnose pneumonia, obstruction, or ileus. Abdominal ultrasound is useful in assessment of pyloric stenosis, ectopic pregnancy, or appendicitis.[13] Abdominal CT scan may be diagnostic with abdominal masses and appendicitis.[14]
- In some cases dehydration and electrolyte abnormalities may require correction with oral or intravenous rehydration. Pediatric surgical consultation may also be needed in specific cases.

REFERENCES

1. Moir CR: Abdominal pain in infants and children. *Mayo Clin Proc* 71:984, 1996.
2. Mason JD: The evaluation of acute abdominal pain in children. *Emerg Med Clin North Am* 14:629, 1996.
3. Vinton NE: Gastrointestinal bleeding in infancy and childhood. *Gastroenterol Clin North Am* 23:93, 1994.
4. Andrassy RJ, Mahour GH: Malrotation of the midgut in infants and children. *Arch Surg* 116:158, 1981.
5. Yamamoto LG, Morita SY, Boychuk RB, et al: Stool appearance in intussusception: Assessing the value of the term "currant jelly." *Am J Emerg Med* 15:292, 1997.
6. Winslow BT, Westfall JM, Nicholas RA: Intussusception [review]. *Am Fam Physician* 54:213, 1996.
7. Conway EE Jr: Central nervous system findings and intussusception: How are they related? *Pediatr Emerg Care* 9:15, 1993.
8. Kirks DR: Air intussusception reduction: "The winds of change." *Pediatr Radiol* 25:89, 1985.
9. Puri P, O'Donnell B: Appendicitis in infancy. *J Pediatr Surg* 13:173, 1978.
10. Horwitz JR, Gursoy M, Jaksic T, Lally KP: Importance of diarrhea as a presenting symptom of appendicitis in very young children. *Am J Surg* 173:80, 1997.
11. Lowe LH, Penney MW, Stein SM, et al: Unenhanced limited CT for the abdomen in the diagnosis of appendicitis in children: comparison with sonography. *Am J Roentgenol* 176:31, 2001.
12. Teo EL, Tan KP, Lam SL, et al: Ultrasonography and computed tomography in a clinical algorithm for the evaluation of suspected acute appendicitis in children. *Singapore Med J* 41: 387, 2000.
13. Gupta H, Dupuy DE: Advances in imaging of the acute abdomen [review]. *Surg Clin North Am* 77:1245, 1997.
14. Johnson GT, Johnson P, Fishman EK: CT evaluation of the acute abdomen: Bowel pathology spectrum of disease. *Crit Rev Diagn Imaging* 37:163, 1996.

For further reading in *Emergency Medicine: A Comprehensive Study Guide*, 6th ed., see Chap. 127, "Pediatric Abdominal Emergencies," by Robert W. Schafermeyer.

78 DIABETIC KETOACIDOSIS IN CHILDREN
David M. Cline

EPIDEMIOLOGY

- Insulin-dependent diabetes mellitus (IDDM) is the most common endocrine disorder of childhood, with an estimated prevalence of 1 in 400.[1]
- As many as 27 to 40% of new-onset diabetics present in diabetic ketoacidosis (DKA).[1,2]
- In known diabetics, DKA is much less common and tends to be clustered in a small subset of patients, with 5% of diabetic children accounting for nearly 60% of DKA episodes.[3]
- DKA is the single most common cause of death in diabetic patients under 24 years of age.[4]

PATHOPHYSIOLOGY

- IDDM is an autoimmune disease caused by destruction of insulin producing β (beta) cells of the islets of Langerhans in the pancreas.[5]
- Genetic predisposition exists for IDDM, although there is no single gene.
- DKA is caused by insulin deficiency. The resultant elevation of counterregulatory hormones (glucagon, cortisol, growth hormone, epinephrine, and norepinephrine) antagonizes the effects of insulin and leads to increased glucose production.[5] Ensuing glucosuria causes an osmotic diuresis, resulting in the loss of fluids and electrolytes. Dehydration, compensatory polydipsia, and hyperosmolality occur as a result of the fluid losses.
- The hormonal interplay of the lack of insulin and excess glucagon levels leads to increased production of ketone bodies from free fatty acids. This increased production of ketone bodies, primarily β-hydroxybutyrate and acetoacetate, exceeds the capacity for peripheral utilization, contributing to the development of metabolic acidosis and compensatory respiratory alkalosis. The presence of increased ketones and acidemia manifest as the classic fruity breath odor of ketosis.

CLINICAL FEATURES

- IDDM is typically characterized by polyuria, polydipsia, and polyphagia; however, other common complaints include failure to gain weight, weight loss, enuresis, anorexia, and changes in vision and school performance.

- DKA is generally defined as a metabolic acidosis (pH <7.25 to 7.3 or serum bicarbonate <15 mEq/L) with hyperglycemia (serum glucose >300 mg/dL) and ketonemia >1:2 dilution.[6,7]
- DKA should be considered in patients with hyperventilation, fruity breath odor of ketosis, dehydration, lethargy, hyperglycemia, vomiting, abdominal pain, or polyuria.
- Physical exam may reveal signs of dehydration (see Chap. 82), mild abdominal tenderness (from vomiting), Kussmaul's respirations, decreased level of consciousness, or coma.
- Cerebral edema is the most dreaded complication and should be suspected in all comatose patients.[6] Mortality rates for children who develop cerebral edema is 40 to 90% and only 14 to 57% of those children affected are left neurologically normal.[4,6]

DIAGNOSIS AND DIFFERENTIAL

- DKA is defined by hyperglycemia (blood glucose >250 mg/dL), ketonemia, and metabolic acidosis (pH <7.2 and plasma bicarbonate level <15 mEq/L), associated with glucosuria and ketonuria.
- Laboratory tests required to manage and diagnose DKA include serum electrolytes, urinalysis, blood pH, and serum ketone determination.
- Children suspected of cerebral edema should have a noncontrast head CT.
- Sepsis should be considered when the cause of DKA is not apparent, and a complete blood count, a chest x-ray, and appropriate cultures should be obtained.
- Other causative factors include trauma, vomiting, noncompliance, and overall stress.

EMERGENCY DEPARTMENT CARE AND DISPOSITION

- The treatment of DKA consists of volume replacement, insulin therapy, correction of electrolyte abnormalities, and a search for a causative factor.
- Patients should be placed on a cardiac monitor, noninvasive blood pressure device, and pulse oximetry, and IV lines established. Initially, hourly monitoring of electrolytes and pH is necessary.
- In general, to calculate the total fluid deficit, compare the patient's presenting weight to a recent weight. If this is not available, assume at least a 10% (100-mL/kg) deficit (see Chap. 82). Volume replacement using a normal saline (NS) infusion of 10 to 20 mL/kg over 1 to 2 hours should be given initially

to most patients. If evidence of shock is present, administer a 20-mL/kg bolus of NS. After initial stabilization is complete, the remaining fluid deficit should be replaced over 24 to 48 hours using 0.45% NS. If serum osmolality remains above 320 mOsm/L, continue NS until the osmolality approaches normal. Monitor glucose levels closely and begin 5% dextrose in 0.45% NS when blood glucose levels are between 300 and 250 mg/dL.
- A regular insulin infusion of 0.1 U/kg/h should be initiated as soon as a glucose level above 250 mg/dL is obtained. There is no need for an insulin bolus, which may produce unwanted hypoglycemia. If the acidosis has not improved after 2 hours of insulin therapy, increase the insulin infusion to 0.15 to 0.2 U/kg/h. Continue both the insulin infusion and 5% dextrose in 0.45% NS until the acidosis is corrected.
- Restoration of sodium levels is accomplished by administration of NS and 0.45% NS fluid. Patients typically reveal sodium deficits of approximately 5 to 10 mEq/kg. Also, the hyperglycemia and hyperlipoidemia associated with DKA cause a falsely low serum sodium level. Monitor serum sodium levels closely, since a decline of the sodium level is sometimes indicative of developing cerebral edema.
- Management of potassium abnormalities is critical to the care of DKA patients. Because of the shift of potassium to the extracellular space secondary to the acidosis of DKA, one may see falsely elevated serum K^+ levels despite total body depletion. If the pH is 7.10 or less and the K^+ level is normal or low, begin replacement therapy immediately by adding 30 to 40 mEq K^+ to each liter of maintenance fluid. Consider higher doses if the potassium level is less than 3.0 mEq/L. If the K^+ level is elevated (greater than 6.0 mEq/L), consider holding K^+ therapy until urine output is present and K^+ is correcting. Use half KCl and half KPO_4. Monitor calcium levels, since excess phosphate can cause hypocalcemia.
- Bicarbonate therapy has not been shown to improve outcome and may lead to cerebral edema, volume overload, hypernatremia, accelerated hypokalemia, and paradoxical central nervous system acidosis.[8] Bicarbonate should be used only in life-threatening situations in which other therapy has failed (including adequate ventilation), such as cardiac dysrhythmias or dysfunction.[8]
- A potentially fatal complication of DKA in children is development of cerebral edema. This typically occurs 6 to 10 hours after initiating therapy and presents as mental status changes progressing to coma. Although the etiology of this complication is unknown, it is felt that several factors may contribute, including overly aggressive fluid therapy, rapid correction of blood glucose levels, bicarbonate therapy, and failure of the

serum sodium level to increase with therapy. Treatment should include mannitol 1 to 2 g/kg, intracranial pressure monitoring, possible intubation with hyperventilation, and fluid restriction.[1]

- Most of these patients will require admission to a critical care or pediatric intensive care unit for monitoring and ongoing therapy. Consultation with the patient's primary care physician and possibly a pediatric endocrinologist should be made early in the course of therapy.

REFERENCES

1. Felner EI, White PC: Improving management of diabetic ketoacidosis in children. *Pediatrics* 108:735, 2001.
2. Smith CP, Firth D, Bennett S, et al: Ketoacidosis occurring in newly diagnosed and established diabetic children. *Acta Paediatr* 87:537, 1998.
3. Rewers A, Chase HP, Mackenzie T, et al: Predictors of acute complications in children with insulin dependent diabetes. *JAMA* 287:2511, 2002.
4. Edge FA, Ford-Adams ME, Dunger DB: Causes of death in children with insulin dependent diabetes 1990-96. *Arch Dis Child* 81:318, 1999.
5. Atkinson MA: The pathogenesis of insulin-dependent diabetes mellitus. *N Engl J Med* 331:1428, 1994.
6. Glaser N, Barnett P, McCaslin I, et al: Risk factors for cerebral edema in children with diabetic ketoacidosis. *N Engl J Med* 344:264, 2001.
7. Linares MY, Schunk JE, Lindsay R: Laboratory presentation in diabetic ketoacidosis and duration of therapy. *Pediatr Emerg Care* 12:347, 1996.
8. Green SM, Rothrock SG, Ho JD, et al: Failure of adjunctive bicarbonate to improve outcome in severe pediatric diabetic ketoacidosis. *Ann Emerg Med* 31:41, 1998.

For further reading in *Emergency Medicine: A Comprehensive Study Guide,* 6th ed., see Chap. 128, "Diabetic Ketoacidosis," by Frederick Place and Thom Mayer.

79   HYPOGLYCEMIA IN CHILDREN

Juan A. March

- Although at times the presentation of hypoglycemia in children may be subtle, especially in the first year of life, prompt diagnosis and treatment may spare an otherwise normal child severe brain damage or even death.

EPIDEMIOLOGY

- Hypoglycemia in children is a relatively rare event, with an incidence of only 6.54 cases per 100,000 pediatric emergency department visits.[1]
- In children presenting to the emergency department, idiopathic ketotic hypoglycemia (IKH) is by far the most common cause of hypoglycemia, and was seen in 58% of cases, while 10% of cases were found to have insulin-dependent diabetes mellitus.[1]
- The most common drugs associated with clinically significant hypoglycemia in children are insulin, sulfonylurea-type medications, and ethanol.

PATHOPHYSIOLOGY

- Young children are predisposed to hypoglycemia because of several factors that include a higher basal metabolic rate, use of glucose for growth and development, greater activity, and relatively smaller glycogen stores.
- The brain is essentially dependent on glucose for its entire metabolism. Since the brain is proportionately much larger in children than adults, glucose use correlates better with brain weight than body weight.
- For children younger than 2 years that are fasting, nearly all endogenously produced glucose is required and used by the brain. If adequate quantities of glucose are not available, then development and growth stop in order to maintain brain metabolism.
- Release of glycogen is normally stimulated by hypoglycemia, and elevated levels of growth hormone, epinephrine, and cortisol.
- As glucose levels fall, a counterregulatory response is generated, which includes the release of glucagon, cortisol, growth hormone, and epinephrine. The release of these substances leads to stimulation of gluconeogenesis. The clinical effects of epinephrine release are called the adrenergic response.
- Calcium channel blockers, β-agonists, and anticholinergic drugs can produce hypoglycemia by suppressing the release of glycogen stores.

CLINICAL FEATURES

- Hypoglycemic patients present with either neuroglycopenic or adrenergic signs and symptoms. Classically, rapid decreases in glucose are associated with more adrenergic type symptoms. Yet a mixture of both neuroglycopenic and adrenergic symptoms is the rule, and not the exception.
- Neurologic symptoms associated with hypoglycemia include confusion, ataxia, depressed consciousness,

blurred vision, focal neurologic deficits, and seizures.

- Adrenergic symptoms associated with hypoglycemia include anxiety, tachycardia, perspiration, tremors, pallor, weakness, abdominal pain, and irritability.
- The symptoms of hypoglycemia in neonates and infants are usually less specific and more difficult to classify. These include poor feeding, jitteriness, emesis, ravenous hunger, lethargy, altered personality, repetitive colic-like symptoms, hypotonia, and hypothermia.
- Hypoglycemia often accompanies a critical illness (eg, meningococcemia) and the features of that illness may dominate the clinical picture, masking the signs of hypoglycemia.
- Hypoglycemia should be suspected in all moderately to severe ill children, and bedside glucose testing should be performed immediately for children with unexplained coma, severe hypothermia, and arrest.

DIAGNOSIS AND DIFFERENTIAL

- Plasma glucose concentration of less than 60 mg/dL constitutes hypoglycemia in school-aged children, adolescents, and adults.[2]
- Although controversial, one should generally consider hypoglycemia for a plasma glucose level of less than 30 mg/dL in the first 24 hours of life. During the remainder of the neonatal period, a plasma glucose level of less than 45 mg/dL should be considered hypoglycemia.[2]
- The differential diagnosis of hypoglycemia differs based on age, and represents an important clinical finding associated with many disorders, illnesses, and ingestions. A partial list of conditions associated with hypoglycemia in infants and children is provided in Table 79-1.

TABLE 79-1   Conditions Associated with Hypoglycemia in Infants and Children*

PERINATAL PERIOD	INFANCY AND CHILDHOOD
Infant of a diabetic mother	Idiopathic ketotic hypoglycemia/starvation
Congenital heart disease	Diabetes mellitus/endocrine disorder
Infection/sepsis	Infection/sepsis
Adrenal hemorrhage	Inborn errors of metabolism
Hypothermia	Hypothermia
Maternal hypoglycemic drug use	Drug induced (salicylates, etc.)
Maternal eclampsia	Hyperinsulinism
Fetal alcohol syndrome	Idiopathic
Hypopituitarism	

*Partial listing, see Chap. 129 in *Emergency Medicine: A Comprehensive Study Guide*, 6th ed. for a complete listing.

- Bedside glucometers have evolved over the years, yet false low readings occur and are associated with abnormal hematocrits, severe dehydration, and hyperosmolar conditions. This is especially true for neonates. Nevertheless, for symptomatic patients treatment should begin based on bedside testing.
- When bedside glucose testing is unavailable, it is better to treat empirically than to delay appropriate treatment, although data suggest that in cases of anoxia and arrest, empirical treatment using dextrose is detrimental due to increased cerebral edema.

EMERGENCY DEPARTMENT CARE AND DISPOSITION

- Although the treatment of hypoglycemia may seem straightforward (ie, administer glucose), there is controversy as to how this is best accomplished. One nationally recognized course (Pediatric Advanced Life Support) recommends that a 5- to 10-mL/kg bolus of 10% dextrose in water ($D_{10}W$) be administered intravenously or intraosseously to hypoglycemic neonates.[3] Older children should receive a bolus of 2 to 4 mL/kg of 25% dextrose in water ($D_{25}W$).[2] Adolescents typically receive the adult dose of 50 mL of 50% dextrose in water ($D_{50}W$). Other sources recommend smaller doses.
- Administration of $D_{25}W$ and $D_{50}W$ is controversial since both are hyperosmolar, cause pain, and increase the risk in smaller veins for phlebitis, extravasation, and surrounding tissue necrosis.
- Use of $D_{25}W$ and $D_{50}W$ may also lead to rebound hypoglycemia due to release of endogenous insulin.
- Hyperosmolar loading in premature neonates is associated with increased risk of intracranial germinal matrix hemorrhage and subsequent periventricular leukomalacia.
- When IV access is unavailable, glucagon 0.03 to 0.05 mg/kg intramuscularly can be considered. Glucagon only works in patients with intact glycogen stores, and its use is controversial in the pediatric population. Thus, intraosseous access should be considered when IV access is not possible.
- When standard therapy fails, hydrocortisone 1 to 2 mg/kg IV, should be considered for those who cannot achieve euglycemia despite adequate dextrose administration. This is especially true of patients with hypopituitarism and adrenal insufficiency.
- Children over age 1 presenting with hypoglycemia, who have normal head circumference, growth, and normal electrolytes, and who recover fully after receiving glucose, do not need as extensive a work-up if the findings are consistent with IKH. On the other hand, infants less than age 1 and neonates should be thoroughly evaluated unless there is a clear cause.

REFERENCES

1. Pershad J, Monroe K, Atchison J: Childhood hypoglycemia in an urban emergency department: Epidemiology and diagnostic approach to the problem. *Pediatr Emerg Care* 14:268, 1998.
2. Reid SR, Losek JD: Hypoglycemia in infants and children. *Pediatr Emerg Med Rep* 5:23, 2000.
3. Chameides L, Hazinski MF: Pediatric Advanced Life Support, Dallas, American Heart Association, 1997, p 6-10.

For further reading in *Emergency Medicine, A Comprehensive Study Guide,* 6th ed., see Chap. 129, "Hypoglycemia," by Randolph Cordle.

80 ALTERED MENTAL STATUS AND HEADACHE IN CHILDREN

Debra G. Perina

ALTERED MENTAL STATUS

EPIDEMIOLOGY

- Altered mental status (AMS) in children is failure to respond to the external environment after appropriate stimulation in a manner consistent with the child's developmental level.
- The etiologies of altered mental status (AMS) in children are quite varied. No epidemiologic data are available that delineate all of the causes.
- In treating children with AMS, aggressive resuscitation, stabilization, diagnosis, and treatment must occur simultaneously to prevent morbidity and death.

PATHOPHYSIOLOGY

- Alterations in mental status result from either depression of both cerebral cortices or localized abnormalities of the reticular activating system in the brainstem and midbrain, and ranges from confusion or delirium to lethargy, stupor, and coma.
- The pathologic conditions that result in AMS can be divided into three broad categories: supratentorial mass lesions, subtentorial mass lesions, and metabolic encephalopathy.[1]
- Supratentorial mass lesions cause AMS by compressing the brainstem and/or diencephalon. Focal motor abnormalities are often present from the onset of the alteration in consciousness. Neurologic dysfunction progresses from rostral to caudal, with sequential failure of midbrain, pontine, and medullary function. Supratentorial lesions cause slow nystagmus toward and fast nystagmus away from a cold stimulus during caloric testing.
- Subtentorial mass lesions lead to dysfunction of the reticular activating system and frequently prompt loss of consciousness. There is a discrete level of dysfunction, with cranial nerve abnormalities and an abnormal respiratory pattern (eg, Cheyne-Stokes respiration, neurogenic hyperventilation, ataxic breathing) frequently seen. With brainstem injury, asymmetric and/or fixed pupils are found. No eye movements occur despite cold stimuli to both auditory canals.
- Metabolic encephalopathy usually causes depressed consciousness before motor signs, which are typically symmetric when present.[2] Respiratory function is involved relatively early, and abnormalities are often secondary to acid-base imbalance. Pupillary reflexes are generally preserved, but pupillary reactivity may be sluggish although intact and symmetric. Pupillary reflexes may be absent in the setting of profound anoxia or in toxicologic effects of exposures to cholinergics, anticholinergics, opiates, and barbiturates.

CLINICAL FEATURES

- A long differential diagnosis list needs to be entertained when an infant or child presents with AMS. Historical data should focus on prodromal events leading to the change in consciousness, including recent illnesses, infectious exposure, toxicologic exposure, and the likelihood of trauma and abuse. Detailed information should be obtained regarding antecedent fever, headaches, head tilt, abdominal pain, vomiting, diarrhea, gait disturbance, seizures, drug ingestion, palpitations, weakness, hematuria, weight loss, and rash. Developmental milestones, past medical history, immunization history, and family history should be assessed.
- The physical examination should initially focus on cardiac and cerebral resuscitation. The objectives of the general examination are to identify occult infectious etiologies, trauma, a specific toxidrome, or metabolic disease.[1,3]
- The neurologic examination should document the child's response to sensory input, motor activity, pupillary reactivity, oculovestibular reflexes, and respiratory pattern, as well as the child's performance on the AVPU (**a**lert, response to **v**erbal stimuli, response to **p**ainful stimuli, **u**nresponsive) coma scale.

DIAGNOSIS AND DIFFERENTIAL

- The differential diagnosis for AMS in children is diverse and differs slightly from that for adults.[3,4] The familiar mnemonic AEIOU TIPS remains a useful tool in organizing diagnostic possibilities (Table 80-1).
- Diagnostic adjuncts should be guided by the clinical situation, but can include analysis of blood, gastric fluid, urine, stool, cerebrospinal fluid (CSF), electrocardiography, or selected radiographic studies. Rapid bedside glucose determination is a universally accepted standard.
- If meningitis or encephalitis is suspected, lumbar puncture and CSF analysis should be done as rapidly as possible after initial resuscitation and stabilization.

EMERGENCY DEPARTMENT CARE AND DISPOSITION

- Initial treatment priorities are airway, breathing, and circulation.
- Oxygenation, fluid resuscitation, bedside glucose determination, control of body temperature, initial control of seizures with benzodiazepines, and restoration of acid-base balance are required for all children with AMS.
- Patients who appear septic should receive empiric antibiotics as quickly as possible, which may be given before lumbar puncture.
- Most infants and children with AMS will require admission and extended observation.

HEADACHE

EPIDEMIOLOGY

- Up to 2% of ED visits are for headache complaints.
- The vast majority of headaches in children have a benign etiology. Occipital location of the headache and the inability of the child to describe the quality of the head pain are associated with serious underlying causes.
- In one study, all patients with neurologic conditions had clear and objective neurologic signs.[5]

PATHOPHYSIOLOGY

- The pathogenesis of headache is unclear. The brain, cranium, and most of the overlying meninges have no pain receptors.[6] Pain is perceived from any structure between the scalp epidermis and the skull periosteum.

TABLE 80-1   AEIOU TIPS Mnemonic for Diagnosing Altered Mental Status

A	**Alcohol.** Changes in mental status can occur with serum levels <100 mg/dL. Concurrent hypoglycemia is common.
	Acid-base and metabolic. Hypotonic and hypertonic dehydration. Hepatic dysfunction, inborn errors of metabolism, diabetic ketoacidosis, primary lung disease, and neurologic dysfunction causing hypercapnia.
	Dysrhythmia (arrhythmia)/cardiogenic. Stokes-Adams, supraventricular tachycardia, aortic stenosis, heart block.
E	**Encephalopathy.** Hypertensive encephalopathy can occur with diastolic pressures of 100–110 mm Hg. Reye's syndrome.
	Endocrinopathy. AMS is rare as a presentation in this category. Addison's disease can present with AMS or psychosis. Thyrotoxicosis can present with ventricular dysrhythmias. Pheochromocytoma can present with hypertensive encephalopathy.
	Electrolytes. Hyponatremia becomes symptomatic around 120 mEq/L. Hypernatremia and disorders of calcium, magnesium, and phosphorus can produce AMS.
I	**Insulin.** AMS from hyperglycemia is rare in children, but diabetic ketoacidosis is the most common cause. Hypoglycemia can be the result of many disorders. Irritability, confusion, seizures, and coma can occur with blood glucose levels <40 mg/dL.
	Intussusception. AMS may be the initial presenting symptom.
O	**Opiates.** Common household exposures are to lomotil, loperamide, diphenoxylate, and dextromethorphan. Clonidine, an α agonist, can also produce similar symptoms.
U	**Uremia.** Encephalopathy occurs in over one third of patients with chronic renal failure. Hemolytic-uremic syndrome can also produce AMS in addition to abdominal pain. Thrombocytopenic purpura and hemolytic anemia can also cause AMS.
T	**Trauma.** Children with blunt trauma are more likely to develop cerebral edema than are adults. The child should be examined for signs of abuse, particularly shaken baby syndrome with retinal hemorrhages.
	Tumor. Primary, metastatic, or meningeal leukemic infiltration.
	Thermal. Hypo- or hyperthermia.
I	**Infection.** One of the most common causes of AMS in children. Meningitis should be high on the differential list.
	Intracerebral vascular disorders. Subarachnoid, intracerebral, or intraventricular hemorrhages can be seen with trauma, ruptured aneurysm, or arteriovenous malformations. Venous thrombosis can follow severe dehydration or pyogenic infection of the mastoid, orbit, middle ear, or sinuses.
P	**Psychogenic.** Rare in the pediatric age group, characterized by decreased responsiveness with normal neurologic examination including oculovestibular reflexes.
	Poisoning. Drugs or toxins can be ingested by accident, through neglect or abuse, or in a suicide gesture.
S	**Seizure.** Generalized motor seizures are often associated with prolonged unresponsiveness in children. Seizure in a young febrile patient suggests intracranial infection.

- Extracranial pain can arise from cervical nerve roots, cranial nerves, or extracranial arteries traversing muscles, leading to pain within specific areas of the head and neck region.
- Intracranial pain can arise from venous sinuses, dural veins or arteries, and arteries around the base of the brain. Posterior fossa pain can be referred to the occiput, ear, or throat, secondary to innervation of the pain nociceptors being innervated by the vagus and glossopharyngeal nerves.

CLINICAL FEATURES

- Headaches can be classified as either primary or secondary. Primary headaches are physiologic (migraine, tension), while secondary headaches have an anatomic basis (vascular malformation, tumor, or infectious). A careful history and physical exam can greatly aid in differentiation between these.
- A history suggestive of secondary headache includes acute onset; morning vomiting; behavioral changes; altered mental status; worst headache ever; awakening from sleep; association with fever, trauma, or toxic exposure; or aggravation by coughing, Valsalva, or lying down. Physical findings suggestive of a secondary headache include blood pressure abnormalities, nuchal rigidity, head tilt, ptosis, retinal hemorrhage or optic nerve distortion, visual field defects, gait disturbances, or focal motor or sensory deficits.

DIAGNOSIS AND DIFFERENTIAL

- There are no evidence-based studies guiding diagnostic work-up. The selection of studies will depend on findings obtained from the history and physical examination.
- Certain presentations such as first headache; worst headache ever; change in pattern of chronic headache; and headaches associated with seizures or fever; or meningeal signs, AMS, or focal neurologic abnormality have a high percentage of positive findings.
- Lumbar puncture is indicated if infection or subarachnoid hemorrhage is suspected.
- Head computed tomography (CT) and magnetic resonance brain imaging may be indicated in trauma or secondary types of headaches.[7,8]

EMERGENCY DEPARTMENT CARE AND DISPOSITION

- Narcotic or non-narcotic analgesics should be given as appropriate for relief of pain according to the disease process and pain level.
- Treatment of the underlying condition identified during diagnostic testing should occur concurrently.
- Potential precipitating factors should be addressed to avoid recurrence of the headache. This may include prophylactic regimens such as β-blockers for migraines.
- Most patients may be discharged after relief of symptoms. Patients with emergent causes of headache such as meningitis, tumor, severe hypertension, or hemorrhage should be admitted for definitive care. Patients with intractable pain may also need admission.

REFERENCES

1. James HC: Emergency management of acute coma in children. *Am Fam Physician* 48:473, 1993.
2. Roth KS: Inborn errors of metabolism: The essentials of clinical diagnosis. *Clin Pediatr* 30:183, 1991.
3. Cantor RM: The unconscious child: Emergency evaluation and management. *Int Pediatr* 4:9, 1989.
4. Rubinstein JS: Initial management of coma and altered consciousness in the pediatric patient. *Pediatr Rev* 15:204, 1994.
5. Lewis DW, Qureshi F: Acute headache in children and adolescents presenting to the emergency department. *Headache* 40:200, 2000.
6. Rosenblum RK, Fischer PG: A guide to children with acute and chronic headaches. *J Pediatr Health Care* 15:229, 2001.
7. Medina LS, Kuntz KM, Pomeroy S: Children with headaches suspected of having a brain tumor: A cost-effective analysis of diagnostic strategies. *Pediatrics* 108:255, 2001.
8. Bulloch B, Tenenbein M: Emergency department management of pediatric migraine. *Pediatr Emerg Care* 16:196, 2000.

For further reading in *Emergency Medicine, A Comprehensive Study Guide,* 6th ed., see Chap. 130, "Altered Mental Status and Headache in Children," by Nancy Pook, Natalie Cullen, and Jonathan Singer.

81 SYNCOPE AND SUDDEN DEATH IN CHILDREN AND ADOLESCENTS

Debra G. Perina

EPIDEMIOLOGY

- Syncope is very common in adolescents and less common in younger children. Between 20 and 50% of adolescents experience at lease one episode of syncope.[1,2] This condition is transient and usually self-limited.

However, 25% of children referred to a cardiologist or neurologist for evaluation are diagnosed with a serious illness.[3]

- The rate of sudden unexpected death in children is 2.3% of all pediatric deaths.[5] Sudden cardiac death makes up about one third of these cases.[6]
- Except for trauma, sudden cardiac death is the most common cause of sports-related deaths,[5] more commonly associated with basketball, football, and track.[7]
- Other causes of sudden cardiac death in children are myocarditis, cardiomyopathy, congenital heart disease, and conduction disturbances.[8,9]
- Hypertrophic cardiomyopathy is the most common cause of sudden cardiac death in adolescents without known cardiac disease.[8]

PATHOPHYSIOLOGY

- Syncope is the temporary loss of consciousness from reversible disruption of cerebral functioning, and usually refers to inadequate cardiac output and cerebral hypoperfusion, resulting in a temporary loss of consciousness.
- Vascular syncope occurs when venous pooling occurs in the legs, leading to a decrease in ventricular preload with a compensatory increase in heart rate and myocardial contractility.
- Neurally-mediated syncope (NMS) or reflex syncope occurs when receptors in the atria, ventricles, and pulmonary arteries sense a decrease in venous return, and an efferent brainstem response via the vagal nerve causes bradycardia, hypotension, or both. NMS is the most common cause of syncope in children.[10] Causes of NMS include vasovagal, orthostatic, situational (urination, coughing), and familial. This type of syncope is usually preceded by sensations of nausea, warmth, or lightheadedness, with a gradual visual grayout.
- Cardiac syncope occurs when there is an interruption of cardiac output from an intrinsic cardiac problem. These causes are divided into tachydysrhythmias, bradydysrhythmias, outflow obstruction, and myocardial dysfunction. Syncope resulting from these causes usually begins and ends abruptly.
- Other known causes of syncope include seizures, breath holding, hyperventilation, hypoglycemia, hysteria, and atypical migraines.
- Any event that causes sufficient cerebral hypoperfusion can lead to sudden death.

CLINICAL FEATURES

- Syncope is the sudden onset of falling, accompanied by a brief episode of loss of consciousness.
- Involuntary motor movements may occur with all

TABLE 81-1   Causes of Syncope in Children and Adolescents

Neurally mediated: most common cause of syncope in children
    Orthostatic: light headedness with standing
    Situational: urination, defecation, coughing, and swallowing may precipitate
    Familial dysautonomia

Cardiac dysrhythmias: events that usually start and end abruptly
    Prolonged QT syndrome
    Wolff-Parkinson-White syndrome
    Sick sinus syndrome: associated with prior heart surgery
    Supraventricular tachycardia
    Atrioventricular block: most common in childen with congenital heart disease
    Pacemaker malfunction

Structural cardiac disease
    Hypertrophic cardiomopathy: exertional syncope most common presentation, but infants can present with congestive heart failure and cyanosis; echocardiography necessary to confirm
    Dilated cardiomyopathy: may be idiopathic, postmyocarditis, or with congenital heart disease
    Congenital heart disease
    Valvular diseases: aortic stenosis usually congenital defect, Ebstein's malformation, or mitral valve prolapse (which is not associated with increased risk of sudden death)
    Dysrhythmogenic right ventricular dysplasia
    Pulmonary hypertension: dyspnea on exertion, exercise intolerance, shortness of breath
    Coronary artery abnormalities: aberrant left main artery causing external compression during physical exercise

Endocrine abnormalities: hyperthyroid, hyperglycemia, adrenal insufficiency

Medications and drugs: antihypertensives, tricyclic antidepressants, cocaine, diuretics, antidysrhythmics

Gastrointestinal disorders: reflux

types of syncopal episodes, but are most common with seizures.[3]

- Two thirds of children experience lightheadedness or dizziness prior to the episode.[3]
- There are many causes of syncope in children. Table 81-1 lists the most common causes of syncope by category.
- Risk factors associated with serious causes of syncope are presented in Table 81-2.

TABLE 81-2   Risk Factors for Serious Causes of Syncope

Exertion preceding the event

History of cardiac disease in patient

Recurrent episodes

Recumbent episode

Family history of sudden death, cardiac disease, deafness

Chest pain, palpitations

Prolonged loss of consciousness

Medications that affect cardiac conduction

TABLE 81-3   Events Mistaken for Syncope

Basilar migraine: headache, loss of consciousness, neurologic symptoms

Seizure: loss of consciousness, simultaneous motor movements, prolonged recovery

Vertigo: no loss of consciousness, spinning or rotating sensation

Hysteria: no loss of consciousness, indifference to the event

Hypoglycemia: confusion, gradual onset associated with diaphoresis

Breath-holding spell: crying prior to the event, age 6–18 months

Hyperventilation: severe hypocapnia can cause syncope

- Events easily mistaken for syncope are presented in Table 81-3 along with common associated symptoms.

DIAGNOSIS AND DIFFERENTIAL

- No specific historical or clinical features reliably distinguish between vasovagal syncope and other causes.[3] However, a thorough history and physical examination can help to arouse suspicion for serious causes. Particular attention should be given to the cardiac examination.
- The most important step in evaluation of children with syncope is a detailed history, including medications, drugs, intake, and food.
- Syncope during exercise suggests a more serious cause. Many of the diseases that cause syncope also cause sudden death in children. Approximately 25% of children who suffer sudden death have a history of syncope. However, syncope is a very common event and a syncopal episode by itself is not associated with an increased risk of sudden death.[4]
- If witnesses note that the patient appeared dead or cardiopulmonary resuscitation was performed, a search for a serious pathologic condition must be undertaken.[11]
- Cardiac dysrhythmia should be suspected if syncope is associated with fright, anger, surprise, or physical exertion.[12]
- The physical examination should include a complete cardiovascular, neurologic, and pulmonary examination. Any abnormalities noted in the cardiovascular examination require an in-depth cardiac work-up.

EMERGENCY DEPARTMENT CARE AND DISPOSITION

- Laboratory assessment is guided by the history, physical examination, and clinical suspicion. Routine laboratory studies are not needed if vasovagal syncope is clearly identified from the history. Those with worri-some associated symptoms should have a chemistry panel and hematocrit, thyroid function tests, chest radiograph, and electrocardiogram (ECG). A pregnancy test should also be done in females of childbearing age. Serum drug screening or alcohol level determination may also be useful if ingestion is suspected.
- An ECG should be done on all patients except those with an unquestionable vasovagal episode.[3,4] The QT interval should be assessed.[13] Patients with hypertrophic cardiomyopathy, prolonged QT interval, or other cardiac dysrhythmias should be referred to a cardiologist.
- An echocardiogram should be obtained in patients with known or suspected cardiac disease.
- Patients resuscitated from sudden death must have a complete evaluation including a creatinine phosphokinase level (CPK-MB) unless a clear cause of the arrest is apparent. One should be alert for complications resulting from the arrest. All such patients should be admitted to a pediatric intensive care unit.
- If no clear cause is found for the syncopal episode, the child may be discharged to be further evaluated and followed by the primary care physician, unless there are cardiac risk factors or exercise-induced symptoms, in which case referral to a cardiologist is warranted.
- Children with documented dysrhythmias should be admitted with continuous cardiac monitoring. Patients with a normal ECG but a history suggesting a dysrhythmic event are candidates for outpatient monitoring and cardiac work-up.

REFERENCES

1. Kudenchuk PJ, McAnulty JH: Syncope: Evaluation and treatment. *Mod Concepts Cardiovasc Dis* 54:25, 1985.
2. Manolis AS: Evaluation of patients with syncope: Focus of age-related differences. *Am Coll Cardiol Curr J Rev* 3:13, 1994.
3. McHarg ML, Shinnar S, Rascoff H, Walsh CA: Syncope in childhood. *Pediatr Cardiol* 18:367, 1997.
4. Gutgesell HP, Barst RJ, Humes RA, et al: Common cardiovascular problems in the young: Part 1. *Am Fam Physician* 56:1825, 1997.
5. Driscoll DJ, Jacobsen SJ, Porter CJ, Wollan PC: Syncope in children and adolescents. *J Am Coll Cardiol* 29:1039, 1997.
6. Maron BJ, Epstein SE, Roberts WC: Causes of sudden death in competitive athletes. *J Am Coll Cardiol* 7:204, 1986.
7. Kuisma M, Suominen P, Korpela R: Pediatric out-of-hospital cardiac arrests: Epidemiology and outcome. *Resuscitation* 30:141, 1995.
8. Klitzer TS: Sudden cardiac death in children. *Circulation* 82:629, 1990.

9. McCaffrey FM, Braden DS, Strong WB: Sudden cardiac death in young athletes: A review. *Am J Dis Child* 145:177, 1991.

10. Pratt JL, Fleisher GR: Syncope in children and adolescents. *Pediatr Emerg Care* 5:80, 1989.

11. Maron BJ, Shirani J, Poliac LC, et al: Sudden death in young competitive athletes. *JAMA* 276:199, 1996.

12. Moss A, Schwartz PJ, Crampton RS, et al: The long QT syndrome: Prospective longitudinal study of 328 families. *Circulation* 84:1136, 1991.

13. Jancin B: Long QT syndrome tracked to a genetic cause. *Pediatr News* 30:8, 1996.

For further reading in *Emergency Medicine: A Comprehensive Study Guide,* 6th ed., see Chap. 131, "Syncope and Sudden Death," by William E. Hauda II and Thom Mayer.

82   FLUID AND ELECTROLYTE DISORDERS IN CHILDREN

Lance Brown

- Fluid and electrolyte disturbances in infants and young children presenting to the emergency department occur most commonly in the setting of acute gastroenteritis.
- Inappropriate home remedies for vomiting and diarrheal illnesses may also contribute to fluid and electrolyte imbalances in infants and young children (for more information on gastroenteritis see Chap. 76).

EPIDEMIOLOGY

- The incidence of fluid imbalance and electrolyte disturbances in children is unknown. However, there are about 3 million physician visits, 220,000 hospitalizations, and between 325 and 425 deaths each year in the United States due to gastroenteritis and the resultant fluid and electrolyte disturbances.[1]

PATHOPHYSIOLOGY

- During the first 2 years of life, there are tremendous caloric and water maintenance requirements. Rapidly growing infants need an enormous amount of calories and water relative to their body weight. The relative daily free water turnover is three to four times that of an adult.

- Young infants are at risk for cardiovascular compromise from sudden fluid losses (eg, vomiting and diarrhea). Factors contributing to this include extensive daily free water turnover, very large relative body surface area, insensible electrolyte free losses from the skin and respiratory tract (especially with fever), a relative inability to concentrate urine, and a relatively large percentage of total body water in the extracellular space.

- In an acute dehydrating illness, the extracellular space is disproportionately depleted. Sodium is the dominant extracellular cation. Dehydration is classified according to the relative balance between water and sodium. In general, dehydration can be classified as isotonic, hypernatremic, and hyponatremic.

- Isotonic dehydration is most common and results from a proportionately equal loss of sodium and water. The serum sodium will remain within the normal range (130 to 145 mEq/L). The most common cause of isotonic dehydration is diarrhea.

- Hypernatremic dehydration results from a relatively greater loss of free water than sodium. The serum sodium is typically greater than 150 mEq/L. Hypernatremic dehydration typically occurs when a young patient with gastroenteritis is fed salt-rich solutions (eg, inappropriately mixed formula, boiled skim milk, chicken broth). Rapid rehydration can lead to an influx of water into brain cells and subsequent brain edema.

- Hyponatremic dehydration is characterized by a serum sodium less than 130 mEq/L. Typically this state develops when acute fluid losses from vomiting and diarrhea are replaced with free water (eg, tea, diluted formula). Hyponatremia may also occur in the setting of increased total body water relative to sodium (eg, syndrome of inappropriate secretion of antidiuretic hormone [SIADH], edema-forming states [nephrotic syndrome and cirrhosis], psychogenic or infantile water intoxication). Conditions that lead to a rapid reduction in serum sodium negatively affect the central nervous system. Irritability, lethargy, and seizures are characteristically seen.

- Although rehydration is generally well tolerated, very rapid correction of profound hyponatremia may result in osmotic demyelination syndrome (central pontine myelinolysis).

CLINICAL FEATURES

- The clinical appearance of patients with dehydration and fluid and electrolyte disturbances depends on the degree of dehydration, the rate at which the fluid was lost, and the age of the patient.
- With prolonged diarrheal illness, older children may tolerate a slow total body water loss as large as 40% of the preillness intracellular volume.

TABLE 82-1   Clinical Estimate of Pediatric Dehydration

CLINICAL CHARACTERISTIC	NONE TO MILD DEHYDRATION	MODERATE DEHYDRATION	SEVERE DEHYDRATION
Percent dehydrated*	<5%	5%–10%	>10%
Overall appearance	Active and playful	Restless and fussy	Limp and sleepy
Eyes	Not sunken	Somewhat sunken	Clearly sunken
Tears	Present when cries	May be absent when cries	Absent when cries
Mouth	Moist mucous membranes	Somewhat dry mucous membranes	Dry mucous membranes
Thirst	Not particularly thirsty	Drinks eagerly	Too sick to drink
Skin pinch	Returns immediately	Returns somewhat slow	Returns slowly

*The number used to calculate the fluid deficit.

- Rapid and large volume loss as is seen in some cases of rotavirus diarrhea (or cholera), can cause young infants to rapidly deteriorate to the point of cardiovascular collapse.

- Because acute fluid (water) loss can be measured as lost weight (1 L water = 1 kg), the gold standard for assessing dehydration is comparison of a very recent preillness weight with weight at presentation on the same scale. From this comparison, the percentage dehydration (as represented by percentage weight loss) can be calculated. Unfortunately, this comparison is almost never available in the emergency department. However, physical examination has been shown to provide a reliable estimation of the degree of dehydration.[2] The dehydration state is classified as either mild, moderate, or severe (Table 82-1).

- An exception to this general pattern occurs in hypernatremic dehydration, in which fluid is drawn from the interstitial and intracellular spaces in the face of the increased serum osmolarity. This process protects the circulating blood volume. Peripheral perfusion and vital signs may be deceptively normal. The skin may reveal a characteristic doughy feel.

DIAGNOSIS AND DIFFERENTIAL

- In the absence of a reliable preillness comparison weight, the diagnosis of dehydration is primarily based on historical data and physical exam findings. Laboratory values may be helpful in some cases, but are not generally needed in mild to moderate cases of dehydration.

- Laboratory data lend supporting evidence, help classify the type of dehydration (eg, isotonic, hypernatremic, or hyponatremic), and identifies related problems (eg, renal failure, ketotic hypoglycemia, diabetic ketoacidosis).

- The serum bicarbonate level (or total CO_2) has been shown to be inversely related to the degree of dehydration (ie, the lower the serum bicarbonate, the greater the degree of dehydration).[2–4]

- The most common cause of dehydration and fluid and electrolyte imbalance in infants and young children is viral gastroenteritis. The most common enteropathogens identified in the United States are rotavirus and enteric adenoviruses.[5]

- Other important causes of fluid and electrolyte disturbances in children include burns, diabetic complications, inappropriate formula administration (mixed incorrectly), inappropriate feedings (eg, extensive juice drinking, bottles of water offered to small infants, chicken broth, boiled milk, etc.), diabetes insipidus, adrenal insufficiency, renal tubular acidosis, anorexia due to febrile illnesses, respiratory illnesses interfering with adequate oral intake, and cystic fibrosis.

- Pyloric stenosis has historically been identified with a hypochloremic metabolic alkalosis. However, with earlier identification of pyloric stenosis, this presentation is becoming increasingly rare.[6]

- Inborn errors of metabolism should be included in the differential diagnosis of a metabolic acidosis with an elevated anion gap in infants, in addition to those conditions seen in adults (ie, renal failure, lactic acidosis, ketoacidosis, and toxic ingestions). The emergency department presentation of infants with inborn errors of metabolism may include vomiting, abnormal tone, seizures, and coma.[7]

EMERGENCY DEPARTMENT CARE AND DISPOSITION

- The management of fluid and electrolyte disturbances in infants and young children revolves around a few basic principles: (1) Identify and treat shock, (2) identify and treat causes that have a specific treatment (eg, diabetic ketoacidosis, pyloric stenosis, respiratory distress), and (3) administer appropriate fluids to replace maintenance fluids, fluids already lost, and ongoing fluid losses.

- Hypovolemic shock should be treated with 20-mL/kg boluses of intravenous (or intraosseous) isotonic crystalloid (eg, 0.9% normal saline [NS] or lactated

Ringer's solution) until improved mental status, vital signs, and peripheral perfusion are noted.

- Maintenance fluids are calculated as follows: for children ≤10 kg administer 100 mL/kg/day over 24 hours; for children 11 to 20 kg administer 1000 mL + 50 mL/kg for each kg >10 over 24 hours; for children >20 kg administer 1500 mL + 20 mL/kg for each kg >20 over 24 hours. Standard solutions for maintenance fluids are $D_5 0.2$ NS (ie, 1\4 NS) for young infants and $D_5 0.45$ NS (ie, 1\2 NS) for older infants and children. Potassium chloride, 20 mEq/L, is typically added after adequate urine output is established.

- Fluid deficit is determined from the clinical appearance and estimated percentage of dehydration (see Table 82-1). Standard solutions for deficit fluid replacement are the same as those for maintenance fluids. The calculations are performed in the following manner: If the patient weighs 15 kg on presentation and is estimated to be 10% dehydrated, then it is estimated that 15 × 10% = 1.5 kg of water has been lost; 1.5 kg of water equals 1.5 L of water, therefore 1500 mL is the estimated deficit. Half of this total is given over the first 8 hours and the remaining half is given over the following 16 hours. The hourly IV fluid rate is determined by the sum of maintenance and deficit fluid requirements for the patient.[8]

- In an attempt to avoid cerebral edema, the fluid deficit is replaced much more slowly in the setting of hypernatremic dehydration. After the fluid deficit calculation, the first half is given over 16 hours instead of 8 hours and the second half is given over 32 hours instead of 16 hours. Oral rehydration has been shown to be as effective as intravenous therapy for rehydrating infants and children, and may be administered by having the patient drink or instilling through a nasogastric tube. There is debate as to what the appropriate sodium content of the rehydration solution should be. The replacement is performed by administering 50 mL/kg orally over 4 hours to mildly dehydrated patients and 100 mL/kg to moderately dehydrated patients.[9–12] Vomiting is not a contraindication to attempting oral rehydration.

- Antiemetics are not typically advocated for use in infants and young children with vomiting.[13] As new classes of antiemetics become available, these recommendations may change.[14]

REFERENCES

1. Glass RI, Lew JF, Gangarosa RE, et al: Estimates of morbidity and mortality rates for diarrheal diseases in American children. *J Pediatr* 118:S27, 1991.
2. Teach SJ, Yates EW, Feld LG: Laboratory predictors of fluid deficit in acutely dehydrated children. *Clin Pediatr* 36:395, 1997.
3. Vega RM, Avner JR: A prospective study of the usefulness of clinical and laboratory parameters for predicting percentage of dehydration in children. *Pediatr Emerg Care* 13:179, 1997.
4. Reid SR, Bonadio WA: Outpatient rapid intravenous rehydration to correct dehydration and resolve vomiting in children with acute gastroenteritis. *Ann Emerg Med* 28:318, 1996.
5. Gastanaduy AS, Begue RE: Acute gastroenteritis. *Clin Pediatrics* 38:1, 1999.
6. Papadakis K, Chen EA, Luks FI, et al: The changing presentation of pyloric stenosis. *Am J Emerg Med* 17:67, 1999.
7. Harrison HE: Dehydration in infancy: Hospital treatment. *Pediatr Rev* 11:139, 1989.
8. Calvo M, Artuch R, Macia E, et al: Diagnostic approach to inborn errors of metabolism in an emergency unit. *Pediatr Emerg Care* 16:405, 2000.
9. Santosham M, Faysd I, Abu Zikri M, et al: A double blind clinical trial comparing World Health Organization oral rehydration solution with a reduced osmolarity solution containing equal amounts of sodium and glucose. *J Pediatr* 128: 45, 1996.
10. Mackenzie A, Barnes G: Randomized controlled trial comparing oral and intravenous rehydration therapy in children with diarrhea. *BMJ* 303:393, 1991.
11. El-Mougi M, Henadawi A, Koura H, et al: Efficacy of standard glucose based and reduced osmolarity maltodextrin based oral rehydration solutions: Effect of sugar malabsorption. *Bull WHO* 74:471, 1996.
12. Cohen MB, Mezoff AG, Laney DW Jr, et al: Use of a single solution for oral rehydration and maintenance therapy of infants with diarrhea and mild to moderate dehydration. *Pediatrics* 95:639, 1995.
13. American Academy of Pediatrics. Practice parameter: The management of acute gastroenteritis in young children. *Pediatrics* 97:424, 1996.
14. Ramsook C, Sahagun-Carreon I, Kozinetz CA, et al: A randomized clinical trial comparing oral ondansetron with placebo in children with vomiting from acute gastroenteritis. *Ann Emerg Med* 39:397, 2002.

For further reading in *Emergency Medicine, A Comprehensive Study Guide,* 6th, ed., see Chap. 132, "Fluid and Electrolyte Therapy," by William Ahrens.

83 UPPER RESPIRATORY EMERGENCIES

Juan A. March

EPIDEMIOLOGY

- Diseases that cause upper respiratory tract (URT) obstruction account for a significant percentage of pediatric emergency department visits. While some diseases of the URT are common and quite benign, others, although rare, are life threatening.

PATHOPHYSIOLOGY

- The physical sign common to all causes of upper respiratory tract (URT) obstruction is stridor.
- Stridor is due to Venturi effects created by somewhat linear airflow through a semicollapsible tube, the airway. When one inhales, the relative pressure in the center of the tube becomes greater than at the edges. The pressure differential leads to collapse of the airway walls and thus obstruction.[1]
- As air progresses from the supraglottic to the glottic and subglottic areas and finally the trachea, there is an increase in physiologic support and therefore a decrease in the amount of collapse that occurs upon inspiration.
- Both inspiratory and expiratory stridor are associated with obstruction at the supraglottic, glottic, and subglottic levels, trachea, and primary bronchi.
- Supraglottic obstruction typically causes inspiratory stridor with marked inspiratory and expiratory variation. Stridor on inspiration is thus indicative of obstruction at or above the larynx.
- Glottic and subglottic obstruction commonly cause both inspiratory and expiratory stridor of lesser magnitudes. Obstruction at the level of the trachea and primary bronchi may be associated with inspiratory or expiratory stridor, but usually to a much lesser degree.
- Expiratory stridor usually means obstruction below the carina. Expiratory stridor, or wheeze, is common in distal airways since intrathoracic pressure may become much greater than atmospheric pressure during expiration. The pressure differential creates high relative laminar flow through semicollapsible bronchi, resulting in wheezes.

CLINICAL FEATURES

- Hypoxia may be present without cyanosis. The presence of cyanosis is dependent on the hemoglobin level and the peripheral circulation. Cyanosis is an ominous sign.
- Tachypnea, chest retractions, and nasal flaring are the triad of labored respirations.
- Signs of labored respirations appear early in the course of the illness and worsen, thus serving as a prognostic as well as a diagnostic sign.
- The physical sign common to all upper respiratory tract obstruction is stridor.
- Chest retractions and nasal flaring are more specific for respiratory tract disorders than is tachypnea.

- Grunting is a valuable diagnostic sign as it localizes disease to the lower respiratory tract and correlates with disease severity.
- Tachypnea is not specific for respiratory tract disease. It can be seen in cardiac disorders and diseases that cause metabolic acidosis.

DIAGNOSIS AND DIFFERENTIAL

- The differential diagnosis is made easier by considering the age of the patient and the duration of symptoms.
- Children less than 6 months old with a long duration of symptoms characteristically have a congenital cause of stridor. Common congenital causes of stridor are laryngomalacia and vocal cord paralysis, with Arnold-Chiari malformations a less common cause.
- Patients over 6 months old with a short duration of symptoms characteristically have an acquired cause of stridor (viral croup, epiglottitis, foreign body aspiration, peritonsillar abscess, or retropharyngeal abscess).

LARYNGOMALACIA

CLINICAL FEATURES

- Laryngomalacia accounts for 60% of all neonatal laryngeal problems.[2]
- Caused by a developmentally weak larynx, airway collapse occurs during inspiration at the epiglottis, aryepiglottic folds, and arytenoids.
- Stridor worsens with crying or if the patient is agitated. Stridor improves with neck extension or when prone.
- This is usually a self-limited disorder that resolves in 90% of cases by age 2.

DIAGNOSIS AND DIFFERENTIAL

- Definitive diagnosis is made by fiberscopic laryngeal exam.
- Less commonly the trachea is less well supported than the larynx, and a diagnosis is made of tracheomalacia.

EMERGENCY DEPARTMENT CARE AND DISPOSITION

- Laryngomalacia is usually a self-limiting disease and is only rarely associated with respiratory failure, failure to thrive, apnea, or feeding problems. Rarely is tracheotomy needed.

- Albuterol may exacerbate symptoms.
- Hypoxic patients or patients showing signs of tiring should be admitted.

VOCAL CORD PARALYSIS

CLINICAL FEATURES

- After tracheomalacia, vocal cord paralysis and paresis are the most common causes of neonatal stridor.
- Most infants will have a history of birth trauma, shoulder dystocia, macrosomia, forceps delivery, or other intrathoracic anomaly.

DIAGNOSIS AND DIFFERENTIAL

- Diagnosis is usually with flexible fiberoptic laryngoscopy with visualization of the cords while the patient is crying.

EMERGENCY DEPARTMENT CARE AND DISPOSITION

- For emergent respiratory failure, endotracheal intubation (ETI) can be quite difficult in a child with bilateral cord paralysis. Placing the bevel of the tube parallel to the small remaining glottic opening and rotating the tube one-quarter turn with gentle pressure may facilitate passing the tube. Force should never be applied since this may cause damage to laryngeal structures.
- Use of an laryngeal mask airway (LMA) is also not advised due to abnormal or obstructed airway structures. For this same reason, retrograde intubation with a guidewire maybe difficult.

ARNOLD-CHIARI (CHIARI II) MALFORMATION

CLINICAL FEATURES

- Arnold-Chiari should be considered in all children that present with stridor, and have trisomy 21, myelomeningocele, hydrocephalus, sacral dimple, or other neurologic abnormalities.
- As the brainstem and cerebellum develop, they partially herniate. As herniation progresses, compression of the cerebellar tonsils, pons, medulla, and upper spinal cord can lead to apnea and stridor.

DIAGNOSIS AND DIFFERENTIAL

- Recognizing this as a possible cause of stridor in children with neurologic abnormalities is critical, since movement of the head and neck can lead to further compression of the vital central nervous system (CNS) structures.

EMERGENCY DEPARTMENT CARE AND DISPOSITION

- ETI should be performed with in-line stabilization to prevent head and neck movement, which could otherwise further compress vital CNS structures.
- Urgent neurosurgical consultation and likely decompression are required.

EPIGLOTTITIS

CLINICAL FEATURES

- Epiglottitis is life threatening and can occur at any age. Since the introduction of *Haemophilus influenzae* vaccine the incidence and demographics have changed remarkably, with less than 25% of cases caused by *Haemophilus,* and a median age of presentation shifting to older children and adults.[3]
- In immunized children, most cases are due to gram-positive organisms, including *Streptococcus pyogenes, Staphylococcus aureus,* and *Streptococcus pneumoniae.*
- In the immunocompromised child, herpes, *Candida,* and varicella must be considered.
- Classically there is abrupt onset of high fever, sore throat, stridor, dysphagia, and drooling, developing over 2 days.
- The presentation in older children and adults is much more subtle. The only complaint may be severe sore throat, with or without stridor.
- The diagnosis is suggested by severe sore throat, with a normal-appearing oropharynx, and a striking tenderness with gentle movement of the hyoid.

DIAGNOSIS AND DIFFERENTIAL

- If the patient is moved to an x-ray suite, a physician trained in airway management should be at the bedside. X-rays are usually unnecessary in patients with a classic presentation.
- If the diagnosis is uncertain, then lateral neck films must be taken with the neck extended during inspiration. The epiglottis is normally tall and thin, but in

epiglottitis it is very swollen and appears squat and flat like a thumbprint.
- False-negative radiographic evaluations do occur, and if suspicion still exists, direct visualization of the epiglottis is necessary to exclude the diagnosis. Blood cultures are positive in up to 90% of patients, while cultures from the epiglottis are less sensitive.

EMERGENCY DEPARTMENT CARE AND DISPOSITION

- If total airway obstruction or apnea does occur, children with epiglottitis can sometimes be effectively bagged.
- Supportive therapy may include humidified oxygen and nebulized epinephrine. Heliox can also be attempted.
- Intubation is usually made by the most experienced individual as soon as the diagnosis is made. Sedation, paralytics, and vagolytics are used as indicated. Use of a tube one size smaller than usual prevents postextubation stridor.
- Only after airway management is accomplished should intravenous antibiotics be considered. These include use of cefuroxime 50 mg/kg IV per dose, cefotaxime 50 mg/kg per dose IV, or ceftriaxone 80 to 100 mg/kg per dose IV, and in regions with increased cephalosporin resistance vancomycin or nafcillin should be added.

VIRAL CROUP (LARYNGOTRACHEOBRONCHITIS)

CLINICAL FEATURES

- Viral croup is responsible for most cases of stridor after the neonatal period. It is usually a benign, self-limited disease caused by marked edema and inflammation of the subglottic area.
- Children ages 6 months to 3 years are most commonly affected, with a peak at age 12 to 24 months.
- It occurs mainly in late fall and early winter, with parainfluenza viruses (I, II and III) being the most common etiology.
- Typically there is a 1 to 5 day prodrome of cough and coryza, which is followed by a 3 to 4 day period of classic barking cough. Symptoms peak on days 3 to 4.
- Physical examination classically reveals a biphasic stridor, although the inspiratory component usually is much greater.

DIAGNOSIS AND DIFFERENTIAL

- The differential diagnosis should include epiglottitis, bacterial tracheitis, or foreign body aspiration. Croup can usually be diagnosed on clinical grounds.

- Radiographs are not necessary, unless other causes are being considered.
- A lateral neck and chest radiograph may demonstrate that the normally squared shoulders of the subglottic tracheal air shadow is shaped like a pencil tip, hourglass, or steeple.

EMERGENCY DEPARTMENT CARE AND DISPOSITION

- Patients should be monitored with pulse oximetry and treated with cool mist and oxygen.
- Administer dexamethasone 0.6 mg/kg PO or IM,[4,5] or an equivalent dose of prednisone or prednisolone (1 to 2 mg/kg).[6] Nebulized budesonide may be clinically useful in moderate to severe cases.[7]
- Nebulized epinephrine, 0.05 mL/kg/dose up to 5 mL of 2.25% solution, should be used to treat moderate to severe cases. Children with stridor only after agitation do not need epinephrine.[8]
- Helium plus oxygen (Heliox) in a 60:40 mixture may prevent the need for intubation.[9] However, if the patient requires greater than 40% supplemental oxygen, Heliox should not be given.
- Although intubation should be performed whenever clinically indicated, if treated aggressively, less than 1% of admitted patients require intubation.
- Discharge criteria include the following: at least 3 hours since the last dose of epinephrine,[8] nontoxic appearance, no clinical signs of dehydration, room air oxygen saturation greater than 90%, age greater than 6 to 12 months, parents able to recognize change in patient's condition, and there are no social concerns with access to telephone and relatively short transit time to hospital.

BACTERIAL TRACHEITIS

CLINICAL FEATURES

- Bacterial tracheitis (membranous laryngotracheobronchitis), a more severe form of croup, is usually rare and caused by bacterial superinfection of a preceding viral upper respiratory infection.
- It is typically seen in children under age 3, but cases are seen in children aged 3 months to 13 years. It is usually caused by *S. aureus, S. pneumoniae,* or β-lactamase-producing gram-negative organisms (*H. influenzae* and *Moraxella catarrhalis*).
- Patients with bacterial tracheobronchitis have more respiratory distress than patients with croup.
- Children appear septic and present similarly to epiglottitis with the following exceptions: severe

inspiratory and expiratory stridor, occasionally with thick sputum production, and a raspy hoarse voice but no dysphagia.

DIAGNOSIS AND DIFFERENTIAL

• Radiographs of the lateral neck and chest usually demonstrate subglottic narrowing of the trachea, and irregular densities may be seen within the trachea, and its borders may appear ragged and indistinct.

EMERGENCY DEPARTMENT CARE AND DISPOSITION

• Management is similar to that of epiglottitis, with greater than 85% of these patients requiring intubation. Ideally these patients should go to the operating room for sedation, paralysis, intubation, and bronchoscopy. Cultures and Gram's stain at that time may help guide antibiotic therapy.
• Empirical antibiotic therapy includes vancomycin 10 mg/kg IV every 6 hours and a third-generation cephalosporin, such as ceftriaxone 80 to 100 mg/kg per dose IV.

FOREIGN BODY ASPIRATION

CLINICAL FEATURES

• Foreign body (FB) aspirations cause over 3000 deaths each year, and have a peak incidence between ages 12 and 36 months, with 90% occurring in children under 4 years of age. In children under 6 months of age, the cause is usually secondary to a feeding by a well-meaning sibling.
• Commonly aspirated foreign bodies usually fall into one of two groups, foods and toys.
• The most commonly aspirated foreign bodies are peanuts, sunflower seeds, raisins, grapes, hot dogs, and small sausages, but almost any object may be aspirated.
• The most dangerous objects are small, smooth, and round.
• Unlike small round metal objects, aspirated vegetable matter commonly causes intense pneumonitis and subsequent pneumonia and suppurative bronchitis.
• At presentation many patients will be completely asymptomatic.
• Patients may have a variety of signs, depending on the location of the FB and the degree of obstruction.
• Classic teaching is that a FB in the laryngotracheal

area causes stridor, whereas a bronchial FB causes wheezing. There is significant overlap in symptoms, and wheeze is present in 30% of laryngotracheal FB aspirations, and stridor in up to 10% of bronchial aspirations,[10] although those with immediate severe-onset stridor and cardiac arrest usually do have laryngotracheal aspirations.
• A significant portion of patients present without cough, wheeze, or stridor.
• Since as many as one third of the aspirations are not witnessed or remembered by the parent, FB aspirations should be considered in all children with unilateral wheezing.

DIAGNOSIS AND DIFFERENTIAL

• A high index of suspicion is required to diagnose a FB aspiration since 36% of patients have fever, 35% wheezes, and 38% have crackles.
• Since many children present 24 hours or more postaspiration, the diagnosis is often difficult.
• Unfortunately, in up to a third of cases plain radiographs are normal, thus a single negative x-ray does not rule out a FB.
• In cases of complete obstruction, atelectasis may be found. In partial obstructions a ball-valve effect occurs, with air trapping caused by the FB leading to hyperinflation of the obstructed lung. Thus, in a stable, cooperative child, inspiratory and expiratory posteroanterior chest radiographs may be helpful. In a stable but noncooperative child, decubitus films may be used, but are less sensitive than fluoroscopy.
• FB aspiration is definitively diagnosed preoperatively in only one third of cases, and thus, if it is clinically suspected, laryngoscopy is indicated.
• Although an upper esophageal FB can impinge on the posterior aspect of the trachea and may present with stridor, they typically have dysphagia and are usually radiopaque.
• Radiographically, flat foreign bodies such as coins are usually oriented in the sagittal plane when located in the trachea (ie, appears as a thick line in an antero-posterior chest x-ray), and in the coronal plane when in the esophagus (ie, appears round on an anteroposterior chest x-ray).

EMERGENCY DEPARTMENT CARE AND DISPOSITION

• If FB aspiration or airway obstruction is clearly present, a protocol for obstructed airway should be implemented immediately .

- Use of racemic epinephrine or Heliox may be considered.
- Ideally, treatment of an airway foreign body is usually with laryngoscopy or rigid bronchoscopy in the operating room under anesthesia.

PERITONSILLAR ABSCESS

CLINICAL FEATURES

- Peritonsillar abscess in children most commonly presents in adolescents with an antecedent sore throat.
- The patients usually appear acutely ill with fevers, chills, dysphagia, trismus, drooling, and a muffled "hot potato" voice.
- The uvula is displaced away from the affected side. As a rule the affected tonsil is anteriorly and medially displaced.

DIAGNOSIS AND DIFFERENTIAL

- Careful visualization of the oral cavity can reliably rule out peritonsillar abscess in many cases. If uvular deviation, marked soft palate displacement, severe trismus, airway compromise, or localized areas of fluctuance are noted, the diagnosis of peritonsillar abscess can be made with confidence and no imaging studies are required.
- In cases without the above mentioned physical findings, differentiation with peritonsillar cellulitis maybe difficult. In toxic-appearing patients or those with inconsistent findings a computed tomography (CT) or ultrasound (US) study is indicated.[11]
- In younger children with trismus, visualization of the oral cavity may not be possible. In these cases some suggest obtaining a CT scan, but due to airway concerns others recommend bedside US.[11]

EMERGENCY DEPARTMENT CARE AND DISPOSITION

- The majority of cases of peritonsillar abscess can be safely treated as outpatients with needle aspiration, antibiotics, and pain control.
- Antibiotic choices include clindamycin 25 to 40 mg/kg IV divided every 6 hours or ampicillin-sulbactam 200 mg/kg/day divided every 6 hours. Definitive follow-up is essential in all cases.
- Formal incision and drainage in the operating room is sometimes necessary, especially in young or uncooperative patients.

RETROPHARYNGEAL ABSCESS

CLINICAL FEATURES

- Retropharyngeal abscesses, although rare, are the second most commonly seen deep neck infections, usually occurring in children aged 6 months to 4 years.
- Patients usually appear toxic, presenting with fever, drooling, dysphagia, and inspiratory stridor.
- Dysphagia and refusal to feed occur before significant respiratory distress.
- Patients may have rapidly fatal airway obstruction from sudden rupture of the abscess pocket.
- Aspiration pneumonia, empyema, infection into the mediastinum, and erosion into the jugular vein and carotid artery have been reported.

DIAGNOSIS AND DIFFERENTIAL

- Physical examination of the pharynx may show a retropharyngeal mass. Although palpation will commonly demonstrate fluctuance, this could lead to rupture of the abscess.
- A lateral neck x-ray performed during inspiration may show a widened retropharyngeal space.
- CT scan of the neck is thought to be near 100% sensitive and very helpful in differentiation between cellulitis and abscess.[12]

EMERGENCY DEPARTMENT CARE AND DISPOSTION

- Immediate airway stabilization should be the first priority. Unstable patients should be intubated before performing a CT scan.
- Antibiotic choice is controversial since most retropharyngeal abscesses contain mixed flora. Broad-spectrum coverage can be accomplished with ampicillin-sulbactam, 200 mg/kg/day divided every 6 hours, and/or clindamycin 25 to 40 mg/kg IV divided every 6 hours. If penicillin allergic, clindamycin and a third-generation cephalosporin are recommended.
- Consultation with an otolaryngologist for operative incision and drainage is indicated. Although cellulitis and some very small abscesses may do well with antibiotics alone, most require surgery.

REFERENCES

1. Rothrock SG, Perkin R: Stridor: A review, update, and current management recommendations. *Pediatr Emerg Med Rep* 1:29, 1996.

2. Mancuso RF: Stridor in neonates. *Pediatr Clin North Am* 43:1339, 1996.

3. Gorelick MH, Baker MD: Epiglottitis in children, 1979-1992: Effects of *Haemophilus influenzae* type B immunization. *Arch Pediatr Adolesc Med* 148:47, 1994.

4. Rittichier KK, Ledwith CA: Outpatient treatment of moderate croup with dexamethasone: intramuscular versus oral dosing. *Pediatrics* 106:1344, 2000.

5. Cruz MN, Stewart G, Rosenberg N: Use of dexamethasone in outpatient management of acute laryngotracheitis. *Pediatrics* 96:220, 1995.

6. Tibbals J, Shann FA, Landau LI: Placebo-controlled trial of prednisolone in children intubated for croup. *Lancet* 340:745, 1992.

7. Klassen TP, Craig WR, Moher D, et al: Nebulized budesonide and oral dexamethasone for treatment of coup: A randomized controlled trial. *JAMA* 279:1629, 1998.

8. Ledwith CA, Shea LM, Mauro RD: Safety and efficacy of nebulized racemic epinephrine in conjunction with oral dexamethasone and mist in the outpatient treatment of croup. *Ann Emerg Med* 25:331, 1995.

9. Weber JE, Chudnofsky CR, Younger JG, et al: A randomized comparison of helium-oxygen mixture (Heliox) and racemic epinephrine for the treatment of moderate to severe croup. *Pediatrics* 107:E96, 2001.

10. Laks Y, Barzilay Z: Foreign body aspiration in childhood. *Pediatr Emerg Care* 4:102, 1988.

11. Scott PM, Loftus WK, Kew J, et al: Diagnosis of peritonsillar infections: A prospective study of ultrasound, computerized tomography, and clinical diagnosis. *J Laryngol Otol* 113:229, 1999.

12. Ravindranath T, Janakiraman N, Harris V: Computed tomography in diagnosing retropharyngeal abscess in children. *Clin Pediatr* 32:242, 1993.

For further reading in *Emergency Medicine: A Comprehensive Study Guide,* 6th ed., see Chap. 133, "Upper Respiratory Emergencies," by Randolph Cordle.

84 PEDIATRIC EXANTHEMS

Lance Brown

- Essential information to make the diagnosis of rash in a child includes the signs and symptoms which preceded or presented with the exanthem, immunization history, human and animal contacts, and environmental exposures.
- Pediatric exanthems can be broadly classified as bacterial, rickettsial, viral, and those of unclear etiology. Potential bioterrorism agents such as cutaneous anthrax and variola (smallpox) are discussed in Chaps. 96 and 98, respectively.

EPIDEMICS OF NONSPECIFIC RASHES

- Since October 2001 there have been multiple epidemics of nonspecific rashes in the United States and Canada.[1] These rashes have been reported to affect nearly half of all children in some schools.
- The distribution of these rashes is primarily on the cheeks and arms. The descriptions of these rashes have been variable, but the lesions are described as pruritic and erythematous, or as a migratory urticaria.
- There are no associated systemic symptoms and the etiologic agent remains unknown.

BACTERIAL INFECTIONS

BULLOUS IMPETIGO

- This exanthem typically occurs in infants and young children.
- Lesions are superficial, thin-walled bullae that characteristically occur on the extremities, rupture easily, leave a denuded base, dry to a shiny coating, and contain fluid which harbors staphylococci.
- Diagnosis is usually made by the appearance of the characteristic bullae (Fig. 84-1).
- Treatment includes local wound cleaning in addition to oral antistaphylococcal agents such as cephalexin or dicloxacillin, and topical agents such as mupirocin.

IMPETIGO CONTAGIOSUM

- This exanthem is a superficial skin infection typically caused by group A β-hemolytic streptococci or *Staphylococcus aureus.*
- The lesions usually occur in small children, often in areas of insect bites or minor trauma. The lesions start as

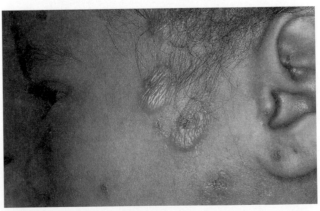

FIG. 84-1. Bullous impetigo. A child with impetiginous lesions on the face. Note the formation of bullae. (Courtesy of Anne W. Lucky, MD.)

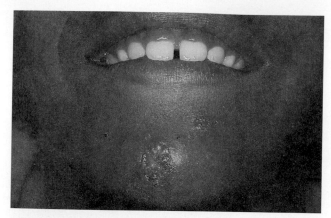

FIG. 84-2. Impetigo. Young girl with crusting impetiginous lesions on her chin. (Courtesy of Michael J. Nowicki, MD.)

red macules and papules which then form vesicles and pustules. Rupture of the vesicles results in the formation of a golden crust. The lesions may become confluent.
- With the exception of lymphadenopathy, fever and systemic signs are rare.
- Most commonly affected areas include the face, neck, and extremities.
- Diagnosis is based on the appearance of the rash (Fig. 84-2).
- Appropriate antibiotic choices include cephalexin, erythromycin, clindamycin, amoxicillin-clavulanate, and dicloxacillin. Further treatment includes local wound cleaning and topical mupirocin.

ERYSIPELAS

- This is a cellulitis and lymphangitis of the skin due to group A β-hemolytic streptococci.
- Fever, chills, malaise, headache, and vomiting are common.
- The face is the most common site and the lesion typically forms in the area of a skin wound or pimple.
- The rash starts as a red plaque which rapidly enlarges. Increased warmth to the touch, swelling, and a raised, sharply demarcated, indurated border are typical.
- Diagnosis is by history and the appearance of the rash.
- A brief course of parenteral penicillin is usually warranted and rapid clinical improvement is expected after treatment has begun.

MYCOPLASMA INFECTIONS

- Rashes associated with mycoplasma infections typically occur in the setting of an acute respiratory illness in a school-aged child (5 to 19 years of age).

- Associated symptoms are typically fever, cough, sore throat, malaise, headache, chills, and rash.
- Mycoplasma should be suspected in school-aged children with pneumonia and a rash.
- The rash is typically on the trunk and is red and maculopapular. Also seen is erythema multiforme and occasionally Stevens-Johnson syndrome.
- The treatment is a macrolide antibiotic (eg, erythromycin).

SCARLET FEVER

- A distinctive rash is seen with scarlet fever. The etiologic agent is typically group A β-hemolytic streptococci (recently group C streptococci have been implicated as well).
- Scarlet fever typically occurs in school-aged children and is diagnosed by the presence of exudative pharyngitis, fever, and the characteristic rash. Associated symptoms include sore throat, fever, headache, vomiting, and abdominal pain.
- The rash typically starts in the neck, groin, and axillae, with accentuation at the flexural creases (Pastia's lines). The rash is red and punctate, blanches with pressure, and has a rough sandpaper feel (Fig. 84-3). In the early course of the illness the tongue has a white coating through which hypertrophic, red papillae project (the "white strawberry tongue"). Hemorrhagic spots may be seen on the soft palate. The rash typically develops 1 to 2 days after the illness onset. Facial flushing and circumoral pallor are characteristic. Desquamation occurs with healing at about 2 weeks after the onset of symptoms.
- The diagnosis is generally made on clinical grounds. Throat culture typically reveals group A β-hemolytic streptococci or group C streptococci.
- Treatment is with penicillin (or erythromycin in the penicillin-allergic patient). Antibiotic treatment shortens the course of the illness and reduces the incidence of rheumatic fever and nephritis.

RICKETTSIAL INFECTIONS

ROCKY MOUNTAIN SPOTTED FEVER
- The etiologic agent for Rocky Mountain spotted fever (RMSF) is *Rickettsia rickettsii,* which is transmitted by ticks.
- The major clinical features include headache, fever, toxicity, myalgias, and rash. The rash of RMSF typically appears on the second or third day of illness. The initial lesions typically appear on the ankles and wrists and spread centrally to the trunk. The palms and soles are usually involved. The lesions begin as

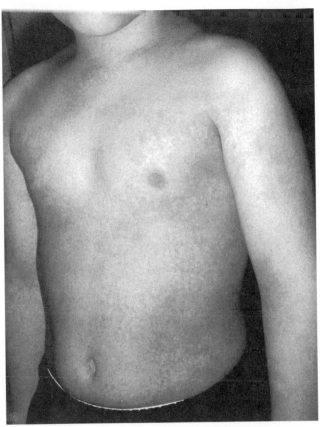

FIG. 84-3. Scarlatina. Erythematous scarlatiniform rash of scarlet fever. (Courtesy of Lawrence B. Stack, MD.)

blanching erythematous macules, but rapidly become maculopapular and petechial.
- Laboratory confirmation of the diagnosis is challenging. Diagnosis and treatment are usually initiated based on the clinical features.
- Appropriate antibiotics for the treatment of RMSF include tetracycline, doxycycline, and chloramphenicol (see Chap. 96).
- The mortality of RMSF is 3 to 6%.

VIRAL INFECTIONS

ENTEROVIRUSES

- Enteroviruses are a group of common, small, single-stranded RNA viruses. Included in this group are coxsackieviruses and echoviruses that can produce a wide range of clinical presentations. These infections typically occur in the summer and early fall. Also included in this group are polioviruses.
- Many enteroviral infections lack characteristic features. Clinical presentation of an enteroviral infection may include nonspecific febrile illnesses, upper respi-

ratory tract infections, parotitis, croup, bronchitis, pneumonia, bronchiolitis, vomiting, diarrhea, abdominal pain, hepatitis, pancreatitis, conjunctivitis, pericarditis, myocarditis, orchitis, nephritis, arthritis, meningitis, and encephalitis.
- The rashes of enteroviral infections may also have a variety of appearances. These include macular eruptions, morbilliform erythema, vesicular lesions, petechial and puerperal eruptions, rubelliform rash, roseola-like rash, and scarlatiniform eruptions.
- One of the enterovirus infections which is both common and has distinctive features is hand-foot-and-mouth disease. At the outset, the patient typically has fever, anorexia, malaise, and a sore mouth. Oral lesions appear on day 2 or 3 of illness, followed by skin lesions. The oral lesions start as very painful vesicles on an erythematous base which then ulcerate. The typical location of the oral lesions is on the buccal mucosa, tongue, soft palate, and gingiva. The skin lesions start as red papules that change to gray vesicles that ultimately heal in 7 to 10 days. The typical locations of the skin lesions include the palms, soles, and buttocks.
- Management of presumed enteroviral infections typically involves symptomatic therapy, assuring adequate hydration, antipyretics, and intraoral analgesics.

ERYTHEMA INFECTIOSUM

- Erythema infectiosum (also known as fifth disease) is a febrile illness, typically appearing in the spring, caused by infection with parvovirus, a single-stranded DNA virus. School-aged children 5 to 15 years old are most commonly affected.
- The rash typically starts as an abrupt-onset bright red rash on the cheeks, giving the so-called "slapped-cheek" appearance (Fig. 84-4). The lesions are closely grouped tiny papules on a erythematous base with slightly raised edges. The eyelids and chin are characteristically spared. Circumoral pallor is typical. This rash fades after 4 to 5 days.
- As the illness progresses, and 1 to 2 days after the facial rash appears, a nonpruritic erythematous macular or maculopapular rash appears on the trunk and limbs. This rash may last for 1 week and is not pruritic. As the rash fades, central clearing of the lesions occurs, leaving a lacy appearance to the rash. Palms and soles are rarely affected.
- This rash may recur intermittently in the weeks following the onset of illness. This may be exacerbated by sun exposure or hot baths.
- Associated symptoms include fever, malaise, headache, sore throat, cough, coryza, nausea, vomiting, diarrhea, and myalgias. There is no specific therapy beyond symptomatic therapy.

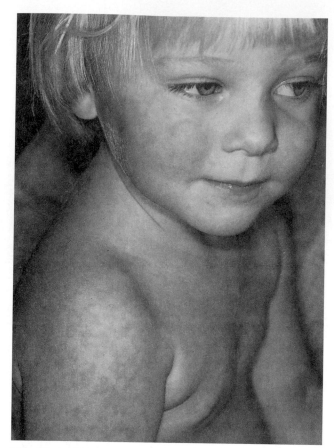

FIG. 84-4. Fifth disease. Toddler with the classic slapped-cheek appearance of fifth disease caused by parvovirus B19. Also note the lacy reticular macular rash on the shoulder and upper extremity. (Courtesy of Anne W. Lucky, MD.)

MEASLES

- Due to immunizations, measles is no longer common. Local epidemics do occur. This myxovirus infection typically occurs in the winter and spring.
- The incubation period is 10 days. A 3-day prodrome of upper respiratory symptoms followed by malaise, fever, coryza, conjunctivitis, photophobia, and cough is typical. Ill appearance is expected.
- Just prior to the development of a rash, Koplik's spots, tiny white spots on the buccal mucosa, may be seen. These spots give a "grains of sand" appearance and are pathognomonic for measles.
- The rash develops 14 days after exposure. Initially a red, blanching, maculopapular rash develops. The rash progresses from the head to the feet. The rash rapidly coalesces on the face. The duration of the rash is about 1 week.
- As the rash resolves, a coppery brown discoloration may be seen and desquamation may occur.
- Measles is self-limited. Treatment is supportive.

INFECTIOUS MONONUCLEOSIS

- The etiologic agent for infectious mononucleosis is the Epstein-Barr virus. The disease primarily affects children and young adults.
- Systemic symptoms include fever, malaise, fatigue, and sore throat. The pharynx is often inflamed with exudate present. Lymphadenopathy typically affects both anterior and posterior cervical chains, but may be generalized.
- A generalized erythematous maculopapular rash with soft palate petechiae is seen in 5% of patients. Nearly all patients who are treated with ampicillin or other related penicillins (eg, amoxicillin) develop an erythematous maculopapular rash.
- The Monospot test is less reliable in children under 5 years of age. Treatment is supportive. Of note is the splenic enlargement that occurs with infectious mononucleosis. If a child participates in contact sports or sustains an injury to the left upper quadrant of the abdomen, splenic rupture may occur.

RUBELLA

- Now quite rare due to immunizations, rubella (German measles) can be seen in teenagers, typically in the spring. The incubation period is 12 to 25 days.
- The prodromal symptoms include fever, malaise, headache, sore throat, and upper respiratory tract symptoms.
- The rash develops as fine, irregular pink macules and papules on the face, which then spread to the neck, trunk, and arms in a centrifugal distribution. The rash coalesces on the face as the eruption reaches the lower extremities and then clears in the same order as it appeared.
- Lymphadenopathy typically involves the suboccipital and posterior auricular nodes. Treatment is supportive.

VARICELLA (CHICKENPOX)

- Due to immunizations, the incidence of varicella has declined dramatically. The etiologic agent is the varicella-zoster virus, a herpes virus.[2]
- It typically occurs in children less than 10 years of age, but it may occur in all ages. Varicella occurs most often in the late winter and early spring.
- Patients are highly contagious from the prodrome phase of the illness until all lesions are crusted over.
- The rash starts as faint red macules on the scalp or

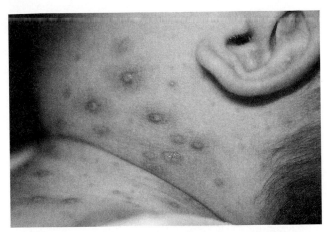

FIG. 84-5. Varicella (chickenpox). Multiple umbilicated cloudy vesicles of varicella. (Courtesy of Lawrence B. Stack, MD.)

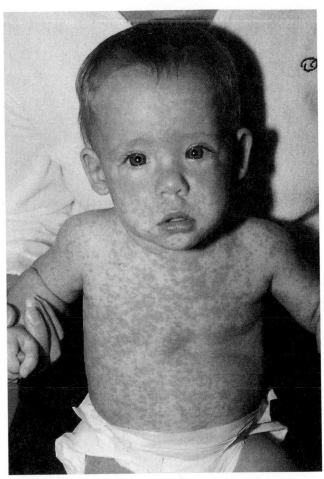

FIG. 84-6. Roseola infantum (exanthem subitum). Toddler with maculopapular eruption of roseola. (Courtesy of Raymond C. Baker, MD.)

trunk. Within the first day the lesions begin to vesiculate and develop a red base, giving the characteristic appearance (Fig. 84-5). Over the next few days, groups of lesions develop, giving the appearance of simultaneous multiple stages of development. Over the next 1 to 2 weeks, the lesions become dry and crusted. The rash typically spreads centrifugally (outward from the center). The palms and soles are spared.

- Low-grade fever, malaise, and headache are frequently seen but are typically mild.
- Treatment is symptomatic (eg, diphenhydramine for itching, acetaminophen for fever) Although not needed in previously healthy children, varicella-zoster immune globulin and acyclovir may be needed for immunocompromised children.

ROSEOLA INFANTUM (EXANTHEM SUBITUM)

- Common acute febrile illness in young children. The most common age group affected is between 6 months and 3 years of age. Roseola is thought to be most commonly caused by human herpesvirus 6.
- Roseola initially starts with an abrupt-onset high fever for 3 to 5 days. Associated symptoms are typically mild and may include irritability when the fever is highest, cough, coryza, anorexia, and abdominal discomfort. Febrile seizures may occur. As the fever begins to resolve, blanching macular or maculopapular rose-colored or pink discrete lesions develop. The areas typically involved with rash include the neck, trunk, and buttocks, but may also include the face and proximal extremities (Fig. 84-6). Mucous membranes

are not involved. The rash lasts 1 to 2 days and rapidly fades. The treatment is symptomatic.

UNCLEAR ETIOLOGY

ERYTHEMA NODOSUM

- Erythema nodosum is an inflammatory exanthem which is associated with medications (eg, oral contraceptives), sarcoidosis, *Yersinia* infections, inflammatory bowel disease, leukemia, vasculitis, tuberculosis, fungal diseases, and streptococcal infections.
- The lesions of erythema nodosum are distinctive, tender nodules up to 5 cm in size on the shins and extensor prominences. The skin overlying the lesions is red, smooth, and shiny. Ulceration is not seen.
- Other symptoms include fever, arthralgias, myalgias, and fatigue.
- The lesions last several weeks. There is no known treatment except analgesia.

KAWASAKI'S DISEASE

- Kawasaki's disease (mucocutaneous lymph node syndrome) is a generalized vasculitis of unknown cause that typically occurs in children under 9 years of age.[3,4]
- Diagnosis depends on the following clinical findings. The patient should have several days of fever, and the illness must not be explained by another known disease process. Then, four of the following five criteria must be met: (1) conjunctivitis; (2) rash; (3) lymphadenopathy; (4) oropharyngeal changes, including injection of the pharynx and lips with prominent papillae of the tongue (strawberry tongue); and (5) extremity erythema and edema.
- Typical rash appearances have been described as erythematous, morbilliform, urticarial, scarlatiniform, or erythema multiforme–like. Perineal rash is not uncommon.
- Associated findings may include leukocytosis, elevation of acute-phase reactants (eg, erythrocyte sedimentation rate, C-reactive protein), elevated liver function tests, arthritis, arthralgia, and irritability. Later in the illness, findings may include a rise in the platelet count, desquamation of the fingers and toes, and coronary artery aneurysms. One to two percent of patients with coronary artery aneurysms develop sudden cardiac death.
- Treatment consists of intravenous gamma globulin and aspirin. The use of steroids is controversial.

PITYRIASIS ROSEA

- Pityriasis rosea is characteristically seen in older school-aged children and young adults in the spring and fall. It does not appear to occur in epidemics and is not contagious.
- The rash evolves over weeks. The rash begins with a herald patch, one red lesion with a raised border on the trunk. Then 1 to 2 weeks later, a widespread eruption of pink maculopapular oval patches erupts on the trunk in a pattern following the ribs (the so-called "Christmas tree distribution"). There may be mucous membrane involvement.
- Pityriasis rosea typically lasts 3 to 8 weeks. Testing for secondary syphilis is commonly done as secondary syphilis may look like pityriasis rosea.
- Treatment is symptomatic and includes antihistamines for itching.

REFERENCES

1. Update: Rashes among schoolchildren. *MMWR* 51:524, 2002.
2. Seward J, Watson B, Peterson C, et al: Varicella disease after introduction of varicella vaccine in the United States, 1995-2000. *JAMA* 287:606, 2002.
3. Brogan P, Bose A, Burgner D, et al: Kawasaki disease: an evidence based approach to diagnosis, treatment, and proposals for future research. *Arch Dis Child* 86:286, 2002.
4. Fukunishi M, Kikkawa M, Hamana H, et al: Prediction of nonresponsiveness to intravenous high dose gamma globulin therapy in patients with Kawasaki disease at onset. *J Pediatr* 137:172, 2000.

For further reading in *Emergency Medicine, A Comprehensive Study Guide,* 6th ed., see Chap. 135. "Pediatric Exanthems," by Michael S. Weinstock and Alexander M. Rosenau.

85 MUSCULOSKELETAL DISORDERS IN CHILDREN

David M. Cline

PATHOPHYSIOLOGY

- The long bones of children are generally less dense and more porous than the long bones of adults. The resulting increased compliance contributes to the tendency of children's long bones to respond to mechanical stress by bowing and buckling, rather than fracturing through and through, as in adult fracture patterns.
- The periosteum of the diaphysis and the metaphysis is thicker in children and is continuous from the metaphysis to the epiphysis, surrounding and protecting the mechanically weaker physis. This physeal weakness is related to the reduced oxygen tension found in the hypertrophic zone of the physis, a location of frequent fractures within the physis.
- The ligaments of children are stronger and more compliant than those of adults.

CHILDHOOD PATTERNS OF INJURY

- The growth plate (physis) is the weakest point in children's long bones and the frequent site of fractures. The ligaments and periosteum are stronger than the physis, tolerating mechanical forces at the expense of physeal injury.
- The blood supply to the physis arises from the epiphysis, so separation of the physis from the epiphysis may be disastrous for future growth.
- The Salter-Harris classification is widely used to describe fractures involving the growth plate (Fig. 85-1).

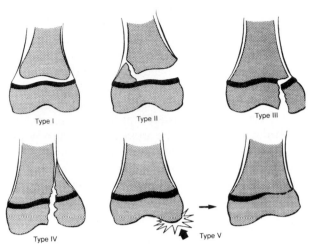

FIG. 85-1. Salter-Harris classification of physeal injuries. (Reproduced with permission from Tolo VT, Wood B: *Pediatric Orthopedics in Primary Care.* Baltimore: Williams & Wilkins, 1994.)

TYPE I PHYSEAL FRACTURE

- In type I physcal fracture (6% of all physeal injuries), the epiphysis separates from the metaphysis. The reproductive cells of the physis stay with the epiphysis. There are no bony fragments. Bone growth is undisturbed.
- Diagnosis of this injury is suspected clinically in children with point tenderness over a growth plate. On x-ray, the only abnormality may be an associated joint effusion. There may be epiphyseal displacement from the metaphysis.
- Treatment consists of splint immobilization, ice, elevation, and referral.

TYPE II PHYSEAL FRACTURE

- Type II physeal fracture is the most common (75%) physeal fracture.
- The fracture goes through the physis and out through the metaphysis. The periosteum remains intact over the metaphyseal fragment, but is torn on the opposite side. Growth is preserved since the physis remains with the epiphysis.
- Treatment is closed reduction with analgesia and sedation followed by cast immobilization.

TYPE III PHYSEAL FRACTURE

- The hallmark of type III physeal fracture is an intra-articular fracture of the epiphysis with the cleavage plane continuing along the physis. This injury usually involves the proximal or distal tibia.

- The prognosis for bone growth depends on the circulation to the epiphyseal bone fragment and is usually favorable.
- Reduction of the unstable fragment with anatomic alignment of the articular surface is critical. Open reduction is often required.

TYPE IV PHYSEAL FRACTURE

- The fracture line of type IV physeal fractures begins at the articular surface and extends through the epiphysis, physis, and metaphysis.
- This most often involves the distal humerus.
- Open reduction is required to reduce the risk of premature bone growth arrest.

TYPE V PHYSEAL FRACTURE

- Type V physeal fracture is a rare pattern usually involving the knee or ankle. The physis is essentially crushed by severe compressive forces. There is no epiphyseal displacement.
- The diagnosis is often difficult. An initial diagnosis of sprain or type I injury may prove incorrect when later growth arrest occurs. X-rays may look normal or demonstrate focal narrowing of the epiphyseal plate. There is usually an associated joint effusion.
- Treatment consists of cast immobilization, no weight bearing, and close orthopedic follow-up in anticipation of focal bone growth arrest.

TORUS FRACTURES

- Children's long bones are more compliant than those of adults and tend to bow and bend under forces where an adult's might fracture. Torus (also called cortical or buckle) fractures involve a bulging or buckling of the bony cortex, usually of the metaphysis.
- Patients have point tenderness over the fracture site and soft tissue swelling. Radiographs may be subtle but show cortical disruption.
- Torus fractures are not typically angulated, rotated, or displaced, so reduction is rarely necessary. Splinting or casting in a position of function for 3 to 4 weeks with orthopedic follow-up is recommended.

GREENSTICK FRACTURES

- In greenstick fracture, the cortex and periosteum are disrupted on one side of the bone, but intact on the other.
- Treatment is closed reduction and immobilization.

PLASTIC DEFORMITIES

- Plastic deformities are seen in the forearm and lower leg in combination with a completed fracture in the companion bone. The diaphyseal cortex is deformed, but the periosteum is intact.

FRACTURES ASSOCIATED WITH CHILD ABUSE

- Certain injury patterns are consistently seen in abused children,[1] particularly multiple fractures in various stages of healing.
- Twisting injuries create spiral fractures in long bones, highly specific for abuse in nonambulatory children. In ambulatory children, spiral fractures may occur from unintentional injury, the classic example being the spiral fracture of the lower third of the tibia (toddler's fracture), but such fractures can also be seen with abuse.
- The injury pattern most closely associated with abuse is the chip fracture of the metaphysis. The tight attachment of the periosteum to the metaphysis will cause avulsion of little chips of the bone with pulling. There is exuberant callus formation and periosteal new bone formation. With direct trauma, subperiosteal hemorrhage characteristically lifts the periosteum off the bone, where it appears as an opacified line.
- Fragmentation of the clavicle and acromion and separation of the costochondral junctions of the ribs are very suggestive of abuse.
- Bony injuries from shaking are similar to twisting injuries, but also include spinal compression fractures and other vertebral injuries.
- Distraction injuries to the long bones cause hemorrhagic separation of the distal metaphysis, creating a lucency proximal to the physis (bucket-handle fracture).
- Squeezing injuries create rib fractures that are highly suggestive of abuse.

SELECTED PEDIATRIC INJURIES

CLAVICLE FRACTURE

- A clavicle fracture is the most common fracture in children.
- Fractures may occur in the newborn during a difficult delivery. Babies may have nonuse of the arm. If the fracture was not initially appreciated, parents may notice a bony callus at 2 to 3 weeks of age.
- In older infants and children, the usual mechanism is a fall onto the outstretched arm or shoulder.
- Care of the patient with a clavicle fracture is directed towards pain control. Even if anatomic alignment is not achieved in the emergency department (ED), displaced fractures usually heal well, although patients may have a residual bump at the fracture site.
- Figure-of-eight shoulder abduction restraints have been the traditional treatment, but many patients have more pain with this device. A simple sling or shoulder immobilizer are equally as effective and less painful. Orthopedic follow-up can be arranged in the next week.
- Orthopedic consultation in the ED is required for an open fracture (which also requires antibiotics), anterior or posterior displacement of the medial clavicle, or a skin-tenting fracture fragment that has the potential to convert to an open fracture.

SUPRACONDYLAR FRACTURES

- The most common elbow fracture in childhood is the supracondylar fracture of the distal humerus. The mechanism is a fall on an outstretched arm.
- The close proximity of the brachial artery to the fracture predisposes the artery to injury. Subsequent arterial spasm or compression by casts may further compromise distal circulation. A forearm compartment syndrome, Volkmann's ischemic contracture, may occur.
- Symptoms include pain in the proximal forearm upon passive finger extension, stocking-glove anesthesia of the hand, and hard forearm swelling. Children complain of pain on passive elbow flexion and maintain the forearm pronated.
- Pulses may remain palpable at the wrist despite serious vascular impairment.
- Injuries to the ulnar, median, and radial nerves are common too, occurring in 5 to 10% of all supracondylar fractures.
- X-rays show the injury, but the findings may be subtle.[2] A posterior fat pad sign is indicative of intra-articular effusion and thus fracture. Normally, the anterior humeral line, a line drawn along the anterior distal humeral shaft, should bisect the posterior two thirds of the capitellum on the lateral view. In subtle supracondylar fractures, the line often lies more anteriorly.
- In cases of neurovascular compromise, immediate fracture reduction is indicated. If an ischemic forearm compartment is suspected after reduction, surgical decompression or arterial exploration may be indicated.[3]
- Admission is recommended for patients with displaced fractures or significant soft tissue swelling. Open reduction is often required.
- Outpatient treatment is acceptable for nondisplaced fractures with minimal swelling; however, telephone consultation with an orthopedic surgeon will provide the preferred splinting technique. Such children need orthopedic reassessment within 24 hours.

• Lateral and medial condylar fractures and intercondylar and transcondylar fractures carry risks of neurovascular compromise, especially to the ulnar nerve. These patients have soft tissue swelling and tenderness, maintaining the arm in flexion. Most patients require open reduction.

RADIAL HEAD SUBLUXATION ("NURSEMAID'S ELBOW")

• Radial head subluxation is a very common injury that is seen most often in children between the ages of 1 and 4. The typical history is that the child was lifted up by an adult pulling on the hand or wrist. Sometimes there is a history of trauma, and sometimes there is no memorable event at all, but the child refuses to use the arm.

• The arm is held close to the body, flexed at the elbow with the forearm pronated. Gentle exam reveals no tenderness to direct palpation, but any attempts to supinate the forearm or move the elbow cause pain.

• If the history and exam are classical, radiographs are not needed, but if the history is atypical or there is a point tenderness or signs of trauma, x-rays should be taken.

• There are two maneuvers for reduction. The supination technique is performed by holding the patient's elbow at 90 degrees with one hand, then firmly supinating the wrist and simultaneously flexing the elbow so the wrist is directed to the ipsilateral shoulder. There may be a "click" with reduction and the child may transiently scream and resist.

• The hyperpronation technique is reported to be more successful, and it can used primarily or as a back-up when supination fails.[4] The hyperpronation technique is performed by holding the child's elbow at 90 degrees in one hand, then firmly pronating the wrist. Usually the child will resume normal activity in 15 to 30 minutes if reduction is achieved. If the child is not better after a second reduction attempt, alternate diagnoses and radiographs should be considered. No specific therapy is needed after successful reduction. Parents should be reminded to avoid linear traction on the arm, as there is an increased risk of recurrence.

SLIPPED CAPITAL FEMORAL EPIPHYSIS (SCFE)

• Slipped capital femoral epiphysis (SCFE) is more common in boys, with peak incidence between ages 12 and 15, and in girls between ages 10 and 13.

• With a chronic SCFE, children complain of dull pain in the groin, anteromedial thigh, and knee, which becomes worse with activity. With walking, the leg is externally rotated and the gait is antalgic. Hip flexion is restricted and accompanied by external rotation of the thigh.

• Acute SCFE is due to trauma or may occur in a patient with pre-existing chronic SCFE. Patients are in great pain, with marked external rotation of the thigh and leg shortening. The hip should not be forced through full range of motion, as this may displace the epiphysis further.

• The differential includes septic arthritis, toxic synovitis, Legg-Calvé-Perthes' disease, and other hip fractures.

• Children with SCFE are not febrile or toxic and have normal white blood cell counts (WBCs) and erythrocyte sedimentation rates (ESRs).

• On x-ray, medial slips of the femoral epiphysis will be seen on anteroposterior (AP) views, while frog-leg views detect posterior slips. In the AP view, a line along the superior femoral neck should transect the lateral quarter of the femoral epiphysis, but not if the epiphysis is slipped.

• The management of SCFE is operative. The main long-term complication is avascular necrosis of the femoral head.

SELECTED NONTRAUMATIC MUSCULOSKELETAL DISORDERS OF CHILDHOOD

• Kawasaki's disease is discussed in Chap. 84.

ACUTE SUPPURATIVE ARTHRITIS

• Septic arthritis occurs in all ages, but especially in children under 3 years old.

• The hip is most often affected, followed by the knee and elbow.

• The diagnosis is critical, because left untreated, purulent joint infection leads to total joint destruction. Bacteria access the joint hematogenously, by direct extension from adjacent osteomyelitis, or from inoculation as in arthrocentesis or femoral venipuncture.

• In the neonate where maternal transmission is possible, group B *Streptococcus,* and *Neisseria gonorrhoeae* are a concern. In all age groups, *Staphylococcus aureus,* gram-negative bacilli, and *Streptococcus* species should be considered. *Haemophilus influenzae* has diminished due to widespread vaccination.

• Although systemic symptoms can be subtle in the newborn, older children will appear ill, with high fever and irritability. The affected joint is very painful and shows warmth, swelling, and severe tenderness to palpation and movement.

• Children with hip or knee infection will limp or not

walk at all, and will maintain an infected hip in flexion, abduction, and external rotation.

- X-rays show joint effusion, but this is nonspecific.
- The differential includes osteomyelitis, transient tenosynovitis, cellulitis, septic bursitis, acute pauciarticular juvenile rheumatoid arthritis (JRA), acute rheumatic fever, hemarthrosis, and SCFE.
- Distinguishing septic arthritis from osteomyelitis may be quite difficult. Osteomyelitis is more tender over the metaphysis, whereas septic arthritis is more tender over the joint line. Joint motion is much more limited in septic arthritis.
- Prompt arthrocentesis is the key to diagnosis, either at the bedside, or in the case of the hip, in the operating room or under ultrasound. Synovial fluid shows WBCs and organisms.
- Prompt joint drainage is critical, either in the operating room in the case of the hip, or arthroscopically or via arthrocentesis in more superficial joints.
- In the neonate, administer oxacillin 37 mg/kg IV every 6 hours plus cefotaxime 50 mg/kg IV every 8 hours. In the infant over 3 months or a child, administer nafcillin 37 mg/kg IV every 6 hours plus cefotaxime 50 mg/kg IV every 8 hours. If resistant organisms are suspected, use vancomycin 10 to 15 mg/kg every 6 hours.
- The prognosis depends on the length of time between symptom appearance and treatment, which joint is involved (worse for the hip), presence of associated osteomyelitis (worse prognosis), and the patient's age (worse for youngest children).

JUVENILE RHEUMATOID ARTHRITIS (JRA)

- The group of diseases comprising JRA share the findings of chronic noninfectious synovitis and arthritis, with systemic manifestations.
- Pauciarticular disease is the most common form, usually involving a single large joint such as the knee. Permanent joint damage occurs infrequently.
- Polyarticular disease occurs in one third of cases. Both large and small joints are affected, and there may be progressive joint damage.
- Systemic JRA occurs in 20% of patients. This form is associated with high fevers and chills.
- Extra-articular manifestations are common, including a red macular coalescent rash, hepatosplenomegaly, and serositis. The arthritis in this form may progress to permanent joint damage.
- In the ED, lab tests focus mostly on excluding other diagnoses. Complete blood count (CBC), ESR, and C-reactive protein (CRP) may be normal. Arthrocentesis may be necessary to exclude septic arthritis, particularly in pauciarticular disease.

- X-rays initially show joint effusions but are nonspecific. The diagnosis of JRA will likely not be made in the ED.
- Initial therapy for patients with an established diagnosis includes aspirin or nonsteroidal anti-inflammatory drugs (NSAIDs). Glucocorticoids are occasionally used, for example for unresponsive uveitis or decompensated pericarditis or myocarditis.

HENOCH-SCHÖNLEIN PURPURA

- Henoch-Schönlein purpura (HSP) is a self-limited generalized leukocytoclastic vasculitis mediated by immune complexes.
- Palpable purpura, the classic vasculitic rash, appears on the trunk, buttocks, and legs.
- HSP also involves the glomeruli, with resulting hematuria and proteinuria.
- Involvement of the bowel wall causes colicky abdominal pain and may lead to melena, hematochezia, or intussusception.
- A polymigratory periarticulitis occurs in most children.
- HSP is largely a clinical diagnosis; useful lab tests include urinalysis, CBC, tests of renal function, and sometimes tests for collagen vascular disease.
- Hospital admission is indicated when the diagnosis is in doubt, dehydration occurs, or when gastrointestinal or renal complications require close observation.
- Therapy with intravenous steroids (1 to 2 mg/kg per day) may improve GI symptoms, but when required is best directed by the admitting pediatrician. Arthritis, when present as an isolated symptom, can be treated with NSAIDs.
- Chronic renal damage, sometimes requiring dialysis, occurs in 7 to 9% of children with HSP.

LEGG-CALVÉ-PERTHES' DISEASE

- Legg-Calvé-Perthes' disease is essentially avascular necrosis of the femoral head with subchondral stress fracture. Collapse and flattening of the femoral head ensues, with potential of subluxation.
- The hip is painful with limited range of motion, muscle spasm, and soft tissue contractures. Onset of symptoms is between ages 4 and 9. The disease is bilateral in 10% of patients. Children have a limp and chronic dull pain in the groin, thigh, and knee, which becomes worse with activity. Systemic symptoms are absent.
- Hip motion is restricted; there may be a flexion-abduction contracture and thigh muscle atrophy.
- Initial radiographs (in the first 1 to 3 months) show widening of the cartilage space in the affected hip and

diminished ossific nucleus of the femoral head. The second sign is subchondral stress fracture of the femoral head. The third finding is increased femoral head opacification. Finally, deformity of the femoral head occurs, with subluxation and protrusion of the femoral head from the acetabulum.

- Bone scan and magnetic resonance imaging are very helpful in making this diagnosis, showing bone abnormalities well before plain films.
- The differential diagnosis includes toxic tenosynovitis, tuberculous arthritis, tumors, and bone dyscrasias.
- In the ED, the most important thing is to consider this chronic but potentially crippling condition. Nearly all children are hospitalized initially for traction.

OSGOOD-SCHLATTER'S DISEASE

- Osgood-Schlatter's disease is a common syndrome that affects preteen boys more than girls. Repetitive stress on the tibial tuberosity by the quadriceps muscle initiates inflammation of the tibial tuberosity, without avascular necrosis.
- Children have pain and tenderness over the anterior knee, which becomes worse with knee bending and better with rest.
- The patellar tendon is thick and tender, with the tibial tuberosity enlarged and indurated.
- X-rays show soft-tissue swelling over the tuberosity and patellar tendon thickening without knee effusion. Normally, the ossification site at the tubercle at this age will be irregular, but the prominence of the tubercle is characteristic of Osgood-Schlatter's disease.
- The disorder is self-limited. Acute symptoms improve after restriction of physical activities involving knee bending for 3 months. Crutches may be necessary, though a knee immobilizer or cylinder cast are only rarely needed. Exercises to stretch taut and hypertrophied quadriceps muscles are also helpful.

POSTSTREPTOCOCCAL REACTIVE ARTHRITIS

- Because of increased group A β-hemolytic streptococcal infections, poststreptococcal reactive arthritis (PSRA) is also increasing.[6] PSRA is a sterile inflammatory nonmigratory mono- or oligoarthritis occurring with infection at a distant site with β-hemolytic streptococci and also *Staphylococcus* and *Salmonella* species.
- Unlike acute rheumatic fever, PSRA is not associated with carditis, and in general is a milder illness. However, the arthritis in PSRA is more severe and prolonged compared to acute rheumatic fever, and may be resistant to salicylates.

- To establish the diagnosis of PSRA, antecedent infection with group A streptococci must be established, either with throat culture or fourfold rise in antistreptolysin O (ASO) or anti-DNase B titer.
- PSRA is responsive to NSAIDs.[6] The issue of penicillin prophylaxis, a mainstay of therapy in acute rheumatic fever, is controversial in PSRA. However, if group A *Streptococcus* is recovered from the throat, treatment with penicillin or erythromycin should be instituted.

ACUTE RHEUMATIC FEVER

- Acute rheumatic fever (ARF) is an acute inflammatory multisystem illness affecting primarily school-age children. It is not common in the United States, but there have been recent epidemics.
- ARF is preceded by infection with certain strains of group A β-hemolytic *Streptococcus,* which stimulates antibody production to host tissues. Children develop ARF 2 to 6 weeks after symptomatic or asymptomatic streptococcal pharyngitis.
- Arthritis, which occurs in most initial attacks, is migratory and polyarticular, primarily affecting the large joints.
- Carditis occurs in one third of patients, and can affect valves, muscle, and pericardium. Carditis confers greatest mortality and morbidity.
- Sydenham's chorea occurs in 10% of patients and may occur months after the initial infection. Manifestations include sudden, aimless, irregular movements and muscle weakness.
- The rash, erythema marginatum, is fleeting, faint, and serpiginous, usually accompanying carditis. Subcutaneous nodules, found on the extensor surfaces of extremities, are quite rare.
- Laboratory tests are used to confirm prior streptococcal infection (throat culture and streptococcal serology) or to assess carditis (electrocardiogram, chest x-ray, and echocardiogram).
- The differential includes JRA, septic arthritis, Kawasaki's disease, leukemia, and other cardiomyopathies and vasculitides.
- Significant carditis is managed with prednisone 1 to 2 mg/kg/day initially. Arthritis is treated with high-dose aspirin (75 to 100 mg/kg/day) to start.
- All children with ARF are treated with penicillin (PCN): benzathine PCN 1.2 million U intramuscularly, procaine PCN G 600,000 U intramuscularly daily for 10 days, or oral PCN VK 25 to 50 mg/kg/day divided four times a day for 10 days. Use erythromycin if the patient is PCN allergic.
- Long-term prophylaxis is indicated for patients with ARF, and lifelong prophylaxis is recommended for patients with carditis.

TRANSIENT TENOSYNOVITIS OF THE HIP

- Transient tenosynovitis is the most common cause of hip pain in children less than age 10.[5] The peak age is 3 to 6 years, with boys affected more than girls. The cause is unknown.
- Symptoms may be acute or gradual. Patients have pain in the hip, thigh, and knee, and an antalgic gait. Pain limits the hip's range of motion. There may be a low-grade fever, and patients do not appear toxic.
- The WBC and ESR are usually normal. Radiographs of the hip are normal or show a mild-to-moderate effusion. The main concern is differentiation from septic arthritis, particularly if the patient is febrile, with elevation of WBC or ESR and effusion.
- Diagnostic arthrocentesis is required, either with fluoroscopic or ultrasound guidance or in the operating room. The fluid in transient tenosynovitis is a sterile clear transudate.
- Once septic arthritis and hip fracture have been ruled out, patients can be treated with crutches to avoid weight bearing, anti-inflammatory agents such as ibuprofen 10 mg/kg, and close follow-up.

REFERENCES

1. Swischuk LE: Radiographic signs of skeletal trauma, in Ludwig S, Kornber AE (eds.): *Child Abuse,* 2nd ed. New York: Churchill Livingstone, 1992, p. 151.
2. Skaggs DL: Elbow fractures in children: Diagnosis and management. *J Am Acad Orthop Surg* 5:303, 1997.
3. Wu J, Perron AD, Miller ME, et al: Orthopedic pitfalls in the ED: Pediatric supracondylar humerus fractures. *Am J Emerg Med* 20:544, 2002.
4. Macias CG, Botherner J, Wiebe R: A comparison of supination flexion to hyperpronation in the reduction of radial head subluxations. *Pediatrics* 102:110, 1998.
5. Warren RW, Perez MD, Wilking AP, Myones BL: Pediatric rheumatic diseases. *Pediatr Clin North Am* 41:783, 1994.
6. Jasen TL, Janssen M, Van Riel PL: Acute rheumatic fever or post-streptococcal reactive arthritis: A clinical problem revisited. *Br J Rheumatol* 37:335, 1998.

For further reading in *Emergency Medicine: A Comprehensive Study Guide,* 6th ed., see Chap. 136, "Musculoskeletal Disorders in Children," by Courtney Hopkins-Mann, David Leader, Donna Moro-Sutherland, and Richard A. Christoph.

86 SICKLE CELL ANEMIA IN CHILDREN

Douglas R. Trocinski

- Sickle cell emergencies in children include vaso-occlusive crises, hematologic crises, and infections. All children with sickle cell disease (SCD) presenting with fever, pain, respiratory distress, or a change in neurologic function require a rapid and thorough emergency department (ED) evaluation.

EPIDEMIOLOGY

- SCD is among the most common pediatric genetic conditions encountered in emergency medicine.
- In the United States about 8% of the African-American population carries the hemoglobin (HgbS) gene and about 0.15% (approximately 1/500) are homozygous (HgbSS).[1]
- SCD is associated with a significant mortality rate: 20 to 30% of all deaths from SCD occur before 5 years of age, with a mean age at death of 14 years.[1]
- The highest mortality occurs in children between 1 and 3 years of age, with sepsis being the leading cause of death.[2]
- Clinical effects of the disorder can begin in infancy but usually are not seen until 5 to 6 months of age, because high levels of fetal hemoglobin are present following birth, and the β-Hgb subunit is not predominant until about 3 months of age.

PATHOPHYSIOLOGY

- The genetic abnormality responsible for the sickling process is caused by a single amino acid substitution of valine for glutamic acid in the β subunit of the hemoglobin molecule.
- HgbS strands, in response to deoxygenation, polymerize abnormally, tending to coalesce and stretch into long monofilaments, distorting the red blood cell membrane into a characteristic sickle shape. This process results in repeated cycles of sickling, eventually leading to irreversibly distorted cells that diminish blood viscosity, causing hemolysis and obstruction of the microcirculation of end-organ tissues (vaso-occlusive phenomenon).
- The National Heart, Lung, and Blood Institute published management guidelines in 2002 which summarize current understanding of the many presenting complications of this disease.[3]

VASO-OCLUSIVE CRISES

- Vaso-occlusive sickle episodes are due to intravascular sickling, which leads to tissue ischemia and infarction. Bones, soft tissue, viscera, and the central nervous system may all be affected.

PAIN CRISES

CLINICAL FEATURES
- The classic sickle cell pain crisis is usually typical in location, character, and severity of pain. The crisis may be triggered by stress, extremes of cold, dehydration, hypoxia, or infection, but most often occur without a specific cause.
- Often there are no physical findings, although pain, local tenderness, swelling, and warmth may occur.
- It is rare for clinical symptoms of the disease to appear before 5 to 6 months of age. Dactylitis, swelling of hands or feet and low grade temperature, thought secondary to ischemia and infarction of bone marrow, may be the initial presenting manifestation of sickle cell disease in infants. As children age, the array of presentations may expand from the extremities to the abdomen, chest, and lumbrosacral area.

DIAGNOSIS AND DIFFERENTIAL
- Painful crises can be associated with low-grade fever and leukocytosis, but temperatures greater than 38.3°C (101°F) are more likely to be due to an infectious cause than to tissue ischemia.
- Vaso-occlusive pain crises usually present in a stereotypical fashion. Atypical character or locations of pain warrant further investigation for infectious sources or complications of sickle cell disease. Osteomyelitis or septic arthritis should be considered in the differential diagnosis.
- Abdominal pain crises are common and are characterized by abrupt onset, lack of localization, and recurrent nature.
- It is important to determine whether the abdominal pain in SCD patients has substantially changed in character, quality, duration, severity, and associated symptoms. If such changes are present, infection or other related diagnoses, such as cholecystitis, appendicitis, pancreatitis, hepatitis, perforated viscus, pelvic inflammatory disease or other gynecologic pathology, should be considered and explored.

EMERGENCY DEPARTMENT CARE AND DISPOSITION
- Aggressive hydration may be accomplished with oral fluids or age-appropriate IV maintenance fluids (5% dextrose [D_5] in 0.25 normal saline solution [NS] or $D_5$0.45 NS) at a rate 1½ times maintenance. Lactated Ringer's or normal saline are indicated in the hypotensive patient, with careful attention paid to avoid fluid overload.
- Mild to moderate pain can often be managed with oral hydration and analgesics, such as narcotic-acetaminophen combinations and nonsteroidal anti-inflammatory drugs (NSAIDs).
- Parenteral, long-acting narcotics, morphine 0.1 to 0.15 mg/kg IV or hydromorphone 0.015 mg/kg IV, are indicated if oral regimens are inadequate.[4]
- Admission is warranted for poor pain control or inadequate oral fluid intake.

ACUTE CHEST SYNDROME

- Acute chest syndrome is believed to be attributable to a combination of pneumonia, pulmonary infarction, and pulmonary emboli from necrotic bone marrow.[5,6]

CLINICAL FEATURES
- Acute chest syndrome should be considered in all patients with SCD who present with complaints of chest pain, especially when it is associated with tachypnea, dyspnea, cough, and other symptoms of respiratory distress. Significant hypoxia and rapid deterioration to respiratory failure can occur.[5,6]

DIAGNOSIS AND DIFFERENTIAL
- Chest x-rays should be obtained, but may be normal during the first hours to days. There are no specific laboratory abnormalities typical of acute chest syndrome; however, a complete blood count (CBC), reticulocyte count, and blood culture should be obtained.
- Noninvasive pulse oximetry should be instituted, and arterial blood gas analysis is indicated in the presence of significant oxygen desaturation or respiratory distress.

EMERGENCY DEPARTMENT CARE AND DISPOSITION
- All children in whom the diagnosis of acute chest syndrome is being considered should be monitored closely for changes in work of breathing and oxygenation, as deterioration can be rapid.
- Supplemental oxygen should be provided if respiratory distress is present or if oxygen saturation is persistently less than or equal to 94%.
- Adequate analgesia for chest pain should be provided (see above), as well as IV hydration with D_5½ NS at 1 to 1½ times maintenance.
- Treat potential underlying bacterial pneumonia with empiric antibiotic therapy such as ceftriaxone 75 mg/kg/day or cefotaxime 50 to 75 mg/kg/day divided every 8 hours.

- Transfusion decisions should be made early and in consultation with a pediatric hematologist.
- All children with suspected acute chest syndrome warrant hospital admission.

ACUTE CENTRAL NERVOUS SYSTEM EVENTS

CLINICAL FEATURES

- Acute central nervous system (CNS) crisis should be considered in any patient with SCD who presents with sudden-onset headache or neurologic changes, including hemiparesis, seizures, speech defects, sensory hearing loss, visual disturbances, transient ischemic attacks, dizziness, vertigo, cranial nerve palsies, paresthesias, or inexplicable coma.

DIAGNOSIS AND DIFFERENTIAL

- When CNS vaso-occlusion is suspected, a computed tomography (CT) scan or magnetic resonance imaging (MRI) scan of the brain should be obtained.
- A lumbar puncture may be necessary to exclude subarachnoid hemorrhage.
- No specific hematologic changes are associated with CNS vaso-occlusion; however, a CBC and reticulocyte count should be obtained, and blood typing and screening should be ordered in case an exchange transfusion is necessary.

EMERGENCY DEPARTMENT CARE AND DISPOSITION

- Suspected CNS vaso-occlusion necessitates immediate stabilization and careful monitoring.
- A pediatric neurosurgeon should be consulted once intracranial bleeding has been confirmed. All children with diagnosed or suspected CNS vaso-occlusion should be admitted to the pediatric intensive care unit for close monitoring and further care.

PRIAPISM

- Priapism, a painful sustained erection in the absence of sexual stimulation, occurs when sickled cells accumulate in the corpora cavernosa. It can affect all males with SCD regardless of age, and severe prolonged attacks can cause impotence.[7]
- Patients with priapism should receive IV hydration with $D_5 0.45NS$ at 1½ to 2 times maintenance, appropriate analgesia, and bladder catheterization if the patient is unable to void spontaneously.
- Treatment options include oral α-adrenergic agonists (eg, terbutaline or pseudoephedrine), intrapenile injection of vasodilators (eg, hydralazine) or dilute epinephrine, and/or needle aspiration of the corpora cav-

ernosa. Management and admission decisions should be made promptly in consultation with a urologist and pediatric hematologist.

HEMATOLOGICAL CRISES

ACUTE SEQUESTRATION CRISES

CLINICAL FEATURES

- Sequestration crises are the second most common cause of death in children with SCD under the age of 5 years.[1]
- The spleen of a young child with sickle cell disease can massively enlarge, trapping a considerable portion of the circulation blood volume. This condition can quickly progress to hypotension, shock, and death. Such crises are often preceded by a viral infection, particularly parvovirus B19.[8]
- Classically, children present with sudden-onset left upper quadrant pain, pallor, and lethargy; a markedly enlarged, tender, and firm spleen on abdominal exam; and signs of cardiovascular collapse, including hypotension and tachycardia.

DIAGNOSIS AND DIFFERENTIAL

- A CBC reveals a profound anemia (hemoglobin drops to less than 6 g/dL or 3 g/dL lower than the patient's baseline level).
- Minor episodes can occur with insidious onset of abdominal pain, slowly progressive splenomegaly, and a more minor fall in hemoglobin level (generally the hemoglobin level remains above 6 g/dL).
- Splenic sequestration crises may be characterized by thrombocytopenia and higher-than-normal reticulocyte counts.
- Less commonly, sequestration can occur in the liver. Clinical features include an enlarged and tender liver with associated hyperbilirubinemia, severe anemia, and elevated reticulocyte count. Cardiovascular collapse is rare in this condition.

EMERGENCY DEPARTMENT CARE AND DISPOSITION

- Early recognition and prompt initiation of treatment are the keys to successful management.
- Transfusion with packed red blood cells (PRBCs) or exchange transfusion is often required and should be instituted immediately. Even children with minor episodes should be admitted to the hospital.

APLASTIC EPISODES

- Potentially life-threatening, aplastic episodes are precipitated primarily by viral infections, but can also be

caused by bacterial infections, folic acid deficiency, or bone-marrow-suppressive or toxic drugs.
- Patients usually present with gradual onset of pallor, dyspnea, fatigue, and jaundice.
- CBC reveals an unusually low hematocrit (10% or lower) with decreased or absent reticulocytosis. White blood cell and platelet counts generally remain stable.
- Pain is not a hallmark of this crisis unless there is an associated vaso-occlusive crisis.
- If anemia is severe, admit for red blood cell transfusion in order to avoid secondary cardiopulmonary complications.

HEMOLYTIC CRISES

- Bacterial and viral infections in children with SCD can also precipitate an increasing degree of active hemolysis.
- The onset is usually sudden. A CBC reveals a hemoglobin level decreased from baseline, with markedly increased reticulocytosis. Increased jaundice and pallor are noticed on physical examination, in addition to other signs and symptoms of the precipitating infection.
- Specific therapy is rarely required. Hematologic values return to normal as the infectious process resolves. Care should be directed toward treating the underlying infection. Close follow-up to monitor hemoglobin and reticulocyte count should be arranged at discharge.

INFECTIONS

CLINICAL FEATURES
- Children with SCD are functionally asplenic and have deficient antibody production and impaired phagocytosis. Therefore bacterial infections, especially with encapsulated organisms, pose a serious and potentially fatal threat to young children with SCD.[9]
- Since sepsis can be rapid, overwhelming, and fatal, particularly in children less than 5 years of age, all children with SCD and fever should be quickly and carefully examined and managed aggressively.
- SCD children should routinely receive *Haemophilus influenzae* and pneumococcal vaccination and be maintained on penicillin prophylaxis.

DIAGNOSIS AND DIFFERENTIAL
- A CBC, reticulocyte count, and blood cultures should be obtained for all children with SCD and fever or history of fever. Clinical signs and symptoms should direct the remainder of the work-up, including lumbar puncture as indicated.

- Knowledge regarding the child's immunization status (particularly whether he or she has been immunized against *H. influenzae* type B and/or pneumococcus) and compliance with their home penicillin prophylaxis is helpful.

EMERGENCY DEPARTMENT CARE AND DISPOSITION
- Children who are ill appearing on presentation should be treated parenterally with an antibiotic with activity against *Streptococcus pneumoniae* and *H. influenzae* (eg, ceftriaxone 50 mg/kg IV or IM) before evaluation is complete and test results are available.
- Fever without a source must be treated aggressively in SCD in consultation with a pediatric hematologist.

DISPOSITION GUIDELINES

- Hospital admission is warranted for the following:
  - Temperature greater than 38.4°C with WBCs greater than 30,000, left shift, or hematologic parameters markedly altered from patient baseline.
  - Any signs of respiratory distress, hypoxia, and/or lobar infiltrate on chest x-ray.
  - Splenic or liver sequestration or aplastic crisis.
  - Any new CNS findings or presentations.
  - Evidence of acute abdomen.
  - Prolonged priapism.
  - Any vaso-occlusive crises not responsive to analgesia and hydration (usually after 4 to 6 hours of therapy).
  - Inability to maintain adequate hydration.
  - Uncertain diagnosis.
  - Inadequate follow-up assurance.
- Blood transfusions are often necessary in children undergoing splenic sequestration crisis and severe aplastic crisis. They may be required for management of cerebrovascular accident (CVA), priapism, or perioperative management prior to surgery. Consider transfusion for hemoglobin <6, reticulocyte count <20% or less than 250,000/μL, evidence of heart failure, hypotension resistant to fluids and oxygen therapy, or marked fatigue. In cases of acute deterioration, a PRBC transfusion is indicated while arranging for exchange transfusion.

VARIANTS OF SICKLE CELL DISEASE

- **Sickle cell trait** is the carrier state of SCD and the most common variant. These patients are asymptomatic and hematologically normal. They will have sickling and concomitant vaso-occlusive complications only in the presence of extreme hypoxia or high altitude.[10] They have minimal complications, the most common being hematuria (1%), most likely due to papillary necrosis in the renal medullary tissue.

- **Sickle cell hemoglobin-C disease** is a heterozygous condition characterized by mild to moderate anemia and mild reticulocytosis. Their smear reveals abundant target cells and few sickled cells. Many adults have splenomegaly and these patients are at risk for pain crisis and organ infarcts. Most patients, however, have few clinical complications.
- **Sickle cell-β thalassemia disease** is a heterozygous condition with varying degrees of severity of symptoms, dependent on the amount of normal β-hemoglobin chains that are produced. The severity can range from mild symptoms to a syndrome similar to SCD.

REFERENCES

1. Davis H, Schoendorf KC, Gergen PJ, Moore RM Jr: National trends in the mortality of children with sickle cell disease, 1968 through 1992. *Am J Public Health* 87:1317, 1997.
2. Gill FM, Sleeper LA, Weiner SJ, et al: Clinical events in the first decade in a cohort of infants with sickle cell disease. Cooperative study of sickle cell disease. *Blood* 86:776, 1995.
3. National Heart, Lung, and Blood Institute: The Management of Sickle Cell Disease, National Institutes of Health, Publication 02-2112. Bethesda, MD: NHLBI, 2002.
4. Pollack CV, Sanders DY, Severance HW: Emergency department analgesia without narcotics for adults with acute sickle cell pain crisis: Case reports and review of crisis management. *J Emerg Med* 9:445, 1991.
5. Vichinsky EP, Neumayr LD, Earles AN, et al: Causes and outcomes of the acute chest syndrome in sickle cell disease. *N Engl J Med* 342:1855, 2000.
6. Vinchinsky EP, Styles LA, Cloangelo LH, et al: Acute chest syndrome in sickle cell disease: Clinical presentation and course. *Blood* 89:1787, 1997.
7. Mantadakis E, Cavender JD, Rogers ZR, et al: Prevalence of priapism in children and adolescents with sickle cell anemia. *Am J Pediatr Hematol Oncol* 21:518, 1999.
8. Malloh AA, Quadah A: Acute splenic sequestration together with aplastic crisis caused by human parvovirus B19 in patients with sickle cell disease. *J Pediatr* 122:593, 1993.
9. Zarkowsky HS, Gallagher D, Gill FM, et al: Bacteremia in sickle hemoglobinopathies. *J Pediatr* 109:579, 1986.
10. Pollack CV Jr: Emergencies in sickle cell disease. *Emerg Med Clin North Am* 11:365, 1993.

For further reading in *Emergency Medicine: A Comprehensive Study Guide*, 6th ed., see Chap. 137, "Sickle Cell Disease," by Peter J. Paganussi, Thom Mayer, and Maybelle Kou.

87 PEDIATRIC URINARY TRACT INFECTIONS

Lance Brown

EPIDEMIOLOGY

- Pediatric urinary tract infections (UTI) occur in 4 to 7% of febrile infants,[1] 2% of children 1 to 5 years of age, and up to 3 to 5% of school-aged girls.[2]

PATHOPHYSIOLOGY

- UTI typically develops from retrograde contamination of the lower urinary tract with organisms from the perineum and periurethral area. In neonates, however, UTI typically develops after seeding of the renal parenchyma from hematogenous spread.
- Factors influencing the development of UTI include virulence of the pathogen, host immunity, congenital urinary tract abnormalities, vesicoureteral reflux, urolithiasis, poor hygiene, voluntary urinary retention, circumcision, and constipation.[3–9]

CLINICAL FEATURES

- Clinical features vary markedly by age.
- Neonatal UTI may present with a septic-like appearance. Features may include fever, jaundice, poor feeding, irritability, and lethargy.
- Infants and young children typically present with gastrointestinal complaints, which may include fever, abdominal pain, vomiting, and change in appetite.
- In older school-aged children and adolescents, cystitis and urethritis (lower tract disease) typically presents with urinary frequency, urgency, hesitancy, and dysuria. Pyelonephritis (upper tract disease) typically presents with fever, chills, back pain, vomiting, and dehydration.

DIAGNOSIS AND DIFFERENTIAL

- Urine culture is the gold standard in the diagnosis of UTI.[2]
- Of isolated organisms, *Escherichia coli* accounts for the vast majority of infections. Other important pathogens include *Klebsiella, Proteus,* and *Enterobacter* species. *Enterococcus* species, *Staphylococcus aureus,* and group B streptococci are the most common gram-positive organisms and are more common in neonates. *Chlamydia trachomatis* may be present in

adolescents with urinary tract symptoms and micro-hematuria.[10] Adenovirus may cause culture-negative acute cystitis in young boys.

- Because urine culture results are not available to the emergency physician during the initial visit, urine chemical test strips that can detect leukocyte esterase and urinary nitrites in conjunction with microscopic urinalysis are often employed to aid in the diagnosis of UTI.

- A negative urine test strip does not rule out UTI. The sensitivities of a positive leukocyte esterase test or nitrite test for a positive urine culture are less than 50%, particularly in neonates and young infants who may not mount sufficient pyuria to have a positive test strip. Combining pyuria (>5 white blood cells [WBCs] per high power field) and bacteriuria on urinary microanalysis yields a sensitivity of 65% and positive predictive value of about 80%.

- Pyuria, hematuria, and proteinuria are very commonly found in UTIs, but are also commonly present in the absence of infection.

- The method of specimen collection impacts directly on how a urinary tract infection is defined. Bag specimens are inappropriate for culture because of a high degree of contamination.

- In infants and young children who are not yet toilet trained, bladder catheterization is the preferred method. A positive urine culture is defined as $\geq 5 \times 10^4$ colony-forming units (CFU)/mL of a single urinary pathogen.[11] Suprapubic aspiration, although invasive, is also an acceptable means of obtaining a cultured specimen. Growth of a urinary pathogen in any number from a suprapubic aspiration is considered a positive culture.[11]

- In toilet trained preschoolers and older children, a midstream clean catch specimen is preferred.[5] Symptomatic patients with $\geq 10^5$ CFU/mL of a single urinary pathogen are considered to have a positive urine culture.[11]

EMERGENCY DEPARTMENT CARE AND DISPOSITION

- Treatment and disposition depends on the age of the patient and severity of the illness.

- Physicians should be familiar with the local susceptibilities of the common urinary pathogens in their geographic region. Medications listed below are generally acceptable, but emerging resistance is a continuing problem.

- Neonates and infants less than 3 months of age with fever and UTI are usually hospitalized and given intravenous antibiotics. Neonates are typically treated with intravenous ampicillin (50 mg/kg per dose) and cefotaxime (50 mg/kg per dose). Infants from 1 to 3 months of age are treated with intravenous cefotaxime or ceftriaxone (50 mg/kg per dose).

- Older infants and children with fever and UTI complicated by vomiting, dehydration, any suspicion of sepsis, or inability to take oral antibiotics are hospitalized for intravenous cefotaxime (50 mg/kg per dose) until they are afebrile and able to take oral medications.

- Older infants and children with fever and uncomplicated UTI (can tolerate oral medication, are not dehydrated, are not immunocompromised, appear well) may receive a single dose of intramuscular or intravenous ceftriaxone (50 mg/kg) in the emergency department and start on outpatient oral antibiotics (cephalexin 25 mg/kg per dose given three times per day) with close primary care follow-up.

- Older infants and children with cystitis (afebrile UTI) are treated for 5 to 7 days with oral cephalexin (25 mg/kg per dose given three times per day) or amoxicillin-clavulanate (20 mg/kg per dose given twice daily) with close outpatient follow-up.

- Adolescent girls with cystitis may be treated like adults with a 3-day oral antibiotic regimen (eg, cephalexin 500 mg given three times per day).

- In addition to those listed above, commonly used parenteral antibiotic regimens for treating urinary tract infections include ampicillin (50 mg/kg per dose) and gentamicin (2.5 mg/kg per dose) in neonates. In older children parenteral cefotaxime, ceftriaxone, or cefepime may be used (all dosed at 50 mg/kg per dose). Commonly used oral antibiotics include amoxicillin (15 mg/kg per dose given three times per day), amoxicillin clavulanate (20 mg/kg per dose given twice daily), trimethoprim-sulfamethoxazole (5 mg/kg per dose given twice daily), cephalexin (25 mg/kg per dose given three times per day), or cefixime (4 mg/kg per dose given twice daily).

- Historically, an important part of the follow-up of children with UTI has been evaluation for vesicoureteral reflux, renal scarring, active renal infection or other anatomic anomalies utilizing renal cortical scans, voiding cystourethrogram, isotope cystogram, and renal ultrasound.[12–15] This testing is arranged as an outpatient or performed during hospitalization and is not typically arranged from the emergency department. The necessity of this renal imaging in all young children with first febrile urinary tract infections has recently been challenged.[16]

REFERENCES

1. Hoberman A, Chao HP, Keller DM, et al: Prevalence of urinary tract infections in febrile infants. *J Pediatr* 23:17, 1993.
2. Gonzalez R: Urinary tract infections, in Behrman R, Klieman R, Arvin A, et al (eds.): *Nelson's Textbook of Pediatrics,* 16th ed. Philadelphia: Saunders, 2002.

3. American Academy of Pediatrics Committee on Quality Improvements. Subcommittee on Urinary Tract Infection: Practice parameter: The diagnosis, treatment, and evaluation of the initial urinary tract infection in febrile infants and young children. *Pediatrics* 103:843, 1999.

4. Bock GH: Urinary tract infections, in Hockerman R, (ed.): *Primary Pediatric Care,* 3rd ed. St. Louis: Mosby-Year Book, 1997, p. 1640.

5. Gearhart P, Herzberg G, Jeffs RD, et al: Childhood urolithiasis: Experiences and advances. *Pediatrics* 87:445, 1991.

6. Smellie JM, Normand ICS, Katz G: Children with urinary tract infection: A comparison of those with and those without vesicoureteric reflux. *Kidney Int* 20:717, 1981.

7. Smellie JM, Normand ICS: Urinary tract infections in children. *Postgrad Med* 61:895, 1985.

8. Bethyn AJ, Jenkins HR, Roberts R, et al: Radiologic evidence of constipation in urinary tract infection. *Am J Dis Child* 73:534, 1995.

9. Nayir A: Circumcision for the prevention of significant bacteriuria in boys. *Pediatr Nephrol* 16:1129, 2001.

10. Meglic A, Cavic M, Hren-Vencelj H, et al: Chlamydial infection of the urinary tract in children and adolescents with hematuria. *Pediatr Nephrol* 15:132, 2000.

11. Hellerstein S: Urinary tract infections: Old and new concepts. *Pediatr Clin North Am* 42:1433, 1995.

12. Conway J, Cohn R: Evolving role of nuclear medicine for diagnosis and management of urinary tract infections. *J Pediatr* 124:87, 1994.

13. Goldraich N, Coldraich I: Update on dimercaptosuccinic acid renal scanning in children with urinary tract infection. *Pediatr Nephrol* 9:221, 1995.

14. Dick PT, Feldman W: Routine diagnostic imaging for childhood urinary tract infection: A systematic overview. *J Pediatr* 128:15, 1996.

15. Andrich MP, Majd M: Diagnostic imaging in the evaluation of the first urinary tract infection in infants and young children. *Pediatrics* 90:436, 1992.

16. Hoberman A, Charron M, Hickey RW, et al: Imaging studies after a first febrile urinary tract infection in young children. *N Engl J Med* 348:195, 2003.

For further reading in *Emergency Medicine, A Comprehensive Study Guide,* 6th ed., see Chap. 140, "Pediatric Urinary Tract Infections," by Michael F. Altieri, Mary Camarca, and Thom Mayer.

88 SEXUALLY TRANSMITTED DISEASES

Gregory S. Hall

- This chapter covers the major sexually transmitted diseases in the United States with the exception of HIV (AIDS) (see Chap. 91). Vaginitis and pelvic inflammatory disease (PID) are covered separately in Chaps. 64 and 65, respectively.

CHLAMYDIAL INFECTIONS

- *Chlamydia trachomatis* is an obligate intracellular bacteria that can cause urethritis, epididymitis-orchitis, proctitis, and Reiter's syndrome (urethritis, conjunctivitis, and rash) in men; urethritis, cervicitis, PID, and infertility in women, and conjunctivitis in both sexes.
- Asymptomatic infection in both sexes is common—patients with chlamydia have a high incidence of coinfection with gonorrhea.
- The incubation period varies from 1 to 3 weeks, with symptoms including mild urinary burning, purulent or mucoid urethral discharge, vaginal discharge, vaginal irritation or pain, scrotal pain with or without swelling (epididymitis-orchitis), abdominal/pelvic pain (PID), and even peritonitis.
- Diagnosis is usually achieved via mucosal swabs utilizing direct immunofluorescence, enzyme-linked immunosorbent assays (ELISA), or DNA probes for *Chlamydia;* all have sensitivities in the range of 70 to 95%.[1] The Centers for Disease Control (CDC) recommends that a nucleic acid amplification test (NAAT) be used as a screening tool.[2] Direct culture of

the organism is possible but has a relatively low yield.
- Treatments of choice for uncomplicated chlamydial infections (not PID) include azithromycin 1 g PO single dose (considered safe in pregnancy) or doxycycline 100 mg PO twice daily for 7 days (see Table 88-1 for alternatives).[1] Patients should be counseled to avoid sexual contact for 7 days (regardless of whether the 1- or 7-day drug regimen is prescribed) and sexual contacts from the preceding 60 days should be treated as well.
- Treatment should also be given for possible coinfection with gonorrhea and pregnant women should be re-evaluated in 3 weeks with repeat testing.

GONOCOCCAL INFECTIONS

- *Neisseria gonorrhoeae* (GC), a gram-negative diplococcus, causes urethritis, cervicitis, PID, and infertility in women, and urethritis, epididymitis-orchitis, and prostatitis in men.[3] Symptomatic pharyngitis, conjunctivitis, and proctitis are unusual but may occur.
- Symptoms can include dysuria, purulent urethral discharge, vaginal discharge, scrotal/epididymal pain with or without swelling, abdominal/pelvic pain, and on occasion peritonitis.
- Rectal infection/proctitis and pharyngeal colonization (usually asymptomatic) can occur in both sexes.
- The incubation period ranges from 7 to 14 days in women, who commonly present with vague nonspecific lower abdominal discomfort and mucopurulent cervicitis—asymptomatic infection is common.
- Eighty to ninety percent of men develop symptoms within 2 weeks, most commonly dysuria and purulent penile discharge (urethritis).
- Dissemination of gonorrhea occurs in 2% of patients with untreated primary infection (most are women),

TABLE 88-1   Antimicrobial Therapy for STDs

DISEASE	FIRST-LINE TREATMENT	ALTERNATE(S)
Chlamydia	Azithromycin 1 g PO single dose *or* Doxycycline 100 mg PO bid × 7 d	Erythromycin 500 mg PO qid × 7 d *or* Ofloxacin 300 mg PO bid × 7 d *or* Levofloxacin 500 mg PO qd × 7 d
Gonorrhea	Cefixime 400 mg PO single dose *or* Ceftriaxone 125 mg IM single dose *or* Ciprofloxacin 500 mg PO single dose *or* Ofloxacin 400 mg PO single dose *or* Levofloxacin 250 mg PO single dose	Spectinomycin 2 g IM single dose *or* Norfloxacin 800 mg PO single dose *or* Gatifloxacin 400 mg PO single dose
Trichomoniasis	Metronidazole 2 g PO single dose	Metronidazole 500 mg PO bid × 7 d
Bacterial vaginosis	Metronidazole 500 mg PO bid × 7 d *or* Metronidazole vaginal gel 0.75% qd for 5 d	Clindamycin 2% cream intravaginally qhs × 7 d
Syphilis (primary, secondary, early tertiary)	Benzathine penicillin G 2.4 million units IM in a single dose	Doxycycline 100 mg PO bid × 14 d
Syphilis (latent, tertiary)	Benzathine penicillin G 2.4 million units IM weekly × 3 weeks	
Herpes simplex virus (primary)	Acyclovir 400 mg PO tid × 7–10 d *or* Famciclovir 250 mg PO tid × 7–10 d *or* Valacyclovir 1 g PO bid × 7–10 d	Acyclovir 200 mg PO 5 times a day × 7–10 d
Herpes simplex virus (recurrent)	Acyclovir 400 mg PO tid × 5 d *or* Famciclovir 125 mg PO bid × 5 d *or* Valacyclovir 500 mg PO bid × 5 d	Acyclovir 800 mg PO bid × 5 days *or* Valacyclovir 1 g PO qd × 5 days
Chancroid	Azithromycin 1 g PO single dose Ceftriaxone 250 mg IM single dose *or* Ciprofloxacin 500 mg PO bid × 3 d	Erythromycin base 500 mg PO qid × 7 d
Lymphogranuloma venereum	Doxycycline 100 mg PO bid × 3 weeks	Erythromycin base 500 mg PO qid × 3 weeks
Donovanosis	Doxycycline 100 mg PO bid × 3 weeks *or* Trimethoprim-sulfamethoxazole DS PO bid × 3 weeks	Ciprofloxacin 750 mg PO bid × 3 weeks *or* Azithromycin 1 g PO weekly × 3 weeks *or* Erythromycin base 500 mg PO qid × 3 weeks

SOURCE: Adapted from the Centers for Disease Control and Prevention: Sexually transmitted diseases treatment guidelines—2002. *MMWR* 51:(RR-6), 2002.

and presents with an initial febrile bacteremic stage with multiple scattered skin lesions (tender pustules on a red or hemorrhagic base or petechial lesions), primarily on the extremities (including palms and soles), tenosynovitis, and myalgias.

• During the second phase of disseminated GC the initial symptoms subside, and are followed by mono- or oligoarticular arthritis, with purulent synovial fluid. Orthopedic consultation is needed as surgical drainage and irrigation may be required.

• Diagnosis of uncomplicated gonorrhea is usually es-

tablished via cervical or urethral swab with culture on a selective medium (sensitivity of 80 to 90%). If proper transport and storage conditions for culture media are not practicable, the CDC recommends that a nucleic acid amplification test (NAAT) be performed on endocervical or urethral swab specimens or on a urine specimen, as a screening tool.[2] Gram's stain of a urethral smear showing intracellular gram-negative diplococci is sensitive and specific in men, but much less useful in women.

• Diagnosis of disseminated GC is often clinical; culture of blood, skin lesions, or synovial fluid is positive in only 20 to 50% of patients (cultures of cervix, rectum, and/or pharynx may improve the yield).

- Effective therapy for uncomplicated gonorrhea (not PID) includes single-dose regimens of oral cefixime or a fluoroquinolone or IM ceftriaxone (see Table 88-1 for treatment regimens). Quinolone resistance has emerged in *Neisseria gonorrhoeae* (QRNG) originating from Asia, the Pacific, and in the U.S., California and Hawaii. The CDC recommends avoiding the use of quinolones for gonococcal infections acquired in these regions.[1,4]
- Disseminated gonorrhea is treated initially with parenteral ceftriaxone (up to 1 g/day).
- Pregnant women should be treated with a cephalosporin, or if allergic, 2 g spectinomycin IM as a single dose.
- Treatment for possible coinfection with *Chlamydia* should also be given, and patients should be advised to avoid sexual contact for at least 7 days and to have contacts from the previous 2 months see a doctor for treatment.

TRICHOMONIASIS

- *Trichomonas vaginalis* is a flagellated protozoan that causes vaginitis with discharge, urethritis with dysuria, and occasionally abdominal pain.
- The majority of men (>90%) infected with *Trichomonas* are asymptomatic, but some have dysuria. Women can also have asymptomatic infection.
- Pregnant women with trichomoniasis are at increased risk for premature rupture of membranes, preterm delivery, and low birth weight. Unfortunately, data from multiple studies do not indicate that treatment for asymptomatic infection prevents these adverse outcomes.
- The incubation period ranges from 3 to 28 days and diagnosis is made by microscopic examination of saline wet preparations of urethral or vaginal discharge or spun urine samples, revealing the classic flagellated motile parasites. Sensitivity of wet prep exam is only 60 to 70% and culture is more sensitive but difficult to perform.
- Metronidazole (2 g PO as a single dose) is the treatment of choice for men and women; alternatively it may be given for 7 days at 500 mg PO twice daily.
- Oral metronidazole is still considered a class C drug in pregnancy by many sources and many clinicians avoid oral treatment in the first trimester. However, several studies suggest that the use of metronidazole in pregnancy has not demonstrated a consistent association with teratogenic or mutagenic effects above the baseline population rate. CDC guidelines indicate

that pregnant women may be treated with a single 2-g dose of metronidazole.[1]
- Metronidazole gel (vaginal) is available, but has an effectiveness of less than 50% compared with oral preparations.

GENITAL WARTS

- Human papillomaviruses (HPV) are DNA viruses that are transmitted by direct contact and cause venereal or anogenital warts.
- The incubation period from contact to appearance of warts varies from 1 to 8 months.
- Genital warts begin as flesh-colored papules or cauliflower-like projections that may eventually coalesce to form condyloma acuminata. They may take on a flat appearance on the cervix.
- Venereal warts commonly occur at the urethra, frenulum, coronal sulcus of the penis, and perianal regions in men, and in women they are common at the posterior introitus and adjacent labia, in the vagina, on the cervix, and often spread to other parts of the perineum (vulva and anus).
- Diagnosis is often clinical, but may be confirmed by skin biopsy and histologic methods or by soaking the suspected skin with dilute acetic acid for 3 minutes; normal skin remains shiny white in color, while areas of wart-neoplasia become dull gray-white in color.
- Treatment is not usually attempted acutely in the ED setting, most often it includes topical podophyllin, imiquimod cream, or cryotherapy in a physician's office or outpatient setting. Refer patients to a dermatologist, urologist, or ob-gyn specialist.

SYPHILIS

- Syphilis is caused by the spirochete *Treponema pallidum,* which is transmitted through direct contact at mucous membranes or nonintact skin.
- Classically syphilis infection is divided into three stages: primary, secondary, and tertiary (or latent).
- Primary syphilis is characterized by a painless chancre or ulcer with indurated borders on the penis, vulva, or other areas of sexual contact, and appears approximately 3 weeks after acquisition. The primary chancre heals spontaneously over the next 3 to 6 weeks; generally there are no constitutional symptoms in this stage.
- Secondary syphilis occurs 3 to 6 weeks after the primary chancre heals, and includes lymphadenopathy and a nonpruritic, polymorphous rash (most often dull, red, and papular or maculopapular, similar to that of pityriasis rosea), which starts on the trunk or

flexor surfaces of the extremities and spreads to involve the palms and soles.

- Constitutional symptoms are common during the secondary stage and may include fever, malaise, headache, and sore throat (mucous membrane involvement with oral lesions), and condyloma lata (wart-like growths) in the anogenital region may also occur.
- The secondary stage (including the rash) resolves spontaneously and may be followed years later by the tertiary (latent) stage of syphilis (now uncommon in the United States). Tertiary syphilis classically develops in about one third of patients with untreated latent secondary syphilis.
- Specific features of tertiary syphilis include peripheral neuropathy (tabes dorsalis), meningitis, dementia, aortitis with aortic valve insufficiency, and thoracic aortic aneurysm formation.
- During the early stages, diagnosis may be made by dark-field microscopic identification of treponemes on a specimen obtained from the primary chancre or secondary oral or condylomata lesions.
- Serologic diagnosis may be made with nontreponemal tests (rapid plasma reagin [RPR] or Venereal Disease Research Laboratory [VDRL]), which become positive about 14 days after the primary chancre appears (false-positive rate of 1 to 2% in the general population), or with specific treponemal tests (fluorescent treponemal antibody absorption [FTA-ABS]), which are more sensitive and specific but technically more difficult to perform.
- Syphilis in all of its stages remains uniformly sensitive to penicillin, the drug of choice (see treatment regimens in Table 88-1). All patients must be referred for follow-up serology testing to determine that adequate treatment has been given so as to prevent progression to secondary or tertiary stages.

HERPES SIMPLEX INFECTIONS

- Herpes simplex virus type 2 (HSV-2) or less commonly type 1 (HSV-1) can cause genital infection via transmission through direct contact with mucosal surfaces or nonintact skin.
- Primary infections present after an incubation period of 7 to 10 days, with painful clusters of vesicular or pustular lesions on a red base, which after 3 to 5 days ulcerate and/or coalesce, and are often accompanied by inguinal adenopathy (80%).
- Systemic symptoms are commonly seen in primary genital herpes infection and may include fever, headache, myalgias, tender inguinal adenopathy, and dysuria; urinary retention and aseptic meningitis can also occur.

- Left untreated, the primary illness lasts 2 to 3 weeks with complete healing of skin lesions, but the virus usually remains latent and is shed in urogenital tract secretions (even in asymptomatic patients). Recurrent or secondary infection, usually of milder and shorter duration (with fewer or no systemic symptoms), occurs in 60 to 90% of patients.
- Diagnosis is usually made on clinical grounds based on the characteristic appearance of the skin lesions, but the virus may be cultured from vesicular fluid (more reliable than the Tzanck prep exam of vesicular fluid for characteristic intranuclear inclusions).
- Treatment for primary genital herpes is acyclovir, famciclovir, or valacyclovir for 7 to 10 days. In those cases severe enough to require hospitalization, treatment with IV acyclovir 5 to 10 mg/kg body weight every 8 hours may be given (see Table 88-1 for specific treatment regimens).
- Treatment for episodes of recurrent genital herpes with a 5-day course of oral acyclovir, valacyclovir, or famciclovir, if started at the onset of symptoms may reduce the severity and duration of the episode.

CHANCROID

- Chancroid is caused by *Haemophilus ducreyi,* a gram-negative bacillus, and is more commonly seen in the tropics, but has shown an increasing incidence in the United States in recent years. Of infected patients in the U.S., 10% are coinfected with HSV or *T. pallidum,* and chancroid appears to be a cofactor for HIV transmission.
- Following an incubation period of 4 to 10 days, a tender papule on an erythematous base appears on the external genitalia. It then enlarges to form a painful, purulent ulcer with irregular edges (multiple ulcers may be present in 50%). Autoinoculation of adjacent skin may lead to formation of "kissing lesions."
- Painful inguinal adenopathy (usually unilateral) develops in about half of untreated patients 1 to 2 weeks after primary infection—sometimes forming a mass of matted lymph nodes (bubo) that may spontaneously suppurate and drain. Otherwise, constitutional symptoms are rare.
- Diagnosis is usually clinical (with care to exclude syphilis), but sometimes the organism can be cultured from a swab of a lesion or pus from the ulcer or bubo (requires special media).
- Treatment regimens include ceftriaxone, azithromycin, ciprofloxacin, or erythromycin (see Table 88-1 for regimens). Buboes may be aspirated to relieve pain from swelling but should not be excised.

LYMPHOGRANULOMA VENEREUM

- Lymphogranuloma venereum (LGV) is caused by three serotypes of *Chlamydia trachomatis,* which are endemic to some regions of the world, but still uncommon in the United States.
- The primary lesion of LGV consists of a painless small papule or vesicle on the genitals, which forms 5 to 21 days after exposure, often goes unnoticed, and heals spontaneously, usually after only 2 to 3 days.
- With anal intercourse, primary LGV may present as painful mucopurulent or bloody proctitis.
- Several weeks to months after the primary lesion heals, painful inguinal adenopathy (unilateral in 60%) develops. The lymph nodes become matted together to form an inguinal mass (bubo), often with the overlying skin taking on a purplish hue. The bubo may spontaneously suppurate and drain. Scarring of the bubo may leave a linear depression parallel to the inguinal ligament ("groove sign").
- Associated systemic symptoms such as fever, chills, arthralgias, erythema nodosum, and rarely meningoencephalitis, may be seen.
- Diagnosis is achieved through serologic testing targeted at the specific chlamydial serovars for LGV and/or culture from aspirated material taken from a bubo. A complement fixation titer for LGV of >1:64 is consistent with infection.
- Doxycycline 100 mg PO twice daily for 21 days is the treatment of choice (see Table 88-1). Buboes may require drainage. Mild untreated cases may resolve spontaneously in 8 to 12 weeks. Late sequelae include scarring; urethral, vaginal, and anal strictures; and occasionally lymphatic obstruction.

DONOVANOSIS

- Granuloma inguinale (donovanosis) is caused by *Calymmatobacterium granulomatis,* a gram-negative intracellular bacterium which is rare in the U.S. but endemic in India, southern Africa, and Pacific nations.
- There is a variable incubation period of 2 weeks to 6 months, after which the patient develops subcutaneous nodular lesions, generally on the penis or labia/vulvar area. These areas evolve to painless ulcers which are highly vascular, friable, and beefy red. The infection may then spread to adjacent areas (including the inguinal region) by subcutaneous extension, giving the appearance of a bubo; however, true lymphadenopathy is rare.
- Diagnosis depends on visualization of the characteristic intracellular Donovan bodies on biopsy or crushed tissue preparation. The organism is difficult to culture.

- Treatment is with doxycycline 100 mg orally twice or trimethoprim-sulfamethoxazole DS orally twice daily for 3 weeks. This will stop the progression of the lesions, but longer treatment may be needed to facilitate complete healing. Ciprofloxacin and azithromycin are alternatives.

REFERENCES

1. Centers for Disease Control and Prevention: 2002 Guidelines for treatment of sexually transmitted diseases. *MMWR* 47:(RR-06), 2002.
2. Centers for Disease Control and Prevention: Screening tests to detect Chlamydia trachomatis and Neisseria gonorrhea infections. *MMWR* 51:(RR-15), 2002.
3. Adimora AA, Hamilton H, Holmes KK, et al: *Sexually Transmitted Diseases: Companion Handbook.* New York: McGraw-Hill, 1994.
4. Hooper DC: New uses for new and old quinolones and the challenge of resistance. *Clin Infect Dis* 30:243, 2000.

For further reading in *Emergency Medicine: A Comprehensive Study Guide,* 6th ed., see Chap. 141, "Sexually Transmitted Diseases," by Joel Kravitz and Susan B. Promes.

89 TOXIC SHOCK
Kevin J. Corcoran

TOXIC SHOCK SYNDROME

EPIDEMIOLOGY

- Toxic shock syndrome (TSS) is a severe life-threatening syndrome that initially was associated with the use of tampons by menstruating women.[1] The overall incidence of menstrual-related toxic shock syndrome (MRTSS) and the number of cases associated with the use of tampons has decreased dramatically over the past 20 years.
- Currently 41% of TSS cases are non-menstrual-related (NMRTSS).[2] Nasal packing, contraceptive sponges and diaphragms, and body art and piercing have been identified as some of the pathways for illness.[3]
- One-tenth of the TSS cases are seen in men, with a mortality rate 3.3 times that of menstruating women.

PATHOPHYSIOLOGY

- The majority of TSS cases have been directly associated with colonization or infection with *Staphylococcus aureus*. Toxic shock syndrome toxin (TSST-1) is an exotoxin that has been implicated in many of the symptoms associated with TSS via direct toxic effects or through release of secondary mediators.
- *S. aureus* strains that produce TSST-1 are responsible for 90% of menstrual-related cases; however, TSST-1 is present in less than half of non-menstrual-related cases of TSS. In NMRTSS, biochemically similar enterotoxins have been identified, explaining the analogous clinical presentations between menstrual and NMRTSS.[4]
- Marked vasodilatation and movement of serum proteins and fluids from the intravascular to the extravascular space occurs, resulting in hypotension and edema. The resulting multisystem organ failure may be a reflection of either a direct effect of the toxin on the tissues or the rapid onset of hypotension and decreased perfusion.

CLINICAL FEATURES

- TSS is characterized by high fever, profound hypotension, diffuse erythrodermatous rash, mucous membrane hyperemia, diffuse myalgias, headache, vomiting, diarrhea, and constitutional symptoms that rapidly progress to multisystem dysfunction.
- Hypotension or orthostasis is seen in all cases and patients appear ill.
- Women with MRTSS typically present between the third and fifth day of menses.
- The rash associated with TSS is described as "painless sunburn" that typically fades within 3 days and is followed by full-thickness desquamation.
- Acute respiratory distress syndrome (ARDS) with refractory hypotension has been described as the ultimate end-organ damage secondary to TSS.

DIAGNOSIS AND DIFFERENTIAL

- Diagnostic criteria are listed in Table 89-1. Five of the six clinical findings defines a probable case. A confirmed case requires all six clinical findings including desquamation unless the patient dies prior to desquamation.
- TSS should be considered in any acute febrile illness associated with erythroderma, hypotension, and multiorgan involvement.
- When considering TSS, the evaluation should include arterial blood gases (ABG), complete blood cell count

TABLE 89-1 Diagnostic Criteria for Toxic Shock Syndrome

Fever: temperature $\geq 38.9°C$ ($\geq 102.0°F$)

Rash: diffuse macular erythroderma

Desquamation: 1–2 weeks after onset of illness

Hypotension

Multisystem involvement (three or more of the following):
- Gastrointestinal: vomiting or diarrhea at onset of illness
- Muscular: severe myalgias or creatinine phosphokinase elevation twice normal
- Mucous membrane: vaginal, oropharyngeal, or conjunctival hyperemia
- Renal: blood urea nitrogen or creatinine at least twice the upper limit of normal or laboratory or urinary sediment with pyuria (≥ 5 leukocytes per high-power field) in the absence of urinary tract infection
- Hepatic: total bilirubin, alanine aminotransferase enzyme, or aspartate aminotransferase enzyme levels at least twice the upper limit of normal for laboratory
- Hematologic: platelets $<100,000/mL$
- Central nervous system: disorientation or alterations in consciousness

Laboratory criteria: negative cultures and titers for alternative organisms

(CBC) with differential, electrolytes including $[Mg^{2+}]$ and $[Ca^{2+}]$, coagulation panel, urinalysis (UA), ECG, and chest x-ray (CXR).
- Other syndromes to consider in the differential diagnosis of TSS include streptococcal toxic shock syndrome (STSS), Kawasaki's disease (KD), staphylococcal scalded skin syndrome (SSSS), Rocky Mountain spotted fever (RMSF), and septic shock (SS).

EMERGENCY DEPARTMENT CARE AND DISPOSITION

- The treatment of TSS consists of airway management, aggressive management of circulatory shock, continuous monitoring of vital signs and urinary output, use of antistaphylococcal antimicrobial agents with β-lactamase stability, and the search for a focus of infection.
- Crystalloid IV fluids should be used initially for hypotension and fluid resuscitation. A central venous pressure (CVP) or Swan-Ganz catheter may be necessary for patient monitoring if there is an inadequate response to initial fluid resuscitation. Large volumes of fluid (up to 20 L) may be required over the first 24 hours.
- Culture all potentially infected sites, including blood, prior to initiating antibiotic therapy.
- Tampons or nasal packing should be removed, if present.
- A dopamine infusion may be necessary to augment fluid resuscitation for refractory hypotension.

- Fresh-frozen plasma, packed red blood cells (PRBCs), or platelets may be given to correct any coagulation abnormalities.
- Initiate antistaphylococcal antimicrobial therapy with β-lactamase stability. Nafcillin or oxacillin in doses of 1-2 g IV every 4 hours, or a cephalosporin such as cefazolin given 2 g every 6 hours provides adequate coverage. In penicillin-allergic patients, clindamycin, vancomycin, or potentially cephalosporins may be used.
- Other considerations include the use of methylprednisolone and intravenous immunoglobulin.
- Patients are typically admitted to the ICU.
- Recurrence of TSS can be seen in patients not treated with β-lactamase–stable antibiotics.

STREPTOCOCCAL TOXIC SHOCK SYNDROME

EPIDEMIOLOGY

- Streptococcal toxic shock syndrome (STSS) is defined as any group A streptococcal (GAS) infection associated with invasive soft tissue infection, early onset of shock, and organ failure. STSS is very similar to TSS; however, STSS is associated with a soft tissue infection which is culture-positive for *Streptococcus pyogenes*. While the incidence of TSS has declined, the number of cases of STSS has increased, with an estimated 2000 to 3000 cases per year.
- Labeled the "flesh-eating bacteria" by the news media, GAS infections cause streptococcal necrotizing fasciitis and myositis with mortality rates of 30 to 80%.[5]

PATHOPHYSIOLOGY

- Virulent streptococcal pyogenic exotoxins are produced by 90% of GAS isolates and are felt to be accountable for the multisystem failure seen with STSS.[6]
- The portals of entry of streptococci include the pharynx, vagina, mucosa, and skin in 50% of STSS cases, but the source cannot be identified in most cases.[7]
- Infection may begin with minor local trauma, although disruption of the skin is not required.

CLINICAL FEATURES

- Pain is the most common presenting symptom, while fever is the most common presenting sign, followed closely by shock.
- STSS typically presents with the abrupt onset of se-

TABLE 89-2   Diagnostic Criteria for Streptococcal Toxic Shock Syndrome

Hypotension

Multiorgan involvement characterized by two or more of the following:
- Renal impairment: creatinine level twice normal
- Coagulopathy
- Liver involvement: enzyme or bilirubin level twice normal
- Acute respiratory distress syndrome
- Generalized erythematous macular rash that may desquamate
- Soft tissue necrosis, including necrotizing fasciitis or myositis, or gangrene

vere pain that precedes physical findings.[5] Eighty percent of patients have signs of soft tissue infection, most commonly affecting the extremities.
- The development of vesicles and bullae at the site of soft tissue infection, that progresses to violaceous or blue discoloration, is considered an ominous sign of necrotizing fasciitis or myositis.
- ARDS develops in 55% of patients, usually following the onset of hypotension.
- Patients are usually febrile, hypotensive, confused, and develop multisystem organ dysfunction.
- Diagnostic criteria are listed in Table 89-2. A confirmed case requires the clinical criteria plus a positive culture from a normally sterile site.

DIAGNOSIS AND DIFFERENTIAL

- When considering STSS, look for soft tissue infection and culture the site. Laboratory evaluation includes CBC, ABG, liver function tests, serum electrolytes including magnesium and calcium, coagulation profile, blood cultures, CXR, ECG, and UA.
- Consider TSS as well as other infections caused by GAS, *Clostridium perfringens* and other bacteria, Kawasaki's disease, RMSF, and septic shock.

EMERGENCY DEPARTMENT CARE AND DISPOSITION

- Treatment is similar to that for TSS, with airway management and aggressive fluid resuscitation with vasopressors as needed.
- Begin antistreptococcal antimicrobial therapy with IV penicillin G 24 million U/day in divided doses, and IV clindamycin 900 mg q8h. In penicillin-allergic patients substitute erythromycin 1.0 g IV q6h or ceftriaxone 2 g IV q24h and clindamycin 900 mg IV q8h.
- Obtain immediate surgical consultation, as 70% of patients with STSS require debridement, fasciotomy, or amputation.
- Intravenous immunoglobulin may be considered.

- All patients suspected of having STSS require admission to the ICU.

REFERENCES

1. Todd J: Toxic-shock syndrome associated with phage group-1 staphylococci. *Lancet* 2:1116, 1978.
2. Chesney PJ: Toxic shock syndrome: Management and long-term sequelae. *Ann Intern Med* 96:84, 1984.
3. Tweeten SS: Infectious complications of body piercing. *Clin Infect Dis* 26:735, 1998.
4. Chance TD: Toxic shock syndrome: Role of the environment, the host and the microorganism. *Br J Biomed Sci* 53:284, 1996.
5. Kaul R: Population-based surveillance for group A streptococcal necrotizing fasciitis: Clinical features, prognostic indicators, and microbiologic analysis of seventy-seven cases, Ontario Group A Streptococcal Study. *Am J Med* 103:18, 1997.
6. Hackett SP: Superantigens associated with staphylococcal and streptococcal toxic shock syndrome are potent producers of tumor necrosis factor synthesis. *J Infect Dis* 168:232, 1993.
7. Stevens D: Invasive streptococcal infections (review article). *J Infect Chemother* 7:69, 2001.

For further reading in *Emergency Medicine: A Comprehensive Study Guide,* 6th ed., see Chap. 142, "Toxic Shock Syndrome and Streptococcal Toxic Shock Syndrome," by Shawna J. Perry and Ashley E. Booth.

90 COMMON VIRAL INFECTIONS

Matthew J. Scholer

- Viral illnesses are among the most common reasons that people come to an emergency department. This chapter focuses on the viral illnesses for which antiviral therapy has been developed. Treatment of primary herpes zoster and mononucleosis is discussed in Chap. 84, and genital herpes is discussed in Chap. 88. Treatment of HIV is covered in Chap. 91, and treatment of cytomegalovirus is discussed in Chap. 99.

INFLUENZA A AND B

EPIDEMIOLOGY

- In the United States, flu generally occurs from November to April. Influenza is spread by droplets generated by coughing. During epidemics, attack rates are in the 20 to 30% range, and may be as high as 50% during pandemics.[1]
- After exposure, the incubation period is usually about 2 days. Viral shedding (contagiousness) starts approximately 24 hours before the onset of symptoms, rises to peak levels within 48 hours, and then declines over the next 3 to 7 days.

PATHOPHYSIOLOGY

- Influenza viruses are single-stranded RNA viruses of the orthomyxovirus family.
- Following exposure, the virus enters the columnar cells of the respiratory tract epithelium. The invaded epithelial cells release large numbers of virions before cell death; thus large numbers of virions are available for spread with respiratory secretions.
- Antigenic drift caused by minor mutations in the RNA genome results in a change in antigenicity that facilitates annual epidemics.
- Antigenic shift occurs by genetic reassortment and is responsible for flu pandemics.

CLINICAL FEATURES

- Classic flu symptoms include fever of 38.6° to 39.8°C (101° to 103°F), with chills or rigor, headache, myalgia, and generalized malaise.
- Respiratory symptoms include dry cough, rhinorrhea, and sore throat, frequently with bilateral tender, enlarged cervical lymph nodes.
- The elderly do not usually have classical symptoms and may present only with fever, malaise, confusion, and nasal congestion.
- Almost half of affected children have gastrointestinal symptoms, but these are unusual in adults.
- The fever generally lasts 2 to 4 days, followed by rapid recovery from most of the systemic symptoms. Cough and fatigue may persist for several weeks.

DIAGNOSIS AND DIFFERENTIAL

- A clinical diagnosis of flu during a known outbreak has an accuracy of approximately 85%,[2,3] but bacteremia should also be considered in patients with rigor and myalgia.
- Newer rapid antigen tests are available that may change the approach to flu-like illnesses and decrease the empirical use of antibiotics. Commercially available tests require less than ½ hour to perform and have sensitivities of 57 to 81%, with specificities of 93 to 100%.[4]

EMERGENCY DEPARTMENT CARE AND DISPOSITION

- Amantadine and rimantadine are antiviral drugs currently available for the treatment of influenza A. Neither has activity against influenza B. Oseltamivir and zanamivir are neuraminidase inhibitors that are active against both influenza A and B.
- For maximal effectiveness, these medications need to be started within 48 hours of onset of symptoms and can reduce the duration of systemic symptoms by 1 to 2 days.
- The dose for both amantadine and rimantadine is 100 mg two times daily for 5 days. Amantadine causes an increase in seizure activity in patients with a pre-existing seizure disorder. Rimantadine has a significantly lower incidence of central nervous system (CNS) side effects than does amantadine but is more expensive.
- Zanamivir is an inhaled medicine, dosed twice a day for 5 days. It may cause bronchospasm and should not be given to patients with underlying pulmonary disease.
- Oseltamivir is dosed at 75 mg twice a day orally for 5 days. Nausea is reported frequently with oseltamivir and can be decreased by taking the drug with food.
- All four anti-influenza medicines are effective in preventing flu, with efficacy rates of 70 to 90% when used at treatment doses (as above) for a prolonged duration (zanamivir is not approved by the FDA for this indication).

HERPES SIMPLEX VIRUS 1

EPIDEMIOLOGY

- Transmission of herpes simplex virus (HSV) is via contact of infected secretions (saliva or genital) with mucous membranes or with open skin.

PATHOPHYSIOLOGY

- After exposure, the virus replicates locally in the epithelial cells, causing lysis of the infected cells and producing an inflammatory response. This response results in the characteristic rash of HSV, which is indistinguishable from the rash of varicella zoster virus (VZV).
- Following primary infection, the virus becomes latent in a sensory nerve ganglion.

CLINICAL FEATURES

- HSV-1 primarily causes oral lesions, but may cause genital infection. The primary infection of HSV-1 is often mild or asymptomatic. The lesions are distributed throughout the mouth and consist of small, thin-walled vesicles on an erythematous base, although they do not always become vesicular.
- The primary lesions generally last 1 to 2 weeks.
- In children under age 5, HSV-1 infection may present as a pharyngitis or gingivostomatitis associated with fever and cervical lymphadenopathy.
- Recurrent oral lesions occur in 60 to 90% of infected individuals and are usually milder and generally occur on the lower lip at the outer vermilion border. The recurrences are often triggered by local trauma, sunburn, or stress. The patient may have pain or tingling prior to developing lesions. The lesions may begin as erythematous papules and then become vesicular.
- HSV-2 is spread primarily sexually. It causes identical lesions, primarily genital, but may cause oral lesions.

DIAGNOSIS AND DIFFERENTIAL

- Viral cultures confirm clinical diagnosis but take days to weeks to be performed.
- The diagnosis is largely clinical.

EMERGENCY DEPARTMENT CARE AND DISPOSITION

- Oral acyclovir has been shown to shorten the duration of symptoms in children if begun within the first 72 hours of symptoms.
- Treatment of recurrent oral herpes labialis with oral acyclovir[5] 400 mg five times per day or topical pencyclovir[6] applied every 2 hours for 4 days shortens duration of symptoms in adults.

HERPES ZOSTER

PATHOPHYSIOLOGY

- Herpes zoster (shingles) is the reactivation of a latent herpes zoster virus infection. There is a lifetime incidence of almost 20%, with the majority of cases being among the elderly.

CLINICAL FEATURES

- The lesions of shingles are identical to those of chickenpox, but are limited to a single dermatome in distribution. Thoracic and lumbar dermatomes are most common.

- The disease begins with a prodrome of pain in the affected area for 1 to 3 days, followed by the outbreak of a maculopapular rash that quickly progresses to a vesicular rash. The course of the disease is usually around 2 weeks, but may persist for a full month. Rash involving more than a single dermatome or crossing the midline should raise suspicion of disseminated disease.
- The cranial nerves may be affected as well, with the potential complications of herpes zoster ophthalmicus[7] (HZO) and Ramsay Hunt syndrome.[8]
- HZO is due to involvement of the ocular branch of cranial nerve (CN) V and is a vision-threatening condition.
- HZO induces keratitis and may be followed by involvement of deeper structures. A dendriform corneal ulcer can often be identified with fluorescein staining.
- Involvement of the geniculate ganglion on CN VII results in Ramsay Hunt syndrome, which presents clinically as a facial nerve palsy resembling Bell's palsy.
- The most common complication of shingles is postherpetic neuralgia (PHN). PHN occurs in 10 to 20% of all patients after an episode of acute zoster, but in up to 70% of patients aged 70 years or older. It generally resolves in 1 to 2 months, but may last greater than a year in some patients.

EMERGENCY DEPARTMENT CARE AND DISPOSITION

- The treatment of herpes zoster in the normal host is aimed at decreasing the risk of PHN, since the antivirals have a clinically small, but statistically significant, effect on the duration of the acute disease.
- Treatment should begin as soon as possible, and within 72 hours of disease onset for maximal benefit. Treatment options include famciclovir (500 mg three times a day for 7 days), valacyclovir (1000 mg three times a day for 7 days), or acyclovir (800 mg five times a day for 7 days).
- All three antiherpes agents are more effective than placebo at reducing the duration of PHN, but not at reducing its incidence.[9–11]
- Initial treatment of patients with PHN is typically systemic analgesia, often narcotics. Patients should be referred back to their primary care provider, because first-line agents often fail, and a trial of amitriptyline or carbamazepine may be tried as second-line therapy.
- HZO or suspected HZO mandates an ophthalmologic consultation due to the threat to vision.

REFERENCES

1. Monto AS, Kloumehr F: The Tecumseh Study of Respiratory Illness: IX. Occurrence of influenza in the community. *Am J Epidemiol* 102:553, 1975.
2. Knight V, Fedson D, Baldini J, et al: Amantadine therapy of epidemic influenza. *Infect Immun* 1:200, 1970.
3. VanVoris LP, Betts RF, Roth FK, et al: Successful treatment of naturally occurring influenza A/USSR/77 H1N1. *JAMA* 245:1128, 1981.
4. Anonymous: Rapid diagnostic tests for influenza. *Med Lett Drugs Ther* 41:121, 1999.
5. Kesson AM: Position paper of the Pediatric Special Interest Group of the Australian Society for Infectious Diseases: Use of acyclovir in herpes simplex virus infections. *J Paediatr Child Health* 34:9, 1998.
6. Spruance SL, Rea TL, Thomig C, et al: Penciclovir cream for the treatment of herpes simplex labialis: A randomized, multicenter, double-blind, placebo-controlled trial. *JAMA* 277:1374, 1997.
7. Marsh RJ: Herpes zoster ophthalmicus. *J Roy Soc Med* 90:670, 1997.
8. Rahimi AR: Ramsay Hunt syndrome. *Geriatrics* 53:93, 1998.
9. Jackson JL, Gibbons R, Meyer G, Inouye L: The effect of treating herpes zoster with oral acyclovir in preventing postherpetic neuralgia. *Arch Intern Med* 157:909, 1997.
10. Tyring S, Barbarash RA, Nahlik JE, et al and the Collaborative Famciclovir Herpes Zoster Study Group: Famciclovir for the treatment of acute herpes zoster: Effects on acute disease and postherpetic neuralgia. *Ann Intern Med* 123:89, 1995.
11. Beutner KR, Friedman DJ, Forszpaniak C, et al: Valacyclovir compared with acyclovir for improved therapy for herpes zoster in immunocompetent adults. *Antimicrob Agents Chemother* 39:1546, 1995.

For further reading in *Emergency Medicine: A Comprehensive Study Guide*, 6th ed., see Chap. 143, "Common Viral Infections: Influenzaviruses and Herpesviruses," by Robert A. Brownstein.

91 HIV INFECTIONS AND AIDS

David M. Cline

- The AIDS (acquired immune deficiency syndrome) epidemic is fastest growing in central Asia and Eastern Europe. As of December 2001, approximately 21.8 million individuals had died from AIDS, and an estimated 40 million people were living with HIV (human immunodeficiency virus) infections and/or AIDS.

EPIDEMIOLOGY

- The Joint United Nations Program on AIDS (UN-AIDS) predicts that by 2020, HIV will be responsible for more than one third of all infectious disease–related deaths worldwide.[1]
- In the United States, the Centers for Disease Control and Prevention (CDC) estimate that 40,000 new HIV infections occur each year.[2]
- Risk factors commonly associated with HIV infection include homosexuality or bisexuality, injected drug use, heterosexual exposure, receipt of a blood transfusion prior to 1985, and vertical and horizontal maternal-neonatal transmission.

PATHOPHYSIOLOGY

- HIV is a cytopathic retrovirus that kills infected cells. The viral genes are carried as a single-stranded RNA molecule within the viral particle. Following infection, the virus selectively attacks host cells involved in immune function, primarily CD4 T lymphocytes.
- As a result of infection, immunologic abnormalities eventually occur, including lymphopenia, qualitative CD4 T-lymphocyte function defects, and autoimmune phenomena. Profound defects in cellular immunity ultimately result in a variety of opportunistic infections and neoplasms.
- Transmission of HIV has been shown to occur via semen, vaginal secretions, blood or blood products, breast milk, and transplacental transmission in utero.

CLINICAL FEATURES

- Acute HIV infection, essentially indistinguishable from a flu-like illness, usually goes unrecognized, but is reported to occur in 50 to 90% of patients.[3]
- The time from exposure to onset of symptoms is usually 2 to 4 weeks, and the most common symptoms include fever (>90%), fatigue (70 to 90%), sore throat (>70%), rash (40 to 80%), headache (30 to 80%), and lymphadenopathy (40 to 70%).[4,5]
- Other reported symptoms include myalgias, diarrhea, and weight loss.
- Seroconversion, reflecting detectable antibody response to HIV, usually occurs 3 to 8 weeks after infection. This is followed by a long period of asymptomatic infection during which patients generally have no findings on physical examination except for possible persistent generalized lymphadenopathy.
- The variables most predictive of disease stage are viral burden and CD4 counts, with a steeper decline in CD4 count and a higher viral burden associated with rapid progression and poor outcome.[6]
- The mean incubation time from exposure to the development of AIDS is estimated at 8.23 years for adults, and 1.97 years for children under age 5.
- Early symptomatic infection is characterized by conditions that are more common and more severe in the presence of HIV infection, but by definition are not AIDS-indicator conditions. Examples include thrush, persistent vulvovaginal candidiasis, peripheral neuropathy, cervical dysplasia, recurrent herpes zoster infection, and idiopathic thrombocytopenic purpura. At this time CD4 counts are 200 to 500/μL. As the CD4 count drops below 200 cells/μL, the frequency of opportunistic infections dramatically increases.
- AIDS is defined by the appearance of any indicator condition (Table 91-1), including a CD4 count of less than 200 cells/μL.
- Median survival time after the CD4 count has fallen to less than 200 cells/μL is 3.7 years.[7] Late symptomatic or advanced HIV infection exists in patients with a CD4 count of less than 50 cells/μL or clinical evidence of end-stage disease, including disseminated *Mycobacterium avium* complex or disseminated cytomegalovirus (CMV).

TABLE 91-1   AIDS-Indicator Conditions

CD4 count <200 cells/μL
Cervical cancer (invasive)
Cryptococcosis
Cryptosporidiosis
Cytomegalovirus retinitis
Esophageal candidiasis
Herpes simplex virus
Histoplasmosis, disseminated
HIV encephalopathy
HIV wasting syndrome
Isosporiasis
Kaposi's sarcoma
Lymphoma (brain)
Mycobacterium avium complex
Mycobacterium tuberculosis disease
Pneumocystis carinii pneumonia
Progressive multifocal leukoencephalopathy
Recurrent bacterial pneumonia
Salmonella septicemia (recurrent)
Toxoplasmosis (brain)
Tuberculosis (pulmonary)

ABBREVIATION: HIV = human immunodeficiency virus.

CONSTITUTIONAL SYMPTOMS AND FEBRILE ILLNESSES

- Systemic symptoms, such as fever, weight loss, and malaise, are common in HIV-infected patients and account for the majority of HIV-related emergency department presentations.[8,9]
- Appropriate laboratory investigation includes electrolytes, complete blood count (CBC), blood cultures, urinalysis and culture, liver function tests, chest radiograph, and serologic testing for syphilis, cryptococcosis, toxoplasmosis, CMV, and coccidioidomycosis.
- Lumbar puncture (LP) should be considered if there are neurologic signs or symptoms, or unexplained fever.
- In HIV patients without obvious focalizing signs or symptoms, sources of fever vary by stage of disease. Patients with CD4 counts greater than 500 cells/μL generally have sources of fever similar to nonimmunocompromised patients. Those with CD4 counts between 200 and 500 cells/μL are most likely to have early bacterial respiratory infections.[10]
- For patients with CD4 counts less than 200 cells/μL, likely infections include *Pneumocystis carinii* pneumonia, central line infection, *M. avium* complex, *Mycobacterium tuberculosis,* CMV, drug fever and sinusitis.
- Disseminated *M. avium* complex (MAC) occurs predominantly in patients with CD4 counts less than 100 cells/μL. Persistent fever and night sweats are typical. Associated symptoms include weight loss, diarrhea, malaise, and anorexia. Diagnosis is made with acid-fast stain of stool or other body fluids or culture.
- A more focal and invasive form of MAC has emerged called **immune reconstitution illness to MAC,** which presents with lymphadenitis and follows weeks to months after starting highly active antiretroviral therapy (HAART).[11]
- CMV is the most common cause of serious opportunistic viral disease in HIV-infected patients. Disseminated disease commonly involves the gastrointestinal or pulmonary systems. The most important manifestation is retinitis.
- Infective endocarditis is a concern, especially in IV drug users (see Chap. 92). Non-Hodgkin's lymphomas are the most commonly occurring neoplasm in HIV patients, and typically present as high-grade, rapidly growing mass lesions.

PULMONARY COMPLICATIONS

- Pulmonary presentations are among the most common reasons for emergency department visits by HIV-infected patients. Presenting complaints frequently are nonspecific and include cough, hemoptysis, shortness of breath, and chest pain.
- The most common causes of pulmonary abnormalities in HIV-infected patients include community-acquired bacterial pneumonia, *Pneumocystis carinii* pneumonia (PCP), *Mycobacterium tuberculosis* (MTB), CMV, *Cryptococcus neoformans, Histoplasma capsulatum,* and neoplasms.
- Despite substantial decreases in the incidence of PCP due to effective prophylaxis and the increased use of HAART, PCP continues to be the most common opportunistic infection among AIDS patietnts.[12]
- Evaluation should include pulse oximetry, arterial blood gases (ABG), sputum culture and Gram's stain, acid-fast stain, blood cultures, and chest x-ray.
- The classic presenting symptoms of PCP are fever, cough (typically nonproductive), and shortness of breath (progressing from being present only with exertion to being present at rest). Negative x-rays are reported in 15 to 20% of patients. Hypoxia or increased alveolar-arterial gradient identifies patients at risk.
- Classic pulmonary manifestations of TB include cough with hemoptysis, night sweats, prolonged fevers, weight loss, and anorexia. TB is common in patients with CD4 counts between 200 and 500 cells/μL. Classic upper lobe involvement and cavitary lesions are less common, particularly among late-stage AIDS patients. False-negative purified protein derivative (PPD) TB test results are frequent among AIDS patients due to immunosuppression.
- Nonopportunistic bacterial pneumonias are the most common pulmonary infections in HIV-infected patients early in the course of the disease process. Common pathogens include *Streptococcus pneumoniae, Haemophilus influenzae,* and *Staphylococcus aureus.* Productive cough, leukocytosis, and the presence of a focal infiltrate suggest bacterial pneumonia.

NEUROLOGIC COMPLICATIONS

- Central nervous system (CNS) disease occurs in 90% of patients with AIDS, and 10 to 20% of HIV-infected patients initially present with CNS symptoms. ED evaluation includes computed tomography (CT) scan and LP.[13]
- Cerebrospinal fluid (CSF) studies should include pressures, cell count, glucose, protein, Gram's stain, India ink stain, bacterial, viral and fungal cultures, toxoplasmosis and cryptococcosis antigen, and coccidioidomycosis titer.
- The most common causes of neurologic symptoms include AIDS dementia, *Toxoplasma gondii,* and *Cryptococcus neoformans.* Symptoms may include

headache, fever, focal neurologic deficits, altered mental status, or seizures.

- AIDS dementia complex (also referred to as HIV encephalopathy or subacute encephalitis) is a progressive process commonly heralded by subtle impairment of recent memory and other cognitive deficits caused by direct HIV infection.
- Other, less common CNS infections that should be considered in the presence of neurologic symptoms include bacterial meningitis, histoplasmosis (usually disseminated), CMV, progressive multifocal leukoencephalopathy, herpes simplex virus, neurosyphilis, and TB.
- Fifty percent of HIV patients will experience HIV neuropathy, characterized by painful sensory symptoms of the feet.

GASTROINTESTINAL COMPLICATIONS

- Approximately 50% of AIDS patients will present with gastrointestinal complaints at some time during their illness. The most frequent presenting symptoms include odynophagia, abdominal pain, bleeding, and diarrhea.
- ED evaluation includes stool for leukocytes, ova, parasites, acid-fast staining, and culture.
- Diarrhea is the most frequent gastrointestinal complaint and is estimated to occur in 50 to 90% of AIDS patients.[14] Common causes include bacterial organisms, such as *Shigella, Salmonella*, enterotoxic *Escherichia coli* (ETEC), and *Campylobacter;* parasitic organisms, such as *Giardia, Cryptosporidium, Entamoeba histolytica*, and *Isospora belli;* CMV; *M. avium intracellulare;* and antibiotic therapy.
- Oral candidiasis or thrush affects more than 80% of AIDS patients. The tongue and buccal mucosa are commonly involved, and the plaques characteristically can be easily scraped from an erythematous base.
- Esophageal involvement may occur with *Candida,* herpes simplex, and CMV. Complaints of odynophagia or dysphagia are usually indicative of esophagitis and may be extremely debilitating.
- Hepatomegaly occurs in approximately 50% of AIDS patients. Elevation of alkaline phosphatase levels are frequently seen. Jaundice is rare. Coinfection with hepatitis B and hepatitis C is common, especially among injected drug users.
- Anorectal disease is common in AIDS patients. Proctitis is characterized by painful defecation, rectal discharge, and tenesmus. Common causative organisms include *Neisseria gonorrhoeae, Chlamydia trachomatis,* syphilis, and herpes simplex.

CUTANEOUS MANIFESTATIONS

- Kaposi's sarcoma appears more often in homosexual men than in other risk groups. Clinically, it consists of painless, raised brown-black or purple papules and nodules that do not blanch. Common sites are the face, chest, genitals, and oral cavity; however, widespread dissemination involving internal organs may occur.
- Reactivation of varicella-zoster virus is more common in patients with HIV infection and AIDS than in the general population.[15]
- Herpes simplex virus infections are common. HIV patients may develop bullous impetigo and *Pseudomonas*-associated chronic ulcerations.

OPHTHALMOLOGIC MANIFESTATIONS

- Seventy-five percent of patients with AIDS develop ocular complications.[16]
- CMV retinitis is the most frequent and serious ocular opportunistic infection and the leading cause of blindness in AIDS patients. The prevalence is estimated to be up to 40%.[17]
- The presentation of CMV retinitis is variable. It may be asymptomatic early on, but later causes changes in visual acuity, visual field cuts, photophobia, scotoma, or eye redness or pain.[17]
- Herpes zoster ophthalmicus is anther diagnosis to consider, recognized by the typical zoster rash.

DIAGNOSIS AND DIFFERENTIAL

- The most common assays used to detect viral antibody are an enzyme-linked immunoassay (EIA) and a confirming Western blot test on EIA-positive specimens. EIA is approximately 99% specific and 98.5% sensitive; the Western blot test is nearly 100% sensitive and specific if performed under ideal laboratory circumstances.
- Diagnosis of acute-stage HIV infection is not possible with standard serologic tests, as seroconversion has not yet occurred.
- Methods for earlier detection of HIV-1 include techniques to detect DNA, RNA, or HIV antigens. The single-use diagnostic system (SUDS) is used to screen rapidly for antibodies to HIV-1 in serum or plasma. OraSure manufactures both a saliva-based and a fingerstick blood assay for rapid HIV testing.
- Knowledge of current or recent CD4 counts and a HIV viremia load will help in the management of HIV patients. CD4 counts less than 200 cells/μL and viral load greater than 50,000 is associated with increased risk of progression to AIDS-defining illness.

EMERGENCY DEPARTMENT CARE AND DISPOSITION

- The initial evaluation of HIV-infected and AIDS patients begins with a heightened awareness of the need for universal precautions. All blood and body fluid exposures should be considered infective. Respiratory isolation should be instituted for patients with suspected TB.
- All unstable patients should have airway management as indicated, oxygen, pulse oximetry, cardiac monitoring, and IV access. Shock, with its myriad causes, should be managed in standard fashion.
- Seizures, altered mental status, gastrointestinal bleeding, and coma should be managed with standard protocols.
- Suspected bacterial sepsis and focal bacterial infections should be treated with standard antibiotics.
- Systemic *Mycobacterium avium* should be treated with clarithromycin 500 mg PO twice daily plus ethambutol 15 mg/kg/day PO plus rifabutin 300 mg daily. Treatment of immune reconstitution illness to MAC should be continuation of HAART therapy, antimicrobials as above, and consider steroids.
- Systemic CMV should be treated with ganciclovir 2.5 mg/kg IV every 8 hours or foscarnet 90 mg/kg IV every 12 hours.
- Ophthalmologic CMV is treated with a ganciclovir implant plus oral ganciclovir 1.0 to 1.5 g PO twice daily or 5 mg/kg IV twice daily for 14 to 21 days.
- Pulmonary PCP should be treated with trimethoprim-sulfamethoxazole (TMP-SMX), 15 to 20 mg of TMP/kg/day and 75 to 100 mg of SMX/kg/day PO for 3 weeks. The typical oral dose is TMP-SMX double strength (DS), 2 tabs three times daily. An alternative is pentamidine 4 mg/kg/day IV or IM for 3 weeks. Oral steroids should be given if hypoxic, prednisone 40 mg twice daily for 5 days, then 40 mg daily for 5 days, then 20 mg daily for 11 more days.
- Pulmonary TB may be treated with isoniazid 5 mg/kg/day PO plus rifabutin 5 mg/kg/day PO plus pyrazinamide 15 to 30 mg/kg/day PO plus streptomycin 15 mg/kg/day IM.
- CNS toxoplasmosis can be treated with pyrimethamine 50 to 100 mg/day PO plus sulfadiazine 4.8 mg/kg/day PO plus folinic acid 10 mg/day PO.
- CNS cryptococcosis can be treated with amphotericin B 0.7 mg/kg/day IV. When improved, switch to fluconazole 400 mg daily for 8 to 10 weeks.
- Candidiasis (thrush) can be treated with clotrimazole 10 mg troches 5 times per day or nystatin 500,000 U, gargle five times per day.
- Esophagitis can be treated with fluconazole 100 to 400 mg daily PO.
- Salmonellosis can be treated with ciprofloxacin 500 mg twice daily for 2 to 4 weeks.
- Cutaneous herpes simplex can be treated with acyclovir 1000 mg per day or famciclovir 250 mg PO three times daily for 14 to 21 days.
- Cutaneous herpes zoster can be treated with acyclovir 4000 mg PO per day or valacyclovir 1 g PO twice daily, or famciclovir 500 mg PO three times daily.
- Herpes zoster ophthalmicus should be treated with acyclovir 30 to 36 mg/kg per day IV for at least 7 days, then switch to oral therapy.
- Although rarely started in the ED, antiretroviral therapy is started for CD4 counts less than 350 cells/μL or for a HIV viral load above 55,000 copies/mL. Initial treatment includes two nucleoside reverse-transcriptase inhibitors plus either one or two protease inhibitors or one non-nucleoside reverse-transcriptase inhibitor drug. An updated guide for their use can be found on the CDC website: www.cdc.gov/hiv/pubs/mmwr.
- The decision to admit an AIDS patient should be based on severity of illness, with attention to the following: new presentation of fever of unknown origin, hypoxia worse than baseline or Pao$_2$ below 60 mm Hg, suspected PCP, suspected TB, new CNS symptoms, intractable diarrhea, suspected CMV retinitis, herpes zoster ophthalmicus, or a patient unable to care for him- or herself.

REFERENCES

1. Joint United Nations Program on HIV/AIDS: AIDS Epidemic Update. Available at www.unaids.org; accessed October 2003.
2. Centers for Disease Control and Prevention: A Glance at the HIV Epidemic. Available at www.cdc.gob/hiv/pubs/facts.htm; accessed October 2003.
3. Schacker T, Collier AC, Hughes J, et al: Clinical and epidemiologic features of primary HIV infection. *Ann Intern Med* 125:257, 1996.
4. Perlmutter BL: How to recognize and treat acute HIV syndrome. *Am Fam Phys* 60:535, 1999.
5. Kahn JO, Walker BD: Acute human immunodeficiency virus type 1 infection. *N Engl J Med* 339:33, 1998.
6. O'Brian WA, Hartigan PM, Martin D, et al: Changes in plasma HIV-1 RNA and CD4-lymphocyte counts and the risk of progression to AIDS. *N Engl J Med* 334:42, 1996.
7. Yarchoan R, Venzon DJ, Pluda JM, et al: CD4 count and the risk for death in patients infected with HIV receiving antiretroviral therapy. *Ann Intern Med* 115:184, 1991.
8. Kelen GD, Johnson G, Digiovanna TA, et al: Profile of patients with human immunodeficiency virus infection presenting to an inner-city emergency department: Preliminary report. *Ann Emerg Med* 19:963, 1990.

9. Hauhuce JS, Witt MD, Zeumer CM, et al: Emergency department triage of patients infected with HIV. *Acad Emerg Med* 9:880, 2002.

10. Moylett EH: HIV: Clinical manifestations. *J Allergy Clin Immunol* 110:3, 2002.

11. Shelburne SA, Hamill RJ, Rodriguez-Barradas MC, et al: Immune reconstitution inflammatory syndrome: Emergence of a unique syndrome during highly active antiretroviral therapy. *Medicine* 81:213, 2002.

12. Wolff AJ, O'Donnell AE: Pulmonary manifestations of HIV infection in the era of highly active antiretroviral therapy. *Chest* 120:1888, 2001.

13. Rothman RE, Keyl PM, McArthur JC, et al: A decision guideline for emergency department utilization of noncontrast head computed tomography in HIV-infected patients. *Acad Emerg Med* 6:1010, 1999.

14. Neild PJ, Nelson MR: Management of HIV-related diarrhea. *Int J STD AIDS* 8:286, 1997.

15. Buchbinder SP, Katz MH, Hessal NA, et al: Herpes zoster and human immunodeficiency virus infection. *J Infect Dis* 166:1153, 1992.

16. Greenwood J, Graham EM: The ocular complications of HIV and AIDS. *Int J STD AIDS* 8:358, 1997.

17. Baven ER, Wilson P, Atkins M, et al: Natural history of untreated CMV retinitis. *Lancet* 346:1671, 1995.

For further reading in *Emergency Medicine: A Comprehensive Study Guide,* 6th ed., see Chap. 144, "HIV Infection and AIDS," by Richard E. Rothman, Catherine A. Marco, and Gabor D. Kelen.

92 INFECTIVE ENDOCARDITIS
Chadwick D. Miller

EPIDEMIOLOGY

- The distribution of infective endocarditis (IE) is changing due to a decrease in rheumatic heart disease, increasing degenerative valvular disease from an aging population, and an increasing use of invasive medical procedures.
- The aortic valve overall is affected most often with *Staphylococcus aureus,* the most common infecting bacteria overall.[1]
- Native valve endocarditis represents 59 to 70% of IE, intravenous drug use (IVDU)–associated IE 11 to 16%, and prosthetic valve IE 14 to 30%.[2,3]

PATHOPHYSIOLOGY

- Normal endothelium is resistant to infection or thrombus formation until it is injured by turbulent blood flow or high pressure states from acquired or congenital heart defects, or talc bombardment from IVDU.
- Injured endothelium leads to fibrin and platelet deposition, forming a sterile vegetation. Sterile vegetations are seeded by transient episodes of bacteremia and lead to IE.
- Highly virulent organisms (*S. aureus*) may directly invade the endothelium.[4]
- Native valve endocarditis occurs in patients with predisposing factors such as congenital heart defects, rheumatic heart disease, underlying valvular pathology, invasive medical procedures, poor dentition, or an immunocompromised status.
- Native valve endocarditis is most commonly caused by *Streptococcus* (*S. viridans*), which is characterized by an indolent course. Other common bacteria include *Staphylococcus* (*S. aureus*) and enterococcus.[5] *S. aureus* is characterized by a fulminant course and may occur on normal valves.
- IVDU-associated IE is commonly caused by skin flora, with *S. aureus* causing >50% of cases. The tricuspid valve is most commonly involved and generally has a more favorable prognosis.
- Prosthetic valve IE is divided into early (<6 months from surgery) and late. Early occurring disease is associated with perioperative contamination, *Staphylococcus epidermidis* as an infecting agent, and a higher mortality of 30 to 80%.[6] Late occurring disease has similar characteristics to native valve IE.

CLINICAL FEATURES

- Patients may present on a spectrum from subacute IE with nonspecific symptoms to acute IE with hemodynamic deterioration and death.
- Signs and symptoms are classified as cardiac, or those caused by bacteremia, emboli, or circulating immune complexes.
- Cardiac murmurs occur in 85% of patients with IE and represent cardiac tissue destruction. Acute or progressive congestive heart failure may present as dyspnea, frothy sputum, or chest pain, and is the most common complication, seen in 70% of patients.
- Heart blocks and arrhythmias may occur from infection extension into the intraventricular septum.
- Bacteremia from IE presents as fever (>38°C) in >90% of patients and may cause tachycardia, sepsis, and hemodynamic instability.

TABLE 92-1   Findings from Circulating Immune Complexes in IE

FINDING	LOCATION	DESCRIPTION	FREQUENCY
Petechiae	Buccal mucosa, conjunctiva, extremities	Nonblanching erythematous pinpoint macules	20–40%
Osler's nodes	Pads of fingers and toes	Small tender subcutaneous nodules	25%
Splinter hemorrhages	Under fingernails or toenails	Linear dark streaks	15%
Janeway lesions	Palms and soles	Small painless hemorrhagic plaques	<10%
Roth spots	Retina	Oval retinal hemorrhages with pale centers near optic disc	<10%

- Arterial embolization of valve vegetation fragments is the second most common complication of IE, occurring in >50% of cases. Emboli may affect any body system including the CNS (stroke, meningoencephalitis, retina), renal system (back pain, hematuria, renal failure), and pulmonary system (pneumonia, infarction). Splenic involvement is also common in IE, with splenomegaly seen in up to 60% of patients.
- Circulating immune complexes cause the conditions outlined in Table 92-1.

DIAGNOSIS AND DIFFERENTIAL

- The diagnosis of endocarditis is based on blood culture results and echocardiographic evidence of valvular injury or vegetations.
- Nonspecific laboratory findings that support the diagnosis of endocarditis include leukocytosis, elevated C-reactive protein, positive rheumatoid factor, normocytic anemia, hematuria, and pyuria.
- Patients with the following scenarios require inpatient evaluation for endocarditis:
  - All febrile IVDU patients because of the high incidence of IE (up to 15%)[7–9]

TABLE 92-2   Empiric Therapy of Suspected Bacterial Endocarditis*

PATIENT CHARACTERISTICS	RECOMMENDED AGENTS	INITIAL DOSE
Uncomplicated history	Ceftriaxone	1–2 g IV
	or nafcillin	2 g IV
	plus gentamicin	1–3 mg/kg IV
Injection drug use, congenital heart disease, hospital-acquired, suspected MRSA, or already on oral antibiotics	Nafcillin	2 g IV
	plus gentamicin	1–3 mg/kg IV
	plus vancomycin	15 mg/kg IV
Prosthetic heart valve	Vancomycin	15 mg/kg IV
	plus gentamicin	1–3 mg/kg IV
	plus rifampin	300 mg PO

ABBREVIATION: MRSA = methicillin-resistant *Staphylococcus aureus*.
*Because of controversy in the literature regarding the optimal regimen for empiric treatment, antibiotic selection should be based on patient characteristics, local resistance patterns, and current authoritative recommendations.

- Patients with fever and cardiac prosthesis
- Patients with a new or changed murmur with evidence of vasculitis or embolization.

EMERGENCY DEPARTMENT CARE AND DISPOSITION

- Acute rupture of the mitral or aortic valve should be stabilized with afterload reducers such as sodium nitroprusside (see Chap. 26), with insertion of a Swan-Ganz catheter for monitoring therapy as soon as possible. Prompt surgical evaluation is indicated for patients who may be surgical candidates.[10,11]
- See Table 92-2 for current antibiotic treatment guidelines.[12,13]
- Antibiotic prophylaxis for IE is indicated prior to invasive procedures for high-risk patients including those with prosthetic valves, a history of endocarditis, congenital cardiac abnormalities, mitral valve prolapse with documented regurgitation, hypertrophic cardiomyopathy, and acquired valvular dysfunction. Invasive procedures include dental work, bronchoscopy, cystoscopy, urethral instrumentation, and endoscopic retrograde cholangiopancreatography.
- Acceptable regimens for dental procedures known to cause bleeding include amoxicillin 2 g PO, 1 hour prior to intervention, or ampicillin 2 g IV or IM, 30 minutes prior to intervention, or clindamycin 600 mg PO or IV. For genitourinary interventions, add gentamicin 1.5 mg/kg IV/IM to the regimen above. For incision and drainage of infected tissue, give cefazolin 1.0 g IV/IM 30 minutes before the procedure or cephalexin 2 g PO 1 hour before the procedure.[14,15]

REFERENCES

1. Mylonakis E, Calderwood SB: Infective endocarditis in adults. *N Engl J Med* 345:1318, 2001.
2. Watanakunakorn C, Burkert T: IE at a large community teaching hospital 1980-1990: a review of 210 episodes. *Medicine* 72:90, 1993.

3. Sondre RM, Shafran SD: IE: Review of 135 cases over 9 years. *Clin Infect Dis* 22:27, 1996.

4. Frontera JA, Gradon JD: Right-side endocarditis in injection drug users: Review of proposed mechanisms of pathogenesis. *Clin Infect Dis* 30:374, 2000.

5. Bansal RC: Infective endocarditis. *Med Clin North Am* 79: 1205, 1995.

6. Vongpatanasin W, Hillis L, Lange R: Prosthetic heart valves. *N Engl J Med* 335:407, 1996.

7. Samet JH, Shevitz A, Flower J, et al: Hospitalization decision in febrile intravenous drug users. *Am J Med* 89:53, 1990.

8. Young GP, Hedges JR, Dixon L, et al: Inability to validate a predictive score for IE in febrile intravenous drug users. *J Emer Med* 11:1, 1993.

9. Weisse AB, Heller DR, Schimenti RJ, et al: The febrile parental drug users: a prospective study in 121 patients. *Am J Med* 94:274, 1993.

10. Chamoun AJ, Conti V, Lenihan DJ: Native valve infective endocarditis: What is the optimal timing for surgery? *Am J Med Sci* 320:255, 2000.

11. Ferguson E, Reardon MF, Letsou GV: The surgical management of bacterial valvular endocarditis. *Curr Opin Cardiol* 15:82, 2000.

12. Wilson WR, Karchmer AW, Dajani AS, et al: Antibiotic treatment of adults with infective endocarditis due to streptococci, enterococci, staphylococci, and HACEK microorganisms. *JAMA* 274:1706, 1995.

13. Alestig K, Hogevik H, Olaison L: Infective endocarditis: A diagnostic and therapeutic challenge for the new millennium. *Scand J Infect Dis* 32:343, 2000.

14. Dajani AS, Taubert KA, Wilson W, et al: Prevention of bacterial endocarditis: Recommendations by the American Heart Association. *JAMA* 277:1794, 1997.

15. Osmon DR: Antimicrobial prophylaxis in adults. *Mayo Clin Proc* 75:98, 2000.

For further reading in *Emergency Medicine: A Comprehensive Study Guide,* 6th ed., see Chap. 145, "Infective Endocarditis," by Richard E. Rothman, Samuel Yang, and Catherine A. Marco.

93   TETANUS AND RABIES

C. James Corrall

TETANUS

EPIDEMIOLOGY

- The current annual incidence of tetanus is 0.02 per 100,000 and the average annual incidence in the United States is less than 50 cases per year.[1,2]
- In the United States, the majority of tetanus occurs in temperate areas, with the states of Texas, California, and Florida responsible for the greatest number of reported cases.[2]
- Intravenous and subcutaneous drug users, especially Hispanics in California, are at disproportionate risk of contracting the disease.[2]
- Sixty-three percent of Americans over age 70 lack adequate immunity to tetanus.[3,4]

PATHOPHYSIOLOGY

- Tetanus is an acute, often fatal disease caused by wound contamination with *Clostridium tetani,* an anaerobic gram-positive rod.
- Any factor that lowers the local oxidation-reduction potential, such as crushed, devitalized tissue, a foreign body, or the development of secondary suppuration, favors the development of the vegetative, toxin-producing form of *C. tetani.*[5]
- *C. tetani* produces two exotoxins: tetanolysin, which appears to be clinically insignificant; and tetanospasmin, a potent neurotoxin that is responsible for all the clinical manifestations of tetanus.
- Tetanospasmin acts on the motor end-plates of skeletal muscle, in the spinal cord, in the brain, and in the sympathetic nervous system, preventing the release of the inhibitory neurotransmitters glycine and gamma-aminobutyric acid (GABA), resulting in loss of normal inhibitory control.

CLINICAL FEATURES

- The clinical manifestations of tetanus are generalized muscular rigidity, violent muscular contractions, and instability and inhibitory loss of the autonomic nervous system.
- Wounds that become infected with toxin-producing *C. tetani* are most often puncture wounds,[1] but vary in severity from deep lacerations to minor abrasions.[1,5]
- The incubation period of tetanus (ie, the period from initial inoculation to the onset of symptoms) can range from less than 24 hours to longer than 1 month. The shorter the incubation period, the more severe is the disease and the worse is the prognosis for recovery.[6]
- Local tetanus is manifested by persistent rigidity of the muscles in close proximity to the site of injury and usually resolves after weeks to months without sequelae, but may progress to generalized tetanus.
- Generalized tetanus is the most common form of the disease and frequently follows a puncture wound to the foot from a nail.[1]
- The most frequent presenting complaints of patients with generalized tetanus are pain and stiffness in the

masseter muscles (lockjaw).[7] Nerves with short axons are affected initially; therefore symptoms appear first in the facial muscles, with progression to the neck, trunk, and extremities.[7]

- Disturbances of the autonomic nervous system, generally a hypersympathetic state, occur during the second week of clinical tetanus and present as tachycardia, labile hypertension, profuse sweating, hyperpyrexia, and increased urinary excretion of catecholamines.[8]
- **Cephalic tetanus** follows injuries to the head, and rarely chronic otitis media, resulting in dysfunction of the cranial nerves, most commonly the seventh. The prognosis is poor.
- **Neonatal tetanus** occurs only if the mother is inadequately immunized. Most cases of neonatal tetanus arise from unsterile handling of the umbilical cord at the time of birth or the umbilical stump after birth.[7]

DIAGNOSIS AND DIFFERENTIAL

- Tetanus is diagnosed solely on the basis of clinical evidence.
- There are no confirmatory laboratory or microbiological tests.
- Strychnine poisoning most closely mimics the clinical picture of generalized tetanus.
- The differential diagnosis includes strychnine poisoning, dystonic reactions to the phenothiazines, hypocalcemic tetany, rabies, and temporomandibular joint disease.

EMERGENCY DEPARTMENT CARE AND DISPOSITION

- Patients with tetanus should be managed in an intensive care unit due to the potential for respiratory compromise. Environmental stimuli must be minimized in order to prevent precipitation of reflex convulsive spasms. Identification and débridement of the inciting wound, if present, is necessary to minimize further toxin production.
- Tetanus immune globulin (TIG), 3000 to 6000 U intramuscularly in a single injection should be given. Even though TIG does not ameliorate the clinical symptoms of tetanus, there is evidence that its administration significantly reduces mortality.[9]
- It should be given before any wound débridement, because more exotoxin may be released during wound manipulation.[10]
- Antibiotics are of questionable value in the treatment of tetanus. If warranted, parenteral metronidazole (500 mg intravenously every 6 hours) is the antibiotic

of choice.[11] Penicillin is contraindicated as it may potentiate the effects of tetanospasmin.[6]

- Midazolam (5 to 15 mg IV as a continuous drip to effect) has been extensively used and results in sedation as well as amnesia, but lorazepam (2 mg intravenously to effect), because of its long duration of action, may be superior and the drug of choice.[7]
- Neuromuscular blockade may be required to control ventilation and muscular spasm and to prevent fractures and rhabdomyolysis. In such cases, vecuronium (6 to 8 mg/h intravenously) is the agent of choice because of its minimal cardiovascular side effects.[12] Sedation during neuromuscular blockade is mandatory.
- The combined α- and β-adrenergic blocking agent labetalol (0.25 to 1 mg/min continuous intravenous infusion) has been used to treat the manifestation of sympathetic hyperactivity, but may precipitate myocardial depression.[13,14]
- Magnesium sulfate (70 mg/kg loading dose, then 1 to 4 g/h intravenously) has been advocated as a treatment for this condition as well.[8,15]
- Morphine sulfate (0.5 to 1 mg/kg/h) is also useful and provides sympathetic control without compromising cardiac output. Clonidine (300 μg every 8 hours nasogastrically), an α-receptor agonist, may also be helpful in the management of cardiovascular instability.
- Patients that recover from clinical tetanus **must** undergo active immunization (see Table 93-1 for treatment schedule).[16–18]

RABIES

EPIDEMIOLOGY

- Rabies is primarily a disease of animals.[19]
- In 2000, 49 states, the District of Columbia, and Puerto Rico reported 7369 cases of rabies in animals.[20] Wild animals accounted for almost 94% of the reported cases: raccoons (37.7%); skunks (30.2%); bats (16.8%); foxes (6.2%); and other wild animals including rodents and lagomorphs (2.2%). Rabid domestic animals included cats (3.4%); cattle (1.1%); dogs (1.6%); horses and mules (0.71%); sheep and goats (0.15%); and other animals such as ferrets (0.06%).
- Current epidemiologic patterns of rabies in the United States have been summarized as follows.[18] The annual reports of rabies in wildlife far exceed those of rabies in domestic animals; rabies variants in bats are associated with a disproportionate number of infections in humans (~90%), although bats constitute only about 15% of all reported rabies cases in animals annually.

TABLE 93-1 Summary Guide to Tetanus Prophylaxis in Wound Management

HISTORY OF ADSORBED TETANUS TOXOID (DOSES)	Clean, Minor Wounds		All Other Wounds*	
	Td†, 0.5 mL IM	TIG, 250 U IM	Td†, 0.5 mL IM	TIG, 250 U IM
Unknown or less than three	Yes‡	No	Yes	Yes
Three or more§	No¶	No	Yes**	No

ABBREVIATIONS: DPT = diphtheria-pertussis-tetanus; DT = diphtheria-tetanus toxoids; Td = tetanus-diphtheria; TIG = tetanus immune globulin.
SOURCE: Adapted from the American College of Emergency Physicians[16,17] with permission.
*For example, wounds >6 hours old, contaminated with soil, saliva, feces, or dirt; puncture or crush wounds; avulsions; wounds from missiles, burns, or frostbite.
†DPT for children <7 years of age (DT if pertussis vaccine is contraindicated); Td for persons >7 years of age.
‡The primary immunization series should be completed. Three doses total are required, with the second dose given at least 4 weeks after the first and the third dose 6 months later.
§If only three doses of fluid toxoid have been received, then a fourth dose of *absorbed* toxoid should be given.
¶Yes, if routine immunization schedule has lapsed in a child <7 years of age or if >10 years since last dose.
**Yes, if routine immunization schedule has lapsed in a child <7 years of age or if >5 years since last dose. Boosters more frequent than every 5 years may predispose to side effects.

- Bat exposure even without a documented bite may warrant rabies prophylaxis. Documented transmission from bats has occurred without physical evidence of a bite when the patient was confined in a closed space with a bat.
- Most other cases of human rabies diagnosed in the United States are attributable to infections acquired in areas of enzootic canine rabies outside of the United States; most persons with a case of rabies that originated in the United States have no history of an animal bite.
- Rodents (squirrels, chipmunks, rats, mice, etc.) and lagomorphs (rabbits, hares, and gophers) may be infected by rabies, but no transmission to humans has been documented from these animals.

PATHOPHYSIOLOGY

- Once introduced, the initial infection and multiplication occur within local monocytes for the first 48 to 96 hours.
- Subsequently the virus spreads across the motor endplate, and ascends and replicates along peripheral nervous axoplasm to the dorsal root ganglia, the spinal cord, and the central nervous system (CNS). Following CNS replication in the gray matter, the virus spreads outward by peripheral nerves to virtually all tissues and organ systems.

CLINICAL FEATURES

- The initial symptoms of human rabies are nonspecific and last 1 to 4 days: fever, malaise, headache, anorexia, nausea, sore throat, cough, and pain or paresthesia at the bite site (80%).

- Subsequently, CNS involvement becomes apparent with restlessness and agitation, altered mental status, painful bulbar and peripheral muscular spasms, opisthotonos, and bulbar or focal motor paresis.

DIAGNOSIS AND DIFFERENTIAL

- The diagnosis of rabies in the emergency department (ED) is clinical.
- A final diagnosis is made by postmortem or perimortem analysis of brain tissue. Cerebrospinal fluid (CSF) and serum antibody titers should be sent to laboratories skilled in rabies identification. Elevated CSF protein and a mononuclear pleocytosis are also seen.
- The differential diagnosis includes viral or other infectious encephalitis, polio, tetanus, viral process, meningitis, brain abscess, septic cavernous sinus thrombosis, cholinergic poisoning, the Guillain-Barré syndrome, and tetanus.

EMERGENCY DEPARTMENT CARE AND DISPOSITION

- The treatment of rabies exposure consists of assessment of risk of rabies, public health and animal control notification, and if warranted, the administration of specific immunobiologic products to protect against rabies.
- Local wound care—débridement of devitalized tissue, if any—is important in reducing the viral inoculum. Wounds of special concern should not be sutured as this promotes rabies virus replication.[21]

- Minor bites by bats and awakening in a room with a bat have been associated with the development of rabies. For this reason, the CDC recommends rabies postexposure prophylaxis for all persons who have sustained a bite, scratch, or mucous membrane exposure to a bat unless the bat is available for testing and is negative for evidence of rabies.[22]

- The CDC recommends that a healthy dog, cat, or ferret that bites a person should be confined and observed for 10 days.[23]

- Human rabies immune globulin (HRIG) is administered only once at the outset of therapy. The dose is 20 IU/kg, with half the dose (based upon tissue volume constraints) infiltrated locally at the exposure site and the remainder administered intramuscularly.

- Human diploid cell vaccine (HDCV) for active immunization is available in two formulations of the same vaccine. The HDCV can be administered intramuscularly or intradermally in five 1-mL doses on days 0, 3, 7, 14, and 28. The World Health Organization recommends a sixth dose on day 90, but this is not universally accepted.

- The recommendations for postexposure prophylaxis should be followed **EXACTLY** as given in the package insert. While there have been no failures in the United States, failures in other countries have been due to alterations in method of administration or dosing interval.[19]

- Identification of all hospital personnel who may have cared for an adult or child with suspected rabies is crucial to prevent secondary spread of the disease. The same postexposure prophylaxis as outlined above is imperative as soon as the disease is suspected in the index case.

- Ordinarily, domestic dogs and cats with normal behavior are quarantined for 10 days, which is sufficient for the disease to manifest if the animal is infected. If no signs become apparent, the animal can be considered nonrabid.

- State or local officials should be consulted regarding the possibility of rabies in local animal populations before decisions on initiating rabies prophylaxis are made. This action may not be possible before the first treatment, but may affect subsequent treatments. Animal bites should be reported to the local animal control unit or police departments so that appropriate animals can be captured or quarantined for observation in a timely fashion.

- The Centers for Disease Control and state or county health departments can provide assistance in the management of complications. The most current information available is on the rabies home page, which is produced and updated regularly by the Centers for Disease Control at www.cdc.gov/ncidod/dvrd/rabies.

REFERENCES

1. Izurieta HS, Sutter RW, Strebel PM, et al: Tetanus surveillance: United States, 1991-1994. *MMWR* 46(SS-2):15, 1997.
2. Bardenheier B, Prevots DR, Khetsurian N, et al: Tetanus: Surveillance—United States, 1995-1997. *MMWR* 47(SS-2): 1, 1998.
3. Gergen PJ, McQuillan GM, Kiely M, et al: A population-based serologic survey of immunity to tetanus in the United States. *N Engl J Med* 332:761, 1995.
4. Richardson JP, Knight AL: Prevention of tetanus in the elderly. *Arch Intern Med* 151:1712, 1991.
5. Kefer MP: Tetanus. *Am J Emerg Med* 10:445, 1992.
6. Bleck TP: Tetanus: Pharmacology, management, and prophylaxis. *Dis Mon* 37:551, 1991.
7. Ernst ME, Klepser ME, Fouts M, et al: Tetanus: Pathophysiology and management. *Ann Pharmacother* 31:1507, 1997.
8. Wright DK, Lalloo UG, Nayiager S, et al: Autonomic nervous system dysfunction in severe tetanus: Current perspectives. *Crit Care Med* 17:371, 1989.
9. Blake PA, Feldman TM, Buchanan TM, et al: Serologic therapy of tetanus in the United States, 1965-1971. *JAMA* 235:42, 1976.
10. Alfrey DD, Rauscher LA: Tetanus: A review. *Crit Care Med* 7:176, 1979.
11. Ahmadsyah I, Salim A: Treatment of tetanus: An open study to compare the efficacy of procaine penicillin and metronidazole. *BMJ* 291:648, 1985.
12. Powles AB, Ganta R: Use of vecuronium in the management of tetanus. *Anaesthesia* 40:879, 1985.
13. Buchanan N, Smit L, Cane RD, De Andrade M: Sympathetic overactivity in tetanus: Fatality associated with propranolol. *BMJ* 2:254, 1978.
14. Edmundson RS, Flowers MS: Intensive care in tetanus: Management, complications, and mortality in 100 cases. *BMJ* 1:401, 1979.
15. James MFM, Manson EDM: The use of magnesium sulfate infusions in the management of very severe tetanus. *Intensive Care Med* 11:5, 1985.
16. American College of Emergency Physicians, Scientific Review Committee: Tetanus immunization recommendations for persons seven years of age and older. *Ann Emerg Med* 15: 1111, 1986.
17. American College of Emergency Physicians, Scientific Review Committee: Tetanus immunization recommendations for persons less than seven years old. *Ann Emerg Med* 16: 1181, 1987.
18. Recommendations of the Immunization Practices Advisory Committee (ACIP): Diphtheria, tetanus, and pertussis: Recommendations for vaccine use and other preventive measures. *MMWR* 40(RR-10):1, 1991.
19. Fishbein DB, Robinson LE: Current concepts: Rabies. *N Engl J Med* 329:1632, 1993.
20. Krebs JW, Mondu AM, Rupprecht CE, et al: Rabies surveillance in the United States during 2000. *JAMA* 219:1687, 2001.
21. Weber DJ, Hansen AR: Infections resulting from animal bites. *Infect Dis Clin North Am* 5:663, 1991.

22. Centers for Disease Control and Prevention: Human rabies—Texas and New Jersey, 1997. *MMWR* 47:1, 1998.

23. Centers for Disease Control and Prevention: Compendium of animal rabies control. *MMWR* 48(RR-3):1, 1999.

For further reading in *Emergency Medicine: A Comprehensive Study Guide,* 6th ed., see Chap. 146, "Tetanus," by Donna L. Carden; and Chap. 147, "Rabies," by David J. Weber, David A. Wohl, and William A. Rutala.

94 MALARIA
Gregory S. Hall

- The continued growth in international travel, particularly to the tropics, has resulted in an increase in the number of cases of malaria seen in the United States; indeed the worldwide incidence is also increasing. Of the 1402 cases reported to the Centers for Disease Control and Prevention (CDC) in 2000, 56% were acquired in Africa, 17% in Asia, 16% in the Caribbean, and 4% in South America.[1]
- Malaria must be considered in anyone with a history of travel to an endemic region who subsequently (even months later) develops an unexplained febrile illness. The clinical symptoms are often nonspecific, so a high index of clinical suspicion must be maintained to seek the diagnosis. A travel history should be routinely sought from all patients presenting to the ED.

EPIDEMIOLOGY

- Four species of the protozoa *Plasmodium, P. vivax, P. ovale, P. malariae,* and *P. falciparum,* infect humans via the bite of a carrier female anopheline mosquito.
- Malaria transmission is most prevalent in sub-Saharan Africa, large areas of Central and South America, the Caribbean (especially the Dominican Republic and Haiti), the Indian subcontinent, Southeast Asia, the Middle East, and Oceania (New Guinea, Solomon Islands, etc).[1]
- More than half of all recent cases of malaria in the U.S. reported to the CDC in Atlanta (and the majority of *P. falciparum* cases) were acquired from travels to sub-Saharan Africa.[1]
- *P. falciparum,* which is responsible for the highest mortality rate among malaria victims, has exhibited growing resistance to standard chloroquine therapy as well as Fansidar (pyrimethamine-sulfadoxine), quinine, mefloquine, and doxycycline.[2] Recently, strains of *P. vivax* have been isolated from patients who have failed chloroquine therapy.[3]
- Chemotherapy resistant *P. falciparum* is especially prevalent in Africa, tropical South America, Asia, and Oceania.[2] It accounted for 49% of cases reported to the CDC in 2000.[1]

PATHOPHYSIOLOGY

- Plasmodial sporozoites are injected into a host's bloodstream during the feeding of the female anopheline mosquito, and travel directly to the liver where they invade hepatic parenchymal cells (exoerythrocytic stage). In the liver the parasites undergo asexual reproduction, forming thousands of daughter merozoites, which after an incubation period of one to several weeks rupture their host hepatic cells and are released into the peripheral circulation.
- The merozoites then rapidly invade circulating erythrocytes, where they mature and take on various morphologic forms—early ring forms, trophozoites, and schizonts, which are a mass of new merozoites (erythrocytic stage).
- Eventually the target red blood cell (RBC) lyses, releasing the merozoites to invade additional erythrocytes, continuing the infection. RBC lysis then often recurs at regular 2- to 3-day intervals, corresponding with the classic periodicity of symptoms. This cyclical feature may be absent in *P. falciparum* infection.
- With *P. vivax* or *P. ovale* infection, portions of the intrahepatic forms are not released, remain dormant for months, and can later activate, resulting in a clinical relapse.
- *Plasmodium* infection may also be acquired via transplacental transmission, infected blood during transfusion, or by sharing of IV needles among drug abusers.
- The classic febrile paroxysm of malaria results from hemolysis of infected RBCs and the resulting release of antigenic agents that activate macrophages and produce cytokines.
- Infected RBCs lose their flexibility and thus are prone to cause congestion and obstruction of the capillary microcirculation of various organs, resulting in sequestration of blood in the spleen and anoxic injury to the lungs, kidneys, brain, and other vital organs.
- Hemolysis is often high with *P. falciparum* infection because of its predilection for erythrocytes of all ages (while the other three *Plasmodium* species target young or old RBCs). RBC sequestration accounts for the paucity of observed mature parasites sometimes

seen on the peripheral blood smear in *P. falciparum* infection.

- Immunologic sequelae such as glomerulonephritis, nephrotic syndrome, thrombocytopenia, and polyclonal antibody stimulation may occur. Hypersplenism with subsequent pancytopenia may occur, especially with prolonged untreated malaria.

CLINICAL FEATURES

- The incubation period between infection and onset of clinical features ranges from 1 to 4 weeks, but partial chemoprophylaxis or incomplete immunity of the host can prolong the incubation period to months or even years. For U.S. residents who acquired malaria while traveling abroad in 2000, disease became evident within 1 month after returning home in 80% of *P. falciparum* cases, but in only 40% of *P. vivax* cases, and only 1% became ill more than 1 year after return to the U.S.[1]
- A recurring febrile paroxysm, the hallmark of malaria, occurs in conjunction with the typical 2- to 3-day cycle of RBC lysis by the merozoite forms.
- Most patients develop a nonspecific prodrome of malaise, myalgias, headache, low-grade fever, and chills.[4] In some cases there may be a prominence of chest pain, abdominal pain, nausea/emesis, diarrhea, or arthralgias, leading to misdiagnosis.
- Symptoms progress to cyclical episodes of high fever, severe rigors/chills, diaphoresis, orthostatic dizziness, and extreme weakness/prostration.
- Physical exam findings are nonspecific and may include high fever, tachycardia, tachypnea, pallor of skin or mucous membranes, prostration, and abdominal tenderness with splenomegaly in advanced cases (all plasmodial forms). Hepatomegaly may or may not be present.
- In *P. falciparum* infection, hepatomegaly, icterus, and peripheral edema often occur.
- Typical laboratory features include normochromic normocytic anemia, hemolysis, thrombocytopenia, and abnormal or low WBC count. Hypoglycemia, hyponatremia, elevated blood urea nitrogen and creatinine, lactic dehydrogenase, and erythrocyte sedimentation rate, mildly elevated liver function tests, and a biologically false-positive Venereal Disease Research Laboratory (VDRL) may also be seen.
- Complications can occur rapidly and may include splenic rupture, glomerulonephritis (especially with *P. malariae*), cerebral malaria (somnolence, coma, delirium, and seizures, with mortality of 20%), noncardiogenic pulmonary edema, and metabolic derangements including lactic acidosis and severe hypoglycemia (the last two most often with *P. falciparum*).[5]

- "Blackwater fever" is a severe renal complication seen almost exclusively with *P. falciparum* infections and presents with massive intravascular hemolysis, jaundice, hemoglobinemia, hemoglobinuria (black urine), and acute renal failure.

DIAGNOSIS AND DIFFERENTIAL

- A definitive diagnosis is achieved by identifying the plasmodial parasite within RBCs on Giemsa-stained thin and thick smears of peripheral blood.
- In early infections, particularly with *P. falciparum,* initial attempts to detect the parasite on peripheral blood smears may prove unsuccessful. Parasite load in the peripheral circulation varies over time and is highest during the clinical episodes of high fever and chills, but failure to detect the organism on initial smears is **not** an indication to withhold treatment if malaria is suspected.
- If the initial peripheral smear is negative, repeated smears should be examined at least twice daily for 3 days to fully exclude malaria as the diagnosis. However, the first smear is positive in >90% of cases.[6]
- Of paramount importance is the determination of which species of *Plasmodium* are present in the blood, since patients with *P. falciparum* should be hospitalized for treatment. Mixed infections with multiple species of *Plasmodium* are uncommon, with <1% of cases reported to the CDC in 1999-2000.[1]
- Differential diagnosis includes influenza, hepatitis, viral syndromes, and a wide variety of other infections.

EMERGENCY DEPARTMENT CARE AND DISPOSITION

- The drug of choice for treatment of infection caused by *P. vivax, P. ovale,* and *P. malariae* is chloroquine (Table 94-1).
- Chloroquine has no effect on dormant hepatic forms of *P. vivax* and *P. ovale,* and thus additional treatment with primaquine is required to prevent relapse. (Primaquine must be avoided in patients with glucose 6-phosphate dehydrogenase deficiency due to the possibility of inducing hemolysis.)
- Indications for hospital admission include confirmed or suspected *P. falciparum* infection, parasitemia of >3% on peripheral smear, significant hemolysis, severe or chronic comorbid conditions that may be aggravated by high fever or hemolysis, infants and pregnant women, elderly patients, and those with apparent complications such as renal failure, cerebral malaria, pulmonary edema, lactic acidosis, or hypoglycemia.[6]
- Many patients can be managed adequately in the out-

TABLE 94 1 Treatment Regimens for Malaria

CLINICAL SETTING	DRUG	DOSAGE GUIDELINES	
		ADULTS	CHILDREN
Uncomplicated infection with *P. vivax, P. ovale, P. malariae,* and chloroquine-sensitive *P. falciparum*	Chloroquine phosphate *plus*	1-g load (600-mg base), then 500 mg (300-mg base) in 6 h, then 500 mg (300-mg base) per day for 2 d (total dose 2.5 g)	10-mg/kg base to maximum of 600 mg load, then 5-mg/kg base in 6 h and 5-mg/kg base per day for 2 d
	Primaquine phosphate*	26.3-mg load (15-mg base) per day for 14 d on completion of chloroquine therapy	0.3-mg/kg base for 14 d on completion of chloroquine therapy
Uncomplicated infection with chloroquine-resistant *P. falciparum*	(a) Quinine sulfate *plus*	650 mg PO tid for 3–7 d	8.3 mg/kg PO tid for 3–7 d
	Doxycycline†	100 mg PO bid for 7 d	Contraindicated in children < 8 years of age†
	Plus or minus Pyrimethamine- sulfadoxine (fansidar)‡	3 tablets (75 mg/1500 mg) PO × 1 dose	Over 2 months old >50 kg 3 tabs 30–50 kg 2 tabs 15–29 kg 1 tab 10–14 kg $\frac{1}{2}$ tab 4–9 kg $\frac{1}{4}$ tab
	or (b) Mefloquine *plus* doxycycline§ *or*	750 mg PO initially followed by 500 mg in 6–8 h See above	10–15 mg/kg base followed by 5–10 mg/kg base in 6–8 h See above
	(c) Atovaquone-proguanil (Malarone)	4 adult-strength (250/100) tabs daily × 3 d	>40 kg, adult dose 31–40 kg, 3 adult tablets × 3 d 21–30 kg, 2 adult tablets × 3 d 11–20 kg, 1 adult tablet × 3 d
Complicated infection with chloroquine-resistant *P. falciparum*	Quinidine gluconate	10-mg/kg load over 2 h (maximum 600 mg), then 0.02 mg/kg per min continuous infusion until patient is stabilized and able to tolerate PO therapy (see above)	Same as adults¶
	plus Doxycycline†	100 mg IV q12h until tolerating PO therapy (see above)	Contraindicated in children < 8 years of age†

*Terminal treatment for *P. vivax* and *P. ovale* only.
†Clindamycin is an alternate to doxycycline at dose of 10 mg/kg (max 900 mg) every 8 h for 3–7 days.
‡Optional; of unlikely value if acquisition is with fansidar resistance.
§Optional; many experts feel comfortable with mefloquine alone.
¶Consult an expert in pediatric infectious disease immediately for guidance.

patient setting, provided adequate oral hydration and home care with close follow-up with repeated blood smears to measure treatment response are available.
- Unless the possibility of chloroquine resistance can be absolutely excluded based on geographic exposure history, it is best to assume the infection to be resistant and treat with a combination of quinine and doxycycline with or without pyrimethamine-sulfadoxine (Fansidar). Clindamycin may be substituted for doxycycline in those with contraindications to tetracyclines (allergy, pregnancy, and children). Mefloquine either alone or in combination with doxycycline is very effective against chloroquine-resistant *P. falciparum,* but it should not be used if it was taken as chemoprophylaxis. Atovaquone-proguanil (Malarone) is highly effective with cure rates >95%.[7]
- Supportive care is critical for ill admitted patients, including close hemodynamic monitoring, judicious fluid replacement, correction of metabolic derange-

ments, and additional support as needed (eg, dialysis, mechanical ventilation, etc).
- Recommendations for chemoprophylaxis for travelers can be obtained from the CDC's 24-hour malaria hotline (888-232-3228) or by accessing the CDC's website at http://www.cdc.gov/travel, which provides up-to-date info on resistance patterns in various countries worldwide.

REFERENCES

1. Centers for Disease Control and Prevention: CDC surveillance summaries: Malaria surveillance—United States, 2000. *MMWR* 51:9, 2002.
2. World Health Organization (WHO): *International Travel and Health, 2002.* Geneva: WHO, 2002.

3. Than M, Kyaw MP, Soe AY, et al: Development of resistance to chloroquine by *Plasmodium vivax* in Myanmar. *Trans Roy Soc Trop Med Hyg* 89:307, 1995.

4. Svenson JE, MacLean JD, Gyorkos TW, Keystone J: Imported malaria: Clinical presentation and examination of symptomatic travelers. *Arch Intern Med* 155:861, 1995.

5. Warrell DA, Molyneaux ME, Beales PF: Severe and complicated malaria. *Trans Roy Soc Trop Med Hyg* 84(Suppl):1, 1990.

6. White NJ: The treatment of malaria. *N Engl J Med* 335:800, 1996.

7. Looareesuwan S, Churley JD, Canfield CJ, et al: Malarone (atovaquone and proguanil hydrocholoride): A review of its clinical development for treatment of malaria. Malarone Clinical Trials Study Group. *Am J Trop Med Hyg* 60:533, 1999.

For further reading in *Emergency Medicine: A Comprehensive Study Guide,* 6th ed., see Chap. 148, "Malaria," by Jeffrey D. Band.

95 INFECTIONS FROM HELMINTHS AND OTHER PARASITIC WORMS

Phillip A. Clement

- Parasitic infections are increasingly common in the United States.
- This is due to immigration from Asia, Africa, and Latin America, to increased travel by U.S. citizens to the developing world, and to the rise of parasitic infections among immunosuppressed individuals.[1]
- The agents that cause parasitic diseases belong to three major groups: helminths (worms), protozoa, and arthropods.
- There are approximately 20 species of helminths that are natural parasites of man, and many others which cause zoonoses (primary infections of animals with subsequent infection of man).
- The protozoa are single-celled organisms that cause a variety of diseases ranging from malaria to amebiasis.
- Arthropods are classified as ectoparasites, and are medically important as obligate intermediate hosts and as mechanical vectors in many diseases.
- This chapter reviews infections from helminths. Helminths are multicellular worms and include nematodes (roundworms), cestodes (flatworms), and trematodes (flukes).

EPIDEMIOLOGY

- Parasitic diseases are a significant cause of morbidity and mortality worldwide, and may be acquired through the consumption of infected food or water, walking barefoot on contaminated soil, and from insect bites.
- According to the World Health Organization, 3.5 billion people worldwide harbor intestinal parasites, of which 450 million are symptomatic. There are 1.3 billion cases of *Ascaris* and 902 million cases of *Trichuris* globally.[2]

CLINICAL FEATURES

- Parasitic diseases present with a wide variety of symptoms (Table 95-1) and may be acute or chronic.
- Presentations range from common complaints, such as headache, fever, cough, and malaise, to life-threatening complications such as seizures, hemoptysis, melena, and intestinal obstruction.

TABLE 95-1   Common Symptoms of Helminth Infections*

SYMPTOM	POSSIBLE CAUSE
Abdominal pain	*Ascaris*, hookworm, *Trichuris*, *Schistosoma*, *Clonorchis*, *Fasciola*, *Taenia*, *Hymenolepis*, *Diphyllobothrium*
Anemia	*Diphyllobothrium*, hookworm, *Trichuris*
CNS symptoms	*Hymenolepis*, *Trichinella*, *Paragonimus*, *Echinococcus*, *Tanenia solium*, *Toxocara*, *Strongyloides*
Diarrhea	Hookworms, *Strongloides*, *Trichuris*, *Trichinella*, *Schistosoma*, *Fasciola*, *Fasciolopsis*, *Taenia*, *Hymenolepis*
Eosinophilia	*Strongyloides*, hookworms, *Trichuris*, *Drancunculus*, *Fasciola*, *Toxocara*, *Ascaris*, *Trichinella*, filariae, (*Wuchereria bancrofti*, *Brugia malayi*) *Hymenolepis*, *Schistosoma*, fluke, *Paragonimus westermani*, *C sinensis*, *Fasciolopsis buski*), *Taenia*
Fever	*Ascaris*, *Toxocara*, hookworms, *Trichuris*, *Trichinella*, filariae (*W bancrofti*), *Schistosoma*, fluke (*C sinensis*), *Fasciola*
Hepatomegaly	*Toxocara*, *Schistosoma*, fluke (*C sinensis*, *Opisthorchis viverrini*, *Fasciola*), tapeworm (*Echinococcus*)
Intestinal obstruction	*Ascaris*, *Strongyloides*, fluke (*F buski*), *Taenia*, *Diphyllobothrium*
Jaundice	Fluke (*C sinensis*, *O viverrini*), *Fasciola*
Cardiac symptoms	*Taenia*, *Trichinella*
Nausea and vomiting	*Ascaris*, *Trichuris*, *Trichinella*, *Taenia*
Ocular disease	Filariae (*Onchocerca volvulus*), *Taenia*, *Trichinella*, *Toxocara canis*, *Ascaris*, hookworm, *Echinococcus*
Pruritus	*Enterobius*, *Trichuris*, filariae (*O volvulus*)
Pulmonary symptoms	*Ascaris*, filariae (*W bancrofti*, *B malayi*), fluke (*P westermani*), hookworms, *Strongyloides*, *Trichinella*, *Paragonimus*, *Echinococcus*, *Toxocara*
Dermatological symptoms	*Dracunculus*, hookworm (*Ancylostoma duodenale*), *Toxocara*, *Schistosoma*, *Ascaris*, *Strongyloides*, *Trichinella*, *Fasciola*, *Trichinella*

*For more information, see the Web site of the Centers for Disease Control and Prevention: www.cdc.gov/ncidod/diseases/list_parasites.

Key: CNS = central nervous system.

DIAGNOSIS AND DIFFERENTIAL

- Parasites flourish in warm, moist climates with poor sanitation and nutrition. Ask about travel to or immigration from high-risk areas.
- Children are more often infected than adults because of their poor hygiene, oral behavior, and inability to ward off arthropod vectors.
- The diagnosis is complicated by the fact that the latent period between exposure and symptoms may be months to years.
- Parasitic disease should be considered in any patient with fever, abdominal pain, persistent or bloody diarrhea, skin rash, ulcers, or eosinophilia.
- Most helminth infections can be diagnosed by testing the stool for ova and parasites.
- *Ascaris lumbricoides, Necator americanus, Ancylostoma duodenale,* and *Strongyloides stercoralis* larvae may be found in the sputum.
- For pinworms, a cellophane tape anal swab is the most useful test.
- The larvae of *Strongyloides* may be detected via duodenal aspirate.[3]
- Eosinophilia is present in most helminth infections.
- The enzyme-linked immunosorbent assay (ELISA) technique can be used to make a serologic diagnosis of many parasitic infections.[4]

EMERGENCY DEPARTMENT CARE AND DISPOSITION

- Patients who are dehydrated from gastrointestinal losses or fever should receive intravenous hydration.
- Those patients who appear severely ill, toxic, those who cannot tolerate anything by mouth, those with significant dehydration, and those with multiple organ system involvement (eg, lung, blood, or central nervous system [CNS]) should be admitted for intravenous hydration, further diagnostic evaluation, and antiparasitic drug treatment as indicated.
- For treatment of specific helminths see below.

NEMATODES (ROUNDWORMS)

- Nematodes are cylindrical, unsegmented, elongated white worms.
- Humans are infected by egg ingestion, penetration through the skin, or inoculation by insect bite.
- The intestinal nematodes include hookworm, roundworm, and whipworm, in which a soil phase is needed for fecally passed eggs to develop. These infections occur in areas of poor sanitation.
- Pinworm eggs are infectious when excreted, facilitating person-to-person spread.
- The tissue nematodes include filariae, arthropod-borne worms that induce lymphatic, ocular, and skin disease.

ASCARIS LUMBRICOIDES

- *Ascaris* has a worldwide distribution. Infection is by the ingestion of eggs.
- Larvae migrate through the lungs and mature in the small intestines.
- Adult worms are 25 to 35 cm in length. Eggs are passed via feces.
- Clinical disease is due to pulmonary hypersensitivity or intestinal complications.
- During the lung phase, patients may develop pulmonary infiltrates, fever, cough, dyspnea, hemoptysis, and eosinophilia.
- Adult worms in the gut may be asymptomatic, or may cause abdominal pain and lead to intestinal obstruction in heavy infections. This is especially true in children.
- Worm migration into the biliary tract may cause biliary obstruction and pancreatitis.
- The diagnosis is made by finding eggs or an adult worm in the stool. The chest x-ray may reveal eosinophilic pneumonitis (Loeffler's syndrome). Serologic tests may be helpful.
- Visceral larva migrans is a related infection caused by the ingestion of eggs of *Toxocara,* a parasite of dogs and cats. Widespread larval migration may lead to pathology involving the CNS, eyes, heart, liver, or lungs.
- Treatment is with oral mebendazole 100 mg bid for 3 days, albendazole 400 mg PO once, or pyrantel pamoate 11 mg/kg PO once up to 1 g. Intestinal obstruction may necessitate surgery.

ENTEROBIUS VERMICULARIS (PINWORM)

- *Enterobius* infection is most prevalent in temperate climates during the winter and fall, and most often affects children.
- Infection is by the ingestion of eggs.
- Adult pinworms are small (2 to 5 mm) and reside in the cecum, appendix, ileum, and ascending colon. The gravid female migrates to the anus, especially at night, depositing eggs and causing intense pruritus.
- Autoinfection with hand-to-mouth transmission occurs after scratching.
- A host of problems from vaginitis to enuresis have been attributed to *Enterobius* infections, all without good evidence.
- Organisms can often be seen by direct examination of the anus.
- The diagnosis is confirmed by finding eggs on a cellophane tape swab of the anus.

- Eosinophilia is usually absent.
- All close household contacts should be examined and treated.
- Treat with pyrantel pamoate 11 mg/kg PO once up to 1 g, mebendazole 100 mg PO once, or albendazole 400 mg PO once. Treatment must be repeated in 2 weeks.

STRONGYLOIDES STERCORALIS (THREADWORM)
- Infection is through skin penetration by filariform larvae.
- Adult threadworms reside in the small intestine but migrate through the lungs.
- Entry of the parasite through the skin can lead to allergic manifestations, causing pruritus and an erythematous rash. Larval migration in the skin produces larva currens.
- Cough, dyspnea, and pneumonitis may occur from migration through lung parenchyma.
- The intestinal phase may produce abdominal pain, diarrhea with mucus and blood, and eosinophilia.
- *Strongyloides* is unique in its ability to reproduce within the host. Fatalities may occur due to hyperinfection in the elderly or the immunosuppressed.
- Diagnosis is made by finding larvae in the stool, duodenal contents, or sputum. An ELISA test is also available.
- An upper gastrointestinal series may reveal a deformed duodenal bulb, and may be confused with ulcer disease.
- Treat with ivermectin 200 μg/kg/day PO for 1 to 2 days or thiabendazole 50 mg/kg/day in two doses (maximum of 3 g/day) for 2 days.

NECATOR AMERICANUS, ANCYLOSTOMA DUODENALE (HOOKWORM)
- *Hookworms* prevail in the southern United States and are often seen in immigrants from warmer climates.
- Infection is by filariform larval migration through the skin and is associated with the use of human feces as fertilizer, the lack of shoes, and the lack of latrines.
- Obligate larval lung migration occurs before the organism matures on the intestinal mucosa.
- Infection through the skin may induce rash. There may be pulmonary and gastrointestinal symptoms as the worms migrate. Patients may have a cough, low-grade fever, abdominal pain, diarrhea, weakness, weight loss, heme-positive stools, and eosinophilia.
- This worm also ingests blood, leading to iron-deficiency anemia. Pica and geophagy are often seen in infected children.
- The diagnosis is made by finding ova in the stool.
- Cutaneous larva migrans is a related infection due to the larvae of *Ancylostoma braziliense* (dog or cat hookworm). Larval migration through the skin causes pruritus and a rash described as the "creeping eruption."
- Treatment is the same as for *Ascaris* (above).

TRICHURIS TRICHIURA (WHIPWORM)
- *Trichuris trichiura* is most common in the rural South, and occurs most often in children who play in the soil.
- Infection is by the ingestion of eggs. Adult worms reside in the cecum and reach 3 to 5 cm in length.
- Symptoms are usually gastrointestinal. Patients may complain of anorexia, insomnia, abdominal pain, fever, flatulence, bloody diarrhea, weight loss, and pruritus. There may be an associated eosinophilia and microcytic hypochromic anemia. Large infections can cause tenesmus, colitis, or rectal prolapse in children.
- The diagnosis is made by finding ova in the stool.
- Treatment is as for *Ascaris* (above).

TRICHINELLA SPIRALIS
- Trichinosis occurs in Mexico and the United States and results from the ingestion of pork, bear, or walrus meat containing encysted larvae.
- Symptoms depend on the parasite load and on the site of invasion, and may include nausea, vomiting, diarrhea, urticaria, headache, muscle weakness, fever, stiff neck, CNS manifestations, and psychiatric disturbances.
- In the early (enteric) phase, larvae mature on the intestinal mucosa and gastrointestinal symptoms predominate.
- Larvae later travel to striated muscle, where encystment begins approximately 3 weeks after the initial infection.
- Although encystment occurs only in striated muscle, inflammation may also occur in the heart, lungs, and CNS.
- Patients may present with acute myocarditis, nonsuppurative meningitis, bronchopneumonia, or catarrhal enteritis.
- The triad of periorbital edema, diffuse myalgias, and eosinophilia strongly suggests trichinosis.
- Pathognomonic splinter hemorrhages and subconjunctival hemorrhages may also occur.
- The diagnosis may be confirmed serologically. Biopsy of tender, involved muscle may be helpful after the fourth week. Stool specimens are only helpful early, during the gastrointestinal stage. Laboratory manifestations of trichinosis include leukocytosis, eosinophilia, elevated creatine phosphokinase, and electrocardiographic changes.
- Most cases are mild and resolve with only symptomatic treatment. Mebendazole 200 to 400 mg PO tid for 3 days and then 400 to 500 mg PO tid for 10 days is indicated for the intestinal phase, but may not be effective after encystment. Steroids are indicated for severe infections, such as CNS disease and myocarditis, but are not advocated routinely because their use can increase the number of circulating larvae.

BLOOD AND TISSUE NEMATODES: FILARIAE

- Transmission is by an arthropod vector (usually fly or mosquito).
- The larval stages are microscopic and are found in the cutaneous tissues or the blood.
- Treatment is with diethylcarbamazine or ivermectin.

WUCHERERIA BANCROFTI, BRUGIA MALAYI— (ELEPHANTIASIS)

- Infection is by mosquito transmission of microfilariae.
- The adult filariae localize to the lymphatic system and cause inflammation, leading to lymphangitis, lymphadenitis, and lymphedema due to obstruction.

LOA LOA (AFRICAN EYE WORM)

- Infection is by the bite of a fly of the genus *Chrysops.*
- Transient "calabar swellings" occur due to the migration of adult worms in the subcutaneous tissues or beneath the conjunctiva.

ONCHOCERCA VOLVULUS (RIVER BLINDNESS)

- Infection is by the bite of black flies (*Simulium*).
- Larval migration occurs through ocular tissues and may result in blindness.

DRACUNCULUS MEDINENSIS (FIRE WORM)

- Infection follows ingestion of water containing infected crustaceans.
- Adult worms migrate to the subcutaneous tissues and produce skin ulcers through which the females discharge larvae.
- Adults may reach 1 meter in length and are common in the lower extremities.
- Treatment is by surgical removal or slowly winding the adult worm around a stick over a period of several days.

TREMATODES (FLUKES)

- Trematodes are leaflike, symmetrical flatworms, possessing a ventral sucker to hold their position. They are found in the tropics, and require intermediate hosts such as snails, crabs, or fish. Trematodes shed their eggs from the human host in the feces, urine, or sputum.

SCHISTOSOMIASIS

- Schistosomiasis is the most common fluke-borne illness.
- *Schistosoma mansoni, S. japonicum,* and *S. haematobium* all have freshwater snails as intermediate hosts.
- Cercariae are the free-living larval form, that live in freshwater and directly penetrate the skin, inducing dermatitis.
- Pathology is caused by inflammation induced by the eggs.
- Acute disease may include fever, diarrhea, abdominal pain, melena, cough, hematemesis, lymphadenopathy, hepatosplenomegaly, urticaria, and eosinophilia.
- Chronic disease occurs from egg deposition in the bladder, intestines, and liver, leading to portal hypertension, ascites, liver failure, and obstructive hydroureter.
- Adults of *S. mansoni* and *S. japonicum* reside in mesenteric veins. Eggs are usually passed in the stool.
- Adults of *S. haematobium* reside in vesical, prostatic, and uterine plexuses. Eggs may be found in urine.
- The diagnosis is suggested by a positive immunofluorescent antibody test and confirmed by finding eggs in the feces or urine or on rectal biopsy.
- Treatment is with praziquantel 40 to 60 mg/kg/day PO in two to three doses per day.

SCHISTOSOMAL DERMATITIS (SWIMMERS ITCH)

- Caused by transient skin penetration of cercariae of another animal (eg, birds). Symptoms are self-limited, usually requiring no treatment.

FASCIOLOPSIS BUSKI (INTESTINAL FLUKE)

- Infection acquired by ingestion of metacercariae (larval form) on water chestnuts and bamboo shoots.
- Infection produces malabsorptive diarrhea.

CLONORCHIS SINENSIS, FASCIOLA HEPATICA (LIVER FLUKES)

- *Clonorchis* infection is caused by ingestion of fish containing encysted metacercariae, and is endemic in the Far East.
- *Fasciola* infection is acquired through ingestion of metacercariae on watercress.
- Both can cause hepatic disease secondary to inflammation, biliary obstruction, or portal cirrhosis. Infection is associated with hepatocellular carcinoma.

PARAGONIMUS WESTERMANI (LUNG FLUKE)

- Infection is acquired through the ingestion of metacercariae encysted in crab. Adult worms are encapsulated in cystic structures adjacent to bronchi. Pulmonary symptoms may include hemoptysis. Eggs may be seen in sputum or feces

CESTODES (FLATWORMS)

- The cestodes are flatworms, commonly referred to as tapeworms. They have a scolex, or head, equipped with suckers, or hooks. Cestodes grow by segmentation, extending proglottids from the neck.

HYMENOLEPIS NANA (DWARF TAPEWORM)

- *Hymenolepsis nana* is the most common tapeworm in the United States and occurs most often in children and institutionalized patients.
- Transmission is by the ingestion of eggs.
- Symptoms are mild and may include diarrhea and abdominal discomfort.
- Treatment is with praziquantel 25 mg/kg PO for one dose.

TAENIA SAGINATA (BEEF TAPEWORM)

- Infection is by the consumption of raw beef containing cysticerci (larvae).
- Adult worms live in the small intestine and may reach 9 meters in length.
- Infections may be asymptomatic or may cause gastrointestinal distress, abdominal pain, and weight loss.
- Diagnosis is by stool examination for proglottids.
- Treatment is with praziquantel 10 mg/kg PO for one dose.

TAENIA SOLIUM (PORK TAPEWORM)

- *Taenia solium* is encountered primarily in immigrants or visitors from Central America or the Middle East.
- Infection is by the ingestion of raw or undercooked pork containing cysticerci (larvae) or by the ingestion of food or water containing eggs.
- Ingestion of the cysticerci leads to disease similar to that produced by *Taenia saginata*.
- Infected patients may be asymptomatic or may present with nausea and vomiting, headache, abdominal pain, pruritus, constipation, diarrhea, and intestinal obstruction.
- Ingestion of the eggs leads to the release of larval oncospheres, which may spread by the blood to multiple body tissues. Encysted larvae may be found in subcutaneous tissue, muscle, the eye, the brain, and the heart.
- This larval stage produces the clinical disease cysticercosis, and may lead to seizures and hydrocephalus.
- Consider cysticercosis in patients from endemic areas with new-onset seizures or other neurologic symptoms.
- Radiographs of the soft tissues may reveal curvilinear calcifications indicative of cysts. Cysts may also be seen in the meninges and brain parenchyma on computed tomography (CT) scan.
- The diagnosis is made by finding gravid proglottids in the stool. An ELISA or hemagglutination reaction may be helpful, but results of both can be falsely negative if the cysts are calcified.
- Treatment of the adult (intestinal) stage is with praziquantel 10 mg/kg PO for one dose. The larval (tissue) stage is treated with albendazole. For cysticercosis, albendazole 15 mg/kg/day PO in two to three doses for 8 to 30 days or praziquantel 50 mg/kg/day PO in

three doses for 15 days are recommended. Adjunctive surgery may also be necessary to remove cysts.

DIPHYLLOBOTHRIUM

- The fish tapeworm *Diphyllobothrium latum* occurs in people who eat raw, larvae-encysted fish (eg, sushi, sashimi, and gefilte fish).
- Patients may be asymptomatic or exhibit mild gastrointestinal symptoms.
- Pernicious anemia may occur, presumably by competition by the worm with the host for vitamin B_{12}.
- Treatment is the same as for *Taenia saginata*.

REFERENCES

1. James SL: Emerging parasitic infections. *FEMS Immunol Med Microbiol* 18:313, 1997.
2. World Health Organization, Division of Control of Tropical Disease: Intestinal Parasite Control, available at: http://www.who.int/ctd/html/intest.html, 1998.
3. Rosenblatt JE: Laboratory diagnosis of parasitic infections. *Mayo Clin Proc* 69:779, 1994.
4. Morris AJ, Murray PR, Reller RB: Contemporary testing for enteric pathogens. *J Clin Microbiol* 34:1776, 1996.

For further reading in *Emergency Medicine: A Comprehensive Study Guide,* 6th Ed., see Chap. 149, "Infections from Helminths," by Harold H. Osborn.

96 ZOONOTIC INFECTIONS

Gregory S. Hall

- Zoonoses, or diseases transmitted from vertebrate animals or arthropod vectors to humans, remain common and often underestimated in prevalence in North America. Contact with household pets (or their associated parasites), domesticated or wild animals, their infected tissues or secretions, and arthropods, especially ticks, are all sources of infections in humans.[1,2]
- Most zoonoses in the United States, including those spread by ticks, have their highest incidence in the spring and summer.[3] These diseases are easily mistaken for other nonspecific self-limited diseases and many patients at risk fail to volunteer their exposure history (ie, cannot recall a tick bite).[4] This chapter focuses primarily on tick-borne infections and a few other entities. For information on rabies refer to Chap. 93.

LYME DISEASE

EPIDEMIOLOGY

- Lyme disease remains the leading vector-borne zoonosis in the United States, and is most prevalent in the Northeast, but has been reported in all 48 contiguous states.[4,5]

PATHOPHYSIOLOGY

- *Borrelia burgdorferi,* a spirochete, is the responsible organism and is transmitted to humans by *Ixodes* species ticks, with rabbits, rodents, and deer serving as host reservoir animals. The overall risk of contracting Lyme disease after a deer tick bite is relatively low, about 3% in highly endemic areas.

CLINICAL FEATURES

- Lyme disease is a multiorgan infection divided into three distinct stages, but not all patients suffer all stages; stages may overlap and remissions between stages may occur.
- Erythema chronicum migrans (ECM) skin lesion, the hallmark of stage I, occurs in 60 to 80% of cases and consists of an annular, erythematous skin plaque with central clearing, which forms 2 to 20 days after a tick bite at the inoculation site. Primary pathophysiology of ECM is that of a vasculitis.[6]
- Stage I (the ECM lesion) may be accompanied by (in decreasing order of frequency) generalized malaise and fatigue, headache, fever, chills, stiff neck, arthralgias, and other constitutional symptoms, all of which if left untreated resolve spontaneously in 3 to 4 weeks.[4,7]
- Stage II corresponds to dissemination of the spirochete, resulting in multiple secondary annular skin lesions (ECM), fever, adenopathy, splenomegaly, and flu-like constitutional symptoms.
- Fifteen percent of untreated stage II patients develop neurologic disease, most often cranial neuritis (especially uni- or bilateral facial nerve palsy), or other peripheral neuropathies. Other neurologic symptoms can include periodic headache, neck stiffness, cerebellar ataxia, encephalitis, myelitis, motor or sensory radiculoneuronitis, mononeuritis multiplex, or difficulty with mentation.[5]
- Also asymmetrical oligoarticular arthritis (usually in large joints, especially knees) may develop during the second stage. Cardiac abnormalities occur in approximately 8% of patients and typically present as first-, second-, or third-degree atrioventricular nodal heart block or myocarditis.

- Stage III represents chronic persistent infection, occurs years after the resolution of stage I, and includes chronic intermittent migratory arthritis, myocarditis, encephalopathy, and axonal polyneuropathy.[8]

DIAGNOSIS AND DIFFERENTIAL

- Diagnosis is dependent initially on clinical features, and a two-step serologic test (enzyme immunoassay and Western blot) is used for confirmation. Culture of the organism is difficult and not widely available.

EMERGENCY DEPARTMENT CARE AND DISPOSITION

- Lyme disease responds well to antimicrobial therapy, especially if started early in the course of the infection. Treatment of choice for early Lyme disease is oral doxycycline 100 mg PO twice daily for 14 to 21 days. Acceptable alternatives include amoxicillin, cefuroxime, azithromycin, clarithromycin, ceftriaxone, or cefotaxime.[5,9]
- Serious CNS disease (meningitis, encephalitis, neuropathy), cardiac manifestations, or severe arthritis warrant hospital admission for supportive care and a 14- to 21-day course of IV ceftriaxone.
- Prophylactic treatment for tick bites is not generally recommended. A vaccine is now available for individuals at high risk of contracting Lyme disease.

ROCKY MOUNTAIN SPOTTED FEVER

EPIDEMIOLOGY

- Rocky Mountain spotted fever (RMSF) is caused by *Rickettsia rickettsii,* an obligate intracellular coccobacillus, carried by *Dermacentor* species ticks. Deer, rodents, horses, cattle, cats, and dogs are the usual animal reservoir hosts.

PATHOPHYSIOLOGY

- Transmission of RMSF to humans via tick bite occurs primarily (95% of cases) between April 1 and September 30, with the highest incidence in the mid-Atlantic states (cases have been reported in most of the contiguous states) and two thirds of all cases are reported in children <15 years old.

CLINICAL FEATURES

- RMSF is classically defined by a triad of fever, rash, and history of tick exposure, but only about 50% of afflicted patients can recall a tick bite, and rash may be absent in up to 20% ("spotless RMSF," which is usually seen in African Americans, the elderly, and in severe, fatal cases).[10,11]
- The incubation period following tick bite is usually 4 to 10 days and is followed by abrupt or insidious onset of nonspecific symptoms such as fever, malaise, severe headache, myalgias, nausea and vomiting, diarrhea, anorexia, abdominal pain, and photophobia.
- Additional signs and symptoms may include lymphadenopathy, hepatosplenomegaly, conjunctivitis, confusion, meningismus, renal or respiratory failure, and myocarditis.
- Rash, the hallmark feature, usually begins during the first 2 weeks of illness, is often maculopapular, and typically begins on the extremities around the wrists and ankles (often involving the palms and soles), and spreads centripetally to the trunk, usually sparing the face (it may become petechial and/or purpuric and rarely necrotic).
- Gastrointestinal symptoms are often prominent features, may precede the onset of rash, and often lead to misdiagnosis of gastroenteritis or even acute abdomen.
- RMSF pneumonitis, a common and potentially fatal complication, presents with cough, dyspnea, pulmonary edema, and systemic hypoxia.[12]
- Serious neurologic involvement occurs in about one quarter of cases, with confusion, stupor, ataxia, seizures, and coma.

DIAGNOSIS AND DIFFERENTIAL

- Lab findings are usually nonspecific, but the combination of neutropenia, thrombocytopenia, hyponatremia, and elevated liver function tests (LFTs) should arouse suspicion of RMSF.
- Untreated patients suffer up to 25% mortality. The clinical diagnosis must be presumed in order to start therapy early, since serology to confirm a rise in antibody titer is not reliably positive until 6 to 10 days after onset of symptoms (diagnosis may also be confirmed by skin rash biopsy with immunofluorescent testing).[13]
- Differential diagnosis includes viral illness (measles, rubella, hepatitis, mononucleosis, encephalitis, enteroviral exanthem), gastroenteritis, acute abdomen, disseminated gonorrhea, meningitis (meningococcus), secondary syphilis, leptospirosis, typhoid fever, pneumonia, and streptococcal infection.

EMERGENCY DEPARTMENT CARE AND DISPOSITION

- Therapy for adults includes doxycycline 100 mg PO twice daily, tetracycline 500 mg PO qid, or chloramphenicol 50 to 75 mg/kg/day IV in four divided doses. (It is advisable to consult an infectious disease expert before using chloramphenicol.[14])
- Therapy for children <45 kg (100 lb) includes doxycycline 4.4 mg/kg/day PO in two divided doses on day 1 followed by 2.2 mg/kg/day PO in two divided doses thereafter. Alternatives include tetracycline and IV chloramphenicol.
- Doxycycline has been used for short courses in children without significant staining of teeth, but these cosmetic risks must be balanced against the potentially serious side effects of chloramphenicol. The risks and benefits of either treatment should be discussed with the parents and the child's pediatrician if possible, and informed consent should be obtained.
- Antimicrobial therapy for RMSF is given for 5 to 7 days or until the patient is afebrile and clinically improving for at least 48 hours.
- Patients with nausea and vomiting or significant systemic disease should be admitted to the hospital for supportive care and IV antimicrobial therapy.

TICK PARALYSIS

PATHOPHYSIOLOGY

- Tick paralysis, a relatively uncommon entity, may be fatal (from aspiration or respiratory failure) if undiagnosed, yet is easily cured by careful removal of the offending tick.
- This rare complication has been reported following bites of the dog tick (*Dermacentor variabilis*) and wood tick (*D. andersoni*) in the United States, with incidence highest in spring to late summer, and children most commonly affected.

CLINICAL FEATURES

- Symptoms are believed to result from a neurologic venom secreted from the salivary glands of the female tick, which results in conduction blockade at the motor end-plate of peripheral nerves.
- Clinical symptoms usually begin 4 to 7 days after attachment of the female tick, with an initial prodrome of malaise, irritability, restlessness, and paresthesias of the hand or foot. Fever is usually absent.
- Symptoms progress to include a symmetrical ascending flaccid paralysis (resembling Guillain-Barré syn-

drome), with eventual loss of deep tendon reflexes, dysphagia, involuntary eye movements, cranial nerve palsies, ataxia, and respiratory paralysis. Sensation remains intact.

DIAGNOSIS AND DIFFERENTIAL

- Diagnosis depends on locating the tick (often hidden under hair on the scalp). Cerebrospinal fluid (CSF) remains normal.

EMERGENCY DEPARTMENT CARE AND DIFFERENTIAL

- Prompt and careful removal of the tick is curative along with supportive care (mechanical ventilation if needed). Most patients begin to recover within hours of tick removal, with complete recovery usually within 48 to 72 hours.

TULAREMIA

EPIDEMIOLOGY

- Tularemia (rabbit skinner's disease) is an infection caused by *Francisella tularensis,* a small gram-negative coccobacillus carried by *Dermacentor* and *Amblyomma* species of ticks, as well as the deerfly. The principal animal host reservoirs include rabbits, hares, deer, muskrats, beavers, and dogs.[12]
- Tularemia has been widely reported in the continental United States, but the highest incidence occurs in Arkansas, Missouri, and Oklahoma, with cases reported year-round, but incidence is highest in early winter (adults) and early summer (children).

PATHOPHYSIOLOGY

- Transmission may occur via arthropod bite; animal bite; inoculation of skin, conjunctiva, or oral mucosa by blood or tissue from an infected animal host; and handling or ingestion of contaminated soil, grain, hay, or water. Several distinct clinical syndromes can occur with clinical features that depend on the route of inoculation.

CLINICAL FEATURES

- The average incubation period following exposure is 3 to 5 days, after which sudden-onset fever (which may persist for several days, remit briefly, then recur), chills, headache, anorexia, malaise, and fatigue may be seen. Additional symptoms which may occur include myalgias, cough, vomiting, abdominal pain, diarrhea, and pharyngitis.
- Ulceroglandular fever (most common presentation) follows a tick or animal bite. A papule develops at the bite site and it evolves into a tender necrotic ulcer with painful regional adenopathy. Glandular tularemia consists of tender regional adenopathy without a skin lesion.
- Other forms include oculoglandular tularemia, with painful conjunctivitis and periauricular, submandibular, and cervical adenopathy; pharyngeal tularemia (ingestion of contaminated food or water), with exudative pharyngitis or tonsillitis; and tularemic pneumonitis (inhalation of organisms), with productive cough, pleuritic chest pain, rales, consolidation, and pleuritic rub.
- Typhoidal tularemia (any form of transmission) includes multiorgan signs and symptoms, including fever, headache, vomiting, diarrhea, myalgias, hepatosplenomegaly, cough, and pneumonitis.

DIAGNOSIS AND DIFFERENTIAL

- Clinical diagnosis rests on suggestive clinical features and serologic (enzyme-linked immunosorbent assay; ELISA) studies to determine acute and convalescent titers; culture of organisms from blood, ulcers, lymph nodes, or sputum may be used to confirm the diagnosis. Other laboratory findings are nonspecific.
- Differential diagnosis includes pyogenic bacterial infection, syphilis, anthrax, plague, Q fever, psittacosis, typhoid, brucellosis, and rickettsial infection.

EMERGENCY DEPARTMENT CARE AND DISPOSITION

- Treatment is with streptomycin 7.5 to 10 mg/kg every 12 hours IM or IV (pediatric dose is 30 to 40 mg/kg IM in two divided doses), or gentamicin 3 to 5 mg/kg/day IV in three divided doses. Other alternatives include tobramycin, doxycycline, chloramphenicol, ciprofloxacin, and azithromycin. Therapy is given for 10 to 14 days.[15–17]

EHRLICHIOSIS

EPIDEMIOLOGY

- A zoonotic disease with two clinical subtypes (human granulocytic and human monocytic) caused by

Ehrlichia species, small gram-negative coccobacilli that infect circulating leukocytes. The human monocytic form (*Ehrlichia chaffeensis*) predominates in the U.S.[18]

PATHOPHYSIOLGY

- Transmission occurs via bite or exposure to *Ixodes* and *Amblyomma* species ticks. Animal host reservoirs include deer, dogs, and other mammals.

CLINICAL FEATURES

- The incubation period ranges from 1 to 21 days (median 7 days), followed by onset of nonspecific symptoms such as high fever, headache, nausea and vomiting, malaise, abdominal pain, anorexia, and myalgias.
- In 20% of cases, a maculopapular or petechial rash (which may involve the palms and soles) develops during the initial phase of illness.
- Serious complications develop in a minority of cases and may include renal or respiratory failure, disseminated intravascular coagulopathy, cardiomegaly, and encephalitis.
- The acute phase of illness lasts less than 4 weeks, with most patients recovering and proceeding to a convalescent phase.

DIAGNOSIS AND DIFFERENTIAL

- Diagnosis must rely on clinical features, but serology (antibody titers) can provide confirmation. Laboratory findings (most prominent on fifth through seventh days of illness) include leukopenia, absolute lymphopenia, thrombocytopenia, and elevated serum transaminase and alkaline phosphatase levels (rarely CSF pleocytosis is seen).
- Differential diagnosis includes rickettsial diseases (especially RMSF) and bacterial meningitis.
- Treatment of choice is doxycycline 100 mg PO or IV twice daily for 7 to 14 days. Alternatives include tetracycline and chloramphenicol; there are no current recommendations for children or pregnant women.[18]

COLORADO TICK FEVER

PATHOPHYSIOLOGY

- An acute viral illness caused by an RNA virus of the genus Coltivirus, transmitted to humans via *Dermacentor* ticks (animal reservoir hosts include deer,

marmots, and porcupines), with most cases reported between late May and early July in the mountainous western regions of the United States.

CLINICAL FEATURES

- Symptoms begin suddenly 3 to 6 days following tick bite and include fever, chills, severe headache, photophobia, nausea and vomiting, and myalgias; lymphadenopathy, hepatosplenomegaly, and conjunctivitis may also be seen.
- Symptoms usually persist for 5 to 8 days then spontaneously remit, but 3 days later up to 50% of patients develop a second phase, which includes a transient generalized maculopapular or petechial rash. The secondary phase usually lasts for 2 to 4 days and spontaneously resolves.

DIAGNOSIS AND DIFFERENTIAL

- Diagnosis rests on clinical features but can be confirmed by fluorescent antibody staining of a patient's erythrocytes or mouse innoculation.[19]
- Differential diagnosis includes meningitis (bacterial or viral), and rickettsial infections (especially RMSF).

EMERGENCY DEPARTMENT CARE AND DISPOSITION

- Treatment consists of supportive care, though empiric treatment with antimicrobial therapy to cover bacterial meningitis and rickettsial infection is often used pending confirmation of the diagnosis.

HANTAVIRUS

EPIDEMIOLOGY

- Hantavirus infection is a viral zoonosis identified in 1977. In North America the etiologic agent is the Sin Nombre virus (a member of Bunyaviridae family), and to date at least 10 distinct serotypes have been identified, each with a specific rodent vector, geographic distribution, and clinical manifestation.[20]

PATHOPHYSIOLOGY

- In the United States, the deer mouse is the primary vector, with transmission to humans accomplished via inhalation of dried particulate feces, contact with urine, or by rodent bite.[21]

- Worldwide the majority of hantavirus serotypes have a predilection for the kidney, with a clinical presentation of acute renal failure, thrombocytopenia, ocular abnormalities, and flu-like symptoms.

CLINICAL FEATURES

- In the United States, the most common presentation is that of hantavirus pulmonary syndrome: an initial flu-like prodrome for 3 to 4 days, followed by pulmonary edema, hypoxia, hypotension, tachycardia, dizziness, nausea and vomiting, thrombocytopenia, and metabolic acidosis; cough is generally absent.[20–22]

DIAGNOSIS AND DIFFERENTIAL

- Diagnosis rests on clinical features plus history of exposure, but may be confirmed by an immunofluorescent or immunoblot assay.[2] Differential diagnosis includes bacterial pneumonia, acute respiratory distress syndrome (ARDS), and influenza.

EMERGENCY DEPARTMENT CARE AND DISPOSITION

- Hantavirus pulmonary syndrome has a reported mortality rate of 50 to 70%. Treatment is primarily with supportive care (especially oxygenation and ventilation) and possibly inhaled ribavirin.[20–22]

ANTHRAX

EPIDEMIOLOGY

- Anthrax is an acute bacterial infection caused by *Bacillus anthracis,* an aerobic gram-positive rod that forms central oval spores, and though very rare in North America, remains of concern in part because of its potential use as an agent of biological warfare or terrorism.

PATHOPHYSIOLOGY

- In nature, the disease is most commonly seen in domestic herbivores (cattle, sheep, horses, and goats) and wild herbivores. Human infection can result from inhalation of spores, inoculation of broken skin, arthropod bite (fleas), or ingestion of inadequately cooked infected meat.

CLINICAL FEATURES

- Symptoms depend on the method of transmission. Inhaled or pneumonic anthrax is contracted via handling of unsterilized, imported animal hides or raw wool. Initially patients suffer a flu-like illness that progresses over 3 to 4 days to include marked mediastinal and hilar edema (mediastinitis rather than true pneumonia) and respiratory failure; it is universally fatal.
- Cutaneous anthrax (a.k.a. woolsorter's disease) begins with a small red macule at the site of inoculation, which over the course of a week progresses through papular, vesicular, or pustular forms to result in an ulcer with a black eschar and adjacent brawny edema (once fully developed it may be painless). Spontaneous healing (the eschar usually sloughs off in 2 weeks) usually follows, but a small minority of untreated patients develop rapidly fatal bacteremia.
- Gastrointestinal anthrax exhibits variable symptoms—fever, nausea and vomiting, abdominal pain, bloody diarrhea, ascites, pharyngitis, and tonsillitis.

DIAGNOSIS AND DIFFERENTIAL

- Diagnosis may be established via Gram's stain, direct fluorescent antibody stain, or culture of skin lesions or vesicular fluid, or testing of sera for antibodies to the organism. Blood cultures may also be positive. Lab findings can include normal leukocyte counts (mild cases) or leukocytosis.

EMERGENCY DEPARTMENT CARE AND DISPOSITION

- Treatment includes either ciprofloxacin 750 mg PO twice daily or 400 mg IV, or doxycycline 100 mg PO or IV twice daily; therapy is given for 10 to 14 days. Alternatives include penicillin G, clindamycin, or rifampin.[23]

PLAGUE

EPIDEMIOLOGY

- Plague or *Yersinia pestis* is a gram-negative bacillus of the Enterobacteriaceae family and is endemic to the United States, most often found in rock squirrels and ground rodents of the Southwest, but may also be carried by cats and dogs. The rodent flea is the primary vector.

PATHOPHYSIOLOGY

- Transmission to humans occurs via the bite of a flea from an infected animal host or through handling or ingestion of infected rodents, resulting in three clinical forms of human disease: (1) bubonic or suppurative (most common), (2) pneumonic, or (3) septicemic.

CLINICAL FEATURES

- The incubation period ranges from 2 to 7 days following exposure. Frequently an eschar develops at the bite site, followed by a painful, sometimes suppurative bubo (enlarged regional lymph nodes), often at the groin.
- Associated symptoms may include fever, headache, malaise, abdominal pain, nausea and vomiting, and bloody diarrhea.
- Ten to twenty percent of patients progress to develop secondary pneumonia with multilobar infiltrates, bloody sputum, and respiratory failure. This form is highly contagious and can be transmitted from person to person via aerosolized respiratory secretions (respiratory isolation is required).
- Subclinical disseminated intravascular coagulation (DIC) may also occur in a large number of patients. Untreated bubonic plague may proceed to generalized sepsis, hypotension, and death.

DIAGNOSIS AND DIFFERENTIAL

- Diagnosis must depend on clinical features in a patient with possible contact with fleas or a host animal. Needle aspiration of a bubo with direct staining using Wayson's or Giemsa stain reveals bipolar safety pin–shaped organisms. Fluorescent antibody staining of aspirate or antibody titers of acute and convalescent sera also confirms the diagnosis.
- Laboratory findings are nonspecific and may include leukocytosis, modest elevations of hepatic transaminases, and DIC.

EMERGENCY DEPARTMENT CARE AND DISPOSITION

- Therapy should begin immediately for any suspected case—treat as an inpatient with gentamicin 2.0 mg/kg IV loading dose, then 1.7 mg/kg IV every 8 hours or streptomycin 1.0 g every 12 hours IV or IM. Therapy is continued for 10 to 14 days. Alternatives include a combination of tetracycline and an aminoglycoside or chloramphenicol.[24]

WEST NILE VIRUS ENCEPHALITIS

EPIDEMIOLOGY

- The West Nile virus is a member of the Japanese encephalitis serocomplex of the Flaviviridae family of viruses. It was first isolated in Uganda in 1937 and was subsequently seen in Eastern Europe, West Asia, and the Middle East. It was first detected in the western hemisphere in 1999.

PATHOPHYSIOLOGY

- The mode of transmission involves mosquitoes, primarily the *Culex* species, that feed on infected birds, which serve as a natural reservoir. Over 110 bird species in the U.S. have been found to be infected by WN virus with crows, ravens, and jays being most common. The virus is transmitted to humans and other vertebrate animals via carrier mosquitoes during a blood meal.

CLINICAL FEATURES

- The incubation period varies from 3 to 15 days with about 20% of those bitten developing fever and a flu-like illness, West Nile fever. Classic presentation is that of a mild dengue-like illness with sudden onset of fever, lymphadenopathy, headache, abdominal pain, vomiting, rash, conjunctivitis, eye pain, and anorexia. Duration of symptoms is typically 3 to 6 days.[25]
- Meningoencephalitis develops in approximately 1 in 150 patients infected, and is more common than meningitis. Risk factors include immunocompromised host (HIV, TB, malaria) or advanced age. Complaints of weakness out of proportion to physical exam findings are common and myoclonus is nearly always seen. Complete flaccid paralysis may occur and may be confused with Guillain-Barré syndrome.
- Other neurologic findings may include Parkinsonian-like signs, ataxia, extrapyramidal signs, cranial nerve abnormalities, myelitis, optic neuritis, and seizures.

DIAGNOSIS AND DIFFERENTIAL

- Laboratory findings are often nonspecific. Blood total white blood cell (WBC) count may be normal or slightly elevated. Hyponatremia has been seen in patients with meningoencephalitis. CSF demonstrates mostly lymphocytes, elevated protein, and a normal glucose level. CT scan of the brain usually shows no evidence of acute disease, though cerebral edema may be seen with progressive meningoencephalitis.

Diagnosis is made by identifying the WN virus–specific IgM antibody in serum or CSF specimens. This IgM antibody is an acute phase identifier and may persist in serum for up to 12 months. WN virus IgG antibody is found in the convalescent phase in both serum and CSF. Polymerase chain reaction (PCR) testing is still in the experimental stage. The differential diagnosis must include other causes of febrile illness (bacterial, viral, rickettsial, etc) or meningoencephalitis (viral including herpes and rabies, syphilis, bacterial, etc).

EMERGENCY DEPARTMENT CARE AND DISPOSITION

• Treatment is purely supportive and any patient with signs or findings of meningoencephalitis is probably best managed initially as an inpatient pending confirmation of the diagnosis and to facilitate close monitoring.

REFERENCES

1. Simpson GL: Vector borne and animal associated infections, in Brillman CJ, Quenzer RW (eds.): *Infectious Diseases in Emergency Medicine,* 2nd ed. Philadelphia: Lippincott-Raven, 1998, p. 209.
2. Hart CA, Trees AJ, Duerden BI: Zoonoses: Proceedings of the third Liverpool Tropical School Bayer Symposium on microbial diseases held on 3 February 1996 (Review Article). *J Med Microbiol* 46:4, 1997.
3. Walker DH, Barbour AG, Oliver JH, et al: Emerging bacterial zoonotic and vector-borne diseases: Ecological and epidemiological factors. *JAMA* 275:463, 1996.
4. Doan-Wiggins L: Tick borne diseases. *Emerg Med Clin North Am* 9:303, 1991.
5. Steere AC: Lyme disease. *N Engl J Med* 345:115, 2001.
6. Steere AC: Lyme disease. *N Engl J Med* 321:586, 1989.
7. Wright SW, Trott AT: North American tick-borne diseases. *Ann Emerg Med* 17:964, 1988.
8. Shaddick NA, Phillips CB, Logigian EL, et al: The long term clinical outcomes of Lyme disease: A population based retrospective cohort study. *Ann Intern Med* 121:560, 1994.
9. Centers for Disease Control and Prevention: Lyme disease: United States, 1987 and 1988. *MMWR* 38:668, 1989.
10. Kirkland KK, Sexton DJ: Therapeutic delay in Rocky Mountain spotted fever. *Clin Infect Dis* 12:1118, 1995.
11. Woodward TE: Rocky Mountain spotted fever: Epidemiological and early clinical signs are keys to treatment and reduced mortality. *J Infect Dis* 150:465, 1984.
12. Spach DH, Liles WC, Campbell GL, et al: Tick-borne disease in the United States. *N Engl J Med* 329:936, 1993.
13. Walker DH: Rocky Mountain spotted fever: A seasonal alert. *Clin Infect Dis* 12:1111, 1995.
14. Byrd RP, Vasquez J, Roy TM: Respiratory manifestations of tick-borne diseases in the southeastern United States. *South Med J* 90:1, 1997.
15. Tan JS: Human zoonotic infections transmitted by dogs and cats. *Arch Intern Med* 157:1933, 1997.
16. Goldstein EJC: Household pets and human infections. *Infect Dis Clin North Am* 5:1177, 1991.
17. Elliot DL, Tolle SW, Goldber L, Miller JB: Pet-associated illness. *N Engl J Med* 16:985, 1985.
18. Dawson JE: Human ehrlichiosis in the United States, in Reminton JS, Swartz MN (eds.): *Current Clinical Topics in Infectious Diseases.* Cambridge, MA: Blackwell Science, 1996, p. 164.
19. Emmons RW: An overview of Colorado tick fever. *Prog Clin Biol Res* 178:47, 1985.
20. Clement J, McKenna P, van der Groen G, et al: Hantavirus, in Palmer SR, Soulsby L, Simpson DIH (eds.): *Zoonosis: Biology, Clinical Practice and Public Health Control.* Oxford: Oxford University Press, 1998, p. 331.
21. Centers for Disease Control and Prevention: Hantavirus pulmonary syndrome: Colorado and New Mexico, 1998. *MMWR* 47:249, 1998.
22. Duchin JS, Koster FT, Peters CJ, et al: Hantavirus pulmonary syndrome: Clinical description of seventeen patients with a newly recognized disease. *N Engl J Med* 330:949, 1994.
23. Brachman PS: Inhalation anthrax. *Ann NY Acad Sci* 353:83, 1980.
24. Perry RD, Fetherston JD: *Yersinia pestis:* Etiologic agent of plague. *Clin Microbiol Rev* 10:35, 1997.
25. Petersen LR, Marfin AA: West Nile virus: A primer for the clinician. *Ann Intern Med* 137:173, 2002.

For further reading in *Emergency Medicine: A Comprehensive Study Guide,* 6th ed., see Chap. 151, "Zoonotic Infections," by John T. Meredith.

97 SOFT TISSUE INFECTIONS

Chris Melton

• The spectrum of illness is differentiated by depth of soft tissue necrosis from superficial necrotizing cellulitis to necrotizing fasciitis to gas gangrene.
• Most cases are polymicrobial; however, some *Clostridium* species and group A *Streptococcus* (GAS) can cause single-organism infection.

GAS GANGRENE (CLOSTRIDIAL MYONECROSIS)

• Gas gangrene is the deepest of the necrotizing soft tissue infections.

- Gas production and sepsis are hallmarks of the disease.

PATHOPHYSIOLOGY

- *Clostridium* species are the etiologic organisms, with *Clostridium perfringens* the most common isolate.[1]
- *Clostridium* produces exotoxins that cause cellular death, rapid progression, and systemic toxicity. Other effects secondary to tissue death include the release of myoglobin, creatine phosphokinase, and potassium. Bacteremia is rare.
- The α-toxin has cardiodepressant activity and is considered the most clinically significant exotoxin.
- Mechanisms for infection with *Clostridium* include direct inoculation in open wounds and hematogenous spread in the immunocompromised.
- *Clostridium* thrives in contaminated wounds and wounds that offer an anaerobic environment.

CLINICAL FEATURES

- Also known as clostridial myonecrosis, gas gangrene presents with pain out of proportion to physical findings and a sense of heaviness in the affected part.
- Physical examination may reveal brawny edema, brownish skin, bullae, malodorous discharge, and crepitance.
- Crepitance is a late finding, and its absence does not exclude the diagnosis.
- Low-grade fever and tachycardia out of proportion to the fever are common findings.
- Delirium and irritability may be systemic manifestations of gas gangrene.

DIAGNOSIS AND DIFFERENTIAL

- Findings that may aid in confirming the diagnosis include gas in the soft tissues on plain radiographs, metabolic acidosis, leukocytosis, anemia, thrombocytopenia, myoglobinuria, and renal or hepatic dysfunction.
- If bullae are present, a Gram's stain of the fluid may reveal pleomorphic gram-positive bacilli with or without spores.
- The differential diagnosis includes other gas-forming infections such as necrotizing fasciitis, streptococcal myositis, and clostridial or nonclostridial anaerobic cellulitis.
- Other causes of crepitance should be excluded, including pneumothorax, laryngeal or tracheal fracture, and pneumomediastinum.

EMERGENCY DEPARTMENT CARE AND DISPOSITION

- The patient should be resuscitated with IV fluids as indicated. Packed red blood cells may be needed for resuscitation if there has been significant hemolysis.
- Vasoconstrictors should be avoided because of compromised perfusion in the affected part.
- Antibiotic therapy should be administered using penicillin G 24 million U/day in divided doses. Because mixed infections are common, the addition of an aminoglycoside, such as gentamicin 1 to 1.5 mg/kg every 8 hours, plus either a penicillinase-resistant penicillin such as nafcillin 2 g IV every 4 hours, or vancomycin 1 g IV every 12 hours, is recommended.
- In the penicillin allergic patient, clindamycin 600 to 900 mg IV every 8 hours, metronidazole 15 mg/kg loading dose then 7.5 mg/kg IV every 6 hours, or chloramphenicol may be used.
- Tetanus prophylaxis should be administered as indicated.
- The patient should be admitted for surgical débridement, hyperbaric oxygen (HBO) therapy, and continued IV antibiotics.

GAS GANGRENE (NONCLOSTRIDIAL MYONECROSIS)

PATHOPHYSIOLOGY

- A mixed infection involving aerobic and anaerobic bacteria.
- Clinical presentation, evaluation, and treatment are similar to that for clostridial myonecrosis. Only the differences will be discussed below.
- *Enterococcus* and *Staphylococcus* are the most commonly found organisms in this polymicrobial infection.

CLINICAL FEATURES

- The pain is not as pronounced as with clostridial myonecrosis.
- The higher mortality rate of nonclostridial myonecrosis is thought to be secondary to the lesser pain and subsequent delayed presentation.

EMERGENCY DEPARTMENT CARE AND DISPOSITION

- Broad-spectrum coverage for aerobic gram-positive and gram-negative organisms as well as anaerobes is necessary.

• Current recommendations include penicillin G 24 million U/day in divided doses, plus an aminoglycoside such as gentamicin 1 to 1.5 mg/kg every 8 hours, plus either metronidazole 15 mg/kg loading dose then 7.5 mg/kg IV every 6 hours, or clindamycin 600 to 900 mg IV every 8 hours. Early surgical debridement and HBO therapy as in clostridial myonecrosis is recommended.

NECROTIZING FASCIITIS

PATHOPHYSIOLOGY

• Extensive necrosis of the subcutaneous tissue and fascia.
• Does not spread to the underlying muscle.
• There is a polymicrobial form involving aerobic and anaerobic bacteria and a single-organism form caused by group A *Streptococcus*.
• Predisposing factors include diabetes, peripheral vascular disease, smoking, and IV drug abuse.
• The most common mechanisms for infection are soft tissue trauma and surgery.
• Risk for group A streptococcal disease is increased in concomitant varicella infection, particularly in children, and with use of nonsteroidal anti-inflammatory drugs (NSAIDs).

CLINICAL FEATURES

• Presenting complaint is typically pain out of proportion to physical findings.
• Erythema and edema are present early with vesicles and crepitance developing later.
• Low-grade fever and tachycardia may also be present.
• Can progress rapidly within several hours, especially GAS.
• GAS infections are more prone to bacteremia and toxic shock syndrome.

DIAGNOSIS AND DIFFERENTIAL

• Bedside soft tissue biopsy extending to the fascial plane may assist in the early diagnosis.
• Very early surgical consultation should be obtained in all suspected cases.

EMERGENCY DEPARTMENT CARE AND DISPOSITION

• Aggressive fluid and blood replacement as well as avoidance of vasopressors.

• Antibiotic therapy is the same as for nonclostridial myonecrosis. If group A *Streptococcus* is identified, penicillin G 24 million U/day plus clindamycin 600 to 900 mg IV every 8 hours are adequate coverage.
• Surgical debridement is the mainstay of therapy with subsequent HBO therapy in polymicrobial disease. Group A *Streptococcus* does not respond to hyperbaric oxygen therapy.

CELLULITIS

PATHOPHYSIOLOGY

• Cellulitis results from soft-tissue bacterial invasion, most commonly with *Staphylococcus* and *Streptococcus* in adults, and *Haemophilus influenzae* in nonimmunized children.
• In patients with diabetes mellitus, Enterobacteriaceae and *Clostridia* should be considered as etiologic agents in addition to *Staphylococcus* and *Streptococcus*.
• Local inflammation occurs at the site of infection and is responsible for the clinical manifestations.[2] In patients who are immunosuppressed, systemic involvement including bacteremia, fever, and leukocytosis may occur.

CLINICAL FEATURES

• Features of cellulitis include localized tenderness, warmth, erythema, and induration.
• Cellulitis may progress to lymphangitis and lymphadenitis, which indicate a more severe infection.
• Bacteremia may develop along with fever and chills, and is most commonly seen in immunocompromised patients.

DIAGNOSIS AND DIFFERENTIAL

• Diagnosis is usually based on clinical findings.
• If there is evidence of bacteremia or in patients with immune compromise, blood cultures and leukocyte counts are indicated.
• The differential diagnosis includes any erythematous skin condition.
• Cellulitis may be complicated by deep venous thrombosis. If there is evidence of venous obstruction, a venogram or Doppler study should be performed.

EMERGENCY DEPARTMENT CARE AND DISPOSITION

• Simple cellulitis can be treated in an outpatient setting using PO dicloxacillin 500 mg every 6 hours, amoxicillin-clavulanate 875 mg/125 mg PO every 12 hours, or a macrolide such as clarithromycin 500 mg PO every 12 hours, for 10 days.

- All patients discharged should have close follow-up to evaluate the patient's cellulitis and response to therapy.
- Patients with diabetes mellitus, alcoholism, evidence of bacteremia, or other immunosuppressive disorders, and all patients with significant cellulitis involving the head or neck should be admitted for IV antibiotics.
- IV antibiotics such as a first-generation cephalosporin (cefazolin 1 g IV every 6 hours) or a penicillinase-resistant penicillin (nafcillin 2 g IV every 4 hours) may be used unless the patient has diabetes.
- In patients with diabetes, ceftriaxone 1 to 2 g IV can be used, or in severe cases imipenem 500 mg IV every 6 hours is indicated.
- In patients with diabetes, ceftriaxone may be used, while imipenem may be used in severe cases of cellulitis.[3]

ERYSIPELAS

PATHOPHYSIOLOGY

- Erysipelas is a superficial cellulitis with lymphatic involvement usually caused by group A *Streptococcus.*
- Inoculation occurs through a portal in the skin.
- Peripheral vascular disease is a significant risk factor for erysipelas.
- Most commonly the infection involves the lower extremities.

CLINICAL FEATURES

- Erysipelas has an acute onset with fever, chills, malaise, and nausea.
- A small area of erythema with a burning sensation then develops over the next 1 to 2 days.
- The erythema is sharply demarcated and is tense and painful.
- Lymphangitis and lymphadenitis commonly develop.
- Purpura, bullae, and necrosis may occur with the erythema.

DIAGNOSIS AND DIFFERENTIAL

- Diagnosis is based primarily on physical findings.
- Differential diagnosis includes other types of local cellulitis.

EMERGENCY DEPARTMENT CARE AND DISPOSITION

- Penicillin G 1 to 2 million U IV every 6 hours may be used in nondiabetic patients.
- Penicillinase-resistant penicillins such as nafcillin 2 g IV every 4 hours, or parental second- or third-generation cephalosporins such as ceftriaxone 1 to 2 g/day, should be used in diabetic patients and in those with facial involvement.
- Imipenem 500 mg IV every 6 hours is indicated in severe cases.
- In patients allergic to penicillin, a macrolide may be used, such as azithromycin 500 mg/day IV for 2 days then PO.
- Except in clearly mild cases, patients are admitted for IV antibiotics.

CUTANEOUS ABSCESSES

PATHOPHYSIOLOGY

- Cutaneous abscesses result from the breakdown of the cutaneous barrier and subsequent contamination with bacteria. The bacteria cause necrosis and liquefaction followed by loculation and walling off to form the abscess.
- *Staphylococcal* species are most often the causative organism.
- Streptococci may be the etiologic agent in tissues surrounding the oral and nasal mucosa.
- Intertriginous and perineal skin may become infected with *Escherichia coli, Proteus mirabilis,* and *Klebsiella* species.
- Axillary abscesses are frequently caused by *P. mirabilis.*
- Perirectal abscesses and abscesses in the genital region are frequently mixed anaerobic and aerobic species. *Bacteroides* is the most common anaerobe infecting these regions.
- Abscesses secondary to foreign bodies usually are caused by *S. aureus.*

CLINICAL FEATURES

- Abscesses present with an area of swelling, tenderness, and erythema. This area is usually localized and often fluctuant.

DIAGNOSIS AND DIFFERENTIAL

- The diagnosis is clinical, with findings of a central area of fluctuance correlating with the collection of purulent exudate.

- Occasionally the presence of an abscess will need to be confirmed by needle aspiration.
- Ultrasound or radiography should be considered if there is the possibility of a foreign body.

EMERGENCY DEPARTMENT CARE AND DISPOSITION

- Conscious sedation should be considered in all patients who require incision and drainage (I&D) (see Chap. 12).
- Bartholin's gland abscess is a unilateral infection of the labia. *Neisseria gonorrhoeae* and *Chlamydia trachomatis* are common isolates from these abscesses. Treatment involves I&D along the vaginal mucosal surface of the abscess and then insertion of a Word catheter. Antibiotics are generally not needed unless a sexually transmitted disease is suspected.
- Hidradenitis suppurativa is a recurrent infection of the apocrine sweat glands, typically in the axilla and the groin. The most common isolate is *Staphylococcus,* although *Streptococcus* may also be present. These abscesses are typically multiple and in different stages of development. Treatment in the ED should include I&D of acute abscesses, antibiotics for cellulitis if present, and referral to a surgeon.
- Infected sebaceous cysts occur in sebaceous glands, which are located throughout the skin. I&D is the appropriate treatment, with wound recheck in 2 to 3 days in the ED or surgeon's office.
- Pilonidal abscess presents along the superior gluteal fold. I&D should be performed with iodoform gauze packing. The wound should be rechecked in 2 to 3 days, the packing removed, and the wound repacked. Antibiotics should be given if there is accompanying cellulitis. Surgical referral should be made for definitive treatment.
- Staphylococcal soft tissue abscess may present in several ways. Folliculitis occurs with bacterial invasion and subsequent inflammation of a hair follicle. Folliculitis can usually be treated with warm compresses. If deeper invasion occurs and surrounding soft tissues become infected, a furuncle (boil) is formed. Warm compresses usually promote spontaneous drainage. When several furuncles coalesce, they may form large interconnected sinus tracts and abscesses called a carbuncle. Carbuncles usually require surgical referral for wide excision and are seen more commonly in diabetics.
- Ultrasound or radiography should be considered if there is the possibility of a foreign body.
- In healthy immunocompetent patients antibiotics are not necessary unless there is secondary infection.
- If the patient is immunocompromised, the threshold for antibiotic use should be lowered.

- Patients with secondary cellulitis or systemic symptoms should be given antibiotics.
- Abscesses involving the face and hands should also be given antibiotics.
- Appropriate choices if antibiotics are used include a first-generation cephalosporin such as cephalexin 500 mg PO every 6 hours, clindamycin 300 mg PO every 6 hours, or amoxicillin-clavulanate 875 mg/ 125 mg PO every 12 hours.
- Prophylactic antibiotics should be considered in patients with structural cardiac abnormalities (see Chap. 92).

SPOROTRICHOSIS

PATHOPHYSIOLOGY

- This disease is caused by traumatic inoculation of the fungus *Sporothrix schenckii,* which is found on plants and in the soil.[4]

CLINICAL FEATURES

- The incubation period is 3 weeks.
- Three types of infection may present. The fixed cutaneous type presents as a crusted ulcer or a verrucous plaque at the site of inoculation. The local cutaneous type also is at the site of inoculation, but presents as a subcutaneous nodule or pustule with or without surrounding erythema. The lymphocutaneous type (most common) presents as a painless nodule at the site of inoculation and develops subcutaneous nodules with migration through lymphatic channels.
- All three types of infection tend to be associated with minimal pain, but do not improve until antibiotic therapy is initiated.

DIAGNOSIS AND DIFFERENTIAL

- The diagnosis is based on history and physical examination.
- Tissue biopsy cultures may yield a diagnosis but are of limited use in the ED.
- The differential diagnosis includes tuberculosis, tularemia, cat-scratch disease, leishmaniasis, nocardiosis, and staphylococcal lymphangitis.

EMERGENCY DEPARTMENT CARE AND DISPOSITION

- Itraconazole for 3 to 6 months is effective when treating sporotrichosis.[5]

- If disseminated, sporotrichosis may be treated with IV amphotericin B.
- Most patients with cutaneous sporotrichosis can be treated as outpatients.
- Patients with systemic symptoms should be admitted for treatment with amphotericin B.

REFERENCES

1. Corey E: Non-traumatic gas gangrene: Case report and review of emergency therapeutics. *J Emerg Med* 9:431, 1991.
2. Sachs M: Cutaneous cellulitis. *Arch Dermatol* 127:493, 1991.
3. Sanford J, Gilbert D, Moellering R, et al: *The Sanford Guide to Antimicrobial Therapy,* 31st ed. Dallas: Antimicrobial Therapy, Inc., 2001.
4. Dixon D, Salkin I, Duncan R, et al: Isolation and characterization of *Sporothrix schenckii* from clinical and environmental sources associated with the largest U.S. epidemic of sporotrichosis. *J Clin Microbiol* 29:1106, 1991.
5. Stalkup J, Bell K, Rosen T: Disseminated cutaneous sporotrichosis treated with itraconazole. *Cutis* 69:371, 2002.

For further reading in *Emergency Medicine: A Comprehensive Study Guide,* 6th ed., see Chap. 152, "Soft Tissue Infections," by Steven G. Folstad.

98 BIOTERRORISM

Roy L. Alson

- Because of similar presentations between biological weapons and endemic diseases, detection can be difficult.
- Challenges faced by the clinician include detecting an attack, identification of the agent, lack of familiarity with the diseases, initiating treatment and/or prophylaxis, and dealing with the psychosocial implications of such an attack.[1,2]

RESPONSE PLANNING

- Local resources for sheltering, decontamination, and treatment of multiple patients must be identified prior to the event.[1-3]
- Planning should include how to notify state and federal agencies and how to integrate outside assets such as the National Pharmaceutical Stockpile (NPS) into

the operation, as well as dealing with the potential for large numbers of fatalities. In addition, bioterrorist events are also crime scenes and personnel will have to assist the FBI and other law enforcement agencies. Preplanning should involve emergency management, EMS, fire, law enforcement and the medical community.

DETECTION OF AN ATTACK

- A biological weapon (BW) attack may be difficult to recognize. The signs and symptoms of the agent may be similar to more common or even endemic illnesses in the area. Complicating the issue is a lack of rapid and reliable tests for most BW agents.
- Many tests require specimens to be sent to state or federal laboratories, which can be overwhelmed during a suspected attack (as was seen during the anthrax attack in the U.S. in the fall of 2001).
- Clinicians must be aware of the common presenting signs and symptoms of BWs. When confronted with a cluster of patients who fit the pattern of signs and symptoms, or even a single patient with appropriate findings and history, the clinician should initiate notification of public health authorities and begin appropriate testing and treatment.
- Real-time testing of suspect specimens and specific diagnostic tests for most BWs are still under development. Thus emergency physicians must combine knowledge of specific disease processes with information regarding the characteristics of thc (possible) exposure, in order to stratify the risk to the patient and community. These same factors will determine the initiation of therapy and activation of local responses.

RESPONSE ACTIONS

- All emergency departments (EDs) should have in place a plan to deal with contaminated and/or BW victims.
- Once identified as possibly exposed or infected, the patient should be placed into the appropriate area, based on the suspected agent and mode of transmission. Staff should all wear appropriate personal protective equipment (PPE). At a minimum this should consist of gowns, gloves, eye protection, and a high-efficiency particulate air (HEPA) mask.
- Information collected from patients should include occupation, travel history, social events, recent close contacts, and what steps if any have been taken for treatment and/or decontamination.
- Contact the local health department and hospital epidemiologist, as well as the hospital media relations representative. Accurate information, distributed ap-

propriately to the public, will decrease the number of "worried well" who will seek care and effectively clog up the system. To be effective, the BW response plan must be integrated into both the hospital and community disaster response plan.

SPECIFIC AGENTS

- The Centers for Disease Control and Prevention (CDC) has divided BW agents into three classes based on their ability to impact a community, the ease of dissemination, and requirements for management.
- Class A agents are easily disseminated and cause widespread disease and/or death (Table 98-1).
- Class B agents pose less of a threat, either because of the disease caused or difficulties in dissemination.
- Class C agents are those that can be a threat in the future. Anthrax, plague, and tularemia are discussed in Chap. 96 of this manual. Class B and class C agents are discussed in Chap. 7 of *Emergency Medicine: A Comprehensive Study Guide,* 6th ed.
- Bioweapons agents may either be live, infectious agents or toxins produced by organisms. Toxins be-

have like chemical agents once they enter the body, while infectious organisms induce specific diseases.
- Infectious agents can be classified as contagious or not. Contagious BW agents include smallpox, plague, and viral hemorrhagic fevers (Ebola, Marburg, etc). Many infectious BW agents are zoonoses and veterinarians may be an additional information resource.

SMALLPOX

- Having been eradicated in the wild due to vaccination, it presents a high risk due to suspension of vaccination programs and because prior vaccination does not convey lifelong immunity.
- The virus is transmitted by droplet nuclei with an incubation time of 10 to 14 days. A prodrome of flu-like symptoms, with headache (HA), myalgias, and fevers, is followed 2 to 4 days later with a macular rash.
- The rash can involve palms and soles and unlike chickenpox, all of the lesions appear to be the same age. The rash progresses to vesicles and then pustules, finally scabbing over.

TABLE 98-1 Class A Biological Agents

AGENT	DISEASE	SIGNS AND SYMPTOMS	PROPHYLAXIS	TREATMENT
Variola major	Smallpox	10–14 days incubation; prodrome flu like with fever, myalgias; rash, face to trunk; vesicles to pustules all of same age; contagious until scabs fall off	Vaccine within 3 days protective; mortality 30% if unvaccinated	Supportive treatment
Bacillus anthracis	Cutaneous anthrax	1–14 days until macule or papule developing into eschar	Vaccine available to military; ciprofloxacin for up to 2 months; doxycycline also effective	Respiratory support for inhalational form; ciprofloxacin or doxycycline plus two others: clindamycin, aminoglycoside, vancomycin, streptomycin
	Inhalational anthrax	<1 week (up to 6 weeks); flu-like symptoms, cough, dyspnea; wide mediastinum on x-ray, then cardiovascular collapse and death (see text for info on GI symptoms)		
Yersinia pestis	Bubonic plague	2–8 days incubation; fever, chills, suppurative nodes, buboes	Ciprofloxacin or doxycycline for 7–10 days	Treat sepsis and pulmonary failure; streptomycin or gentamicin; ciprofloxacin also useful
	Pneumonic plague	2–3 days incubation; fever, chills, cough, SOB, becomes septic; contagious		
	Septicemic plague	2–8 days incubation; fever, chills, suppurative nodes; buboes, then becomes septic		
Clostridium botulinum	Food-borne botulism	1–5 days incubation; GI symptoms; N/V, followed by progressive bulbar palsies; descending paralysis	Not applicable	Support ventilation, need may be prolonged; administer antitoxin from CDC
	Inhalational botulism	May not have GI symptoms; will have descending paralysis		
Francisella tularensis	Tularemia	2–5 days incubation followed by febrile illness which can progress to pneumonitis; may have ulcerative skin lesions	Investigational vaccine; ciprofloxacin or doxycycline for 14 days	Streptomycin or ciprofloxacin or doxycycline
Filoviruses and arenavirus	Viral hemorrhagic fevers	2 days to 3 weeks incubation; flu-like illness with fever, progresses to GI bleeding, shock and death; contagious	None	Supportive care; 90% mortality; Ribavirin may be helpful

ABBREVIATIONS: CDC = Centers for Disease Control; GI = gastrointestinal; N/V = nausea and vomiting; SOB = shortness of breath.

- The patient is contagious until the scabs slough (17 to 21 days).
- Vaccine (vaccinia) given within 3 days of exposure is protective.
- Exposed persons should be quarantined for 18 days.
- Care of infected patient is supportive. Mortality of unvaccinated persons is about 30%, with flat and hemorrhagic forms having higher mortality.

BOTULISM

- Botulinum toxin is produced by *Clostridium botulinum,* a spore-forming obligate anaerobe found throughout the world.[4]
- The toxin (with seven different antigenic types) blocks acetylcholine release at the synapse, causing a flaccid paralysis.
- Natural cases are either food-borne (consumption of toxin) or wound or intestinal infection. Inhalation of toxin can occur and is felt to be the best route for weaponization.
- Symptoms begin 12 to 72 hours postinhalation and from 1 to 4 days after oral intake. The patient, who remains alert, is afebrile and develops multiple cranial nerve palsies.
- Care is symptomatic, as death is usually from respiratory failure. Antitoxin should be given. Avoid aminoglycosides, which can worsen paralysis.

RICIN

- Ricin is a by-product of the extraction of castor oil from the castor bean (*Ricinus communis*).
- It can be inhaled or ingested and has been used as an injected assassination weapon. It causes cell destruction by interfering with protein synthesis.
- Symptom onset varies with route of exposure. Inhalation (the most likely weaponized route) causes fever, cough, chest tightness, and weakness, leading to pulmonary edema and cardiovascular collapse.
- With ingestion, GI symptoms predominate. Death follows in 36 to 48 hours. No known antidote exists.
- Treatment is supportive.

EBOLA AND MARBURG VIRUSES

- Viral hemorrhagic fevers (*Filovirus* and *Arenavirus*) such as Ebola and Marburg are highly contagious via person-to-person contact.
- Following a 3- to 21-day incubation period, a prodrome of high fever and myalgias is followed by GI

and other mucosal bleeding, petechiae, edema, hypotension, and finally cardiovascular collapse.
- Mortality approaches 90%.
- Strict isolation in a negative pressure room plus the use of HEPA masks and gowns are key to limiting spread.
- Ribavirin may be effective postexposure against Argentine hemorrhagic fever.

MANAGEMENT ISSUES

- Decontamination of exposed persons who may have agents on them is important to limit spread.[1,3] Removal of contaminated clothing followed by showering with soap and water is effective.
- Bag clothing as evidence.
- The use of dilute hypochlorite bleach should be limited to decontaminating surfaces and equipment.
- Staff will need to wear appropriate protective equipment. Be aware that prolonged wearing of such gear can cause both physical and psychological stress on staff members.
- As this field is evolving rapidly, additional information can be found at these websites: CDC: http://www.bt.cdc.gov, the *Journal of the American Medical Association:* http://pubs.ama-assn.org/bioterror.html, and the U.S. Army Research Institute for Infectious Diseases: http://www.usamriid.army.mil.

REFERENCES

1. Kiem M, Kaufman A: Principles of emergency response to bioterrorism. *Ann Emerg Med* 34:177, 1991.
2. Association for Professionals in Infection Control and Epidemiology Bioterrorism Taskforce: Bioterrorism Readiness Plan: A Template for Healthcare Facilities, April 1991, available at www.apic.org/educ/readiness.cfm
3. U.S. Army Medical Research Institute for Infectious Diseases: Medical Management of Biologic Casualties Handbook, USAMRIID. Fort Dietrick, MD: 2001.
4. Arnon S et al: Botulinum toxin as a biological weapon. *JAMA* 285:1097, 2001.

For further reading in *Emergency Medicine: A Comprehensive Study Guide,* 6th ed., see Chap. 7, "Bioterrorism Response: Implications for the Emergency Clinician," by Anthony G. Macintyre and Joseph A. Barbera.

99 THE TRANSPLANT PATIENT

David M. Cline

- Compromised response to infection and other side effects of immunosuppressive medication are common to all transplant recipients. Disorders specific to the transplanted organ are manifestations of acute rejection, surgical complications specific to the procedure performed, and altered physiology (most important in cardiac transplantation). Also the management of routine injuries or illnesses may be complicated by the patient's immunosuppressed state of medication.

POSTTRANSPLANT INFECTIOUS COMPLICATIONS

CLINICAL FEATURES

- Infection is the most common cause of mortality and morbidity for transplant patients in the first year.[1,2]
- Predisposing factors to posttransplant infections include ongoing immunosuppression in all patients and the presence of diabetes mellitus, advanced age, obesity, and other host factors in some.
- Table 99-1 displays the broad array of potential infections and the time after transplant they are most apt to occur.[2,3]
- The most common infection in recipients of solid organs, especially in bone marrow graft recipients, is cytomegalovirus (CMV). This infection may manifest with daily fever and malaise in its mildest form. Progressively more serious disease manifestations include leukopenia, hepatopathy (elevated transaminase enzymes), enteropathy (epigastric pain and diarrhea), and pneumonitis. Mortality associated with CMV pneumonitis exceeds 50%.
- During active CMV infection, immunosuppression is maintained at the minimum possible level and, if liver, gut, or pulmonary involvement is documented, intravenous ganciclovir therapy, often in conjunction with immune globulin, is prescribed.
- The initial presentation of a potentially life-threatening infectious illness may be quite subtle in transplant recipients. The transplant recipient receiving glucocorticoids may not mount an impressive febrile response.
- Central nervous system (CNS) infections are more common in transplant recipients than in other patients. Common etiologies include *Listeria monocytogenes* and cryptococci.
- A significant subset of renal transplant recipients have undergone intentional splenectomy to improve

TABLE 99-1 Infectious Complications of Whole-Organ Transplantation

FIRST MONTH POSTTRANSPLANT
Bacterial
Wound infection (*Staphylococcus aureus*, *S. epidermidis*, gram-negative bacilli)
Pneumonia (gram-negative bacilli)
Urinary tract infection (gram-negative bacilli, enterococcus)
Line-related sepsis (*S. aureus*, *S. epidermidis*, gram-negative bacilli)
Intra-abdominal infections (liver transplant)
Viral
HSV
Fungal
Candidal pharyngitis, esophagitis, cystitis
SECOND TO SIXTH MONTH POSTTRANSPLANT
Bacterial
Pneumonia: pneumococcal and other community acquired
Meningitis (*Listeria monocytogenes*)
Urinary tract infection
Nocardial infection
Listeriosis
Viral
Cytomegalovirus, EBV, HSV, varicella zoster
Adenovirus
Hepatitis A, B, C
Fungal
Aspergillosis
Candidal pharyngitis, esophagitis, cystitis
Other opportunistic infections
Pneumocystis carinii pneumonia, tuberculosis, toxoplasmosis
BEYOND SIXTH MONTH POSTTRANSPLANT
Bacterial
Pneumonia: pneumococcal and other community acquired
Urinary tract infection
Listeriosis
Viral
Cytomegalovirus chorioretinitis
Varicella zoster
Hepatitis C, B
Fungal
Cryptococcal
Other opportunistic infections
P. carinii pneumonia

ABBREVIATIONS: HSV = herpes simplex virus; EBV = Epstein-Barr virus.

allograft survival. Although this procedure is no longer routinely practiced, these patients, as in other postsplenectomy patients, are at particularly high risk for overwhelming sepsis caused by encapsulated bacteria such as pneumococci or meningococci.
- Liver transplant patients are especially susceptible to intra-abdominal infections during the first postoperative month.
- Lung transplant patients are especially prone to pneumonia during the first 3 postoperative months.
- Cardiac transplant patients may develop mediastinitis during the first postoperative month.

DIAGNOSIS AND DIFFERENTIAL

- A patient presenting with a febrile illness should have as part of their assessment a complete blood cell count, chest radiograph, and measurement of renal and liver function.
- Therefore, complaints of recurrent headaches, with or without fever, should be investigated vigorously, first with a structural study to exclude a mass lesion (CNS lymphomas occur with increased frequency), then with a lumbar puncture.
- A nonproductive cough with few or no findings on physical examination may be the only clue to emerging *Pneumocystis carinii* pneumonia or CMV pneumonia. The threshold for obtaining chest radiographs for these patients should be low.
- Viral infections produce significant morbidity and mortality in transplant recipients, and pose difficult diagnostic challenges because cultures are not very sensitive.[4]

EMERGENCY DEPARTMENT CARE AND DISPOSITION

- Drug choice, dose, and ultimate management should be accomplished in consultation with the transplant team.
- For skin and superficial wounds, probable offending organisms are gram-positive cocci, especially *Staphylococcus aureus,* and treatment should be with a penicillinase-resistant penicillin such as nafcillin or oxacillin 1 to 2 g IV every 4 hours, or a first-generation cephalosporin such as cefazolin, 2 g IV every 8 hours.
- If there is suspicion of methicillin-resistant organisms or sensitivity to β-lactams, vancomycin 1 g IV every 12 hours should be used.
- Nosocomial pneumonia is likely due to gram-negative organisms such as *Escherichia coli, Enterobacter,* or *Pseudomonas.* Treatment options include imipenem 500 mg IV every 6 hours, meropenem 1 g IV every 8 hours, cefotaxime 1 to 2 g IV every 6 to 8 hours plus gentamicin 1 to 2 mg/kg IV every 8 hours, or piperacillin-tazobactam 3.375 g IV every 6 hours. Community-acquired pneumonia should be treated as such with a fluoroquinolone such as levofloxacin 500 mg IV every day, with the proviso that opportunistic infection may also be present.
- Intra-abdominal infection may be due to enterococci, gram-negative bacilli, or anaerobes, and sometimes *S. aureus.* Triple coverage may be necessary empirically, with ampicillin 500 mg IV every 6 hours or vancomycin plus an aminoglycoside such as gentamicin to treat enterococci; a broad-spectrum penicillin or second- or third-generation cephalosporin such as piperacillin or cefotaxime and clindamycin 900 mg IV every 8 hours to treat gram-negative organisms; or metronidazole 500 mg IV every 12 hours to treat anaerobes. Penicillins with β-lactamase inhibitors such as ticarcillin-sulbactam 3.1 g IV every 6 hours or ampicillin-sulbactam 3 g IV every 6 hours have broad coverage against gram-positive cocci, gram-negative bacilli, and anaerobes.
- Meningitis is frequently due to *Listeria monocytogenes,* and patients with suspected meningitis should be treated with ampicillin 2 g IV every 4 hours plus cefotaxime 2 g IV every 6 hours. Consider adding vancomycin.
- The mainstay of fungal treatment has been amphotericin B 0.7 mg/kg/day IV; however, fluconazole 400 mg daily IV is an alternative. *Candida albicans* can be treated first with fluconazole 100 mg/day PO.
- Viral therapy depends on the disease syndrome and the offending agent. CMV disease is treated with ganciclovir, with a dose of 5 mg/kg IV twice daily.
- Varicella and herpes simplex virus are typically treated with acyclovir 800 mg IV five times per day for dissemination or ocular involvement. Acyclovir has renal excretion and the dose must be adjusted for renal insufficiency. Epstein-Barr virus (EBV) is typically treated with a reduction in the immunosuppressive regimen.
- Treatment of choice for *P. carinii* pneumonia is with trimethoprim-sulfamethoxazole (TMP-SMX), 15 mg of TMP component/kg/day IV divided every 8 hours while critically ill. Prednisone should be given before TMP-SMX. Oral therapy is TMP-SMX double strength, 2 tabs PO every 8 hours for 3 weeks total therapy. Pentamidine, 4 mg/kg/day IV or IM for 3 weeks, is reserved as an alternative therapy if TMP-SMX is not tolerated.
- Toxoplasmosis can be treated initially with pyrimethamine 50 to 100 mg PO plus sulfadiazine 1 to 1.5 g PO plus folinic acid 10 mg PO.
- Urinary tract infections, invasive gastroenteritis (due to *Salmonella, Campylobacter,* and *Listeria*), and diverticulitis can be treated with the usual antimicrobial agents.

COMPLICATIONS OF IMMUNOSUPPRESSIVE AGENTS

- Therapeutic immunosuppression is accompanied by a number of side effects and complications (Table 99-2). Combined toxicities can produce or worsen pre-existing renal insufficiency, hypertension, and hyperglycemia.
- Elevated cyclosporine levels cause renal arteriolar constriction, which reduces glomerular blood flow and stimulates the renin-angiotensin system, and elevates blood pressure.

TABLE 99-2   Antirejection Medication Side Effects

Cyclosporine
  Nephrotoxicity
  Neurotoxicity
  Hyperkalemia
  Hypomagnesemia
  Hyperuricemia
  Hypertension
  Anorexia
  Hyperbilirubinemia
  Cholestasis
  Gastric dysmotility
  Hirsutism
  Hypercholesterolemia

Tacrolimus
  Nephrotoxicity
  Neurotoxicity
  Hyperkalemia
  Hypomagnesemia
  Hyperglycemia
  Anemia
  Headache
  Diarrhea
  Hypertension
  Nausea

Azathioprine
  Leukopenia
  Thrombocytopenia
  Cholestatic jaundice
  Alopecia

Mycophenolate mofetil
  Diarrhea
  Abdominal pain
  Vomiting
  Leukopenia
  Anemia
  Peripheral edema

Prednisone
  Cushing's syndrome
  Osteoporosis
  Adrenal suppression
  Hypertension
  Hyperglycemia
  Peptic ulcer disease
  Myopathy
  Cataracts
  Poor wound healing

- Glucocorticoids promote renal salt and water retention, which further aggravate hypertension.
- A headache syndrome often indistinguishable from migraine is common in transplant recipients and usually develops within the first 2 months of immunosuppression. An important differential must include infectious causes and malignancy when headache first presents, and usually requires a head computed tomography (CT) scan with subsequent biochemical analysis of cerebrospinal fluid.[5]
- Recently, the newer immunosuppressive agents tacrolimus and mycophenolate mofetil have been used in place of cyclosporine and azathioprine, respectively.[6,7] The most common side effects of tacrolimus are similar to those of cyclosporine. The most common side effects of mycophenolate mofetil are diarrhea, vomiting, leukopenia, and increased opportunistic infections, especially CMV.[8]

- Sirolimus is the newest macrolide antibiotic with immunosuppressive effects (similar to tacrolimus). Unlike tacrolimus, it does not induce hypertension, diabetes, or neurologic adverse effects. The major side effects are bone marrow suppression and hyperlipidemia.[9]
- Overall, the risk of coronary artery disease posttransplant is three- to fivefold that for age- and sex-matched control subjects.[10]
- Any illness that prevents transplant patients from taking or retaining their immunosuppressive therapy warrants hospital admission for intravenous therapy, preferably at a transplant center.
- Starting even simple medications can precipitate complications. For example, nonsteroidal anti-inflammatory drugs may increase nephrotoxicity. In general, any new medications should be discussed with a representative of the patient's transplant team.

CARDIAC TRANSPLANTATION

- Transplantation results in a denervated heart that does not respond with centrally medicated tachycardia in response to stress or exercise, but does respond to circulating catecholamines and increased preload.[11] Patients may complain of fatigue or shortness of breath with the onset of exercise, which resolves with continued exertion as an appropriate tachycardia develops.
- The donor heart is implanted with its sinus node intact to preserve normal atrioventricular conduction. The normal heart rate for a transplanted heart is 90 to 100 beats per minute.
- The technique of cardiac transplantation also results in the preservation of the recipient's sinus node at the superior cavoatrial junction. The atrial suture line renders the two sinus nodes electrically isolated from each other. Thus electrocardiograms (ECGs) will frequently have two distinct P waves. The sinus node of the donor heart is easily identified by its constant 1:1 relationship to the QRS complex, whereas the native P wave marches through the donor heart rhythm independently.

CLINICAL FEATURES

- Because the heart is denervated, myocardial ischemia does not present with angina. Instead, recipients present with heart failure secondary to silent myocardial infarctions or with sudden death.

- Transplant recipients who present with new-onset shortness of breath, chest fullness, or symptoms of congestive heart failure (CHF) should be evaluated in routine fashion with ECG and serial cardiac enzyme levels for the presence of myocardial ischemia or infarction.
- Although most episodes of acute rejection are asymptomatic, symptoms can occur. The most common presenting symptoms are dysrhythmias and generalized fatigue. The development of either atrial or ventricular dysrhythmias in a cardiac transplant recipient (or CHF) must be assumed due to acute rejection until proven otherwise.
- In children, rejection may present with low-grade fever, fussiness, and poor feeding.

EMERGENCY DEPARTMENT CARE AND DISPOSITION

- Consultation: Differentiating rejection from other acute illnesses in the transplant patient can be difficult. Treatment for rejection without biopsy confirmation is contraindicated except when patients are hemodynamically unstable.
- Rejection: Management of acute rejection is 1 g of methylprednisolone IV, after consultation with a representative from the transplant center.
- Dysrhythmias: If patients are hemodynamically compromised by dysrhythmias, empiric therapy for rejection with methylprednisolone 1 g IV may be given after consultation. Atropine has no effect on the denervated heart; isoproterenol is the drug of choice for bradydysrhythmias in these patients.[11] Patients who present in extremis should be treated with standard cardiopulmonary resuscitation measures.
- Hypotension: Low-output syndrome, or hypotension, should be treated with inotropic agents such as dopamine or dobutamine when specific treatment for rejection is instituted.
- Hospitalization: Transplant patients suspected of having rejection or acute illness should be hospitalized, preferably at the transplant center if stable for transfer.

LUNG TRANSPLANTATION

CLINICAL FEATURES

- Clinically, patients with rejection may have cough, chest tightness, fatigue, and fever (>0.5°C above baseline).[12] Acute rejection may manifest with frightening rapidity, causing a severe decline in patient status in only a day.
- Isolated fever may be the only finding; in contrast, spirometry may show a 15% drop in forced expiratory volume in 1 second (FEV_1), and examination may reveal rales and adventitious sounds.
- Chest radiograph may demonstrate bilateral interstitial infiltrates, septal lines, and effusions. The radiograph may be normal, however, when rejection occurs late in the course. The longer the period of time a patient is from transplant, the less classic a chest x-ray may appear for acute rejection.
- Infection, such as interstitial pneumonia, may present with a clinical picture similar to acute rejection. Diagnostically, bronchoscopy with transbronchial biopsy is usually needed, not only to confirm rejection, but to exclude infection.
- Two late complications of lung transplant are obliterative bronchiolitis and posttransplant lymphoproliferative disease (PTLD).[13,14] Obliterative bronchiolitis presents with episodes of recurrent bronchitis, small airway obliteration, wheezing, and eventually respiratory failure. PTLD is associated with Epstein-Barr virus and presents with painful lymphadenopathy and otitis media (due to tonsillar involvement), or may present with malaise, fever, and myalgia.
- Evaluation of the lung transplant patient should include chest radiograph, arterial blood gas analysis, complete blood cell count (CBC), serum electrolytes, creatinine, magnesium levels, and appropriate drug levels.

EMERGENCY DEPARTMENT CARE AND DISPOSITION

- Consultation: Communication should be made directly with the transplant center (often a nurse coordinator). Coordinators should have the patients' current medication doses, recent infection history, and knowledge of complications for which patients may be at risk.
- Rejection: If clinically indicated (ie, infection is excluded), methylprednisolone 500 to 1000 mg IV should be given. Patients who have a history of seizures associated with the administration of high-dose glucocorticoids will also need concurrent benzodiazepines to prevent further seizure episodes.
- Late complications: Obliterative bronchiolitis is treated with increased immunosuppression, whereas PTLD is treated with reduced immunosuppression. These decisions should be made by specialists from the transplant center.

RENAL TRANSPLANT

CLINICAL FEATURES

- Diagnosis and treatment of acute rejection is most critical. Without timely recognition and intervention, allograft function may deteriorate irreversibly in a few days.[15] When symptomatic from acute rejection, renal transplant recipients complain of vague tenderness over the allograft (in the left or right iliac fossa).

- Patients may also describe decreased urine output, rapid weight gain (from fluid retention), low-grade fever, and generalized malaise.[16]

- Physical examination may disclose worsening hypertension, allograft tenderness, and peripheral edema.

- However, the absence of these symptoms and signs does not exclude the possibility of acute rejection.

- With improved methods of maintenance immunosuppression, the only clue may be an asymptomatic decline in renal function. Even a change in creatinine levels from 1.0 mg/dL to 1.2 or 1.3 mg/dL may be important. When such changes in creatinine levels are reproducible, a careful work-up consists of complete urinalysis, renal ultrasonography, and a trough level of cyclosporine (if appropriate), in addition to a careful history and examination. It is critical to interpret changes in renal function in the context of prior data (eg, trends of recent serum creatinine levels, recent history of rejection, or other causes of allograft dysfunction).

- Evaluation should consider the multiple etiologies of decreased renal function in the renal transplant recipient. The two most common causes, apart from acute rejection causing an increase in creatinine, are volume contraction and cyclosporine-induced nephrotoxicity.

EMERGENCY DEPARTMENT CARE AND DISPOSITION

- Consultation: Communication should be made directly with the transplant center (often a nurse coordinator). Coordinators should have the patients' current medication doses, recent infection history, and knowledge of complications for which patients may be at risk.

- Rejection: Treatment of allograft rejection consists of high-dose glucocorticoids, typically methylprednisolone (250 to 500 mg IV).

LIVER TRANSPLANT

CLINICAL FEATURES

- Though frequently subtle in presentation, a syndrome of acute rejection includes fever, liver tenderness, lymphocytosis, eosinophilia, liver enzyme elevation, and a change in bile color or production.

- In the perioperative period, the differential diagnosis must include infection, acute biliary obstruction, or vascular insufficiency.

- Diagnosis can be made with certainty only by hepatic ultrasound and biopsy, which usually requires referral back to the transplant center for management and follow-up.

- Three possible surgical complications in liver transplant patients are biliary obstruction, biliary leakage, and hepatic artery thrombosis.[17]

- Biliary obstruction follows three typical presentations. The most common is intermittent episodes of fever and fluctuating liver function tests. The second is a gradual worsening of liver function tests without symptoms. Finally, obstruction may present as acute bacterial cholangitis with fever, chills, abdominal pain, jaundice, and bacteremia.

- It can be difficult to distinguish clinically from rejection, hepatic artery thrombosis, CMV infection, or a recurrence of a pre-existing disease, especially hepatitis.

- Patients most often have peritoneal signs and fever, but these signs may be masked by concomitant use of steroids and immunosuppressive agents.

- Presentation is signaled by elevated PT and transaminase levels and little or no bile production, but this complication may also present as acute graft failure, liver abscess, unexplained sepsis, or a biliary tract problem (leak, obstruction, abscess, or breakdown of the anastomosis).

- If a biliary complication is suspected, all patients should have a CBC; serum chemistry levels; liver function tests; amylase and lipase levels; cultures of blood, urine, bile, and ascites, if present; chest x-ray; and abdominal ultrasound.

- Ultrasound rules out the presence of fluid collections, screens for the presence of thrombosis of the hepatic artery or portal vein, and identifies any dilatation of the biliary tree.

- Biliary leakage is associated with 50% mortality. It occurs most frequently in the third or fourth postoperative week.[17]

EMERGENCY DEPARTMENT CARE AND DISPOSITION

- Consultation: Communication should be made directly with the transplant center (often a nurse coordinator). Coordinators should have the patients' current medication doses, recent infection history, and knowledge of complications for which patients may be at risk.[18]

- Rejection: Acute rejection is managed with high-dose glucocorticoid bolus.[18]

- Surgical complications are best managed at the transplant center. Biliary obstruction is managed with balloon dilatation, and all patients should receive broad-spectrum antibiotics (such as ticarcillin-sulbactam

3.1 g IV every 6 hours or ampicillin-sulbactam 3 g IV every 6 hours) against gram-negative and -positive enteric organisms. Biliary leakage is treated with reoperation, and hepatic artery thrombosis is treated with retransplantation.[19]

REFERENCES

1. Tanphaichit NT, Brennan DC: Infectious complications in renal transplant recipients. *Adv Ren Replace Ther* 7:131, 2000.
2. Fishman J, Rubin R: Infection in organ-transplant recipients. *N Engl J Med* 338:1741, 1998.
3. Patel R: Infections in recipients of kidney transplants. *Infect Dis Clin North Am* 15:901, 2001.
4. Smith SR: Viral infection after renal transplantation. *Am J Kidney Dis* 37:659, 2001.
5. Zetterman R: Primary care management of the liver transplant patient. *Am J Med* 96:10S, 1994.
6. Kelly PA, Burckart GJ, Venkatarmanan R: Tacrolimus: A new immunosuppressive agent. *Am J Health Syst Pharm* 52:1521, 1995.
7. Hood KA, Zarembski DG: Mycophenolate mofetil: A unique immunosuppressive agent. *Am J Health Syst Pharm* 54:285, 1997.
8. Kirklin JK, Bourge RC, Naftel DC, et al: Treatment of recurrent heart rejection with mycophenolate mofetil (RS-61443): Initial clinical experience. *J Heart Lung Transplant* 13:444, 1994.
9. Nashan B: Early clinical experience with a novel rapamycin derivative. *Ther Drug Monit* 24:53, 2002.
10. Kasiske BL: Epidemiology of cardiovascular disease after renal transplantation. *Transplantation* 72(6 Suppl):S5, 2001.
11. Farrell TG, Camm AJ: Action of drugs in the denervated heart. *Semin Thorac Cardiovasc Surg* 2:279, 1990.
12. Speich R, Boehler A, Zalunardo MP, et al: Improved results after lung transplantation: Analysis of factors. *Swiss Med Wkly* 131:238, 2001.
13. Estenne J, Hertz MI: Bronchiolitis obliterans after human lung transplantation. *Am J Respir Crit Care Med* 166:440, 2002.
14. Dharnidharka VR, Tejani AH, Ho PL, Harmon WE: Post-transplant lymphoproliferative disorders in the United States: Young Caucasian males are at highest risk. *Am J Transpl* 2: 993, 2002.
15. Cecka JM, Terasaki PI: Early rejection episodes. *Clin Transplant* 1:425, 1989.
16. Bromberg JS, Grossman RA: Care of the organ transplant recipient. *J Am Board Fam Pract* 6:563, 1993.
17. Greif F, Bronsther O, Van Thiel D, et al: The incidence, timing and management of biliary tract complications after orthotopic liver transplantation. *Ann Surg* 219:40, 1994.
18. Savitsky E, Uner A, Votey S: Evaluation of orthotopic liver transplant recipients presenting to the emergency department. *Ann Emerg Med* 31:507, 1998.
19. Porayko M, Kondo M, Steers J: Liver transplantation: Late complications of the biliary tract and their management. *Semin Liver Dis* 15:139, 1995.

For further reading in *Emergency Medicine: A Comprehensive Study Guide,* 6th ed., see Chap. 60, "Cardiac Transplantation," by Michael R. Mill and Michelle S. Mill; Chap. 70, "The Lung Transplant Patient," by Thomas P. Noeller; Chap. 90, "The Liver Transplant Patient," by Steven Kronick; and Chap. 99, "The Renal Transplant Patient," by Richard Sinert and Mert Erogul.

TOXICOLOGY AND PHARMACOLOGY

100 GENERAL MANAGEMENT OF THE POISONED PATIENT

Sandra L. Najarian

EPIDEMIOLOGY

- Poisonings are the third leading cause of death in the United States. The incidence has increased approximately 300% in recent years.
- The majority of accidental exposures are preventable through increased awareness and education.

PATHOPHYSIOLOGY

- Poisons affect the body by inhibiting normal cellular function, changing normal organ function, or by changing the normal uptake or transport of substances into or within the organism.
- Routes of exposure include inhalation, insufflation, ingestion, injection, and cutaneous and mucous membrane exposure.

CLINICAL FEATURES

- A detailed history of the poisoning is essential. Every attempt should be made to ascertain the number of persons exposed, as well as the timing, type, amount, and route of exposure.
- Details about the environment in which the patient was found (eg, the presence of pill bottles or empty containers, drug paraphernalia, unusual odors or smells, or presence of a suicide note) should be gathered, as these may provide clues to identifying the poison.

- Caution should be used when searching the patient's clothing for substances. Attention to vital signs, general appearance, skin, pupils, mucous membranes, and heart, lung, gastrointestinal, and neurologic examinations is important since exposure to certain substances results in specific clinical signs and symptoms called **toxidromes** (Table 100-1).

DIAGNOSIS AND DIFFERENTIAL

- Diagnosis is based on history and clinical presentation. If there is a question of a toxic ingestion, having the actual container, pill remnants, or liquids is very important.
- Laboratory studies may be useful, but often serve only to confirm the diagnosis. Toxicologic drug screens also may be useful for certain ingestions, but rarely alter management.
- Acetaminophen and aspirin are common co-ingestants in suicide attempts; consideration should be given to performing routine testing for these medications. Other tests that may be useful include electrocardiogram (ECG), arterial blood gas analysis, urine pregnancy test, and electrolyte and glucose levels.
- If the toxin is unknown, recognition of toxidromes can assist the physician in narrowing the differential diagnosis (Table 100-2).

EMERGENCY DEPARTMENT CARE AND DISPOSITION

- Attention to airway, breathing, and circulation (ABCs) always takes precedence in managing the poisoned patient. Patients require oxygen administration, cardiac monitoring, and IV access.

TABLE 100-1 Toxidromes

TOXIDROME	REPRESENTATIVE AGENT(S)	MOST COMMON FINDINGS	ADDITIONAL SIGNS AND SYMPTOMS	POTENTIAL INTERVENTIONS
Opioid	Heroin Morphine	CNS depression, miosis, respiratory depression	Hypothermia, bradycardia Death may result from respiratory arrest, pulmonary edema	Ventilation or naloxone
Sympathomimetic	Cocaine Amphetamine	Psychomotor agitation, mydriasis, diaphoresis, tachycardia, hypertension, hyperthermia	Seizures, rhabdomyolysis, myocardial infarction Death may result from seizures, cardiac arrest, hyperthermia	Cooling, sedation with benzodiazepines, hydration
Cholinergic	Organophosphate insecticides Carbamate insecticides	Salivation, lacrimation, diaphoresis, nausea, vomiting, urination, defecation, muscle fasciculations, weakness, bronchorrhea	Bradycardia, miosis/mydriasis, seizures, respiratory failure, paralysis Death may result from respiratory arrest secondary to paralysis and/or bronchorrhea, seizures	Airway protection and ventilation, atropine, pralidoxime
Anticholinergic	Scopolamine Atropine	Altered mental status, mydriasis, dry/flushed skin, urinary retention, decreased bowel sounds, hyperthermia, dry mucous membranes	Seizures, dysrhythmias, rhabdomyolysis Death may result from hyperthermia and dysrhythmias	Physostigmine (if appropriate), sedation with benzodiazepines, cooling, supportive management
Salicylates	Aspirin Oil of wintergreen	Altered mental status, respiratory alkalosis, metabolic acidosis, tinnitus, hyperpnea, tachycardia, diaphoresis, nausea, vomiting	Low-grade fever, ketonuria Death may result from pulmonary edema, cardiorespiratory arrest	MDAC, alkalinization of the urine with potassium repletion, hemodialysis, hydration
Hypoglycemia	Sulfonylureas Insulin	Altered mental status, diaphoresis, tachycardia, hypertension	Paralysis, slurring of speech, bizarre behavior, seizures Death may result from seizures, altered behavior	Glucose-containing solution intravenously, and oral feedings if able, frequent capillary blood for glucose measurement
Serotonin syndrome	Meperidine/ dextromethorphan + MAOI, SSRI + TCA, SSRI/TCA/ MAOI + amphetamine, SSRI overdose	Altered mental status, increased muscle tone, hyperreflexia, hyperthermia	"Wet dog shakes" (intermittent whole body tremor) Death may result from hyperthermia	Cooling, sedation with benzodiazepines, supportive management, theoretical benefit—cyproheptadine

ABBREVIATIONS: CNS = central nervous system; MDAD = multidose activated charcoal; MAOI = monoamine oxidase inhibitor; SSRI = selective serotonin reuptake inhibitor; TCA = tricyclic antidepressant.

- Once the ABCs are secured, decontamination, elimination of the toxin, and administration of the antidote should take place (Table 100-3).
- Primary evaluation includes assessment of airway patency and quality of respirations. Early endotracheal intubation should be considered, especially if gastric lavage is indicated in a patient with a depressed level of consciousness.
- Respiratory status should be continuously monitored. Abnormalities in breathing are not usually the direct effect of a toxin, but rather a result of the patient's altered level of consciousness.
- Hypotension should be corrected with IV fluids; pressors are rarely required. Ventricular dysrhythmias should be treated according to standard Advanced Cardiac Life Support (ACLS) protocol unless treatment of a particular toxin dictates an alternative treatment. Atropine should be used for bradyarrhythmias; cardiac pacing may be necessary.
- For those patients found unresponsive or with altered mental status, administration of naloxone (0.2 to 2.0 mg IV in adults), glucose (50 mL 50% dextrose IV), and thiamine (100 mg IV) should be considered after taking into account the history, vital signs, and initial laboratory data. Administration of naloxone, a competitive opioid antagonist, may precipitate acute withdrawal syndrome, especially if large doses are given.
- Routine use of flumazenil, a benzodiazepine antagonist, is not recommended.

TABLE 100 2   Agents that May Alter Presenting Signs or Symptoms*

DRUGS	SEIZURES	CHANGE IN BLOOD PRESSURE	CHANGE IN VENTILATION	CHANGE IN HEART RATE	TEMPERATURE CHANGE
Alcohol withdrawal	✓	↑	↑	↑	↑
Amphetamines	✓	↑	↑	↑	↑
Anticholinergic	✓	↑	↑	↑	↑
Baclofen	✓	↓	↓	↑	↓
Caffeine	✓	↑	↑	↑	
Camphor	✓				
Cocaine	✓	↑	↑	↑	↑
Gyromitra esculenta (mushroom)	✓				
Isoniazid	✓				
Lithium	✓				
Methaqualone	✓	↑	↓	↑	
Serotonin syndrome	✓	↑	↑	↑	↑
Theophylline	✓	↑	↑	↑	
Tricyclic antidepressants	✓	↑	↓	↑	
β-Adrenergic antagonists	✓	↓		↓	
Calcium channel blockers		↓		↓	
Clonidine		↓	↓	↓	↓
Ethanol		↓	↓	↑	↓
Phenothiazines		↓	↓	↑	
Opioids		↓	↓	↓	↓
Organophosphates	✓	↓	↓	↓	
Meprobamate		↓	↓		
Monoamine oxidase inhibitor overdose	✓	↑	↑	↑	↓
Phencyclidine		↑	↓	↑	↓
Sedative hypnotic withdrawal	✓	↑	↑		↑
Phenylpropanolamine		↑	↑	↑	
Barbiturates		↓	↓	↓	↓
Ethchlorvynol		↓	↓	↓	
Glutethimide		↓	↓		
Salicylates		↓	↑	↑	↑
Nicotine	✓	↑	↑	↑	
Hydrocarbons		↓	↑	↑	
Toxic alcohols	✓	↓	↑	↑	
Iron	✓	↓	↑	↑	

*Listed are the most common or most classically seen with the agent.

- Seizures should be treated with benzodiazepines (lorazepam 2 mg IV) initially, followed by phenobarbital if necessary.
- Physical and chemical restraints should be considered in the agitated patient. Short-acting benzodiazepines or haloperidol may be useful.
- Decontamination of the poisoned patient is the mainstay of therapy. Gross (surface) decontamination is the initial step. If patients are being contaminated by a toxin through dermal contact, they should be removed from the toxic substance; this includes undressing patients completely and washing their skin with copious amounts of water. Properly gowned staff should assist the patient in an isolated area so as to avoid contamination of other patients and staff.
- With ocular exposure, the eyes must be immediately flushed with irrigation solution until the pH of the eyes returns to a physiologic range.

TABLE 100-3   Antidotes to Some Common Poisons

ANTIDOTE	Dose — CHILD	Dose — ADULT	POISON
N-acetylcysteine	140 mg/kg PO load, followed by 70 mg/kg PO q4h for 18 total doses		Acetaminophen
Activated charcoal	1 g/kg PO		Most ingested poisons
Antivenin Fab	4–6 vials IV initially over 1 h may be repeated; 2 vials every 6 h for 18 h.		Envenomation by *Crotalidae*
Calcium gluconate 10% (9 mg/mL elemental calcium)	0.6–0.8 mL/kg IV	30 mL IV	Hypermagnesemia, hypocalcemia (ethylene glycol, hydrofluoric acid), calcium channel antagonists, black widow spider venom
Calcium chloride 10% (27.2 mg/mL elemental calcium)	0.2–0.25 mL/kg IV	10 mL IV	
Cyanide antidote kit			
Amyl nitrate	Not typically used	1 ampule in oxygen chamber of ambu-bag 30 seconds on/ 30 seconds off	Cyanide poisoning
Sodium nitrite	0.33 mL/kg IV (3% solution)	10 mL (3% solution)	Hydrogen sulfide (use only sodium nitrate)
Thiosulfate	1.65 mL/kg IV	12.5 g IV	
Deferoxamine	90 mg/kg IM (1 g max) or 15 mg/kg/h IV (1 g max)	2 g IM or 15 mg/kg/h (6–8 g/d max)	Iron
Dextrose	1–1.5 g/kg IV		Hypoglycemia
Digoxin Fab			
Acute	5–10 vials IV		Digoxin and cardiac glycosides
Chronic	1–2 vials IV	3–6 vials IV	
Ethanol			
10% for IV	0.8 g/kg = 8 mL/kg load; then 1/10 per h		Ethylene glycol, methanol
20% PO	0.8 g/kg = 4 mL/kg, then 1/10 per q1h		
Folic acid/leucovorin	1–2 mg/kg q4–6h IV		Methanol, methotrexate (only leucovorin)
Fomepizole	15 mg/kg IV, then 10 mg/kg q12h		Methanol, ethylene glycol, disulfiram
Glucagon	50 μg/kg	1–10 mg IV	Calcium channel blocker, β-blocker
Methylene blue	1–2 mg/kg Neonates: 0.3–1 mg/kg	1–2 mg/kg	Oxidizing chemicals (eg, nitrites, benzocaine, sulfonamides)
Octreotide	1 μg/kg q6h SC	50 μg SC q6h	Refractory hypoglycemia after oral hypoglycemic agent ingestion
Naloxone	As much as is needed; typical starting dose 0.4–10 mg IV		Opioid, clonidine
Physostigmine	0.02 mg/kg IV	1–2 mg IV	Anticholinergic substances (not TCAs)
Pralidoxime (2-PAM)	20–40 mg/kg IV	1–2 g IV	Cholinergic substances
Protamine	1 mg neutralizes 100 U of administered heparin; 0.6 mg/kg administered over 15 min	25–50 mg IV; empiric	Heparin
Pyridoxine	Gram-for-gram dose if amount of INH is known 70 mg/kg IV	5 g IV	INH, *Gyromitra esculenta,* rocket fuel
Sodium bicarbonate	1–2 mEq/kg IV bolus, followed by 2 mEq/kg/h		Sodium channel blockers, alkalinization of urine or serum
Thiamine	10–100 mg IV	100 mg IV	Ethylene glycol, Wernicke's syndrome, "Wet" beri-beri
Vitamin K_1	2–5 mg/d PO	25–50 mg TID	Anticoagulants
Whole bowel irrigation	0.5 L/h PO	1.5–2 l/h PO	Multiple indications (eg, sustained-release products, body packers)

- Gastric decontamination includes gastric emptying, adsorption of the toxin in the gut, and irrigation of the bowel. Selecting the appropriate method is dependent upon the toxin, timing of exposure, and clinical status of the patient.
- Gastric lavage is the preferred method of gastric emptying. Ipecac is contraindicated. Gastric lavage should be reserved for patients with a recent ingestion (usually within 60 minutes) of a potentially life-threatening toxin.[1] When performed, a large-bore orogastric tube with connections for infusion and drainage should be used. The patient should be placed in the left lateral decubitus position with the head lower than the feet.
- Prior to removing the tube, activated charcoal (1 g/kg) should be administered to help bind any remaining toxin. Activated charcoal may be given orally or per nasogastric tube when gastric lavage is not indicated.
- Osmotic cathartics (1 g/kg of 70% sorbitol or 4 mg/kg of 10% magnesium citrate) may be given with activated charcoal to reduce transit time through the GI tract.[2,3]
- Multiple-dose activated charcoal is an option usually reserved for very large ingestions, life-threatening toxins known to slow gut motility, or slow-release toxins.[4]
- Whole bowel irrigation may be useful in eliminating sustained-release preparations, toxins not known to be adsorbed by activated charcoal, or packages of toxic drugs (body packers). Polyethylene glycol 2 L/h should be administered in adults (50 to 250 mL/kg/h in pediatric patients) until rectal effluent is clear.
- Once decontamination is underway, specific antidotes or other special treatment may be given. Enhancing elimination of certain toxins may be indicated; these methods include urinary alkalization, hemoperfusion, or hemodialysis for specific toxins.
- Disposition of patients depends on the nature of the exposure and underlying conditions. Consideration should be given to delayed effects and absorption of toxins.
- Psychiatric consultation should be obtained for all intentional overdoses. Poisonings in children over 5 years old should be considered suspicious and warrant social work consultation or law enforcement involvement.

REFERENCES

1. Kulig KW, Bar-Or D, Cantrill SV, et al: Management of acutely poisoned patients without gastric emptying. *Ann Emerg Med* 14:562, 1985.
2. Krenzelok EP, Keller R, Stewart RD: Gastrointestinal transit times of cathartics combined with charcoal. *Ann Emerg Med* 14:1152, 1985.
3. Harchelroad F, Cottington E, and Krenzelok EP: Gastrointestinal transit times of a charcoal/sorbitol slurry in overdose patients. *J Toxicol Clin Toxicol* 27:91, 1989.
4. Roberge RJ, Martin TG: Whole bowel irrigation in an acute oral lead intoxication. *Am J Emerg Med* 10:577, 1992.

For further reading in *Emergency Medicine: A Comprehensive Study Guide*, 6th ed., see Chap. 156, "General Management of Poisoned Patients," by Jason B. Hack and Robert S. Hoffman.

101 ANTICHOLINERGIC TOXICITY
O. John Ma

EPIDEMIOLOGY

- Anticholinergic toxicity is frequently encountered because of the common use of tricyclic antidepressants, phenothiazines, antihistamines, and antiparkinsonian drugs.
- Jimsonweed is the most common plant associated with anticholinergic toxicity.

PATHOPHYSIOLOGY

- The mechanism of action involves cholinergic blockade of either muscarinic receptors (primarily in the brain), or nicotinic receptors, or both. The expected clinical effects of these agents are modulated through disturbances in the parasympathetic nervous system (peripheral effects) and the brain (central effects).
- Drug absorption can occur after ingestion, smoking, or ocular use.
- Table 101-1 lists the important anticholinergic agents and the classes to which they belong.

CLINICAL EFFECTS

- Clinical findings include mydriasis, hypo- or hypertension, hypoactive or absent bowel sounds, tachycardia, flushed skin, disorientation, urinary retention, hyperthermia, dry skin and mucous membranes, confusion, agitation, and auditory or visual hallucinations.
- Findings can be remembered using the mnemonic: Hot as Hades, Blind as a Bat, Dry as a Bone, Red as a Beet, and Mad as a Hatter.

TABLE 101-1 Anticholinergic Substances

Antihistamines
  Ethanolamines
    Dimenhydrinate (Dramamine)
    Diphenhydramine (Benadryl)
  Ethylenediamines
    Tripelennamine (pyribenzamine)
  Alkylamines
    Chlorpheniramine (Teldrin)
  Piperazines
    Astemizole (Hismanal)
    Terfenadine (Seldane)
    Loratadine (Claritin)
    Cyclizine (Marezine)
    Meclizine (Antivert)
  Phenothiazines
    Prochlorperazine (Compazine)
    Promethazine (Phenergan)

Antiparkinsonian drugs
  Benztropine mesylate (Cogentin)
  Biperiden (Akineton)
  Ethopropazine (Parsidol)
  Trihexyphenidyl (Artane)
  Procyclidine (Kemadrin)

Antipsychotics
  Phenothiazines
    Chlorpromazine (Thorazine)
    Thioridazine (Mellaril)
    Perphenazine (Trilafon)
  Nonphenothiazines
    Clozaril (Clozapine)
    Molindone (Moban)
    Loxapine (Loxitane)

Antispasmodics
  Clidinium bromide (Quarzan, Librax)
  Dicyclomine (Bentyl)
  Methantheline bromide (Banthine)
  Propantheline bromide (Pro-Banthine)
  Tridihexethyl chloride (Pathilon)

Plants
  Deadly nightshade
  Mandrake
  Jimsonweed

Belladonna alkaloids, synthetic cogeners
  Atropine (Hyoscyamine)
  Belladonna alkaloid mixtures
  Glycopyrrolate (Robinul)
  Homatropine (Dia-Quel, Malcotran)
  Methscopolamine bromide (Pamine)
  Scopolamine hydrobromide (Hyoscine)

Cyclic antidepressants
  Amitriptyline hydrochloride (Elavil, Amitril, Endep)
  Desipramine hydrochloride (Norpramin, Pertofrane)
  Doxepin hydrochloride (Sinequan, Adapin)
  Imipramine hydrochloride (Tofranil, Pramine)
  Nortriptyline hydrochloride (Aventyl, Pamelor)
  Protriptyline hydrochloride (Vivactil)
  Trimipramine (Surmontil)
  Maprotiline hydrochloride (Ludiomil)
  Zimelidine hydrochloride
  Fluoxetine (Prozac)
  Amoxapine (Asendin)

Ophthalmic products
  Atropine and scopolamine solutions
  Cyclopentolate hydrochloride (Cyclogyl)
  Tropicamide (Mydriacyl)

OTC medications (including antihistamines and belladonna alkaloids)
  Analgesics: Excedrin PM, Percogesic
  Cold remedies: Actifed, Allerest, Coricidin, Dristan, Flavihist, Romex, Sine-Off
  Hypnotics: Compoz, Sleep-Eze, Sominex
  Menstrual products: Pamprin, Premesyn PMS

Skeletal muscle relaxants
  Orphenadrine citrate (Norflex)
  Cyclobenzaprine hydrochloride (Flexeril)

Mushrooms
  Amanita muscaria
  Amanita pantherina

Other
  Diphenidol (Cephadol, Vontrol)

SOURCE: Adapted from Goldfrank et al., with permission.

- The most common electrocardiogram (ECG) finding is sinus tachycardia. Also, QRS-interval prolongation, bundle-branch blocks, atrioventricular dissociation, and atrial and ventricular tachycardias may be seen.[1]

DIAGNOSIS AND DIFFERENTIAL

- Diagnosis is primarily clinical. In isolated anticholinergic toxicity, routine laboratory studies should be normal, and toxicology screening is of little value. Nonetheless, electrolytes, glucose level, and pulse oximetry should be obtained in the presence of altered mental status.
- In contrast, sympathomimetic toxicity and delirium tremens will show moist skin and active bowel sounds. Acute psychiatric disorders may have tachycardia and tachypnea, but the physical examination is otherwise unremarkable.
- The differential diagnosis includes viral encephalitis, Reye's syndrome, head trauma, other intoxications, neuroleptic malignant syndrome, delirium tremens, acute psychiatric disorders, and sympathomimetic toxicity.

EMERGENCY DEPARTMENT CARE AND DISPOSITION

- Treatment is primarily supportive. The patient should be placed on a cardiac monitor and intravenous access secured.

- Gastric lavage may be useful within 1 hour of ingestion. Activated charcoal may decrease drug absorption. Whole-bowel irrigation is recommended for jimsonweed ingestion up to 12 to 24 hours after ingestion due to delayed gastric emptying of the seeds.
- Hyperthermia and seizures should be treated conventionally.
- Standard antiarrhythmics are usually effective, but class Ia medications should be avoided. Dysrhythmias, widened QRS complexes, and hypotension from sodium blocking agents (eg, cyclic antidepressants) can be treated with intravenous sodium bicarbonate.
- Agitation should be treated with benzodiazepines (lorazepam 2 to 4 mg IV). Phenothiazines should be avoided.
- Physostigmine treatment is controversial. It is indicated only if conventional therapy fails to control seizures, agitation, unstable dysrhythmias, coma with respiratory depression, malignant hypertension, or hypotension. The initial dose is 0.5 to 2 mg IV, slowly administered over 5 minutes. When effective, a significant decrease in agitation may be apparent within 15 to 20 minutes.
- Physostigmine may worsen cyclic antidepressant toxicity and lead to bradycardia and asystole. It is contraindicated in patients with cardiovascular or peripheral vascular disease, bronchospasm, intestinal obstruction, heart block, or bladder obstruction. The patient should be observed for cholinergic excess.[2]
- Patients with mild anticholinergic toxicity can be discharged after 6 hours of observation if their symptoms are improving. More symptomatic patients should be admitted for 24 hours of observation. Patients receiving physostigmine usually require at least a 24-hour admission.

REFERENCES

1. Holger JS, Harris CR, Engebretsen KM: Physostigmine, sodium bicarbonate, or hypertonic saline to treat diphenhydramine toxicity. *Vet Hum Toxicol* 44:1, 2002.
2. Burns MJ, Linden C, Graudins A, et al: A comparison of physostigmine and benzodiazepines for the treatment of anticholinergic poisoning. *Ann Emerg Med* 35:374, 2000.

For further reading in *Emergency Medicine: A Comprehensive Study Guide,* 6th ed., see Chap. 183, "Anticholinergic Toxicity," by Paul M. Wax.

102 PSYCHOPHARMACOLOGIC AGENTS
C. Crawford Mechem

SEROTONIN SYNDROME

PATHOPHYSIOLOGY

- Serotonin syndrome is a rare idiosyncratic complication of antidepressant therapy, characterized by cognitive impairment and autonomic and neuromuscular dysfunction.
- It may be caused by any drug or combination of drugs that increases central serotonin transmission. Most cases occur at therapeutic drug levels.

CLINICAL FEATURES

- The diagnosis is made on clinical grounds. Cognitive and behavioral findings may include confusion, agitation, coma, anxiety, hypomania, lethargy, seizures, insomnia, hallucinations, and dizziness.
- Autonomic signs may include hyperthermia, diaphoresis, sinus tachycardia, hypertension, tachypnea, dilated or unreactive pupils, flushed skin, hypotension, diarrhea, abdominal cramps, and salivation.
- Neuromuscular findings include myoclonus, hyperreflexia, muscle rigidity, tremor, hyperactivity, ataxia, shivering, Babinski's sign, nystagmus, teeth chattering, opisthotonus, and trismus.

EMERGENCY DEPARTMENT CARE AND DISPOSITION

- Therapy involves discontinuing all serotoninergic agents and providing supportive care.
- Antiserotoninergic agents may have a role. Most experience has been with cyproheptadine, 4 to 8 mg PO, repeated in 2 hours if no response is noted. Additional dosing should be discontinued if the patient fails to respond to 16 mg. Patients who do respond are then given 4 mg PO every 6 hours for 48 hours.
- Benzodiazepines may be used to relieve muscle rigidity and discomfort.
- Patients with muscle rigidity, seizures, or hyperthermia should be monitored for development of rhabdomyolysis and/or metabolic acidosis. All patients require admission.

TRICYCLIC ANTIDEPRESSANTS

EPIDEMIOLOGY

- Tricyclic antidepressants (TCAs) cause more drug-related deaths than any other class of prescription medication.[1]
- There are approximately 18,000 annual reported exposures to TCAs, resulting in 110 deaths.

PATHOPHYSIOLOGY

- The clinical and toxic effects of TCAs relate to their antimuscarinic and antihistaminic effects, their inhibition of reuptake of amines including norepinephrine and serotonin, and inhibition of α-adrenergic receptors.[2]
- TCA-mediated blockade of sodium channels results in cardiotoxicity, the single most important factor contributing to mortality.[3]
- TCAs also cause potassium channel antagonism and GABA-A receptor antagonism.

CLINICAL FEATURES

- Mild to moderate TCA toxicity may present with drowsiness, confusion, slurred speech, ataxia, dry mucous membranes, sinus tachycardia, urinary retention, myoclonus, hyperreflexia, decreased bowel sounds, and ileus.
- Serious toxicity almost always manifests within 6 hours of major ingestion and consists of cardiac conduction delays, supraventricular tachycardia, premature ventricular contractions, ventricular tachycardia, hypotension, coma, respiratory depression, and seizures.[4]
- Secondary complications include aspiration pneumonia, anoxic encephalopathy, hyperthermia, rhabdomyolysis, and pulmonary edema.

DIAGNOSIS AND DIFFERENTIAL

- Diagnosis is made on clinical grounds. Most cases of serious toxicity are associated with elevated TCA plasma levels, but the results are rarely available to the emergency physician.
- Electrocardiographic (ECG) abnormalities are common and may be useful in identifying patients at risk for seizures and ventricular dysrhythmias.
- Classic ECG findings in TCA toxicity include sinus tachycardia, right axis deviation (RAD) of the terminal 40 ms (a positive terminal R wave in lead aVR and a negative S wave in lead I), and prolongation of PR,

QRS, and QTc intervals. Life-threatening complications are more likely when the QRS interval is greater than 100 ms or with RAD of the terminal 40 ms.
- Complications can occur in the absence of significant ECG abnormalities.[5]
- The differential diagnosis includes toxicity due to carbamazepine, cyclobenzaprine, diphenhydramine, phenothiazines, class Ia and Ic antiarrhythmics, propranolol, propoxyphene, cocaine, lithium, and hyperkalemia.

EMERGENCY DEPARTMENT CARE AND DISPOSITION

- All patients should be promptly evaluated for altered mental status, hemodynamic instability, and respiratory impairment. IV access and cardiac monitoring should be initiated.
- All patients should receive activated charcoal 1 g/kg PO or per nasogastric tube.
- Gastric lavage is indicated early (<2 hours) after ingestion.
- Sodium bicarbonate, 1 to 2 mEq/kg IV bolus, is given for a QRS interval greater than 100 ms, hypotension refractory to hydration, terminal rightward axis in aVR, or ventricular dysrhythmias.
- Sodium bicarbonate may be repeated until the patient improves or until the serum pH is 7.50 to 7.55. As an alternative to repeat boluses, an IV infusion may be mixed by adding 3 ampules to 1 L D_5W and run at 2 to 3 mL/kg/h. Serum potassium should be closely monitored.
- Ventricular dysrhythmias refractory to sodium bicarbonate should be treated with lidocaine. Synchronized cardioversion is indicated for unstable patients. Torsades de pointes should be treated initially with 2 g of IV magnesium sulfate.
- Thiamine and naloxone are warranted for altered mental status, and a fingerstick serum glucose level should be obtained.
- Seizures should be controlled with IV lorazepam or diazepam.
- Refractory seizure cases are treated with phenobarbital at an initial loading dose of 15 mg/kg IV.
- Hypotension and respiratory depression should be anticipated. If neuromuscular blockade and endotracheal intubation prove necessary, electroencephalographic (EEG) monitoring and continued anticonvulsant therapy are required.
- Crystalloid IV fluids should be administered in increments of 10 mL/kg for hypotension and the patient closely watched for signs of pulmonary edema.
- Norepinephrine is the vasopressor of choice in cases refractory to IV fluids and sodium bicarbonate.

- Patients who remain asymptomatic 6 hours after ingestion may be medically cleared. Psychiatric consultation should be considered, based on the circumstances.
- All symptomatic patients require admission to a monitored setting.

NEWER ANTIDEPRESSANTS AND SEROTONIN SYNDROME

PATHOPHYSIOLOGY

- The mechanism of action is believed to relate to inhibition of neurotransmitter reuptake (except mirtazapine).
- Unlike TCAs, these agents do not significantly inhibit sodium, potassium, or calcium channels.
- They do not inhibit monoamine oxidase and do not cause tyramine-like reactions.
- They lack the antimuscarinic effects of TCAs and have negligible effects on dopamine or GABA.

TRAZODONE AND NEFAZODONE

CLINICAL FEATURES

- Adverse effects due to trazodone include orthostatic hypotension, drowsiness, dizziness, dry mouth, nausea, vomiting, liver toxicity, and priapism.
- Cardiac dysrhythmias may include sinus bradycardia, atrial fibrillation, sinus arrest, atrioventricular (AV) blocks, premature ventricular contractions, and torsades de pointes.
- Nefazodone toxicity may produce headache, dizziness, drowsiness, asthenia, tremor, dry mouth, nausea, constipation, and blurred vision.
- Nefazodone can inhibit metabolism of terfenadine, astemizole, cisapride, and pimozide, resulting in QTc interval prolongation and torsades de pointes.
- Nefazodone also potentiates central nervous system (CNS) depression caused by benzodiazepines.
- Its use is less commonly associated with orthostatic hypotension and priapism than is the case with trazodone.
- In acute trazodone overdose, serious toxicity is rare at doses less than 2 g. Manifestations include CNS depression, orthostatic hypotension, nausea, vomiting, abdominal pain, muscle weakness, priapism, ataxia, dizziness, seizures, and coma.
- Respiratory depression is rarely seen. On ECG, QTc-interval prolongation may be seen, rarely leading to torsades de pointes.
- In acute nefazodone overdose, nausea, vomiting, and somnolence have been reported.

EMERGENCY DEPARTMENT CARE AND DISPOSITION

- In most trazodone or nefazodone overdoses, supportive care is sufficient.
- The patient should be assessed for respiratory or hemodynamic compromise from a co-ingestion and an acetaminophen level obtained.
- An IV line should be started and cardiac monitoring initiated for all patients.
- Activated charcoal, 1 g/kg, should be administered. Gastric lavage is unnecessary unless there is a clear history of life-threatening co-ingestion.
- Hypotension is best treated initially with crystalloid IV fluids. In refractory cases, norepinephrine is the vasopressor of choice.
- Patients who remain asymptomatic 6 hours after ingestion can be medically cleared. Symptomatic patients should be admitted to a monitored setting.

BUPROPION

CLINICAL FEATURES

- Adverse effects include dry mouth, dizziness, agitation, nausea, headache, constipation, tremor, anxiety, confusion, blurred vision, and increased motor activity.
- It rarely causes catatonia, hallucinations, psychosis, and paranoia.
- Bupropion has a low toxic-to-therapeutic ratio. Toxicity may be seen at doses at, or just above, the maximum therapeutic dose of 450 mg/day.
- Findings include sinus tachycardia, lethargy, tremor, seizures, confusion, vomiting, and mild hyperthermia. The hallmark of overdose is seizures, which usually develop within the first 4 hours, often without associated signs of toxicity.[6]
- Sustained-release preparations may causes seizures up to 14 hours postingestion.

EMERGENCY DEPARTMENT CARE AND DISPOSITION

- Seizures should be anticipated in all patients. Significant cardiotoxicity is unlikely except in mixed overdoses.
- IV access should be established and the patient placed on a cardiac monitor.
- Gastric lavage for acute ingestions (<1 hour) and activated charcoal, 1 g/kg, are recommended.
- Seizures should be controlled with benzodiazepines and phenobarbital.
- Admission to a monitored setting is indicated for patients with sinus tachycardia, lethargy, or seizures.
- Patients who remain asymptomatic 8 hours after ingestion of regular-release bupropion may be medically cleared. Ingestion of more than 450 mg of a sustained-release preparation warrants admission for further monitoring.

MIRTAZAPINE

CLINICAL FEATURES
- Adverse effects include weight gain and somnolence.
- Mirtazapine has limited toxicity in acute overdose.
- The patient may present with sedation, confusion, sinus tachycardia, and mild hypertension. Respiratory depression or coma may be seen at higher doses or when combined with another CNS depressant.

EMERGENCY DEPARTMENT CARE AND DISPOSITION
- Experience with mirtazapine overdose is limited, so early consultation with a poison control center is recommended. Supportive care is usually sufficient.
- Activated charcoal, 1 g/kg, should be administered. Gastric lavage may be indicated early after large overdoses or with significant co-ingestants.
- Symptomatic patients should be admitted to a monitored bed. Asymptomatic patients may be medically cleared after 8 hours of observation.

SELECTIVE SEROTONIN REUPTAKE INHIBITORS (SSRIs)

CLINICAL FEATURES
- The selective serotonin reuptake inhibitors (SSRIs) have a high therapeutic-to-toxic ratio. The most serious adverse effect is development of serotonin syndrome.
- Other effects include headache, sedation, insomnia, dizziness, fatigue, tremor, and nervousness. Seizures occur rarely.
- Dystonic reactions, akathisia, dyskinesia, hypokinesia, and Parkinsonism have been reported.
- Other adverse effects include nausea, vomiting, diarrhea, constipation, anorexia, dry mouth, increased sweating, blurred vision, priapism, hyponatremia, and hypoglycemia.
- In acute overdose, patients may present with nausea, vomiting, sedation, tremor, and sinus tachycardia. Less commonly, mydriasis, seizures, diarrhea, agitation, hallucinations, hypertension, and hypotension may be noted.
- While cardiotoxicity is uncommon, sinus bradycardia may be observed in fluvoxamine overdoses, and citalopram may cause QRS interval widening and QTc interval prolongation.

EMERGENCY DEPARTMENT CARE AND DISPOSITION
- Pure SSRI overdoses are rarely associated with serious toxicity. However, the patient should be carefully observed for the development of seizures or serotonin syndrome.

- All patients should have IV access and cardiac monitoring.
- Activated charcoal, 1 g/kg, should be administered. Gastric lavage is only indicated in the setting of very large overdoses or mixed ingestions.
- Sodium bicarbonate should be used to treat QRS interval prolongation.
- Benzodiazepines are recommended as initial anticonvulsant therapy.
- All patients should be observed for 6 hours postingestion. Patients who continue to manifest toxicity, such as tachycardia or lethargy, should be admitted for further monitoring.

VENLAFAXINE

CLINICAL FEATURES
- Adverse effects are similar to those of SSRIs, including development of serotonin syndrome.[7] It also produces hypertension in doses exceeding 225 mg/day.
- In acute overdose, signs and symptoms include tachycardia, hypertension, diaphoresis, tremor, and mydriasis. CNS depression and generalized seizures are common. Severe hypotension requiring vasopressors has been reported.
- ECG findings include sinus tachycardia, QRS interval widening, and QTc interval prolongation.

EMERGENCY DEPARTMENT CARE AND DISPOSITION
- Venlafaxine has greater toxicity in overdose than SSRIs, and onset of symptoms may be precipitous.
- All patients should have IV access and be placed on a cardiac monitor.
- Early gastric lavage should be strongly considered. Activated charcoal, 1 g/kg, should be administered to all patients.
- Benzodiazepines are the anticonvulsants of choice.
- Hypertension and tachycardia may require pharmacologic management. Administration of a β-blocker should be considered.
- IV sodium bicarbonate should be considered for QRS interval greater than 100 ms.
- Patients should be observed for 6 hours postingestion. Symptomatic patients should be admitted to a monitored bed.

MONOAMINE OXIDASE INHIBITORS

EPIDEMIOLOGY
- In the past decade there have been approximately 6000 reported monoamine oxidase inhibitor (MAOI) exposures and 58 deaths.

• The mortality rate may be higher in intentional overdoses.

PATHOPHYSIOLOGY

• MAO removes amine groups from biogenic amines such as norepinephrine, dopamine, and serotonin, resulting in their deactivation.
• MAO also decreases systemic availability of absorbed dietary biogenic amines such as tyramine.
• Inhibition of MAO results in accumulation of neurotransmitters in the presynaptic nerve terminals as well as increased systemic availability of dietary amines.
• Tyramine is a dietary amine found in aged meats, cheeses, and red wine. Co-ingestion with MAOIs results in release of norepinephrine, epinephrine, serotonin, and dopamine.

CLINICAL FEATURES

• Within 90 minutes of ingestion of tyramine, patients taking MAOIs may develop hypertension, diaphoresis, headache, mydriasis, neck stiffness, neuromuscular excitation, palpitations, and chest pain.[8]
• Symptoms generally resolve within 6 hours but deaths, which are usually due to intracranial hemorrhage or myocardial infarction, have been reported.
• When MAOIs are combined with certain other medications (Table 102-1), several potentially serious types of drug interactions may develop. These include a hyperadrenergic state similar to the tyramine reaction when taken with sympathomimetics.
• MAOIs inhibit the clearance of other drugs, including opiates and sedative-hypnotics. Tranylcypromine and phenelzine stimulate insulin secretion, leading to hypoglycemia in patients on sulfonylureas.
• Serotonin syndrome has been reported, especially when combined with other serotonergic agents such as meperidine, dextromethorphan, or tramadol.
• In acute overdose, toxicity may develop at doses less than 2 mg/kg. A dose of 4 to 6 mg/kg may be fatal.[9]
• Signs and symptoms usually develop 6 to 12 hours postingestion, but may be delayed up to 24 hours.
• Symptoms include headache, agitation, irritability, nausea, palpitations, and tremor.
• Signs include sinus tachycardia, hyperreflexia, hyperactivity, fasciculations, mydriasis, hyperventilation, nystagmus, and generalized flushing.
• Opisthotonus, muscle rigidity, diaphoresis, chest pain, hypertension, diarrhea, hallucinations, combativeness, confusion, marked hyperthermia, and trismus may develop.
• "Ping-pong" gaze, or bilateral wandering horizontal eye movements, may be noted.
• Severe toxicity presents with bradycardia, worsening hyperthermia, papilledema, seizures, coma, and cardiac arrest. Hypotension is associated with a poor prognosis.

TABLE 102-1   Drugs Contraindicated with MAOIs

INDIRECT SYMPATHOMIMETICS	MISCELLANEOUS DRUGS
Benzphetamine	β-Blockers
Bretylium	Bupropion
Cocaine	Buspirone
Dexfenfluramine	Caffeine
Diethylpropion	Carbamazepine
Dopamine	Cyclobenzaprine
Ephedrine	Dextromethorphan
Fenfluramine	Disulfiram
Guanethidine	Ergot alkaloids
Isometheptene	Fentanyl
Mephentermine	Furazolidone
Metaraminol	Ketamine
Methamphetamine	Levodopa (L-dopa)
3,4-Methylenedioxymethamphetamine (MDMA)	Lithium
Methyldopa	Meperidine
Methylphenidate	Mirtazapine
Pemoline	Oral hypoglycemic agents
Phentermine	Phenothiazines
Phencyclidine	Procarbazine
Phenylpropanolamine	St. John's wort
Propylhexedrine	Sumatriptan
Pseudoephedrine	Theophylline
Reserpine	Tramadol
Ritodrine	Tricyclic antidepressants
Tyramine	

DIAGNOSIS AND DIFFERENTIAL

• The diagnosis is a clinical one. Laboratory tests are used to detect complications such as hypoxia, rhabdomyolysis, renal failure, hyperkalemia, metabolic acidosis, hemolysis, and disseminated intravascular coagulation.
• The differential diagnosis for MAOI toxicity includes all causes of a hyperadrenergic state, altered mental status, and/or muscle rigidity (Table 102-2).

EMERGENCY DEPARTMENT CARE AND DISPOSITION

• All patients require IV access, cardiac monitoring, and supplemental oxygen.
• Gastric lavage within 2 hours of significant overdose is recommended.
• A single dose of activated charcoal, 1 g/kg, should be administered.
• Phentolamine, 2.5 to 5 mg IV every 10 to 15 minutes, is used to treat hypertension. An infusion of 0.2 to 5.0 mg/min may be used for maintenance therapy.

TABLE 102-2   Differential Diagnosis of Monoamine Oxidase Inhibitor Overdose

Intoxications	Medical conditions	Adverse drug reactions
Amphetamines	Heat stroke	Dystonic reactions
Antimuscarinics	Hypoglycemia	Malignant hyperthermia
Cathinone	Hyperthyroidism	Serotonin syndrome
Clonidine (early)	Pheochromocytoma	Tyramine reaction
Cocaine		Spontaneous hypertensive crisis
Lysergic acid diethylamide (LSD)		Neuroleptic malignant syndrome
Methylphenidate		
MDMA*		
Nicotine (early)		
Phencyclidine		
Phenylpropanolamine		
Strychnine		
Theophylline		
Tricyclic antidepressants (early)		
Withdrawal states	Infectious diseases	Psychiatric
Ethanol	Encephalitis	Lethal catatonia
(delirium tremens)	Meningitis	
Sedative-hypnotics	Rabies	
Clonidine	Sepsis	
β-Blockers	Tetanus	

*3,4-Methylenedioxymethamphetamine.

Sodium nitroprusside, starting at 0.5 to 1.0 μg/kg/min, is an effective alternative, as is fenoldopam, administered as a titratable infusion starting at 0.05 to 0.1 μg/kg/min.

- Hypotension is treated with crystalloid IV fluid boluses of 10 to 20 mL/kg.
- Norepinephrine is the preferred vasopressor in refractory hypotension.
- Lidocaine, procainamide, and phenytoin are used to treat dysrhythmias. Bradycardia is treated with atropine, isoprotcrcnol, and dobutamine.
- Benzodiazepines are the agents of choice for seizure control. Barbiturates are alternatives but may precipitate hypotension and respiratory depression.
- Hyperthermia is managed with cool mist sprays, fans, or ice baths. Benzodiazepines may be given to minimize muscle hyperactivity and associated heat production. Nondepolarizing neuromuscular blockers or dantrolene, 0.5 to 2.5 mg IV every 6 hours, may be required for muscle relaxation in refractory cases.
- With few exceptions, all patients with MAOI exposures should be monitored for at least 24 hours.
- All intentional overdoses and accidental exposures of greater than 1 mg/kg should be admitted to an intensive care unit (ICU); others can usually be admitted to a monitored floor.

ANTIPSYCHOTICS

EPIDEMIOLOGY
- Deaths due to antipsychotics are rare. In 2000, 23 deaths associated with antipsychotic use were reported to the American Association of Poison Control Centers. In only 6 of these was an antipsychotic the sole agent involved.[1]

PATHOPHYSIOLOGY
- All antipsychotics block dopamine receptors in the limbic system, which is believed to account for their clinical effects.
- Dopamine receptor antagonism in the basal ganglia also occurs, causing disinhibition of cholinergic neurons. This may be responsible for extrapyramidal side effects.
- Antipsychotics block α-adrenergic, muscarinic, and histaminic receptors.
- The newer antipsychotics in addition block serotonin receptors.

CLINICAL FEATURES
- Antipsychotics have a high therapeutic index. However, they have adverse effects related to their anticholinergic, antihistaminic, and antiadrenergic properties.
- They also can cause dystonic reactions, akathisia, bradykinesia, tardive dyskinesia, and neuroleptic malignant syndrome. Neuroleptic malignant syndrome presents with hyperthermia, muscle rigidity, autonomic instability, and altered mental status.[10]
- In acute overdose, patients present with CNS depression, seizures, tachycardia, hypotension, and impaired thermoregulation.
- Cardiac conduction disturbances may develop, ranging from asymptomatic QTc interval prolongation to ventricular dysrhythmias, including torsades de pointes.

EMERGENCY DEPARTMENT CARE AND DISPOSITION
- Management is supportive. All patients require an ECG and continuous cardiac monitoring.
- Patients with altered mental status should receive oxygen and naloxone, and their blood sugar determined at bedside.
- Hypotension is treated with IV crystalloid fluids.
- If vasopressors are required, those with β-adrenergic properties (epinephrine, dopamine, isoproterenol) should be avoided. Norepinephrine is the vasopressor of choice.
- Activated charcoal, 1 g/kg, should be administered. Gastric lavage may be appropriate early after a large overdose.
- Ventricular dysrhythmias are treated with class Ib antidysrhythmics (eg, lidocaine); the Ia agents (quinidine, procainamide, disopyramide) should be avoided.
- Wide complex tachycardias should be treated with sodium bicarbonate, 1 to 2 mEq/kg IV bolus, followed by an infusion of 100 to 150 mEq in 1 L of D_5W, titrated over 4 to 6 hours with a target arterial pH of 7.5.
- Torsades de pointes is treated with 2 to 4 g IV magnesium sulfate or overdrive pacing.
- Seizures may be controlled with benzodiazepines, phenobarbital, or phenytoin.
- Patients with altered mental status or cardiotoxicity should be admitted to an ICU. All patients who have ingested thioridazine or mesoridazine should be monitored for at least 24 hours.
- Other patients may be medically cleared if asymptomatic 6 hours postingestion, their physical examination is normal, and there is no QTc interval widening on ECG.

LITHIUM

EPIDEMIOLOGY
- The true incidence of lithium toxicity is unknown.
- It has been estimated that 75 to 90% of patients who use lithium chronically will develop toxicity.
- Over a recent 5-year period, 25,000 potential toxic exposures were reported to the American Association of Poison Control Centers. Of these, 44 resulted in death.[11]

PATHOPHYSIOLOGY
- Lithium is thought to cause toxicity through several mechanisms.[12] It competes with sodium, potassium, magnesium, and calcium, displacing them from intracellular sites and bone. Therefore, underlying electrolyte disturbances can contribute to lithium toxicity.
- Lithium inhibits adenylate cyclase, decreasing intracellular cyclic adenosine monophosphate (cAMP).

- Lithium interferes with reuptake of norepinephrine at nerve terminals.
- Lithium enhances serotonin release from the hippocampus.

CLINICAL FEATURES
- The most common adverse effects are hand tremor, polyuria, and rash.
- Nephrogenic diabetes insipidus and incomplete distal renal tubular acidosis have been reported.
- Neurologic effects include memory loss, decreased concentration, fatigue, ataxia, and dysarthria.
- Toxicity results from acute or chronic exposure or decreased drug clearance. Patients with renal insufficiency or volume depletion are at increased risk.[13]
- Following an acute overdose, patients with mild toxicity may present with nausea, vomiting, tremor, hyperreflexia, ataxia, agitation, and muscle weakness. With increasing toxicity, patients may manifest depressed mental status, rigidity, and hypotension.
- Severe toxicity may present with coma, seizures, myoclonus, and cardiovascular collapse.
- Serum lithium levels correlate poorly with toxicity in the acute setting.
- Cardiac abnormalities include the presence of U waves, T wave changes, ST-segment depression, QTc interval prolongation, bundle-branch block, junctional rhythms, and bradycardia.
- Patients with chronic toxicity tend to show a preponderance of neurologic symptoms. Serum lithium levels correlate better with chronic toxicity than in the acute setting.

EMERGENCY DEPARTMENT CARE AND DISPOSITION
- Activated charcoal does not bind lithium but may be indicated for co-ingestions. Early gastric lavage or whole bowel irrigation should also be considered.[14]
- Seizures may be controlled with benzodiazepines or phenobarbital.
- Aggressive hydration with IV normal saline enhances lithium elimination.
- Hemodialysis is used in severe cases to reduce the serum lithium level to less than 1 mEq/L. Indications include a level greater than 3.5 mEq/L (4.0 mEq/L in acute overdose), little change in a level of 1.5 to 3.5 mEq/L after 6 hours of hydration, an increasing level, renal failure, or ingestion of sustained-release preparations.[15]
- Sodium polystyrene sulfonate, 15 g PO qid or 30 g rectally, may be useful in clearing lithium in mild to moderate toxicity.[16]
- While serum levels do not correlate well with symptoms, it is recommended that patients with levels greater than 1.5 mEq/L be admitted, as should patients who have ingested sustained-release preparations.

- In acute overdose, patients who remain asymptomatic after 6 hours may be medically cleared.
- In chronic toxicity, patients with mild symptoms and no other risk factors may be hydrated for 4 to 6 hours and discharged if their levels drop below 1.5 mEq/L and there is clinical improvement. Patients with more severe manifestations should be admitted.

REFERENCES

1. Litovitz TI, Klein-Schwartz W, Rodgers GC, et al: 2001 Annual Report of the American Association of Poison Control Centers Toxic Exposure Surveillance System. *Am J Emerg Med* 20:391, 2002.
2. Buckley NA, McManus PR: Can the fatal toxicity of antidepressant drugs be predicted with pharmacological and toxicological data? *Drug Saf* 18:369, 1998.
3. Kolecki PF, Curry SC: Poisoning by sodium channel blocking agents. *Crit Care Clin* 13:829, 1997.
4. Hutten B-A, Adams R, Askenasi R: Predicting severity of tricyclic antidepressant overdose. *Clin Toxicol* 30:161, 1992.
5. Caravati EM, Bossart PJ: Demographic and electrocardiographic factors associated with severe tricyclic antidepressant toxicity. *Clin Toxicol* 29:31, 1991.
6. Spiller HA, Ramoska EA, Krenzelok EP: Bupropion overdose: A 3-year multicenter retrospective analysis. *Am J Emerg Med* 12:43, 1994.
7. Mills KC: Serotonin syndrome: A clinical update. *Crit Care Clin* 13:763, 1997.
8. Brown C, Taniguchi G, Yip K: The monoamine oxidase inhibitor-tyramine interaction. *J Clin Pharmacol* 29:529, 1989.
9. Linden CH, Rumack BH, Strehlke C: Monoamine oxidase inhibitor overdose. *Ann Emerg Med* 13:1137, 1984.
10. Lev R, Clark RF: Neuroleptic malignant syndrome presenting without fever: Case report and review of the literature. *J Emerg Med* 12:49, 1994.
11. Kulig K: Initial management of ingestions of toxic substances. *N Engl J Med* 326:1677, 1992.
12. Shaldubina A, Agam G, Belmaker BH: The mechanism of lithium action: State of the art, ten years later. *Prog Neuropsychopharmacol Biol Psychiatry* 25:855, 2001.
13. Bendz H, Aurell M, Balldin J, et al: Kidney damage in long-term lithium patients: A cross-sectional study of patients with 15 years or more on lithium. *Nephrol Dial Transplant* 9:1250, 1994.
14. Smith SW, Ling LH, Halstenson CE: Whole bowel irrigation as treatment for acute lithium overdose. *Ann Emerg Med* 20:536, 1991.
15. Jaeger A, Sauder P, Kopferschmitt J, et al: When should dialysis be performed in lithium poisoning? A kinetic study in 14 cases of lithium poisoning. *Clin Toxicol* 31:429, 1993.
16. Roberge RJ, Martin TM, Schneider SM: Use of sodium polystyrene sulfonate in a lithium overdose. *Ann Emerg Med* 22:1911, 1993.

For further reading in *Emergency Medicine: A Comprehensive Study Guide,* 6th ed., see Chap. 158, "Tricyclic Antidepressants," Chap. 159, "Newer Antidepressants and Serotonin Syndrome," and Chap. 160, "Monoamine Oxidase Inhibitors," by Kirk C. Mills; Chap. 161, "Antipsychotics," by Richard A. Harrigan and William J. Brady; and Chap. 162, "Lithium," by Sandra M. Schneider and Daniel S. Cobaugh.

103 SEDATIVE-HYPNOTICS
Keith L. Mausner

BARBITURATES

EPIDEMIOLOGY

- Overall, barbiturate abuse has been declining since the 1970s; since 1990, however, increased use among adolescents has been reported.
- Barbiturates are ranked among the top five toxic agents in overdose associated with major complications and fatalities.

PATHOPHYSIOLOGY

- Barbiturates are classified according to their duration of action: long-acting (barbital, phenobarbital, duration of action >6 hours); intermediate-acting (amobarbital, duration of action 3 to 6 hours); short-acting (pentobarbital, secobarbital, duration of action <3 hours); and ultrashort-acting (thiopental, methohexital, duration of action 0.3 hours).
- Long-acting barbiturates are weaker acids (lower pK_a values); in a basic medium they are largely ionized and therefore less lipid soluble. Tissue permeability decreases and the drug is more readily excreted by the kidneys. This is why forced alkaline diuresis is useful in long-acting barbiturate overdose.
- The intermediate-, short-, and ultrashort-acting barbiturates are stronger acids and are not affected by pH in this way; urinary alkalinization is not clinically useful.
- Barbiturates are hepatically metabolized and induce hepatic cytochrome P450 activity. Chronic barbiturate users will have an increased rate of metabolism of oral contraceptives, anticoagulants, and corticosteroids.
- The main action of barbiturates is to depress nerve and muscle cell activity; this occurs mainly through enhancement of the action of the inhibitory neurotransmitter gamma-aminobutyric acid (GABA).

CLINICAL FEATURES

- Mild to moderate intoxication resembles alcohol intoxication; drowsiness, disinhibition, ataxia, slurred speech, and confusion worsen with increasing dose.
- Stupor, coma, or complete neurologic unresponsiveness occur with severe intoxication, as do respiratory depression, hypotension, and hypothermia.
- Heart rate is not diagnostic, and pupil size and reactivity, nystagmus, and deep tendon reflexes are variable.
- Gastrointestinal (GI) motility is slowed, delaying gastric emptying.
- Hypoglycemia may be seen.
- Respiratory depression and hypothermia are centrally mediated.
- Hypotension is due to decreased vascular tone and venous pooling.
- Early death from barbiturate overdose usually results from cardiovascular collapse and respiratory arrest.
- Complications include aspiration pneumonia, noncardiogenic pulmonary edema, and acute respiratory distress syndrome (ARDS).
- Severe poisoning can be assumed if more than 10 times the hypnotic dose is ingested at one time.[1]

DIAGNOSIS AND DIFFERENTIAL

- Barbiturate serum levels may establish the diagnosis, and are useful to distinguish long- from short-acting barbiturates, since the treatment approach is different.
- The differential diagnosis of barbiturate poisoning includes intoxication with other sedative-hypnotics or alcohol, as well as environmental hypothermia and other causes of coma.
- Barbiturates are more likely to produce coma and myocardial depression than benzodiazepines. Chloral hydrate is associated with cardiac arrhythmias.
- Ethchlorvynol may produce a vinyl-like odor and prolonged coma.
- Glutethimide may cause fluctuating central nervous system (CNS) impairment and anticholinergic signs.
- Bedside glucose determination is indicated for all patients with altered level of consciousness, as well as consideration of naloxone and thiamine administration.

EMERGENCY DEPARTMENT CARE AND DISPOSITION

- Emergent priorities remain airway, breathing, and circulation. Cardiac monitoring and an intravenous (IV) line should be instituted.
- Endotracheal intubation is often necessary in severe sedative-hypnotic overdose.

- Volume expansion with isotonic saline is the primary treatment for shock and hypotension. In elderly patients, or those with a history of heart failure or renal failure, 250-mL boluses may be prudent. Dopamine or norepinephrine may be necessary if volume resuscitation is ineffective.
- Activated charcoal 1 to 2 g/kg should be administered since it decreases absorption; the addition of a cathartic such as sorbitol has no proven benefit. The airway should be secured first if there is significant risk of aspiration.
- Multiple dose activated charcoal 25 to 50 g every 4 hours may decrease barbiturate serum levels.[2] There is no evidence of any benefit of gastric lavage over activated charcoal.
- Forced diuresis with saline and furosemide, titrating urine output to 4 to 6 mL/kg/h, is beneficial in phenobarbital poisoning.
- Urinary alkalinization promotes the excretion of long-acting barbiturates. Sodium bicarbonate 1 to 2 mEq/kg IV bolus should be administered. Then, 50 to 100 mEq bicarbonate should be added to 500 mL of D_5W and the drip rate adjusted to maintain an arterial pH of 7.45 to 7.50, urinary pH of 8.0, and urine output of 2 mL/kg/h.
- The serum potassium level must remain at least 4.0 mEq/L for alkalinization to be effective. Electrolytes and effectiveness of therapy should be monitored every 2 to 4 hours.
- Hemodialysis and hemoperfusion are indicated for patients who deteriorate despite aggressive supportive care.
- Close monitoring over 6 to 8 hours and documentation of improvement in neurologic and vital signs may allow patients with mild to moderate toxicity to be discharged to psychiatric care or home if appropriate.
- Severe toxicity requires admission, and toxicology consultation is recommended.
- Barbiturate abstinence syndrome occurs with abrupt withdrawal in chronic users, and produces minor withdrawal findings within 24 hours and major life-threatening manifestations in 2 to 8 days. Short-acting agents produce more severe withdrawal than do long-acting agents.[3]
- Clinical manifestations of barbiturate abstinence syndrome are similar to alcohol withdrawal. Minor findings include anxiety, depression, insomnia, anorexia, nausea, vomiting, muscle twitching, abdominal cramping, and sweating.
- Severe manifestations include psychosis, hallucinations, delirium, seizures, hyperthermia, and cardiovascular collapse.
- Treatment of barbiturate abstinence syndrome consists of aggressive supportive care and IV benzodiazepines or barbiturates, with subsequent tapering of dose.

BENZODIAZEPINES

EPIDEMIOLOGY

- In 2000, there were 49,849 reported benzodiazepine toxic exposures.[4] There is a low mortality rate from isolated benzodiazepine ingestion. However, mixed overdose results in higher morbidity and mortality.

PATHOPHYSIOLOGY

- A specific CNS benzodiazepine receptor has been identified.[5] Interaction of a benzodiazepine and the receptor increases the activity of the inhibitory neurotransmitter GABA.

CLINICAL FEATURES

- Fatal isolated benzodiazepine overdose is more likely with short-acting agents such as triazolam, alprazolam, or temazepam.
- Chronic benzodiazepine users are at risk for a withdrawal syndrome similar to alcohol or barbiturate withdrawal.
- The most significant effects of benzodiazepines are on the CNS, which include drowsiness, dizziness, slurred speech, confusion, and cognitive impairment. Other reported effects are headache, nausea, vomiting, chest pain, arthralgias, diarrhea, and incontinence.
- Rare paradoxical reactions include rage and delirium.
- Respiratory depression and hypotension are more likely to occur with parenteral administration or with co-ingestants.
- The elderly are more susceptible to the adverse effects of benzodiazepines.

DIAGNOSIS AND DIFFERENTIAL

- Toxicology screening may be useful in establishing the diagnosis, but the laboratory may not routinely screen for all available benzodiazepines. It is therefore essential to know the laboratory's limitations.
- Serum benzodiazepine levels are not clinically useful in overdoses.

EMERGENCY DEPARTMENT CARE AND DISPOSITION

- Emergent priorities remain airway, breathing, and circulation.
- Activated charcoal 1 to 2 g/kg should be adminis-

tered; there is no role for multiple dose activated charcoal.
- Flumazenil, a benzodiazepine antagonist, is not indicated for empiric administration in poisoned patients. Seizures may occur in mixed ingestions, especially those involving tricyclic antidepressants, and in patients chronically dependent on benzodiazepines or with underlying seizure disorders.[6]
- Flumazenil is also contraindicated in suspected elevated intracranial pressure or head injury.
- Flumazenil's primary use is in reversing the effects of benzodiazepines administered acutely for sedation. Due to its short half-life (approximately 1 hour), it is mainly effective with short-acting agents such as midazolam.
- Flumazenil is administered 0.2 mg IV every minute to response or a total dose of 3 mg.
- Forced diuresis, urinary alkalinization, hemodialysis, and hemoperfusion are not effective in enhancing benzodiazepine elimination.
- Care for benzodiazepine ingestions is primarily supportive.
- Hospital admission is indicated for significant alterations in mental status, respiratory depression, and hypotension. Psychiatric consultation is indicated for intentional overdoses.

NONBENZODIAZEPINE SEDATIVE-HYPNOTICS

EPIDEMIOLOGY

- Despite rare clinical use, drugs such as ethchlorvynol, meprobamate, glutethimide, and methaqualone continue to be reported in toxic exposures.[7] Newer drugs such as buspirone, zolpidem, and zaleplon are prescribed commonly.
- Gamma-hydroxybutyrate (GHB) is used abroad in the treatment of narcolepsy and cataplexy.
- In the United States, only sodium oxybate (Xyrem), a form of GHB, has been approved for the treatment of cataplexy associated with narcolepsy.
- Intentional misuse and overdose of GHB is increasingly prevalent in raves, circuit parties, and bodybuilder club cultures.[8,9] GHB has been implicated in drug-facilitated sexual assault.[10]

PATHOPHYSIOLOGY

- The nonbenzodiazepine sedative-hypnotics tend to be highly lipophilic and concentrate in the CNS, causing varying degrees of CNS depression.
- Gamma-hydoxybutyrolactone (GBL) and gamma-

1,4-butanediol (GD) are metabolized after ingestion to GHB.

CLINICAL FEATURES

GAMMA-HYDROXYBUTYRATE (GHB)

- Effects are dose dependent. Abrupt onset of aggressive behavior followed by drowsiness, dizziness, euphoria, or coma, with rapid awakening and amnesia may be seen.
- Other findings may include nystagmus, ataxia, apnea, seizure-like activity, and bradycardia.
- Marked agitation on stimulation such as a sternal rub or intubation is common.
- Improperly synthesized GHB may contain sodium hydroxide, causing esophageal burns or pulmonary injury in the event of aspiration.
- Chronic GHB users may be at risk for an abstinence syndrome similar to alcohol withdrawal, which may be severe and last from 5 to 15 days.[11]

BUSPIRONE

- Buspirone is unrelated to the other sedative-hypnotics and does not appear to be addictive.[12]
- Overdoses of up to 3 g (150 times the average anxiolytic dose) have produced no lasting ill effects.
- Symptoms of overdose include drowsiness and dysphoria. Rare findings include hypotension, bradycardia, seizures, GI upset, dystonia, and priapism.
- Hypertensive reactions may occur with co-administration of monoamine oxidase inhibitors.

CHLORAL HYDRATE

- Toxic doses produce severe CNS, respiratory, and cardiovascular depression, as well as resistant ventricular arrhythmias, which are the leading cause of mortality in overdose.[13]
- Clues to ingestion include a combination of a pear-like breath odor, hypotension, and dysrhythmias. It is also a GI irritant and overdose may be associated with GI bleeding or intestinal perforation. Chloral hydrate is radiopaque and abdominal radiographs may be useful in diagnosis and to exclude perforation.

ETHCHLORVYNOL

- CNS effects of overdose include nystagmus, lethargy, and prolonged coma.
- Hypothermia, hypotension, bradycardia, and noncardiogenic pulmonary edema may occur.
- A distinct vinyl-like breath odor may be a clue to diagnosis.

GLUTETHIMIDE

- The manifestations of glutethimide overdose are similar to barbiturate toxicity except for the presence of prominent anticholinergic findings, and a fluctuating, prolonged coma.

MEPROBAMATE

- The CNS manifestations of meprobamate toxicity are similar to those of other sedative-hypnotics.
- Hypotension is a common feature of serious overdose.
- Seizures, cardiac arrhythmias, and pulmonary edema have been reported as well.
- Prolonged fluctuating coma may occur secondary to continued absorption from GI concretions of the drug.
- Abstinence syndromes in individuals physically dependent on meprobamate can be severe, and usually occur within 1 to 2 days of drug discontinuation.
- Meprobamate is the active metabolite of carisoprodol (Soma), a commonly prescribed noncontrolled muscle relaxant.[14]

METHAQUALONE

- Methaqualone has similar CNS, respiratory, and cardiovascular effects to the other sedative hypnotics.
- Unlike the others, it also causes hypertonicity, clonus, hyperreflexia, and muscle twitching.
- It often impairs judgment and impulse control, increasing the risk of morbidity and mortality from trauma.[15]

ZALEPLON AND ZOLPIDEM

- Zaleplon and zolpidem are used for the treatment of insomnia.
- Findings in zolpidem overdose include drowsiness, vomiting, and rarely coma and respiratory depression.
- Flumazenil may reverse some of the effects of zolpidem, but its use is not recommended in most overdose situations for the reasons outlined in the section on benzodiazepines.

EMERGENCY DEPARTMENT CARE AND DISPOSITION

- Emergent priorities remain airway, breathing, and circulation.
- Treatment for nonbenzodiazepine sedative-hypnotic toxicity is primarily supportive.
- Since these agents may cause pulmonary edema, judicious administration of IV fluids along with early vasopressors is indicated to treat hypotension.
- Activated charcoal 1 to 2 g/kg should be administered.
- Because of meprobamate's tendency to form GI concretions, whole bowel irrigation using 2 L/h polyethylene glycol (40 mL/kg/h in children) until rectal effluent is clear may be of benefit once GI perforation is excluded. Forced diuresis is not effective with

the nonbenzodiazepine agents due to limited renal excretion.

- Chloral hydrate–induced arrhythmias may respond to β-blockers. Overdrive pacing may be necessary for ventricular tachycardia.
- β-Adrenergic agents (epinephrine, isoproterenol, and dopamine) may worsen chloral hydrate–induced arrhythmias; if a pressor is needed for hypotension, an α-acting agent such as norepinephrine should be used.
- There should be a low threshold for hospital admission of these patients, especially with any significant CNS or respiratory depression, hypotension, or arrhythmias.
- Glutethimide and meprobamate are of special concern because of the potential for fluctuating or delayed manifestations.

REFERENCES

1. McCarron MM, Schulze BW, Walberg CB, et al: Short-acting barbiturate overdosage: Correlation of intoxication with serum barbiturate concentration. *JAMA* 248:55, 1982.
2. Anonymous: Position statement and practice guidelines on the use of multidose activated charcoal in the treatment of acute poisoning. American Academy of Clinical Toxicology; European Association of Poisons Centres and Clinical Toxicologists. *Clin Toxicol* 37:731, 1999.
3. Khantzian EJ, McKenna GJ: Acute toxic and withdrawal reactions associated with drug use and abuse. *Ann Intern Med* 90:361, 1979.
4. Litovitz TL, Klein-Schwartz W, White S, et al: 2000 Annual Report of the American Association of Poison Control Centers Toxic Exposure Surveillance System. *Am J Emerg Med* 19:337, 2001.
5. Mohler H, Okada T: Benzodiazepine receptor: Demonstration in the central nervous system. *Science* 198:849, 1977.
6. Spivey WH: Flumazenil and seizures: An analysis of 43 cases. *Clin Ther* 14:292, 1992.
7. Litovitz TL, Klein-Schwartz W, Rogers GC Jr, et al: 2001 Annual Report of the American Association of Poison Control Centers Toxic Exposure Surveillance System. *Am J Emerg Med* 20:391, 2002.
8. Weir E: Raves: A review of the culture, the drugs and the prevention of harm. *Can Med Assoc J* 162:1843, 2000.
9. Mansergh G, Colfax GN, Marks G, et al: The circuit party men's health survey: Findings and implications for gay and bisexual men. *Am J Public Health* 91:953, 2001.
10. ElSohly MA, Salamone SJ: Prevalence of drugs used in cases of alleged sexual assault. *J Anal Toxicol* 23:141, 1999.
11. Dyer JE, Roth B, Hyma BA: Gamma-hydroxybutyrate withdrawal syndrome. *Ann Emerg Med* 37:147, 2001.
12. Pecknold JC: A risk-benefit assessment of buspirone in the treatment of anxiety disorders. *Drug Safety* 16:118, 1997.
13. Gaulier JM, Merle G, Lacassie E, et al: Fatal intoxications with chloral hydrate. *J Forensic Sci* 46:1507, 2001.
14. Reeves RR, Carter OS, Pinkofsky HB, et al: Carisoprodol (Soma): Abuse potential and physician unawareness. *J Addict Dis* 18:51, 1999.
15. Wetli CV: Changing patterns of methaqualone abuse: A survey of 246 fatalities. *JAMA* 249:621, 1983.

For further reading in *Emergency Medicine: A Comprehensive Study Guide,* 6th ed., see Chap. 163, "Barbiturates," by R.M. Schears; Chap. 164, "Benzodiazepines," by G.M. Bosse; and Chap. 165, "Nonbenzodiazepine Hypnosedatives," by R.M. Schears.

104 ALCOHOLS
Michael P. Kefer

INTRODUCTION

- An understanding of the osmolal gap is important in discussing the toxicity of the common alcohols. The presence of an osmolal gap suggests the presence of a low-molecular-weight substance such as ethanol, isopropanol, methanol, or ethylene glycol.
- The osmolal gap = osm measured − osm calculated

normal osm gap <10 mOsm/L
osm measured = laboratory determination by freezing point depression
osm calculated = 2 (Na) + BUN/2.8 + glucose/18

ETHANOL

EPIDEMIOLOGY

- Ethanol is the most frequently used and abused intoxicant in the United States and contributes to about 100,000 deaths per year.[1] About 3 percent of all emergency department (ED) visits are related to ethanol use.[2]
- Distilled spirits have ethanol volumes of 40 to 50% (80 to 100 proof), wines 10 to 20%, and beers 2 to 6%.

PATHOPHYSIOLOGY

- Although acute ethanol intoxication may cause death directly from respiratory depression, morbidity and mortality are usually related to accidental injury from impaired cognitive function.

- The major site of absorption is in the proximal small bowel.
- Ethanol is metabolized in the liver by alcohol dehydrogenase, with a small portion excreted unchanged in the lungs and urine.
- On average, nondrinkers eliminate ethanol from the bloodstream at a rate of 15 to 20 mg/dL/h and chronic drinkers at 25 to 35 mg/dL/h.

CLINICAL FEATURES

- Signs and symptoms of ethanol intoxication include slurred speech, disinhibited behavior, central nervous system (CNS) depression, and altered coordination. Lowering of blood pressure with a reflex tachycardia may be seen.
- Manifestations of serious head injury may be identical to, or clouded by, ethanol intoxication.
- Legally, for purposes of operating a motor vehicle, a blood ethanol level of 80 to 100 mg/dL defines intoxication. Clinically, the level correlates poorly because of the development of tolerance. A level of 400 mg/dL may be lethal in the nondrinker, but in the alcoholic there may be no significant signs of intoxication.[3]

DIAGNOSIS AND DIFFERENTIAL

- The diagnosis is based on clinical presentation with confirmation of ethanol intake, usually by obtaining a serum ethanol level.
- The differential diagnosis is wide when one considers other drugs that cause CNS depression such as benzodiazepines, barbiturates, narcotics, and other alcohols. Head injury or hypoglycemia may manifest identical to or be clouded by ethanol intoxication.

EMERGENCY DEPARTMENT CARE AND DISPOSITION

- The mainstay of treatment is observation of the patient until clinically sober. A careful physical examination should be performed to evaluate for complicating injury or illness.
- Hypoglycemia should be excluded by measuring fingerstick glucose. Thiamine 100 mg IV or IM should be administered. If required, IV fluids should contain 5% dextrose, as these patients are often glycogen depleted.
- Any deterioration or lack of improvement during observation should be considered secondary to causes other than ethanol and managed accordingly. The patient can be discharged once intoxication has resolved

to the extent that the patient does not pose a threat to self or others.

ISOPROPANOL

EPIDEMIOLOGY

- Isopropanol is commonly found in rubbing alcohol, solvents, skin and hair products, paint thinners, and antifreeze.

PATHOPHYSIOLOGY

- Most isopropanol is absorbed within 30 minutes of oral ingestion.
- Its CNS depressant effects are twice as potent and twice as long lasting as ethanol.
- Isopropanol is metabolized in the liver to acetone. Acetone is further metabolized to acetate and formate, but not to such a degree as to cause a significant metabolic acidosis.

CLINICAL FEATURES

- Isopropanol intoxication manifests similarly to ethanol intoxication except the duration is longer and the CNS depressant effects are more profound.
- The smell of rubbing alcohol or the fruity odor of ketones may be noted on the patient's breath. Severe poisoning is marked by early onset coma, respiratory depression, and hypotension.
- Hemorrhagic gastritis is a characteristic finding that causes nausea, vomiting, and abdominal pain.
- Upper gastrointestinal (GI) bleeding may be severe. Less common complications include hepatic dysfunction, acute tubular necrosis, and rhabdomyolysis.

DIAGNOSIS AND DIFFERENTIAL

- Calculation of the osmolal gap is useful if isopropanol testing is not immediately available. In addition to an elevated isopropanol level, laboratory investigation may reveal ketonemia and ketonuria from accumulation of acetone, without hyperglycemia or glycosuria, and the presence of an osmolal gap.
- Mild acidosis may be present from acetone metabolism to acetate and formate, or hypotension with resultant lactic acidosis.
- Isopropanol intoxication is characteristically distinguished from that of other common alcohols by the significant osmolal gap without a significant anion gap metabolic acidosis and a negative ethanol level.

EMERGENCY DEPARTMENT CARE AND DISPOSITION

- General supportive measures are indicated. As with any patient who presents with altered mental status, administration of glucose, thiamine, and naloxone should be considered.
- While charcoal does not bind alcohols, it should be administered if there is suspected co-ingestion of an adsorbable substance.
- Hypotension usually responds to IV fluids but vasopressors may be necessary. Severe hemorrhagic gastritis may require transfusion.
- Hemodialysis is indicated for refractory hypotension or when the predicted peak level of isopropanol is >400 mg/dL. Hemodialysis removes both isopropanol and acetone.
- Patients with prolonged CNS depression require admission. Those who are asymptomatic after 6 to 8 hours of observation can be discharged or referred for psychiatric evaluation if indicated.

METHANOL AND ETHYLENE GLYCOL

EPIDEMIOLOGY

- Methanol is commonly found as a solvent in paint products, windshield wiper fluids, and antifreeze.
- Ethylene glycol is commonly used as an antifreeze and preservative, and is found in polishes and detergents.

PATHOPHYSIOLOGY OF METHANOL

- Methanol is metabolized in the liver by alcohol dehydrogenase to the toxic compounds formaldehyde and formic acid. In the presence of folate, formic acid is converted to carbon dioxide and water.
- Methanol accumulation results in a large osmolal gap.
- Formaldehyde accumulation in the retina causes edema and optic papillitis.
- Formic acid accumulation results in a high anion–gap metabolic acidosis.
- Methanol is a potent GI mucosal irritant and causes pancreatitis.

PATHOPHYSIOLOGY OF ETHYLENE GLYCOL

- Ethylene glycol is metabolized in the liver by alcohol dehydrogenase to the toxic compound glycoaldehyde. This is further metabolized in the liver and kidneys to formic acid, glyoxylic acid, and oxalic acid. In the

presence of thiamine or pyridoxine, glyoxylic acid is converted to nontoxic metabolites.
- Ethylene glycol accumulation results in a large osmolal gap.
- Acid metabolite accumulation results in a high anion–gap metabolic acidosis.
- Oxalic acid precipitates with calcium to form calcium oxalate crystals found in the urine.

CLINICAL FEATURES OF METHANOL POISONING

- Symptoms may not appear for 12 to 18 hours after ingestion because its toxic metabolites must accumulate. Time to symptom onset may be longer if ethanol is consumed, as ethanol inhibits methanol metabolism.
- Symptoms include altered sensorium, visual disturbances (classically, feeling as if one is looking at a snowstorm), abdominal pain, nausea, and vomiting.
- The GI symptoms may be due to mucosal irritation or pancreatitis.
- On physical examination, CNS signs can vary from lethargy to coma. Funduscopic examination may show retinal edema or hyperemia of the optic disk caused by formaldehyde.

CLINICAL FEATURES OF ETHYLENE GLYCOL POISONING

- Ethylene glycol poisoning often exhibits three distinct clinical phases after ingestion due to its toxic metabolites.
- First, within 12 hours, CNS effects predominate. The patient appears intoxicated without the odor of ethanol on the breath.
- Second, 12 to 24 hours after ingestion, cardiopulmonary effects predominate. Elevated pulse rate, respiratory rate, and blood pressure are common. Congestive heart failure, acute respiratory distress syndrome, and circulatory collapse are also noted.
- Third, 24 to 72 hours after ingestion, renal effects predominate. Flank pain with costovertebral angle tenderness is noted. Acute tubular necrosis with acute renal failure occurs if appropriate treatment is not received. Calcium oxalate crystals are noted on urinalysis. Elevated creatine phosphokinase (CPK) may be seen.
- Hypocalcemia may result from precipitation of calcium oxalate into tissues and may be severe enough to cause tetany and prolongation of the QT interval.
- The funduscopic examination is normal, which helps to distinguish this from methanol toxicity.

TABLE 104-1   The Differential Diagnosis of an Anion Gap Metabolic Acidosis Is Recalled by the Acronym MUDPILES

Methanol

Uremia

Diabetic ketoacidosis

Paraldehyde

Iron, isoniazid, inhalants

Lactic acidosis

Ethanol, ethylene glycol

Salicylates

DIAGNOSIS AND DIFFERENTIAL

- The diagnosis is based on clinical presentation and laboratory findings of a high anion–gap metabolic acidosis with elevated levels of methanol or ethylene glycol. An elevated osmolal gap is present, and calculation of this is useful if methanol or ethylene glycol testing is not immediately available.
- Other laboratory findings include hypocalcemia, leukocytosis, and calcium oxalate crystals in the urine.
- The differential diagnosis includes other causes of an anion gap metabolic acidosis and can be recalled using the acronym MUDPILES (Table 104-1).
- Ethylene glycol poisoning differs from methanol poisoning in that visual disturbances and funduscopic abnormalities are absent and calcium oxalate crystals are present in the urine.

EMERGENCY DEPARTMENT CARE AND DISPOSITION

- Treatment is based on preventing formation of the toxic metabolites and removing them from the body.
- General supportive measures are indicated, including the administration of glucose, thiamine, and naloxone in the patient with altered mental status.
- Sodium bicarbonate may be required to correct acidosis.
- Fomepizole, when available, is preferred over ethanol to prevent formation of toxic metabolites by alcohol dehydrogenase.[4,5] Fomepizole has 8000 times greater affinity for alcohol dehydrogenase, with fewer side effects compared to ethanol.[6]
- Ethanol has 20 times greater affinity for alcohol dehydrogenase than methanol and 100 times that of ethylene glycol.
- Indications for initiating fomepizole or ethanol treatment include: (1) suspected methanol or ethylene glycol poisoning; (2) the presence of an anion-gap metabolic acidosis; (3) a methanol or ethylene glycol level >20 mg/dL; and (4) any patient requiring dialysis.

- The dose of fomepizole is 15 mg/kg IV load followed by 10 mg/kg every 12 hours for 4 doses.
- The dose of ethanol is 0.8 g/kg IV load followed by 0.11 g/kg/h continuous infusion in the average drinker, and 0.15 g/kg/h in the heavy drinker. The continuous infusion is adjusted accordingly, to keep the blood ethanol level at 100 to 150 mg/dL.
- If necessary, oral treatment with alcoholic beverages can be initiated. The amount of ethanol contained in these is calculated by the formula: grams of ethanol = mL beverage × 0.9 × (proof/200).
- Glucose levels are monitored during treatment with ethanol, especially in children.
- Dialysis eliminates both methanol and ethylene glycol and their toxic metabolites. Indications for dialysis are: (1) signs or symptoms of significant toxicity; (2) the presence of an anion-gap metabolic acidosis; (3) a methanol or ethylene glycol level >20 mg/dL; and (4) signs of ocular toxicity from methanol or nephrotoxicity from ethylene glycol.
- Peritoneal dialysis is considered only when hemodialysis is not available.
- Use of fomepizole or ethanol does not affect indications for dialysis. Both fomepizole and ethanol are dialyzable. Therefore, during dialysis, the dosing interval of fomepizole is increased to every 4 hours. The continuous infusion rate of ethanol is doubled initially and readjusted accordingly, to maintain a level of 100 to 150 mg/dL.
- Treatment with dialysis, fomepizole, or ethanol is continued until the methanol or ethylene glycol level is zero and acidosis has resolved.
- Vitamin therapy is important in treatment. In methanol poisoning, folate 50 mg IV every 4 hours is administered to drive the conversion of formic acid to carbon dioxide and water.
- In ethylene glycol poisoning, pyridoxine 100 mg and thiamine 100 mg IV or IM is administered to drive the conversion of ethylene glycol to nontoxic metabolites.
- Calcium replacement may be necessary due to ethylene glycol toxicity.
- Any patient with serious signs or symptoms of toxicity should be admitted to a facility capable of intensive care and hemodialysis.
- Asymptomatic individuals should be admitted for observation because of possible delayed onset of toxic symptoms.

REFERENCES

1. Secretary of Health and Human Services: Tenth Special Report to the U.S. Congress on Alcohol and Health. Washington, DC: U.S. Dept of Health and Human Services, 2000.

2. Li G, Keyl PM, Rothman R, et al: Epidemiology of alcohol-related emergency department visits. *Acad Emerg Med* 5:788, 1998.

3. Sullivan JB, Hauptman M, Bronstein AC: Lack of observable intoxication in humans with high blood alcohol concentrations. *J Forensic Sci* 32:1660, 1987.

4. Brent J, McMartin KE, Phillips S, et al: Methylpyrazole for Toxic Alcohols Study Group. Fomepizole for the treatment of methanol poisoning. *N Engl J Med* 344:424, 2001.

5. Brent J, McMartin KE, Phillips S, et al: Methylpyrazole for Toxic Alcohols Study Group. Fomepizole for the treatment of ethylene glycol poisoning. *N Engl J Med* 340:832, 1999.

6. Sivilotti MLA, Burns MJ, McMartin KE, et al: Toxicokinetics of ethylene glycol during fomepizole therapy: Implications for management. *Ann Emerg Med* 36:11, 2000.

For further reading in *Emergency Medicine: A Comprehensive Study Guide,* 6th ed., see Chap. 166, "Alcohols," by William A. Burke and Wilma V. Henderson.

105 DRUGS OF ABUSE

Jeffrey N. Glaspy

OPIOIDS

EPIDEMIOLOGY

- The most commonly abused opioids in the U.S. are heroin and methadone.
- Emergency department (ED) visits related to hydrocodone (Vicodin) and oxycodone (Percocet, OxyContin) overdose have almost doubled since 1999.[1]

PATHOPHYSIOLOGY

- The International Union of Pharmacology has adopted new nomenclature for opioid receptors. The μ receptor is now called OP3, the κ is now OP2, and the δ is now the OP1 receptor.
- Opioids act as agonists at the OP3, OP2, and OP1 sites in the central nervous system (CNS), peripheral nervous system (PNS), and the gastrointestinal (GI) tract.
- Stimulation of OP3 receptors, which are further divided into subtypes a and b, results in analgesia, respiratory depression, cough suppression, and euphoria.[2] All currently available opioids have some activity

at the OP3b receptor and result in some degree of respiratory depression.
- The metabolism of codeine, morphine, propoxyphene, oxycodone, meperidine, and methadone is mostly hepatic. Co-ingestion of certain medications, such as antiretroviral agents, can inhibit hepatic metabolism, especially the metabolism of methadone.

CLINICAL FEATURES

- Opioids cause varying degrees of respiratory depression, altered mental status, miosis, orthostatic hypotension, nausea, vomiting, histamine release (resulting in urticaria and bronchospasm), decreased GI motility, and urinary retention.
- Although the classic triad of opioid overdose is coma, miosis, and respiratory depression, miosis is not universally present.
- Normal pupillary size or mydriasis has been reported with the use of meperidine, morphine, propoxyphene, pentazocine, and diphenoxylate.
- Mydriasis also may result from co-ingestants or with severe cerebral hypoxia.
- Opioid withdrawal usually manifests in feelings of anxiety, insomnia, yawning, lacrimation, diaphoresis, rhinorrhea, diffuse myalgias, piloerection, mydriasis, nausea, vomiting, diarrhea, and abdominal cramping. Opioid withdrawal is rarely life threatening.

DIAGNOSIS AND DIFFERENTIAL

- Opioid overdose or withdrawal is a clinical diagnosis.
- The classic triad of coma, miosis, and respiratory depression strongly suggests acute or chronic opioid intoxication.
- Detection of opioids in the urine may aid in diagnosis of opioid overdose; however, there is a high false-negative rate and the results of the urine test are not immediately available to the clinician.
- An acetaminophen level should be obtained in cases of propoxyphene, oxycodone, hydrocodone, tramadol, and codeine overdose, as well as in any intentional suicidal ingestion.
- The differential diagnosis of opioid overdose includes ingestion of clonidine, organophosphates, carbamates, phenothiazines, sedative-hypnotic agents, or gamma-hydroxybutyrate (GHB); carbon monoxide poisoning; hypoglycemia; CNS infection; postictal state; and pontine hemorrhage.
- The diagnosis of opioid withdrawal is established when a constellation of withdrawal symptoms are temporally related to the abrupt cessation of an opioid agent.

The differential diagnosis of opioid withdrawal includes drugs and toxins that promote an adrenergic state, other drug withdrawal, and hyperthyroidism.

EMERGENCY DEPARTMENT CARE AND DISPOSITION

- Airway management is the most crucial aspect in the initial treatment of opioid overdose. Bag-valve-mask support may be needed to maintain oxygenation while naloxone and/or endotracheal intubation are being prepared.
- Naloxone is a pure competitive antagonist at all opioid receptors, with particular affinity for the OP3 receptor. It can be given intravenously, intratracheally, intramuscularly, subcutaneously, and intralingually. Onset after IV administration is 1 to 2 minutes; it has a 20- to 60-minute duration of action.
- For patients presenting with significant respiratory depression, a 2-mg IV dose should be given. Repeated doses of 2 mg IV every 3 minutes are then administered until respiratory depression is reversed or until a maximum dose of 10 mg has been reached.
- Propoxyphene, fentanyl, pentazocine, dextromethorphan, and sustained preparations of oxycodone may require administration of serial 2-mg doses.
- For opioid-dependent individuals without respiratory depression, smaller doses of naloxone (such as 0.05 mg IV) may be used to prevent opioid withdrawal. For non–opioid dependent individuals without respiratory depression, an initial dose of 0.4 mg IV may be given initially.
- A continuous naloxone infusion should be administered only if the patient has required multiple boluses of naloxone. The IV infusion dosage is two thirds of the total reversal dose per hour.
- Patients on naloxone infusions may require additional bolus doses and/or upward (for respiratory depression) or downward (for opioid withdrawal) adjustments in the infusion rate, and should be admitted to an intensive care unit or monitored setting.[3]
- Activated charcoal should be administered if large amounts of opioids have been ingested or if co-ingestion is a possibility. Multiple dose activated charcoal administration is indicated in diphenoxylate hydrochloride-atropine sulfate (Lomotil) ingestion and in cases of large ingestions of sustained-release preparations.
- An ED observation period of 4 to 6 hours is recommended for most cases of opioid intoxication.
- For longer-acting opioids (propoxyphene, methadone) or for sustained-release preparations, a 24- to 48-hour hospital admission is indicated.
- Opioid withdrawal is rarely life threatening. Supportive care with clonidine 0.1 to 0.2 mg PO, antiemetics, and antidiarrheals may alleviate discomfort.

SPECIAL CONSIDERATIONS

- Meperidine and its metabolite normeperidine are proconvulsive agents. Normeperidine is largely renally excreted and may accumulate in patients with impaired renal function, increasing the risk of seizures.
- Patients with meperidine-induced seizures should undergo a full seizure work-up and be observed in the hospital for 24 to 48 hours.
- The combination of meperidine or dextromethorphan with monoamine oxidase inhibitors can result in serotonin syndrome.
- Propoxyphene and its metabolite norpropoxyphene are cardiotoxic and neurotoxic. Propoxyphene overdose has been associated with intraventricular conduction disturbances, heart block, prolonged QT interval, ventricular bigeminy, and seizures.
- Patients with propoxyphene overdose should have an ECG ordered, be observed with cardiac monitoring for 6 hours, and be administered 1 mEq/kg of sodium bicarbonate if cardiotoxic effects are seen.
- Acute lung injury can occur immediately or be delayed up to 24 hours following heroin or methadone abuse. Treatment includes adequate oxygenation, intubation, and use of positive end-expiratory pressure ventilation. Naloxone, diuretics, and digoxin are usually not indicated.

COCAINE, AMPHETAMINES, AND OTHER STIMULANTS

EPIDEMIOLOGY

- Cocaine use is highest among persons 18 to 25 years of age, and the incidence appears to be climbing.
- ED visits by cocaine-abusing patients have tripled since 1988.

PATHOPHYSIOLOGY

COCAINE
- Cocaine is a water-soluble hydrochloride salt that is rapidly absorbed across all mucous membranes. Ether extraction yields crack cocaine, which is stable to pyrolysis and commonly smoked.
- The nasal route of ingestion causes a peak effect in 30 minutes and a duration of effect of 1 to 3 hours. Both the IV and inhalational routes produce rapid (1 to 2 minutes) effect and short (15 to 30 minutes) duration.

- Cocaine has quinidine-like effects on cardiac conduction, which may cause a wide QRS complex and QT interval prolongation. In large doses, myocardial toxicity may result in negative inotropy, wide complex dysrhythmia, bradycardia, and hypotension.
- Central effects are mediated through activation of the sympathetic nervous system, which produce characteristic effects of mydriasis, tachycardia, hypertension, and diaphoresis. These effects predispose the user to dysrhythmias, seizures, and hyperthermia.

AMPHETAMINES

- Methamphetamine is abused by ingestion, IV injection, inhalation, or insufflation. Peak effects occur rapidly with inhalation, insufflation, and IV injection.
- Amphetamines enhance the release and block the reuptake of catecholamines, and may directly stimulate catecholamine receptors. Some amphetamine metabolites inhibit monoamine oxidase.
- Stimulants such as ephedrine and phenylpropanolamine produce toxic effects similar to cocaine and amphetamines. Ephedrine has been linked to significant cardiovascular and neurologic toxicity, psychosis, severe hypertension, and death.

CLINICAL FEATURES

- Cocaine induces dysrhythmias, myocarditis, cardiomyopathy, myocardial ischemia and infarction, aortic rupture, and aortic and coronary artery dissection. Even at low doses, it can produce coronary artery vasoconstriction.[4]
- Animal data demonstrate increased platelet aggregation, thrombogenesis, accelerated atherosclerosis, myocardial toxicity, and increased myocardial oxygen demand.
- Any route of cocaine administration may induce Q wave and non–Q wave myocardial infarction in patients, even those without coronary artery disease.
- Cocaine abuse during pregnancy increases risk for spontaneous abortion, abruptio placentae, fetal prematurity, and intrauterine growth retardation.[5,6]
- Cocaine, amphetamine, phenylpropanolamine, and ephedrine abuse have been associated with significant neurologic syndromes, including seizure, intracranial infarctions, and hemorrhages.
- Crack cocaine use has been associated with pulmonary hemorrhage, pneumonitis, asthma, pulmonary edema, pneumomediastinum, pneumothorax, and pneumopericardium.
- "Body stuffers" (those who ingest small, poorly wrapped bags) and "body packers" (those who ingest large amounts of well-packaged bags) may die or demonstrate signs of severe cocaine toxicity if even a single bag ruptures.

- Intestinal ischemia, bowel necrosis, ischemic colitis, GI bleeding, bowel perforation, and splenic infarction may be induced by cocaine.
- Mortality from amphetamine toxicity is most commonly the result of hyperthermia, dysrhythmias, seizures, hypertension that results in intracranial infarction or hemorrhage, and encephalopathy.
- Methamphetamine abuse during pregnancy also has detrimental effects on fetal growth.
- Rhabdomyolysis also may occur with cocaine or amphetamine use.
- The cocaine- or amphetamine-intoxicated patient may demonstrate tachycardia, tachypnea, hypertension, hyperthermia, and any degree of altered mental status. Common symptoms include chest pain, palpitations, dyspnea, headache, and focal neurologic complaints.

DIAGNOSIS AND DIFFERENTIAL

- Diagnosis of cocaine, amphetamine, and stimulant intoxication is usually made clinically.
- Urine drug screening for the cocaine metabolite benzoylecgonine will be positive in most cases if cocaine use has occurred within the past 72 hours. This test is fairly specific and exhibits little cross-reactivity.
- Urine drug screens for amphetamines, however, are not specific and have high false-negative and false-positive results.
- Patients with hyperthermia and agitation should have a chemistry panel, blood urea nitrogen, creatinine, and creatine kinase (CK) screen for metabolic acidosis, renal failure, and rhabdomyolysis. An electrocardiogram (ECG), chest radiograph, and cardiac enzymes should be considered in cocaine- or amphetamine-intoxicated patients presenting with chest pain.
- Traumatic injury and hypoglycemia should be included in the differential diagnosis.
- Concomitant use of substances such as alcohol or opioids may significantly alter the presentation.

EMERGENCY DEPARTMENT CARE AND DISPOSITION

- Treatment of cocaine and amphetamine toxicity involves adequate sedation and assessment of vital signs. Benzodiazepines, such as lorazepam 2 mg IV or diazepam 5 mg IV, will often improve tachycardia and hypertension.
- Active cooling with mist spray and fanning is used to treat moderate or severe hyperthermia.
- Seizures should also be treated with benzodiazepines; however, phenobarbital loading or neuromuscular blockade may be necessary for status epilepticus.

- Cardiac ischemia or infarction should be treated with aspirin, nitrates, morphine, and benzodiazepines.
- β-Blockers are contraindicated due to unopposed α-receptor stimulation. Fibrinolytic therapy should be used with great caution since cocaine-associated intracranial hemorrhage and aortic or coronary artery dissection is a contraindication to thrombolysis.
- Cocaine-induced wide complex tachydysrhythmias and QRS interval prolongation should be treated by alkalinizing the serum to a pH of 7.45 to 7.5 with sodium bicarbonate. Acidification of the urine for amphetamine intoxication is not recommended.
- Hypertensive emergencies should be treated with nitroprusside or phentolamine.
- Asymptomatic body packers should be given one dose of activated charcoal, followed by polyethylene glycol electrolyte solution (GoLYTELY). If symptomatic, these patients should be given benzodiazepines and have immediate surgical consultation for laparotomy and packet removal.
- Amphetamines have a longer duration of effect than cocaine; therefore intoxication may require longer periods of observation or hospital admission.
- Patients with significantly increased CK levels, hyperthermia, myoglobinuria, or ECG changes consistent with myocardial ischemia should be hospitalized in an intensive care unit setting.

HALLUCINOGENS

EPIDEMIOLOGY

- The classic hallucinogens include the indole alkylamines [lysergic acid diethylamide (LSD), psilocybin] and phenylethylamine ("ecstasy," mescaline); however, other drugs [phencyclidine (PCP), marijuana] are also frequently abused for the purpose of alteration of sensory perception.

PATHOPHYSIOLOGY

- Table 105-1 summarizes the classification, mechanism, typical dose, duration of action, features, complications, and specific treatments of commonly abused hallucinogens.

CLINICAL FEATURES

- Massive overdose of LSD may produce coma, respiratory arrest, hyperthermia, and coagulopathy.[7]
- Symptom onset after psilocybin ingestion is about 30 minutes and duration of action is 4 to 6 hours. Serious

medical side effects are rare, but seizures and hyperthermia have been reported.
- Mescaline causes hallucinogenic effects similar to, but weaker than, LSD. These effects usually begin several hours after ingestion and persist for 6 to 12 hours. Significant morbidity and mortality due to mescaline abuse is rare.
- Methylenedioxymethamphetamine, also known as MDMA or "ecstasy," is structurally related to both amphetamines and mescaline. Effects last about 4 to 6 hours and include intensification of sensory stimuli and hallucinations. Mydriasis and mild elevations of pulse and blood pressure are common, although fatal arrhythmias and death have been reported.
- PCP is a piperidine derivative and a commonly abused street drug that is structurally related to ketamine. Unlike the classic hallucinogens it causes clouding of the sensorium.
- PCP can be smoked, snorted, ingested, or injected. Patients may present with CNS stimulation or depression, violent behavior, catatonia, and sympathomimetic effects. Rhabdomyolysis, renal failure, seizure, ataxia, muscle rigidity, hypoglycemia, hypertension, and elevated CPK levels are not uncommon.
- Marijuana use most commonly causes drowsiness, euphoria, heightened sensory awareness, paranoia, and distortions of time and space.

DIAGNOSIS AND DIFFERENTIAL

- Diagnosis of LSD abuse is based on history of use and presence of sympathomimetic signs.
- Routine drug screens will not detect psilocybin or mescaline.
- Urine tests for PCP may be falsely negative in acute intoxication or falsely positive weeks after use in chronic abusers.[8]
- Traumatic injuries, hypoglycemia, elevated CK level, and rhabdomyolysis should be ruled out in suspected cases of PCP intoxication.
- Urine tests for marijuana are unreliable indicators of acute use since patients may be positive for days to weeks after their last use.
- The differential diagnosis of hallucinogen intoxication includes alcohol and benzodiazepine withdrawal, hypoglycemia, anticholinergic poisoning, thyrotoxicosis, CNS infections, structural CNS lesions, and acute psychosis.

EMERGENCY DEPARTMENT CARE AND DISPOSITION

- Initial management of patients with hallucinogen intoxication is support of airway, breathing, and

TABLE 105-1   Characteristics of Hallucinogens

DRUG	CHEMICAL CLASSIFICATION	MECHANISM OF ACTION	TYPICAL DOSE	DURATION OF ACTION	CLINICAL FEATURES	COMPLICATIONS	SPECIFIC TREATMENT
LSD	Indole alkylamine	5-HT$_2$ agonist	50–300 μg	8–12 h	Mydriasis Sympathomimetic symptoms Nausea Muscle tension	Persistent psychosis Hallucinogen persisting perception disorder	Supportive Benzodiazepines
Psilocybin	Indole alkylamine	5-HT$_2$ agonist	5–100 mushrooms, 4–6 mg of psilocybin	4–6 h	Mydriasis Sympathomimetic symptoms Nausea	Seizures (rare) Hyperthermia (rare)	Supportive Benzodiazepines
Mescaline	Phenylethylamine	5-HT$_2$ agonist	3–12 "buttons," 200–500 mg of mescaline	6–12 h	Mydriasis Abdominal pain Vomiting Dizziness Sympathomimetic symptoms	Rare	Supportive Benzodiazepines
MDMA ("ecstasy")	Phenylethylamine	5-HT release	50–200 mg	4–6 h	Mydriasis Sympathomimetic symptoms Bruxism Jaw tension Ataxia	Arrhythmias Hypertension Seizures Hyperthermia Rhabdomyolysis DIC Chronic neuropsychiatric problems	Benzodiazepines Hydration Active cooling
Phencyclidine (PCP)	Piperadine derivative	Glutamate antagonist at NMDA receptor	1–9 mg	4–6 h	Miosis or midsized pupils Nystagmus Hypertension Sympathomimetic, anticholinergic, and cholinergic symptoms	Coma Seizures Hyperthermia Rhabdomyolysis Hypertension Hypoglycemia	Benzodiazepines Hydration Active cooling Multiple doses of activated charcoal Alkalinize urine (for rhabdomyolysis)
Marijuana	Cannabinoid	Binds cannabinoid receptor	5–15 mg of THC	2–4 h	Tachycardia Conjunctival injection Impaired motor coordination	Rare	Supportive Benzodiazepines

ABBREVIATIONS: DIC = disseminated intravascular coagulation; NMDA = N-methyl-D-aspartate; THC = tetrahydrocannabinol.

circulation. Hypoxia and hypoglycemia must be diagnosed and treated immediately.

- Supportive care is usually all that is needed to manage a patient with LSD intoxication. IV benzodiazepines may be given for extremely agitated patients.
- Haloperidol should be considered as a second-line therapy since it may lower the seizure threshold. Most patients may be safely discharged after a period of observation, although patients with symptoms lasting more than 8 to 12 hours may require hospital admission.
- Management of patients with psilocybin intoxication and mescaline ingestion is supportive. Co-ingestion of abused substances should be considered.
- Treatment of ecstasy use includes activated charcoal if ingestion was recent and standard treatment of arrhythmias. Benzodiazepines may alleviate hypertension and tachycardia, although nitroprusside or phentolamine should be used for severe cases.
- Management of the PCP-intoxicated patient is generally supportive. If possible, activated charcoal should be given to patients with large or recent use.
- Sedation with benzodiazepines is preferred over physical restraint of PCP-intoxicated patients. Seizures should be controlled with benzodiazepines, but may require additional therapy.
- Hypertensive emergencies related to PCP use may require use of nitroprusside. Rhabdomyolysis should be treated in the typical fashion. Patients with significant medical complications should be admitted to the hospital.
- Most patients with hallucinogen intoxication can be safely discharged from the ED after a period of observation.
- Patients with serious medical complications, such as severe hyperthermia or hypertension, seizures, or rhabdomyolysis should be admitted to the hospital.

REFERENCES

1. Substance Abuse and Mental Health Services Administration Office of Applied Studies: *Emergency Department Trends from the Drug Abuse Warning Network, Final Estimates 1994-2001,* DAWN Series D-21, DHHS Publication No. (SMA) 02-3635. Rockville, MD: 2002.
2. Dhawan BN, Cesselin F, Raghubir R, et al: International Union of Pharmacology XII. Classification of opioid receptors. *Pharmacol Rev* 48:567, 1996.
3. Moore PA, Rumack BH, Conner CS, et al: Naloxone under-dosage after narcotic poisoning. *Am J Dis Child* 134:156, 1981.
4. Lange RA, Cigarroa RG, Yancy CW, et al: Cocaine-induced coronary artery vasoconstriction. *N Engl J Med* 321:1557, 1989.
5. Ness RB, Grisso JA, Hirschinger N, et al: Cocaine and tobacco use and the risk of spontaneous abortion. *N Engl J Med* 340:333, 1999.
6. Plessinger MA, Woods JR: Cocaine in pregnancy: Recent data on maternal and fetal risks. *Obstet Gynecol Clin North Am* 25: 99, 1998.
7. Klock JC, Boerner U, Becker CE: Coma, hyperthermia and bleeding associated with massive LSD overdose: A case report of eight cases. *Clin Toxicol* 8:191, 1975.
8. Simpson GM, Khajawall AM, Alatore E, et al: Urinary phencyclidine excretion in chronic abusers. *J Toxicol Clin Toxicol* 19:1051, 1982.

For further reading in *Emergency Medicine: A Comprehensive Study Guide,* 6th ed., see Chap. 167, "Opioids," by Suzanne Doyon; Chap. 168, "Cocaine, Amphetamines, and Other Stimulants," by Jeanmarie Perrone and Robert S. Hoffman; and Chap. 169, "Hallucinogens," by Karen N. Hansen and Katherine M. Prybys.

106 ANALGESICS

Keith L. Mausner

SALICYLATES

EPIDEMIOLOGY

- In 2000, aspirin was involved in 20,892 toxic exposures, with over 12,000 treated at a health care facility. There were 45 deaths (0.2% of cases) attributed to salicylate toxicity.[1]
- Many over-the-counter medications [eg, Pepto-Bismol, oil of wintergreen (methyl salicylate), liniments used in vaporizers] contain large amounts of salicylates, and ingestion or application can lead to inadvertent salicylate toxicity.

PATHOPHYSIOLOGY

- Absorption of salicylate may be delayed or erratic. Peak serum levels may be significantly delayed, but toxic levels are usually apparent within 6 hours. Peak levels from ingestion of enteric-coated or sustained-release aspirin have been reported up to 60 hours after ingestion.[2]
- Aspirin may form a gelatinous gastric mass, and large amounts of aspirin may remain in the stomach long

after an overdose. In addition, aspirin has an inhibitory effect on gastric emptying.

- After absorption, aspirin is hydrolyzed to salicylate; toxicity depends on cellular salicylate concentration.
- At physiologic pH (7.40), essentially all salicylate molecules are ionized. A decrease in pH (acidosis) increases the proportion of nonionized salicylate. Nonionized salicylate molecules cross cell membranes, including the blood-brain barrier. Therefore, acidemia increases intracellular salicylate concentration.
- Mortality from salicylate toxicity correlates directly with brain salicylate concentration.[3]
- A urinary pH above 8.0 will ionize the salicylate in the urine and impair reabsorption of salicylate across the urinary tubules, resulting in enhanced urinary elimination.[4]
- Salicylate toxicity causes respiratory alkalosis due to an initially increased respiratory rate through a direct effect on the medullary respiratory center.[5]
- Salicylate toxicity causes uncoupling of oxidative phosphorylation and inhibition of various Krebs' cycle enzymes. This results in increased catabolism and elevated carbon dioxide and heat production, increased glycolysis and demand for glucose, and production of organic acids including lactate, pyruvate, and ketoacids, which contribute to the metabolic acidosis of salicylate poisoning.
- Salicylate toxicity causes alterations of central and peripheral glucose metabolism.
- Normoglycemia, hyperglycemia, or hypoglycemia may be seen. Hypoglycemia in brain cells may occur despite normal serum glucose levels.[6]
- Chronic administration of large doses of salicylates when the serum salicylate level is greater than 60 mg/dL results in hypoprothrombinemia and an elevated prothrombin time (PT).

CLINICAL FEATURES

- The clinical manifestations of salicylate toxicity depend on the dose, whether exposure is acute or chronic, and the patient's age.
- Acute ingestion of less than 150 mg/kg usually produces mild toxicity with nausea, vomiting, and gastrointestinal (GI) irritation.
- Acute ingestion of 150 to 300 mg/kg usually results in moderate toxicity with vomiting, hyperventilation, sweating, and tinnitus. In adults, these findings often coincide with salicylate levels above 30 mg/dL.
- Toxicity from ingestion of more than 300 mg/kg is usually severe.
- The pathognomonic acid-base disturbance of salicylate toxicity is increased anion gap metabolic acidosis, metabolic alkalosis (due to volume contraction), and respiratory alkalosis.

- The most common clinical picture is combined respiratory alkalosis and increased anion gap metabolic acidosis. In addition, co-ingestion of sedative drugs may impair the respiratory drive and result in respiratory acidosis.
- Only one other single clinical entity, sepsis, produces a similar triple acid-base disturbance (lactic acidosis, contraction metabolic acidosis, and respiratory alkalosis).
- Uncommon manifestations of severe acute salicylate toxicity include fever, neurologic dysfunction, renal failure, pulmonary edema, and acute respiratory distress syndrome (ARDS). Rarely, rhabdomyolysis, gastric perforation, and GI hemorrhage occur.
- Fatality is more likely with advanced age.
- Unconsciousness, fever, severe acidosis, seizures, and dysrhythmias are also associated with increased mortality risk.
- Chronic salicylate toxicity (associated with long-term therapeutic use) is usually seen in elderly patients with underlying medical problems. It may present with hyperventilation, tremor, papilledema, agitation, paranoia, bizarre behavior, memory loss, confusion, and stupor.
- Chronic salicylism should be considered in any patient with unexplained nonfocal neurologic and behavioral abnormalities, especially with coexisting acid-base disturbance, tachypnea, dyspnea, or noncardiogenic pulmonary edema.
- Patients taking carbonic anhydrase inhibitors to treat glaucoma are at increased risk for chronic salicylism. The carbonic anhydrase inhibitor produces a metabolic acidosis, which increases the volume of distribution of salicylates, leading to increased central nervous system (CNS) salicylate levels and possible toxicity despite a "therapeutic" serum salicylate level.
- In children, acute salicylate overdoses generally present within a few hours of ingestion.
- Children under age 4 years tend to develop metabolic acidosis (pH <7.38), whereas children over age 4 years usually have mixed acid-base disturbance as in adults.
- In children, chronic (repeated dose) salicylate toxicity is usually more serious than acute toxicity, and more likely to be lethal.[7,8]
- It may take several days for symptoms to appear, and there may be an underlying illness that triggered the salicylate administration.
- Chronic salicylism may be mistaken for an infectious process. A child may present with hyperventilation, volume depletion, acidosis, marked hypokalemia, and CNS disturbances.
- Fever indicates a worse prognosis. Renal failure is a severe complication. Pulmonary edema is rare in pediatric patients.

DIAGNOSIS AND DIFFERENTIAL

- Salicylate levels should be interpreted cautiously since severe toxicity may be present despite a "therapeutic" or declining level.
- The use of the Done nomogram, which was developed to predict toxicity after acute ingestion within a known time frame, may be misleading and is no longer recommended.
- Enteric-coated aspirin may be visible on plain radiographs; however, a negative radiograph does not exclude the ingestion.
- The differential diagnosis of salicylate toxicity includes theophylline toxicity, caffeine overdose, acute iron poisoning, Reye's syndrome, diabetic ketoacidosis, sepsis, and meningitis.

EMERGENCY DEPARTMENT CARE AND DISPOSITION

- Emergent priorities remain airway, breathing, and circulation. Cardiac monitoring and an intravenous (IV) line should be instituted.
- Activated charcoal 1 g/kg should be administered to minimize absorption and hasten elimination. Multiple doses are probably not beneficial.
- Whole bowel irrigation may be effective when toxicity is due to sustained-release or enteric-coated aspirin.
- Intravenous normal saline should be administered to patients with evidence of volume depletion. Except for the initial saline resuscitation, all subsequent fluids should contain at least 5% dextrose; if hypoglycemia or neurologic symptoms are present, then administration of IV fluids with 10% dextrose should be considered.
- After adequate urine output (1 to 2 mL/kg/h) is established, and if not contraindicated by initial electrolyte and renal function test results, potassium 40 mEq/L should be added to the patient's IV fluids.
- Alkalinization of the serum and urine enhances salicylate protein binding and urinary elimination. This may be accomplished with a second IV concurrent with volume resuscitation.
- A bolus of 1 to 2 mEq/kg of sodium bicarbonate should be administered. Then, 150 mEq (3 ampules) of sodium bicarbonate should be added to a liter of D_5W and infused at 1.5 to 2.0 times the patient's maintenance rate; the infusion should be adjusted to maintain urine pH above 7.5.
- Severe salicylate toxicity may result in significant volume depletion and metabolic abnormalities; during resuscitation frequent clinical evaluation as well as at least hourly monitoring of urine pH, salicylate level, electrolytes, glucose, and acid-base status is indicated.

- Bicarbonate administration will further exacerbate hypokalemia; potassium levels should be closely followed.
- A sudden drop in serum pH due to respiratory failure may acutely worsen salicylate toxicity; early intubation and controlled ventilation is indicated in the event of impending respiratory failure.
- Hemodialysis is indicated for clinical deterioration despite supportive care and alkalinization, renal insufficiency or failure, severe acid-base disturbance, altered mental status, or ARDS.
- Hemorrhage due to elevated PT in chronic salicylism is rarely seen, but may be treated with fresh frozen plasma.
- Dysrhythmias should be treated by correcting metabolic abnormalities and with standard antiarrhythmics.
- In significant ingestions, patients should undergo serial examinations and the salicylate levels should be checked every 2 hours until the peak occurs, and then checked every 4 to 6 hours until the level is nontoxic.
- In severe ingestions, hourly levels correlated with clinical status are indicated.
- Except with ingestion of enteric-coated or sustained-release formulations, a patient may be discharged from the emergency department (ED) if there is progressive clinical improvement, no significant acid-base abnormality, and a decline in serial salicylate levels toward the therapeutic range. In deliberate overdoses, a psychiatric consultation should be obtained prior to discharge.
- With enteric-coated and sustained-release salicylates, peak serum levels may not occur until 10 to 60 hours after ingestion.
- In potentially large ingestions, the patient should be admitted and observed for at least 24 hours to assure declining serial salicylate levels and improving clinical status.

ACETAMINOPHEN

EPIDEMIOLOGY

- Acetaminophen is the most popular over-the-counter analgesic in the United States. In 2000, acetaminophen accounted for 5 percent of all toxic exposures and for 23 percent of reported fatalities.[1]

PATHOPHYSIOLOGY

- Acetaminophen is rapidly absorbed from the GI tract. In overdose, peak serum levels usually occur within 2 hours. However, delayed absorption may occur with acetaminophen preparations containing propoxyphene or diphenhydramine and with Tylenol Arthritis Pain Extended Relief.

- Acetaminophen is mainly metabolized by the liver through sulfation and glucuronidation; only a small percentage (<5%) undergoes direct renal elimination.
- A small percentage of acetaminophen is also oxidized by cytochrome P-450 to a toxic metabolite, *n*-acetyl-*p*-benzoquinoneimine (NAPQI). NAPQI is detoxified by hepatic glutathione to a nontoxic compound that undergoes renal elimination.
- In acetaminophen overdose, hepatic glucuronidation and sulfation are quickly saturated, and a higher percentage of acetaminophen is metabolized by cytochrome P-450 to NAPQI. When hepatic glutathione stores are depleted to less than 30 percent of normal, NAPQI accumulates, and hepatic toxicity occurs.
- NAPQI causes hepatocellular injury, and typically produces hepatic centrilobular necrosis.
- Patients with low glutathione stores (alcoholics and AIDS patients), and those with induced cytochrome P-450 activity (alcoholics and individuals on anticonvulsant or antituberculosis drugs) are at greater risk of developing acetaminophen toxicity.
- N-acetylcysteine (NAC) is a specific antidote for acetaminophen. Among other actions, NAC inhibits binding of NAPQI to hepatic proteins, it may act as a glutathione precursor or substitute, and it may directly reduce NAPQI back to acetaminophen.

CLINICAL FEATURES

- Acute acetaminophen toxicity presents in four stages. During the first 24 hours, the patient may be asymptomatic or have nonspecific symptoms such as anorexia, nausea, vomiting, and malaise.
- On days 2 and 3, nausea and vomiting may improve, but evidence of hepatotoxicity, such as right upper quadrant abdominal pain and tenderness with elevated transaminases and bilirubin, may be present.
- On days 3 and 4, there may be progression to fulminant hepatic failure with lactic acidosis, coagulopathy, renal failure, and encephalopathy, as well as recurrent nausea and vomiting.
- Those who survive hepatic failure will begin to recover over the next weeks with complete resolution of hepatic dysfunction.
- Massive acetaminophen ingestion (4-hour acetaminophen level >800 μg/mL) may be associated with acute onset of either coma or agitation and lactic acidosis.

DIAGNOSIS AND DIFFERENTIAL

- Acetaminophen toxicity may occur with acute ingestion of more than 140 mg/kg or when more than 7.5 g are ingested by an adult in a 24-hour period. The diagnosis of a significant ingestion depends on laboratory testing, since symptoms may initially be absent or nonspecific.
- An acetaminophen level should be measured in all patients presenting with any drug overdose since acetaminophen is a common co-ingestant.[9]
- An acetaminophen level, drawn as soon as possible within 4 to 24 hours of ingestion, will guide subsequent ED management. In a single large overdose, the Rumack-Matthew nomogram (Fig. 106-1) accurately predicts acetaminophen toxicity based on the serum acetaminophen level measured 4 to 24 hours after the estimated time of ingestion.[10]

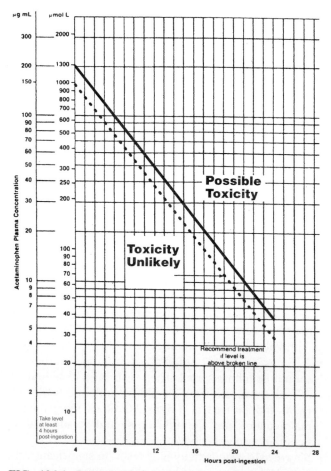

FIG. 106-1. Rumack-Matthew nomogram. (Reproduced with permission from Rumack BH, Matthew H: Acetaminophen poisoning and toxicity. *Pediatrics* 55:871, 1975.)

- The nomogram is not useful outside of this 4 to 24 hour window.
- A 4-hour level greater than 150 μg/dL is usually toxic. After 24 hours, a detectable acetaminophen level or the presence of elevated transaminases may predict toxicity.
- When multiple ingestions have occurred over a period of time, assessment is problematic. One approach is to assume a single ingestion at the earliest possible point in time and use the Rumack-Matthew nomogram accordingly.
- Clinical experience with Tylenol Arthritis Pain Extended Relief ingestion is limited. If a 4 to 8 hour level is in the toxic range, then therapy should be initiated. If the 4 to 8 hour level is elevated but below the toxicity cutoff on the nomogram, then a second level 4 to 6 hours later should be obtained and therapy initiated if the second level is in the toxic range.[11]
- The differential diagnosis of acetaminophen toxicity includes viral and alcoholic hepatitis, other drug- or toxin-induced hepatitides, and hepatobiliary disease.
- Acute acetaminophen poisoning can often be distinguished from other forms of hepatitis by its acute onset, rapid progression, and markedly elevated transaminase levels.

EMERGENCY DEPARTMENT CARE AND DISPOSITION

- Emergent priorities remain airway, breathing, and circulation. Cardiac monitoring and an IV line should be instituted.
- Activated charcoal 1 g/kg is indicated for GI decontamination and in case of co-ingestion of other drugs.
- NAC is the specific antidote. It effectively prevents toxicity if administered within 8 hours of ingestion, significantly reduces hepatotoxicity if administered within 24 hours of ingestion, and may be of value even after 24 hours.[12]
- If the acetaminophen level is not going to be available within 8 hours of ingestion, then NAC therapy should be initiated and continued if indicated based on the subsequent acetaminophen level.
- NAC is administered orally or by nasogastric tube as a 140 mg/kg loading dose, followed by 70 mg/kg every 4 hours for 17 additional doses.
- NAC may be administered immediately after activated charcoal; there is no evidence that activated charcoal decreases NAC's effectiveness.
- NAC is safe in pregnancy.
- Nausea and vomiting during NAC therapy may be reduced by diluting NAC in a beverage and by adminis-

tration of antiemetics such as metoclopramide or ondansetron.
- Intravenous NAC therapy is not approved in the United States, but may be used in consultation with a toxicologist for patients unable to tolerate or receive oral therapy.[13]
- Treatment of fulminant hepatic failure includes NAC therapy, correction of coagulopathy and acidosis, treatment of cerebral edema, supportive measures for multi–organ system failure, and early referral to a liver transplant center.
- Patients with nontoxic acetaminophen levels based on the Rumack-Matthew nomogram may be discharged from the ED if there is no evidence of other drug ingestion. In deliberate overdoses, a psychiatric evaluation should be obtained prior to discharge.
- All patients receiving NAC therapy should be admitted.

NONSTEROIDAL ANTI-INFLAMMATORY DRUGS

EPIDEMIOLOGY

- Between 1997 and 2000 the American Association of Poison Control Centers reported 290,031 nonsteroidal anti-inflammatory drug (NSAIDs) toxic exposures resulting in 35 deaths; this is compared with 62,076 aspirin toxic exposures resulting in 175 deaths and 269,143 acetaminophen toxic exposures resulting in 287 deaths.
- NSAID morbidity at therapeutic doses is far more significant than morbidity from overdoses.
- NSAID-related GI bleeding is estimated to lead to 103,000 hospitalizations and 16,500 deaths annually in the United States.[14] NSAIDs have also been implicated in a significant proportion of cases of drug-induced renal failure.

PATHOPHYSIOLOGY

- NSAIDs inhibit the enzyme cyclooxygenase (COX), which produces prostaglandins from arachidonic acid. There are at least two forms of cyclooxygenase, COX-1 and COX-2. COX-1 is probably responsible for most of the adverse effects of NSAIDs.
- There are three types of cyclooxygenase inhibitors: nonselective, which inhibit both COX-1 and COX-2 (the majority of NSAIDs are in this class); partially selective, which preferentially inhibit COX-2 only at low doses (etodolac and meloxicam); and selective, which preferentially inhibit COX-2 (valdecoxib, rofecoxib, and celecoxib).

- NSAIDs are rapidly absorbed from the GI tract. Most NSAIDs undergo at least partial hepatic metabolism before elimination in the urine or feces.
- Plasma half-lives of NSAIDs range from 2 to 4 hours for ibuprofen, to approximately 15 hours for the new COX-2 inhibitors, and to longer than 50 hours for piroxicam and phenylbutazone.

CLINICAL FEATURES

- Phenylbutazone and naproxen may displace warfarin from plasma proteins, resulting in elevated PT times. Phenylbutazone also decreases the elimination of warfarin. The selective COX-2 inhibitors have been reported to slightly elevate the PT at therapeutic doses.
- Other NSAIDs do not interact in these ways with warfarin, but nonselective NSAID use is contraindicated with warfarin because NSAID platelet aggregation inhibition may significantly increase the risk of bleeding.
- NSAIDs may decrease the effectiveness of antihypertensives, including diuretics, α-adrenergic blockers, angiotensin-converting enzyme inhibitors, and β-adrenergic blockers.[15]
- NSAIDs inhibit the renal clearance of lithium and methotrexate and may cause toxicity from these drugs.
- Toxicity associated with therapeutic use of NSAIDs is more common than acute overdose. The most frequent problems are GI bleeding and renal insufficiency.
- CNS effects such as headache, mental status changes, and aseptic meningitis may be seen.[16] Seizures have been seen with large ingestions, especially of mefenamic acid.
- Pulmonary manifestations such as bronchospasm and hypersensitivity pneumonitis have been reported.
- Hepatic dysfunction may occur, especially in the elderly and in patients with autoimmune disease.
- Inhibition of platelet aggregation may lead to bleeding. The COX-2 inhibitors (eg, rofecoxib, celecoxib) have less antiplatelet effect than conventional NSAIDs; the lack of platelet inhibition with COX-2 inhibitors may increase the risk of acute coronary syndrome or thromboembolic stroke in at-risk patients who were previously on conventional NSAIDs.[17]
- Bone marrow suppression, including aplastic anemia, has been reported.
- NSAIDs account for approximately 10 percent of cutaneous drug reactions, ranging from benign rashes and phototoxic reactions to severe Stevens-Johnson syndrome and toxic epidermal necrolysis.[18,19]
- Fetal NSAID exposure may lead to premature closure of the ductus arteriosus, oligohydramnios, renal dysfunction, necrotizing enterocolitis, and CNS hemorrhage.

- Acute NSAID overdose generally has low morbidity, and usually becomes clinically apparent within 4 hours of ingestion.
- Abdominal pain, nausea, and vomiting may occur.
- CNS manifestations include altered mental status, diplopia, nystagmus, headache, and rarely, seizures. Hypotension and bradydysrhythmias have been reported.
- Renal failure may occur and be associated with serum electrolyte abnormalities and volume overload.

DIAGNOSIS AND DIFFERENTIAL

- The manifestations of NSAID toxicity are nonspecific.
- NSAID levels are not readily available and are not clinically useful in assessing toxicity.
- Acetaminophen and salicylate levels will exclude co-ingestion of these agents.

EMERGENCY DEPARTMENT CARE AND DISPOSITION

- Emergent priorities remain airway, breathing, and circulation. Cardiac monitoring and an IV line should be instituted.
- Activated charcoal 1 g/kg is indicated for GI decontamination.
- Volume resuscitation, correction of acid-base and electrolyte disorders, and standard treatment of other complications such as seizures, dysrhythmias, and renal failure are performed as indicated.
- Patients with asymptomatic NSAID ingestions may be safely discharged from the ED after screening for co-ingestants and a 4 to 6 hour observation period. In deliberate overdoses, a psychiatric consultation should be obtained prior to discharge.

REFERENCES

1. Litovitz TL, Klein-Schwartz W, White S, et al: 2000 Annual Report of the American Association of Poison Control Centers Toxic Exposure Surveillance System. *Am J Emerg Med* 19:337, 2001.
2. Wortzman DJ, Grunfeld A: Delayed absorption following enteric-coated aspirin overdose. *Ann Emerg Med* 16:434, 1987.
3. Hill JB: Salicylate intoxication. *N Engl J Med* 288:1110, 1973.
4. Smith PK, Gleason HL, Stoll CG, et al: Studies on the pharmacology of salicylates. *J Pharmacol Exp Ther* 87:237, 1946.
5. Tenny SM, Miller RM: The respiratory and circulatory actions of salicylate. *Am J Med* 19:498, 1955.

6. Thurston JH, Pollock PG, Warren SK, et al: Reduced brain glucose with normal plasma glucose in salicylate poisoning. *J Clin Invest* 49:2139, 1970.

7. Gaudreault P, Temple AR, Lovejoy FH: The relative severity of acute versus chronic salicylate poisoning in children: A clinical comparison. *Pediatrics* 70:566, 1982.

8. Snodgrass W: Salicylate toxicity following therapeutic doses in young children. *Clin Toxicol* 18:247, 1981.

9. Ashbourne JF, Olson KR, Khayam-Bashi H: Value of rapid screening for acetaminophen in all patients with intentional drug overdose. *Ann Emerg Med* 18:1035, 1989.

10. Rumack BH, Matthew H: Acetaminophen poisoning and toxicity. *Pediatrics* 55:871, 1975.

11. Cetaruk EW, Dart RC, Hurlbut KM, et al: Tylenol Extended Relief overdose. *Ann Emerg Med* 30:104, 1997.

12. Smilkstein MJ, Knapp GL, Kulig KW, et al: Efficacy of oral N-acetylcysteine in the treatment of acetaminophen overdose. *N Engl J Med* 319:1557, 1988.

13. Yip L, Dart RC, Hurlbut KM: Intravenous administration of oral N-acetylcysteine. *Crit Care Med* 26:40, 1998.

14. Singh G, Triadafilopoulous G: Epidemiology of NSAID-induced GI complications. *J Rheumatol* 26(Suppl):18, 1999.

15. Houston MC: Nonsteroidal anti-inflammatory drugs and antihypertensives. *Am J Med* 90(5A):42S, 1991.

16. Hoppman RA, Peden JG, Ober SK: Central nervous system side effects of nonsteroidal anti-inflammatory drugs. *Arch Intern Med* 151:1309, 1991.

17. Singh G, Ramey DR, Morfeld D, Fries JF: Comparative toxicity of nonsteroidal anti-inflammatory agents. *Pharmacol Ther* 62:175, 1994.

18. Roujeau JC, Stern RS: Severe adverse cutaneous reactions to drugs. *N Engl J Med* 331:1272, 1994.

19. Roujeau JC, Kelly JP, Naldi L, et al: Medication use and the risk of Stevens-Johnson syndrome or toxic epidermal necrolysis. *N Engl J Med* 333:1600, 1995.

For further reading in *Emergency Medicine: A Comprehensive Study Guide*, 6th ed., see Chap. 170, "Salicylates," by L. Yip; Chap. 171, "Acetaminophen," by O. Hung and L. Nelson; and Chap. 172, "Nonsteroidal Antiinflammatory Drugs," by G.R. Bruno and W.A. Carter.

107 THEOPHYLLINE

Mark B. Rogers

EPIDEMIOLOGY

- The elderly with concomitant medical problems are more susceptible to life-threatening toxicity after chronic overmedication than are younger patients after an acute overdose.[1]

- Although theophylline toxicity can be life threatening, elevated theophylline levels are common and most patients tolerate them with only minor effects.[2]
- Toxicity is rarely the result of intentional overdose.

PATHOPHYSIOLOGY

- Theophylline's mechanism of action has not been entirely elucidated but includes inhibition of phosphodiesterase and antagonism of adenosine.
- Theophylline's elimination (85 to 90%) occurs via the hepatic cytochrome P450 system and undergoes hepatobiliary enteric circulation.
- Factors that increase theophylline's half-life include smoking cessation; disease states such as cirrhosis, congestive heart failure, and chronic obstructive pulmonary disease; and medications such as cimetidine, quinolones, and erythromycin.

CLINICAL FEATURES

- Theophylline toxicity can cause life-threatening cardiac, neurologic, and metabolic abnormalities.
- Life-threatening effects may occur suddenly and before minor symptoms are evident.
- Caffeine produces many of the same toxic effects as theophylline.
- Cardiac side effects include sinus tachycardia, premature atrial contractions, atrial flutter, and atrial fibrillation. Premature ventricular contractions and ventricular tachycardia are seen, particularly in the elderly with chronic overdoses and levels of 40 to 60 μg/mL. Younger patients with acute ingestions may tolerate levels above 100 μg/mL.
- Neurologic side effects include agitation, headache, irritability, sleeplessness, tremors, and seizures. Seizures are seen in patients with high serum levels or with a history of epilepsy. Hallucinations and psychosis may be seen.
- Metabolic side effects include an increase in catecholamine, glucose, free fatty acid, and insulin levels. Hypokalemia may occur and be worsened by β-agonist therapy.
- Gastrointestinal (GI) effects commonly include nausea and vomiting. GI bleeding and epigastric pain may occur.

DIAGNOSIS AND DIFFERENTIAL

- Therapeutic serum theophylline levels of 10 to 20 μg/mL may produce toxic effects and some patients may remain asymptomatic at higher levels.[3]

In chronic exposures, minor symptoms are not predictive of elevated serum levels.[4]

EMERGENCY DEPARTMENT CARE AND DISPOSITION

- Treatment of theophylline toxicity consists of initial stabilization, gastric decontamination and elimination, treatment of life-threatening toxic effects, and in severe cases, hemoperfusion or dialysis.
- Patients should be placed on a cardiac monitor, non-invasive blood pressure device, and pulse-oximeter. An IV line should be inserted.
- Gastric lavage should be considered for acute ingestions of toxic doses within 2 to 4 hours. Ipecac should not be used.
- Multiple doses of oral activated charcoal (1 g/kg), mixed with a cathartic such as sorbitol, should be administered every 2 to 4 hour in the first 24 hours due to hepatobiliary enteric circulation.
- Ranitidine 50 mg IV is useful for the nausea and vomiting associated with toxicity.
- Seizure activity may be treated with diazepam, phenobarbital, or phenytoin.
- Hypotension initially should be treated with IV isotonic crystalloid. In patients unresponsive to IV fluids or conventional vasopressors, an α-adrenergic agent such as phenylephrine should be considered.
- Cardiac arrhythmias may be treated cautiously with β-blockers such as metoprolol or esmolol, or a calcium channel blocker such as diltiazem.[5] Ventricular dysrhythmias have been treated with lidocaine, phenytoin, and digoxin.
- Adenosine for supraventricular tachycardia may induce bronchospasm. Hypokalemia should be considered in recurrent dysrhythmias and treated.
- Indications for hemoperfusion or hemodialysis remain controversial and are listed in Table 107-1.[6]

- Patients with seizures or ventricular dysrhythmias should be monitored until their levels normalize.[7]
- Patients with mild symptoms or levels below 25 μg/mL do not require specific treatment or admission, but their medication dosing should be decreased or discontinued.
- Patients with levels above 30 μg/mL should be treated with oral activated charcoal and monitored for toxic side effects.

REFERENCES

1. Shannon M: Predictors of major toxicity after theophylline overdose. *Ann Intern Med* 119:1161, 1993.
2. Emerman CL, Devlin C, Connors AF: Risk of toxicity in patients with elevated theophylline levels. *Ann Emerg Med* 19: 643, 1990.
3. Bertino JS, Walker JW: Reassessment of theophylline toxicity: Serum concentrations, clinical course, and treatment. *Arch Intern Med* 147:757, 1987.
4. Melamed J, Beaucher WN: Minor symptoms are not predictive of elevated theophylline levels in adults on chronic therapy. *Ann Allergy Asthma Immunol* 75:516, 1995.
5. Seneff M, Schott J, Friedman B, Smith M: Acute theophylline toxicity and the use of esmolol to reverse cardiovascular instability. *Ann Emerg Med* 19:67, 1990.
6. Shannon M: Comparative efficacy of hemodialysis and hemoperfusion in severe theophylline intoxication. *Acad Emerg Med* 4:674, 1997.
7. Sessler CN: Theophylline toxicity: Clinical features of 116 consecutive cases. *Am J Med* 88:567, 1990.

For further reading in *Emergency Medicine: A Comprehensive Study Guide,* 6th ed., see Chap. 173, "Theophylline," by Heather Marshall and Charles L. Emerman.

TABLE 107-1   Indications for Hemoperfusion/Hemodialysis

CLINICAL CONDITIONS	RECOMMENDATION
Life-threatening toxicity (ie, seizures, tachydysrhythmias) not responsive to other therapy	Indicated
Acute overdose with level ≥100 μg/mL	Possibly indicated
Chronic overdose with level ≥60 μg/mL	Possibly indicated
Elderly patient with known prolonged theophylline half-life, severe liver or severe cardiac disease, or level ≥40 μg/mL	Controversial
Theophylline level ≤30 μg/mL	Not indicated

108   CARDIAC MEDICATIONS
C. Crawford Mechem

DIGITALIS GLYCOSIDES

EPIDEMIOLOGY

- According to the American Association of Poison Control Centers, 2977 exposures to cardiac glycosides were reported in 2001. Of these patients, 652 demonstrated moderate or major morbidity and 13 died.

PATHOPHYSIOLOGY

- Digitalis inactivates the sodium-potassium-adenosine triphosphate (Na^+,K^+-ATPase) pump.[1] Accumulated intracellular sodium is exchanged for calcium. Increased calcium in the sarcoplasmic reticulum is responsible for the positive inotropic effect of digitalis.[2]
- Digitalis increases vagal tone and decreases conduction through the atrioventricular node. In toxic doses, these result in bradydysrhythmias.[3]

CLINICAL FEATURES

- Toxicity results from accidental ingestion, intentional overdose, or chronic therapy.
- At increased risk are the elderly and patients with underlying conditions such as chronic obstructive pulmonary disease (COPD), cardiac or hepatic disease, or hypokalemia.[4]
- Drug interactions, such as those involving class IA antidysrhythmics, may potentiate toxicity.
- Acute overdose presents with cardiac dysrhythmias such as supraventricular tachycardia with atrioventricular (AV) block, bradycardia, and ventricular dysrhythmias.[3] Patients may develop nausea, vomiting, and mental status changes.
- Chronic toxicity is more common in elderly patients with renal insufficiency or those taking diuretics, and presents with gastrointestinal (GI) symptoms, weakness, altered mental status, seizures, and cardiac dysrhythmias.

DIAGNOSIS AND DIFFERENTIAL

- Hyperkalemia is often seen in acute poisoning but may be absent in chronic toxicity.
- Serum digoxin levels are neither sensitive nor specific for toxicity.[5] However, the higher the serum level, the more likely the patient will experience toxicity.
- The differential diagnosis includes sinus node disease or toxicity from calcium channel blockers, β-blockers, class IA antidysrhythmics (quinidine, procainamide), clonidine, organophosphates, or cardiotoxic plants such as rhododendron or yew berry.

EMERGENCY DEPARTMENT CARE AND DISPOSITION

- Management includes supportive care, prevention of further absorption, treatment of complications, and antidote administration. All patients require continuous cardiac monitoring, IV access, and frequent re-evaluation.
- Activated charcoal, 1 g/kg initially followed by 0.5 g/kg every 4 to 6 hours, should be administered.[6]
- Atropine, 0.5 to 2.0 mg IV, and cardiac pacing may be used to treat bradydysrhythmias.
- Ventricular dysrhythmias are treated with phenytoin, 15 mg/kg, infused no faster than 25 mg/min; lidocaine, 1 mg/kg; or magnesium sulfate, 2 to 4 g IV.
- Electrocardioversion may induce refractory ventricular dysrhythmias and should be considered only as a last resort. The initial setting should be 10 to 25 J.
- Hyperkalemia is treated with glucose followed by insulin; other options are sodium bicarbonate, potassium-binding resin, or hemodialysis. Calcium chloride should be avoided.[7]
- Digoxin-specific Fab is indicated for ventricular dysrhythmias, hemodynamically significant bradydysrhythmias unresponsive to standard therapy, and hyperkalemia greater than 5.5 mEq/L. Dosage is based on the estimated total-body load of digoxin. If this is unknown, 5 to 10 vials are recommended as the initial dose in severe cases.
- Patients with signs of toxicity or with a history of a large overdose should be admitted to a monitored setting. Patients receiving Fab fragments should be admitted to an intensive care unit (ICU).
- Patients who are asymptomatic after 12 hours of observation may be medically cleared.[5]

BETA-BLOCKERS

EPIDEMIOLOGY

- From 1985 to 1995, 52,156 exposures to β-blockers were recorded by the American Association of Poison Centers Toxic Exposure Surveillance System, with 164 fatalities.

PATHOPHYSIOLOGY

- The β-receptor in the cell membrane is a glycoprotein coupled to cyclic adenosine monophosphate (cAMP).
- Three types of β-receptors exist: the β_1 receptor is found in the myocardium; the β_2 receptor in the liver, pancreas, adipose tissue, and muscle; and the β_3 receptor in adipose tissue.
- When catecholamines bind to β-receptors, adenyl cyclase is activated, leading to increased cAMP and calcium entry into cells.[8]
- β-Blockade prevents the formation of cAMP. Potential consequences include negative inotropy and

chronotropy, vasoconstriction, bronchospasm, and hypoglycemia.

CLINICAL FEATURES

- Toxicity usually develops within 2 to 4 hours of acute ingestion. In the case of sustained-release preparations, toxicity has not been reported more than 6 hours postingestion.[9]
- Cardiac manifestations include hypotension, bradycardia, conduction abnormalities, cardiogenic shock, and asystole.[10]
- Sotalol, unlike other β-blockers, is a class III antidysrhythmic. As such, it may cause QT-interval prolongation and ventricular tachycardia, torsades de pointes, and ventricular fibrillation. Noncardiac manifestations of toxicity include altered mental status, psychosis, seizures, hypoglycemia, bronchospasm, and respiratory depression.

DIAGNOSIS AND DIFFERENTIAL

- The diagnosis is made on clinical grounds. Drug levels correlate poorly with clinical effects.
- Laboratory studies are directed at identifying underlying medical conditions or complications.
- The differential diagnosis includes overdose of calcium channel blockers, centrally acting α-agonists, digoxin, organophosphates, cyanide, hydrogen sulfide, plants such as oleander and rhododendron, and Chinese herbal preparations containing cardiac glycosides.

EMERGENCY DEPARTMENT CARE AND DISPOSITION

- The goal of specific cardiovascular drug therapy is restoration of perfusion to critical organs by increasing heart rate and myocardial contractility.
- All patients require supportive care, continuous cardiac monitoring, and IV access. Oxygen should be administered to correct hypoxia. IV crystalloid boluses are appropriate to treat hypotension.
- Bedside serum glucose determination is warranted in the setting of altered mental status.
- Activated charcoal, 1 g/kg, should be administered. Gastric lavage prior to administration of charcoal may be beneficial if performed within 1 to 2 hours of ingestion.
- Glucagon has both positive inotropic and chronotropic effects and is a first-line agent. It is administered as an IV bolus of 0.05 to 0.15 mg/kg. This is followed by a continuous infusion of 1 to 10 mg/h.[11]

- Amrinone, given as a 1 mg/kg bolus over 2 minutes followed by a continuous infusion of 5 to 20 μg/kg/min, may be used if glucagon is unavailable.
- Atropine is unlikely to treat β-blocker–induced bradycardia or hypotension.
- Epinephrine is used for refractory hypotension.
- Cardiac pacing may be used to treat bradycardia refractory to other measures, but is not always successful and may not reverse hypotension.
- Lidocaine, magnesium sulfate, isoproterenol, and overdrive pacing are used to treat sotalol-induced ventricular dysrhythmias.[12]
- Patients who develop bradycardia, hypotension, conduction disturbances, or altered mental status should be managed in an ICU.
- Patients who have ingested multiple cardioactive agents or a sustained-release preparation should be admitted to a monitored setting due to concern for delayed toxicity.
- Those patients who remain asymptomatic 6 hours following ingestion can in most cases be medically cleared. However, this period may need to be extended in cases of sotalol ingestion.

CALCIUM CHANNEL BLOCKERS

EPIDEMIOLOGY

- More than 4500 cases of calcium channel blocker poisoning are treated in health care facilities annually.
- Over the past 5 years, calcium channel blockers have accounted for more poisoning deaths than any other cardiovascular drug.

PATHOPHYSIOLOGY

- Intracellular calcium is the stimulus for muscle contraction and for impulse formation in the sinoatrial pacemaker cells. Calcium channel blockers prevent entry of calcium into cells, resulting in smooth muscle relaxation, decreased cardiac contractility, blunted cardiac automaticity, and intracardiac conduction delay.[13]
- The three classes of calcium channel blockers are the phenylalkylamines (eg, verapamil), benzothiazepines (eg, diltiazem), and dihydropyridines (eg, nifedipine and most newer agents). Verapamil has the greatest cardiotoxic effect.

CLINICAL FEATURES

- Cardiac manifestations of toxicity consist of sinus bradycardia, AV block, and hypotension.[14]

- In dihydropyridine overdose, reflex tachycardia is common.
- In severe cases, all classes of calcium channel blockers can cause complete heart block, depressed myocardial contractility, and vasodilatation ultimately resulting in cardiovascular collapse.
- Noncardiac consequences include hyperglycemia, lactic acidosis, hypokalemia, noncardiogenic pulmonary edema, seizures, delirium, and coma.
- Altered mental status is usually due to hypoperfusion. If noted in the setting of a normal blood pressure, other causes should be sought.

DIAGNOSIS AND DIFFERENTIAL

- A careful history should be obtained in all cases, including the agent taken, whether it is a sustained-release preparation, any co-ingestants, and time of ingestion.
- In the setting of dihydropyridine overdose, vasodilatation may result in flushed skin, hypotension, and tachycardia.
- Lactic acidosis manifesting with an elevated anion gap and low serum bicarbonate may be noted.
- Hyperglycemia is common and helps to distinguish calcium channel blocker from β-blocker toxicity, which is often associated with hypoglycemia.
- Hypokalemia may be seen in severe overdoses.
- Serum acetaminophen and aspirin levels should be obtained in all patients following a suicide attempt by overdose.
- The differential diagnosis for bradycardia and hypotension includes hypothermia, acute coronary syndrome, hyperkalemia, and toxicity due to cardiac glycosides, β-blockers, class IA and IC antidysrhythmics, and central α-adrenergic agonists (clonidine).

EMERGENCY DEPARTMENT CARE AND DISPOSITION

- All patients require supplemental oxygen, cardiac monitoring, and IV access. Patients with altered mental status should receive an opiate antagonist and have a bedside serum glucose determination.
- The end point of treatment of bradycardia and hypotension is adequate end-organ perfusion.
- Gastric lavage is indicated for all patients presenting within 60 minutes of a potentially life-threatening calcium channel blocker overdose and for those patients requiring endotracheal intubation. Because of the associated risk of aspiration with gastric lavage, definitive airway management is often required.

- Activated charcoal, 1 g/kg, is indicated for all patients. Whole bowel irrigation has been advocated for sustained-release preparations.
- Crystalloid IV fluids should be administered for hypotension, with care taken to avoid fluid overload.
- Hypotension refractory to IV fluids is treated with a 1- to 3-g IV bolus of calcium chloride, repeated as needed or administered as an infusion of 2 to 6 g/h. Care should be exercised in avoiding extravasation, which may result in tissue necrosis.
- Calcium gluconate is an alternative therapy but provides one third the amount of calcium on a weight-to-weight basis.[15]
- Glucagon is a first-line agent for moderate to severe calcium channel blocker toxicity. It is administered as a 0.05 mg/kg bolus, which may be repeated every 10 minutes to a total dose of 0.15 mg/kg. Patients who respond should be started on an infusion of 0.075 to 0.15 mg/kg/h.
- Since glucagon may cause vomiting, prophylactic endotracheal intubation should be considered.
- Dopamine, epinephrine, norepinephrine, amrinone, or milrinone may be used to treat refractory hypotension.
- Anecdotal evidence supports the co-administration of regular insulin and dextrose to patients with a severe overdose who fail to respond to other measures.
- After checking the serum glucose level, regular insulin is administered as a 1.0 μm/kg IV bolus followed by an infusion of 0.5 to 1.0 μm/kg/h. A 10% dextrose infusion is run at 200 to 300 mL/h (15 to 20 mL/kg/h in children), and blood sugar and potassium levels monitored every 20 minutes. The target blood sugar range is 150 to 300 mg/dL.[16]
- Symptomatic patients should be admitted to a monitored setting or ICU. Patients who have taken a sustained-release preparation should be admitted to a monitored setting for 24 hours.[17]
- Patients who are asymptomatic, have received charcoal decontamination, and have normal vital signs following a 6-hour observation period after ingestion of a non–sustained-release product may be medically cleared.

ANTIHYPERTENSIVES

DIURETICS

- Diuretics include **thiazides** (hydrochlorothiazide), **loop diuretics** (furosemide, bumetanide, ethacrynic acid, torsemide), **potassium-sparing diuretics** (spironolactone, triamterene, amiloride), **carbonic anhydrase inhibitors** (acetazolamide), and **osmotic agents** (mannitol).

CLINICAL FEATURES

Thiazides and Loop Diuretics

- Patients may present with hypotension, tachycardia, altered mental status, hyponatremia, hypokalemia, hypocalcemia (loop diuretics), hypomagnesemia, hyperuricemia (thiazides), and hypochloremic metabolic alkalosis.
- Patients may also develop rash, pruritus, hearing loss, leukopenia, and thrombocytopenia.

Potassium-Sparing Diuretics

- Toxicity manifests with volume depletion, hyperkalemia, hyponatremia, and hypochloremia.

Carbonic Anhydrase Inhibitors

- Overdose results in volume depletion, electrolyte disturbances, and non–anion-gap metabolic acidosis.

Osmotic Agents

- Signs of toxicity include volume depletion and electrolyte imbalances.
- Pulmonary edema, anaphylaxis, and acute renal failure also have been reported.

EMERGENCY DEPARTMENT CARE AND DISPOSITION

- Management is supportive and includes fluid resuscitation and correction of electrolyte and pH abnormalities. All patients require continuous cardiac monitoring and IV access.
- IV normal saline is used to correct hypovolemia, hyponatremia, and alkalosis.
- Dopamine is used for hypotension refractory to volume resuscitation.
- Potassium abnormalities should be aggressively corrected using standard measures. Patients with severe hyperkalemia from potassium-sparing diuretics may require dialysis.
- Most asymptomatic patients can be medically cleared after therapy and observation.
- Patients with electrolyte abnormalities may require admission.

CLONIDINE AND OTHER CENTRALLY ACTING AGENTS

CLINICAL FEATURES

- Clonidine toxicity causes hypotension and bradycardia, leading to myocardial ischemia and congestive heart failure.
- Other findings include respiratory depression, hypothermia, mental status changes, miosis, and seizures.
- Guanabenz, guanfacine, methyldopa, and reserpine can cause hypotension, symptomatic bradycardia, dry mouth, and mental status changes.

EMERGENCY DEPARTMENT CARE AND DISPOSITION

- Recurrent apnea from clonidine, most commonly seen in children, may warrant endotracheal intubation. All patients require continuous cardiac monitoring and IV access.
- IV crystalloid should be administered for hypotension.
- Dopamine or norepinephrine is used for hypotension refractory to fluid resuscitation.
- Atropine is indicated for management of symptomatic bradycardia.
- Naloxone may be effective for cases of refractory hypotension or altered mental status.[18]
- Tolazoline, 10 mg IV titrated every 15 minutes to a total of 40 mg, is recommended for treatment of clonidine-induced cardiovascular effects that fail to respond to fluids, dopamine, atropine, and naloxone.
- Seizures are controlled with standard anticonvulsants.
- Dialysis may be warranted in severe cases of methyldopa toxicity.
- Symptoms of clonidine toxicity can persist for up to 72 hours, so admission should be considered for any patient suspected of clonidine overdose.

PERIPHERAL α_1-ADRENERGIC RECEPTOR ANTAGONISTS

- Agents include doxazosin, prazosin, terazosin, and phenoxybenzamine.
- Toxicity is uncommon but may include hypotension and tachycardia. Syncope, headache, paresthesias, vertigo, gastrointestinal discomfort, and weakness have also been reported.
- Treatment is supportive and includes IV fluid administration, vasopressors if needed, and inpatient cardiac monitoring.

DIRECT VASODILATORS

CLINICAL FEATURES

- Toxicity from hydralazine is uncommon. Hypotension is the most common presentation. Symptomatic tachycardia may also be noted.
- Minoxidil causes hypotension and tachycardia.
- Toxicity from sodium nitroprusside includes hypotension, altered mental status, and dysrhythmias, and is more common after prolonged infusion and in patients with hepatic or renal failure.
- Less commonly, thiocyanate toxicity with tinnitus, altered mental status, nausea, and abdominal pain may develop.

- Rarely, cyanide toxicity presents with acidosis, coma, and respiratory arrest. In very rare cases, methemoglobinemia and cellular hypoxia develop.

EMERGENCY DEPARTMENT CARE AND DISPOSITION

- IV fluids are used to treat hypotension. Hypotension from sodium nitroprusside infusion is best avoided by careful monitoring and titration of dosage.
- Vasopressors can induce dysrhythmias in cases of hydralazine-induced hypotension, so it should be used with caution. Dopamine is the preferred agent.
- For minoxidil-induced hypotension, dopamine or phenylephrine should be considered, as vasopressors such as epinephrine that have β-adrenergic activity can result in excessive cardiac stimulation.
- β-Blockers can be used to treat symptomatic tachycardias.
- Thiocyanate toxicity may be avoided by limiting the duration of infusion and restricting the use of nitroprusside in patients with renal insufficiency. In severe cases, thiocyanate may be removed by dialysis.
- Cyanide toxicity is avoided by co-administration of sodium thiosulfate or by limiting the duration of infusion.

DOPAMINE AGONISTS

- Fenoldopam is used to treat acute, severe hypertension and is an alternative to sodium nitroprusside in patients with renal insufficiency.
- Experience with this agent is limited, but toxicity may theoretically result in hypotension.
- Care is supportive. Hypotension is best treated with IV fluids and vasopressors such as dopamine or norepinephrine.

ANGIOTENSIN-CONVERTING ENZYME INHIBITORS

- Hypotension is the most common concern in overdose.
- Care is supportive. Hypotension may be treated with IV normal saline, followed by vasopressors such as dopamine.
- Naloxone has been reported to reverse captopril-induced hypotension, but its mechanism of action is unknown.

ANGIOTENSIN II RECEPTOR ANTAGONISTS

- Experience with toxicity is limited, but hypotension and tachycardia are the most common toxic effects.

- Vagally-mediated bradycardia may occur.
- Hyperkalemia has also been reported.
- Therapy is supportive and includes IV fluid administration, correction of electrolyte disturbances, and cardiac monitoring for at least 6 hours.

REFERENCES

1. Smith TW: Digitalis: Mechanisms of action and clinical use. *N Engl J Med* 318:358, 1988.
2. Sagawa T, Sagawa K, Kelly JE, et al: Activation of cardiac ryanodine receptors by cardiac glycosides. *Am J Physiol Heart Circ Physiol* 282:1118, 2001.
3. Moorman JR, Pritchett EL: The arrhythmias of digitalis intoxication. *Arch Intern Med* 145:1289, 1985.
4. Wofford JL, Ettinger WH: Risk factors and manifestations of digoxin toxicity in the elderly. *Am J Emerg Med* 9:11, 1991.
5. Seltzer A: Role of serum digoxin assay in patient management. *J Am Coll Cardiol* 5:106, 1985.
6. Lalonde RL, Deshpande R, Hamilton PP, et al: Acceleration of digoxin clearance by activated charcoal. *Clin Pharmacol Ther* 37:367, 1985.
7. Antman EM, Wenger TL, Butler VP, et al: Treatment of 150 cases of life-threatening digitalis intoxication with digoxin-specific Fab antibody fragments: Final report of a multicenter study. *Circulation* 81:1744, 1990.
8. Kerns W, Kline J, Ford M: Beta-blocker and calcium blocker toxicity. *Emerg Med Clin North Am* 12:365, 1994.
9. Love JN. β-Blocker toxicity after overdose: When do symptoms develop in adults? *J Emerg Med* 12:799, 1994.
10. Love JN, Litovitz TL, Howell JM, Clancy C: Characterization of fatal beta-blocker ingestion: A review of the American Association of Poison Control Centers data from 1985 to 1995. *J Toxicol Clin Toxicol* 35:353, 1997.
11. White CM: A review of potential cardiovascular uses of intravenous glucagon administration. *J Clin Pharmacol* 39:442, 1999.
12. Leatham EW, Holt DW, McKenna WJ: Class III antiarrhythmics in overdose: Presenting features and management principles. *Drug Saf* 9:450, 1993.
13. Abernethy DR, Schwartz JB: Calcium antagonist drugs. *N Engl J Med* 341:1447, 1999.
14. Ramoska EA, Spiller HA, Winter M, Borys D: A one-year evaluation of calcium channel blocker overdoses: Toxicity and treatment. *Ann Emerg Med* 22:196, 1993.
15. Henry M, Kay MM, Viccellio P: Cardiogenic shock associated with calcium-channel and beta blockers: Reversal with intravenous calcium chloride. *Am J Emerg Med* 3:334, 1985.
16. Boyer EW, Shannon M: Treatment of calcium-channel-blocker intoxication with insulin infusion. *N Engl J Med* 344:1721, 2001.
17. Tom PA, Morrow CT, Kelen GD: Delayed hypotension after overdose of sustained release verapamil. *J Emerg Med* 12:621, 1994.
18. Kulig K, Duffy J, Rumack BH, et al: Naloxone for treatment of clonidine overdose. *JAMA* 247:1697, 1982.

For further reading in *Emergency Medicine: A Comprehensive Study Guide*, 6th ed., see Chap. 174, "Digitalis Glycosides," by William Dribben and Mark Kirk; Chap. 175, "Beta-Blocker Toxicity," by Teresa Carlin; Chap. 176, "Calcium Channel Blockers," by Kennon Heard and Jeffrey A. Kline; and Chap. 177, "Antihypertensives," by Arjun Chanmugam and Keith Thomasset.

109 PHENYTOIN AND FOSPHENYTOIN TOXICITY

Mark B. Rogers

EPIDEMIOLOGY

- Most phenytoin-related deaths have been caused by rapid IV administration and hypersensitivity reactions.

PATHOPHYSIOLOGY

- Phenytoin works by blocking sodium channels in neurons.
- Peak levels occur anywhere from 3 to 12 hours after a single oral dose.
- Phenytoin is extensively protein-bound (90%). The free, unbound form is active. Patients who have hypoalbuminemia (eg, in cirrhosis, nephrosis, malnutrition, or burns) or take drugs that displace phenytoin from binding sites (eg, salicylate, valproate, or sulfisoxazole) may exhibit toxic signs while in the therapeutic range.
- Drugs that inhibit or enhance hepatic microsomal activity may result in an increase or decrease of phenytoin level, respectively.
- Toxicity depends upon the duration of exposure, dosage taken, and most importantly, route of administration.
- An acute oral overdose is typically dose related and usually presents with nystagmus, nausea, vomiting, ataxia, dysarthria, choreoathetosis, opisthotonos, and central nervous system (CNS) depression or excitation. Death from oral overdose alone is extremely rare.[1]
- Propylene glycol, the diluent in the IV preparation, is a strong myocardial depressant and vasodilator, and increases vagal tone.[2]
- Life-threatening effects such as hypotension, bradycardia, and asystole can be seen with IV administra-

tion, and are secondary to propylene glycol.[2] This morbidity can be avoided by slowing the rate of administration.
- Fosphenytoin, a prodrug of phenytoin, is more soluble and less irritating to tissues. Intravenous fosphenytoin can cause pruritus and hypotension.
- Blood pressure and cardiac monitoring are recommended when loading fosphenytoin intravenously but not intramuscularly. The adverse and toxic effects of fosphenytoin are the same as for phenytoin, except the toxic effects of propylene glycol are not present.[3]

CLINICAL FEATURES

- CNS toxicity begins with horizontal nystagmus; however, vertical, bidirectional, or alternating nystagmus may occur with severe intoxication. A depressed level of consciousness is common, with sedation, lethargy, ataxic gait, and dysarthria progressing to confusion, seizures, coma, and apnea in a large overdose.
- Depressed or hyperactive deep tendon reflexes, clonus, and extensor toe responses may be noted. Acute dystonia and movement disorders, such as opisthotonos and choreoathetosis, may occur. Peripheral neuropathy and ataxia may persist for months.
- Cardiovascular toxicity is usually associated with IV administration only. In an otherwise healthy patient, cardiac toxicity has never been reported after an oral overdose of phenytoin; when observed, this requires assessment for other causes.
- Cardiovascular toxicity includes hypotension, bradycardia, conduction delays (which may progress to complete atrioventricular nodal block), ventricular tachycardia, ventricular fibrillation, and asystole.
- Electrocardiographic changes include increased PR interval, widened QRS interval, and altered ST-wave and T-wave segments. Bradycardia, hypotension, and syncope in healthy volunteers have been reported after small IV doses. Most of these side effects are due to the propylene glycol.
- Phenytoin causes significant soft tissue toxicity. Intramuscular injection can result in localized crystallization of the drug, hematoma, sterile abscess, and myonecrosis.
- Reported complications of extravasation after IV infusion have included skin and soft tissue necrosis, compartment syndrome, gangrene, and death. Fosphenytoin is well tolerated intramuscularly or intravenously.[4]
- Hypersensitivity reactions usually occur within 1 to 6 weeks of initiation of phenytoin therapy. Reactions can include systemic lupus erythematosus, erythema multiforme, toxic epidermal necrolysis, Stevens-Johnson syndrome, hepatitis, rhabdomyolysis, acute

interstitial pneumonitis, lymphadenopathy, leukopenia, disseminated intravascular coagulation, and renal failure.
- Gingival hyperplasia is a common side effect of phenytoin and its absence may suggest poor compliance.
- Phenytoin is teratogenic and should never be initiated in a pregnant patient without consulting a neurologist and obstetrician.

DIAGNOSIS AND DIFFERENTIAL

- Therapeutic levels are between 10 and 20 μg/mL (40 to 80 μmol/L). Some patients require levels above 20 μg/mL for adequate seizure control. Patients with underlying brain disease are predisposed to toxicity and may become toxic at low levels.
- Toxicity generally correlates with increasing plasma levels (Table 109-1). Due to erratic absorption, serial phenytoin levels should be obtained to ensure the level has peaked.
- Almost any CNS-active drug, such as ethanol, carbamazepine, benzodiazepines, barbiturates, and lithium, can mimic phenytoin toxicity.
- Disease states that resemble phenytoin toxicity include hypoglycemia, Wernicke's encephalopathy, and posterior fossa hemorrhage or tumor.
- Seizures caused by phenytoin toxicity are uncommon, and other causes should be investigated such as trauma or alcohol withdrawal.

EMERGENCY DEPARTMENT CARE AND DISPOSITION

- Supplemental oxygen should be administered to maintain an adequate pulse oximetry reading. Respiratory acidosis should be avoided. Patients should be placed on a cardiac monitor, noninvasive blood pressure device, and pulse oximeter. An IV line should be established.

TABLE 109-1   Correlation of Plasma Phenytoin Level and Side Effects

PLASMA LEVEL (μg/mL)	SIDE EFFECTS
<10	Usually none
10–20	Occasional mild nystagmus
20–30	Nystagmus
30–40	Ataxia, slurred speech, nausea and vomiting
40–50	Lethargy, confusion
>50	Coma, seizures

- Hypotension from IV administration of phenytoin should be treated with IV isotonic crystalloid and the discontinuation of the infusion.
- For an acute oral overdose, multiple doses of oral activated charcoal (1 g/kg), mixed with a cathartic such as sorbitol, should be given every 2 to 4 hours in the first 24 hours due to the extended absorptive phase.[5]
- Bradydysrhythmias may require atropine or cardiac pacing.
- Seizures may be treated with a benzodiazepine or phenobarbital.
- Hemodialysis and hemoperfusion are of no benefit.
- Following an oral ingestion, patients with serious complications (eg, seizures, coma, altered mental status, and ataxia) should be admitted.
- With mild symptoms, the patient may be treated with activated charcoal in the emergency department and discharged home if repeat serum levels return to normal and the patient is not actively suicidal.
- Patients with symptomatic chronic intoxication should be admitted for observation unless the toxic effects are minimal, adequate care can be obtained at home, and they are 8 to 12 hours from their last dose.
- Following IV administration of phenytoin, patients with significant or persistent complications should be admitted for observation on a telemetry unit. Those with transient effects can be discharged.

REFERENCES

1. Mellick LB, Morgan JA, Mellick GA: Presentations of acute phenytoin overdose. *Am J Emerg Med* 7:61, 1989.
2. Gross DR, Kitzman JV, Adams HR: Cardiovascular effects of intravenous administration of propylene glycol in calves. *Am J Vet Res* 40:783, 1979.
3. Dean JC, Smith KR: Safety, tolerance, and pharmacokinetics of intramuscular fosphenytoin in neurosurgical patients. *Epilepsia* 34:111, 1993.
4. Hanna DR: Purple glove syndrome: a complication of intravenous phenytoin. *J Neurosci Nurs* 24:340, 1992.
5. Howard CE, Roberts S, Ely DS: Use of multiple-dose activated charcoal in phenytoin toxicity. *Ann Pharmacother* 28:201, 1994.

For further reading in *Emergency Medicine: A Comprehensive Study Guide*, 6th ed., see Chap. 178, "Phenytoin and Fosphenytoin Toxicity," by Harold H. Osborn.

110 IRON

O. John Ma

EPIDEMIOLOGY

- Iron toxicity from an intentional or accidental ingestion is a common poisoning. Approximately 30,000 calls related to iron supplement ingestion were made to U.S. poison centers in 2000.[1]

PATHOPHYSIOLOGY

- Iron is a direct gastrointestinal (GI) irritant and causes vomiting, diarrhea, abdominal pain, mucosal ulceration, and GI bleeding after a significant ingestion.
- Vomiting and diarrhea from iron toxicity may lead to hypovolemia, which in turn may produce hypotension, tissue hypoperfusion, and metabolic acidosis.
- When transferrin's ability to combine with iron is exhausted, free iron becomes available to enter mitochondria, where it inhibits oxidative phosphorylation and results in metabolic acidosis.

CLINICAL FEATURES

- When determining a patient's potential for experiencing toxicity, elemental iron must be used in calculations. Ferrous sulfate contains 20% elemental iron and pediatric multivitamins typically contain 10 to 18 mg of elemental iron per tablet.
- Based on clinical findings, iron poisoning can be divided into five stages. Patients can die in any stage of iron poisoning.
- The first stage develops within the first few hours after the ingestion. The direct irritative effects of iron on the GI tract produce abdominal pain, vomiting, and diarrhea. Hematemesis is not unusual. Vomiting is the clinical sign most consistently associated with acute iron toxicity. The absence of these symptoms within 6 hours of ingestion essentially excludes a diagnosis of significant iron toxicity.[2–4]
- During the second stage, which may continue for up to 24 hours following ingestion, the patient's GI symptoms may resolve, thereby giving a false sense of security despite toxic amounts of iron being absorbed into the body. Patients may not be symptomatic but will still appear ill, and may have abnormal vital signs and evidence of poor tissue perfusion be-

cause of ongoing volume loss and worsening metabolic acidosis.
- The third stage may appear either early or develop hours after the second stage. Shock and a metabolic acidosis develop. Iron-induced coagulopathy may worsen bleeding and hypovolemia. Hepatic dysfunction, cardiomyopathy, and renal failure also may occur.
- The fourth stage develops 2 to 5 days after ingestion. It manifests as elevation of aminotransferase and may progress to hepatic failure.
- The fifth stage, which occurs 4 to 6 weeks after ingestion, involves gastric outlet obstruction secondary to the corrosive effects of iron on the pyloric mucosa.

DIAGNOSIS AND DIFFERENTIAL

- The diagnosis of iron poisoning is based on the clinical picture and the history provided by the patient, significant others, or out-of-hospital care providers.
- Toxic effects have been reported following oral doses as low as 10 to 20 mg/kg elemental iron. Moderate toxicity occurs at doses of 20 to 60 mg/kg elemental iron, and severe toxicity can be expected following doses of >60 mg/kg elemental iron.[5]
- Laboratory work should be sent for serum electrolytes, blood urea nitrogen, serum glucose, coagulation studies, complete blood count, hepatic enzymes, and serum iron level.
- It is crucial to note that the determination of a single serum iron level does not reflect what iron levels have been previously, what direction they are going, or the degree of iron toxicity in the tissues. A single low serum level does not exclude the diagnosis of iron toxicity since there are variable times to peak level following ingestion of different iron preparations.
- Serum iron levels have limited use in directing management since excess iron is toxic intracellularly and not in the blood.
- In general, serum iron levels between 300 and 500 μg/dL correlate with mild systemic toxicity, and iron levels between 500 and 1000 μg/dL correlate with moderate systemic toxicity. Levels greater than 1000 μg/dL are associated with significant morbidity.
- The total iron binding capacity (TIBC) is now thought to have little value in the assessment of iron-poisoned patients because it becomes falsely elevated in the presence of elevated serum iron levels or deferoxamine.[6]
- A plain radiograph of the kidneys, ureters, and

bladder (KUB) may reveal iron in the GI tract; however, many iron preparations are not routinely detected, so negative radiographs do not exclude iron ingestion.[4]

EMERGENCY DEPARTMENT CARE AND DISPOSITION

- Patients who have remained asymptomatic for 6 hours after ingestion of iron and who have a normal physical examination do not require medical treatment for iron toxicity.
- Patients whose symptoms resolve after a short period of time, and who have normal vital signs, usually have mild toxicity and require only supportive care. This subset of patients still requires an observation period.
- Patients who are symptomatic or demonstrate signs of hemodynamic instability after iron ingestion should be managed aggressively in the ED.
- They should receive supplemental oxygen, be placed on a cardiac monitor, and have two large-bore IVs established.
- Patients should receive vigorous IV crystalloid infusion to help correct hypovolemia and tissue hypoperfusion.
- Patients who present within 2 hours of ingestion should undergo gastric lavage. Activated charcoal does not bind iron and its use is not recommended.
- Whole bowel irrigation with polyethylene glycol solution has been demonstrated to be efficacious. Administration of 250 to 500 mL/h in children and 2 L/h in adults via nasogastric tube may clear the GI tract of iron pills before absorption occurs.
- Antiemetics such as promethazine (25 mg IM in adults; 0.25 to 0.5 mg/kg IM in pediatric patients) or ondansetron (4 mg IV in adults; 0.1 mg/kg to a maximum dose of 4 mg in pediatric patients) should be administered.
- Coagulopathy should be corrected with vitamin K_1 (5 to 25 mg SC) and fresh frozen plasma (10 to 25 mL/kg in adults; 10 mL/kg in pediatric patients). Blood should be typed and screened or cross-matched, as necessary.
- Deferoxamine is a chelating agent that can remove iron from tissues and free iron from plasma. Deferoxamine combines with iron to form water-soluble ferrioxamine, which is excreted in the urine. Deferoxamine is safe to administer to children and pregnant women.
- Patients with mild iron toxicity may be treated with deferoxamine 90 mg/kg IM, up to 1 g in children and 2 g in adults. The dose may be repeated every 4 to 6 hours, as clinically indicated.
- For patients with more severe iron toxicity, the preferred route of deferoxamine administration is as an

IV infusion. Since hypotension is the rate-limiting factor for IV infusion, it is recommended to begin with a slow IV infusion at 5 mg/kg/h. The deferoxamine infusion rate can be increased to 15 mg/kg/h, as tolerated, within the first hour of treatment. It is recommended not to exceed a total daily dose of 6 to 8 g. In a clinically ill patient with a known acute ingestion of iron, deferoxamine therapy should be initiated without waiting for the serum iron level result.
- Determining the efficacy of deferoxamine involves evaluating serial urine samples. As ferrioxamine is excreted, the urine changes to the classic vin rose appearance. Clinical recovery of the patient is probably the most important factor in terminating deferoxamine therapy.[5]
- Patients who remain asymptomatic after 6 hours of observation and have a reliable history of an insignificant ingestion may be considered for discharge. Patients initially symptomatic who become asymptomatic should still be admitted since this may represent the second stage.
- Patients who receive deferoxamine therapy should be admitted to an intensive care setting. All patients should be assessed for suicide risk. Child abuse or neglect should be considered in pediatric cases.

REFERENCES

1. Litovitz T, Klein-Schwartz W, White S, et al: 2000 Annual Report of the American Association of Poison Control Centers Toxic Exposure Surveillance System. *Am J Emerg Med* 19: 337, 2001
2. Lacouture PG, Wason S, Temple AR, et al: Emergency assessment of severity in iron overdose by clinical and laboratory methods. *J Pediatr* 99:89, 1981.
3. Chyka PA, Butler AY: Assessment of acute iron poisoning by laboratory and clinical observations. *Am J Emerg Med* 11:99, 1993.
4. Palatnick W, Tenenbein M: Leukocytosis, hyperglycemia, vomiting, and positive x-rays are not indicators of severity of iron poisoning. *Am J Emerg Med* 14:454, 1996.
5. Schauben JL, Augustein WL, Cox J, et al: Iron poisoning: Report of three cases and a review of therapeutic intervention. *J Emerg Med* 8:309, 1990.
6. Bentur Y, St Louis P, Klein J, et al: Misinterpretation of iron-binding capacity in the presence of deferoxamine. *J Pediatr* 118:139, 1991.

For further reading in *Emergency Medicine: A Comprehensive Study Guide,* 6th ed., see Chap. 179, "Iron," by Joseph G. Rella and Lewis S. Nelson.

111 HYDROCARBONS AND VOLATILE SUBSTANCES

J. Christian Fox

EPIDEMIOLOGY

- Between 3 and 10% of all unintentional childhood ingestions are related to hydrocarbons.
- Approximately 3.5 to 10% of young people have tried volatile substance inhalation.[1]

PATHOPHYSIOLOGY

- Products containing hydrocarbons are found in many household and work place settings; these include fuels, lighter fluids, paint removers, pesticides, polishers, degreasers, and lubricants.
- Volatile substances containing hydrocarbons such as glue, propellants, and gasoline are occasionally used for abuse.
- Pulmonary toxicity presents as a chemical pneumonitis caused by direct parenchymal injury and altered surfactant function. This results either from aspiration of a low-viscosity compound or inhalation of a high-volatility compound.
- Central nervous system (CNS) toxicity results from a direct response to the systematically absorbed hydrocarbon or indirectly from the hypoxia due to pulmonary toxicity.
- Peripheral neuropathy secondary to demyelination and retrograde axonal degeneration results from the P450 metabolism of six-carbon hydrocarbons to the toxic metabolite 2,5-hexanedione.[2]
- Free radical metabolism of halogenated hydrocarbons causes hepatocellular damage by lipid peroxidation.[3]
- With methylene chloride exposure, carbon monoxide formation may continue after cessation of exposure; this is caused by slow release of methylene chloride from the tissues prior to its metabolism to carbon monoxide.[4]

CLINICAL FEATURES

- Toxicity depends on the route of exposure (ingestion, inhalation, or dermal), physical characteristics (volatility, viscosity, and surface tension), chemical characteristics (aliphatic, aromatic, or hydrogenated), and the presence of toxic additives (eg, lead or pesticides).
- Pulmonary and cardiac toxicity are the most common. Toxicity is reviewed by chemical composition in Table 111-1.
- Chemical pneumonitis, the most common pulmonary complication, results from aspiration of the highly volatile aliphatic substances such as gasoline, kerosene, methane, or butane. Additional complications include pneumomediastinum, pneumothorax, and pneumatocele.
- Patients present with coughing, dyspnea, choking, and gasping. Physical examination findings include tachypnea, wheezing, grunting, and decreased breath sounds.
- Chest radiographic findings lag behind the clinical picture by 4 to 6 hours.
- Toxicity of the CNS is most common with the volatile petroleum distillates such as toluene and tri-

TABLE 111-1 Chemical Toxicity

CHEMICAL COMPOSITION	EXAMPLE	COMMERCIAL USE	TOXICITY
Aliphatic (open chain)	*Short chain:* methane, butane, propane	Fuel	Pulmonary, negligible GI absorption
	Intermediate chain: gasoline, kerosene mineral seal oil	Motor fuel, stove fuel, furniture polish	Hemolysis
	Long chain: N-hexane, ketone	Tar, rubber cement	Polyneuropathy
Aromatic (benzene ring)	Benzene, toluene, xylene	Gasoline, airplane glue, cleaning agent, degreaser	Dysrhythmias, aplastic anemia, chronic myelogenous leukemia
Halogenated (substituted halogen group)	Carbon-tetrachloride, chloroform, trichloroethylene, Trichloroethane	Refrigerant, propellant, solvent, spot remover, degreaser	Dysrhythmias, hepatic toxicity, acute renal failure, hemolysis

chloroethane. Symptoms range from giddiness, slurred speech, ataxia, and hallucinations to seizures, lethargy, obtundation, and coma. Chronic exposure may cause cerebellar ataxia and mood lability.

- Cardiac toxicity from aromatic and halogenated hydrocarbons is due to the sensitization of the myocardium to catecholamines. This may cause serious dysrhythmias (ventricular tachycardia or fibrillation), decreased contractility, bradycardia, and heart blocks.
- Hepatic toxicity from halogenated hydrocarbons such as carbon tetrachloride and chloroform cause hepatocellular injury. Liver enzymes may be elevated within 24 hours, and right upper quadrant abdominal pain and jaundice develop within 48 to 96 hours. Chronic exposure causes cirrhosis and hepatoma.
- Hematologic toxicity due to gasoline, kerosene, and trichloroethane can cause hemolysis.[5] Chronic benzene abuse can cause aplastic anemia and hematologic malignancies.
- Dermal toxicity includes rashes (erythema, papules, vesicles, or scarlatiniform rash), eczematous dermatitis, and burns.
- Carbon monoxide poisoning from methylene chloride metabolism may result in a metabolic acidosis.

DIAGNOSIS AND DIFFERENTIAL

- Diagnosis is made by the history and accompanying physical examination findings.
- Laboratory tests that should be ordered include arterial blood gas, liver function panel, blood urea nitrogen (BUN), creatinine, hematocrit, and carboxyhemoglobin level (in methylene chloride exposure).
- A chest radiograph should be ordered to evaluate for pneumonitis.
- A kidney, ureter, and bladder (KUB) radiograph may show the presence of chlorinated hydrocarbons (eg, carbon tetrachloride) in the gastrointestinal (GI) tract because of the radiopaque nature of these polyhalogenated substances.[6]

EMERGENCY DEPARTMENT CARE AND DISPOSITION

- All symptomatic patients should be administered supplemental oxygen and placed on a cardiac monitor.
- Strong consideration for endotracheal intubation should be given to patients having respiratory distress. Positive end-expiratory pressure may be added if necessary, but pneumothorax or pneumatocele are potential complications.
- In severe pulmonary aspiration resulting in refractory hypoxemia, treatment with extracorporeal membrane oxygenation and high-frequency jet ventilation has proved to be successful.
- Decontamination of the patient should follow standard HAZMAT measures, which preferably should occur in the out-of-hospital setting.
- Hypotension should be treated with IV crystalloid infusion. Catecholamines may precipitate life-threatening dysrhythmias and should be avoided, except in cases of cardiac arrest.
- Tachydysrhythmias may be treated with propranolol (1 mg IV; may repeat if blood pressure is stable). Seizures should be managed using standard regimens.
- Some hydrocarbons, such as the CHAMP (camphor, halogenated, aromatic, metals, pesticides) agents and wood distillates (turpentine or pine oil), get absorbed through the GI tract; patients with these ingestions should undergo GI decontamination.
- The majority of hydrocarbon ingestions, which consist of aliphatic mixtures, do not require GI decontamination. Aliphatic hydrocarbons are poorly absorbed from the GI tract and carry a risk of aspiration during GI decontamination measures.
- Activated charcoal and cathartics are of no benefit with any hydrocarbon ingestion.
- Hyperbaric oxygen therapy may be indicated for patients who develop significant carbon monoxide toxicity after exposure to methylene chloride.
- Because most fatalities occur in the first 24 to 48 hours, all patients who are symptomatic at the time of evaluation should be admitted. Patients exposed to significant amounts of methemoglobinemia-producing hydrocarbons should also be admitted.
- Asymptomatic patients with a normal chest radiograph who remain symptom-free after 6 hours of observation may be discharged. All discharged patients should receive close follow-up since delayed toxicity (>18 hours) has been reported.

REFERENCES

1. Ramsey J, Anderson HR, Bloor K, et al: An introduction to the practice, prevalence and chemical toxicology of volatile substance abuse. *Hum Toxicol* 8:261, 1989.
2. Herskowitz A, Ishii N, Schaumburg H: *N*-Hexane neuropathy: A syndrome occurring as a result of industrial exposure. *N Engl J Med* 285:82, 1971.
3. Baerg RD, Kimberg DV: Centrilobular hepatic necrosis and acute renal failure in solvent sniffers. *Ann Intern Med* 73:713, 1970.
4. Leikin JB, Kaufman D, Lipscomb JW, et al: Methylene chloride: Report of five exposures and two deaths. *Am J Emerg Med* 8:534, 1990.

5. Algren JT, Rodgers CYC: Intravascular hemolysis associated with hydrocarbon poisoning. *Pediatr Emerg Care* 8:34, 1992.
6. Kleinschmidt K, Goto GS, Roth B: Multiple small volume subcutaneous WD-40 injections with severe local and systemic toxicity. *J Toxicol Clin Toxicol* 37:653, 1999.

For further reading in *Emergency Medicine: A Comprehensive Study Guide*, 6th ed., see Chap. 180, "Hydrocarbons and Volatile Substances," by Paul M. Wax.

112 CAUSTICS
Christian A. Tomaszewski

EPIDEMIOLOGY

- The American Association of Poison Control Centers reports approximately 100,000 caustic exposures each year in the U.S.[1] Very few exposures result in death (less than 100 in 2002) partly because most are unintentional and involve children.
- Alkali exposures mainly result from household cleaners, such as sodium hydroxide for drain opening and sodium tripolyphosphate in automatic dishwasher detergent. Acid exposures involve household and toilet cleaners, like sulfuric and hydrochloric acid, and the more dangerous and insidious chemical, hydrofluoric acid, which is potentially lethal through dermal exposure.
- The most common caustic exposure is household bleach, with approximately 50,000 exposures annually. It combines a mild acid and sodium hypochlorite, stabilized with a strong alkali (potassium or sodium hydroxide). Although potentially lethal in intentionally large overdoses, it rarely results in any morbidity among the countless incidental pediatric exposures each year.[2]

PATHOPHYSIOLOGY

- The strength of a caustic and the duration of exposure determine its ability to cause damage. Although concentration, pH, and pK_a are important, the titratable alkaline (or acid) reserve may predict potential damage better.[3] This is the measure of the amount of acid or alkali necessary to restore neutrality to a caustic solution.
- Alkalis penetrate deeply into tissue through liquefaction necrosis. Liquid alkali ingestions cause more proximal damage to the esophagus, rather than to the stomach; they eventually lead to stricture formation if the exposure is severe. Granular forms of alkalis produce even more proximal damage, typically focal burns in the oropharynx and esophagus.

- Strong acids tend to produce coagulation necrosis. The early formation of eschar generally protects against deeper injury in the esophagus. Regardless, both esophageal and gastric injury can occur.[4]
- Hydrofluoric acid is unique in that although it is a weak acid ($pK_a = 3.8$), it can cause delayed morbidity and mortality. The fluoride component of the acid penetrates deeply and complexes with calcium and magnesium. This results in local cell death as well as systemic hypocalcemia and ventricular dysrhythmias. This can occur after a dermal exposure, with as little as a 2.5% body surface area burn at a concentration of 100%.

CLINICAL FEATURES

- Alkalis are relatively tasteless and odorless. When swallowed, alkalis can lead to esophageal perforation or delayed stricture.
- Nausea, vomiting, dysphagia, and epigastric pain may mark gastrointestinal (GI) injury. More severe injury may present days later as chest pain from esophageal perforation and mediastinitis, or peritonitis from gastric perforation.
- Acids tend to be foul smelling and tasting, as well as strong irritants. Although acids can cause damage to the esophagus, they also tend to pool in the stomach, leading to gastric hemorrhage, necrosis, and perforation.[4] In addition, acids that are absorbed by the patient can cause metabolic acidosis, hemolysis, and renal failure.
- Caustic ingestions can cause distal GI injury without necessarily causing oral or facial burns.[5] More distal injury may lead to vomiting, dysphagia, odynophagia, and epigastric pain. Laryngotracheal injury is usually marked by dysphonia, drooling, stridor, and respiratory distress.
- Dermal exposures to caustics usually only produce local pain and irritation. However, sodium hydrofluoric acid differs in its ability to cause deep, often delayed, tissue necrosis accompanied by hypocalcemia and hypomagnesemia, which may lead to death from ventricular dysrhythmias.
- Dermal exposures to this acid are unique in that the patient can present hours later with tremendous pain with soft tissue erythema and edema.
- Caustic exposures to the cornea are particularly serious if they involve alkalis. Acid exposures tend to be superficial and do not usually lead to perforation or scarring as can be seen with alkali exposure.

DIAGNOSIS AND DIFFERENTIAL

- Clinically, it is difficult to exclude esophageal or gastric injury. The absence of burns to the mouth or oropharynx does not necessarily exclude significant esophageal or gastric injury.[5]
- Patients with serious esophageal injuries from alkali ingestions usually are symptomatic.[6]
- Laboratory tests are not generally useful in caustic ingestions. In serious cases (particularly after acid ingestion) where the patient is symptomatic, arterial blood gas and electrolytes may be useful.
- In hydrofluoric acid exposures, calcium and magnesium levels, as well as an electrocardiogram (ECG), may be useful.
- An upright chest radiograph will evaluate for aspiration, pneumomediastinum, or pneumoperitoneum from gastric perforation.
- Endoscopy is the diagnostic test of choice in evaluating for serious esophageal or gastric injury.[7] It is indicated in all patients with signs or symptoms of serious injury—vomiting, drooling, dyspnea, or stridor—or severe oropharyngeal burns.
- The presence of a third-degree burn reliably predicts the formation of stricture, regardless of treatment.[8]
- Second-degree burns (deep ulcerations without necrosis) may warrant the use of steroids in an attempt to prevent esophageal stricture and the need for replacement.[9]
- Asymptomatic patients who intentionally ingest strong acids may also benefit from endoscopy to exclude occult gastric injury. Early endoscopy, within several hours of ingestion, can be safe and useful in determining the extent of injury as well as the need for admission.
- Computed tomography may be a useful screening test in patients with symptoms referable to the GI tract distal to the stomach. Ultrasonography can be used to follow-up gastric injury after caustic ingestion.

EMERGENCY DEPARTMENT CARE AND DISPOSITION

- One hundred percent oxygen should be administered to any patient with respiratory symptoms, followed by endotracheal intubation under direct visualization for any patient with respiratory distress. A cardiac monitor and pulse oximetry should be applied.
- Gastric decontamination in the form of activated charcoal, ipecac, or gastric lavage is contraindicated.
- Only in cases of strong acid ingestions may a nasogastric tube (NGT) be inserted for removal of excessive acid in the stomach. This is especially true for hydrofluoric acid, where fluoride binding can be effected with milk (8 ounces) orally or magnesium citrate 300 mL by NGT.
- Dilution is indicated only for solid alkali ingestions; particles should be washed away with water or milk. For other caustic ingestions, dilution is contraindicated because it can precipitate vomiting. Neutralization cannot be routinely recommended.
- Steroids are controversial in alkali ingestions.[8] They may be indicated within the first 6 hours of ingestion for patients at risk of esophageal strictures, particularly those with deep, discrete, or circumferential ulcerations, but without evidence of necrosis. Dexamethasone 0.1 mg/kg or methylprednisolone 1 mg/kg IV bolus is recommended.
- Antibiotics (eg, ampicillin 500 mg IV every 6 hours) are reserved for patients placed on IV steroids or who have suspected esophageal or gastric perforation.
- Emergent GI consultation should be obtained for any caustic ingestion other than an unintentional, benign ingestion. Patients who experienced unintentional ingestions can usually be discharged home after a few hours of observation if they remain asymptomatic and tolerate liquids well.[7]
- Intentional ingestion warrants endoscopy and admission regardless of symptoms. Psychiatric consultation should be initiated as well.
- Ocular exposures should be treated with copious irrigation for at least 20 to 30 minutes with 1 to 2 L of normal saline. Alkali exposures usually require more prolonged irrigation. The final pH of the conjunctivae should be below 8.0 before ceasing irrigation.
- Dermal exposures to caustics usually only require copious irrigation with water.
- Hydrofluoric acid dermal exposures require additional treatment. Small areas of skin can initially be treated with topical application of calcium gluconate gel (3.5 g mixed with 5 ounces of water-soluble surgical lubricant) every 4 to 8 hours, dictated by pain relief. In nondigital areas, if no relief is obtained or an extensive area is involved, then intradermal calcium gluconate 10% (0.5 mL/cm^2) should be administered. In digits, intra-arterial calcium gluconate (10 mL of 10% in 50 mL of D_5W over 4 hours) should be administered into the radial artery of the affected extremity.[10]
- Oral ingestions of hydrofluoric acid and ammonium bifluoride and severe dermal exposures (>20% concentration) usually require systemic treatment as well. Known or suspected hypocalcemia can be treated with calcium chloride 10% 0.02 to 0.04 mL/kg in adults (0.1 to 0.3 mL/kg in children). Alternatively, calcium gluconate 10% can be used at three times the dose, with less concern for local tissue necrosis if infiltrated.

- Prolonged QT interval or ventricular dysrhythmias can also be treated with magnesium sulfate 2 to 4 g IV (25 to 50 mg/kg in children).
- Suspected disc battery ingestions require a chest radiograph to exclude esophageal lodgment.[11] If it is discovered in the esophagus, then immediate endoscopic removal is indicated to help prevent esophageal perforation.

REFERENCES

1. Litovitz TL, Klein-Schwartz W, Rodgers GC, et al: Annual Report of the American Association of Poison Control Centers Toxic Exposure Surveillance System. *Am J Emerg Med* 20:391, 2002.
2. Racioppi F, Daskaleros PA, Besbelli N, et al: Household bleaches based on sodium hypochlorite: review of acute toxicology and poison control center experience. *Food Chem Tox* 32:845, 1994.
3. Hoffman RS, Howland MA, Kamerow HN, et al: Comparison of titratable acid/alkaline reserve and pH in potentially caustic household products. *J Toxicol Clin Toxicol* 27:241, 1989.
4. Zargar SA, Kochhar R, Nagi B: Ingestion of corrosive acids: Spectrum of injury to the upper gastrointestinal tract and natural history. *Gastroenterology* 97:702, 1989.
5. Previtera C, Giusti F, Guglielmi M: Predictive value of visible lesions (cheeks, lips, oropharynx) in suspected caustic ingestion: May endoscopy reasonably be omitted in completely negative pediatric patients? *J Pediatr Emerg Care* 6:176, 1990.
6. Gorman RL, Khin-Maung-Gyi MT, Klein-Schwartz W, et al: Initial symptoms as predictors of esophageal injury in alkaline corrosive ingestions. *Am J Emerg Med* 10:189, 1992.
7. Christesen HB: Prediction of complications following unintentional caustic ingestion in children. Is endoscopy always necessary? *Acta Paediatrica* 84:1177, 1995.
8. Anderson KD, Rouse TM, Randolph JG: A controlled trial of corticosteroids in children with corrosive injury of the esophagus. *N Engl J Med* 323:637, 1990.
9. Howell JM, Dalsey WC, Hartsell FW, Butzin CA: Steroids for the treatment of corrosive esophageal injury: a statistical analysis of past studies. *Am J Emerg Med* 10:421, 1992.
10. Vance MV, Curry SC, Kunkel DB, et al: Digital hydrofluoric acid burns: Treatment with intra-arterial calcium infusion. *Ann Emerg Med* 15:890, 1986.
11. Litovitz TL, Schmitz BF: Ingestion of cylindrical and button batteries: An analysis of 2382 cases. *Pediatrics* 89:747, 1992.

For further reading in *Emergency Medicine: A Comprehensive Study Guide,* 6th ed., see Chap. 181, "Caustics," by G. Richard Bruno and Wallace A. Carter.

113 INSECTICIDES, HERBICIDES, AND RODENTICIDES

Christian A. Tomaszewski

EPIDEMIOLOGY

- In 2001, over 90,000 pesticide exposures were reported to poison control centers, with approximately 50% of them in children <6 years of age and 19,495 receiving treatment in a health care facility.[1]
- Many pesticides contain inactive ingredients, such as petroleum distillates, that are harmful as well.
- Organophosphorus insecticides are the most common cause of major toxicity among all pesticides.
- Mass poisoning may be seen, particularly with organophosphates, in the setting of terrorist activity or chemical warfare.

PATHOPHYSIOLOGY

- Organophosphates bind irreversibly to and inhibit cholinesterases in the nervous system, which leads to the accumulation of neurotransmitters at the nerve synapses and neuromuscular junctions.
- Organophosphate toxicity is manifested systemically as cholinergic excess in muscarinic, nicotinic, and central nervous system (CNS) overstimulation.[2]

CLINICAL FEATURES

INSECTICIDES

ORGANOPHOSPHATES
- Patients usually become symptomatic within 8 hours of dermal exposure to organophosphates; nerve gas agents (eg, VX gas) can cause immediate effects via dermal or inhalation routes. The main exceptions are the fat-soluble agents (eg, fenthion), which can cause delayed or persistent symptoms.
- Muscarinic overstimulation results in the **SLUDGE** syndrome (**S**alivation, **L**acrimation, **U**rination, **D**efecation, **G**astrointestinal, **E**mesis) along with the **killer "B"s** (bradycardia, bronchospasm, and bronchorrhea). In addition, especially with nerve gas agents, the patient may have blurred vision associated with miosis.
- Nicotinic stimulation leads to fasciculations and muscle weakness, which is most pronounced in the pulmonary system already compromised by muscarinic effects.

- Nicotinic effects can also lead to paradoxical tachycardia and mydriasis.
- CNS effects, which often predominate in children, include tremor, restlessness, confusion, seizures, and coma.
- An intermediate syndrome, which occurs 1 to 4 days after acute poisoning, may present with paralysis or weakness of neck, facial, and respiratory muscles. This can result in respiratory arrest if not treated.[3]
- Organophosphate-induced delayed neuropathy occurs 1 to 3 weeks after acute poisoning. By inhibiting neuronal esterase, the patient develops a distal motor-sensory polyneuropathy.[4]
- Carbamates produce a similar cholinergic toxidrome to that of organophosphates, but of shorter duration and with less CNS symptomatology.[5]

ORGANOCHLORINES
- Organochlorines [eg, DDT (dichlorodiphenyltrichloroethane)] are represented by methoxychlor, endosulfan, toxaphene, and the therapeutic agent lindane.
- Acute poisoning with organochlorines primarily produces CNS stimulation, with headache, excitability, myoclonus, and seizures.[6] Excessive dermal application of lindane has produced toxicity.

PYRETHRINS
- Pyrethroids, synthetic derivatives of pyrethrins, are probably the safest insecticides. In massive ingestion, however, they may cause gastrointestinal (GI) distress, and rarely seizures.
- The main issue with pyrethrins and pyrethroids is the occasional allergic response, which can include contact dermatitis, rhinitis, and refractory asthma.

DEET
- N,N-diethyl-3-methylbenzamide (DEET), an extensively used insect repellent, can lead to neuronal toxicity after ingestion or multiple applications, particularly in small children.
- Clinical manifestations of DEET toxicity include restlessness, confusion, ataxia, lethargy, seizures, or coma.

HERBICIDES

- Topical exposure causes local irritation, and ingestion may result in vomiting, diarrhea, and pulmonary edema.
- Chlorophenoxy compounds (eg, 2,4-dichlorophenoxyacetic acid) may cause tachycardia, dysrhythmias, and hypotension along with muscle toxicity manifested by muscle pain, fasciculations, and rhabdomyolysis.

- Paraquat is especially toxic, with caustic effects resulting in severe dermal, corneal, and mucous membrane burns, including that of the respiratory and GI epithelium. Cardiovascular collapse may occur early, especially in the case of large ingestions.
- If patients survive the initial insult, they can develop liver and renal necrosis, followed by irreversible pulmonary fibrosis weeks later.[7]
- Diquat is very similar in toxicity to paraquat, although it lacks the pulmonary toxicity, but is more prone to produce brainstem hemorrhage.
- A cross between organophosphates and herbicides is glyphosate, which generally causes only mild dermatitis and mucosal irritation on contact. Massive ingestions of concentrated solution have caused widespread organ dysfunction, including pulmonary edema, acidosis, and hyperkalemia.

RODENTICIDES

SEVERE TOXICITY
- Sodium monofluoroacetate and related compounds typically demonstrate delayed toxicity until metabolites block aerobic metabolic pathways, which leads to lactic acidosis. Patients exhibit nausea and anxiety followed by respiratory depression, pulmonary edema, cardiovascular collapse, coma, and seizures.[8]
- Strychnine toxicity blocks the spinal cord inhibitor glycine and results in "awake seizures," which are characterized by facial grimacing, muscle twitching, severe extensor spasms, and opisthotonos. This can lead to rhabdomyolysis, hyperthermia, and lactic acidosis.
- Exposure to thallium sulfate initially causes GI hemorrhage and vomiting, which are followed by neurologic sequelae days later. Patients can develop painful paresthesias, weakness, tremors, ataxia, seizures, and coma. Death is typically due to respiratory failure and dysrhythmias.
- Zinc phosphide ingestion results in the liberation of phosphine gas that subsequently causes GI irritation, hepatocellular toxicity, pulmonary edema, altered mental status, seizures, and cardiovascular collapse; hypomagnesemia and hypocalcemia also can result.
- Yellow phosphorus causes severe topical burns and also may cause jaundice, seizures, and cardiovascular collapse.
- Within hours of ingestion, barium carbonate poisoning can cause GI distress with dysrhythmias, hypokalemia, respiratory failure, weakness, and paralysis.
- N-3-pyridylmethyl-N-p-nitrophenyl urea (vacor) has the unique ability to induce insulin deficiency and peripheral neuropathy. Mortality or morbidity may result from GI perforation, diabetic ketoacidosis, or cardiac dysrhythmias.

- Arsenic poisoning may present initially with nausea and vomiting, hypotension, bloody diarrhea, altered mental status, and seizures. If the patient survives, peripheral neuropathies ensue with weakness and muscle wasting.

MODERATE TOXICITY

- α-Naphthyl-thiourea (ANTU) poisoning exhibits primarily pulmonary effects with dyspnea, pleuritic chest pain, and noncardiogenic pulmonary edema.
- Cholecalciferol causes the typical symptoms of vitamin D excess.

LOW TOXICITY

- Red squill poisoning can present with severe GI distress and cardiac dysrhythmias due to digitalis effect.
- After large deliberate ingestions, bromethalin can cause headache, confusion, tremors, seizures, and coma.
- Norbromide poisoning causes dermatitis from chronic handling.

SUPERWARFARINS

- The most common rodenticide exposures are due to superwarfarins (eg, brodifacoum), which are present in a variety of grain-based rodent baits.
- Because of their extraordinary half-lives, exposures may come to attention months later with symptoms of unexplained coagulopathy.
- This coagulopathy may manifest itself when the patient experiences hematuria, epistaxis, GI hemorrhage, spontaneous hemoperitoneum, or fatal intracranial hemorrhage.[9]

DIAGNOSIS AND DIFFERENTIAL

- The diagnosis of pesticide poisoning is made clinically in the overwhelming majority of cases.
- In the case of organophosphate poisoning, clues at the bedside include the odor of garlic or hydrocarbons.
- A positive response to atropine and pralidoxime (2-PAM) will usually confirm the diagnosis of organophosphate poisoning.
- For delayed confirmation of organophosphate poisoning, an assay of either plasma (easier to obtain) or red blood cell (more accurate) cholinesterase activity can be obtained for diagnosis and treatment guidance.[10]
- Qualitative and quantitative assays of blood and urine for paraquat may at times be clinically useful in confirming exposure and prognostication.
- In deliberate or massive ingestions of superwarfarins, a 48-hour postingestion prothrombin time (PT) is needed.[11]
- Other routine laboratory testing is nondiagnostic, but may reveal hyperglycemia, electrolyte abnormalities, metabolic acidosis, leukocytosis, hyperamylasemia, or liver enzyme abnormalities.
- In cases involving severe respiratory distress, a chest radiograph may show signs of pulmonary edema.
- Electrocardiographic findings are variable and may include tachydysrhythmia, ventricular blocks, bradydysrhythmia, or QT-interval prolongation with ensuing torsades de pointes.[12]
- Pesticide poisoning can easily be mistaken for routine illnesses. Bronchospasm and pulmonary edema may be attributed to asthma or congestive heart failure exacerbations. Vomiting and diarrhea could be mistaken for gastroenteritis.
- The differential diagnosis for organophosphate poisoning includes these illnesses along with a variety of cardiopulmonary and neurologic emergencies.
- Other toxic agents may mimic the same effects of organophosphates: muscarinic effects may arise from bethanecol or the mushrooms *Clitocybe* and *Inocybe;* agitation and diaphoresis may arise from sympathomimetics like cocaine; nicotinic effects may arise from tobacco toxicity; and seizures may be due to a variety of toxins.

EMERGENCY DEPARTMENT CARE AND DISPOSITION

- Prior to encountering the pesticide-poisoned patient (especially involving organophosphates), health care workers should at least gown and glove (neoprene or nitrile) to prevent secondary contamination.
- Symptomatic patients require emergent attention to airway protection and ventilation. Supplemental oxygen should be administered to maintain oxygen saturation greater than 95%.
- Endotracheal intubation and mechanical ventilation may be necessary in severe poisoning; the effects of succinylcholine may exacerbate certain conditions and its use should be carefully considered during rapid sequence intubation.
- Decontamination in dermal exposures can be performed using soap and water or with dilute bleach.
- In recent significant ingestions, aspiration of gastric contents with a nasogastric tube and administration of activated charcoal may be helpful, especially if a coingestion may be involved.
- The mainstay of treatment for pesticide exposure is identification of the specific agent involved, supportive monitoring, and treatment. Maintenance of intravascular volume and urine output should be assured.
- Cardiac dysrhythmias should be treated in standard fashion.

TABLE 113-1   Pesticides and Specific Antidotes

PESTICIDE	ANIDOTE	DOSING
Organophosphates	Atropine	0.05 mg/kg up to 1–2 mg IV initially q 5–15 min; consider IV infusion and titrate to effect (drying secretions)
	2-PAM	20–40 mg/kg up to 1 g IV; may repeat in 1–2 h, then every 6–8 h for 48 h
Carbamates	Atropine 2-PAM	As for organophosphates; use is controversial
Zinc phosphide	NaHCO$_3$ Calcium gluconate	50–100 mEq (1 ampule) for intragastric alkalinization 10 mL of 10% IV (for hypocalcemia)
Yellow phosphorus	K permanganate or H$_2$O$_2$	1:5000 dilution used for gastric lavage
Sodium monofluoroacetate	Ethanol	10 mL/kg of 10% IV bolus, then 1.5 mL/kg/h
PNU (Vacor)	Niacinamide	500 mg IV
Arsenic	BAL DMSA	3–5 mg/kg IM every 4 h 10 mg/kg PO every 8 h
Red squill	Fab fragments	May start with 5 vials in severe toxicity
Superwarfarins	Vitamin K$_1$	Up to 20 mg IV, repeated and titrated to effect

ABBREVIATIONS: 2-PAM = pralidoxime; NaHCO$_3$ = sodium bicarbonate; H$_2$O$_2$ − hydrogen peroxide; BAL − dimercaprol (British Anti-Lewisite); DMSA = succimer (dimercaptosuccinic acid).

- Benzodiazepines (eg, lorazepam 2 mg IV) remain the initial therapy for seizures.[13]
- If the PT/INR is elevated after superwarfarin ingestion, vitamin K$_1$ 10 to 20 mg SC or IV can be administered; if serious bleeding is present, fresh frozen plasma (FFP) also may be required.
- Administration of a specific antidote may be appropriate for selected agents (Table 113-1).
- Asymptomatic patients with a history of contact with a pesticide may require decontamination and a 4 to 6 hour observation period. Close follow-up should be arranged for exposures to rodenticides that produce delayed symptoms.
- A low threshold for admission should be maintained for patients with intentional ingestions or symptoms. Any patient with a history of paraquat or diquat exposure should be admitted because of the extreme lethality of these compounds.

REFERENCES

1. Litovitz TL, Klein-Schwartz W, Rodgers GC, et al: 2001 Annual Report of the American Association of Poison Control Centers Toxic Exposure Surveillance System. *Am J Emerg Med* 20:391, 2002.
2. Agarwal SB: A clinical, biochemical, neurobehavioral, and sociopsychological study of 190 patients admitted to hospital as a result of acute organophosphorus poisoning. *Environ Res* 62:63, 1993.
3. Senanayake N, Karalliedde L: Neurotoxic effects of organophosphorus insecticides: An intermediate syndrome. *N Engl J Med* 316:761, 1987.
4. Steenland K, Jenkins B, Ames RG, et al: Chronic neurological sequelae to organophosphate pesticide poisoning. *Am J Public Health* 84:731, 1994.
5. Lifshitz M, Rotenberg M, Sofer S, et al: Carbamate poisoning and oxime treatment in children: A clinical and laboratory study. *Pediatrics* 93:652, 1994.
6. Kilburn KH, Thornton JC: Protracted neurotoxicity from chlordane sprayed to kill termites. *Environ Health Perspect* 103:691, 1995.
7. Vale JA, Meredith TJ, Buckley BM: Paraquat poisoning: clinical features and immediate general management. *Hum Toxicol* 6:41, 1987.
8. Chi CH, Chen KW, Chan SH, et al: Clinical presentation and prognostic factors in sodium monofluoroacetate intoxication. *J Toxicol Clin Toxicol* 34:707, 1996.
9. Morgan B, Tomaszewski C, Rotker I: Spontaneous hemoperitoneum from brodifacoum overdose. *Am J Emerg Med* 14:656-659, 1996.
10. Nouira S, Abroug F, Elatrous S, et al: Prognostic value of serum cholinesterase in acute organophosphate poisoning. *Chest* 106:1811, 1994.
11. Ingels M, Lai C, Tai W, et al: A prospective study of acute, unintentional, pediatric superwarfarin ingestions managed without decontamination. *Ann Emerg Med* 40:73, 2002.
12. Chuang FR, Jang SW, Lin JL, et al: QTc prolongation indicates a poor prognosis in patients with organophosphate poisoning. *Am J Emerg Med* 14:451, 1996.
13. Murphy MR, Blick DW, Dunn MA, et al: Diazepam as a treatment for nerve gas poisoning in primates. *Aviat Space Environ Med* 64:110, 1993.

For further reading in *Emergency Medicine: A Comprehensive Study Guide,* 6th ed., see Chap. 182, "Insecticides, Herbicides, and Rodenticides," by Walter C. Robey III and William J. Meggs.

114 METALS AND METALLOIDS
Lance H. Hoffman

LEAD

EPIDEMIOLOGY

- Lead is the most common cause of chronic metal poisoning, with approximately 890,000 children between the ages of 1 and 5 years having a blood lead level of at least 10 μg/dL.[1]
- Lead exposure may occur through occupational, recreational, or environmental exposure.

PATHOPHYSIOLOGY

- Lead injures the astrocytes and microvasculature of the central nervous system (CNS), demyelinates peripheral nerves, disrupts porphyrin metabolism, and impairs proximal renal tubule function.

CLINICAL FEATURES

- Lead poisoning should be suspected in any individual, especially a child, demonstrating CNS symptoms (delirium, seizures, coma, and memory deficit), abdominal symptoms (colicky pain, constipation, diarrhea), or anemia (hypoproliferative or hemolytic).
- Lead poisoning manifests as signs and symptoms affecting a variety of organ systems (Table 114-1).

DIAGNOSIS AND DIFFERENTIAL

- Serum lead levels of greater than 10 μg/dL are diagnostic of lead toxicity. An elevated serum lead level confirms the diagnosis, but the results of this test are often delayed in the emergency department.
- Radiographic evidence of lead toxicity includes horizontal metaphyseal bands in long bones, especially involving the knee, and radiopaque material in the alimentary tract.
- Another finding suggestive of lead poisoning is basophilic stippling of erythrocytes.

TABLE 114-1   Common Signs and Symptoms of Lead Poisoning

SYSTEM	CLINICAL MANIFESTATIONS
Central nervous system	Acute: encephalopathy, seizures, altered mental status, papilledema, optic neuritis, ataxia Chronic: headache, irritability, depression, fatigue, mood and behavioral changes, memory deficit, sleep disturbance
Peripheral nervous system	Paresthesias, motor weakness (classic wrist drop) depressed or absent DTRs, sensory function intact
Gastrointestinal	Abdominal pain (mostly with acute poisoning), constipation, diarrhea
Renal	Acute: Fanconi's syndrome (aminoaciduria, glucosuria, phosphaturia) renal tubular acidosis Chronic: interstitial nephritis, renal insufficiency, hypertension, gout
Hematologic	Hypoproliferative and/or hemolytic anemia; basophilic stippling (rare and nonspecific)
Reproductive	Decreased libido, impotence, sterility, abortions, premature births, decreased or abnormal sperm production

ABBREVIATIONS: DTRs = deep tendon reflexes.

EMERGENCY DEPARTMENT CARE AND DISPOSITION

- Gastrointestinal (GI) decontamination with whole bowel irrigation using polyethylene glycol solution is indicated for lead ingestion. The adult rate of instillation is 500 to 2000 mL/h, and the pediatric rate of instillation is 100 to 500 mL/h.
- Chelation therapy is indicated in all symptomatic individuals, and adults with a serum lead level of 70 μg/dL or more and children with a serum lead level of 45 μg/dL or more.
- Symptomatic individuals should receive dimercaprol (British Anti-Lewisite or BAL) 50 to 75 mg/m^2 IM followed in 4 hours with a continuous IV infusion of CaNa$_2$-EDTA 1500 mg/m^2/d, with higher dosing being reserved for patients with encephalopathy.
- Adults with a serum lead level of 70 to 100 μg/dL or children with a serum lead level of 45 to 69 μg/dL and with few or no symptoms should receive succimer (dimercaptosuccinic acid or DMSA) 350 mg/m^2 PO tid for 5 days, then bid for 14 days.
- Chelation therapy is not indicated for asymptomatic adults with a serum lead level less than 70 μg/dL or children with a serum lead level less than 45 μg/dL. Only removal from the exposure is needed in these cases.
- Patients requiring parenteral chelation therapy or whose only option is to return to the environment producing the lead exposure should be admitted to the hospital.

ARSENIC

EPIDEMIOLOGY

- Arsenic is the most common cause of acute metal poisoning and the second most common cause of chronic metal poisoning. It is found in agricultural chemicals, contaminated well water, and mining and smelting operations.

PATHOPHYSIOLOGY

- Arsenic inhibits pyruvate dehydrogenase, interferes with the cellular uptake of glucose, and uncouples oxidative phosphorylation.[2]

CLINICAL FEATURES

- Acute ingestion results in a profound gastroenteritis within hours of exposure. Hypotension and tachycardia may be present secondary to intravascular volume depletion and direct myocardial dysfunction.
- Encephalopathy, pulmonary edema, acute renal failure, and rhabdomyolysis have also been described.
- Chronic poisoning causes stocking glove peripheral neuropathies, morbilliform skin rash, malaise, myalgia, abdominal pain, memory loss, and personality changes.

DIAGNOSIS AND DIFFERENTIAL

- Acutely, the electrocardiogram (ECG) may demonstrate a prolonged QT interval or tachydysrhythmia, and abdominal radiographs may reveal radiopaque arsenic in the alimentary tract.[3,4]
- The diagnosis is confirmed by demonstrating an elevated 24-hour urine arsenic level.
- Other diagnoses to consider include septic shock, encephalopathy, peripheral neuropathy, Addison's disease, hypo- and hyperthyroidism, porphyria, and other metal poisonings.
- Transverse white lines of the nails (Mees' lines) may be evident 4 to 6 weeks postingestion.

EMERGENCY DEPARTMENT CARE AND DISPOSITION

- Hypotension should be treated with volume resuscitation and vasopressors. Dysrhythmias are managed by Advanced Cardiac Life Support (ACLS) protocol, with the need to avoid antiarrhythmia agents that prolong the QT interval (class IA, IC, and III agents).

- Whole bowel irrigation with polyethylene glycol solution is indicated for patients with an arsenic ingestion and an abdominal radiograph demonstrating radiopaque foreign bodies in the alimentary tract.
- Chelation therapy with BAL 3 to 5 mg/kg IM every 4 hours should be administered in severe arsenic poisonings.
- Succimer (350 mg/m² PO tid for 5 days, then bid for 14 days) is the preferred chelating agent for patients who are able to tolerate oral intake, are hemodynamically stable, and can be treated as outpatients without risk of repeated exposure to arsenic.

MERCURY

CLINICAL FEATURES

- Short-chained alkyl mercury (methyl, dimethyl, and ethyl) and elemental mercury produce a constellation of neurologic abnormalities collectively referred to as erethism (anxiety, depression, irritability, mania, sleep disturbances, and memory loss).[5] Tremor is also common.[6]
- Ingestion of mercury salts results in a severe gastroenteritis and acute tubular necrosis, while not affecting the CNS.
- Acrodynia is the term used to describe an immune-mediated condition that affects children exposed to mercury. Features include a generalized rash, fever, irritability, splenomegaly, and hypotonia.
- Inhalation of elemental mercury can result in pneumonitis, acute respiratory distress syndrome, and pulmonary fibrosis.[7]

DIAGNOSIS AND DIFFERENTIAL

- An elevated 24-hour urine mercury level confirms the diagnosis for all forms of mercury except the short-chained alkyl mercury compounds, which are excreted in the bile, undergo extensive enterohepatic recirculation, and accumulate in erythrocytes. An elevated whole blood mercury level must be used to confirm poisoning from these types of mercury compounds.
- The differential diagnosis of symptoms caused by mercury poisoning is extensive and includes all the causes of encephalopathy or tremor.
- Alternative causes of corrosive gastroenteritis (ingestion of iron, arsenic, phosphorus, acids, and alkalis) should be considered if mercury salt ingestion is suspected.

EMERGENCY DEPARTMENT CARE AND DISPOSITION

- Although BAL is contraindicated in short-chained alkyl mercury poisoning because it may exacerbate the CNS symptoms, it is the chelator of choice for mercury salts. BAL is administered as 3 to 5 mg/kg IM every 4 hours, in addition to initial GI decontamination.
- Succimer (DMSA) 10 mg/kg PO every 8 hours is the agent of choice in short-chained alkyl mercury poisonings.[8]

REFERENCES

1. Pirkle JL, Brody DJ, Gunter EW, et al: The decline of blood lead levels in the United States: The National Health and Nutrition Examination Surveys. *JAMA* 272:284, 1994.
2. Leibl B, Muckter H, Doklea E, et al: Reversal of oxyphenyl-arsine-induced inhibition of glucose uptake in MDCK cells. *Fundam Appl Toxicol* 27:1, 1995.
3. Beckman KJ, Bauman LJ, Pimental PA, et al: Arsenic-induced torsades de pointes. *Crit Care Med* 19:290, 1991.
4. Hilfer RJ, Mandel A: Acute arsenic intoxication diagnosed by roentgenograms. *N Engl J Med* 266:633, 1962.
5. Eto K: Pathology of Minamata disease. *Toxicol Pathol* 25:614, 1997.
6. Taueg C, Sanfilippo DJ, Rowens B, et al: Acute and chronic poisoning from residential exposures to elemental mercury—Michigan 1989-1990. *J Toxicol Clin Toxicol* 30:63, 1992.
7. Lim HE, Shim JJ, Lee SY, et al: Mercury inhalation poisoning and acute lung injury. *Korean J Intern Med* 13:127, 1998.
8. Roels HA, Boeckx M, Ceulemans E, et al: Urinary excretion of mercury after occupational exposure to mercury vapour and influence of the chelating agent meso-2,3-dimercaptosuccinic acid (DMSA). *Br J Ind Med* 48:247, 1991.

For further reading in *Emergency Medicine: A Comprehensive Study Guide,* 6th ed., see Chap. 184, "Metals and Metalloids," by Heather Long and Lewis S. Nelson.

115 HAZARDOUS MATERIALS

Christian A. Tomaszewski

EPIDEMIOLOGY

- A hazardous material is any substance (chemical, biological, or nuclear) that poses a risk to health, safety, property, or the environment.

- Well over a half million potentially toxic compounds have been produced, ranging from industrial chemicals to hazardous nuclear, biological, and chemical agents, known as weapons of mass destruction (WMD).
- The National Response Center logged over 34,000 hazardous oil and chemical incidents during 2001, with 80% at fixed facilities, 20% transportation related, and over 10% within hospitals and schools.[1]
- Ten to thirty percent of hazardous material incidents involve fatalities as a result of traumatic injuries, burns, or respiratory compromise.[2,3]
- Most injuries and deaths are agricultural related and are associated with exposure to chlorine, ammonia, nitrogen fertilizer, or hydrochloric acid.[4]
- Sources for chemical data include regional poison centers, material safety data sheets, transportation-specific markings (Department of Transportation placards, shipping papers, bills of lading), private agencies (Chemtrec), government agencies (Nuclear Regulatory Commission, U.S. Environmental Protection Agency, Centers for Disease Control, Agency for Toxic Substances and Disease Registry, Radiation Emergency Assistance Center/Training Site), and computerized databases (Micromedex, ToxNet).[5]

DECONTAMINATION

- The goal of decontamination is to decrease further exposure to victims and to prevent secondary contamination of health care workers.
- Decontamination is performed in three "zones." The **hot zone** is the area at the scene or outside the hospital where contaminated patients are held and where only immediate life-threatening conditions are addressed.
- The **warm zone** is the area outside (or physically isolated from) the hospital where decontamination occurs along with further stabilization of the patient.
- The **cold zone** is where fully decontaminated victims are transferred. There should be no movement of health care personnel between zones.
- Because of the risk of contamination, access to the hot and warm zones is restricted to personnel with suitable protective clothing. Level A attire (fully encapsulated chemical-resistant suit and self-contained breathing apparatus) is recommended by the Environmental Protection Agency when the concentration or identity of toxins is unknown (most hazardous incidents).[6]
- The minimum personal protection available for hospital personnel caring for contaminated patients is level C: splash protection with chemical-resistant clothing (eg, Tyvek or Saranex) and full-faced, air purifying

canister-equipped respirator. Higher levels of protection are available, but are not generally practical for hospital personnel.[6]

- Triage should occur outside the hospital, where both urgency of care and adequacy of decontamination are assessed.
- Contaminated patients should not be allowed to enter the hospital premises. Personnel without appropriate personal protective gear should not be allowed into the decontamination/triage area.
- Medical stabilization prior to decontamination is limited to opening the airway, cervical spine stabilization, oxygen administration, ventilatory support, and application of direct pressure to arterial bleeding.
- As patients are triaged, decontamination commences in the warm zone by removing all of the victims' clothing and brushing away gross particulate matter. Ocular and wound contamination is initiated by focused irrigation of those sites.
- Whole body irrigation is performed by using copious amounts of water and mild soap or detergent, beginning at the hands and head; this is followed by showering for 3 to 5 minutes.
- A variety of chemicals require special irrigation. Dilute household bleach (1 part to 9 parts water) will inactivate organophosphate pesticides, nerve agents, and most biological agents.
- Water-reactive metals such as sodium, lithium, and potassium should initially be covered with mineral or vegetable oil, removed or brushed off, and then irrigated with water.
- Other water-reactive substances include acetic anhydride, chlorosulfonic acid, dry lime (calcium oxide), hydrides (boranes and silanes), titanium tetrachloride, and organometallics (alkylaluminums, zinc phosphide).
- In the absence of proper decontamination solutions for these agents, especially in critically ill patients, large volumes of water may be considered once the agents are mechanically removed as much as possible.
- White phosphorus ignites in air; burns from it should be kept continuously moist with water or saline dressings.
- Tar burns cannot be readily debrided and usually will benefit from repeated application of Neosporin cream, petroleum jelly, or mayonnaise.
- Vomiting by the contaminated patient may also be a source of secondary contamination. This is especially true for organophosphates.
- Some materials, such as sodium azide, react to produce toxic gases, namely hydrogen cyanide, when combined with stomach acid. Gastric emptying or activated charcoal should be considered early in such ingestions.
- Following decontamination, patients can be wrapped in clean blankets and transferred to the cold zone, where medical assessment and treatment can be completed. The secondary survey can be carried out with the goal of identifying the specific hazardous material toxidrome, which may require a specific antidote.

EMERGENCY DEPARTMENT CARE AND DISPOSITION

INHALED TOXINS

- Inhaled toxins include gases, dusts, fumes, and aerosols, and generally result in either upper airway damage or pulmonary toxicity.
- Agents greater than 10 μm in particle size or highly water-soluble agents are deposited primarily in the upper airway. Water-soluble gases include ammonia, sulfur dioxide, and various acids such as hydrochloric acid. These patients develop symptoms rapidly and complain of mucous membrane irritation accompanied by coughing and wheezing.
- Smaller particles or non–water-soluble agents, like phosgene, ozone, or nitrogen oxides reach deeper into the pulmonary system and tend to inflict delayed effects.
- A gas of intermediate solubility like chlorine gas can cause early upper respiratory irritant symptoms followed by delayed pulmonary edema.
- Systemic toxicity from carbon monoxide and cyanide toxicity should be considered if a history of combustion is present.
- The mainstay of treatment in inhaled toxins is to administer 100% oxygen, consider bronchodilators, and examine the upper airway for signs of compromise. Patients should be intubated early if they develop respiratory distress or airway edema.

NEUROTOXINS

- Hydrocarbon inhalation victims may present with headache, dizziness, confusion, lethargy, and coma.
- Central nervous system (CNS) stimulants (eg, organophosphates or nitrophenols) can cause agitation, seizures, and hyperthermia. Some inhaled agents, such as carbon monoxide, hydrogen sulfide, methanol, certain metals, and pesticides, can cause serious delayed neurotoxic effects.
- Simple asphyxiants (eg, nitrogen, carbon dioxide, or natural gas) can cause dramatic loss of consciousness in an enclosed space. Prior to this, patients may experience headache, dizziness, nausea, or confusion.
- Treatment for neurotoxins is 100% oxygen after removal from the environment.

DERMAL TOXINS

- Solvents and heat exposure may increase the dermal absorption of toxins, particularly organophosphate or organochlorine pesticides.
- Systemic toxicity can result from any of the following agents that can also be readily absorbed through intact skin: acrylamide, acetonitrile, aniline, chlordane, dinitrophenol, hydrogen cyanide, hydrofluoric acid, organic mercury, methyl bromide, nerve agents, nitrobenzene, and phenol.
- Corrosive effects from hazardous materials may be immediately obvious in the case of mineral acids or delayed after alkaline corrosives or hydrofluoric acid.
- Alkaline burns can be particularly problematic because of the deeper penetration associated with liquefaction necrosis, as opposed to the coagulation necrosis seen with acids.
- Another dermal effect from hazardous materials is frostbite from liquid phosphine, phosgene, ammonia, chlorine, hydrogen sulfide, or propane.
- Hydrocarbons further promote the absorption of hazardous material because of their ability to defat in addition to burning.
- Treatment of acid or alkaline burns consists of copious irrigation with pH monitoring of the skin.
- Phenols can cause skin destruction, facilitating its absorption into the circulation. This may lead to CNS depression, intravascular hemolysis, pulmonary edema, and hepatorenal dysfunction.
- Phenol absorption is enhanced by water; however, copious irrigation should obviate this problem. Alternatively, the burn area may be soaked with gauze impregnated with polyethylene glycol.
- Hydrofluoric acid burns also require special therapy with topical, systemic, and intradermal calcium salts.

OCULAR EXPOSURES

- Ocular chemical burns are marked by conjunctival injection, blepharospasm, and clouding of the cornea. The main threat is ulceration and globe perforation.[7]
- Ocular exposures demand emergent irrigation with large volumes of water. In stable patients, immediate prehospital irrigation for up to 20 minutes prior to transport is recommended.
- Gross particulate matter should be brushed away from the eye and contact lenses should be removed.
- Absence of pain may not indicate cessation of ocular damage; irrigation should continue until ocular pH returns to 7.4.

METABOLIC TOXINS

- Hydrogen sulfide is a colorless gas used in industry and encountered in sewage treatment or manure collections. Although it has a distinct "rotten egg" odor, this olfactory warning is lost with extended exposure or high concentrations.
- Hydrogen sulfide causes cellular asphyxia with production of lactate and ensuing metabolic acidosis.
- In high concentrations, rapid loss of consciousness, seizures, and death may occur after a few breaths.
- Survivors may develop pulmonary edema and corneal damage from irritant effects.
- Other similar metabolic poisons are carbon monoxide and hydrogen cyanide.
- After decontamination, the patient may benefit from sodium nitrite administration.

MYOCARDIAL TOXINS

- Certain solvents—Freon and halogenated and aromatic hydrocarbons—can sensitize the myocardium to dysrhythmic effects of catecholamines. Refraining from the use of sympathomimetic drugs may decrease the chance of inducing fatal ventricular tachydysrhythmias.
- In cases of hydrocarbon exposure, if the patient is soaked, countershocking may need to be avoided because of flammability issues.
- Cases of hydrofluoric acid exposure can present with dysrhythmias from hypocalcemia and hypomagnesemia. Intravenous calcium therapy may be life saving.

HEMATOLOGIC TOXINS

- Hemolysis or methemoglobinemia can result from a variety of chemical oxidants, usually from aniline or nitrites.
- Other agents that can induce hemolysis or methemoglobinemia include chlorates, benzene, acetanilide, nitrogen oxides, phenols, nitrophenols, and sulfonamides.

POSTINCIDENT RESPONSE

- Prolonged observation in the emergency department or hospital admission should be considered for exposures to certain hazardous materials. For example, the nitriles can form cyanide; methylene chloride can be metabolized to carbon monoxide; aniline can cause hemolysis; and delayed pulmonary edema can result from cadmium, chlorine, halogenated solvents,

methyl bromide, nitrogen oxides, ozone, paraquat, phosgene, phosphine, and zinc phosphide.
• Ethylene oxide and metals can cause hepatorenal toxicity.
• In many cases, patients require follow-up for symptomatic care as well as counseling for post-traumatic stress and fears of carcinogenic or harmful reproductive side effects. Hepatic and renal tests may reveal delayed toxicity.[8]

REFERENCES

1. National Response Center, 2002.
2. Kales SN, Polyhronpoulos GN, Castrol MJ, et al: Injuries caused by hazardous materials accidents. *Ann Emerg Med* 42:546, 2000.
3. Hall HI, Chara VR, Price-Green PA, et al: Surveillance for emergency events involving hazardous substances: United States, 1990-1992. *MMWR* 43:1, 1994.
4. Burgess JL, Kovalchick DF, Harter L, et al: Hazardous materials events: An industrial comparison. *J Occup Environ Med* 42:546, 2000.
5. Burgess JL, Keifer MC, Barnhart S, et al: Hazardous materials exposure information service: Development, analysis, and medical implications. *Ann Emerg Med* 29:248, 1997.
6. Hick JL, Hanfling D, Burstein JL, et al: Protective equipment for health care facility decontamination personnel: Regulations, risks, and recommendations. *Ann Emerg Med* 42:370, 2003.
7. Saari KM, Leinonen J, Aine E: Management of chemical eye injuries with prolonged irritation. *Acta Ophthalmol Suppl* 161:52, 1984.
8. Burgess JL, Kovalchick DF, Lymp JF, et al: Risk factors for adverse health effects following hazardous materials incidents. *J Occup Environ Med* 39:760, 1997.

For further reading in *Emergency Medicine: A Comprehensive Study Guide,* 6th ed., see Chap. 185, "Hazardous Materials Exposure," by Suzanne R. White and Col. Edward M. Eitzen, Jr.

116 HERBALS AND VITAMINS
Christian A. Tomaszewski

EPIDEMIOLOGY

• Sales of over-the-counter herbal preparations exceeded $1.5 billion in 1997, all without FDA control except for label wording.

• Many of these products can induce significant toxicity, particularly if used in excess. In 2001, there were 5530 vitamin and 7182 dietary supplement exposure patients who sought treatment at health care facilities.[1]
• The biggest threats among dietary supplements are herbal medicines, which were associated with 12 deaths in 2001.[1] The FDA allows herbal medicines to be marketed for intended, but not clinically proven, symptomatic effects.

CLINICAL FEATURES

VITAMINS

VITAMIN A
• The daily recommended doses of vitamin A for adult men and women are 5000 IU and 4000 IU, respectively.
• Hypervitaminosis A usually occurs when children are given excessive amounts of high-potency supplements. Dialysis patients are also at risk for bone resorption with resulting hypercalcemia.
• Patients with vitamin A toxicity may have dry or abnormally pigmented skin, pruritus, and loss of hair.
• Central nervous system complaints can include blurred vision and headache; pseudotumor cerebri may develop.
• Because of storage of vitamin A in the liver, patients may develop hepatomegaly. Hypercalcemia from toxicity can cause ectopic calcifications and bone pain.

VITAMIN D
• Vitamin D is associated with hypercalcemia at doses greater than 1000 IU/kg, although infants may experience toxic effects at 2000 IU.
• Patients may present with anorexia, nausea, abdominal pain, lethargy, weight loss, polyuria, constipation, and confusion. Eventually, high calcium levels can lead to ectopic bone formation and renal failure.

VITAMIN E
• Although nontoxic at daily doses up to 600 IU, higher doses of vitamin E can antagonize vitamin K production. This can be important as a potential cause of bleeding, particularly for patients on anticoagulants.
• Chronic use of large doses of vitamin E can lead to nausea, fatigue, headache, weakness, and blurred vision.

VITAMIN K
• Vitamin K, in spite of being fat soluble, does not tend to accumulate in the body and is readily excreted in the urine.
• At low doses, it is required for maintenance of clotting function; at higher doses, vitamin K_3 (menadione) can

cause hemolytic anemia, kernicterus, and hemoglobin-uria in infants.

- There are rare reports of cardiovascular collapse with rapid intravenous (IV) injection of vitamin K_1 (phytonadione).

VITAMIN B₃

- Vitamin B_3 (niacin) consists of water-soluble nicotinic acid and its active metabolite nicotinamide. Acute ingestion of as little as 100 mg of nicotinic acid can cause "niacin flush," which is characterized by burning, itching, and redness of the face, neck, and chest due to histamine release.
- Higher doses can cause nausea, abdominal cramps, diarrhea, and headache.
- Chronic toxicity from high doses (more than 2000 mg per day) can cause elevated liver enzymes, impaired glucose tolerance, hyperuricemia, and skin dryness and discoloration.

VITAMIN B₆

- Vitamin B_6 (pyridoxine) in chronic high doses can cause a sensory axonal neuropathy. Typically, more than 5 g/day must be taken over several weeks.
- Patients may present with unstable gait and numbness of the feet. This can progress to similar symptoms in the upper extremities accompanied by loss of position and vibratory senses.
- A unique interaction of vitamin B_6 is the inactivation of levodopa, which may pose problems for Parkinson's disease patients.

OTHER WATER-SOLUBLE VITAMINS

- Excessive doses of the water-soluble vitamins B_1 (thiamine), B_2 (riboflavin), B_{12}, biotin, and folic acid do not cause medical problems.
- High doses of vitamin C can precipitate gout and nephrolithiasis in susceptible patients; diarrhea and abdominal cramps also may ensue.

HERBAL AGENTS

- Chaparral, derived from the creosote bush and used for cancer and pain relief, can be hepatotoxic.[2,3] By adding 2 to 4 teaspoons of nutmeg, enterprising individuals may experience hallucinations.
- High doses of chaparral can cause gastrointestinal upset, agitation, miosis, coma, and hypertension.
- Ephedra, used for weight loss, contains ephedrine and can cause sympathomimetic toxicity, particularly in large doses. It has been associated with deaths from stroke, seizures, and cardiac toxicity.[4]
- Yohimbine, an α_2-adrenergic receptor antagonist, can cause sympathomimetic excess, especially when taken with phenylpropanolamine, a decongestant that was taken off the market because of its association with hemorrhagic stroke. Toxic effects include hallucinations, weakness, hypertension, and paralysis.
- Distributed as a European liquor, absinthe (wormwood) contains volatile oils that can cause psychosis, intellectual deterioration, ataxia, headache, and vomiting.[5]
- Black (or blue) cohosh, used to treat menopause, can induce nausea, vomiting, dizziness, and weakness.[5]
- Juniper, used as a diuretic, can cause renal toxicity, nausea, and vomiting.[5]
- Lobelia, used for asthma, can produce anticholinergic syndrome.[5]
- Chamomile and echinacea have been associated with anaphylaxis.
- Garlic, ginkgo, and ginseng all have antithrombotic activity, which may precipitate bleeding in patients on warfarin.
- St. John's wort, in conjunction with other antidepressants, may precipitate serotonin syndrome.

DIAGNOSIS AND DIFFERENTIAL

- Diagnosis of vitamin or herbal toxicity usually is made clinically.

EMERGENCY DEPARTMENT CARE AND DISPOSITION

- Discontinuation of the vitamin, particularly water-soluble ones, or the herbal preparation is usually all that is needed if a patient presents with mild toxicity.
- In vitamin A overdoses, gastric decontamination with activated charcoal 1 g/kg orally is indicated for acute ingestions of more than 300,000 IU in children or 1,000,000 IU in adults.
- Only deliberate massive overdoses of vitamin D, such as 100 or more multivitamin tablets, should be considered for decontamination.
- Hypercalcemia, from either vitamin A or D ingestion, can be treated with IV fluids, prednisone, and furosemide. In addition, lumbar puncture may be useful in pseudotumor cerebri from massive vitamin A ingestion.
- Diphenhydramine 25 to 50 mg IV or orally can be given to patients with "niacin flush" symptoms.
- Administration of N-acetylcysteine, 140 mg/kg orally or IV, should be considered for treating severe hepatotoxicity from herbal preparations such as chaparral or pennroyal oil.

REFERENCES

1. Litovitz TL, Klein-Schwartz W, Rodgers GC, et al: 2001 Annual Report of the American Association of Poison Control Centers Toxic Exposure Surveillance System. *Am J Emerg Med* 20:5, 2002.
2. Perharic L, Shaw D, Murray F: Toxic effects of herbal medicines and food supplements. *Lancet* 342:180, 1993.
3. Anonymous: Chaparral-Induced Toxic Hepatitis—California and Texas, 1992. *MMWR* 41:812, 1992.
4. Shekelle PG, Hardy ML, Morton SC, et al: Efficacy and safety of ephedra and ephedrine for weight loss and athletic performance: a meta-analysis. *JAMA* 289:1537, 2003.
5. Ko RJ: Causes, epidemiology, and clinical evaluation of suspected herbal poisoning. *J Clin Tox* 37:697, 1999.

For further reading in *Emergency Medicine: A Comprehensive Study Guide,* 6th ed., see Chap. 186, "Herbals and Vitamins," by G. Richard Braen.

117 ANTIMICROBIALS

Christian A. Tomaszewski

- In 2001, of the 61,215 exposures to antimicrobials reported to the American Association of Poison Control Centers (AAPCC), there were 365 (0.6%) cases of significant morbidity and 13 fatalities (0.02%).[1]
- Most adverse effects occur at therapeutic doses and include hypersensitivity reactions, alterations in microbial flora, drug interactions, and cutaneous drug interactions.[2,3]

ISONIAZID

EPIDEMIOLOGY

- AAPCC data show that isoniazid (INH) accounts for one fourth of all major morbidity from antibiotic exposures.

PATHOPHYSIOLOGY

- Therapeutic doses (5 mg/kg) can cause neuropathy and hepatic injury.
- In overdose, INH depletes vitamin B_6; this decreases the activity of coenzyme pyridoxal 5-phosphate, which in turn impairs the synthesis of the central neuroinhibitory neurotransmitter gamma-aminobutyric acid (GABA).

CLINICAL FEATURES

- The initial features of INH overdose include nausea, vomiting, and altered mental status.
- Severe signs include seizures, coma, and lactic acidosis. Seizures are usually seen within 1 hour of acute ingestions of more than 30 mg/kg.

DIAGNOSIS AND DIFFERENTIAL

- Generally, the diagnosis of INH overdose is made clinically and should be considered in any patient with refractory seizures.[4]
- A serum INH level can be used for confirmation.
- Acute INH overdose usually presents with an anion gap metabolic acidosis.
- In severe cases with prolonged seizure activity, serial arterial blood gas analysis to follow lactic acidosis and serial creatine phosphokinase (CPK) levels to exclude rhabdomyolysis may be helpful.
- Hepatic profile may be useful in cases of chronic use.

EMERGENCY DEPARTMENT CARE AND DISPOSITION

- In addition to managing seizure activity or coma in the standard approach, the emergency physician should treat the patient with pyridoxine (vitamin B_6) at a dose of 1 gram for every gram of INH ingested. If the amount is unknown, then 5 g (70 mg/kg in children) IV over 30 minutes should be administered.[5] Further doses of 1 g every 2 to 3 minutes can be administered until seizures resolve.[6]
- Most patients will manifest serious symptoms within 2 hours, and can be discharged after 6 hours if they remain asymptomatic.

ANTIMALARIAL DRUGS

EPIDEMIOLOGY

- Although infrequently used, antimalarials are the antimicrobial agents most likely to cause severe toxic effects. The most common antimalarial agents are quinine, chloroquine, mefloquine, and primaquine.

PATHOPHYSIOLOGY

- Use of quinine and chloroquine result in severe central nervous system (CNS) and cardiac abnormalities.

CLINICAL FEATURES

- Quinine and chloroquine can cause headache, altered mental status, and seizures. Both medications can cause prolonged intervals on electrocardiogram (ECG) and hypotension.
- Quinine has the unique property of causing blindness.

DIAGNOSIS AND DIFFERENTIAL

- Quinine should also be considered in the differential diagnosis of hypoglycemia.
- Use of chloroquine can lead to hypokalemia.
- Patients who have overdosed on dapsone, chloroquine, or primaquine may benefit from a methemoglobinemia determination if they are cyanotic or dyspneic.[3]

EMERGENCY DEPARTMENT CARE AND DISPOSITION

- Attention to early intubation, gastric decontamination, and sedation with benzodiazepines may decrease mortality in serious overdoses.[7]
- The pressor of choice for hypotension is epinephrine starting at 0.25 μg/kg/min IV.
- Sodium bicarbonate 50 mEq IV (1 mEq/kg in children) push can be used for prolonged QRS interval, particularly in the face of hypotension.
- Multiple dose activated charcoal may be helpful in overdoses of dapsone and chloroquine.[2,3]
- Any ingestion of more than a daily therapeutic dose, especially in children, warrants at least 6 hours of observation on a cardiac monitor.

PENICILLINS AND THE β-LACTAM AGENTS

PATHOPHYSIOLOGY

- Most overdoses of penicillins and β-lactams are relatively benign.

CLINICAL FEATURES

- High-dose penicillin G, cephalosporins, and imipenem have caused confusion, agitation, myoclonic jerking, and seizures.
- Amoxicillin has been associated with renal failure.

DIAGNOSIS AND DIFFERENTIAL

- CNS toxicity from β-lactams usually only occurs in renal failure patients receiving high doses who have underlying CNS abnormalities.
- Renal function tests and electrolytes may be indicated in large symptomatic overdoses.

EMERGENCY DEPARTMENT CARE AND DISPOSITION

- Seizures should be treated in the standard fashion, starting with lorazepam 2 mg IV or IM (0.05 mg/kg in children).

AMINOGLYCOSIDES

CLINICAL FEATURES

- Because no oral formulations exist, aminoglycoside overdoses are usually iatrogenic and occur in neonates.
- These toxic exposures can result in ototoxicity and nephrotoxicity.

DIAGNOSIS AND DIFFERENTIAL

- The potential for hearing loss is associated with prolonged or high-dose therapy, with neomycin being the worst offender.
- The risk for nephrotoxicity is due to a combination of factors: dose, duration, hydration, and extremes of age.

EMERGENCY DEPARTMENT CARE AND DISPOSITION

- Intravenous hydration (3 to 6 mL/kg/h) with monitoring of renal and hearing function is the main approach to most acute toxic exposures.
- Hemodialysis should only be considered in patients with renal failure.

REFERENCES

1. Litovitz TL, Klein-Schwartz W, Rodgers GC, Cobaugh DJ, et al: 2001 Annual Report of the American Association of Poison Control Centers Toxic Exposure Surveillance System. *Am J Emerg Med* 20:391, 2002.

2. American Academy of Clinical Toxicology; European Association of Poisons Centres and Clinical Toxicologists. Position statement and practice guidelines on the use of multi-dose activated charcoal in the treatment of acute poisoning. *Clin Toxicol* 37:731, 1999.

3. Sin DD, Shafran SD: Dapsone- and primaquine-induced methemoglobinemia in HIV-infected individuals. *J Acquir Immune Defic Syndr Hum Retrovirol* 12:477, 1996.

4. Sullivan EA, Geoffroy P, Weisman R, Hoffman R, Frieden TR: Isoniazid poisonings in New York City. *J Emerg Med* 16:57, 1998.

5. Brent J, Nguyen V, Kulig K, et al: Reversal of prolonged isoniazid-induced coma by pyridoxine. *Arch Intern Med* 150:1751, 1990.

6. Wason S, Lacouture PG, Lovejoy FH: Single high-dose pyridoxine treatment of isoniazid overdose. *JAMA* 246:1102, 1981.

7. Clemessy JL, Taboulet P, Hoffman JR, et al: Treatment of acute chloroquine poisoning: a 5-year experience. *Crit Care Med* 24:1189, 1996.

For further reading in *Emergency Medicine: A Comprehensive Study Guide,* 6th ed., see Chap. 187, "Antimicrobials," by G. Richard Bruno and Wallace A. Carter.

---

118 CYANIDE

Mark E. Hoffmann

EPIDEMIOLOGY

- Cyanide poisonings occur in occupational settings; inadvertent, suicidal, or homicidal ingestions of cyanide or cyanide by-products;[1] ingestion of plant products containing cyanogenic glycosides;[2] inhalation of smoke from burning plastics in closed-space fires;[3–5] and from infusion of nitroprusside.[6]
- Elevated cyanide levels, often associated with elevated carbon monoxide levels, are implicated in fire-related fatalities.[3–5,7]
- Cyanide poisoning in children may result from ingestion of acetonitrile-containing products present in artificial nail remover and other cosmetic solvents.[8]

PATHOPHYSIOLOGY

- Cyanide disrupts oxidative phosphorylation in the production of adenosine triphosphate (ATP) in aero-

bic metabolism by binding to the cytochrome AA3 complex.[9]
- Cyanide forces conversion from aerobic to anaerobic metabolism, resulting in excessive lactate production, an anion gap metabolic acidosis, and tissue hypoxia.
- Sulfurtransferase metabolism to form thiocyanate is critical for detoxification.[10]

CLINICAL FEATURES

- An occupational history, particularly in a suicidal patient, may provide a clue to the possibility of cyanide poisoning.
- Symptoms begin immediately after inhalation of cyanide gas. Ingestion of cyanide salts may cause toxicity within minutes.[11]
- Ingestion of cyanogenic compounds (eg, acetonitrile in nail removal solvents, amygdaline in apricot pits) may take hours to develop symptoms.[1]
- Patients with cyanide toxicity may complain of mucous membrane irritation, anxiety, headache, dyspnea, confusion, seizures, and coma. Early tachycardia, hypertension, and tachypnea are replaced by bradycardia, hypotension, apnea, and asystole.
- Mydriasis, cherry red retinal vessels, oral burns, the smell of bitter almonds, and dyspnea with high venous oxygen saturations are clues to the diagnosis.
- A metabolic acidosis with high lactate levels and a wide anion gap is commonly encountered. The hallmark of cyanide poisoning is apparent hypoxia without cyanosis.[1]

DIAGNOSIS AND DIFFERENTIAL

- The diagnosis of cyanide toxicity should be considered in patients with profound high anion gap metabolic acidosis with a normal partial pressure of arterial oxygen (PaO$_2$).
- The differential diagnosis includes poisonings that accumulate lactate (iron, methemoglobin inducers, methanol, biguanides, strychnine), other cellular toxins or asphyxiants (salicylates, carbon monoxide, hydrogen sulfide, azides, arsine, phosphine, nerve agents, organophosphates), and seizure-inducing agents (cocaine and other stimulants, theophylline, camphor, cicutoxin).

EMERGENCY DEPARTMENT CARE AND DISPOSITION

- All patients with suspected cyanide toxicity should be placed on continuous cardiac monitoring with frequent blood pressure monitoring, 100% oxygen, and have adequate IV access. Airway management and resuscitation should always take priority over decontamination.

- Those with altered mental status must be considered for IV glucose, thiamine, and naloxone administration.
- Decontamination should include copious irrigation of dermal exposures and gastric lavage followed by activated charcoal for acute ingestions.
- Specific antidote therapy with nitrite-thiosulfate in the form of a kit from Taylor Pharmaceuticals should be considered in symptomatic patients (Table 118-1).
- Due to the potential side effects of hypotension and induction of methemoglobinemia, patients who are hypotensive and acidotic and without a clear history of cyanide toxicity or smoke inhalation should receive IV sodium thiosulfate only.[12]
- Hydroxocobalamin, which has orphan drug status in the United States, will be an ideal agent in this setting.[4]
- All patients who receive antidotal therapy or patients who have ingested a substance that may result in delayed toxicity should be admitted to a monitored bed.

TABLE 118-1   Treatment of Cyanide Poisoning

Adults
1. 100% oxygen.
2. Amyl nitrite: crack vial and inhale for 30 seconds.*
3. Sodium nitrite (3% $NaNO_2$): 10 mL IV (10-mL ampule 3% solution = 300 mg).†
4. Sodium thiosulfate (25% $Na_2S_2O_3$): 50 mL IV (50-mL ampule 25% solution = 12.5 g).
5. May repeat at half dose if symptoms persist.

Children
1. 100% oxygen.
2. Administration of IV sodium nitrite and sodium thiosulfate:

Hb (g/dl)	3% $NaNO_2$ (mL/kg)	25% $Na_2S_2O_3$ (mL/kg)
7	0.19	1.65
8	0.22	1.65
9	0.25	1.65
10	0.27	1.65
11	0.30	1.65
12	0.33	1.65
13	0.36	1.65
14	0.39	1.65

3. May repeat once at half dose if symptoms persist.
4. Monitor methemoglobin to keep level less than 30%.

*Not necessary if IV is in place.
†Avoid nitrites in the presence of severe hypotension if diagnosis is unclear.

REFERENCES

1. Borron SW, Baud FJ: Acute cyanide poisoning: Clinical spectrum, diagnosis, and treatment. *Arch Hig Rada Toksikol* 47:307, 1996.
2. Braico KT, Humbert JR, Terplan KL, et al: Laetrile intoxication. *N Engl J Med* 300:238, 1979.
3. Kirk MA, Gerace R, Kulig KW: Cyanide and methemoglobin kinetics in smoke inhalation victims treated with the cyanide antidote kit. *Ann Emerg Med* 22:1413, 1993.
4. Kulig K: Cyanide antidotes and fire toxicity. *N Engl J Med* 325:1801, 1991.
5. Baud FJ, Barriot P, Toffis V, et al: Elevated blood cyanide concentrations in victims of smoke inhalation. *N Engl J Med* 325:1761, 1991.
6. Curry SC, Arnold-Capell P: Toxic effects of drugs used in the ICU: Nitroprusside, nitroglycerin, and angiotensin-converting enzyme inhibitors. *Crit Care Clin* 7:555, 1991.
7. Silverman SH, Purdue GF, Hunt JL, et al: Cyanide toxicity in burned patients. *J Trauma* 28:171, 1998.
8. Losek JD, Rock AL, Boldt RR: Cyanide poisoning from a cosmetic nail remover. *Pediatrics* 88:337, 1991.
9. Baud FJ, Borron SW, Bavoux E, et al: Relation between plasma lactate and blood cyanide concentrations in acute cyanide poisoning. *BMJ* 312:26, 1996.
10. Isom GE, Johnson JD: Sulphur donors in cyanide intoxication,. in Ballantyne B, Marrs TC, (eds.): *Clinical and Experimental Toxicology of Cyanides.* Bristol, England: IOP Publishers, pp. 414-418, 1987.
11. Hall AH, Rumack BH: Clinical toxicology of cyanide. *Ann Emerg Med* 15:1067, 1986.
12. Way JL: Cyanide intoxication and its mechanism of antagonism. *Rev Pharmacol Toxicol* 24:451, 1984.

For further reading in *Emergency Medicine: A Comprehensive Study Guide*, 6th ed., see Chap. 188, "Cyanide," by Larissa Velez and Kathleen Delaney.

119   DYSHEMOGLOBINEMIAS
Howard E. Jarvis III

METHEMOGLOBINEMIA

PATHOPHYSIOLOGY

- Methemoglobinemia is acquired when an oxidant stress, such as a drug or chemical, overwhelms normal mechanisms to eliminate methemoglobin. Hemoglobin becomes structurally altered and can no longer carry oxygen.

- Medications that may precipitate this condition include phenazopyridine (Pyridium), benzocaine (a topical anesthetic), and dapsone (an antibiotic often used in HIV-related therapy). There may be significant time delays from exposure to symptoms with some agents.
- Nitrates (in well water and vegetables) and nitrite salts may cause epidemic methemoglobinemia.[1]
- All age groups are affected but neonates and infants are more susceptible due to an underdeveloped methemoglobin reduction mechanism. Gastroenteritis may precipitate methemoglobinemia in infants.[2]

CLINICAL FEATURES

- The clinical suspicion of methemoglobinemia should be raised when the pulse oximetry approaches 80 to 85% and there is no response to supplemental oxygen. The patient may display brownish-blue skin.
- "Chocolate brown" blood discoloration typically is noted on venipuncture.[3]
- Patients with normal hemoglobin concentrations do not develop clinically significant effects until methemoglobin levels rise above 20% of the total hemoglobin.
- Patients may seek evaluation for cyanosis that occurs when the methemoglobin level approaches 1.5 g/dL; this is approximately 10% of the total hemoglobin in normal individuals.
- Patients with anemia require a higher percentage as it is the absolute concentration (1.5 g/dL) that determines cyanosis.
- When levels reach 20 to 30%, symptoms may include anxiety, headache, weakness, and lightheadedness. Tachypnea and sinus tachycardia may occur.
- Methemoglobin concentrations of 50 to 60% impair oxygen delivery to vital tissues, causing myocardial ischemia, dysrhythmias, depressed mental status (including coma), seizures, and lactic acidosis.
- Levels above 70% are largely incompatible with life.
- Patients with anemia and those with pre-existing diseases that impair oxygen delivery (eg, emphysema, congestive heart failure) may be symptomatic at lower concentrations of methemoglobin.

DIAGNOSIS AND DIFFERENTIAL

- The diagnosis of methemoglobinemia must be considered in any cyanotic patient, especially if the cyanosis is unresponsive to oxygen.
- Pulse oximetry must be interpreted with caution, as it cannot properly differentiate oxyhemoglobin from methemoglobin. Pulse oximetry trends toward 80 to 85% in those with methemoglobinemia, and it will

suggest a falsely high oxygen saturation in those with methemoglobin levels above 20%.[4]
- The oxygen saturation obtained from an arterial blood gas analysis will also be falsely normal, as it is calculated from dissolved oxygen tension, which is appropriately normal.
- Definitive identification of methemoglobin relies on co-oximetry, which is a widely available test and requires only venous blood (although arterial blood can be used). It can differentiate oxyhemoglobin, deoxyhemoglobin, carboxyhemoglobin, and methemoglobin species.

EMERGENCY DEPARTMENT CARE AND DISPOSITION

- Patients with methemoglobinemia require optimal supportive measures to ensure oxygen delivery.
- The effectiveness of gastric decontamination is limited since there is often a substantial time from exposure to development of methemoglobin. If an ongoing source of exposure exists, a single dose of oral activated charcoal 1 g/kg PO is indicated.
- Antidotal therapy with methylene blue is reserved for those with documented methemoglobinemia or a high clinical suspicion of disease. Unstable patients should receive methylene blue, but may require blood transfusion or exchange transfusion for immediate enhancement of oxygen delivery.
- The initial dose of methylene blue is 1 to 2 mg/kg IV and its effect should be seen within 20 minutes. Repeat dosing of methylene blue is acceptable, but high doses (>7 mg/kg) may actually induce methemoglobin formation.
- Treatment failures occur in some patients, including those with glucose-6-phosphate dehydrogenase (G6PD) deficiency[5] and other enzyme deficiencies, and may occur in the presence of hemolysis. Hemolysis is seen with some inducers of methemoglobinemia, such as chlorates.
- Agents with long half-lives, such as dapsone, may require repetitive dosing of methylene blue.
- Patients with methemoglobinemia unresponsive to methylene blue should be treated supportively. If the patient is clinically unstable, the use of blood transfusions or exchange transfusions is indicated. If newly transfused red blood cell hemoglobin undergoes oxidation, it will likely respond to methylene blue therapy.

SULFHEMOGLOBINEMIA

- Sulfhemoglobinemia is caused by many of the same agents that cause methemoglobinemia, though it is clinically less concerning.

- Cyanosis may occur at levels of 0.5 g/dL due to increased pigmentation.
- Sulfhemoglobin is differentiated from methemoglobin by the addition of cyanide to the laboratory cooximetry sample.
- Failure to eliminate the methemoglobin peak with the addition of cyanide confirms the diagnosis of sulfhemoglobinemia.
- Patients with sulfhemoglobinemia do not respond to methylene blue and should be treated supportively. They may require blood transfusions in cases of severe toxicity.

REFERENCES

1. Shih RD, Marcus SM, Genese CA, et al: Methemoglobinemia attributable to nitrite contamination of potable water through boiler fluid additives—New Jersey, 1992 and 1996. *MMWR* 46:202, 1997.
2. Pollack ES, Pollack CV: Incidence of subclinical methemoglobinemia in infants with diarrhea. *Ann Emerg Med* 24:652, 1994.
3. Henretig RM, Gribetz B, Kearney T, et al: Interpretation of color change in blood with varying degree of methemoglobinemia. *J Toxicol Clin Toxicol* 26:293, 1988.
4. Barker SJ, Tremper KK, Hyatt J: Effects of methemoglobinemia on pulse oximetry and mixed venous oximetry. *Anesthesiology* 70:112, 1989.
5. Rosen PJ, Johnson C, McGehee WG: Failure of methylene blue treatment in toxic methemoglobinemia: Association with glucose-6-phosphate dehydrogenase deficiency. *Ann Intern Med* 75:83, 1971.

For further reading in *Emergency Medicine: A Comprehensive Study Guide*, 6th ed., see Chap. 189, "Dyshemoglobinemias," by Sean M. Rees and Lewis S. Nelson.

120   HYPOGLYCEMIC AGENTS

Christian A. Tomaszewski

EPIDEMIOLOGY

- Because diabetes is the most common endocrine disorder, there are numerous poisonings each year from hypoglycemic agents, both intentional and unintentional. In 2001, there were over 1000 symptomatic exposures with almost 30 deaths.[1]
- Although tighter glycemic control delays the onset and progression of microvascular and neurologic complications in patients with type I diabetes, there are at least 61 episodes of hypoglycemia requiring treatment per 100 patient-years.[2]

PATHOPHYSIOLOGY

- Hypoglycemia is the failure to maintain a serum glucose level above 60 mg/dL.
- The initial physiologic response to hypoglycemia is autonomic, with the release of catecholamines and glucagon.
- Chronic ethanol abuse, extremes of age, and medications that blunt counterregulatory mechanisms (eg, β-blockers) all impair the ability to avoid hypoglycemic spells.

CLINICAL FEATURES

- The body's autonomic response to hypoglycemia consists of diaphoresis, anxiety, nausea, tremors, and palpitations.
- The organ most dependent on a constant supply of glucose is the brain. Neurologic symptoms and signs of hypoglycemia include dizziness, confusion, headache, diplopia, dysarthria, lethargy, coma, and seizures.[3]
- Patients also may present with focal neurologic deficits as profound as hemiparesis.
- The only parenteral hypoglycemic agent, and the most commonly involved with severe symptomatic hypoglycemia, is insulin.
- The duration of action of insulin is usually based on the form taken; however, a large subcutaneous injection of regular insulin may behave like a long-acting formulation, thus resulting in delayed or prolonged hypoglycemia.
- The most common oral agents for diabetes are the sulfonylureas; as a result, they are most often implicated in hypoglycemia cases. These agents cause the release of insulin from the pancreas, reduce hepatic glucose production, and increase peripheral insulin sensitivity.
- Second-generation sulfonylureas have supplanted the first-generation agents primarily because they are not solely dependent on renal elimination. Nonetheless, they have a long duration of action, particularly after overdose, which can lead to delayed hypoglycemia as late as 16 hours after ingestion.[4]
- More popular agents for initial control of diabetes are the biguanides, represented by metformin. It suppresses glucose output by the liver while stimulating its uptake by muscle.
- Although metformin does not specifically cause hypoglycemia, it can increase this risk in patients on concomitant sulfonylureas or insulin.
- The more serious adverse effect of metformin is lactic

acidosis, which is partly due to inhibition of gluconeogenesis. It can occur after overdose, but more commonly is associated with renal insufficiency or the administration of intravascular iodinated contrast media.[5]

- Thiazolidinediones are becoming as popular as sulfonylureas because of their ability to ameliorate hyperglycemia without increasing insulin secretion.
- In addition to increasing insulin sensitivity, thiazolidinediones decrease hepatic glucose output and increase muscle glucose uptake. Hepatically metabolized, there have been rare cases of liver failure associated with these agents.
- The benzoic acid derivative repaglinide increases insulin secretion. Like sulfonylureas, the risk of developing hypoglycemia exists even though overdose experience is lacking.
- Another group of diabetic agents that have not been associated with hypoglycemia are the α-glucosidase inhibitor agents. Acarbose, miglitol, and voglibose all decrease gastrointestinal absorption of carbohydrates.
- Adverse effects of α-glucosidase inhibitors include flatulence, bloating, and malabsorption; rare cases of hepatic toxicity have occurred with acarbose.

DIAGNOSIS AND DIFFERENTIAL

- Hypoglycemia should be considered in all patients with altered mental status. In addition, all patients with stroke-like symptoms, seizures, or hypothermia should be screened.
- Rapid glucose determination can be done with a reagent strip or glucometer at the bedside, with confirmation by formal laboratory testing if hypoglycemia is still suspected.
- Angiotensin-converting enzyme inhibitors, chloramphenicol, disopyramide, pentamidine, salicylates, quinidine, and streptozocin have been implicated with patients experiencing hypoglycemic episodes.
- Ethanol, especially in the presence of malnutrition, can induce hypoglycemia.
- Medical causes of hypoglycemia include insulinoma, endocrine insufficiency, hepatic disease, sepsis, and autoimmune disease.

EMERGENCY DEPARTMENT CARE AND DISPOSITION

- Once hypoglycemia is suspected or determined, a 50-mL IV bolus of dextrose 50% solution should be given. Children may receive dextrose 25% at 2 mL/kg, and neonates dextrose 10% at 2 mL/kg.
- A repeat glucose determination should be performed every 30 to 60 minutes after the initial dextrose administration.
- If hypoglycemia recurs or is expected to recur, then the patient can be rebolused with 50 mL IV of dextrose 50% solution or started on a continuous infusion of $D_{10}W$ at 1 to 2 mL/kg/h.
- If IV access cannot be established, glucagon 1 to 2 mg IM or SQ (0.1 mg/kg in children, up to 2 mg) can be administered. Glucagon will not work well in patients with depleted glycogen stores or after sulfonylurea toxicity.
- Diazoxide, 300 mg IV, has been used successfully in sulfonylurea overdose. Because it can cause hypotension and does not work well in insulin overdoses, its use is limited.[6]
- In cases of sulfonylurea overdose with extreme glucose requirements, octreotide 50 μg SQ every 6 hours can be used.[7]
- Gastric decontamination with activated charcoal, 1 g/kg PO, may be indicated early after oral overdoses of hypoglycemic agents.
- Whole bowel irrigation with polyethylene glycol based electrolyte solutions may benefit massive overdoses of sustained-release preparations.
- Urine alkalinization will increase the clearance of chlorpropamide.[8]
- Thiamine, 100 mg IV, may be warranted when administering glucose to patients who are hypoglycemic secondary to ethanol abuse or malnutrition.
- Metformin overdoses should be monitored for lactic acidosis. Aggressive treatment of acidosis should be instituted with sodium bicarbonate therapy, while reserving hemodialysis for refractory cases.
- Patients with unintentional hypoglycemia from a short- or intermediate-acting insulin can be discharged after several hours of observation, particularly if they have eaten, have not had a recurrence of hypoglycemia, and have a reliable individual who lives with them.
- Because of their long duration of action, patients with symptomatic overdoses of sulfonylureas should be admitted for regular glucose monitoring. This includes patients with an episode of hypoglycemia from a therapeutic dose of their sulfonylurea agent.
- Asymptomatic patients should be observed for at least 12 to 16 hours after an overdose, depending on the particular sulfonylurea they have taken, because of the danger of delayed hypoglycemia.

REFERENCES

1. Litovitz TL, Klein-Scwartz W, Rodgers GC, et al: 2001 Annual Report of the American Association of Poison Control Centers toxic exposure surveillance system. *Am J Emerg Med* 20:5, 2002.
2. Diabetic Control and Complications Trial Research Group: Hypoglycemic Control in the Diabetes Control and Complications Trial. *Diabetes* 46:271, 1997.

3. Service FJ: Hypoglycemic disorders. *N Engl J Med* 332:1144, 1995.

4. Spiller HA, Villalobos D, Krenzelok EP, et al: Prospective multicenter study of sulfonylurea ingestion in children. *J Pediatr* 131:141, 1997.

5. Stang MR, Wysowski DK, Butler-Jones D: Incidence of lactic acidosis in metformin users. *Diabetes Care* 22:925, 1999.

6. Palatnick W, Meatherall RC, Tenenbein M: Clinical spectrum of sulfonylurea overdose and experience with diazoxide therapy. *Arch Intern Med* 151:1859, 1991.

7. McLaughlin SA, Crandall CS, McKinney PE: Octreotide: An antidote for sulfonylurea-induced hypoglycemia. *Ann Emerg Med* 36:133, 2000.

8. Neuvonen PJ, Karkkainen S: Effects of charcoal, sodium bicarbonate, and ammonium chloride on chlorpropamide kinetics. *Clin Pharmacol Ther* 33:386, 1983.

For further reading in *Emergency Medicine: A Comprehensive Study Guide,* 6th ed., see Chap. 190, "Hypoglycemic Agents," by Joseph G. Rella and Lewis S. Nelson.

121 FROSTBITE AND HYPOTHERMIA

Mark E. Hoffmann

EPIDEMIOLOGY

- In the United States, more than 700 people die from hypothermia each year; one-half of those who die are older than 65 years.[1]
- People at the extremes of age are at risk for developing hypothermia.
- Alcohol and drug-intoxicated persons, along with psychiatric patients, account for the majority of frostbite cases in the United States.[2]

PATHOPHYSIOLOGY

- Body temperature falls as a result of heat loss by conduction, convection, radiation, or evaporation.
- Heat conservation is controlled by the hypothalamus. Heat is conserved by shivering, peripheral vasoconstriction, and behavioral responses (ie, dressing appropriately and seeking shelter).
- Exposure to cold environments, depressed metabolic rate, central nervous system (CNS) dysfunction, sepsis, dermal disease, and drug use can lead to hypothermia.
- The initial excitatory response to hypothermia consists of a rise in heart rate, blood pressure, and cardiac output, and vasoconstriction with shivering.
- Hypothermia impairs platelet function. It also produces a leftward shift of the oxyhemoglobin dissociation curve, which results in impaired oxygen release to the tissues.

- Local cold injury and frostbite occur when hypothermia causes increased blood viscosity, extracellular ice crystal formation, intracellular dehydration, and lysis. This occurs when freezing temperatures are reached.[3,4]

CLINICAL FEATURES

- Mild hypothermia, 32°C (89.6°F) to 35°C (95°F), presents with shivering, tachycardia, and elevated blood pressure.
- Shivering ceases as both heart rate and blood pressure fall when core temperatures drop below 32°C (89.6°F). Mentation slows and there is a loss of cough and gag reflexes. Aspiration is a common complication.
- Hypothermia impairs renal concentrating ability and leads to a "cold diuresis" that may result in dehydration.
- With progressively lower core temperatures, patients become lethargic and comatose.
- Prolonged immobility increases the risk of rhabdomyolysis and acute renal failure.
- Hemoconcentration and volume depletion may lead to intravascular thrombosis and disseminated intravascular coagulation.
- Hyperglycemia is common; however, up to 40% of patients are hypoglycemic. Acid-base disturbances are usually present but do not follow a uniform pattern.
- The electrocardiogram (ECG) may show PR-, QRS-, and QT-interval prolongations and Osborn J waves.
- The cardiac rhythm progresses from tachycardia to bradycardia to atrial fibrillation with a slow ventricular rate to ventricular fibrillation and finally to asystole, as the core temperature falls.
- First-degree and second-degree frostbite are superficial injuries that present with edema, burning, and erythema; blistering is present in second-degree frostbite (Table 121-1).

TABLE 121-1 Classification of Cold Injury According to Severity

CLASSIFICATION	SYMPTOMS
SUPERFICIAL	
First degree: partial skin freezing Erythema, edema, hyperemia No blisters or necrosis Occasional skin desquamation (5–10 d later)	Transient stinging and burning Throbbing and aching possible May have hyperhidrosis
Second degree: full-thickness injury Erythema, substantial edema, vesicles with clear fluid Blisters that desquamate and form blackened eschar	Numbness Vasomotor disturbances in severe cases
DEEP	
Third degree: full-thickness skin and subcutaneous freezing Violaceous or hemorrhagic blisters Skin necrosis Blue-gray discoloration	Initially, no sensation Tissue feels like "block of wood" Later, shooting pains, burning, throbbing, aching
Fourth degree: full-thickness skin, subcutaneous tissue, muscle, tendon, and bone freezing Little edema Initially mottled, deep red, or cyanotic Eventually dry, black, mummified	Possible joint discomfort

SOURCE: From Britt LD et al[8] with permission.

- Third-degree injury is characterized by freezing damage that involves the deeper subdermal plexus. Hemorrhagic blisters, necrosis, and blue-gray discoloration of the involved extremity are common.
- Fourth-degree injury is characterized by deep injuries involving the subcutaneous tissue, muscle, tendon, and bone. There is little edema. Patients present with cyanotic insensate tissue that may have hemorrhagic blisters and skin necrosis that later appears mummified.[5]
- Frostnip is a less severe form of frostbite that resolves with rewarming and involves no tissue loss.
- Trench foot results from cooling of tissue in a wet environment at above-freezing temperatures over several hours to days. Long-term hyperhidrosis and cold insensitivity are common.
- Chilblains (pernio) presents with painful and inflamed skin lesions caused by chronic, intermittent exposure to damp, nonfreezing ambient temperatures.[6] Once affected by chilblains, frostnip, or frostbite, the involved body part becomes more susceptible to reinjury.

DIAGNOSIS AND DIFFERENTIAL

- Hypothermia is diagnosed when the core body temperature is below 35°C (95°F).

- Other underlying disease states that may result in hypothermia include thyroid deficiency, adrenal insufficiency, CNS dysfunction, infection, sepsis, dermal disease, drug intoxication, and metabolic derangements.

EMERGENCY DEPARTMENT CARE AND DISPOSITION

- Chilblains and trench foot should be managed with elevation, warming, and bandaging of the affected tissues. Nifedipine 20 mg PO tid, topical corticosteroids, prednisone, and prostaglandin E_1 (limaprost 20 μg PO tid) may be helpful.[7]
- Rapid rewarming with circulating water at 42°C (107°F) for 10 to 30 minutes results in thawing of frostbitten extremities.
- Dry air rewarming may cause further tissue injury and should be avoided.
- Patients should receive narcotics, ibuprofen, and aloe vera. Penicillin G 500,000 units every 6 hours for 48 to 72 hours has been shown to be beneficial.[8]
- Clear blisters rich in prostaglandins and thromboxane should be debrided or aspirated. Hemorrhagic blisters should be left intact.
- Rewarming techniques include passive rewarming, active external rewarming, and active core rewarming (Table 121-2).
- Patients with mild hypothermia may be warmed passively by removal from the cold environment and with the use of insulating blankets.
- Patients with more severe hypothermia should be placed on pulse oximetry, cardiac monitor, and continued core temperature monitoring (rectal or esophageal probe).
- Attention should be placed on the ABCs and initial resuscitation. If there is no cardiovascular instability,

TABLE 121-2 Rewarming Techniques

Passive rewarming:
  Removal from cold environment
  Insulation

Active external rewarming:
  Warm water immersion
  Heating blankets set at 40°C
  Radiant heat
  Forced air

Active core rewarming at 40°C:
  Inhalation rewarming
  Heated IV fluids
  GI tract lavage
  Bladder lavage
  Peritoneal lavage
  Pleural lavage
  Extracorporeal rewarming
  Mediastinal lavage via thoracotomy

active external warming may be applied (radiant heat, warmed blankets, warm water immersion, and heated objects) in conjunction with warmed IV fluids and warmed humidified oxygen.

- If cardiovascular instability is present, more aggressive active core rewarming is required (gastric, bladder, peritoneal, and pleural lavage). These lavage fluids should be heated to 42°C (107°F).[9]
- Patients with suspected thiamine depletion and alcoholism should receive thiamine 100 mg IV or IM and 50% glucose 50 to 100 mL IV if rapid glucose testing is not available or if glucose is low.
- Patients with suspected hypothyroidism or adrenal insufficiency may require IV thyroxine and hydrocortisone (100 mg).
- Ventricular fibrillation is usually refractory to defibrillation until a temperature of 30°C (86°F) is obtained, although three countershocks should be attempted.
- Rewarming through an extracorporeal circuit is the method of choice in the severely hypothermic patient in cardiac arrest.[10] If this equipment is not available, resuscitative thoracotomy with internal cardiac message and mediastinal lavage is an acceptable alternative.
- All patients with more than isolated superficial frostbite or mild hypothermia should be admitted to the hospital. A patient should not be discharged unless they can return to a warm environment.

REFERENCES

1. Centers for Disease Control and Prevention: Hypothermia-related deaths—Georgia, January 1996–December 1997, and United States, 1979–1995. *MMWR* 47:1037, 1998.
2. Smith DJ, Robson MC, Heggers JP: Frostbite and other cold-related injuries, in Auerbach PS, Geehr EC (eds): *Management of Wilderness and Environmental Injuries,* 3rd ed. St Louis: Mosby, 1995, p. 129.
3. Vogel EJ, Dellon AL: Frostbite injuries of the hand. *Clin Plast Surg* 16:565, 1989.
4. Jackson D: The diagnosis of the depth of burning. *Br J Surg* 40:588, 1953.
5. Heggers JP, Robson MC, Manaualen K, et al: Experimental and clinical observations on frostbite. *Ann Emerg Med* 16:1056, 1987.
6. Carruther R: Chilblains (pernosis). *Aust Fam Physician* 17:968, 1988.
7. Saito S, Shimada H: Effect of prostaglandin E₁ analogue administration on peripheral skin temperature at high altitude. *Angiology* 45:455, 1994.
8. Britt LD, Dacombe W, Rodriquez A: Frostbite treatment summary. *Surg Clin North Am* 71:359, 1991.
9. Otto RJ, Metzler MH: Rewarming from experimental hypothermia: Comparison of heated aerosol inhalation, peritoneal lavage, and pleural lavage. *Crit Care Med* 16:869, 1988.
10. Lazar HL: The treatment of hypothermia. *N Engl J Med* 337:1545, 1997.

For further reading in *Emergency Medicine: A Comprehensive Study Guide,* 6th ed., see Chap. 191, "Frostbite and Other Localized Cold-Related Injuries," by Mark B. Rabold; and Chap. 192, "Hypothermia," by Howard A. Bessen.

122 HEAT EMERGENCIES

T. Paul Tran

EPIDEMIOLOGY

- Heat-related illnesses cause approximately 400 deaths annually in the U.S.[1]
- Risks for heat-related deaths are highest among children and the elderly, those with predisposing medical conditions, and those on medications that interfere with the thermoregulatory response.[1,2]
- Heat-related illnesses and deaths are preventable and are closely correlated with high environmental temperature and urban heat waves, which are defined as three or more consecutive days with ambient temperatures >32.2°C.[3]

PATHOPHYSIOLOGY

- Body heat generated by metabolism and heat gained from the hot environment must be dissipated to maintain body temperature at or near 37°C.
- Externally, body heat is thermodynamically dissipated through radiation, convection, evaporation, and conduction.
- While radiation is the primary mechanism for heat loss in a cold environment (accounting for 65% of total heat loss), evaporation becomes the primary mechanism for heat dissipation in a hot environment.[3]
- Internally, thermoregulatory homeostasis is accomplished via the body's thermoregulatory response, acute phase response, and heat shock protein response.[3,4]
- Upon exposure to heat stress, cardiac output is augmented, core blood circulation is shifted to the peripheral circulation, vasodilatation occurs, and thermal sweating is enhanced.
- Several inflammatory cytokines and heat shock proteins are released to improve tissue repair and protect against tissue injury and protein denaturation.

- Heat stroke is a life-threatening injury characterized by hyperthermia and central nervous system (CNS) dysfunction.[3] It is the result of interplay among thermoregulatory response failure, exaggerated acute phase response, and altered heat shock protein response.
- The end result of heat stroke is endothelial injury, coagulation disorder, microcirculatory failure, and ultimately multiorgan failure.

CLINICAL FEATURES

- Patients with heat stroke have an alteration in mental status and an elevated body temperature. A history of environmental or occupational heat exposure can usually be discerned.
- Core temperature ranges from 40° to 47°C.
- Neurologic abnormalities include ataxia, confusion, bizarre behavior, agitation, seizures, obtundation, and coma. Anhidrosis is not invariably present.
- Risk factors for heat-related injuries include extremes of age (<4 years and >75 years), predisposing conditions (heart failure, psychiatric illnesses, alcohol abuse, dehydration, poverty, social isolation), certain medications (anticholinergics, β-blockers, calcium channel blockers), and persons who lack access to air conditioning, have poor physical conditioning, and are poorly acclimatized to hot weather.

DIAGNOSIS AND DIFFERENTIAL

- Heat stroke is a true time-dependent medical emergency and should be considered in the clinical context of environmental heat stress, hyperthermia, and altered mental status.
- Patients are tachycardic, hyperventilating, and have respiratory alkalosis.
- About 20% of heat stroke patients are hypotensive.[3]
- In contrast to classic heat stroke, patients with exertional heat stroke may have both respiratory alkalosis and lactic acidosis.
- Exertional heat stroke patients may present with rhabdomyolysis, hyperkalemia, hyperphosphatemia, and hypocalcemia.
- Neuroimaging studies and other evaluation (eg, septic work-up) can be individualized as clinically indicated.
- The differential diagnosis includes infection (sepsis, meningitis, encephalitis, malaria, typhoid fever), toxins (serotonin syndrome, anticholinergics, phenothiazine, salicylate, PCP, sympathomimetic abuse, alcohol withdrawal), metabolic and endocrinologic emergencies (thyrotoxicosis, diabetic ketoacidosis), CNS disorders (status epilepticus, stroke syndrome), neuroleptic malignant syndrome, and malignant hyperthermia.[5-7]

EMERGENCY DEPARTMENT CARE AND DISPOSITION

- Emergent priorities remain airway, breathing, and circulation. Cardiac monitoring and an IV line should be established.
- High flow supplemental oxygen should be administered. Patients with significantly altered mental status, diminished gag reflex, or hypoxia should undergo endotracheal intubation.
- Core temperature should immediately be obtained with a rectal (or bladder) probe and continuously monitored.
- Volume-depleted patients should be rehydrated with IV normal saline or lactated Ringer's solution to maintain mean arterial pressure >60 mm Hg. Care should be exercised not to volume overload the patient.
- A central venous catheter line or pulmonary artery catheter may be required to guide fluid therapy. Inotropic support and pressors may be required.
- Evaporative cooling is the most efficient and practical means of cooling hyperthermic patients in the emergency department (ED). Fans are positioned near the completely disrobed patient, who is then sprayed with tepid water.
- Spraying with ice water should be avoided since this may cause shivering, which induces thermogenesis.
- Excessive shivering can be treated with benzodiazepines (midazolam 2 mg IV). The goal is to bring the core temperature below 40°C.
- Other methods of cooling such as immersion cooling, cold water gastric and urinary bladder lavage, thoracostomy lavage, and cardiopulmonary bypass may be considered as clinically indicated and logistically feasible.
- Seizures can be treated with benzodiazepines.
- Rhabdomyolysis can be treated with IV hydration, diuretics (furosemide 40 mg IV), sodium bicarbonate (3 ampules in 1 liter of D_5W at 250 mL/h).
- Hyperkalemia should be treated with standard regimens. The patient's electrolytes should be monitored every hour initially.
- Heat stroke patients need to be admitted to an intensive care unit for further observation and monitoring.

OTHER HEAT ILLNESSES

HEAT EXHAUSTION

- Heat exhaustion is a clinical syndrome that results from heat exposure.
- It is characterized by nonspecific signs and symptoms, including malaise, fatigue, weakness, dizziness, syncope, headache, nausea, vomiting, myalgias,

diaphoresis, tachypnea, tachycardia, and orthostatic hypotension.

- Core body temperature is frequently elevated, but may be normal.
- Although patients may complain of neurologic symptoms, the patient's sensorium and neurologic examination should be normal.
- Laboratory examination usually demonstrates hemoconcentration. A creatinine kinase level should be checked to exclude rhabdomyolysis.
- Treatment consists of rest, evaporative cooling, and administration of IV normal saline or oral electrolyte solution, depending upon the clinical situation.
- Since heat exhaustion has the potential to evolve into heat stroke, patients should be aggressively treated and observed until symptoms resolve.
- The majority of patients can be discharged home. Those patients with significant comorbid conditions (heart failure, poor social support) or severe electrolyte abnormality may require hospitalization.

HEAT SYNCOPE

- Heat syncope results from volume depletion, peripheral vasodilation, and decreased vasomotor tone.
- It occurs most commonly in the elderly and poorly acclimatized individuals.
- Postural vital signs may or may not be demonstrable on presentation to the ED.
- Patients should be evaluated for any trauma resulting from a fall.
- Potentially serious causes of syncope (eg, cardiovascular, neurologic, infectious, endocrine, and electrolyte abnormalities) should be investigated, especially in the elderly.
- Treatment for heat syncope consists of rest and oral or IV rehydration.

HEAT CRAMPS

- Heat cramps are characterized by painful muscle spasms, especially in the calves, thighs, and shoulders.
- Common during athletic events, they are thought to result from dilutional hyponatremia as individuals replace evaporative losses with free water but not salt.
- Core body temperature may be normal or elevated.
- Treatment consists of rest and administration of oral electrolyte solution or IV normal saline. Patients should be instructed to replace future fluid losses with a balanced electrolyte solution.

HEAT TETANY

- Heat tetany is due to the effects of respiratory alkalosis that result when an individual hyperventilates in response to an intense heat stress.
- Patients may complain of paresthesia of the extremities, circumoral paresthesia, and carpopedal spasm. Muscle cramps are minimal or nonexistent.
- Treatment consists of removal from the heat stress and self-rebreathing through a paper bag.

HEAT EDEMA

- Heat edema is a self-limited, mild swelling of dependent extremities (hands and feet) that occurs in the first few days of exposure to a new hot environment.
- It is due to cutaneous vasodilation and pooling of interstitial fluid in dependent extremities.
- Treatment consists of elevation of the extremities, and in severe cases, application of compressive stockings. Administration of diuretics may exacerbate volume depletion and should be avoided.

HEAT RASH

- Heat rash (prickly heat) is a maculopapular eruption that is most commonly found over clothed areas of the body.
- It results from inflammation and obstruction of sweat ducts.
- Early stages present with a pruritic, erythematous rash best treated with antihistamines and chlorhexidine cream or lotion.
- Continued blockage of pores results in a nonpruritic, nonerythematous, whitish papular rash known as the profunda stage of prickly heat.
- This is best treated with antistaphylococcal antibiotics and application of 1% salicylic acid to affected areas tid.

REFERENCES

1. Centers for Disease Control and Prevention: Heat-related deaths—Four states, July-August 2000, and United States, 1979-1999. *MMWR* 61:567, 2002.
2. Wexler RK: Evaluation and treatment of heat-related illnesses. *Am Fam Physician* 65:2307, 2002.
3. Bouchama A, Knochel JP: Heat stroke. *N Engl J Med* 346: 1978, 2002.
4. Mackowiak PA: Concepts of fever. *Arch Intern Med* 158:1870, 1998.

5. Lappin RI, Auchincloss EL: Treatment of the serotonin syndrome with cyproheptadine. *N Engl J Med* 331:1021, 1994.

6. Martinez M, Devenport L, Saussy J: Drug-associated heat stroke. *South Med J* 95:799, 2002.

7. Marzuk PM, Tardiff K, Leon AC, et al: Ambient temperature and mortality from unintentional cocaine overdose. *JAMA* 279: 1795, 1998.

For further reading in *Emergency Medicine: A Comprehensive Study Guide*, 6th ed., see Chap. 193, "Heat Emergencies," by James S. Walker and David E. Hogan.

123 BITES AND STINGS

Burton Bentley II

HYMENOPTERA

CLINICAL FEATURES

- Wasps, bees, and stinging ants are members of the order Hymenoptera. Both local and generalized reactions may occur in response to an encounter.
- Most of the allergic reactions reported each year from Hymenoptera occur from Vespidae (wasp, hornet, and yellow jacket) stings.
- The most common response to Hymenoptera venom is pain, slight erythema, edema, and pruritus at the sting site. Although it may involve neighboring joints, local reactions cause no systemic symptoms.
- Severe local reactions increase the likelihood of serious systemic reactions if the patient is exposed again at a later time.
- Toxic reactions are a nonantigenic response to multiple stings. They have many of the same features that are seen in true systemic (allergic) reactions, but there is a greater frequency of gastrointestinal (GI) disturbances, while bronchospasm and urticaria do not occur.
- Systemic or anaphylactic reactions are true allergic reactions that range from mild to fatal. In general, the shorter the interval between the sting and the onset of symptoms, the more severe the reaction.
- Initial symptoms of anaphylactic reactions usually consist of itchy eyes, urticaria, and cough. As the reaction progresses, patients may experience respiratory failure and cardiovascular collapse.

- The majority of anaphylactic reactions occur within the first 15 minutes and nearly all occur within 6 hours. There is no correlation between a systemic reaction and the number of stings.
- Delayed reactions may appear 10 to 14 days after a sting. Symptoms of delayed reactions resemble serum sickness and include fever, malaise, headache, urticaria, lymphadenopathy, and polyarthritis.

EMERGENCY DEPARTMENT CARE AND DISPOSITION

- The treatment of all Hymenoptera encounters is the same. Any bee stinger remaining in the patient must be removed immediately and the wound should be cleansed.
- Erythema and swelling seen in local reactions may be difficult to distinguish from cellulitis. As a general rule, infection is present in a minority of cases.
- For minor local reactions, oral antihistamines and analgesics may be the only treatment needed.
- Severe reactions require treatment with 1:1000 epinephrine subcutaneously (SC); 0.3 mL to 0.5 mL for an adult and 0.01 mL/kg for a child (0.3 mL maximum). Some patients may require a second epinephrine injection in 10 to 15 minutes.
- Parenteral H_1- and H_2-receptor antagonists (eg, diphenhydramine and ranitidine) and steroids (eg, methylprednisolone) should be rapidly administered.
- Bronchospasm responds to courses of inhaled β-agonists (eg, albuterol).
- Hypotension should be treated aggressively with crystalloid, although dopamine and epinephrine infusions may be required.
- Patients with minor symptoms who respond well to conservative measures may be discharged after monitoring for several hours. Severe reactions require admission to the hospital.
- All patients with Hymenoptera reactions should be referred to an allergist for further evaluation and prescribed a premeasured epinephrine injector (EpiPen).

ANTS (FORMICIDAE)

- The fire ant sting results in a papule that evolves to a sterile pustule over 6 to 24 hours. Local necrosis, scarring, and systemic reactions may also occur.
- Treatment is the same as for Hymenoptera stings; appropriate referral should be made for desensitization therapy.

ARACHNIDS (SPIDERS, SCABIES, CHIGGERS, AND SCORPIONS)

BROWN RECLUSE SPIDERS (*LOXOSCELES RECLUSA*)

CLINICAL FEATURES
- The bite of the brown recluse causes a mildly erythematous lesion that may become firm and heal over several days to weeks. Occasionally, a severe reaction with immediate pain, blister formation, and bluish discoloration may occur.
- These lesions often become necrotic over the next 3 to 4 days and form an eschar from 1 to 30 cm in diameter.
- Loxoscelism is a systemic reaction that may occur 1 to 2 days after envenomation. Signs and symptoms may include fever, chills, vomiting, arthralgias, myalgias, petechiae, and hemolysis; severe cases progress to seizure, renal failure, disseminated intravascular coagulation (DIC), and death.[1]
- The diagnosis of *L. reclusa* envenomation may need to be made on clinical grounds since the bite is often unwitnessed.

EMERGENCY DEPARTMENT CARE AND DISPOSITION
- Treatment of the brown recluse spider bite includes the usual supportive measures. Currently, there is no commercially available antivenin. Tetanus prophylaxis, analgesics, and antibiotics may be offered when appropriate.
- Surgery is reserved for lesions greater than 2 cm in size and is deferred for 2 to 3 weeks following the bite.
- The role of dapsone (50 to 200 mg per day) and hyperbaric oxygen has recently been challenged, but these may prevent some ongoing local necrosis.
- Patients with systemic reactions and hemolysis must be hospitalized for consideration of blood transfusion and hemodialysis.

HOBO SPIDERS (*TEGENARIA AGRESTIS*)

- The hobo spider bite causes clinical signs and symptoms that are quite similar to those of the brown recluse spider bite.
- The skin site is initially painless before developing induration, erythema, blistering, and necrosis. Victims also may experience headache, vomiting, and fatigue.
- There is no specific diagnostic test or therapeutic intervention for hobo spider bites. Surgical repair may be required, though it must be delayed until the necrotizing process is complete.

BLACK WIDOW SPIDERS

CLINICAL FEATURES
- Black widow spider bites induce an immediate pinprick sensation that often allows the victim to identify the offending spider.
- Within 1 hour, the patient may experience erythematous skin lesions (often target-shaped), swelling, and diffuse muscle cramps.
- Large muscle groups are involved, resulting in painful cramping of the abdominal wall musculature that may mimic peritonitis. Severe pain may wax and wane for up to 3 days, but muscle weakness and spasm can persist for weeks to months.[2]
- Serious acute complications include hypertension, respiratory failure, shock, and coma.

EMERGENCY DEPARTMENT CARE AND DISPOSITION
- Initial therapy includes local wound treatment and supportive care. Analgesics and benzodiazepines will relieve pain and cramping.
- For severe envenomations, hospitalization is required for parenteral pain medication and antivenin therapy.
- The antivenin, derived from horse serum, is rapidly effective for severe envenomation. If the patient tolerates placement of a standard cutaneous test dose, the usual IV dose is 1 to 2 diluted vials delivered over 30 minutes.[3]

TARANTULAS

- When threatened, tarantulas may flick barbed hairs into their victim. These hairs can embed deeply into the conjunctiva and cornea and result in a local or generalized ocular inflammatory response.
- Tarantulas may also render a painful bite, resulting in erythema, swelling, and local joint stiffness.
- Any patient complaining of ocular symptoms after exposure to a tarantula should undergo a thorough slitlamp examination.
- Treatment includes topical steroids and consultation with an ophthalmologist for surgical removal of the hairs.
- The tarantula bite only requires local wound care and appropriate analgesia.

SCORPIONS

CLINICAL FEATURES
- Of all North American scorpions, only the bark scorpion (*Centruroides exilicauda*) of the western United States is capable of producing systemic toxicity.

- *C exilicauda* venom causes immediate burning and stinging although no local injury is visible. Systemic effects are infrequent, and mainly occur at the extremes of patient age.
- Findings may include tachycardia, excessive secretions, roving eye movements, opisthotonos, and fasciculations.
- The diagnosis may be elusive if the scorpion is not seen. Roving eye movements are pathognomonic. A positive "tap test" (ie, exquisite local tenderness when the area is lightly tapped) is also suggestive.

EMERGENCY DEPARTMENT CARE AND DISPOSITION
- Treatment includes local wound care and reassurance to allay misconceptions about the lethality of scorpion stings.
- The application of ice often provides immediate relief of local pain. Muscle spasm and fasciculations respond promptly to benzodiazepines.
- Severe toxicity may warrant scorpion antivenin. One to two vials of this goat-derived product affords immediate symptomatic resolution.

SCABIES

CLINICAL FEATURES
- Scabies are caused by the mite *Sarcoptes scabei,* and are concentrated in the web spaces between fingers and toes. Other common areas include the penis, children's faces and scalps, and the female nipple.
- Transmission is typically by direct contact.
- The distinctive feature of scabies infestation is intense pruritus with burrows. These white, thread-like channels form zigzag patterns with small gray spots at the closed end, where the mite rests.
- Undisturbed burrows can be traced with a hand lens and the female mite is easily scraped out with a blade edge. Associated vesicles, papules, crusts, and eczematization may obscure the diagnosis.

EMERGENCY DEPARTMENT CARE AND DISPOSITION
- Adult treatment of scabies infestation consists of a thorough application of permethrin (Elimite) from the neck down; infants may require additional application to the scalp, temple, and forehead.
- Reapplication is only necessary if mites are found 2 weeks following treatment, though the pruritus may last for several weeks after successful therapy.

CHIGGERS

CLINICAL FEATURES
- Chiggers are tiny mite larvae that cause intense pruritus when they feed on host epidermal cells.

- Itchiness begins within a few hours, followed by a papule that enlarges to a nodule over the next 1 to 2 days. Single bites can also cause soft tissue edema, while infestation has been associated with fever and erythema multiforme.
- Children who have been sitting on lawns are prone to chigger lesions in the genital area.
- The diagnosis of chigger bites is based on typical skin lesions in the context of a known outdoor exposure.

EMERGENCY DEPARTMENT CARE AND DISPOSITION
- Treatment consists of symptomatic relief with oral or topical antihistamines; oral steroids may be required in more severe cases.
- Annihilation of the mites requires topical application of lindane (Kwell), permethrin, or crotamiton (Eurax).

FLEAS

- Flea bites cause intensely pruritic zigzag lines, especially on the legs and waist area. The lesions have hemorrhagic puncta surrounded by erythematous and urticarial patches.
- Oral antihistamines, starch baths, calamine lotion, and topical steroids relieve discomfort. If secondary infection develops, topical or oral antibiotics may be needed.

LICE

- Body lice concentrate around the waist, shoulders, axillae, and neck. Pubic lice are spread by sexual contact.
- Their bites induce intensely pruritic papules and wheals. Reactions to louse saliva and feces may cause fever, malaise, and lymphadenopathy.
- Permethrin is the primary treatment of body lice infestation. Treatment of hair infestation requires a thorough application of pyrethrin with piperonyl butoxide; reapplication is mandatory in 10 days.
- Clothing, bedding, and personal articles must be sterilized in hot (>52°C) water to prevent reinfestation.

KISSING BUGS AND BEDBUGS (*HEMIPTERA*)

- Kissing bugs (conenose beetles) and bedbugs feed on blood as they attack the exposed surface of a sleeping victim.[4]
- The initial bite is painless; wheals, hemorrhagic papules, and bullae may follow. Anaphylaxis is common in the sensitized individual.

- Treatment consists of local wound care and analgesics. Allergic reactions must be treated as previously outlined for Hymenoptera envenomation.

PUSS CATERPILLARS (*MEGALOPYGE OPERCULARIS*)

- The puss caterpillar has stinging spines on its body that provoke immediate, intense, and rhythmic pain. Local edema is often followed by pruritus vesicles and papules.
- Fever, muscle cramps, anxiety, and shock-like symptoms may occur. Lymphadenopathy with local desquamation may develop in a few days.
- Treatment consists of immediate spine removal with cellophane tape.
- IV calcium gluconate is effective in relieving pain. Mild cases may respond to an antihistamine.

BLISTER BEETLES

- Blister beetles induce local irritation and blistering within hours of contact.
- Intense GI disturbances occur if ingested.
- Treatment consists of local wound care and drainage of large bullae. Application of steroid creams may also speed recovery.

CROTALIDAE (PIT VIPERS)

EPIDEMIOLOGY
- There are approximately 8000 venomous snakebites each year in the United States, but only about 10 deaths result. Twenty-five percent of bites are "dry strikes" with no effect from the venom.
- Except for imported species and coral snakes, the only venomous North American snakes are members of the Crotalidae family (eg, rattlesnakes, copperheads, water moccasins, and massasaugas).
- Crotalid snakes, commonly known as pit vipers, are identified by their two retractable fangs and by the heat-sensitive depressions (pits) located bilaterally between each eye and nostril.

CLINICAL FEATURES
- The effects of Crotalid envenomation depend on the size and species of snake, the age and size of the victim, the time elapsed since the bite, and the characteristics of the bite itself.
- The hallmark of pit viper envenomation is fang marks with local pain and swelling.[5]
- There are three classes of criteria that determine the severity of a rattlesnake bite: (1) degree of local

injury (swelling, pain, ecchymosis), (2) degree of systemic involvement (hypotension, tachycardia, paresthesia), and (3) evolving coagulopathy (thrombocytopenia, elevated prothrombin time, hypofibrinogenemia). Abnormalities in any of these three areas indicate that envenomation has occurred.
- Conversely, the absence of any clinical findings after 8 to 12 hours effectively rules out venom injection.
- Since the degree of poisoning following an encounter is variable, it is crucial to remember that initially benign-appearing bites may still evolve with devastating complications.

DIAGNOSIS AND DIFFERENTIAL
- The diagnosis of crotalid envenomation is based on the clinical findings and corroborating laboratory data.
- In general, all envenomated patients will have swelling within 30 minutes, although some may take up to 12 hours.
- The degree of envenomation is graded on a progressive continuum.
- Minimal envenomation describes cases with local swelling, no systemic signs, and no laboratory abnormalities.
- Moderate envenomation causes increased swelling that spreads from the site. These patients may also have systemic signs such as nausea, paresthesia, hypotension, and tachycardia. Coagulation parameters may be abnormal, but there is no significant bleeding.
- Severe envenomation causes extensive swelling, potentially life-threatening systemic signs (eg, hypotension, altered mental status, respiratory distress), and markedly abnormal coagulation parameters that may result in hemorrhage.

EMERGENCY DEPARTMENT CARE AND DISPOSITION
- All patients bitten by a pit viper must be evaluated at a medical facility; first aid measures must not delay definitive care. The patient should minimize physical activity, remain calm, and immobilize any bitten extremity in a neutral position below the level of the heart.
- Local wound care and tetanus immunization should be given, but prophylactic antibiotics and steroids have no proven benefit.[6]
- Limb circumference at several sites above and below the wound should be checked every 30 minutes, and the border of advancing edema should be marked.
- Any patient with progressive local swelling, systemic effects, or coagulopathy should immediately receive antivenin therapy.
- Polyvalent Crotalidae immune Fab (CroFab), a new sheep-derived antivenin, has generally replaced antivenin (Crotalidae) polyvalent, an equine-derived product.[7,8] Polyvalent Crotalidae immune Fab is

administered as an initial dose of 4 to 6 vials IV; there is no need for a prior intradermal skin test.

- The initial dose of polyvalent Crotalidae immune Fab is diluted in 250 mL of normal saline and infused IV over 60 minutes. Since allergic reactions may occur, the infusion should proceed at a slow rate of 25 to 50 mL/h for the first 10 minutes. If the patient remains stable, the infusion rate may be increased to the full 250-mL/h rate.
- Since the goal of therapy is to neutralize the existing venom, dosing regimens are exactly the same for both children and adults (although the amount of diluent will need proper adjustment).
- One hour after the initial dose has been administered, the patient must be re-examined to determine if local swelling has been arrested, coagulation tests have normalized, and systemic symptoms have abated. If the initial dose was ineffective in any of these three areas, then a repeat dose of 4 to 6 vials should be administered.
- Laboratory determinations are repeated every 4 hours or after each course of antivenin, whichever is more frequent.
- Since the end point of antivenin therapy is the arrest of progressive symptoms and coagulopathy, the administration of antivenin must continue until complete control of the envenomation is achieved.
- Once initial control has been achieved, the protocol is completed by administering additional 2-vial doses every 6 hours for an additional 18 hours (ie, three more doses).
- Compartment syndromes may occur secondary to envenomation. Repeated dosing of antivenin is the most effective therapy for elevated compartment pressures. Limb elevation, IV mannitol, and surgical fasciotomy may be required.
- The mainstay of uncomplicated coagulopathy remains antivenin therapy. Severe active bleeding due to coagulopathy may require the transfusion of blood products.
- All patients with a pit viper bite must be observed for at least 8 hours. Patients with no evidence of envenomation after 8 to 12 hours may be discharged.
- Serum sickness occurs in 16% of patients within 1 to 2 weeks of receiving polyvalent Crotalidae immune Fab antivenin. Oral prednisone is the standard treatment.

CORAL SNAKES

CLINICAL FEATURES
- All true coral snakes have their yellow bands directly touching the red bands; nonpoisonous impostors have an intervening black band. This distinctive pattern establishes the mnemonic for North American snakes: "Red on yellow, kill a fellow; red on black, venom lack."

- Only the bite of the eastern coral snake (*Micrurus fulvius fulvius*) requires significant treatment; the bite of the Sonoran (Arizona) coral snake is mild and only needs local care.
- Eastern coral snake venom is a potent neurotoxin capable of causing tremor, salivation, respiratory paralysis, seizures, and bulbar palsies (eg, dysarthria, diplopia, and dysphagia).

EMERGENCY DEPARTMENT CARE AND DISPOSITION
- Patients with possible envenomation must be admitted to the hospital for 24 to 48 hours of observation.
- The toxic effects of coral snake venom may be preventable, but they are not easily reversed.[9]
- All patients who have potential envenomation should receive 3 vials of antivenin (*Micrurus fulvius*).
- Additional doses are required if symptoms appear and these patients must be admitted to an intensive care unit.

GILA MONSTERS

- Gila monsters are slow-moving poisonous lizards that are indigenous to the desert of the southwestern United States.
- Gila monsters have a tenacious bite and may be difficult to remove from the bitten extremity. Most bites result in local pain and swelling that worsens over several hours before subsiding.
- Patients rarely may experience systemic toxicity, including weakness, lightheadedness, paresthesia, diaphoresis, or severe hypertension.
- Treatment involves removal of the reptile from the bite site. The Gila monster will often loosen its grip when no longer suspended in midair. Other reported methods include submersion, cast spreaders, or application of an irritating flame.
- The only requisite treatment is local wound care with a careful search for implanted teeth.

REFERENCES

1. Sams HH, Dunnick CA, Smith ML, King LE: Necrotic arachnidism. *J Am Acad Dermatol* 44:561, 2001.
2. Clark RF, Werthern-Kestner S, Vance MV, Gerkin R: Clinical presentation and treatment of black widow spider envenomation: A review of 163 cases. *Ann Emerg Med* 21:782, 1992.
3. Clark RF: The safety and efficacy of antivenin *Lactrodectus mactans*. *J Clin Toxicol* 39:125, 2001.
4. Vetter R: Kissing bugs (*Triatoma*) and the skin. *Dermatol Online J* 7:6, 2001.

5. Gold BS, Dart RC, Barish RA: Bites of venomous snakes. *N Engl J Med* 347:347, 2002.

6. Tagwireyi DD, Ball DE, Nhachi CF: Routine prophylactic antibiotic use in the management of snakebite. *BMC Clin Pharmacol* 1:4, 2001.

7. Dart RC, McNally J: Efficacy, safety, and use of snake antivenoms in the United States. *Ann Emerg Med* 37:181, 2001.

8. Ruha A-M, Curry AC, Beuhler M: Initial postmarketing experience with Crotalidae Polyvalent Immune Fab for treatment of rattlesnake envenomation. *Ann Emerg Med* 39:609, 2002.

9. Kitchens CS, Van Mierop LHS: Envenomation by the eastern coral snake (*Micrurus fulvius fulvius*): A study of 39 victims. *JAMA* 258:1615, 1987.

For further reading in *Emergency Medicine, A Comprehensive Study Guide,* 6th ed., see Chap. 194, "Arthropod Bites and Stings," by Richard F. Clark and Aaron B. Schneir; and Chap. 195, "Reptile Bites," by Richard C. Dart and Frank F.S. Daly.

124 TRAUMA AND ENVENOMATION FROM MARINE FAUNA
Christian A. Tomaszewski

EPIDEMIOLOGY

- The most common aquatic animal exposures are jellyfish and venomous fish stings, particularly stingrays.[1]

PATHOPHYSIOLOGY

- Fatalities are rare and often involve the more painful jellyfish, such as the box jellyfish (*Chironex fleckeri* and *Chiropsalmus*) and Portuguese man-of-war (*Physalia physalis*).[2]

CLINICAL FEATURES

- Marine animals reported in attacks include sharks, great barracudas, moray eels, giant groupers, sea lions, seals, crocodiles, alligators, needlefish, wahoos, piranhas, and triggerfish.
- Marine animals have inflicted abrasions, puncture wounds, lacerations, and crush injuries. With shark bites, there is the added issue of substantial tissue loss associated with hemorrhagic shock, hypothermia, and near drowning.

- Coral cuts and scrapes are the most common underwater injury, and cause local stinging pain, erythema, urticaria, and pruritus. This may progress to cellulitis with lymphangitis and, in worse cases, ulceration and wound necrosis.
- Ocean water contains many potentially pathogenic bacteria including *Aeromonas hydrophila, Bacteroides fragilis, Chromobacterium violaceum, Clostridium perfringens, Escherichia coli, Salmonella enteritidis, Staphylococcus aureus,* and *Streptococcus* species.
- Among the most serious infections are those due to the species from the genera *Vibrio* and *Aeromonas* (both gram-negative rods).
- *Vibrio* infections are some of the most virulent, causing rapid infections marked by pain, swelling, hemorrhagic bullae, vasculitis, necrotizing fasciitis and sepsis. Immunosuppressed patients, particularly those with chronic liver disease, are especially susceptible to sepsis and death (up to 60%) with *Vibrio vulnificus* infections.[3]
- *Erysipelothrix rhusiopathiae,* the bacterium implicated in fish handler's disease, causes painful, marginating plaques on the hand following a cutaneous puncture wound.
- Another unique marine bacterium is *Mycobacterium marinum,* an acid-fast bacillus that can cause a chronic cutaneous granuloma 3 to 4 weeks after exposure.
- Numerous invertebrate and vertebrate marine species are venomous. These venoms can be cytotoxic, hematoxic, myotoxic, and neurotoxic. Most are heat labile.
- The invertebrates consist of five phyla: Cnidaria, Porifera, Echinodermata, Annelida, and Mollusca.
- The Cnidaria include true jellyfish (Scyphozoa), box jellyfish (Cubozoa), anemones (Anthozoa), fire corals, and Portuguese man-of-war (Hydrozoa). Most of these organisms have tentacles with nematocysts or stinging cells that release venom upon contact.
- Most reactions are localized, with resulting pain, erythema, and urticaria.[4,5]
- *Physalia physalis* (the Portuguese man-of-war) also causes severe pain and respiratory distress, and even death (possibly due to anaphylaxis).[2]
- The deadliest cnidarians are the box jellyfish, particularly *Chironex fleckeri* in Australia and *Chiropsalmus,* which even exists in the Gulf of Mexico. Death is rapid due to cardiovascular failure.[2]
- Another Australian box jellyfish, *Carukia barnesi,* can cause the Irukandji syndrome, which is characterized by diffuse pain, hypertension, tachycardia, diaphoresis, and pulmonary edema.
- Porifera are sponges that produce a stinging dermatitis. In addition, spicules of silica or calcium carbonate carried by the sponge may become embedded in the

skin. In severe cases, chronic inflammatory changes may develop and result in a papulovesicular rash and erythema multiforme.

- Echinodermata include sea urchins, sea stars, and sea cucumbers. Sea urchin spines produce immediate pain, followed by erythema, myalgia, and local swelling. Delayed effects consist of granulomas from retained spines.
- Systemic envenomation from sea urchins rarely occurs, and is manifested by nausea, paresthesia, paralysis, abdominal pain, syncope, respiratory distress, and hypotension.
- The most notorious sea star, *Acanthaster planci* (crown-of-thorns starfish), has sharp, rigid spines that cause burning pain and local inflammation. Although uncommon, severe envenomation can cause nausea, vomiting, paresthesia, and paralysis.
- Annelida include bristleworms, which embed bristles in the skin, causing pain and erythema.
- The Indo-Pacific cone shell, *Conus magus,* has a poison dart with envenomation similar to bee stings; however, it may induce muscle paralysis and respiratory failure within 30 minutes.
- The blue ringed octopus, *Hapalochalena,* can inject tetrodotoxin and cause paresthesias, flaccid paralysis, and respiratory failure.
- Vertebrate envenomations are primarily due to stingrays (order Rajiformes), with an occasional sting from venomous spined fish and bites from sea snakes.
- The stingray has a venomous spine which punctures or lacerates the skin and causes an intense painful local reaction. The spine sheath and even the spine itself may break off as a retained body.
- Systemic manifestations from stingray exposure may include weakness, nausea, vomiting, diarrhea, syncope, seizures, paralysis, hypotension, and dysrhythmias.
- There are a variety of spined venomous fish, including scorpionfish (popular in aquariums), rockfish, catfish, weeverfish, toadfish, ratfish, rabbitfish, stargazers, and scats. All of them have spines associated with venom glands, but only cause severe local pain, erythema, and edema, with an occasional retained spine.
- The most venomous is the Indo-Pacific stonefish (*Synaceja*), which in addition to severe local effects can cause diaphoresis, nausea, and hypotension.
- Sea snakes, which live in tropical Indo-Pacific oceans, have venom that contains a paralyzing neurotoxin and myotoxin.
- Symptoms, occurring 30 minutes to 4 hours after a sea snake bite, include myalgia, ophthalmoplegia, ascending paralysis, and respiratory failure; myoglobinuria and elevated liver enzymes may be found. If death occurs, it is usually due to ventilatory failure that occurs within 6 hours.

EMERGENCY DEPARTMENT CARE AND DISPOSITION

- Lacerations should be copiously irrigated, explored for foreign matter, and débrided of devitalized tissue. Soft tissue radiographs may help locate foreign bodies.
- Most wounds should undergo delayed primary closure. Tetanus prophylaxis should be updated as appropriate.
- Empiric antibiotic therapy is not indicated for routine minor wounds in healthy patients.
- Patients who are immunocompromised and have liver disease or with grossly contaminated or extensive lacerations require antibiotics; in high-risk patients the initial dose should be parenteral.
- Aerobic and anaerobic cultures should be ordered and the lab alerted since special media may be needed.
- Antibiotic therapy should cover *Staphylococcus* and *Streptococcus* species; in ocean-related infections, *Vibrio* species should be covered with a third-generation cephalosporin or quinolone.
- Granulomas from *Mycobacterium marinum* require several months of treatment with clarithromycin, or rifampin plus ethambutol for deep-seated infections.
- For Cnidaria envenomation, the wound should be rinsed with saline; fresh water should be avoided since this may cause further envenomation.
- To deactivate attached nematocysts, particularly from the deadly box jellyfish and Portuguese man-of-war, 5% acetic acid (vinegar) should be applied for 30 minutes or until pain is resolved. Greater clinical success is achieved by immersing the wound of a Hawaiian box jellyfish (*Carybdea alata*) in hot water (>40°C);[6] wounds of some other species of true jellyfish should be immersed in a slurry of sodium bicarbonate.
- Retained tentacles and nematocysts can be picked off with gloved hands or scraped off. Chronic inflammatory problems can be treated with topical steroids.
- Corneal envenomation should be irrigated copiously; persistent symptoms may require topical steroids.
- Patients with systemic symptoms should be observed for at least 8 hours. There is an antivenin for systemic symptoms from the box jellyfish *Chironex* venom.
- Sponge-induced dermatitis should be treated with gentle drying of the skin and removal of spicules with adhesive tape. Antihistamines and topical steroids may be beneficial in chronic inflammatory reactions.
- Echinodermata envenomation should be treated by removing gross spines and with hot water immersion (45°C) for 30 to 90 minutes. In Annelida envenomation, bristles should be removed with adhesive tape or forceps.
- With stingray, scorpionfish, and other vertebrate envenomations, the affected area should be immersed in

hot water, spines removed, and the wound explored and debrided as necessary. The patient for should be observed for 4 hours to exclude systemic toxicity.

- With sea snake bites, the injured area should be kept immobilized and dependent; the application of local pressure such as an elastic bandage may help sequester the venom.
- Sea snake antivenin, either monovalent (for the beaked sea snake in southeast Asia) or polyvalent, is indicated for any systemic symptoms and may be beneficial up to 36 hours after envenomation. If no symptoms develop after 8 hours, then envenomation can be excluded.

References

1. Hanley M, Tomaszewski C, Kerns W: The epidemiology of aquatic envenomations in the U.S.: Most common symptoms and animals. *J Toxicol Clin Toxicol* 38:512, 2000.
2. Fenner PH, Williamson JA: Worldwide deaths and severe envenomation from jellyfish stings. *Med J Aust* 165:658, 1996.
3. Strom MS, Paranjpye RN: Epidemiology and pathogenesis of *Vibrio vulnificus. Microbes Infect* 2:177, 2000.
4. Lotan A, Fishman L, Zlotkin E: Toxin compartmentation and delivery in the Cnidaria: The nematocyst's tubule as a multi-headed poisonous arrow. *J Exp Zool* 275:444, 1996.
5. Burnett JW, Calton GJ: Jellyfish envenomation syndromes updates. *Ann Emerg Med* 16:1000, 1987.
6. Nomura JT, Sato RL, Ahern RM, et al: A randomized paired comparison trial of cutaneous treatments for acute jellyfish (*Carybdea alata*) stings. *Am J Emerg Med* 20:624, 2002.

For further reading in *Emergency Medicine: A Comprehensive Study Guide,* 6th ed., see Chap. 196, "Trauma and Envenomation from Marine Fauna," by Geoffrey K. Isbister and David G. Caldicott.

125 HIGH ALTITUDE MEDICAL PROBLEMS

Keith L. Mausner

EPIDEMIOLOGY

- The incidence of acute mountain sickness (AMS), as well as high altitude cerebral edema (HACE) and high altitude pulmonary edema (HAPE), is influenced primarily by the rapidity of ascent and sleeping altitude.

- An AMS incidence between 17 and 40% has been reported at resorts with altitudes between 2200 and 2700 m (7200 and 9000 ft).[1]
- The incidence of HAPE is much lower than that of AMS. HAPE has been reported in less than 1 in 10,000 skiers in Colorado, and 2 to 3% of climbers on Mt. McKinley. The incidence of HACE is lower than that of HAPE.

PATHOPHYSIOLOGY

- AMS is caused by hypobaric hypoxia, and HAPE and HACE can be viewed as extreme progressions of the same pathophysiology.
- Hypobaric hypoxemia increases cerebral blood flow and cerebral capillary hydrostatic pressure, contributing to fluid shifts and either mild cerebral edema in AMS or severe cerebral edema in HACE. In addition, increased permeability of capillaries as a result of inflammatory endothelial activation may also play a role, especially in the brain.
- Hypoxemia elevates sympathetic nervous system activity, which promotes uneven pulmonary vasoconstriction, and increases pulmonary capillary pressure.
- Increased sympathetic nervous system activity is associated with decreased urine output, mediated by increased renin-angiotensin, aldosterone, and antidiuretic hormone (ADH). This leads to fluid retention and results in elevated capillary hydrostatic pressure in lungs, brain, and peripheral tissues.[2]
- Susceptibility to AMS is linked to a low hypoxic ventilatory response and low vital capacity; susceptible individuals are prone to recurrence on return to high altitude.
- Partially acclimatized individuals who live at intermediate altitudes of 1000 to 2000 m are less likely to develop AMS on ascent to higher altitude.

CLINICAL FEATURES

- AMS is usually seen in unacclimated people making a rapid ascent to over 2000 m (6600 ft) above sea level. The earliest symptoms are light-headedness and mild breathlessness.
- Symptoms similar to a hangover may develop within 6 hours after arrival at altitude, but may be delayed as long as 1 day. These include bifrontal headache, anorexia, nausea, weakness, and fatigue.
- Worsening headache, vomiting, oliguria, dyspnea, and weakness indicate progression of AMS.
- There are few specific physical examination findings in AMS. Postural hypotension and peripheral and facial edema may occur. Localized rales are noted in

20% of cases. Funduscopy reveals tortuous and dilated veins; retinal hemorrhages are common at altitudes over 5000 m.

- HACE is an extreme progression of AMS, and is usually associated with pulmonary edema. It presents with altered mental status, ataxia, stupor, and progression to coma. Focal neurologic signs such as third and sixth cranial nerve palsies may be present.
- HAPE is the most lethal of the high altitude syndromes. Risk factors include heavy exertion, rapid ascent, cold exposure, excessive salt intake, use of sleeping medications, and previous history of HAPE.
- Individuals with pulmonary hypertension as well as children with acute respiratory infections may be more susceptible to HAPE.
- Early findings of HAPE include a dry cough, impaired exercise capacity, and localized rales, usually in the right mid-lung field.
- Progression of HAPE leads to tachycardia, tachypnea, resting dyspnea, severe weakness, productive cough, cyanosis, and generalized rales. Low grade fever is common.
- As hypoxemia worsens, consciousness is impaired, and without treatment coma and death usually follow.
- Other findings of HAPE may include signs of pulmonary hypertension such as a prominent P_2 and right ventricular heave on cardiac examination, as well as right axis deviation and a right ventricular strain pattern on electrocardiogram (ECG).
- Early recognition of HAPE, and descent and treatment are essential to prevent progression.
- High altitude may adversely affect patients with chronic obstructive pulmonary disease (COPD), heart disease, sickle cell disease, and pregnancy.
- COPD patients may require supplemental O_2 or an increase in their usual O_2 flow rate.
- Patients with atherosclerotic heart disease do surprisingly well at high altitude, but there may be a risk of earlier onset of angina and worsening of heart failure.[3]
- Ascent to 1500 to 2000 m may cause a vaso-occlusive crisis in individuals with sickle cell disease or sickle thalassemia.
- Individuals with sickle cell trait usually do well at altitude, but splenic infarction has been reported during heavy exercise.
- Pregnant long-term high altitude residents have an increased risk of hypertension, low birth weight infants, and neonatal jaundice, but no increase in pregnancy complications has been reported in pregnant visitors to high altitude who engage in reasonable activities.
- It is reasonable to advise pregnant women to avoid altitudes above which oxygen saturation falls below 85%; this corresponds to a sleeping altitude of approximately 10,000 ft.

DIAGNOSIS AND DIFFERENTIAL

- The differential diagnosis of the high altitude syndromes includes hypothermia, carbon monoxide poisoning, pulmonary or central nervous system infections, dehydration, and exhaustion.
- HACE may be difficult to distinguish in the field from other high altitude neurologic syndromes.
- Strokes due to arterial or venous thrombosis or arterial hemorrhage have been reported at high altitude in individuals without classic risk factors.
- Reversible focal neurologic signs or symptoms may occur and may be due to vasospasm, migraine headache, or transient ischemic attack. These syndromes typically have more focal findings than HACE.
- Previously asymptomatic brain tumors may be unmasked by ascent to high altitude.
- Underlying epilepsy may be worsened by hyperventilation, which is part of the normal acclimatization response.
- HAPE must be distinguished from pulmonary embolus, cardiogenic pulmonary edema, and pneumonia. Low-grade fever is common in HAPE and may make it difficult to distinguish from pneumonia.
- A key to diagnosis is the clinical response to treatment.

CARE AND DISPOSITION IN THE FIELD AND EMERGENCY DEPARTMENT

- Gradual ascent is effective at preventing AMS. A reasonable recommendation for sea level dwellers is to spend a night at 1500 to 2000 m before sleeping at altitudes above 2500 m.
- High altitude trekkers should allow two nights for each 1000-m gain in sleeping altitude starting at 3000 m.
- Eating a high carbohydrate diet and avoiding overexertion, alcohol, and respiratory depressants may also help prevent AMS.
- Mild AMS usually improves or resolves in 12 to 36 hours if further ascent is delayed and acclimatization is allowed. A decrease in altitude of 500 to 1000 m may provide prompt relief of symptoms.
- Oxygen relieves symptoms of mild AMS, and nocturnal low-flow O_2 (0.5 to 1 L/min) is helpful.
- Patients with mild AMS should not ascend to a higher sleeping elevation. Descent is indicated if symptoms persist or worsen.
- Immediate descent and treatment is indicated if there is a change in the level of consciousness, or if there is ataxia, or pulmonary edema.
- Acetazolamide causes a bicarbonate diuresis, leading to a mild metabolic acidosis. This stimulates ventilation

and pharmacologically produces an acclimatization response. It is effective in prophylaxis and treatment.

- Specific indications for acetazolamide are: (1) prior history of altitude illness; (2) abrupt ascent to over 3000 m (10,000 ft); (3) treatment of AMS; and (4) symptomatic periodic breathing during sleep at altitude.
- The adult dose of acetazolamide is 125 mg PO bid, or alternately 5 mg/kg per day in 2 or 3 divided doses; it is continued until symptoms resolve or started 24 hours before ascent and continued for 2 days at altitude as prophylaxis.
- Acetazolamide should be restarted if symptoms recur.[2] Acetazolamide is contraindicated in sulfa-allergic patients.
- Dexamethasone (4 mg PO, IM, or IV every 6 hours) is effective in moderate to severe AMS. Tapering of the dose over several days may be necessary to prevent rebound.
- Aspirin or acetaminophen may improve headache in AMS. Prochlorperazine (5 to 10 mg IM, IV, or PO) may help with nausea and vomiting.
- Diuretics may be useful for treating fluid retention, but should be used with caution to avoid intravascular volume depletion.
- HACE mandates immediate descent or evacuation. Oxygen and dexamethasone (8 mg PO, IM, or IV, then 4 mg every 6 hours) should be administered.
- Furosemide (40 to 80 mg) may help reduce brain edema in HACE.
- Intubation and hyperventilation are necessary in severe cases of HACE. Careful monitoring of arterial blood gases is needed to prevent excessive lowering of P_{CO_2} (below 30 mm Hg), which may cause cerebral ischemia. Mannitol should also be administered.
- HAPE should also be treated with immediate descent. Oxygen may be life-saving if descent is delayed. The patient should be kept warm and exertion minimized.
- For HAPE, drugs are second-line treatment after descent and oxygen. Nifedipine (10 mg PO every 4 to 6 hours, or 30 mg extended release every 12 hours), as well as morphine and furosemide, may be effective.
- HAPE patients are usually volume depleted, and care should be taken to avoid precipitating drug-induced hypotension.
- An expiratory positive airway pressure (EPAP) mask may be useful in the field, and without supplemental O_2 can increase oxygen saturation by 10 to 20%.
- Portable fabric inflatable hyperbaric chambers may be effective in the field when immediate descent is not possible.
- In individuals with prior episodes of HAPE, nifedipine 20 mg (slow-release preparation) every 8 hours during ascent may be effective as prophylaxis.[4]
- Inhaled salmeterol twice a day may also help prevent recurrent HAPE.[5]

MISCELLANEOUS HIGH ALTITUDE SYNDROMES

- Acute hypoxia may occur with decompression of an aircraft or failure of a mountaineer's oxygen delivery system. Symptoms include dizziness, light-headedness, and dimming of vision progressing to loss of consciousness.
- A sudden drop in oxygen saturation to 50 or 60% will usually result in unconsciousness. Deliberate hyperventilation may increase the period of useful consciousness in the setting of acute hypoxia.
- High altitude retinopathy includes retinal edema, tortuous and dilated retinal veins, disc hyperemia, retinal hemorrhages, and less frequently, cotton wool exudates.
- Except for macular hemorrhages, retinal hemorrhages are usually asymptomatic and descent is not indicated unless visual changes occur; hemorrhages usually resolve in 10 to 14 days.
- High altitude pharyngitis and bronchitis are due to local irritation and drying of mucus membranes from breathing high volumes of cold, dry air. Severe coughing spasms and bronchospasm may be present. Symptomatic treatment as well as hydration, lozenges to encourage salivation, and breathing of steam or through a scarf to trap moisture and heat may provide some relief.
- Chronic mountain polycythemia in long-term high altitude residents may be attributed in half of patients to underlying diseases such as COPD or sleep apnea that worsen hypoxia at altitude, or may be linked to idiopathic hypoventilation due to a diminished respiratory drive.
- Symptoms of chronic mountain polycythemia include impaired cognition, sleep, and peripheral circulation, as well as headache, drowsiness, and chest congestion, along with an abnormally elevated hemoglobin, usually over 20 to 22 g/dL.
- Treatment options for chronic mountain polycythemia include moving to a lower altitude, phlebotomy, home oxygen, and respiratory stimulants such as acetazolamide and medroxyprogesterone.
- Ultraviolet keratitis (snow blindness) may affect unprotected eyes in as little as 1 hour at high altitude. The usual findings are severe pain, photophobia, tearing, conjunctival erythema, chemosis, and eyelid swelling.
- Cold compresses, analgesics, and occasionally eye patching are generally adequate symptomatic treatment for ultraviolet keratitis; the keratitis usually heals in 24 hours. Prevention with adequate sunglasses that transmit less than 10% of UVB light is essential.

REFERENCES

1. Honigman B, Theis MK, Koziol-McLain J, et al: Acute mountain sickness in a general tourist population at moderate altitudes. *Ann Intern Med* 118:587, 1993.
2. Hackett P, Roach RC: High-altitude illness. *N Engl J Med* 345: 107, 2001.
3. Levine B, Zuckerman J, de Filippi C: Effect of high-altitude exposure in the elderly: The Tenth Mountain Division Study. *Circulation* 96:1224, 1997.
4. Bartsch P, Maggiorini M, Ritter M, et al: Prevention of high-altitude pulmonary edema by nifedipine. *N Engl J Med* 325: 1284, 1991.
5. Sartori C, Allemann Y, Duplain H, et al: Salmeterol for the prevention of high-altitude pulmonary edema. *N Engl J Med* 346:1631, 2002.

For further reading in *Emergency Medicine: A Comprehensive Study Guide*, 6th ed., see Chap. 207, "High Altitude Medical Problems," by Peter H. Hackett.

126 DYSBARISM AND COMPLICATIONS OF DIVING

Christian A. Tomaszewski

PATHOPHYSIOLOGY

- Dysbarism is usually encountered in scuba divers and refers to complications associated with changes in environmental ambient pressure and with breathing compressed gases.[1] These effects are governed by the gas laws.
- Boyle's law states that at a constant temperature, the pressure and volume of a gas are inversely related. This is the basic mechanism for barotrauma, which results when divers are unable to equalize pressures in air-filled cavities with ambient environmental pressure. The end result is overexpansion of the lungs when divers hold their breath.
- Henry's law states that at equilibrium the quantity of gas in solution is proportional to the partial pressure of the gas with which it is in equilibrium.
- Decompression sickness occurs because of the increased ambient pressure during descent; this causes an increase in the partial pressure of the inspired nitrogen in the breathing air. Due to Henry's law, nitrogen dissolves and accumulates in tissues. If ascent is too rapid, nitrogen comes out of solution abruptly, leading to bubble formation.

CLINICAL FEATURES

- Barotrauma, the most common diving-related affliction, is caused by the direct mechanical effects of pressure, as gas-filled cavities in the body contract with pressure.
- Middle ear squeeze, or barotitis media, is the most frequently seen form of barotrauma.
- Middle ear squeeze occurs secondary to eustachian tube dysfunction during descent.[2] If the dive is not aborted or pressure not otherwise equalized, then the eardrum may rupture. The diver may experience a sensation of air bubbles escaping from the ear that is associated with nausea and vertigo.
- The patient with barotitis media may complain of ear pain or fullness on presentation. On physical examination, there may be blood behind the tympanic membrane or within the canal, mild conductive hearing loss, and tympanic membrane perforation.
- If the sinus ostia are occluded on descent, an impending squeeze can cause bleeding from the maxillary or frontal sinuses with subsequent pain and epistaxis.
- Middle ear squeeze may also manifest as subconjunctival hemorrhage if a diver does not exhale into his mask and equalize pressure during descent.
- Inner ear barotrauma typically occurs during rapid descent, when the diver does an overly forceful Valsalva maneuver. Instead of clearing his ears or rupturing the tympanic membrane, pressure is transmitted through the vestibular and cochlear structures. This may lead to serious inner ear damage, including rupture of the oval or round window, fistula formation, or rupture of Reissner's membrane.
- Inner ear barotrauma may present with roaring tinnitus, vertigo, sensorineural hearing loss, a feeling of ear fullness, nausea, and vomiting. Insufflation of the tympanic membrane on the affected side may cause contralateral eye deviation, known as a positive fistula test.
- Barotrauma during ascent is due to expansion of gas in body cavities. "Reverse squeeze" may affect the ear or sinuses during ascent with rupture.
- Alternobaric vertigo (ABV) can temporarily occur during ascent due to unbalanced vestibular stimulation from unequal middle ear pressures.
- Tooth squeeze may be noted during ascent due to air-filled dental cavities.
- Gastrointestinal barotrauma presents with abdominal fullness, colicky abdominal pain, belching, and flatulence. Severe cases of air swallowing have resulted in stomach rupture on ascent.
- Pulmonary overpressurization syndrome (POPS) may occur during ascent, resulting in mediastinal and subcutaneous emphysema.[3]
- Although rapid ascents without exhalation are the usual cause of POPS, patients with obstructive lung

disease and congenital cysts may have air trapping as well.

- After the dive, patients with POPS may experience gradual onset of increasing hoarseness, neck fullness, substernal chest pain, dyspnea, and dysphagia; in severe cases, syncope and pneumothorax may occur.
- Air embolism is the most severe form of pulmonary barotrauma. Gas bubbles may enter the pulmonary venous circulation and embolize to the brain, causing cerebral arterial gas embolism.[4]
- Air embolism typically presents acutely in a diver surfacing after a rapid ascent. This can also occur in patients with central venous catheters or on cardiac bypass, when an inadvertent air embolus enters the right side of the heart and crosses over into the left atrium via a patent foramen ovale.
- Cerebral arterial gas embolism can result in immediate apnea and death, as seen in 4% of dive-related cases.
- If the patient survives the acute air embolism insult, they usually present within an hour of their dive with syncope, seizure, disorientation, or hemiplegia. Milder cases may present with sensory disturbances, confusion, or vertigo.
- Decompression sickness (DCS) is not a form of barotrauma. It is due to gas bubble formation as inert gas comes out of solution in blood and tissues when ascent is too rapid, without adequate time for decompression.
- In conventional compressed air diving, the culprit in DCS is nitrogen.
- DCS is a multi–organ system disorder that results from the direct effects of nitrogen bubbles on circulation and cells, as well as to secondary inflammatory responses and activation of clotting mechanisms.
- Type I DCS (pain only) typically involves the joints, extremities, and the skin, which exhibits purple mottling.
- Type II DCS is more serious and involves the central nervous system, typically the spine, and occasionally the vestibular ("staggers") and cardiopulmonary ("chokes") systems.
- The most common initial symptoms of DCS may be nonspecific; they include fatigue, headache, nausea, and dizziness.
- Divers with type I DCS typically have deep pain in the knee or shoulder that is relieved with movement.
- Type II DCS may present with vague patchy paresthesias. On physical examination, the patient may have ataxia, bladder dysfunction, and partial paralysis.
- In pulmonary DCS, the patient may present with cough, hemoptysis, dyspnea, and substernal chest pain.
- Vestibular DCS, which may be mistaken for inner ear barotrauma, can present with vertigo, hearing loss, tinnitus, and dysequilibrium.

DIAGNOSIS AND DIFFERENTIAL

- The time of symptom onset in relation to the dive profile—depth, duration, and repetitiveness—and in relation to descent or ascent are the most useful historical factors in distinguishing decompression illness from other disorders.
- During descent, the most common maladies are the squeeze syndromes.
- During the ascent phase, barotrauma or ABV are most likely to occur. DCS, if severe, may become symptomatic during ascent.
- Onset of severe symptoms within 10 minutes of surfacing is an air embolism until proven otherwise.
- POPS and other forms of barotrauma also usually present shortly after ascent.
- DCS tends to be less catastrophic initially, developing more severe symptoms 1 to 6 hours after surfacing, but symptoms may be delayed for up to 48 hours.
- The differential diagnosis for decompression illnesses is broad. Musculoskeletal complaints could be due to joint strain or a newly symptomatic herniated cervical disk. Chest pain may be due to cardiac ischemia from overexertion.
- Acute pulmonary edema from cardiogenic causes has occurred in young people during strenuous dives, particularly in cold water.[5]
- Sudden loss of consciousness or seizure may be idiopathic or from subarachnoid hemorrhage. Paresthesias, particularly hot-cold sensation reversal, may occur within a day of eating a ciguatoxin-contaminated predatory fish.
- In challenging cases, patients with these diverse symptoms may deserve a trial of pressure within a hyperbaric chamber, which would result in dramatic clinical improvement if symptoms are DCS-related.

EMERGENCY DEPARTMENT CARE AND DISPOSITION

- Attention should be focused on airway, breathing, circulation, treatment of life-threatening injuries, and correction of hypothermia. High-flow oxygen should be administered.
- If air embolism is suspected, the patient should be placed in a supine position; the left lateral decubitus position may be used if vomiting occurs, but Trendelenburg is no longer recommended.
- Lidocaine, 1 mg/kg bolus, may be given followed by a continuous infusion at a 1 mg/min.[6] There is no support for the use of heparin, aspirin, or corticosteroids at this time.[7]
- If air embolism or DCS is suspected, recompression chamber therapy should be initiated as quickly as

possible.[8] Aeromedical transport should be at an altitude of less than 1000 ft or in an aircraft that can be pressurized to 1 atmosphere absolute.

- Most DCS patients are volume depleted; IV fluids should be administered if not otherwise contraindicated.
- Patients with middle ear and other squeeze syndromes should stop diving until symptoms resolve. Decongestants and analgesics may be helpful.
- Antibiotics such as amoxicillin are indicated if the eardrum is ruptured; diving is contraindicated until it has healed.
- Sinus squeeze is treated similarly to middle ear squeeze; antibiotics are optional.
- Inner ear barotrauma usually mandates ENT consultation since surgical repair may be indicated.
- These patients should avoid straining, be prescribed medications for nausea and vertigo, and be placed on bed rest with the head elevated.
- POPS may require needle decompression or tube thoracostomy if a pneumothorax develops. POPS usually resolves with rest and supplemental oxygen, and rarely requires recompression therapy.

REFERENCES

1. Strauss MB, Borer RC: Diving medicine: contemporary topics and their controversies. *Am J Emerg Med* 19:232, 2001.
2. Becker GD, Parell GJ: Barotrauma of the ears and sinuses after scuba diving. *Euro Arch Otorhinolaryngol* 258;159, 2001.
3. Harker CP, Neuman TS, Olson LK, et al: The roentgenographic findings associated with air embolism in sport SCUBA divers. *J Emerg Med* 11:443, 1993.
4. Neuman TS: Arterial gas embolism and decompression sickness. *News Physiol Sci* 17:77, 2001.
5. Hampson NB, Dunford RG: Pulmonary edema of scuba divers. *Undersea Hyper Med* 24:29, 1997.
6. Mitchell SJ: Lidocaine for the treatment of decompression illness: A review of the literature. *Undersea Hyper Med* 28:165, 2001.
7. Catron PW, Flynn ET: Adjuvant drug therapy for decompression sickness: A review. *Undersea Biomed Res* 9:161, 1982.
8. Martin JD, Thom SR: Vascular leukocyte sequestration in decompression sickness and prophylactic hyperbaric oxygen therapy in rats. *Aviat Space Environ Med* 73:565, 2002.

For further reading in *Emergency Medicine: A Comprehensive Study Guide,* 6th ed., see Chap. 197, "Dysbarism and Complications of Diving," by Brain Snyder and Tom Neuman.

127 NEAR DROWNING
Richard A. Walker

EPIDEMIOLOGY

- Drowning is the third leading cause of accidental death.[1]
- Drowning rates are highest for males, children less than 5 years of age, and young adults 15 to 24 years of age.[1]
- The elderly are at increased risk of bathtub drowning.
- Freshwater drowning is more common than salt water drowning, even in coastal areas.

PATHOPHYSIOLOGY

- Near drowning is defined as survival longer than 24 hours after a submersion event, and tends to occur in otherwise healthy young individuals.
- Transient protection from parasympathetic activation of the diving reflex (bradycardia, apnea, peripheral vasoconstriction, and central shunting of blood flow) may occur during submersion and is strongest in young infants, but the effects decrease with age.[2]
- Cerebral protection in cold water submersions may result from rapid central nervous system (CNS) cooling.
- "Dry drowning" results from laryngospasm that causes hypoxemia and varying degrees of neurologic insult, and represents up to 20% of submersion injuries.
- "Wet drowning" consists of aspiration of water into the lungs, causing washout of surfactant, which results in diminished alveolar gas transfer, atelectasis, and ventilation-perfusion mismatch.

CLINICAL FEATURES

- Noncardiogenic pulmonary edema results from moderate to severe aspiration of water in "wet drowning" cases.
- Physical examination may reveal clear lungs, rales, rhonchi, or wheezes.
- Mental status may range from normal to comatose.
- Patients are at risk for hypothermia, even in warm water submersions.[3]

DIAGNOSIS AND DIFFERENTIAL

- Spinal cord injuries may occur in association with diving or surfing injuries or in boating accidents.[4,5]

- Syncope, seizures, hypoglycemia, and underlying heart disease, including acute myocardial infarction and dysrhythmias, have been associated with near drowning.[4,5]
- Laboratory findings may include metabolic acidosis and electrolyte abnormalities if there is associated renal injury from hypoxemia, hemoglobinuria, or myoglobinuria.[6,7]
- Massive hemolysis may occur with very large volumes of aspirated fresh water.
- Disseminated intravascular coagulation is rare.
- The chest radiograph may show generalized pulmonary edema or perihilar infiltrates or be normal.
- Since the chest radiograph may not correlate with the arterial Po_2, an arterial blood gas (ABG) analysis to assess oxygen saturation and metabolic acidosis is important.

EMERGENCY DEPARTMENT CARE AND DISPOSITION

- All patients should have their airway, ventilation, and oxygenation status assessed, and the cervical spine should be stabilized and evaluated in cases of diving accidents, multiple trauma, or if the circumstances are unknown.
- Warmed IV normal saline and warming adjuncts (overhead warmer, bear hugger, etc) should be used if the patient is hypothermic. The patient's core temperature should be monitored.
- Patients with a Glasgow Coma Scale (GCS) score ≥14 should receive supplemental oxygen to maintain oxygen saturation (Sao_2) >95%. They may be discharged home after a 4- to 6-hour observation period as long as their pulmonary and neurologic examinations and Sao_2 remain normal.
- The patient with an oxygen requirement or abnormal examination after 4 to 6 hours should be admitted.
- Patients with a GCS <14 should be administered supplemental oxygen. Intubation and mechanical ventilation are indicated if the Pao_2 cannot be maintained >60 mm Hg in adults or >80 mm Hg in children, despite high-flow oxygen (40 to 60%).
- Childhood victims of fresh water near drowning rarely develop dilutional hyponatremia and seizures, which are usually easily controlled by correction of the electrolyte abnormality.
- Prophylactic antibiotics are not indicated since the development of bacterial pneumonia is rare.
- Efforts at "brain resuscitation," including the use of mannitol, loop diuretics, hypertonic saline, fluid restriction, mechanical hyperventilation, controlled hypothermia, barbiturate coma, and intracranial pressure monitoring have not shown benefit.[6,8]
- Asystole in the out-of-hospital arena or in the emergency department is a poor prognostic sign in pediatric warm-water submersion injuries, but there are anecdotal reports of neurologic recovery.[6] Patients with short warm-water submersion time and short transport time should undergo vigorous resuscitation attempts.
- Continuous infusion of vasopressors may be required in the postresuscitation phase.
- Consideration should be given to withholding resuscitation in patients with prolonged submersion and transport.
- Reports of complete and near complete neurologic recovery after asystole in adults and children have been reported in prolonged icy-water submersion.
- Hypothermic victims of cold-water submersion in cardiac arrest should undergo prolonged and aggressive resuscitation maneuvers until they are normothermic or considered not viable.

REFERENCES

1. Drownings in a Private Lake—North Carolina, 1981–1990. *MMWR* 41;329, 1991.
2. Goksor E, Rosengren L, Wennergren G: Bradycardic response during submersion in infant swimming. *Acta Paediatr* 1:307, 2002.
3. Steinman A, Geisbrecht G: Immersion into cold water, in Auerbach PS, (ed.): *Wilderness Medicine,* 4th ed. St. Louis: Mosby, 2001, p. 197.
4. Hwang V, Shofer FS, Durbin DR, et al: Prevalence of traumatic injuries in drowning and near drowning in children and adolescents. *Arch Pediatr Adolesc Med* 157:50, 2003.
5. Watson RS, Cummings P, Quan L, et al: Cervical spine injuries among submersion victims. *J Trauma* 51:658, 2001.
6. Ibsen LM, Koch T: Submersion and asphyxial injury. *Crit Care Med* 30:S402, 2002.
7. Orlowski JP, Szpilman D: Drowning. Rescue, resuscitation, and reanimation. *Pediatr Clin North Am* 48:627, 2001.
8. Spack L, Gedeit R, Splaingard M: Failure of aggressive therapy to alter outcome in pediatric near-drowning. *Pediatr Emerg Care* 13:98, 1997.

For further reading in *Emergency Medicine: A Comprehensive Study Guide,* 6th ed., Chap. 198, "Near Drowning," by Alan L. Causey and Mark A. Nichter.

128 THERMAL AND CHEMICAL BURNS

Robert J. French

THERMAL BURNS

EPIDEMIOLOGY

- The American Burn Association estimates that approximately 1 million burn injuries occur each year, which result in 700,000 emergency department (ED) visits, 45,000 hospitalizations, and 4500 deaths.[1]
- Nearly 70% of pediatric burn injuries are due to scalds. Flame injuries are more common in working-age adults. Up to 20% of pediatric burn injuries result from child abuse.[2]
- The risk of burns is highest in the 18- to 35-year-old age group. The death rate in patients over 65 years of age is much higher than in the overall burn population.[3,4]
- The risk of death from a major burn is associated with increased burn size, increased age, concomitant inhalation injury, and female sex.[4]
- Significant advances in burn management have decreased the mortality rate for major thermal burns to 4%.[5]

PATHOPHYSIOLOGY

- Local effects of thermal injury include both direct tissue coagulation and microvascular reactions that lead to the release of vasoactive substances such as histamine, serotonin, arachidonic acid metabolites, and free oxygen radicals.
- These vasoactive substances increase capillary permeability and lead to egress of fluid from the intravascular space to interstitial areas adjacent to the burn wound. In larger burns, this extravascular fluid shift, coupled with evaporative water loss, causes hypovolemic shock.
- Burn size greater than 20% of body surface area (BSA) results in a systemic response, with interstitial edema developing in distant organs and soft tissues.[2] This systemic response occurs secondary to wound release of vasoactive mediators and hypoproteinemia.[2] The intensity of this systemic response is proportional to the size of the burn.
- After successful fluid resuscitation, a hypermetabolic response occurs with a near doubling of the cardiac output and basal metabolic rate.[2]
- A full-thickness burn is described as having three concentric zones of tissue injury. Extending peripherally from the central zone, these areas are: (1) the zones of coagulation, where tissue is irreversibly destroyed by thrombosis of blood vessels; (2) the zones of stasis, where tissue is viable but there is stagnation of the microcirculation; and (3) the zones of hyperemia, where tissue is viable and there is increased blood flow.
- Transformation of the zone of stasis to coagulation is attributed to the degree of dermal ischemia and reflects inadequate resuscitation.

CLINICAL FEATURES

- Burns are categorized by their size and depth. Burn size is calculated as the percentage of total BSA involved.[6]
- The most common method to estimate the percentage of BSA burned is the "rule of nines" (Figure 128-1).
- A more accurate tool to determine the percentage of BSA burned, especially in infants and children, is the Lund and Browder burn diagram (Figure 128-2). This chart accounts for age-specific differences in body part proportions.
- For smaller burns, the patient's hand can be used as a "ruler" to estimate percent BSA. This area represents approximately 1% of the patient's BSA.
- Burn depth has historically been described in degrees: first, second, third, and fourth.[7]
- A more clinically relevant classification scheme used to determine the need for surgical intervention categorizes burns as: superficial partial-thickness, deep partial-thickness, and full-thickness.[2]

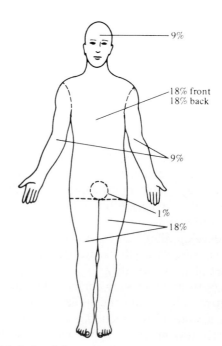

FIG. 128-1. Rule of nines to estimate percentage of burn.

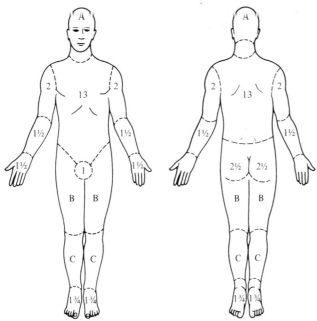

Relative Percentages of Areas Affected by Growth (Age in Years)

	0	1	5	10	15	Adult
A: half of head	9½	8½	6½	5½	4½	3½
B: half of thigh	2¾	3¼	4	4¼	4½	4¾
C: half of leg	2½	2½	2¾	3	3¼	3½

Second-degree _____ and

Third-degree _____ =

Total percent burned ____

FIG. 128-2. Lund and Browder diagram to estimate percentage of pediatric burn.

- Superficial partial-thickness burns blister and cause pain. The exposed dermis is red and moist with intact capillary refill. Healing occurs in 14 to 21 days with little or no scar formation.
- Deep partial-thickness burns are white to yellow in color. Pressure applied to the skin can be felt, but two-point discrimination is diminished. Capillary refill and pain sensation are absent.
- Deep partial-thickness burns are difficult to differentiate from full-thickness burns. Healing occurs in 3 weeks to 3 months and scarring is common.
- Full-thickness burns are charred, pale, leathery, and painless. These injuries do not heal spontaneously since all dermal elements are destroyed. Surgical repair and skin grafting is needed.
- Smoke inhalation injury occurs most frequently in closed-space fires and in patients with decreased cognition (eg, alcohol intoxication, drug abuse, head injury, dementia).
- Smoke inhalation injury can occur to both the upper and lower airways due to exposure from heat, particulate matter, and toxic gases.[8]

- Upper airway edema, secondary to thermal injury, can result in acute airway compromise.
- Signs of pulmonary smoke inhalation injury are often delayed by 12 to 24 hours and include cough, wheezing, and respiratory distress.
- Clinical indicators of smoke inhalation injury include facial burns, singed nasal hair, soot in the nose or mouth, hoarseness, carbonaceous sputum, and wheezing.
- Carbon monoxide poisoning should be suspected in all patients with smoke inhalation injury. Clinical signs include headache, vomiting, confusion, lethargy, and coma.

DIAGNOSIS AND DIFFERENTIAL

- Burns can be classified as major, moderate, or minor.
- Examples of major burns include: (1) partial-thickness burns >20% BSA in adults or >10% BSA in children (<10 years old) or older adults (>50 years old), (2) full-thickness burns >5% BSA, (3) significant burns to face, eyes, ears, genitalia, hands, feet, or major joints, and (4) concomitant smoke inhalation or major trauma.
- Examples of minor burns include: (1) partial-thickness burns <10% BSA in adults or <5% BSA in children or older adults and (2) full-thickness burns <2% BSA.
- Moderate burns are those not meeting criteria for either major or minor burns.
- The diagnosis of smoke inhalation injury is primarily made on clinical history of enclosed-space fire with exam findings of facial burns, singed nasal hairs, carbonaceous sputum, soot in mouth and nose, and/or wheezing.
- The chest radiograph in smoke inhalation injury may be normal initially. Flexible fiberoptic bronchoscopy can confirm the diagnosis.[9]
- Carboxyhemoglobin levels should be obtained if carbon monoxide poisoning is suspected.

EMERGENCY DEPARTMENT CARE AND DISPOSITION

- Emergent priorities remain airway, breathing, and circulation. High-flow oxygen should be administered.
- If there are signs of airway compromise or an airway burn, then the patient should undergo endotracheal intubation for airway protection.
- Indicators for emergent intubation include oral/perioral burns, circumferential neck burns, stridor, depressed mental status, or respiratory distress.
- At least two IV lines should be established over unburned areas.

- Initial fluid resuscitation, which should be guided by the Parkland formula, is 2 to 4 mL/kg times the percentage of BSA burned per 24 hours. Half the calculated amount is given in the first 8 hours postinjury and the remainder over the next 16 hours. Lactated Ringer's solution is recommended.
- The 24-hour time interval begins from the time the patient sustained the burn injuries, not the time of resuscitation onset. The percentage BSA used in this calculation should include only second- and third-degree burns.
- A Foley catheter should be placed and urine output maintained at 0.5 to 1 mL/kg/h. Other physiologic resuscitative guides include mental status, capillary refill, blood pressure, pulse rate, and base deficit.
- Burns should be immediately cooled by immersion in cold water or application of a cool compress. Immediate cooling of small wounds helps limit burn depth and decrease release of damaging inflammatory mediators.
- Prolonged cooling of larger-BSA burns for greater than 30 minutes can result in severe hypothermia. Ice should not be applied directly to the wound because it can cause tissue injury from frostbite.
- Intravenous narcotic analgesia should be administered early and titrated to the patient's pain. Anxiolytic agents should be used as an adjuvant in pain management.
- Minor burns can be treated as an outpatient. Large blisters (>2 cm) or those involving mobile joints should be drained or debrided.[10,11] Small blisters on non-mobile areas should be left intact.
- Topical antibiotics should be used to prevent wound infection and sepsis.[2,6] The most common agent is 1% silver sulfadiazine, which has low systemic toxicity, broad antibiotic spectrum, and can be applied painlessly.
- Alternate topical agents such as bacitracin or triple-antibiotic (neomycin, polymyxin B, and bacitracin zinc) ointment can be used.
- Synthetic occlusive dressings instead of topical agents are another method of managing partial-thickness wounds as an outpatient.
- Moderate and major burns require inpatient admission. These patients should generally be referred to a hospital with a burn center.
- The American Burn Association's burn unit referral criteria are listed in Table 128-1.
- After evaluation and resuscitation, sterile drapes should be placed over the burns. Topical antibiotic agents should not be used until the admitting service evaluates the burn wound.
- Empiric IV antibiotics for moderate and major burns are not recommended.
- Patients with circumferential burns of the limbs may develop compromise of the distal circulation. Circumferential burns of the chest and neck may cause

TABLE 128-1 American Burn Association Burn Unit Referral Criteria

Partial-thickness burns greater than 10% total body surface area (BSA)

Burns that involve the face, hand, feet, genitalia, perineum, or major joints

Third-degree burns in any age group

Electrical burns, including lightning injury

Chemical burns

Inhalation injury

Burn injury in patients with pre-existing medical disorders that could complicate management, prolong recovery, or affect mortality

Any patients with burns and concomitant trauma (such as fractures) in which the burn injury poses the greatest risk of morbidity or mortality

Burned children in hospitals without qualified personnel or equipment for the care of children

Burn injury in patients who will require special social, emotional, or long-term rehabilitative intervention

SOURCE: American Burn Association, www.ameriburn.org.

mechanical ventilatory restriction. Escharotomy may be needed in these cases.
- Treatment of inhalation injury may include humidified oxygen, endotracheal intubation and mechanical ventilation, bronchodilators, and pulmonary toilet.
- Hyperbaric oxygen therapy is used for severe carbon monoxide poisoning.
- Routine tetanus toxoid prophylaxis should be administered based on the patient's immunization history. Tetanus immune globulin should be given in patients without primary immunization.

CHEMICAL BURNS

EPIDEMIOLOGY

- Chemical burn injuries account for 5 to 10% of burn center admissions. Common household chemical burns are caused by lye (drain cleaner), halogenated hydrocarbons (paint removers), phenols (deodorizers, disinfectants), sodium hypochlorite (bleach), and sulfuric acid (toilet bowl cleaner).
- Body sites most often burned by chemicals are the face, eyes, and extremities.
- Although chemical burns are smaller and have a lower mortality rate than thermal burns, wound healing and length of hospital stay are longer.

PATHOPHYSIOLOGY

- Contact with chemical agents can result in burns, irritant contact dermatitis, allergic reaction, thermal injury, or systemic toxicity.

- Skin damage by chemicals can be similar to thermal injury, ranging from superficial erythema to full-thickness loss. Chemical burns may initially appear deceptively mild, but progress to more extensive skin damage and systemic toxicity.
- The majority of chemical burns are caused by acids or alkalis. Alkalis usually produce far more tissue damage than acids.
- Most acid burns cause a coagulation necrosis with protein precipitation and formation of leathery eschar. This eschar forms a barrier which helps limit the penetration of the acid.
- Alkalis (lye, lime, Portland cement) combine with protein and fat in skin tissue to form soluble protein complexes and soaps. The resulting liquefaction necrosis permits the passage of hydroxyl ions into deep tissues.

CLINICAL FEATURES

- Skin damage from chemical burns depends on the type of agent, concentration, volume, and duration of exposure.
- Hydrochloric and sulfuric acid, if not decontaminated early, can produce a coagulation necrosis that results in dark brown or black skin discoloration.
- Hydrofluoric (HF) acid emulates alkali burns in that it rapidly penetrates the skin and can cause progressive pain and tissue destruction. The onset of pain can be delayed up to 12 hours postexposure.
- The presenting complaint of acute topical HF acid exposure is pain, often in the absence of any physical evidence of burn. As tissue injury progresses, the involved skin may develop a blue-gray appearance with surrounding erythema.
- Since alkalis cause liquefaction necrosis, deep tissue destruction may result. Soft, gelatinous, brownish eschars may form. Wounds that initially appear superficial may progress to full-thickness.
- Airbags deploy by ignition of a solid propellant (sodium azide) that creates an exothermic reaction and certain corrosive by-products (sodium hydroxide, nitric oxide, and ammonia).
- Airbag deployment may cause a combination of friction, thermal, and chemical burns.[12–14]
- Chemical burns of the eye are true ocular emergencies and cause redness, pain, and tearing.
- Acid ocular burns quickly precipitate proteins in the superficial eye structures, resulting in the typical "ground glass" appearance.
- Alkali ocular burns are more severe due to deeper penetration secondary to liquefaction necrosis. Severe chemosis, blanched conjunctiva, and an opacified cornea that obscures the view of the iris and lens can occur.

- Blindness can result from retinal penetration with destruction of sensory elements.
- Lacrimators (tear gas) such as chloroacetophenone (CN), chlorobenzylidenemalonitrile (CS), dibenzoxazepine (CR), and trichloronitromethane (pepper mace) can cause ocular, mucous membrane, and pulmonary irritation.

DIAGNOSIS AND DIFFERENTIAL

- For ocular exposures, pH paper can help distinguish alkali from acid exposure.

EMERGENCY DEPARTMENT CARE AND DISPOSITION

- The first priority in treatment of chemical burns is to terminate the burning process. This is accomplished by removal of garments and copious irrigation.
- Dry chemical particles should be manually removed before irrigation.
- Elemental metals (sodium, lithium, calcium, magnesium) can ignite spontaneously when exposed to air.
- Water should not be used to extinguish burning particles because of the explosive exothermic reaction that results. These burning elemental metal particles should be covered with mineral oil or extinguished with a class D fire extinguisher.
- In cases of ocular exposure to alkalis, acids, or lacrimators, eye irrigation with 1 to 2 L of normal saline for a minimum of 1 hour is needed.
- With alkali or acid ocular exposure, return of the pH to neutral (pH 7.4) is a measurable end point for irrigation. Visual acuity check should follow, not precede, ocular irrigation.
- Phenol and phenolic compounds should be irrigated with water immediately. Water lavage may be ineffective since the phenol compound may become entrapped beneath the water-impermeable necrotic eschar. In these cases, phenol should be decontaminated with a polyethylene glycol solution (PEG 300 or PEG 400), glycerol, or isopropyl alcohol.
- In addition to copious irrigation, HF acid burns often require calcium gluconate to bind fluoride and neutralize its toxic effects.
- Calcium gluconate can be administered as: (1) calcium gluconate gel applied topically (mixed with Surgilube or dimethyl sulfoxide to a concentration of 2.5 to 10%), (2) subcutaneous and intradermal injection of 5% calcium gluconate via 30-gauge needle with a maximum dose of 1 mL for each square centimeter of burned tissue, and (3) intra-arterial infusion of calcium gluconate.[15]

- Systemic toxicity can result from topical exposure of certain chemical agents such as: (1) acids (acidosis, hypotension, and shock), (2) oxalic and HF acid (hypocalcemia, hypomagnesemia, hyperkalemia, cardiac arrhythmias, and sudden death), (3) tannic, formic, and chromic acid (hepatic necrosis and nephrotoxicity), and (4) phenol and creosol (methemoglobinemia, massive hemolysis, and multisystem organ failure).
- After initial measures, treatment is similar to that of thermal burns, with IV fluid resuscitation, analgesia, and tetanus immunoprophylaxis.

REFERENCES

1. American Burn Association: Burn incidence fact sheet. Accessed at www.ameriburn.org, June 13, 2003.
2. Sheridan RL: Burns. *Crit Care Med* 30(11 Suppl):S500, 2002.
3. Ryan CM, Schoenfeld DA, Thorpe WP, et al: Objective estimates of the probability of death from burn injuries. *N Engl J Med* 338:362, 1988.
4. Mueller MJ, Pegg SP, et al: Determination of death following burn injury. *Br J Surg* 88:583, 2001.
5. Saffle JR, Davis B, Williams P, American Burn Association Registry Participant Group: Recent outcome of burn injury in the United States: A report from the American Burn Association Patient Registry. *J Burn Care Rehabil* 16:219, 1995.
6. Saffle J: *Practice Guidelines for Burn Care.* Chicago: American Burn Association, 2001, p. 175.
7. Hendricks WM: The classification of burns. *J Am Acad Dermatol* 22:853, 1998.
8. Hartzel GE: Overview of combustion toxicology. *Toxicology* 115:7, 1996.
9. Becker DG, Himmel HN, et al: Salvage of a patient with burn inhalation injury and pancreatitis. *Burns* 19:444, 1993.
10. Jordan BS, Harrington DT: Management of the burn wound in burn management. *Nurs Clin North Am* 32:251, 1997.
11. Robson MC, et al: Acute management of the burned patient. *Plast Reconstr Surg* 89:1155, 1992.
12. Swanson-Bierman B: Air-bags: lifesaving with toxic potential? *Am J Emerg Med* 11:38, 1993.
13. Hallock GG: Mechanism of burn injury secondary to airbag deployment. *Ann Plast Surg* 39:111, 1997.
14. Ulrich D, et al: Burn injuries caused by airbag deployment. *Burns* 27:196, 2001.
15. Vance MV, et al: Digital hydrofluoric acid burn treatment with intra-arterial calcium infusion. *Ann Emerg Med* 15:890, 1988.

For further reading in *Emergency Medicine: A Comprehensive Study Guide,* 6th ed., see Chap. 199, "Thermal Burns," by Lawrence R. Schwartz and Chenicheri Balakrishnan; and Chap. 200, "Chemical Burns," by Fred P. Harchelroad, Jr. and David M. Rottinghaus.

129 ELECTRICAL AND LIGHTNING INJURIES

Howard E. Jarvis III

ELECTRICAL INJURIES

EPIDEMIOLOGY

- An estimated 17,000 patients per year are treated in emergency departments for electrical injury. In 1998, 550 electrocution deaths were reported in the U.S.[1]
- Toddlers (with electrical cords and appliances), teenagers (with risk-taking behavior), and professionals working with electricity are groups at increased risk.

PATHOPHYSIOLOGY

- Electrical current flow is measured in amperes (A). Current flows when there is a potential difference between two locations; this is measured in volts (V). The intervening material resists the flow of current; this is measured in ohms of resistance (R).
- Current can either be continuous in one direction (direct current, DC) or in alternating directions (alternating current, AC).
- Factors associated with severity of electrical injuries include the amount, duration, type (AC or DC), the current path through the body, and environmental factors (eg, water immersion).
- Electrical energy in tissues can cause burns (entry and exit), thermal heating, flash and arc burns, blunt trauma, and muscular tetany.
- Low-voltage AC current will cause muscular tetany, causing the injured person to continually grasp the source, increasing contact time.
- High-voltage AC and DC currents cause a single violent muscular contraction, which tends to throw the victim from the source, thus increasing the risk of blunt trauma and blast injuries.
- Electricity causes damage by direct effects of current upon cells and by thermal damage from the heat generated by the resistance of tissues.
- Energy is greatest at the contact point; thus the skin often has the greatest visible damage.
- The exit wound is often larger than the entrance site.

CLINICAL FEATURES

- As current flows through the body, the greatest damage is sustained by nerves, blood vessels, and muscles.

- This may result in coagulation necrosis, neuronal death, and damage to blood vessels. As a result, the overall picture often resembles a crush injury more than a thermal burn.
- Traumatic injuries frequently accompany electrical injuries.
- Specific complications of electrical injuries are summarized in Table 129-1.
- Low-voltage AC current tends to cause ventricular fibrillation while high-voltage AC and DC current tend to cause asystole and respiratory arrest.
- Oral burns in children may have delayed labial artery bleeding (up to 2 weeks later).

DIAGNOSIS AND DIFFERENTIAL

- Diagnosis of electrical injury is usually based on history.
- The type of current (high-tension wires produce the greatest injury), and surrounding circumstances, such as falls or intoxication, should be noted.
- In unclear cases, characteristic skin lesions or oral lesions in children may be helpful.
- The creatine kinase (CK-MB) may be elevated without myocardial damage due to extensive muscle injury.

- Computed tomographic (CT) scanning of the head is indicated for those with severe head injury, coma, or unresolving mental status changes.

EMERGENCY DEPARTMENT CARE AND DISPOSITION

- The airway, breathing, and circulation should be stabilized. Spinal immobilization should be instituted for any unwitnessed events or when there is a potential for spine injury.
- High-flow oxygen should be administered by face mask.
- Patients should have continuous cardiac monitoring, pulse oximetry, noninvasive blood pressure monitoring, and preferably two large-bore IV lines.
- Ventricular fibrillation, asystole, or ventricular tachycardia should be treated by standard Advanced Cardiac Life Support (ACLS) protocols. Other dysrhythmias are usually transient and do not need immediate therapy.
- IV crystalloid fluid should be given with an initial bolus of 20 to 40 mL/kg over the first hour. Fluid requirements are generally higher than those of thermal burn patients.

TABLE 129-1 Complications of Electrical Injuries

Cardiovascular	Sudden death (ventricular fibrillation, asystole), chest pain, dysrhythmias, ST-T segment abnormalities, bundle-branch block, myocardial damage, ventricular dysfunction, myocardial infarction (rare), hypotension (volume depletion), hypertension (catecholamine release)
Neurologic	Altered mental status, agitation, coma, seizures, cerebral edema, hypoxic encephalopathy, headache, aphasia, weakness, paraplegia, quadriplegia, spinal cord dysfunction (may be delayed), peripheral neuropathy, cognitive impairment, insomnia, emotional lability
Cutaneous	Electrothermal contact injuries, noncontact arc and "flash" burns, secondary thermal burns (clothing ignition, heating of metal)
Vascular	Thrombosis, coagulation necrosis, disseminated intravascular coagulation, delayed vessel rupture, aneurysm, compartment syndrome
Pulmonary	Respiratory arrest (central or peripheral; eg, muscular tetany), aspiration pneumonia, pulmonary edema, pulmonary contusion, inhalation injury
Renal/metabolic	Acute renal failure (due to heme pigment deposition and hypovolemia), myoglobinuria, metabolic (lactic) acidosis, hypokalemia, hypocalcemia, hyperglycemia
Gastrointestinal	Perforation, stress ulcer (Curling's ulcer), GI bleeding, GI tract dysfunction, various reports of lethal injuries at autopsy
Muscular	Myonecrosis, compartment syndrome
Skeletal	Vertebral compression fractures, long bone fractures, shoulder dislocations (anterior and posterior), scapular fractures
Ophthalmologic	Corneal burns, delayed cataracts, intraocular hemorrhage or thrombosis, uveitis, retinal detachment, orbital fracture
Auditory	Hearing loss, tinnitus, tympanic membrane perforation (rare), delayed mastoiditis or meningitis
Oral burns	Delayed labial artery hemorrhage, scarring and facial deformity, delayed speech development, impaired mandibular/dentition development
Obstetric	Spontaneous abortion, fetal death

TABLE 129-2   Indications for Admission for Patients with Electrical Injuries

High voltage >600 V

Symptoms suggestive of systemic injury
   Cardiovascular: chest pain, palpitations
   Neurologic: loss of consciousness, confusion, weakness, headache, paresthesias
   Respiratory: dyspnea
   Gastrointestinal: abdominal pain, vomiting

Evidence of neurologic or vascular injury to a digit or extremity

Burns with evidence of subcutaneous tissue damage

Dysrhythmia or abnormal electrocardiogram

Suspected foul play, abuse, suicidal intent, or unreliable social situation

High-risk exposures

Associated injuries requiring admission

Comorbid diseases (cardiac, renal, neurologic)

- If evidence of rhabdomyolysis is present, then fluid loading is desirable to prevent renal failure.
- Tetanus prophylaxis should be given. Prophylactic antibiotics are not necessary initially unless large open wounds are present.
- Seizures are treated with standard therapy.
- It is appropriate to consult a general surgeon if there is evidence of systemic or deep tissue injury. These patients may require formal wound exploration, débridement, fasciotomy, and long-term care.
- Children with oral injuries should be evaluated by an ENT specialist or plastic surgeon.
- All pregnant patients should undergo obstetric consultation for admission and fetal monitoring.
- Table 129-2 summarizes admission criteria. Patients with an unclear history of exposure or degree of injury should be admitted.
- Children with isolated oral injuries or isolated hand wounds can usually be discharged. Parents should be given instructions for controlling delayed labial artery bleeding.[2]
- Asymptomatic patients with household voltage exposure (110 to 220 volts), a normal electrocardiogram (ECG), and a normal examination may be discharged.

LIGHTNING INJURIES

EPIDEMIOLOGY

- There are about 300 lightning injuries reported each year in the United States, with approximately 100 deaths.[3]
- Unlike electrical injuries, extensive tissue damage and renal failure are rare, though as many as 75% of survivors sustain significant morbidity and permanent sequelae.[4]

- Sports, particularly water sports, and transportation are associated with increased risk of lightning injury.

PATHOPHYSIOLOGY

- Lightning is DC current imparting a single extremely high-voltage discharge of energy.
- Lightning injures can result via direct strike, side flash (current flows over from another struck object), contact strike (a person touching a struck object), ground current (passing through the ground and transferred to a standing person), or step potential (ground strike passes up a person's leg and down through the other leg).

CLINICAL FEATURES

- Lightning injuries can vary in severity depending on the circumstances of the strike, and range from minor injuries to cardiac arrest.
- Minor injuries produce a stunned patient. They may have signs of confusion, amnesia, and short-term memory problems. Other symptoms include headache, muscle pain, paresthesias, and temporary visual or auditory problems.
- Most patients with minor lightning injuries have a gradual improvement and few long-term sequelae.
- Complications associated with lightning injuries are summarized in Table 129-3.

DIAGNOSIS AND DIFFERENTIAL

- The diagnosis of lightning injury is based on history and should be considered in a patient found unconscious or in arrest who was outside during appropriate weather conditions.
- Pupillary dilatation or anisocoria may occur and have no prognostic value.
- Ruptured tympanic membranes or fern-like erythematous skin markings should alert the physician to potential lightning injury.
- Misdiagnoses include stroke or intracranial hemorrhage, seizure disorder, and cerebral, spinal cord, or other neurologic trauma.

EMERGENCY DEPARTMENT CARE AND DISPOSITION

- Aggressive resuscitation measures are indicated, as survival has been reported after prolonged respiratory arrest.[5,6]

TABLE 129-3   Complications Associated with Lightning Injuries

SYSTEM	INJURY
Cardiovascular	Dysrhythmias (asystole, ventricular fibrillation/tachycardia, premature ventricular contractions), electrocardiographic changes, myocardial infarction (unusual)
Neurologic	(Immediate or delayed, permanent or transient). Loss of consciousness, confusion, amnesia, intracranial hemorrhage, hemiplegia, amnesia, respiratory center paralysis, cerebral edema, neuritis, seizures, Parkinsonian syndromes, cerebral infarction, myelopathy, progressive muscular atrophy, progressive cerebellar syndrome, transient paralysis, paresthesias, myelopathy, autonomic dysfunction
Cutaneous	Burns (first- to third-degree), scars, contractures
Ophthalmologic	Cataracts (often delayed), corneal lesions, uveitis, iridocyclitis, vitreous hemorrhage, macular degeneration, optic atrophy, diplopia, chorioretinitis, retinal detachment, hyphema
Otologic	Tympanic membrane rupture, temporary or permanent deafness, tinnitus, ataxia, vertigo, nystagmus
Renal	Myoglobinuria, hemoglobinuria, renal failure (rare)
Obstetric	Fetal death, placental abruption
Miscellaneous	Secondary blunt trauma, compartment syndrome, disseminated intravascular coagulation

- Spinal immobilization should be used in unwitnessed events or when there is potential spine injury.
- Continuous cardiac monitoring, pulse oximetry, non-invasive blood pressure monitoring, and at least one large-bore IV should be utilized.
- Hypotension is unexpected and should prompt investigation for hemorrhage.
- High-flow oxygen should be administered by face mask.
- Ventricular tachycardia or fibrillation and asystole should be treated with standard ACLS protocols.
- Fluid resuscitation is usually unnecessary.
- Tetanus prophylaxis should be given.
- Seizures may be treated with standard therapy.
- Those with moderate or severe injuries should be admitted to a critical care unit with appropriate consultation.
- Most patients with minor injuries should be admitted for close monitoring of cardiac and neurologic status.
- All pregnant patients should be admitted and undergo fetal monitoring.

REFERENCES

1. Hiser S: 1998 Electrocutions associated with consumer products. Washington, D.C.: U.S. Consumer Product Safety Commission, 2001. http://www.cpsc.gov/library/shock98.pdf.
2. Garcia CT, Smith GA, Cohen DM, et al: Electrical injuries in a pediatric emergency department. *Ann Emerg Med* 26:604, 1995.
3. Centers for Disease Control: Lightning-associated injuries and deaths among military personnel—United States 1998–2001. *MMWR* 51:859, 2002.
4. Muehlberger T, Vogt PM, Munster AM: The long-term consequences of lightning injuries. *Burns* 27:829, 2001.
5. Cooper MA: Emergent care of lightning and electrical injuries. *Semin Neurol* 15:268, 1995.
6. European Resuscitation Council: Part 8: Advanced Challenges in Resuscitation. Section 3: Special challenges in ECG. 3G: Electric shock and lightning strikes. *Resuscitation* 46:297, 2000.

For further reading in *Emergency Medicine: A Comprehensive Study Guide*, 6th ed., see Chap. 201, "Electrical Injuries"; and Chap. 202, "Lightning Injuries," by Raymond M. Fish.

130   CARBON MONOXIDE

Christian A. Tomaszewski

EPIDEMIOLOGY

- Carbon monoxide is responsible for greater morbidity and mortality than any other toxin.[1]
- Carbon monoxide is formed from the incomplete combustion of any fossil fuel (eg, gasoline, kerosene, natural gas, charcoal) or tobacco, and as a metabolite of methylene chloride (paint remover).
- Carbon monoxide toxicity is more common in northern climates and during winter months.

PATHOPHYSIOLOGY

- Carbon monoxide is an odorless, nonirritating, colorless gas with the capability to cause clinical problems with ambient levels as low as 200 parts per million (ppm).
- Carbon monoxide competes with oxygen at binding sites on hemoglobin, myoglobin, and cytochrome aa_3, thus interfering with oxygen delivery and utilization.
- Carbon monoxide binds to hemoglobin about 240 times more tenaciously than oxygen. The binding of carbon monoxide to hemoglobin shifts the oxyhemoglobin dissociation curve to the left. Therefore carboxyhemoglobin (COHb) holds on to oxygen at lower oxygen tensions.
- When carbon monoxide binds to mitochondrial cytochromes, it stops the electron chain reaction and prevents oxidative phosphorylation.[2]
- Poisoning of the myocardial myoglobin reduces cardiac contractility, cardiac output, and oxygen delivery.
- The combination of decreased oxygen utilization and hypotension can cause ischemic reperfusion injury during recovery from carbon monoxide poisoning.
- White blood cells adhere to the endothelium, particularly of the brain microvasculature. Oxidation free radicals and excitatory neurotransmitters are then produced during reperfusion, leading to lipid peroxidation and subsequent neuronal cell death.[3]

CLINICAL FEATURES

- Clinical symptoms and signs of carbon monoxide poisoning primarily relate to the cardiovascular and neurologic systems.
- Patients initially present with flu-like symptoms: headache, dizziness, nausea, and vomiting.
- With increasing exposure, the patient may develop dyspnea, altered mental status, coma, seizures, and respiratory arrest.
- Cardiovascular signs and symptoms include chest pain from myocardial ischemia, palpitations from dysrhythmias, hypotension, and ultimately, cardiac arrest.
- Patients occasionally may develop rhabdomyolysis and subsequent renal failure if unconscious for a prolonged period.
- Survivors of acute carbon monoxide poisoning are still susceptible to secondary problems, primarily from the ischemic reperfusion injury.
- They may develop persistent or delayed neurologic sequelae, resulting in deficiencies in learning and memory, chronic headaches, and parkinsonism.
- Early predictors of such sequelae are alterations in mental status or cerebellar dysfunction (abnormal past-pointing or ataxia).[4]
- Fetuses and neonates are particularly susceptible to the toxic effects of carbon monoxide due to the presence of fetal hemoglobin and an oxygen dissociation curve that is already shifted to the left. The result is an increase in stillbirths and cranial and limb malformations.[5]

DIAGNOSIS AND DIFFERENTIAL

- Any patient with flu-like illness, particularly in winter with any carbonaceous heating source, should be considered for COHb determination.
- COHb determination can be done by co-oximeter on venous blood, even hours old, provided it has been drawn in a closed heparinized tube.
- Although COHb levels confirm exposure, they do not correlate with symptoms or prognosis, partly because of variability in initial treatment with oxygen and delay to testing. Generally, a level greater than 10% confirms poisoning in smokers; greater than 5% in nonsmokers.
- Pulse oximetry, although useful if abnormal, overestimates the oxygen saturation of hemoglobin. It confuses COHb for oxyhemoglobin, providing false reassurance.[6]
- The half-life of COHb is 3 to 4 hours when the patient breathes room air, 60 minutes when breathing 100% room pressure oxygen, and 23 minutes when breathing 100% hyperbaric oxygen (HBO) at 2.8 atmospheres absolute of pressure.[7]
- Although COHb may help confirm exposure, careful neurologic examination will help determine seriousness of poisoning and potential need for HBO therapy.[8,9]
- A bedside mini-mental status examination may reveal memory and learning deficits. In addition, patients may have cerebellar dysfunction manifested by abnormal past-pointing or ataxia.
- Arterial blood gas may be useful to determine base deficit.
- In susceptible patients complaining of chest pain or who may be unconscious, electrocardiogram (ECG) and cardiac enzyme determinations are recommended.
- Chest radiographs are generally obtained for smoke inhalation victims.
- In comatose patients with poor prognosis, computed tomography (CT) scan or magnetic resonance imaging (MRI) of the brain may identify generalized cerebral edema or specific lesions, particularly lesions of the basal ganglia, which bodes a poor prognosis.[10]
- The differential diagnosis for carbon monoxide poisoning is extremely broad because of the wide spectrum of disease entities associated with dizziness, headache, or nausea. A variety of toxins, infectious agents, and cardiac diseases may account for the signs and symptoms of carbon monoxide poisoning.
- Smoke inhalation victims, particularly if enclosed during exposure, should be evaluated specifically for carbon monoxide poisoning.

TABLE 130-1   Indications for Hyperbaric Oxygen Treatment Within 24 Hours of Acute Carbon Monoxide Poisoning

DEFINITE INDICATION	RELATIVE INDICATION
Abnormal neurological examination (ie, altered mental status, coma)	Persistent neurological symptoms (eg, headache or dizziness) after 4 hours of 100% normobaric oxygen
Syncope	Carboxyhemoglobin level >25%
Seizure	Persistent metabolic acidosis (base deficit >2 mmol/L)
Cerebellar dysfunction (eg, abnormal past-pointing, ataxia)	Pregnancy (particularly if symptomatic with elevated level >10% or fetal distress)
	Myocardial ischemia

EMERGENCY DEPARTMENT CARE AND DISPOSITION

- Initially, patients must be removed from the source of exposure and immediate attention focused on the airway, breathing, and circulation.
- High-flow 100% oxygen should be administered with a tight-fitting mask and reservoir; cardiac monitoring and IV access should be established. Oxygen therapy should be continued until the patient becomes asymptomatic.
- HBO therapy is indicated for severe poisoning based upon clinical findings and the COHb level (Table 130-1).
- COHb levels over 25% and base deficit of greater than 2 mmol/L are also worrisome.
- The goal of treatment is not only amelioration of the acute event, but more importantly, prevention of delayed neuropsychiatric sequelae.[8,11]
- HBO therapy should be strongly considered for patients at the extremes of age and in pregnancy, which is not a contraindication to treatment.

REFERENCES

1. Mah JC: Non-fire carbon monoxide deaths associated with the use of consumer products. 1998 annual estimates. Bethesda, MD: Consumer Product Safety Commission, 1998.
2. Brown SD, Piantadosi CA.: Recovery of energy metabolism in rat brain after carbon monoxide hypoxia. *Ann Neurol* 89:666, 1992.
3. Thom SR, Fisher D, Manevich Y: Roles for platelet-activating factor and nitric oxide-derived oxidants causing neutrophil adherence after CO poisoning. *Am J Physiol Heart Circ Physiol* 281:H923, 2001.
4. Choi HS: Delayed neurological sequelae in carbon monoxide intoxication. *Arch Neurol* 40:435, 1983.
5. Koren G, Sharav T, Pastuszak S, et al: A multicenter, prospective study of fetal outcome following accidental carbon monoxide poisoning in pregnancy. *Reprod Toxicol* 3:397, 1991.
6. Bozeman WP, Myers RA, Barish RA: Confirmation of the pulse oximetry gap in carbon monoxide poisoning. *Ann Emerg Med* 30:608, 1997.
7. Tomaszewski C: Carbon monoxide, in, Ford M, Delaney KA, Ling LJ, Erickson T (eds.): *Clinical Toxicology*. Philadelphia: WB Saunders, 2001, p. 657.
8. Weaver LK, Hopkins RO, Chan KJ, et al: Hyperbaric oxygen for acute carbon monoxide poisoning. *N Engl J Med* 347: 1057, 2002.
9. Messier LD, Myers RA: A neuropsychological screening battery for emergency assessment of carbon monoxide poisoning. *J Clin Psychol* 47:675, 1991.
10. Pracyk JB, Stolp BW, Fife CE, et al: Brain computed tomography after hyperbaric oxygen therapy for carbon monoxide poisoning. *Undersea Hyperbaric Med* 22:1, 1995.
11. Thom SR, Taber RL, Mendiguren II, et al: Delayed neuropsychologic sequelae after carbon monoxide poisoning: prevention by treatment with hyperbaric oxygen. *Ann Emerg Med* 25:474, 1995.

For further reading in *Emergency Medicine: A Comprehensive Study Guide*, 6th ed., see Chap. 203, "Carbon Monoxide Poisoning," by Keith W. Van Meter.

131   POISONOUS PLANTS AND MUSHROOMS

Sandra L. Najarian

EPIDEMIOLOGY

- Mushrooms are among the more common toxic exposures, with approximately 5 ingestions for every 100,000 people in 1996.[1]
- *Amanita* species are responsible for 95% of fatalities associated with mushrooms in the United States.
- Young children account for 70 to 80% of all plant-related exposures.

PATHOPHYSIOLOGY

- Various toxins found in plants and mushrooms produce effects ranging from mild gastrointestinal (GI) symptoms to organ failure and death.
- Mushrooms with psilocybin- and psilocin-containing toxins have neuroactive chemicals similar to lysergic acid diethylamide (LSD), which produce hallucinogenic effects; they are often intentionally ingested for their mind-altering effects.

- Gyromitrin is a volatile, heat-labile toxin hydrolyzed in the stomach. It is converted to a free radical in the liver that causes local hepatic necrosis and inhibits the activity of the cytochrome P450 system, glutathione, and other hepatic enzyme systems.[2]
- Amatoxins are absorbed in the intestines and enter the enterohepatic circulation; they bind to hepatocytes and inhibit formation of messenger RNA.[3]
- Ricin, a potent toxalbumin found in castor beans, produces severe cytotoxic effects in multiple organ systems.
- Amygdalin, found in the pits of peaches, apricots, pears, crab apples, and hydrangea, is metabolized to hydrocyanic acid, and can lead to acute cyanide poisoning if ingested in sufficient quantities.

CLINICAL FEATURES

- Nausea, vomiting, hematemesis, abdominal pain, and diarrhea (at times bloody) may follow ingestion of *Actaea* (baneberry), *Abrus,* aloe, *Cicuta maculata* (water hemlock), *Conium* (poison hemlock), *Convallaria* (lily of the valley), *Daphne, Euphorbia* (poinsettia), *Ilex* (holly), *Phytolacca* (pokeweed), rhododendron, *Ricinus, Solanum* (nightshades), and *Taxus* (yews). Fatalities occur from electrolyte abnormalities.
- Cicutoxin, found in water hemlock, produces severe GI symptoms, followed by delirium, seizures, and death.
- Direct irritation and chemical burns to the oropharynx have been reported after ingestion of *Actaea, Abrus* (rosary pea), *Capsicum* (ornamental peppers), *Daphne, Dieffenbachia,* and rhododendron.
- Cardiovascular symptoms, including hypotension, dysrhythmias, and conduction defects, have been reported after ingestion of *Convallaria, Taxus,* rhododendron, and oleander, and may be life-threatening.
- Jimson weed contains atropine-like alkaloids that can cause an acute anticholinergic crisis.
- Urushiol, found in *Toxicodendron* species (poison ivy, oak, and sumac), produces a contact dermatitis in sensitized individuals.
- Andromedotoxin, in *Rhododendron* species, produces a cholinergic syndrome.
- Hallucinations have been reported with *Actaea* ingestion.
- Seizures may be seen after ingestion of *Conium, Actaea,* and *Ricinus.*
- Early toxicity of mushroom poisoning (within 1 hour of ingestion) generally indicates a benign course.
- Delayed toxicity of mushroom poisoning (greater than 6 hours) suggests a more toxic ingestion, which can lead to hepatic failure, renal failure, and even death (Table 131-1).
- Ingestion of *Gyromitra* and *Amanita* species of mushrooms produces delayed onset of GI symptoms 6 to 48 hours after ingestion. Manifestations of hepatic failure, intestinal necrosis, and renal failure develop 1 to 3 days after exposure.
- Cortinarius species of mushroom contain the nephrotoxic compounds orellanine and orelline, which result in delayed onset of GI symptoms 1 to 3 days after ingestion and delayed renal failure 3 to 20 days after ingestion.
- Consuming alcohol after ingestion of coprine-containing mushrooms will result in a disulfiram-like reaction. Facial flushing, nausea and vomiting, diaphoresis, palpitations, hypotension, and weakness can be observed 2 to 72 hours after ingestion.
- Mushrooms with ibotenic acid and muscimol present with early-onset anticholinergic symptoms.
- *Inocybe* and *Clitocybe* species containing muscarine cause early-onset cholinergic and muscarinic effects, characterized by the SLUDGE syndrome (**S**alivation, **L**acrimation, **U**rination, **D**efecation, **G**astrointestinal hypermotility, and **E**mesis).

DIAGNOSIS AND DIFFERENTIAL

- Diagnosis of plant and mushroom poisoning is clinical, based on history of ingestion and onset of symptoms, and should be considered in patients at risk who present with gastroenteritis.
- Physical examination should include a search for evidence of cholinergic, anticholinergic, or sympathetic nervous system stimulation.
- If symptoms suggest cytotoxic mushroom poisoning, electrolytes, blood urea nitrogen, creatinine, liver enzymes, and coagulation studies should be obtained.

EMERGENCY DEPARTMENT CARE AND DISPOSITION

- Initial treatment for plant-related and mushroom poisoning is supportive, with priority given to airway management, ventilation, and fluid resuscitation.
- Activated charcoal should be administered to decontaminate the GI tract.
- Whole bowel irrigation is indicated for patients who may have ingested cytotoxic mushrooms and present within 24 hours.
- High-dose penicillin therapy (0.3 to 1.0 million units/kg/day of penicillin G) is the most effective therapy for amatoxin poisoning; it blocks the uptake of amatoxin into the liver.[4]
- High-dose cimetidine (10 g/day) also has been found to be effective for amatoxin poisoning.[5] Hemodialysis and hemoperfusion, once thought to be the standard of care, have limited use.

TABLE 131 1 Mushrooms: Symptoms, Toxicity, and Treatment

SYMPTOMS	MUSHROOMS	TOXICITY	TREATMENT
Gastrointestinal symptoms Onset <2 h	*Chlorophyllum molybdites* *Omphalotus illudens* *Cantharellus cibarius* *Amanita caesarea*	Nausea, vomiting, diarrhea (occasionaly bloody)	IV hydration Antiemetics
Onset 6–24 h	*Gyromitra esculenta:* fall season *Amanita phalloides, Amanita verna,* and *Amanita virosa:* spring season	Initial: nausea, vomiting, diarrhea Day 2: rise in AST, ALT Day 3: hepatic failure	IV hydration, glucose, monitor AST, ALT, PT, PTT, bilirubin, BUN, creatinine For *Amanita:* activated charcoal Penicillin G 300,000–1,000,000 units/kg per day Silymarin 20–40 mg/kg per day Consider cimetidine 4–10 g/day Hyperbaric oxygen
Muscarinic syndrome Onset <30 min	*Inocybe* *Clitocybe*	SLUDGE	Supportive atropine 0.01 mg/kg repeated as needed for severe secretions
CNS excitement Onset <30 min	*Amanita muscaria* *Amanita pantherina*	Intoxication, dizziness, ataxia, visual disturbances, seizures, tachycardia, hypertension, warm dry skin, dry mouth, mydriasis (anticholinergic effects)	Supportive sedation with phenobarbital 30 mg IV or diazepam 2–5 mg IV as needed for adults
Hallucinations Onset <30 min	*Psilocybe* *Gymnopilus*	Visual hallucinations, ataxia	Supportive sedation with phenobarbital 0.5 mg/kg or, for adults 30–60 mg IV, or diazepam 0.1 mg/kg or 5 mg IV for adults
Disulfiram 2–72 h after mushroom, and <30 min after alcohol	*Coprinus*	Headache, flushing, tachycardia, hyperventilation, shortness of breath, palpitations	Supportive IV hydration β-blockers for supraventricular tachycardia Norepinephrine for refractory hypotension

ABBREVIATIONS: ALT = alanine aminotransferase; AST = aspartate aminotransferase; BUN = blood urea nitrogen; CNS = central nervous system; PT = prothrombin time; PTT = partial thromboplastin time; SLUDGE syndrome = salivation, lacrimation, urination, defecation, gastrointestinal hypermotility, and emesis.

- Emergent liver transplant is indicated for patients with an aspartate aminotransferase (AST) level >2000 IU, grade 2 hepatic encephalopathy, and prothrombin time >50 seconds despite therapy.[6]
- High-dose pyridoxine (25 mg/kg) is recommended for patients presenting with neurologic symptoms associated with gyromitrin.
- Fluid and electrolyte replacement and hemodialysis are the mainstays of treatment for orellanine/orelline toxicity.
- Atropine should be administered to patients with severe muscarinic symptoms.
- Patients with potential amatoxin, gyromitrin, or orellanine/orelline poisoning, or those with refractory symptoms, require admission and monitoring for at least 48 hours. All other patients who are asymptomatic after 4 to 6 hours of treatment and observation can be discharged.

REFERENCES

1. Litovitz TL, Smilkstein M, Felberg L, et al: Annual report of the American Association of Poison Control Centers Toxic Exposure Surveillance System. *Am J Emerg Med* 15:447, 1997.
2. Michelot S, Toth B: Poisoning by *Gyromitra esculenta:* A review. *J Appl Toxicol* 11:235, 1991.
3. Lindell TJ, Weinberg F, Morris PW, et al: Specific inhibition of nuclear RNA polymerase II by alpha-amanitin. *Science* 170:447, 1970.
4. Floersheim GL, Schneeberger J, Buschner K: Curative potencies of penicillin in experimental *Amanita phalloides* poisoning. *Agents Actions* 2:138, 1971.
5. Schneider SM, Borochovitz D, Krenzelok EP: Cimetidine protection against alpha-amanitin hepatotoxicity in mice: A potential model for the treatment of *Amanita phalloides* poisoning. *Ann Emerg Med* 16:1136, 1987.
6. Fanatozzi R, Ledda F, Caramelli L, et al: Clinical findings and follow-up evaluation of an outbreak of mushroom poisoning: Survey of *Amanita phalloides* poisoning. *Klin Wochenschr* 64: 38, 1986.

For further reading in *Emergency Medicine: A Comprehensive Study Guide,* 6th ed., see Chap. 204, "Mushroom Poisoning," by Sandra M. Schneider and Anne Brayer; and Chap. 205, "Poisonous Plants," by Mark A. Hostetler and Sandra M. Schneider.

132 DIABETIC EMERGENCIES

Michael P. Kefer

HYPOGLYCEMIA

EPIDEMIOLOGY

- Patients on insulin or oral hypoglycemic agents are especially at risk for hypoglycemia. Up to 20% of these individuals will experience hypoglycemia that requires emergency department care.[1-3] Patients with alcoholism, sepsis, adrenal insufficiency, or malnutrition are also at risk.
- Repaglinide and nateglinide increase insulin secretion. These are known to cause hypoglycemia.
- Metformin increases insulin effects and decreases glucose production. Acarbose and miglitol decrease the gastrointestinal absorption of carbohydrates. Rosiglitazone and pioglitazone decrease insulin resistance and glucose production. None of these agents used alone are associated with hypoglycemia.

PATHOPHYSIOLOGY

- Glucose is the main energy source of the brain. Severe hypoglycemia can cause brain damage or death.
- Serum glucose is dependent upon hormonal balance between insulin and the counterregulatory hormones epinephrine, glucagon, cortisol, and growth hormone. Excess insulin, either relative or absolute, will result in decreased glucose production and utilization.

CLINICAL FEATURES

- Typical symptoms of hypoglycemia include sweating, shakiness, anxiety, nausea, dizziness, confusion, blurred vision, headache, and lethargy.
- Typical signs include diaphoresis, tachycardia, and almost any neurologic finding, ranging from altered mental status or tremor to focal neurologic deficit or seizure.

DIAGNOSIS AND DIFFERENTIAL

- The diagnosis is based on a low serum glucose level in conjunction with the clinical features.
- The differential diagnosis is wide due to the nonspecific signs and symptoms manifested in patients with hypoglycemia. It can easily be misdiagnosed as a primary neurologic, psychiatric, or cardiovascular condition.

EMERGENCY DEPARTMENT CARE AND DISPOSITION

- Glucose should be administered orally or intravenously as the condition warrants. IV treatment begins with 1 g/kg of dextrose as a 50% solution.
- A continuous infusion of 10% dextrose solution may be required to maintain the serum glucose level above 100 mg/dL.
- Hypoglycemia refractory to glucose administration may require hydrocortisone 100 mg IV or glucagon 1 mg IV.
- Glucagon 1 mg intramuscularly (IM) or subcutaneously (SC) may be required if IV access cannot be obtained.

- Octreotide, a somatostatin analogue, has been used in preventing recurrent sulfonylurea-induced hypoglycemia.[4]
- Factors to be considered in determining disposition include the patient's response to treatment, etiology of hypoglycemia, existing comorbid conditions, and social situation.
- Most diabetics with insulin reactions respond rapidly to treatment. They can be discharged with instructions to continue oral intake of carbohydrates and to closely monitor their fingerstick glucose level.
- Patients with prolonged or recurrent hypoglycemia, which can result from use of the sulfonylureas, should be admitted.

DIABETIC KETOACIDOSIS

EPIDEMIOLOGY

- Diabetic ketoacidosis (DKA) occurs predominantly in type 1 insulin-dependent diabetics, but does occur in type 2 non–insulin-dependent diabetics.[5]
- New-onset diabetes mellitus presents as DKA in 25% of cases.[6]
- Mortality is 5%, and it is higher in the elderly.[6]

PATHOPHYSIOLOGY

- DKA is precipitated by noncompliance with insulin therapy or any type of physiologic stress such as infection, stroke, myocardial infarction, trauma, or pregnancy.
- DKA results from a relative insulin deficiency and counterregulatory hormone excess, resulting in cellular starvation.
- Insulin acts on the liver to promote glucose storage as glycogen, on adipose tissue to promote storage of triglycerides, and on skeletal muscle to promote protein synthesis. Although serum glucose levels are high, cells cannot use glucose as fuel in the absence of insulin.
- The counterregulatory hormones epinephrine, glucagon, cortisol, and growth hormone have the opposite effect of insulin. Glycogenolysis releases glucose stores. Proteolysis and lipolysis result in release of amino acids and glycerol, respectively, for gluconeogenesis to synthesize more glucose.
- Free fatty acids are metabolized in the liver to the ketone bodies β-hydroxybutyrate, acetoacetate, and acetone. However, these also are unable to be used as fuel by cells in the absence of insulin.
- Hyperglycemia results in an osmotic diuresis with volume depletion and electrolyte loss.

- Ketonemia results in a high anion-gap metabolic acidosis with myocardial depression, vasodilation, and compensatory hyperpnea (Kussmaul's respiration).

CLINICAL FEATURES

- Clinical manifestations are directly related to metabolic derangements.
- Hyperglycemia causes an osmotic diuresis with dehydration, hypotension, and tachycardia.
- Ketonemia causes an acidosis with myocardial depression, vasodilation, and compensatory Kussmaul's respiration. Nausea, vomiting, and abdominal pain are also common.
- Inappropriate normothermia is seen clinically, so infection must be considered even in the absence of fever.

DIAGNOSIS AND DIFFERENTIAL

- The diagnosis of DKA is based on the clinical presentation and laboratory values of a glucose above 250 mg/dL, bicarbonate level below 15 mEq/L, pH below 7.3, and the presence of a moderate ketonemia.[6,7]
- β-Hydroxybutyrate is the reduced form of acetoacetate. In DKA, reduction of acetoacetate to β-hydroxybutyrate is favored. As a result, in advanced cases, acetoacetate levels are low and β-hydroxybutyrate levels are high.
- If the nitroprusside test is used to detect serum or urine ketones, results may be falsely low or negative because this test detects acetoacetate and not β-hydroxybutyrate.
- Sodium, chloride, calcium, phosphorus, and magnesium levels may be low from osmotic diuresis.
- Pseudohyponatremia is common: for each 100 mg/dL increase in the glucose level, there is a 1.6 mEq/L decrease in sodium.
- Serum potassium may be low (from osmotic diuresis and vomiting), normal, or high (from acidosis since acidosis drives potassium out of cells). The patient who is acidotic with a normal or low potassium level has a marked depletion of total body potassium.
- Ketonemia results in an anion-gap metabolic acidosis $[Na^+ - (Cl^- + HCO_3^-) > 12 \pm 4 \text{ mEq/L}]$.
- The differential diagnosis includes other causes of an anion-gap metabolic acidosis recalled by the acronym "MUDPILES" (see Table 104-1). Hypoglycemia and hyperosmolar hyperglycemic state also should be considered.

EMERGENCY DEPARTMENT CARE AND DISPOSITION

- The goal of treatment is to correct hypovolemia, ketonemia, acidosis, and electrolyte abnormalities, and treat the underlying cause.
- Isotonic fluid resuscitation is the most important initial step to restore intravascular volume and tissue perfusion. The average patient in DKA has a body water deficit of 5 to 10 L. The first liter should be administered over 30 to 60 minutes.
- Once intravascular volume is restored, or if the serum sodium is above 155 mEq/L, hypotonic solution should be infused to provide free water for intracellular volume replacement.6 Patients with heart disease may need invasive monitoring to avoid congestive heart failure.
- Insulin is required to shut off ketosis and resume glucose utilization. Insulin should be administered by continuous infusion. This allows close control of effect, compared to the IM or SC route, where absorption may be erratic or delayed in an unstable patient.
- The half-life of regular insulin is 5 minutes when administered IV and 2 hours when administered IM or SC. Initiating a continuous infusion of insulin at 0.1 U/kg/h is recommended. A loading dose of 0.1 U/kg IV is optional.[6–8] If there is no response within the first hour of treatment, insulin resistance is suggested and the infusion rate is doubled each hour until a response is obtained.
- Hyperglycemia is controlled much more rapidly with insulin than is ketoacidosis. To reverse ketoacidosis, insulin treatment must continue despite decreasing serum glucose. Therefore, to prevent hypoglycemia, glucose infusion will be necessary when the serum glucose level falls below 300 mg/dL.
- Potassium should be administered to maintain normal serum levels. Upon initiating treatment for DKA, potassium levels will fall due to dilution from volume replacement, correction of acidosis, renal excretion, and the insulin effect of driving potassium intracellularly.
- To avoid the dangerous effects of hypokalemia, if the potassium level is below 3.3 mEq/L, potassium replacement should begin 30 minutes before insulin is administered, and immediately if the level is between 3.3 and 5 mEq/L and urine output is adequate.
- To avoid the dangerous effects of hyperkalemia, potassium should not be administered until the level is below 5 mEq/L. Potassium chloride 10 to 20 mEq may be added to each liter of IV fluid as required by close monitoring of serum potassium.
- Potassium phosphate 10 to 20 mEq may be used if phosphorus supplementation is also required. Phosphorus replacement is recommended if the serum level is below 1 mg/dL.
- Phosphorus has an important role in energy production (ATP), oxygen delivery (2,3-DPG), and enzymatic reactions. Acute deficiency has been associated with all types of muscle dysfunction.
- Magnesium is administered if levels are low or the patient has symptoms of hypomagnesemia.
- Bicarbonate therapy remains controversial as to when the benefits of correcting the effects of acidosis (vasodilation, depression of cardiac contractility and respiration, central nervous system depression) outweigh the risks of bicarbonate treatment (paradoxical cerebrospinal fluid acidosis, hypokalemia, impaired oxyhemoglobin dissociation, rebound alkalosis, sodium overload). This therapy is recommended as a last resort in the face of severe acidosis.[8,9]
- The serum glucose, anion gap, potassium, and bicarbonate levels should be monitored hourly until recovery is well established.
- Cerebral edema occurs predominantly in children. It tends to develop 4 to 12 hours into treatment and manifests as a deterioration in neurologic function.[10]
- Cerebral edema has been associated with rehydration rates exceeding 50 mL/kg in the first 4 hours of treatment, so this rate serves as a guideline.[11] Treatment with mannitol 1 g/kg should be initiated before the diagnosis is confirmed by computed tomography.

HYPEROSMOLAR HYPERGLYCEMIC STATE

EPIDEMIOLOGY

- The American Diabetes Association recommends hyperosmolar hyperglycemic state (HHS) as the current terminology for the condition previously referred to as nonketotic hyperosmolar coma.
- HHS occurs in poorly-controlled type 2 diabetics. Like DKA, it is a relatively common presentation of new-onset diabetes mellitus. Precipitating factors are the same as those for DKA.
- The mortality rate of HHS is 15 to 30% compared to 5% for DKA.[6]

PATHOPHYSIOLOGY

- HHS occurs in the type 2 diabetic when insulin resistance results in decreased utilization of glucose.
- Serum glucose increases, which results in an osmotic diuresis causing glucosuria and volume depletion.
- Initially, a contraction metabolic alkalosis occurs. With progressive hypovolemia, a metabolic acidosis develops from azotemia and lactic acidosis.

CLINICAL FEATURES

- The typical patient is elderly with type 2 diabetes, presents with complaints of weakness or mental status changes, and has pre-existing renal or heart disease. Because metabolic changes progress slowly, symptoms often signal advanced HHS.
- Physical examination reveals signs of dehydration with orthostasis, dry skin and mucous membranes, and altered mental status. Kussmaul's respiration and the smell of acetone on the breath are not present.
- Mental status changes range from confusion to coma. Focal deficits and focal or generalized seizures also occur.

DIAGNOSIS AND DIFFERENTIAL

- The diagnosis is based on clinical and laboratory findings. HHS is differentiated from DKA by a greater degree of hyperglycemia, a lesser degree of acidosis, and absent or minimal serum and urine ketones.
- Laboratory findings include serum glucose above 600 mg/dL, bicarbonate level above 15 mEq/dL, and pH above 7.3. Ketosis is absent or mild.
- Sodium, potassium, chloride, calcium, phosphorus, and magnesium levels may be low from osmotic diuresis. Pseudohyponatremia is common.

EMERGENCY DEPARTMENT CARE AND DISPOSITION

- The goal of treatment is to correct hypovolemia and electrolyte abnormalities and treat the underlying cause.
- Isotonic 0.9% NS should be used initially to restore intravascular volume. This should be followed by hypotonic 0.45% NS to provide free water to restore intracellular volume.[6]
- The average fluid deficit is 8 to 12 L. One half of the deficit should be replaced over 12 hours and the other half over the next 24 hours.
- Particularly in children, a rehydration rate of slower than 50 mL/kg in the first 4 hours is recommended to avoid cerebral edema.
- Potassium, magnesium, and phosphorus replacement principles are identical to those of DKA.
- An insulin drip 0.1 U/kg/h can be initiated. In less severe cases the patient will correct with fluids alone or may require 1 to 2 bolus doses of regular insulin 0.1 U/kg in conjunction with fluid therapy.

REFERENCES

1. Hayward RA, Manning WG, Kaplan SH, et al: Starting insulin therapy in patients with type 2 diabetes: Effectiveness, complications, and resource utilization. *JAMA* 278:1663, 1997.
2. Anonymous: Hypoglycemia in the Diabetes Control and Complications Trial: The Diabetes Control and Complications Trial Research Group. *Diabetes* 46:271, 1997.
3. Shorr RI, Ray WA, Daugherty JR, Griffin MR: Incidence and risk factors for serious hypoglycemia in older persons using insulin or sulfonylureas. *Arch Intern Med* 157:1681, 1997.
4. MacLaughlin SA, Crandell CS, McKinney PE: Octreotide: An antidote for sulfonylurea-induced hypoglycemia. *Ann Emerg Med* 36:133, 2000.
5. Westphal SA: The occurrence of diabetic ketoacidosis in non-insulin-dependent diabetes and newly diagnosed diabetic adults. *Am J Med* 101:19, 1996.
6. American Diabetes Association: Hyperglycemic crises in patients with diabetes mellitus. *Diabetes Care* 25:S100, 2002.
7. Umpierrez GE, Khajavi M, Kitabchi AE: Review: Diabetic ketoacidosis and hyperosmolar hyperosmolar nonketotic syndrome. *Am J Med Sci* 310:225, 1996.
8. Levobitz HE: Diabetic ketoacidosis. *Lancet* 345:767, 1995.
9. Viallon A, Zeni F, Lafond P, et al: Does bicarbonate therapy improve the management of severe diabetic ketoacidosis? *Crit Care Med* 27:2690, 1999.
10. Edge J: Cerebral oedema during treatment of diabetic ketoacidosis: Are we any nearer finding a cause? *Diabetes Metab Res Rev* 16:316, 2000.
11. Hoffman WH, Steinhart CM, Gammal TE, et al: Cranial CT in children and adolescents with diabetic ketoacidosis. *AJNR Am J Neuroradiol* 9:733, 1988.

For further reading in *Emergency Medicine: A Comprehensive Study Guide*, 6th ed., see Chap. 210, "Hypoglycemia," by William Brady and Richard A. Harrigan; Chap. 211, "Diabetic Ketoacidosis," by Michael E. Chansky and Cary L. Lubilin; and Chap. 214, "Hyperosmolar Hyperglycemic State," by Charles S. Graffeo.

133 ALCOHOLIC KETOACIDOSIS
Michael P. Kefer

EPIDEMIOLOGY

- Alcoholic ketoacidosis (AKA) can occur in either first-time drinkers or chronic alcoholics. Recurrence has been reported in up to 23% of patients.[1]

PATHOPHYSIOLOGY

- AKA results from heavy ethanol intake, either acute or chronic, and minimal to no food intake. Glycogen stores become depleted and insulin secretion is suppressed.
- To maintain a supply of glucose, the counterregulatory hormones glucagon, growth hormone, cortisol, and epinephrine are released.
- Fat and ethanol oxidation become the body's primary substrate for energy production, resulting in the formation of the ketone bodies β-hydroxybutyrate, acetoacetate, and acetone.
- Acetone is rapidly excreted. Acetoacetate and β-hydroxybutyrate accumulate, resulting in a metabolic acidosis.
- β-Hydroxybutyrate is the reduced form of acetoacetate. In AKA, the reduction of acetoacetate to β-hydroxybutyrate is favored. As a result, in advanced cases, acetoacetate levels are low and β-hydroxybutyrate levels are high.
- If the nitroprusside test is used to detect serum or urine ketones, results may be falsely low or negative because this test only detects acetoacetate and not β-hydroxybutyrate.[2]

CLINICAL FEATURES

- The patient with alcoholic ketoacidosis typically presents with complaints of nausea, vomiting, orthostasis, and abdominal pain 24 to 72 hours after the last alcohol intake.
- Physical examination reveals the patient to be acutely ill and dehydrated with a tender abdomen. Abdominal tenderness is typically diffuse and nonspecific or is a result of other causes associated with the use of alcohol, such as gastritis, hepatitis, or pancreatitis.
- The presentation may be confounded by other complications of alcoholism, such as infection or alcohol withdrawal.

DIAGNOSIS AND DIFFERENTIAL

- Laboratory investigation reveals an anion-gap ($Na^+ - [Cl^- + HCO_3^-] > 12 \pm 4$ mEq/L) metabolic acidosis.
- The serum pH may be low, normal, or high, as these patients often have mixed acid-base disorders, such as a metabolic acidosis from alcoholic ketoacidosis and a metabolic alkalosis from vomiting and volume depletion.
- Blood glucose ranges from low to mildly elevated.

- The alcohol level is usually low or zero, as vomiting and abdominal pain limit intake.
- Serum ketones, acetoacetate, and β-hydroxybutyrate are elevated. Although ketones are usually detected in significant amounts, the redox state may be such that most or all acetoacetate is reduced to β-hydroxybutyrate, resulting in a false negative or falsely low estimate of the severity of ketoacidosis.
- If the diagnosis is unclear, serum levels of acetoacetate and β-hydroxybutyrate can be measured directly.
- Approximately 15% of patients with AKA will have a negative urine nitroprusside test.[1]
- The diagnosis of alcoholic ketoacidosis is established in the patient with a history of recent heavy alcohol consumption, decreased food intake, vomiting, abdominal pain, and laboratory findings of an anion-gap metabolic acidosis, a positive nitroprusside test for ketones, and a low to mildly elevated glucose.
- The differential diagnosis includes other causes of an anion-gap metabolic acidosis, commonly recalled by the acronym MUDPILES (see Table 104-1).

EMERGENCY DEPARTMENT CARE AND DISPOSITION

- Treatment of alcoholic ketoacidosis consists of IV infusion of D_5NS. The crystalloid solution restores intravascular volume.
- Glucose administration stimulates insulin release, which inhibits ketosis. Unlike treatment for diabetic ketoacidosis, insulin administration is not necessary, as endogenous insulin secretion occurs normally with restoration of volume and glucose administration.
- Administration of thiamine 50 to 100 mg IV is recommended before glucose administration to prevent precipitation of Wernicke's disease.
- Other electrolytes and vitamins should be supplemented as the condition warrants.
- Treatment should be continued until the acidosis is reversed, which is usually within 12 to 18 hours, and the patient is tolerating oral intake.

REFERENCES

1. Wrenn KD, Slovis CM, Minion GE, et al: The syndrome of alcoholic ketoacidosis. *Am J Med* 91:119, 1991.
2. Umpierrez GE, DiGirolamo M, Tuvlin JA, et al: Differences in metabolic and hormonal milieu in diabetic and alcohol induced ketoacidosis. *J Crit Care* 15:52, 2000.

For further reading in *Emergency Medicine: A Comprehensive Study Guide,* 6th ed., see Chap. 213, "Alcoholic Ketoacidosis," by William A. Woods and Debra G. Perina.

134   THYROID DISEASE EMERGENCIES

Matthew A. Bridges

NORMAL THYROID STATE

- Synthesis and release of thyroid hormone are controlled by thyroid-stimulating hormone (TSH) from the anterior pituitary. Release of TSH is regulated by thyroid-releasing hormone from the hypothalamus.
- Circulating levels of thyroxine (T_4) and L-triiodothyronine (T_3) provide feedback regulation.
- Thyroid hormone is reversibly bound to thyronine-binding globulin and other circulating proteins.
- Unbound hormone is biologically active, predominantly as T_4. T_4 is deiodinated in the periphery to T_3, a more active hormone with a shorter half-life than T_4.

HYPERTHYROIDISM

- Hyperthyroidism is uncommon under the age of 15, and is 10 times more common in women.
- Graves' disease is the most common cause of hyperthyroidism, followed by toxic multinodular and toxic nodular goiters. Graves' disease is common in the third and fourth decades of life.
- Clinical features of Graves' disease include diffuse goiter, ophthalmopathy, and dermopathy.
- Symptoms of hyperthyroidism include heat intolerance, palpitations, weight loss, sweating, tremors, nervousness, weakness, and fatigue.
- Laboratory tests reveal an elevated free T_4 and low or undetectable TSH level. Occasionally, in Graves' disease, the T_4 may be normal and TSH decreased. A T_3 level should be checked to exclude T_3 toxicosis.

THYROID STORM

PATHOPHYSIOLOGY

- Thyroid storm is a life-threatening hypermetabolic state due to hyperthyroidism. It is most often seen in patients with unrecognized or undertreated hyperthyroidism.
- Mortality is high (10 to 75%) despite treatment.
- Precipitants of thyroid storm include infection, trauma, diabetic ketoacidosis (DKA), myocardial infarction, stroke, pulmonary embolism, surgery, withdrawal of thyroid medication, iodine administration, palpation of the thyroid gland, ingestion of thyroid hormone, and idiopathic causes (20 to 25%).
- Generally, thyroid hormone levels do not help to differentiate between symptomatic, uncomplicated hyperthyroidism, and thyroid storm.

CLINICAL FEATURES

- The signs and symptoms associated with thyroid storm are related to enhanced sympathetic nervous system activity. The most common signs are fever, tachycardia, altered mental status, and diaphoresis.[1]
- Clues to the diagnosis include a history of hyperthyroidism, exophthalmos, a widened pulse pressure, and a palpable goiter.
- Central nervous system (CNS) disturbances are common and include confusion, delirium, seizure, and coma.
- Cardiovascular abnormalities are often present, with sinus tachycardia most common. Other dysrhythmias include atrial fibrillation and premature ventricular contractions. Patients may present with signs and symptoms of congestive heart failure.
- Gastrointestinal (GI) symptoms such as diarrhea and hyperdefecation occur in most patients. Apathetic thyrotoxicosis is a distinct presentation seen in elderly patients, in which the characteristic symptoms are absent, and lethargy, slowed mentation, and apathetic facies are seen. Goiter, weight loss, and proximal muscle weakness are present.

DIAGNOSIS AND DIFFERENTIAL

- Thyroid storm is a clinical diagnosis, as laboratory tests do not help to distinguish it from thyrotoxicosis.
- Diagnostic criteria include fever; tachycardia out of proportion to fever; dysfunction of the CNS, cardiovascular, and/or GI systems; and exaggerated peripheral manifestations of thyrotoxicosis.
- In this clinical setting, an elevated T_4 level and a suppressed TSH level confirm the diagnosis.
- The differential diagnosis includes sepsis, other causes of congestive heart failure, stroke, complications of diabetes (eg, DKA or hypoglycemia), heat stroke, delirium tremens, malignant hyperthermia, neuroleptic malignant syndrome, pheochromocytoma, medication withdrawal, and sympathomimetic drug overdose.

TABLE 134-1   Drug Treatment of Thyroid Storm

Decrease de novo synthesis:

Propylthiouracil	600–1000 mg PO initially, followed by 200–250 mg q4h
Methimazole	40 mg PO initial dose, then 25 mg PO q6h

Prevent release of hormone (after synthesis blockade initiated):

Iodine	Iapanoic acid (Telepaque) 1 g IV q8h for the first 24 h, then 500 mg IV bid *or*
	Potassium iodide (SSKI) 5 drops PO q6h *or*
	Lugol solution 8–10 drops PO q6h
Lithium carbonate	800–1200 mg PO per day

Prevent peripheral effects:

β-blockade	Propranolol (IV) titrate 1 to 2 mg q5min prn (may need 240–480 mg PO per day) *or*
	Esmolol (IV) 500 μg/kg IV bolus, then 50–200 μg/kg per min maintenance
Guanethidine	30–40 mg PO q6h
Reserpine	2.5–5 mg IM q4–6h

Other considerations:

Corticosteroids	Hydrocortisone 100 mg IV q8h *or* Dexamethasone 2 mg IV q6h
Antipyretics	Cooling blanket Acetaminophen 650 mg PO q4h

EMERGENCY DEPARTMENT CARE AND DISPOSITION

- Treatment can be divided into five areas: general supportive care, inhibition of thyroid hormone synthesis, retardation of thyroid hormone release, blockade of peripheral thyroid hormone effects, and identification and treatment of precipitating events.
- Airway stabilization, supplemental oxygen, intravenous fluids, and cardiac monitoring are indicated.
- The pharmacologic treatment of thyroid storm is summarized in Table 134-1.
- Appropriate cultures and antibiotics may be indicated.
- In cases in which clinical deterioration occurs despite appropriate therapy, direct removal by exchange transfusion, plasma transfusion, plasmapheresis, and charcoal plasma perfusion may successfully remove thyroid hormone.
- All patients should be monitored closely and admitted to the intensive care unit.

HYPOTHYROIDISM

PATHOPHYSIOLOGY

- Hypothyroidism occurs with insufficient hormone production or secretion and is more common in women than in men.
- The most common etiologies are primary thyroid failure due to autoimmune disease (Hashimoto's thyroiditis), idiopathic causes, ablative surgery, or iodine deficiency.

- Postpartum thyroiditis occurs within 3 to 6 months postpartum and occurs in 2 to 16% of women.
- Secondary hypothyroidism is due to pituitary tumors, infiltrative disease, or hemorrhage. Tertiary hypothyroidism is due to hypothalamic disease.
- Medications that cause hypothyroidism include amiodarone (due to release of iodine during metabolism of the drug), and lithium, which mimics iodine and inhibits thyroid hormone release.

CLINICAL FEATURES

- The typical symptoms of hypothyroidism include fatigue, weakness, cold intolerance, constipation, weight gain, and deepening of voice.
- Cutaneous signs include dry, scaly, yellow skin; nonpitting, waxy edema of the face and extremities (myxedema); and thinning eyebrows.
- Cardiac findings include bradycardia, enlarged heart, and low-voltage electrocardiogram (ECG).
- Paresthesia, ataxia, and prolongation of the deep tendon reflexes are characteristic neurologic findings.
- A thyroidectomy scar may be present, but a goiter is uncommon.

EMERGENCY DEPARTMENT CARE AND DISPOSITION

- Most patients with uncomplicated symptomatic hypothyroidism may be referred to their primary care physician for further evaluation and initiation of treatment.
- Thyroid hormone therapy may exacerbate some secondary etiologies and therefore is rarely initiated in the emergency department.

MYXEDEMA COMA

CLINICAL FEATURES

- Myxedema coma is a rare, life-threatening expression of severe hypothyroidism.
- Myxedema coma is most often seen during the winter months in elderly women with undiagnosed or undertreated hypothyroidism.
- Precipitating events of myxedema coma include infection, congestive heart failure, drugs, trauma, and exposure to a cold environment.
- In addition to all of the features of hypothyroidism, the patient with myxedema coma may present with hypothermia, altered mental status, hyponatremia, hypoglycemia, hypotension, and bradycardia.
- Respiratory failure with hypoventilation, hypercapnia, and hypoxia is common.

- Delusions and psychosis (myxedema madness) may occur.
- Cardiac findings include bradycardia, enlarged heart, and a low-voltage ECG.

DIAGNOSIS AND DIFFERENTIAL

- The diagnosis of myxedema coma must be suspected based upon the clinical presentation.
- Confirmatory thyroid tests will typically demonstrate a low free T_4 level and elevated TSH.
- The patient's core temperature will be low.
- The differential diagnosis of myxedema coma includes coma secondary to respiratory failure, hyponatremia, hypothermia, congestive heart failure, stroke, and drug overdose.

EMERGENCY DEPARTMENT CARE AND DISPOSITION

- Airway stabilization and establishment of adequate oxygenation and ventilation are vital. Cardiovascular status should be supported and monitored.
- Hypothermic patients should be gradually rewarmed.
- Hyponatremia typically responds to fluid restriction, but may require hypertonic saline solution and furosemide in severe cases.
- Vasopressors are usually ineffective in this setting and should be used only for severe hypotension.
- Sedating drugs, such as phenothiazines, generally should be avoided.
- Precipitating causes should be sought and treated. Antibiotics are indicated for underlying infection.
- Hydrocortisone 100 mg IV every 8 hours should be administered.
- Thyroid hormone is the most specific therapy for myxedema coma. Intravenous levothyroxine in an initial dose of 300 to 500 μg should be given by slow IV infusion; this is followed by 50 to 100 μg IV daily.
- Alternative treatment consists of L-triiodothyronine 25 μg IV or orally every 8 hours.
- L-triiodothyronine dosage should be halved in patients with cardiovascular disease.
- Patients should be admitted to a monitored setting.

REFERENCES

1. Ringel M: Management of hypothyroidism and hyperthyroidism in the intensive care unit. *Crit Care Clin* 17:115, 2001.
2. Lindsay RS, Toft AD: Hypothyroidism. *Lancet* 349:413, 1997.

For further reading in *Emergency Medicine: A Comprehensive Study Guide*, 6th ed., see Chap. 215, "Hyperthyroidism and Thyroid Storm," and Chap. 216, "Hypothyroidism and Myxedema Coma," by Horace K. Liang.

135 ADRENAL INSUFFICIENCY AND ADRENAL CRISIS
Michael P. Kefer

PATHOPHYSIOLOGY

- Adrenal insufficiency may be acute or chronic, and results when the physiologic demand for glucocorticoids and mineralocorticoids exceeds the supply from the adrenal cortex.
- The hypothalamus secretes corticotropin-releasing factor (CRF), which stimulates the pituitary to secrete adrenocorticotropic hormone (ACTH) and associated melanocyte-stimulating hormone (MSH).
- ACTH stimulates the adrenal cortex to secrete cortisol (and aldosterone to a minor degree). Cortisol has negative feedback on the pituitary to inhibit secretion of ACTH and MSH.
- Cortisol is the major glucocorticoid. It has a key role in maintaining blood glucose levels by decreasing glucose uptake and stimulating proteolysis and lipolysis for gluconeogenesis. Cortisol is necessary for the proper function of catecholamines on cardiac muscle and arterioles. Cortisol also controls body water balance.
- Aldosterone is the major mineralocorticoid. The renin-angiotensin system and serum potassium regulate its secretion. ACTH has a minor effect.
- The adrenal cortex as a source of androgens is much more important in women than men.
- Adrenal insufficiency is described as primary, secondary, or tertiary, based on whether the insufficiency occurs at the level of the adrenal glands, pituitary, or hypothalamus, respectively.

CLINICAL FEATURES

- Manifestations of primary adrenal insufficiency are due to cortisol and aldosterone deficiency and include weakness, dehydration, hypotension, anorexia, nausea, vomiting, weight loss, and abdominal pain.
- Hyperpigmentation of both exposed and nonexposed skin and mucous membranes occurs as a result of uninhibited MSH secretion in conjunction with ACTH.

- Androgen deficiency in women manifests as thinning of pubic and axillary hair.
- Secondary and tertiary adrenal insufficiency results from inadequate secretion of ACTH (which is accompanied by MSH) and CRF, respectively, with resultant cortisol deficiency. Aldosterone levels are not significantly affected because of regulation through the renin-angiotensin system. Therefore, hyperpigmentation and hyperkalemia are not seen.
- Adrenal crisis is the acute, life-threatening form of adrenal insufficiency. Clinical features are as described above, but to the extreme and accompanied by shock and altered mental status.

DIAGNOSIS AND DIFFERENTIAL

- The diagnosis of adrenal insufficiency can be made in the emergency department based on the presence of the clinical features and performing a cosyntropin (synthetic ACTH) stimulation test. The cosyntropin stimulation test is performed by drawing a baseline cortisol level, then administering cosyntropin 0.25 mg IM or IV. After 60 minutes, a repeat cortisol level is drawn and should be double the baseline.
- In primary adrenal insufficiency, the diseased adrenal cortex does not respond to ACTH and will not increase the cortisol level. In secondary and tertiary adrenal insufficiency, the adrenal cortex does respond to ACTH and will increase the cortisol level.
- For primary adrenal insufficiency, laboratory investigation reveals varying degrees of hyponatremia, hyperkalemia, hypoglycemia, anemia, metabolic acidosis, and prerenal azotemia. All patients with adrenal insufficiency have low plasma cortisol levels.
- The most common cause of adrenal insufficiency and adrenal crisis is adrenal suppression from prolonged steroid use with either abrupt steroid withdrawal or exposure to increased physiologic stress such as injury, illness, or surgery.
- Adrenal suppression can occur with steroids given by any route (oral, topical, intrathecal, or inhaled).
- In general, there is no adrenal suppression regardless of the daily dose of steroids if the duration of use is less than 3 weeks, and regardless of duration of use if the daily dose does not exceed 5 mg.[1]
- It may take up to 1 year for the hypothalamic-pituitary-adrenal axis to recover following prolonged suppression with steroid treatment.

- Other causes of adrenal insufficiency include autoimmune, idiopathic, metastatic cancer, sarcoidosis, ketoconazole use, bilateral adrenal hemorrhage associated with meningococcemia (Waterhouse-Friderichsen syndrome) or heparin therapy, and pituitary hemorrhage from head trauma or postpartum necrosis (Sheehan's syndrome).
- Of infectious causes, tuberculosis is the most common worldwide and HIV the most common in the United States.[2]

EMERGENCY DEPARTMENT CARE AND DISPOSITION

- Outpatient management of stable patients with known or suspected adrenal insufficiency consists of steroid replacement therapy and is best managed by the consultant.
- Treatment of adrenal crisis includes resuscitation with crystalloid fluids, glucocorticoids, and mineralocorticoids to correct volume, glucose, and sodium deficits.
- D_5NS is the initial fluid of choice.
- Hydrocortisone 100 to 300 mg IV every 6 to 8 hours provides adequate glucocorticoid and mineralocorticoid activity.
- If a cosyntropin stimulation test is being performed, then dexamethasone 4 mg IV should be substituted for hydrocortisone so as not to give a false positive test.
- In refractory cases, additional hydrocortisone or vasopressors may be necessary.

REFERENCES

1. Zaloga GP, Marik P: Hypothalamic-pituitary-adrenal insufficiency. *Crit Care Clin* 17:25, 2001.
2. Coursin DB, Wood KE: Corticosteroid supplementation for adrenal insufficiency. *JAMA* 287:236, 2002.

For further reading in *Emergency Medicine: A Comprehensive Study Guide*, 6th ed., see Chap. 217, "Adrenal Insufficiency," by Charles N. Shoenfeld.

136 EVALUATION OF ANEMIA AND THE BLEEDING PATIENT

Sandra L. Najarian

PATHOPHYSIOLOGY

- Anemia is due to loss of red blood cells (RBCs) by hemorrhage, increased destruction of RBCs, or impaired production of RBCs.
- Bleeding disorders from congenital or acquired abnormalities in the hemostatic system can result in excessive hemorrhage, excessive clot formation, or both.

CLINICAL FEATURES

- The rate of the development of the anemia, the extent of the anemia, and the ability of the cardiovascular system to compensate for the decreased oxygen-carrying capacity determine the severity of the patient's symptoms and clinical presentation.
- Patients may complain of palpitations, dizziness, postural faintness, easy fatigability, exertional intolerance, and tinnitus.
- On physical examination, patients may have pale conjunctiva, skin, and nail beds.
- Tachycardia, hyperdynamic precordium, and systolic murmurs may be present. Tachypnea at rest and hypotension are late signs.
- Use of ethanol, prescription drugs, and recreational drugs may alter the patient's ability to compensate for the anemia.
- Risk factors for underlying bleeding disorders include a family history of bleeding disorder, history of liver disease, and use of aspirin, nonsteroidal anti-inflammatory drugs, ethanol, warfarin, or certain antibiotics.
- Signs of platelet disorders include mucocutaneous bleeding (including petechiae, ecchymoses, purpura, and epistaxis), gastrointestinal or genitourinary bleeding, or heavy menstrual bleeding.
- Signs of coagulation factor deficiencies include delayed bleeding, hemarthrosis, or bleeding into potential spaces (eg, retroperitoneum).
- Patients with combined abnormalities of platelets and coagulation factors, such as disseminated intravascular coagulation, present with both mucocutaneous and deep space bleeding.

DIAGNOSIS AND DIFFERENTIAL

- Decreased red blood cell (RBC) count, hemoglobin, and hematocrit are diagnostic of anemia. Hemoccult examination, complete blood cell count, reticulocyte count, review of RBC indices, and examination of peripheral blood smear are necessary for the initial evaluation of the patient with anemia (Table 136-1).
- The mean cellular volume and reticulocyte count can assist in classifying the anemia and can aid in differential diagnosis (Fig. 136-1).
- Complete blood cell count, platelet count, prothrombin time, and partial thromboplastin time are necessary for the initial evaluation of the patient with a suspected bleeding disorder (Table 136-2).

EMERGENCY DEPARTMENT CARE AND DISPOSITION

- Emergent priorities remain airway, breathing and circulation. Hemorrhage should be controlled with direct pressure.

TABLE 136-1   Tests in the Evaluation of Anemia

TEST	INTERPRETATION	CLINICAL CORRELATION
MCV (mean corpuscular volume)	Measure of the average red blood cell size	Decreased MCV (microcytosis) is seen in chronic iron deficiency, thalassemia, anemia of chronic disease Increased MCV (macrocytosis) is seen in B_{12} or folate deficiency, alcohol abuse, liver disease, disease, phenytoin, some HIV drugs
MCH (mean corpuscular hemoglobin)	Measure of the amount of hemoglobin in average red blood cell	
MCHC (mean corpuscular hemoglobin concentration)	Measure of hemoglobin concentration in average red blood cell	
Reticulocyte count	These red blood cells of intermediate maturity are a marker of production by the bone marrow	Decreased reticulocyte count reflects impaired red blood cell production Increased counts are a marker of accelerated red cell production
Peripheral blood smear	Allows visualization of the red blood cell morphology Allows evaluation for abnormal cell shapes Allows examination of the white blood cells and platelets	
Direct and indirect Coombs test	Diirect Coombs test is used to detect antibodies on red blood cells Indirect Coombs test is used to detect antibodies in the sera	Direct Coombs test is positive in autoimmune hemolytic anemias, transfusion reactions, and some drug-induced hemolytic anemias Indirect Coombs test is routinely used in compatibility testing prior to transfusion

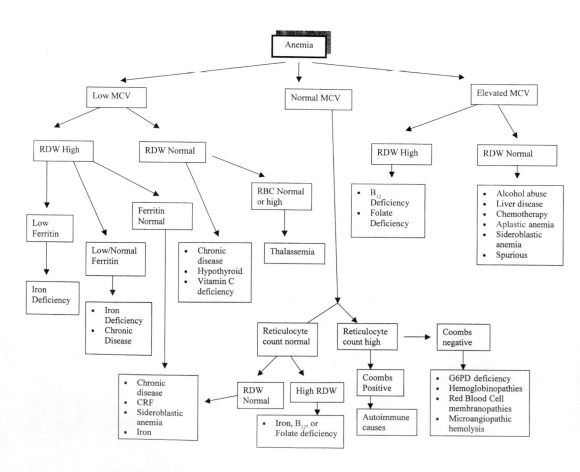

FIG. 136-1. Flow chart for the evaluation of anemia. CRF = chronic renal failure; G6PD = glucose-6-phosphate dehydrogenase; MCV = mean corpuscular volume; RDW = red blood cell distribution width index.

TABLE 136-2   Tests of Hemostasis

SCREENING TESTS	NORMAL VALUE	MEASURES	CLINICAL CORRELATIONS
PRIMARY HEMOSTASIS			
Platelet count	150,000–300,000/μL	Number of platelets per μL	Decreased platelet count (thrombocytopenia)—bleeding usually not a problem until platelet count <50,000/mL; high risk of spontaneous bleeding including CNS with count <10,000/μL; usually due to decreased production or increased destruction Elevated platelet count (thrombocytosis)—commonly reactive to inflammation or malignancy, or in polycythemia vera; can be associated with hemorrhage or thrombosis
Bleeding time (BT)	2.5–10 min (template BT)	Interaction between platelets and the subendothelium	Prolonged BT caused by: Thrombocytopenia (platelet count <50,000/μL) Abnormal platelet function (vWD, ASA, NSAIDs, uremia, liver disease)
SECONDARY HEMOSTASIS			
Prothrombin time (PT) and International Normalized Ratio (INR)	11–13 s, depending on reagent; INR 1.0	Extrinsic system and common pathway—factors VII, X, V, prothrombin, and fibrinogen	*Prolonged PT*—most commonly caused by: Use of warfarin (inhibits vitamin K–dependent factors II, VII, IX, and X) Liver disease with decreased factor synthesis Antibiotics, some cephalosporins, (moxalactam, cefamandole, cefotaxime, cefoperazone) that inhibit vitamin K–dependent factors
Activated partial thromboplastin time (aPTT)	22–34 s Depends on type of thromboplastin used; "activated" with Kaolin	Intrinsic system and common pathway including factors XII, XI, IX, VIII, X, V, prothrombin, and fibrinogen	*Prolongation of aPTT* most commonly caused by: Heparin therapy Factor deficiencies; factor levels have to be >30% of normal to cause prolongation
Thrombin clotting time (TCT)	10–12 s	Conversion of fibrinogen to fibrin monomer	*Prolonged TCT* caused by: Low fibrinogen level (DIC) Abnormal fibrinogen molecule (liver disease) Presence of heparin, FDPs or a paraprotein (multiple myeloma); these interfere with the conversion Very high fibrinogen level (acute phase reactant)
"Mixes"	Variable	Performed when one or more of the above screening tests is prolonged; the patient's plasma ("abnormal") is mixed with "normal" plasma and the screening test is repeated	*If the "mix" corrects* the screening test, one or more factor deficiencies are present. *If the "mix" does not correct the screening test,* an inhibitor is present
OTHER HEMOSTATIC TESTS			
Fibrin degradation products and D-dimer (evaluate fibrinolysis)	Variable	*FDPs* measure breakdown products from fibrinogen and fibrin monomer; normal <2.5 μg/L *D-Dimer* measures breakdown products of cross-linked fibrin; normal <500 μg/L	Levels of these are elevated in DIC, thrombosis, pulmonary embolus, liver disease
Factor level assays	60–130% (0.60–1.30 units/mL)	Measures the percent activity of a specified factor compared to normal	Used to identify specific factor deficiencies and in therapeutic management of patients with deficiencies
Inhibitor screens	Variable	Verifies the presence or absence of antibodies directed against one or more of the coagulation factors	*Specific inhibitors*—directed against one coagulation factor, most commonly against factor VIII; can be in patients with congenital or acquired deficiency *Nonspecific inhibitors*—directed against more than one of the coagulation factors; example is lupus-type anticoagulant

ABBREVIATIONS: ASA = aspirin; CNS = central nervous system; DIC = disseminated intravascular coagulation; FDPs = fibrin degradation products; NSAIDs = nonsteroidal anti-inflammatory drugs; vWD = von Willebrand disease.

- Type- and cross-matched blood should be ordered if blood transfusion is anticipated. Packed RBCs should be transfused in symptomatic patients and those who are hemodynamically unstable.
- Patients with anemia and ongoing blood loss should be admitted to the hospital for further evaluation and treatment.
- Patients with chronic anemia or newly diagnosed anemia with unclear etiology require admission if they are hemodynamically unstable, hypoxic, or acidotic, or demonstrate cardiac ischemia.
- Hematology consultation is warranted in patients with suspected bleeding disorders and anemia of unclear etiology.

BIBLIOGRAPHY

Beutter E: The common anemias. *JAMA* 259:2433, 1988.

Goldhill D, Boralessa H: Anemia and red cell transfusion in the critically ill. *Anaesthesia* 57:527, 2002.

Hemphill RR: Hematologic emergencies and life-threatening bleeding disorders: Differential diagnosis, evaluation and management. *Emerg Med Report* 22:183, 2001.

Hermiston ML, Mentzer WC: A practical approach to the evaluation of the anemic child. *Pediair Clin North Am* 49:877, 2002.

Sallah S, Kato G: Evaluation of bleeding disorders. A detailed history and laboratory tests provide clues. *Postgrad Med* 103:209, 1998.

For further reading in *Emergency Medicine: A Comprehensive Study Guide,* 6th ed., see Chap. 218, "Evaluation of Anemia and the Bleeding Patient," by Robin R. Hemphill.

137   ACQUIRED BLEEDING DISORDERS

Matthew A. Bridges

BLEEDING DUE TO PLATELET ABNORMALITIES

PATHOPHYSIOLOGY

- Acquired platelet abnormalities include both qualitative (functional) and quantitative platelet defects.
- Quantitative platelet disorders begin at levels below 50,000/μL and can be caused by decreased platelet production, increased platelet destruction, increased platelet loss, and splenic sequestration.[1]
- Causes of decreased platelet production include marrow infiltration, aplastic anemia, drugs, and viral infections.
- Causes of increased platelet destruction include idiopathic thrombocytopenic purpura (ITP), thrombotic thrombocytopenic purpura (TTP), hemolytic-uremic syndrome (HUS), disseminated intravascular coagulation (DIC), and viral infection.[2,3]
- Causes of increased platelet loss include hemorrhage and hemodialysis.
- Qualitative disorders result in excessive bleeding regardless of the number of available platelets; common causes include liver disease, medications, antiplatelet antibodies, DIC, and uremia.

EMERGENCY DEPARTMENT CARE AND DISPOSITION

- Platelet transfusion is warranted in all patients with a platelet count <10,000/μL, regardless of etiology or symptomatology.[4]
- Patients with serious bleeding problems and platelet counts below 50,000/μL should receive transfusions. However, hematologic consultation should be obtained, as some conditions, such as DIC and TTP, may be worsened by platelet transfusion.
- The patient with ITP should be started on prednisone.

BLEEDING DUE TO WARFARIN USE OR VITAMIN K DEFICIENCY

PATHOPHYSIOLOGY

- Vitamin K is a necessary cofactor in the production of factors II, VII, IX, and X, as well as the anticoagulants protein C and protein S.
- Warfarin inhibits the production of vitamin K–dependent factors, resulting in anticoagulation.[5]
- Patients with liver disease, those with vitamin K deficiency due to poor nutrition or malabsorption, and patients taking warfarin are at increased risk of bleeding.

EMERGENCY DEPARTMENT CARE AND DISPOSITION

- Guidelines for treatment of warfarin-related bleeding are summarized in Table 137-1.

TABLE 137-1   Warfarin Reversal Guidelines

INR VALUE	BLEEDING	RECOMMENDATIONS
Any elevation	Major to life threatening	• Withhold warfarin • Replace coagulation factors with FFP or factor complex concentrates • Vitamin K 5–10 mg IV (dose dependent on INR)
Any elevation	Mild to moderate	• Withhold warfarin • Vitamin K 2–4 mg PO (dose dependent on INR)
<5	None	• Withhold warfarin until INR therapeutic and then restart at same or lower dose
5–9	None	• Withhold warfarin • Vitamin K 1–2 mg PO
>9	None	• Withhold warfarin • Vitamin K 2–4 mg PO

ABBREVIATIONS: FFP = fresh frozen plasma; INR = International Normalized Ratio.

BLEEDING DUE TO HEPARIN USE OR FIBRINOLYTIC THERAPY

PATHOPHYSIOLOGY

- Bleeding is the most common side effect of the use of heparin or fibrinolytic therapy.
- All fibrinolytic agents have similar rates of major and minor bleeding complications, including a 1 to 2% risk of intracranial hemorrhage.

EMERGENCY DEPARTMENT CARE AND DISPOSITION

- Heparin or fibrinolytic therapy should be discontinued if bleeding cannot be controlled by local measures.
- Protamine can be used to neutralize heparin at a dose of 1 mg IV per 100 U of infused heparin in the previous 4 hours.
- Protamine is partially effective in reversing the effects of low–molecular weight heparin.
- Bleeding or thrombosis associated with heparin-induced thrombocytopenia should be treated with discontinuation of heparin and anticoagulation with a different agent (eg, danaparoid, ancrod, or hirudin).[6] Low molecular weight heparins should not be used.[7]
- Massive bleeding associated with fibrinolytic therapy should be treated with cryoprecipitate (10 U IV). If bleeding persists, treatment with fresh frozen plasma (FFP), 2 U IV, should be initiated.
- Further treatment for bleeding associated with fibrinolytic therapy should be in conjunction with a hematologist, but may include platelet transfusion or aminocaproic acid administration.

BLEEDING IN LIVER DISEASE

PATHOPHYSIOLOGY

- Liver disease places patients at risk for hemostatic abnormalities by multiple mechanisms, including decreased coagulation factor production due to hepatocyte dysfunction or vitamin K deficiency, thrombocytopenia (most often due to splenic sequestration from portal hypertension), and increased fibrinolysis.

EMERGENCY DEPARTMENT CARE AND DISPOSITION

- All patients with liver disease and active bleeding should receive vitamin K (10 mg SC or IM).
- Patients with severe bleeding should receive FFP to rapidly replace coagulation factors.
- Platelet transfusion can be used in severe bleeding with associated thrombocytopenia.
- Desmopressin (DDAVP 0.3 μg/kg SC or IV) may shorten bleeding times in some patients.
- Cryoprecipitate may be beneficial in patients with active bleeding and fibrinogen levels <100 mg/dL.

BLEEDING IN RENAL DISEASE

PATHOPHYSIOLOGY

- The bleeding tendency exhibited by patients with renal disease is related to the degree and duration of uremia.
- Bleeding is the result of platelet dysfunction, deficiency of coagulation factors, and thrombocytopenia.[8]

EMERGENCY DEPARTMENT CARE AND DISPOSITION

- Transfusion of packed red blood cells (PRBCs) to maintain a hematocrit between 26 and 30 optimizes platelet function.
- Hemodialysis improves platelet function transiently for 1 to 2 days.
- DDAVP (0.3 μg/kg SC or IV) shortens bleeding time in the majority of patients.
- Conjugated estrogens improve bleeding time in most patients.
- Platelet transfusions and cryoprecipitate are indicated for life-threatening bleeding only, and are to be used in conjunction with the previously listed therapies.

BLEEDING IN DISSEMINATED INTRAVASCULAR COAGULATION

PATHOPHYSIOLOGY

- DIC results from the activation of both the coagulation and fibrinolytic systems and is triggered by the activation of tissue factor.[9]
- The most common conditions associated with DIC are listed in Table 137-2.

CLINICAL FEATURES

- The complications of DIC are related to both bleeding and thrombosis, although in an individual patient, one usually predominates.
- Bleeding typically occurs in the skin and mucous membranes. The skin may show signs of petechiae or ecchymoses.
- Bleeding from several sites, including venipuncture sites and surgical wounds, is common.
- Gastrointestinal, urinary tract, and central nervous system bleeding also may occur. Other patients show primarily thrombotic symptoms.
- Depending on the site of the thrombosis, patients may exhibit focal ischemia of the extremities, mental status changes, oliguria, or symptoms of acute respiratory distress syndrome.
- Purpura fulminans develops when there is widespread thrombosis, resulting in gangrene of the extremities and hemorrhagic infarction of the skin.

DIAGNOSIS AND DIFFERENTIAL

- The diagnosis of DIC is based on the clinical setting and characteristic laboratory abnormalities listed in Table 137-3.

TABLE 137-2   Common Conditions Associated with Disseminated Intravascular Coagulation

CLINICAL SETTING	COMMENTS

Infection
  Bacterial
  Viral
  Fungal
	Probably the most common cause of DIC; 10–20% of patients with gram-negative sepsis have DIC; endotoxins stimulate monocytes and endothelial cells to express tissue factor; Rocky Mountain spotted fever causes direct endothelial damage; DIC more likely to develop in asplenic patients or those with cirrhosis; septic patients are more likely to have thrombosis than bleeding

Carcinoma
  Adenocarcinoma
  Lymphoma
	Malignant cells may cause endothelial damage and allow the expression of tissue factor as well as other procoagulant materials; most adenocarcinomas tend to have thrombosis (Trousseau syndrome), except prostate cancer tends to have more bleeding; DIC is often chronic and compensated

Acute leukemia	DIC most common with promyelocytic leukemia; blast cells release procoagulant enzymes, there is excessive release at time of cell lysis (chemotherapy); more likely to have bleeding than thrombosis
Trauma	DIC especially with brain injury, crush injury, burns, hypothermia, hyperthermia, rhabdomyolysis, fat embolism, hypoxia
Liver disease	May have chronic compensated DIC; acute DIC may occur in the setting of acute hepatic failure, tissue factor is released from the injured hepatocytes
Pregnancy	Placental abruption, amniotic fluid embolus, septic abortion, intrauterine fetal death (can be chronic DIC); can get DIC in HELLP (hemolysis, elevated liver enzymes, low platelets) syndrome
Vascular disease	Large aortic aneurysms (chronic DIC can become acute at time of surgery), giant hemangiomas, vasculitis, multiple telangiectasias
Envenomation	DIC can develop with bites of rattlesnakes and other vipers; the venom damages the endothelial cells; bleeding is not as bad as expected from laboratory values
Acute respiratory distress syndrome (ARDS)	Microthrombi are deposited in the small pulmonary vessels, the pulmonary capillary endothelium is damaged; 20% of patients with ARDS develop DIC and 20% of patients with DIC develop ARDS.

Transfusion reactions
  Acute hemolytic reaction
  Massive transfusion
	DIC with severe bleeding, shock, and acute renal failure

TABLE 137-3   Laboratory Abnormalities Characteristic of Disseminated Intravascular Coagulation

STUDIES	RESULT
MOST USEFUL	
Prothrombin time	Prolonged
Platelet count*	Usually low
Fibrinogen level†	Low
HELPFUL	
Activated partial thromboplastin time	Usually prolonged
Thrombin clot time‡	Prolonged
Fragmented red blood cells§	Should be present
FDPs and D-dimers¶	Elevated
*Specific factor assays***	
Factor II	Low
Factor V	Low
Factor VII††	Low
Factor VIII‡‡	Low, normal, high
Factor IX	Low (decreases later than other factors)
Factor X	Low

ABBREVIATIONS: DIC = disseminated intravascular coagulation; FDP = fibrin degradation products.
*Platelet count usually low, most important that it is falling if it started at an elevated level.
†Fibrinogen level correlates best with bleeding complications; it is an acute phase reactant so it may actually start out at an elevated level; fibrinogen level <100 mg/dL correlates with severe DIC.
‡Not a sensitive test, prolonged by many abnormalities.
§Fragmented red blood cells and schistocytes are not specific for DIC.
¶Levels may be chronically elevated in patients with liver or renal disease.
**The factors in the extrinsic pathway are most affected (VII, X, V, and II).
††Factor VII is usually low early because it has the shortest half-life.
‡‡Factor VIII is an acute phase reactant so its level may be normal, low, or elevated in DIC.

EMERGENCY DEPARTMENT CARE AND DISPOSITION

- Hemodynamic stabilization should be provided through IV fluids or PRBC transfusion.
- The underlying medical or surgical illness should be treated.
- If bleeding predominates and the PT is elevated more than 2 seconds, replacement of coagulation factors is indicated.
- FFP is infused 2 U at a time.
- Cryoprecipitate is used to replace fibrinogen; it is typically infused 10 bags at a time.
- If the platelet count is <50,000/μL with active bleeding or <10,000/μL regardless of bleeding, platelet transfusion should be initiated.
- All patients with bleeding due to DIC should also receive vitamin K (10 mg SC or IM) and folate (1 mg IV).
- If thrombosis predominates, heparinization should be considered, although this is controversial.

- Heparin is most likely to be beneficial if the underlying medical condition is carcinoma, acute promyelocytic leukemia, or retained uterine products, or if the patient exhibits signs of purpura fulminans.

BLEEDING DUE TO CIRCULATING ANTICOAGULANTS

PATHOPHYSIOLOGY

- Circulating anticoagulants are antibodies directed against one or more of the coagulation factors.[10]
- The two most common circulating anticoagulants are factor VIII inhibitor (a specific inhibitor directed only against factor VIII) and antiphospholipid antibodies, including lupus anticoagulant and anticardiolipin antibody (nonspecific inhibitors directed against several coagulation factors).

CLINICAL FEATURES

- Patients with factor VIII inhibitor have massive spontaneous bruises, ecchymoses, and hematomas.
- Patients with antiphospholipid antibodies may have thromboses or recurrent fetal loss.[11]
- Bleeding abnormalities are rare in patients with antiphospholipid antibodies.

DIAGNOSIS AND DIFFERENTIAL

- Laboratory studies in patients with factor VIII inhibitor reveal a normal PT, normal thrombin clot time (TCT), and a greatly prolonged partial thromboplastin time (PTT) that does not correct with mixing.
- A factor VIII–specific assay will show low or absent factor VIII activity.
- Patients with antiphospholipid antibodies will have a normal or slightly prolonged PT, a normal TCT, and a moderately prolonged PTT that also does not correct with mixing.
- Factor-specific assays will show a decrease in all factor levels.

EMERGENCY DEPARTMENT CARE AND DISPOSITION

- Patients with factor VIII inhibitor and active bleeding should be managed in conjunction with a hematologist. Treatment options include concentrates of factor VIIa, factor VIII, factor IX, and prothrombin complex, as well as plasmapheresis.

- Patients with antiphospholipid antibodies and arterial or venous thrombosis should be treated with long-term warfarin anticoagulation.

BLEEDING DUE TO INFECTION WITH HUMAN IMMUNODEFICIENCY VIRUS

PATHOPHYSIOLOGY

- Infection with HIV is associated with several abnormalities of hemostasis. Most common are thrombocytopenia and circulating anticoagulants.
- The most common symptoms are easy bruising, petechiae, and mucosal bleeding. Clinically significant bleeding is rare.
- HIV-positive patients with antiphospholipid antibodies have a lower risk of thrombosis than HIV-negative patients.

EMERGENCY DEPARTMENT CARE AND DISPOSITION

- The treatment of the HIV-infected patient with bleeding associated with thrombocytopenia or circulating anticoagulants is identical to the treatment of those conditions in those without HIV, as discussed above.

REFERENCES

1. McCrae KR, Bussel JB, Mannucci PM, et al: Platelets: An update on diagnosis and management of thrombocytopenic disorders. *Hematology* (Am Soc Hematol Educ Program) 20: 282, 2001.
2. Greinacher A, Eicheler P, Lubenow N, Kiefel V: Drug-induced and drug-dependent immune thrombocytopenias. *Rev Clin Exp Hematol* 5:166, 2001.
3. Cines DB, Blanchette VX: Immune thrombocytopenic purpura. *N Engl J Med* 346:995, 2002.
4. Rebulla P: Platelet transfusion trigger in difficult patients. *Transfus Clin Biol* 8:249, 2001.
5. Hirsh J, Dalen J, Anderson D, et al: Oral anticoagulants: Mechanism of action, clinical effectiveness, and optimal therapeutic range. *Chest* 119:8S, 2001.
6. Warkentin TE: Current agents for the treatment of patients with heparin-induced thrombocytopenia. *Curr Opin Pulm Med* 8: 405, 2002.
7. Ginsberg JA, Crowther MA, White RH, Ortel TL: Anticoagulation therapy. *Hematology* 20:339, 2001.
8. Opatrny K: Hemostasis disorders in chronic renal failure. *Kidney Int Suppl* 62:S87, 1997.
9. Levi M, ten Cate H: Disseminated intravascular coagulation. *N Engl J Med* 341:586, 1999.
10. Sallah S: Inhibitors to clotting factors. *Ann Hematol* 75:1, 1997.
11. Levine JS, Branch DW, Rauch J: The antiphospholipid syndrome. *N Engl J Med* 346:752, 2002.

For further reading in *Emergency Medicine: A Comprehensive Study Guide,* 6th ed., see Chap. 219, "Acquired Bleeding Disorders," by Mary A. Wittler and Robin R. Hemphill.

138 HEMOPHILIAS AND VON WILLEBRAND'S DISEASE

Jeffrey N. Glaspy

HEMOPHILIA

EPIDEMIOLOGY

- Hemophilia A (factor VIII deficiency) occurs in about 1:10,000 male births.
- Hemophilia B, or Christmas disease, is a factor IX deficiency and occurs in 1:35,000 male births.
- Spontaneous gene mutation accounts for about 33% and 20% of new cases of hemophilia A and B, respectively.

PATHOPHYSIOLOGY

- Hemophilia is an inherited disorder of a circulating coagulation protein. Hemophilia A and B are X-linked, recessive disorders, and therefore affect males almost exclusively.
- Deficiency or defect of the factor VIII or IX protein results in abnormal intrinsic coagulation pathway function.

CLINICAL FEATURES

- Patients with hemophilia are categorized as having mild (5 to 25% of normal factor function), moderate (1 to 5% of normal function), or severe ($<1\%$ of normal function) disease.
- Hemophilia is characterized by easy bruising and bleeding into the muscles and joints.
- The extent, severity, and frequency of bleeding are dependent on the severity of disease (mild, moderate, or severe).

- Trauma, surgical procedures, and spontaneous retroperitoneal or central nervous system bleeding may be life threatening. Traumatic bleeding may be delayed for several hours.
- Unless there is another underlying disease, patients with hemophilia do not have problems with minor cuts and abrasions.
- Compartment syndrome may result from extremity hematoma.

DIAGNOSIS AND DIFFERENTIAL

- Laboratory testing in patients with hemophilia most often shows a normal prothrombin time (PT), prolonged partial thromboplastin time (PTT), and bleeding time (BT).
- If more than 30% of factor activity is present, the PTT may be normal.
- Specific factor assays may be used to differentiate between the types of hemophilia.
- Approximately 10 to 25% of patients with hemophilia A and 1 to 2% of patients with hemophilia B will develop an inhibitor, which is an antibody against the deficient factor.
- An inhibitor is diagnosed by mixing the patient's plasma 50:50 with plasma of a normal control and finding that the mixture still has a prolonged PTT. The quantity of inhibitor is measured by the Bethesda inhibitor assay (BIA) and is reported in BIA units.

EMERGENCY DEPARTMENT CARE AND DISPOSITION

- For major or life-threatening bleeding, factor replacement with an initial dose of 50 U/kg of factor VIII or 100 U/kg of factor IX during the initial resuscitation is the mainstay of treatment. Further factor replacement is almost always needed, especially in patients with inhibitor.
- The management of less severe bleeding depends on the severity of hemophilia, presence or absence of inhibitor, and site and severity of bleeding.
- For severe bleeding the desired factor level is 80 to 100%. For less severe bleeding the desired factor level is 30 to 50%.
- The amount of factor VIII required is determined by: amount required = weight (kg) $\times$ 0.5 $\times$ (% change in factor activity needed).
- The amount of factor IX required is determined by: amount required = weight (kg) $\times$ 1.0 $\times$ (% change in factor activity needed).
- If factor concentrate is unavailable, or if the type of hemophilia is unknown, fresh frozen plasma (FFP)

should be administered. Each milliliter of FFP contains 1 U of factor VIII and factor IX. Volume constraints make complete replacement with FFP difficult.
- Cryoprecipitate may be used if no factor concentrate is available; however, it does not contain factor IX. Each milliliter of cryoprecipitate contains 6 U of factor VIII.
- Desmopressin (DDAVP) may be used to raise factor VIII levels in patients with mild to moderate hemophilia A and no inhibitor.

VON WILLEBRAND'S DISEASE

EPIDEMIOLOGY

- Von Willebrand's disease is the most common inherited bleeding disorder, occurring in 1% of the population. However, only 1 in 10,000 people manifest a clinically significant bleeding disorder.

PATHOPHYSIOLOGY

- Von Willebrand's factor (vWF) is a cofactor for platelet adhesion as well as a carrier protein for factor VIII, protecting factor VIII from proteolytic degradation.
- When exposed to the subendothelial matrix, vWF undergoes a structural change, allowing it to bind to glycoprotein Ib. This leads to platelet activation and adhesion to other platelets and to the damaged endothelium.

CLINICAL FEATURES

- There are three main types von Willebrand's disease. Type I (80% of patients with von Willebrand's disease) is a mild form with bleeding episodes usually manifesting as epistaxis, easy bruising, menorrhagia, or dental bleeding.
- Type II is a qualitative disorder accounting for about 10% of patients with von Willebrand's disease.
- Type III is a severe form accounting for less than 10% of cases. These patients manifest with severe bleeding episodes that may resemble the hemophilias (hemarthrosis and hematomas).
- Unlike the hemophilias, patients with von Willebrand's disease often present with skin and mucosal bleeding. Hemarthrosis is not typical unless severe disease (type III) is present.
- In mild cases of von Willebrand's disease, the patient may not be aware of their disease until a traumatic episode or surgical procedure.

DIAGNOSIS AND DIFFERENTIAL

- In patients with von Willebrand's disease, the PT and PTT are usually normal. The BT is prolonged and vWF activity is low.
- Occasionally, the PT and factor VIII level may be abnormal, making it difficult to distinguish vWD from hemophilia A.

EMERGENCY DEPARTMENT CARE AND DISPOSITION

- For most patients with von Willebrand's disease, DDAVP is the mainstay of treatment.
- DDAVP works by stimulating endothelial cells to secrete stored vWF, and possibly by promoting hemostasis via additional endothelial effects.
- The dose of DDAVP is 0.3 μg/kg IV or SC over 30 minutes every 12 hours. The dose of the concentrated intranasal form of DDAVP is 1 spray in one nostril (150 μg) for children over 5 years of age and 1 spray in each nostril (300 μg) for adolescents and adults.
- For patients that do not respond to DDAVP or for patients with type II or III disease, factor VIII concentrate is required. The most commonly used factor VIII concentrates are Humate-P and Koate-HP.
- Cryoprecipitate also contains high concentrations of vWF and may be used to treat patients with vWD. There is, however, a greater risk of viral transmission and therefore the purified products like Humate are recommended.
- Platelet transfusions may benefit patients with certain types of vWD (type III) who do not respond to factor VIII concentrates.
- For women with vWD and menorrhagia, birth control pills may help increase the vWF levels and limit the menstrual bleeding.

BIBLIOGRAPHY

Hemphill RR: Hematologic emergencies and life-threatening bleeding disorders: Differential diagnosis, evaluation and management. *Emerg Med Report* 22:183, 2001.

Mannucci PM: Management of inherited von Willebrand's disease. *Best Pract Res Clin Haemotol* 14:462, 2001.

Mannucci PM, Giangrande PL: Choice of replacement therapy for hemophilia. *Hematol J* 1:76, 2000.

Shapiro A: Inhibitor treatment: state of the art. *Semin Hematol* 38:34, 2001.

For further reading in *Emergency Medicine: A Comprehensive Study Guide,* 6th ed., see Chapt.220, "Hemophilias and Von Willebrand's Disease," by Robin R. Hemphill.

139 HEMOLYTIC ANEMIAS

Sandra L. Najarian

HEREDITARY HEMOLYTIC ANEMIAS

EPIDEMIOLOGY

- Sickle cell disease (SCD) is inherited in an autosomal co-dominant pattern.
- Sickle cell trait, the most common variant of SCD, is found in 8% of the U.S. African-American population.
- Painful vaso-occlusive crisis of SCD is the most common reason for emergency department (ED) visits.
- In children, 80% of vasoocclusive events are infection related. In adults, the majorities of crises are unexplained; however, up to one third may be related to infection.
- Acute chest syndrome is currently the leading cause of death from SCD in the U.S.
- Thalassemias are most common in those of Mediterranean, Middle Eastern, African, and Southeast Asian decent.
- Heterozygous hemoglobinopathies, such as hemoglobin C SCD and sickle β-thalassemias, result from the inheritance of a sickle cell gene and an abnormal β-chain gene.
- Glucose-6-phosphate dehydrogenase (G6PD) deficiency, the most common human enzyme defect, is an X-linked disorder. In the U.S. it affects 15% of African-American males.
- Hereditary spherocytosis, a red blood cell (RBC) membrane defect, is the most prevalent hereditary hemolytic anemia among people of northern European descent.

PATHOPHYSIOLOGY

- Hemoglobinopathies are the result of an inherited abnormality of one or more hemoglobins.
- Hemoglobin S, the most common hemoglobin variant, is caused by a single point mutation on the β chain. Deoxygenated hemoglobin S polymerizes, which deforms the RBC and produces the characteristic sickled appearance.

- The distorted RBC results in premature RBC destruction and increases the viscosity of blood, leading to obstruction within the microvasculature.[1]
- Vaso-occlusive crisis occurs from intravascular sickling in the microcirculation; this results in tissue ischemia and infarction that affects most organ systems.
- Acidosis, vascular stasis, dehydration, low oxygen tension, and the presence of increased hemoglobin S can shift the oxygen dissociation curve to the right and promote increased sickling.
- Hydroxyurea has been used to reduce the frequency and severity of painful crises.[2]
- Thalassemias are characterized by defective synthesis of globin chains that results in the inability to produce normal adult hemoglobin.[3]

CLINICAL FEATURES

- SCD is a chronic hemolytic anemia and patients may have flow murmurs, congestive heart failure, cardiomegaly, cor pulmonale, lower extremity ulcerations, icterus, and hepatomegaly.
- Patients with acute chest syndrome will have pulmonary manifestations such as pleuritic chest pain, fever, sudden decrease in pulmonary function, and hypoxia.
- Neurologic manifestations include cerebral infarction in children, cerebral hemorrhage in adults, transient ischemic attack, headache, seizure, and coma.
- Patients with SCD are functionally asplenic after early childhood and are at risk for serious infection from encapsulated organisms.
- Common precipitants of vaso-occlusive crises include cold exposure, dehydration, high altitude, and infections, particularly with encapsulated organisms such as *Haemophilus influenzae* or pneumococci. Patients may present with joint, muscle, or bone pain, or diffuse abdominal pain.[4]
- Hematologic crises present with weakness, dyspnea, fatigue, worsening heart failure, or shock in the setting of a precipitous drop in hemoglobin.
- Acute splenic sequestration of blood and bone marrow suppression (aplastic crisis) are two types of hematologic crisis.
- Other clinical presentations of sickle cell disease include priapism, swelling of the hands or feet due to vaso-occlusion (dactylitis), and infarction of the renal medulla, which is associated with flank pain and hematuria.
- Patients with sickle cell trait have minimal to no complications; sickling is only present under conditions of extreme hypoxia.
- Patients with sickle cell-hemoglobin C disease have mild to moderate hemolytic anemia, mild reticulocytosis, and splenomegaly.
- Patients with sickle cell β-thalassemia vary in clinical presentation from mild hemolytic anemia to vaso-occlusive crises.
- Infection, exposure to oxidant drugs, metabolic acidosis, and ingestion of fava beans can precipitate an acute hemolytic crisis in patients with G6PD deficiency.
- Patients with hemoglobin S have mild hemolytic anemia, splenomegaly, and intermittent jaundice.

DIAGNOSIS AND DIFFERENTIAL

- SCD is usually diagnosed early in the patient's life. Presence of sickling red blood cells (RBCs) on peripheral blood smear is diagnostic.
- For patients suffering an acute crisis, a drop in hemoglobin by 2 g/dL from the patient's baseline suggests hematologic crisis or blood loss. A reticulocyte count is necessary in these patients; a count less than the baseline of 5 to 15% may reflect aplastic crisis.
- Leukocytosis along with a left shift should raise the suspicion of infection.
- Arterial blood gas testing is warranted in patients with respiratory complaints and evidence of hypoxia on pulse oximetry. Patients with sickle cell disease may have a mild to moderate hypoxia; however, a PaO$_2$ of less than 60 mm Hg suggests an acute problem.
- Differential diagnosis for complaints related to SCD is extensive and includes osteomyelitis, acute arthritides, pancreatitis, hepatitis, pelvic inflammatory disease, pyelonephritis, pneumonia, pulmonary embolus, and meningitis.

EMERGENCY DEPARTMENT CARE AND DISPOSITION

- Patients with evidence of dehydration or acute pain should be rehydrated orally if they can tolerate fluids, or with IV fluids such as normal saline at 1.5 times maintenance.
- Narcotics should be promptly administered for severe pain. Patients who present to the ED frequently will benefit from a protocol treatment plan.
- Patients with symptoms of acute infection or with a temperature >38°C should have the appropriate cultures drawn. Broad-spectrum antibiotics, such as cefuroxime or ceftriaxone, should be administered.[5]
- Transfusion for sickle cell crisis or complications is reserved for specific indications, such as aplastic crisis, pregnancy, stroke, respiratory failure, general surgery, and priapism.[6–8]
- Patients with priapism require hydration, analgesia, and immediate urologic consultation.

- Patients with acute bone pain suggestive of osteomyelitis should have cultures drawn and receive IV antibiotic therapy to cover *Streptococcus aureus* and *Salmonella typhimurium*.
- Admission criteria include pulmonary, neurologic, aplastic, or infectious crises; splenic sequestration; intractable pain; persistent nausea and vomiting; or patients with an uncertain diagnosis.
- Discharged patients should receive oral analgesics, close follow-up, and instructions to return immediately for fever >38°C or worsening symptoms.

ACQUIRED HEMOLYTIC ANEMIAS

EPIDEMIOLOGY

- Thrombotic thrombocytopenic purpura (TTP) is more common in women between the ages of 10 and 60.
- Hemolytic-uremic syndrome (HUS) is a disease of infancy and early childhood with peak incidence between 6 months and 4 years of age, often following a viral or bacterial illness.

PATHOPHYSIOLOGY

- Acquired hemolytic anemias are classified according to mechanism: immune-mediated, fragmentation in the microvascular and macrovascular circulation, direct toxic effects, drug induced, mechanical injury, or abnormal splenic function (Table 139-1).
- Pregnancy is the most common precipitating event for TTP. Infection, autoimmune disorders, vaccination, and certain drugs are other triggers.
- TTP and HUS are microangiopathic hemolytic anemias whereby platelet aggregation in the microvascular circulation via mediation of von Willebrand's factor leads to thrombocytopenia and fragmentation of RBCs as they pass through these occluded arterioles and capillaries.[9]
- Deficiency of the von Willebrand's factor–cleaving metalloprotease ADAMTS-13 appears to play a key role in the pathogenesis of TTP.[10]

CLINICAL FEATURES

- Warm-type autoimmune hemolytic anemia is more common in elderly female patients with underlying medical conditions. In children, it can occur after acute infections and immunizations (Table 139-2).
- Patients with warm-type autoimmune hemolytic ane-

TABLE 139-1 Etiologies of Acquired Hemolytic Anemia

Immune-mediated
  Autoimmune
    Warm-type antibody
    Cold-type antibody
      Cold agglutinin syndrome (CAS)
      Paroxysmal cold hemoglobinuria (PCH)
    Mixed-type (warm and cold antibody)
  Alloimmune
    Hemolytic disease of the newborn
    Hemolytic transfusion reaction
  Drug-related
    Autoimmune type
    Drug adsorption type
    Neoantigen type

Microangiopathic
  Thrombotic thrombocytopenic purpura (TTP)
  Hemolytic-uremic syndrome (HUS)
  Pregnancy-associated
    Pre-eclampsia/eclampsia
    HELLP (hemolysis, elevated liver enzymes, and low platelets)
      syndrome
    TTP/HUS
  Disseminated intravascular coagulation
  Malignant hypertension
  Malignancy
  Immune complex vasculitis

Macrovascular
  Prosthetic heart valve
  Intracardiac patch
  Coarctation of the aorta
  Extracorporeal circulation (cardiovascular bypass or hemodialysis)

Toxin-mediated
  Infectious etiology
  Envenomation
  Copper toxicity (Wilson's disease)

Drug-induced (without immune-related mechanism)
  Methemoglobin-mediated

Mechanical damage
  Heat denaturation
  March hemoglobinuria (exertion-related)

mia may present with mild anemia and splenomegaly to life-threatening anemia, splenomegaly, pulmonary edema, mental status changes, and venous thrombosis.
- Cold-type antibody hemolytic anemia presents in two forms. Cold agglutinin syndrome may present as an acute disease in younger people following infections with organisms such as *Mycoplasma pneumoniae*. The anemia is usually mild.
- The chronic form is seen in elderly patients with underlying lymphoproliferative disorders, and involves hemolysis in parts of the body exposed to cold.
- Paroxysmal cold hemoglobinemia is another acute form found in patients with untreated syphilis or viral illnesses, and presents with fever, chills, hemoglobinuria, and pain involving the back, legs, and abdomen.
- Autoimmune hemolytic anemia also can be drug-induced, involving α-methyldopa, penicillin, sulfa drugs, or quinidine.

TABLE 139-2   Causes of Warm-Type Antibody Hemolytic Anemia

Lymphoproliferative disease
   Chronic lymphocytic leukemia
   Lymphoma/Hodgkin's disease
   Waldenström's macroglobulinemia
   Multiple myeloma

Autoimmune disease/collagen-vascular disease
   Systemic lupus erythematosus
   Rheumatoid arthritis
   Polyarteritis nodosa
   Pernicious anemia
   Scleroderma
   Ulcerative colitis/Crohn' disease

Infection (can be associated with warm or cold or often both)
   Infectious mononucleosis
   Cytomegalovirus
   Viral hepatitis
   Malaria
   Pediatric viral respiratory illness

Immunodeficiency syndrome
   Human immunodeficiency virus
   Congenital syndromes
      X-linked agammaglobulinemia
      Common variable immunodeficiency
      IgA deficiency
      Wiskott-Aldrich syndrome
      Dysglobulinemia

Nonlymphoid tumors
   Ovarian carcinoma and dermoid cysts
   Teratomas
   Kaposi's sarcoma
   Thymoma

- Alloimmune hemolytic anemia includes hemolytic disease of the newborn and hemolytic transfusion reactions.
- In hemolytic disease of the newborn, maternal alloantibodies form after RhD-negative maternal RBCs are exposed to RhD-positive fetal blood. These alloantibodies cross the placenta and destroy fetal RBCs, which can lead to mild anemia, fetal hydrops, and intrauterine fetal demise.
- Patients with hemolytic transfusion reactions often have a history of previous transfusion in which sensitization to allogenic RBC antigens occurs. With subsequent transfusions, patients may develop fever, chest and flank pain, tachypnea, tachycardia, hypotension, hemoglobinuria, and oliguria.
- Microangiopathic hemolytic anemia results from fragmentation hemolysis. This includes damage to RBCs from passage through artificial heart valves, calcified aortic valves, or through arterioles and microcirculation damaged by TTP, HUS, pregnancy, vasculitis, malignant hypertension, and certain malignancies.
- TTP more commonly affects women and presents with fever, neurologic changes, hemorrhage, and renal insufficiency.

- HUS is a disease of early childhood and presents with fever, acute renal failure, and neurologic deficits, following a prodromal infection.
- Fragmentation hemolysis in pregnancy is seen in pre-eclampsia, eclampsia, and placental abruption.
- The HELLP syndrome is characterized by hemolysis, elevated liver enzymes, and low platelet counts in the presence of pre-eclampsia, eclampsia, or placental abruption. The clinical and laboratory findings of HELLP syndrome may extend up to 6 days postpartum.[11]
- Direct toxic effects causing hemolysis may result from infection (malaria being most common), and from the venom of bees, wasps, certain spiders, and cobras.
- Oxidative hemolysis of RBCs results from methemoglobin-producing drugs, such as lidocaine and sulfonamides.
- Mechanical damage to RBCs can result in hemolysis and hemoglobinuria. Etiologies include extensive burns and strenuous physical activity.
- Patients who have been on cardiopulmonary bypass can develop hemolysis, fever, and leukopenia, known as postperfusion syndrome. The passage of blood through the oxygenator activates complement, leading to acute intravascular hemolysis.
- Hemolysis as a result of sequestration and destruction of RBCs in the spleen, or hypersplenism, is most commonly seen in portal hypertension, infiltrative disease, and infections.

DIAGNOSIS AND DIFFERENTIAL

- Diagnosis is based on recognition of clinical signs and symptoms and obtaining appropriate laboratory studies. Complete blood cell count will reveal anemia. Review of the peripheral blood smear is vital and often will give keys to the diagnosis.
- Schistocytes (fragmented RBCs) are seen in microangiopathic hemolytic anemia and are the result of direct trauma.
- Spherocytes are evidence of warm antibody immune hemolysis and hereditary spherocytosis. Other laboratory abnormalities include elevations in lactic acid dehydrogenase and indirect bilirubin.
- A decrease in haptoglobin level is another indicator of intravascular hemolysis.
- Patients with evidence of microangiopathic hemolytic anemia and thrombocytopenia must be assumed to have TTP until proven otherwise.
- In TTP, the platelet count is often $<20,000/\mu L$.
- Patients with HUS will have thrombocytopenia, although not to the degree of those with TTP. An elevated blood urea nitrogen and creatinine levels are seen in HUS and TTP.

- An elevated reticulocyte count is the best indicator of normal bone marrow in the setting of hemolysis, and may be as high as 30 to 40%.
- Evidence of an autoantibody against RBCs in the form of a positive direct antigen test (direct Coombs' test) and identification of an autoantibody, either from washing off the antibodies from the patient's RBCs or detecting the autoantibodies present in the patient's serum (indirect Coombs' test), is diagnostic for autoimmune hemolytic anemia.

EMERGENCY DEPARTMENT CARE AND DISPOSITION

- Prednisone (1.0 mg/kg/day) is the initial treatment for warm-type antibody hemolytic anemia and TTP. Azathioprine and cyclophosphamide are occasionally utilized, and splenectomy may be required for those who fail or cannot tolerate steroids.
- Plasma exchange transfusion is the foundation of therapy for TTP. If unavailable, fresh frozen plasma should be infused while arranging transfer to a tertiary care center.
- Except in cases of life-threatening bleeding or intracranial hemorrhage, platelet transfusions should be avoided in TTP because they can aggravate the thrombotic process. Aspirin should be avoided because it may worsen hemorrhagic complications in the face of severe thrombocytopenia.
- Immunotherapy may also be initiated for TTP patients who are refractory to treatment.
- Transfusion of packed RBCs is indicated for angina, heart failure, mental status changes, or hypoxia.
- Patients with cold-type antibody hemolytic anemia should be kept in a warm environment.
- Dialysis should be considered in the management of HUS.
- Prompt delivery of the infant followed by supportive care is mandatory for patients with HELLP syndrome.
- Iron and folate should be given to patients with traumatic hemolysis due to artificial heart valves. If hemolysis is severe, the defective valve may need replacement.

REFERENCES

1. Frenette PS: Sickle cell vasoocclusion: A multistep and multicellular paradigm. *Curr Opin Hematol* 9:101, 2002.
2. Davies S, Olujohungbe A: Hydroxyurea for sickle cell disease. *Cochrane Database Syst Rev* 2:CD003427, 2002.
3. Scjroer SL: Pathophysiology of thalassemia. *Curr Opin Hematol* 9:123, 2002.
4. Smith JA: Bone disorders in sickle cell disease. *Hematol Oncol Clin North Am* 10:1345, 1996.
5. Ballas SK: Sickle anemia: Progress in pathogenesis and treatment. *Drugs* 62:1143, 2002.
6. Telen MJ: Principles and problems of transfusion in sickle cell disease. *Semin Hematol* 38:315, 2001.
7. Riddington C, Williamson L: Preoperative blood transfusions for sickle cell disease. *Cochrane Database Syst Rev* 3: CD003427, 2002.
8. Riddington C, Wang W: Blood transfusion for preventing stroke in people with sickle cell disease. *Cochrane Database Syst Rev* 1:CD003427, 2002.
9. Moake JL: Thrombotic microangiopathies. *N Engl J Med* 347:589, 2002.
10. Elliot MA, Nichols WL: Thrombotic thrombocytopenic purpura and hemolytic uremic syndrome. *Mayo Clin Proc* 76: 1154, 2001.
11. Abraham KA, Connolly G, Farrell J: The HELLP syndrome, a prospective study. *Renal Fail* 23:705, 2001.

For further reading in *Emergency Medicine: A Comprehensive Study Guide,* 6th ed., see Chap. 221, "Hereditary Hemolytic Anemias," by Robin R. Hemphill; and Chap. 222, "Acquired Hemolytic Anemia," by Patty Chu and Robin R. Hemphill.

140 TRANSFUSION THERAPY

Walter N. Simmons

WHOLE BLOOD

- The total blood volume of a 70-kg adult is approximately 75 mL/kg, or 5 L.
- Whole blood has limited usefulness as a transfusion therapy. Although it can provide both volume and oxygen-carrying capacity, this is often better achieved using the individual blood components.
- Disadvantages of whole blood, in part because of degradation during storage, include low levels of clotting factors; frequently elevated levels of potassium, hydrogen ion, and ammonia; and the presence of a large number of antigens.
- A unit of whole blood contains about 500 mL of blood plus a preservative-anticoagulant, usually citrate phosphate dextrose adenine.

PACKED RED BLOOD CELLS

- Red blood cell replacement is usually done with packed red blood cells (PRBCs), primarily to increase oxygen-carrying capacity.[1]

- One unit of PRBCs, about 250 mL in volume, raises an adult's hemoglobin by 1 g/dL, or the hematocrit by 3%, and is usually transfused over 1 to 2 hours unless there is hemodynamic instability.
- The major indications for PRBC transfusion include the following: (1) acute hemorrhage: blood loss greater than 25 to 30% blood volume (1500 mL) in otherwise healthy adults usually requires transfusion of PRBCs to replace oxygen-carrying capacity, and crystalloid infusion to replace volume; (2) surgical blood loss greater than 2 L usually requires transfusion of PRBCs and crystalloid; and (3) in chronic anemia, transfusion may be indicated for symptomatic patients, those with underlying cardiopulmonary disease, and those with hemoglobin levels less than 7 g/dL.[2-4]
- Most patients can be typed (ABO and RhD blood group type) in about 15 minutes.
- A type and cross-match against blood intended for transfusion takes approximately 1 hour.
- RBCs are available as leukocyte poor, frozen, or washed. Leukocyte-poor RBCs have up to 85% of the leukocytes removed and are indicated for transplant recipients or candidates, and for patients with a history of febrile nonhemolytic transfusion reactions.
- Frozen RBCs are a source of rare blood types and provide reduced antigen exposure.
- Washed RBCs are for patients who have hypersensitive reactions to plasma, for neonatal transfusions, and for those with paroxysmal nocturnal hemoglobinuria.

PLATELETS

- Platelet transfusions may be used in thrombocytopenic patients to either prevent bleeding or to help stop active bleeding.[5,6]
- One unit contains 3 to 6×10^{11} platelets in a volume of 250 to 350 mL and are transfused using ABO compatibility.
- Dosing is usually 1 unit per 10 kg (approximately 6 U for an adult), which raises the platelet count about 50,000/μL. ABO- and Rh-compatible platelets are preferable.
- The platelet count should be checked 1 and 24 hours after infusion.
- Transfused platelets survive 3 to 5 days unless there is platelet consumption.
- If the platelet count is above 50,000/μL, bleeding from thrombocytopenia is unlikely unless there is platelet dysfunction.
- Principles for platelet transfusions in adults include the following: (1) maintain the platelet count greater than 50,000/μL in patients undergoing major surgery or with significant bleeding; (2) a platelet count between 10,000 and 50,000/μL increases the risk of bleeding with trauma or invasive procedures, and patients with platelet dysfunction (eg, renal or liver disease) may have spontaneous hemorrhage with these counts; and (3) a platelet count below 10,000/μL presents a high risk for spontaneous bleeding, and prophylactic transfusion is indicated.
- In thrombocytopenia due to platelet destruction, however, platelet transfusion may have little effect.

FRESH FROZEN PLASMA

- Fresh frozen plasma (FFP) is indicated for: (1) acquired coagulopathy with active bleeding or before invasive procedures when there is greater than 1.5 times prolongation of the prothrombin time (PT) or partial thromboplastin time (PTT), or a coagulation factor assay less than 25% of normal; (2) congenital isolated factor deficiencies when specific virally-safe products are not available; (3) thrombotic thrombocytopenic purpura (TTP) patients who are undergoing plasma exchange; (4) patients receiving massive transfusion who develop coagulopathy and active bleeding; and (5) antithrombin III deficiency, when antithrombin III concentrate is not available.[7]
- One bag of FFP contains 200 to 250 mL, 1 U/mL of each coagulation factor, and 1 to 2 mg/mL of fibrinogen.
- FFP should be ABO compatible with a typical starting dose of 8 to 10 mL/kg, or 2 to 4 bags.
- One unit of FFP will increase most coagulation factors by 3 to 5%.

CRYOPRECIPITATE

- Cryoprecipitate is derived from FFP; one bag contains 80 to 100 U factor VIIIC, 80 U von Willebrand's factor, 200 to 300 mg fibrinogen, 40 to 60 U factor XIII, and variable amounts of fibronectin.
- The usual dose is 2 to 4 bags per 10-kg body weight (10 to 20 bags); ABO compatible bags are preferable.
- Indications for cryoprecipitate therapy are: (1) fibrinogen level less than 100 mg/dL associated with disseminated intravascular coagulation or congenital fibrinogen deficiency; (2) von Willebrand's disease with active bleeding when desmopressin is not effective and factor VIII concentrate containing von Willebrand's factor is not available; (3) hemophilia A when virally-inactivated factor VIII concentrates are not available; (4) use as fibrin glue surgical adhesives; and (5) fibronectin replacement.

INTRAVENOUS IMMUNOGLOBULINS

- Indications for intravenous immunoglobulins include the treatment of primary and secondary immunodeficiency and treatment of immune or inflammatory disorders, such as immune thrombocytopenia and Kawasaki's syndrome.
- Adverse reactions include anaphylaxis, febrile reactions, headache, and renal failure.
- There have been some documented cases of patients developing a positive serology to hepatitis C after intravenous immunoglobulin therapy.

ANTITHROMBIN III

- Antithrombin III (ATIII) is a serum protein that inhibits coagulation factors, thrombin, and activated factors IX, X, XI, and XII.

- Deficiency can be congenital or acquired.
- ATIII is mainly used for prophylaxis of thrombosis or to treat thromboembolism in patients with hereditary ATIII deficiency.

ALBUMIN

- Albumin is available for patients with decreased intravascular oncotic pressure.
- Due to cost and lack of proven efficacy, its use is controversial and it is currently used infrequently.[8–9]

SPECIFIC FACTOR REPLACEMENT THERAPY

- Table 140-1 outlines therapy for congenital coagulation factor deficiencies.

TABLE 140-1   Replacement Therapy for Congenital Factor Deficiencies

COAGULATION FACTOR	INCIDENCE*	REPLACEMENT THERAPY
Factor I (fibrinogen)	150 cases	Cryoprecipitate
Factor II (prothrombin)	>30 cases	FFP for minor bleeding episodes Prothrombin complex concentrate† for major bleeding
Factor V	150 cases	FFP
Factor VII	150 cases	FFP for minor bleeding episodes Prothrombin complex concentrates for major bleeding Recombinant factor VII$_A$ (experimental)
Factor VIII	1 in 10,000 males	Factor VIII concentrates (cryoprecipitate or FFP if not available) Desmopressin for those with mild hemophilia
Von Willebrand's disease	up to 1 in 100 persons	Desmopressin (or some factor VIII concentrates or cryoprecipitate)
Factor IX	1 in 30,000 males	Factor IX concentrates
Factor X	1 in 500,000	FFP for minor bleeding episodes Prothrombin complex concentrates for major bleeding
Factor XI†	3 in 10,000 Ashkenazi Jews 1 in 1,000,000 in general	FFP
Factor XII	Several hundred cases	Replacement not required
Factor XIII	>100 cases	FFP or cryoprecipitate

ABBREVIATION: FFP = fresh frozen plasma.
*Incidence as of 1998.
†Factor XI levels correlate poorly with bleeding complications; many patients have low levels, but no bleeding complications.

TABLE 140-2   Acute Transfusion Reactions: Recognition, Management, Evaluation

REACTION TYPE	SIGNS AND SYMPTOMS	MANAGEMENT	EVALUATION
Acute intravascular hemolytic reaction	Fever, chills, low back pain, flushing, dyspnea, tachycardia, shock, hemoglobinuria	Immediately stop transfusion IV hydration to maintain diuresis; diuretics may be necessary Cardiorespiratory support as indicated Can be life threatening	Retype and cross-match Direct and indirect Coombs tests CBC, creatinine, PT, aPTT Haptoglobin, indirect bilirubin, LDH, plasma free hemoglobin Urine for hemoglobin
Acute extravascular hemolytic reaction	Often have low-grade fever but may be entirely asymptomatic	Stop transfusion Rarely causes clinical instability	Hemolytic work-up as above to rule out the possibility of intravascular hemolysis
Febrile nonhemolytic transfusion reaction	Fever, chills	Stop transfusion Manage as in intravascular hemolytic reaction (above) because cannot initially distinguish between the two Can treat fever and chills with acetaminophen and meperidine Usually mild but can be life threatening in patients with tenuous cardiopulmonary status Consider infectious work-up	Hemolytic work-up as above because initially cannot distinguish the etiology
Allergic reaction	If mild, urticaria, pruritus If severe, dyspnea, bronchospasm, hypotension, tachycardia, shock	Stop transfusion If mild, reaction can be treated with diphenhydramine; if symptoms resolve, can restart transfusion If severe, may require cardiopulmonary support; do not restart transfusion	For mild symptoms that resolve with diphenhydramine, no further work-up is necessary, although blood bank should be notified For severe reaction, do hemolytic work-up as above because initially will be indistinguishable from a hemolytic reaction

ABBREVIATIONS: aPTT = activated partial thromboplastin time; CBC = complete blood count; LDH = lactate dehydrogenase; PT = prothrombin time.

COMPLICATIONS OF TRANSFUSIONS

- Adverse reactions occur in up to 20% of transfusions and are usually mild.
- Transfusion reactions can be immediate or delayed.
- Table 140-2 summarizes the types of immediate reactions as well as methods of recognition, management, and evaluation.

DELAYED TRANSFUSION REACTIONS

- Delayed hemolytic reactions can occur 7 to 10 days after transfusion.
- Infection may result from transfusion. There is a small risk of transmission of HIV, hepatitis B and C, cytomegalovirus, parvovirus, and human T-cell lymphotropic viruses I and II.
- Other rare but reported pathogens include Epstein-Barr virus, syphilis, malaria, babesiosis, toxoplasmosis, and trypanosomiasis.
- Hypothermia may occur from rapid transfusions of refrigerated blood.
- Noncardiogenic pulmonary edema may be caused by incompatible passively transferred leukocyte antibodies, and usually occurs within 4 hours of transfusion.

- Clinical findings of noncardiogenic pulmonary edema are respiratory distress, fever, chills, tachycardia, and patchy infiltrates on chest radiograph without cardiomegaly. There is no evidence of fluid overload.
- Electrolyte imbalance may occur. Citrate is part of the preservative solution and chelates calcium. Significant hypocalcemia even with massive transfusion is rare because patients with normal hepatic function readily metabolize citrate into bicarbonate.
- Hypokalemia can occur with large transfusions due to the metabolism of citrate to bicarbonate, leading to alkalosis, which drives potassium ions into the intracellular space.
- Hyperkalemia can occur in patients with renal failure or in neonates.
- Graft-versus-host disease, fatal in greater than 90% of cases, occurs when nonirradiated lymphocytes are inadvertently transfused into an immunocompromised patient.

EMERGENCY TRANSFUSIONS

- Use of type O or type-specific incompletely cross-matched blood may be life-saving but carries the risk of life-threatening transfusion reactions.

- Its use should be limited to the early resuscitation of patients with severe hemorrhage without adequate response to crystalloid infusion.
- Before transfusing, blood for baseline laboratory tests and type and cross-matching should be obtained. Rh-negative blood is preferable when it is not fully cross-matched.

MASSIVE TRANSFUSION

- Massive transfusion is the approximate replacement of a patient's total blood volume within a 24-hour period.
- Complications include bleeding, citrate toxicity, and hypothermia.
- Bleeding may result from thrombocytopenia, platelet dysfunction, disseminated intravascular coagulation, or coagulation factor deficiencies.
- Patients receiving more than 5 U of whole blood, those with liver disease, and neonates are at risk for hypocalcemia from citrate toxicity.
- The QT interval is not a reliable indicator in this setting; an ionized calcium level is necessary.
- Hypocalcemia should be treated with 5 to 10 mL of IV calcium gluconate infused slowly.
- Physicians should be wary of hypothermia when administering 3 U or more of blood rapidly.

BLOOD ADMINISTRATION

- The correct identification of the patient and the unit to be transfused should always be ensured.
- A 16-gauge or larger IV catheter is preferred to prevent hemolysis and to permit rapid infusion. Micropore filters should be used to filter out microaggregates of platelets, fibrin, and leukocytes.
- Normal saline solution is the only crystalloid compatible with PRBCs. Warmed saline solution (39° to 43°C or 102.2° to 109.4°F) may be given concurrently or a blood warmer used to prevent hypothermia. The blood itself will hemolyze if warmed to greater than 40°C (104°F).
- Rapid transfusion may be facilitated by the use of pressure infusion devices.
- Patients at risk for hypervolemia should receive each unit over 3 to 4 hours.

REFERENCES

1. Blajchman MA, Hebert PC: Red blood cell transfusion strategies. *Transfus Clin Biol* 8:207, 2001.

2. Hill SR, Carless PA, Henry DA, et al: Transfusion thresholds and other strategies for guiding allogenic red blood cell transfusion. *Cochrane Database Syst Rev* 2:CD002042, 2002.
3. Carson JL, Hill S, Carless P, et al: Transfusion triggers: A systematic review of the literature. *Transfus Med Rev* 16:187, 2002.
4. Myhre BA: Clinical commentary: The transfusion trigger: The search for a quantitative holy grail. *Ann Clin Lab Sci* 31:359, 2001.
5. Rebulla P: Revisitation of the clinical indication for the transfusion of platelet concentrates. *Rev Clin Exp Hematol* 5:228, 2001.
6. Rebulla P: Platelet transfusion trigger in difficult patients. *Transfus Clin Biol* 8:249, 2001.
7. Fay A, Abinun M: Current management of hereditary angioedema (C-1 esterase inhibitor deficiency). *J Clin Pathol* 55:266, 2002.
8. Wilkes MM, Navickis RJ: Patient survival after human albumin administration. A meta-analysis of randomized, controlled trials. *Ann Intern Med* 135:149, 2001.
9. Alderson P, Bunn F, Lefebvre C, et al: Human albumin solution for resuscitation and volume expansion in critically ill patients. *Cochrane Database Syst Rev* 1:CD001208, 2002.

For further reading in *Emergency Medicine: A Comprehensive Study Guide*, 6th ed., see Chap. 223, "Transfusion Therapy," by Sally A Santen.

141 EXOGENOUS ANTICOAGULANTS AND ANTIPLATELET AGENTS
Robert A. Schwab

ANTITHROMBOTIC AGENTS

ORAL ANTICOAGULANTS

- Oral anticoagulants inhibit thrombus formation or propagation, and reduce the risk of embolization in patients with existing thrombosis.
- Sodium warfarin inhibits synthesis of vitamin K–dependent clotting factors and antithrombotic proteins C and S. Dosing is guided by the International Normalized Ratio (INR), which is derived from the prothrombin time (PT).
- The desired INR is between 2.0 and 2.5.[1]
- Drug interactions and certain disease states can interfere with warfarin absorption or metabolism; these interactions may be clinically significant.
- Warfarin is contraindicated in pregnancy.
- Full anticoagulation occurs 3 to 4 days after initiating therapy.

- During the first 24 to 36 hours, a hypercoagulable state occurs due to variable half-lives of clotting factors and antithrombotic proteins; the effects of this can be minimized by beginning with a warfarin dose of 5 mg/day.
- In situations in which immediate anticoagulation is critical, a heparin product should be used until an adequate INR is achieved.

PARENTERAL ANTICOAGULANTS

- Unfractionated heparin (UFH) is a heterogenous mixture of polysaccharides that binds antithrombin III; this complex inhibits multiple steps in the coagulation cascade.[2]
- A bolus of 70 to 80 U/kg IV is followed by IV infusion at 15 to 18 U/kg/h.
- Therapy is monitored by the partial thromboplastin time (PTT); the therapeutic range is 1.5 to 2.5 times the normal value.
- Low molecular weight heparin (LMWH) fractions (eg, enoxaparin, dalteparin, and ardeparin) are derived from unfractionated heparin.
- Advantages of LMWH over UFH include longer half-life and decreased binding to plasma proteins, endothelial cells, and macrophages.
- LMWH is a much more predictable anticoagulant with fixed dose-response relationships. LMWH can be administered subcutaneously (SC) once to twice daily, and does not require monitoring, except in patients with renal failure and obesity.[3]
- LMWH may be used safely in pregnancy.
- UFH or LMWH is indicated for deep venous thrombosis (DVT) prophylaxis and treatment, pulmonary embolism (PE), unstable angina, and acute myocardial infarction (AMI).
- Only enoxaparin is approved for outpatient management of DVT.

DIRECT THROMBIN INHIBITORS

- Hirudin is a protein derived from leeches that is now prepared using recombinant technology.
- Hirudin and its analogues inhibit both circulating and clot-bound thrombin.
- They are currently approved for use in patients with heparin-induced thrombocytopenia and as anticoagulants during percutaneous coronary intervention.

INHIBITORS OF PLATELET ACTIVATION

- Aspirin is an irreversible inhibitor of cyclooxygenase, an enzyme that produces competing effects on platelet aggregation.

- At low doses of aspirin, inhibitory effects predominate; the recommended antiplatelet dose is usually 81 to 162 mg/day.
- Side effects of aspirin are usually related to the gastrointestinal (GI) tract; active GI bleeding is a contraindication. Patients with guaiac-positive stool and no active bleeding can be treated with careful monitoring.
- Nonsteroidal anti-inflammatory drugs (NSAIDs) reversibly inhibit cyclooxygenase; platelet inhibition usually lasts less than 24 hours.

INHIBITORS OF PLATELET AGGREGATION

- Platelet aggregation involves binding of fibrinogen to the platelet glycoprotein IIb-IIIa receptor.
- Platelet membrane altering agents ticlopidine 250 mg twice daily and clopidogrel 75 mg/day inhibit binding of adenosine diphosphate (ADP) to the receptor, rendering it ineffective.
- These agents should be used in patients with acute coronary syndromes who cannot take aspirin.
- Glycoprotein IIb-IIIa inhibitors (eg, abciximab, eptifibatide, and tirofiban) inhibit aggregation, prevent thrombosis, and may augment fibrinolysis.
- These agents can improve outcomes in selected patients with unstable angina and non–ST elevation myocardial infarction; they should be used in consultation with interventional cardiologists.[4]

FIBRINOLYTIC AGENTS

- Fibrinolytic agents convert plasminogen to plasmin, which dissolves the fibrin in thrombi.
- Streptokinase (SK) and anistreplase (APSAC) are antigenic; retreatment should not occur within 6 months of the initial therapy.
- Tissue plasminogen activator (tPA) is theoretically more "clot specific" than SK or APSAC.
- Reteplase and tenecteplase are modified versions of tPA, designed to improve efficacy and safety.
- Although the side effect profile of these agents is similar, bolus-dose fibrinolytics (APSAC, reteplase, and tenecteplase) result in significantly fewer medication errors.

INDICATIONS FOR ANTITHROMBOTIC THERAPY

ACUTE MYOCARDIAL INFARCTION

- Fibrinolytic therapy should be initiated within 30 minutes or angioplasty within 90 minutes of arrival at the emergency department. Criteria include presentation within 12 hours of symptom onset, ST-segment

TABLE 141-1 Contraindications to Fibrinolytic Therapy*

Absolute
  Active or recent internal bleeding ($\leq$ 14 d)
  CVA <2–6 mo or hemorrhagic CVA†
  Intracranial or intraspinal surgery or trauma $\leq$2 mo
  Intracranial or intraspinal neoplasm, aneurysm, or arteriovenous malformation
  Known severe bleeding diathesis
  On anticoagulants (warfarin, PT > 15 s, heparin, increased aPTT)
  Uncontrolled hypertension (ie, blood pressure > 185/100 mm Hg)
  Suspected aortic dissection or pericarditis
  Pregnancy
Relative
  Active peptic ulcer disease
  Cardiopulmonary resuscitation >10 min
  Hemorrhagic opthalmic conditions
  Puncture of noncompressible vessel <10 d
  Advanced age >75 y
  Significant trauma or major surgery >2 wk and <2 mo
  Advanced kidney or liver disease

*Concurrent menses is *not* a contraindication.
†In ischemic CVA, symptoms longer than 3 hours, severe hemispheric stroke, platelets below 100/mL, and glucose below 50 or above 400 mg/dL are additional contraindications.
Key: aPTT = activated partial thromplastic time, CVA = cardiovascular accident, PT = prothrombin time.

elevation in two or more contiguous leads, or new-onset left bundle-branch block, and absence of contraindications (Table 141-1).
• Angioplasty is preferred in patients with cardiogenic shock.
• Timely initiation of therapy is more important than the specific agent utilized.
• Aspirin should be administered immediately except in patients with aspirin allergy; these patients should receive clopidogrel or ticlopidine.

DEEP VENOUS THROMBOSIS OR PULMONARY EMBOLISM

• Treatment of DVT or PE can be initiated with either UFH or LMWH.
• LMWH is as effective as UFH, with fewer side effects, and allows for outpatient management of selected patients.
• Selected patients may benefit from fibrinolytic therapy.[5,6]

ISCHEMIC STROKE

• tPA may benefit some stroke patients if administered within 3 hours of symptom onset;[7] there is an increased risk of conversion to hemorrhagic stroke.[8]
• Fibrinolytic agents should not be given to patients with hypertension, signs of hemorrhagic stroke, or rapidly improving symptoms.

COMPLICATIONS OF ANTICOAGULATION AND ANTITHROMBOTIC THERAPY

• Treatment for the complications of warfarin, heparin, and fibrinolytic therapy is discussed in Chap. 137.

REFERENCES

1. Ansell J, Hirsh J, Dalen J et al: Managing oral anticoagulant therapy. *Chest* 119:22, 2001.
2. Pineo GF, Hull RD: Unfractionated and low-molecular-weight heparin: Comparisons and current recommendations. *Med Clin North Am* 82:587, 1998.
3. Cohen M, Antman EM, Gurfinkel EP et al: The ESSENCE (Efficacy and Safety of Subcutaneous Enoxaparin in Non-Q-wave Coronary Events) and TIMI IIB Investigators: Enoxaparin in unstable angina/non-ST-segment elevation myocardial infarction: Treatment benefits in prespecified sub-groups. *J Thrombosis Thrombolysis* 12:199, 2001.
4. Braunwald E, Antman EM, Beasley JW et al: ACC/AHA guidelines for the management of patients with unstable angina and non-ST-segment elevation myocardial infarction: A report of the American College of Cardiology/American Heart Association Task Force on Practice Guidelines. *J Am Coll Cardiol* 26:970, 2000.
5. Agnelli G, Becattini C, Kirschstein T: Thrombolysis vs heparin in the treatment of pulmonary embolism: A clinical outcome-based meta-analysis. *Arch Intern Med* 162:2537, 2002.
6. Dalen JE: The uncertain role of thrombolytic therapy in the treatment of pulmonary embolism. *Arch Intern Med* 162: 2521, 2002.
7. Marler JR, Tilley BC, Lu M et al: Earlier treatment associated with better outcome: The NINDS-TPA Stroke Study. *Neurology* 55:1649, 2002.
8. The NINDS-TPA Stroke Study group: Intracerebral hemorrhage after intravenous tPA therapy for ischemic stroke. *Stroke* 28:2109, 1997.

For further reading in *Emergency Medicine: A Comprehensive Study Guide,* 6th ed., see Chap. 224, "Anticoagulants, Antiplatelet Agents, and Fibrinolytics," by Jim Edward Weber, F. Michael Jaggi, and Charles V. Pollack, Jr.

142 EMERGENCY COMPLICATIONS OF MALIGNANCY
T. Paul Tran

BONE EMERGENCIES

EPIDEMIOLOGY

• Carcinomas of the breast, lung, and prostate commonly metastasize to the proximal aspects of the limbs, pelvis, ribs, sternum, and skull to cause bone pain and pathologic fractures. These three cancers account for 80% of all metastatic disease.[1]

PATHOPHYSIOLOGY

- Through hematogenous spread, cancer cells invade bone marrow and secrete stimulating factors, which through various mediators and cytokines may disrupt normal bone homeostasis to favor either osteoblastic or osteolytic activity (osteolytic being more common).
- While certain cancers may cause osteolysis (eg, renal) and osteogenesis (eg, prostate), the majority of cancers may produce simultaneous osteolytic and osteoblastic lesions.

CLINICAL FEATURES

- Patients with a known history of primary cancer may present with bone pain.
- The pain may be vague and insidious in onset, developing over days or weeks, and may even be the first sign of metastatic disease.

DIAGNOSIS AND DIFFERENTIAL

- Clinical examination and plain radiographs are usually sufficient for the initial screening.[1]
- Computed tomography (CT) can be used to evaluate bone integrity and soft tissue extension.
- Older women may suffer from osteoporosis in which cortical bone is preserved. In contrast, cortical bone is destroyed in metastatic bone cancer.

EMERGENCY DEPARTMENT CARE AND DISPOSITION

- Patients with metastatic bone pain without fractures should be administered narcotic analgesics.
- Patients with pathologic fracture should be administered IV narcotics and have the fracture sites immobilized. Most pathologic fractures benefit from surgical intervention.
- Nondisplaced fractures involving non–weight bearing bones can be treated conservatively.
- Indications for hospitalization include hemodynamic instability, irreducible fractures, neurovascular compromise, disabling fractures (eg, fractures of the hip or femur), intractable pain, and inadequate home care.

SPINAL CORD COMPRESSION

EPIDEMIOLOGY

- Up to 1 in 5 patients with vertebral metastases will develop epidural spinal cord compression.[2]

- The thoracic spine is most commonly involved (70%), followed by lumbar (20%), and cervical (10%).[1]
- Breast, lung, unknown primary, lymphoma, multiple myeloma, and prostate cancer are the most common cancers to cause spinal cord compression.[1]

PATHOPHYSIOLOGY

- Neurologic symptoms are caused by direct mechanical effects or infiltration of the tumor on the nerve root or anterior aspects of the spinal cord.

CLINICAL FEATURES

- Patients with epidural spinal cord compression may present with back pain (locally or with radiculopathy), bilateral motor weakness, sensory changes (hyperesthesia or anesthesia), and bladder or bowel retention or incontinence.
- Back pain is progressive, unrelenting, and worsened by recumbency.
- Because the anterior aspect of the spine is more often involved, motor function symptoms such as leg weakness usually precede sensory symptoms such as leg hyperesthesia or anesthesia (anterior cord syndrome).[2]
- Bowel control and bladder symptoms such as urinary retention are a late presentation. Postvoid bladder residual may be greater than 150 mL.
- Physical examination may reveal vertebral percussion tenderness, decreased rectal tone, saddle anesthesia, lower extremity hyporeflexia or areflexia, and absent anal "wink."

DIAGNOSIS AND DIFFERENTIAL

- Intramedullary primary or metastatic disease may present similarly, but the extremity weakness is usually unilateral.
- Plain radiographs (or bone scan) can be ordered to identify the level of vertebral involvement, but a gadolinium-enhanced magnetic resonance imaging (MRI) scan of the whole spine is required to ascertain the diagnosis.

EMERGENCY DEPARTMENT CARE AND DISPOSITION

- If epidural spinal cord compromise is clinically suspected, patients should initially be administered dexamethasone 24 mg IV every 6 hours.[3]

- Emergent consultation with specialists in radiation oncology and neurosurgery should be initiated for acute radiation therapy and/or surgical decompression.

UPPER AIRWAY OBSTRUCTION

PATHOPHYSIOLOGY

- Tumors in the oropharynx, larynx, trachea, thyroid, and lung can cause upper airway obstruction.
- Acute airway obstruction occurs when a vulnerable upper airway is further compromised by foreign body, airway edema, new bleeding, secretions, or infection.

CLINICAL FEATURES

- Patients may complain of dyspnea on exertion, wheezing, voice change, and orthopnea.
- Physical examination signs may include tachycardia, tachypnea, wheezing, stridor, intercostal retraction, and accessory muscle use.
- Stridor is an ominous sign.
- Bradycardia, cyanosis, or obtundation may be the harbingers of cardiac arrest.

DIAGNOSIS AND DIFFERENTIAL

- Metastatic disease, tracheomalacia, oropharyngeal infections (eg, Ludwig's angina and epiglottitis), and lower airway tumors can also produce the clinical syndrome of airway obstruction.
- Bronchoscopy is diagnostic.

EMERGENCY DEPARTMENT CARE AND DISPOSITION

- The airway should be suctioned and supplemental oxygen administered. Heliox[4] (70% nitrogen and 30% oxygen) and laryngeal mask airway may be used as temporizing measures.
- Percutaneous jet ventilation is contraindicated in upper airway obstruction.
- Patients with impending airway obstruction require immediate intervention to create a secure and patent airway. Ideally, this should be accomplished in the operating room by an otolaryngologist.
- In consultation with a pulmonologist, otolaryngologist, or anesthesiologist, emergency department measures include orotracheal intubation with fiberoptic laryngoscopy or bronchoscopy. Surgical airway via cricothyroidotomy or tracheostomy should be performed as clinically indicated.

MALIGNANT PERICARDIAL EFFUSION AND TAMPONADE

EPIDEMIOLOGY

- Up to 10% of dying patients with metastatic disease have cardiac and pericardial involvement.
- Common causes of malignant pericardial effusion include carcinomas of the breast and lung, lymphoma, leukemia, and malignant melanoma. Rarely, pericardial effusions can also be caused by therapeutic irradiation and chemotherapeutic agents (busulphan, cytarabine, and tretinoin).

PATHOPHYSIOLOGY

- The rate of accumulation and distensibility of the pericardial sac determine the degree of hemodynamic instability.
- Sudden or large (>500 mL) effusions may compress on the right ventricle and reduce cardiac output.

CLINICAL FEATURES

- Patients may present with fatigue, chest heaviness, dyspnea, palpitations, cough, and syncope.
- Physical examination findings of tamponade include tachycardia, narrowed pulse pressure, hypotension, distended neck vein, muffled heart tone, and pulsus paradoxus.

DIAGNOSIS AND DIFFERENTIAL

- Chest radiograph may demonstrate an enlarged cardiac silhouette and pleural effusion.
- Electrocardiogram (ECG) may show sinus tachycardia, low QRS amplitude, and pulsus alternans.
- Transthoracic echocardiogram is diagnostic.
- Chemotherapy-induced cardiomyopathy and radiation-induced cardiac disease should be considered in the differential diagnosis.

EMERGENCY DEPARTMENT CARE AND DISPOSITION

- Echocardiography-guided percutaneous pericardiocentesis under local anesthesia (general anesthesia is contraindicated) is the treatment of choice for cardiac tamponade.[5]
- Oxygen, volume expansion with crystalloid, and dopamine, up to 20 μg/kg/min IV, can be initiated as temporizing measures before pericardiocentesis.

- Care of patients with malignant pericardial effusion without tamponade should be discussed with the oncologist.

SUPERIOR VENA CAVA SYNDROME

EPIDEMIOLOGY

- Superior vena cava syndrome is commonly caused by bronchogenic carcinoma, breast carcinoma, lymphoma, and anterior mediastinal tumors (thymoma, thymic carcinoid, and teratoma).

PATHOPHYSIOLOGY

- The pathogenesis of the superior vena cava syndrome is predominantly related to the reduced venous return in the superior vena cava, with subsequent upper body congestion, reduced preload, and reduced cardiac output.[2]
- Expansive tumors and lymph nodes in the fixed space mediastinum can cause extrinsic mass effects on the thin-walled superior vena cava, leading to venous stasis.
- Tracheal compression can cause acute airway difficulty.

CLINICAL FEATURES

- Patients may present with an insidious onset of dyspnea, chest pain, cough, and facial and arm swelling.
- Physical examination signs include distended neck and chest veins, nonpitting edema of the neck, distended arm veins and arm swelling, tongue and facial swelling, and cyanosis.[2,6]

DIAGNOSIS AND DIFFERENTIAL

- Chest radiograph may show a widened mediastinum.
- Contrast-enhanced CT of the chest is diagnostic.

EMERGENCY DEPARTMENT CARE AND DISPOSITION

- Emergency therapy includes supplemental oxygen, sedation, bedrest, and elevation of the head and upper body.
- Increases in intracranial pressure can be treated with either methylprednisolone 125 to 250 mg IV or dexamethasone 20 mg IV.
- Airway compromise should be managed with orotracheal intubation.

- Furosemide once was suggested as a temporizing measure but its efficacy and safety are controversial. Diuresis can further exacerbate the already reduced cardiac output, leading to more hemodynamic instability.[6]
- Intravascular stenting, chemotherapy, and radiotherapy are effective therapeutic measures after the specific tumor type is determined.

THROMBOEMBOLISM

EPIDEMIOLOGY

- Approximately 90% of pulmonary embolisms originate from blood clots embolizing from the deep veins of the pelvis and legs.[4]
- Most thromboembolic diseases are associated with four types of cancers: adenocarcinoma of the lung, pancreas, stomach, and colon.[4]

PATHOPHYSIOLOGY

- Malignancy is associated with a hypercoagulable state. Neoplastic cells and chemotherapy can cause intimal injury. Obstructive tumors often cause venous stasis, which is exacerbated by decreased mobility.[7]
- Significant pulmonary embolism leads to hypoxemia via ventilation-perfusion mismatch and shunting.
- Pulmonary embolism also causes hemodynamic instability via a complex interplay of mechanical obstruction of the pulmonary vascular bed and a compensatory pulmonary vasoconstriction mechanism.[4]

CLINICAL FEATURES

- Patients may present with dyspnea, fever, cough, dyspnea on exertion, pleuritic chest pain, leg pain or swelling, and hemoptysis.
- Low grade fever, tachypnea, tachycardia, pleural rub, and unilateral lower extremity swelling are some of the nonspecific findings that may be present on physical examination.

DIAGNOSIS AND DIFFERENTIAL

- Nonspecific T-wave inversion and tachycardia on ECG are common abnormal findings.
- Alveolar arterial oxygen tension was abnormal in >60% of patients in the PIOPED study.
- The chest radiograph may demonstrate local infiltrates, ipsilateral diaphragm elevation, Westermark's (decreased lung markings from oligemia) or Hampton's signs (wedge infiltrate).

- The D-dimer assay is sensitive, but not specific for pulmonary embolism.[8]
- Ventilation-perfusion scan and spiral CT are often diagnostic, but a pulmonary angiogram occasionally may be necessary to diagnose pulmonary embolism.[8]

EMERGENCY DEPARTMENT CARE AND DISPOSITION

- Resuscitative measures should be initiated on hemodynamically unstable patients along with low molecular weight heparin (enoxaparin 1 mg/kg SC) or heparin therapy.
- Thrombolytic therapy should be considered in selected cases.
- Admission to the hospital should be made in consultation with the patient's oncologist.

HYPERCALCEMIA OF MALIGNANCY

EPIDEMIOLOGY

- Up to 40% of patients with cancer will develop hypercalcemia during their course of the disease.[9]
- Carcinoma of the breast and lung, lymphoma, and multiple myeloma are most commonly associated with hypercalcemia.[9]

PATHOPHYSIOLOGY

- Hypercalcemia associated with malignancy is most often caused by a parathyroid hormone–related peptide secreted by the cancer cells. This hormone activates the parathyroid hormone receptor, stimulating osteoclastic activity and promoting renal reabsorption of calcium.[10]

CLINICAL FEATURES

- Mild hypercalcemia (<12 mg/dL) usually is asymptomatic.
- More severe hypercalcemia (>14 mg/dL) may cause polydipsia, polyuria, generalized weakness, lethargy, anorexia, nausea, vomiting, constipation, abdominal pain, volume depletion, altered mentation, and frank psychosis.[9]

DIAGNOSIS AND DIFFERENTIAL

- ECG may demonstrate shortened QT interval, ST-segment depression, and atrioventricular blocks.

- Total serum calcium level should be corrected for protein binding. Measurement of ionized calcium is confirmatory.
- Medications (diuretics), granulomatous disorders, primary hyperparathyroidism, and other endocrine disorders can also cause hypercalcemia.

EMERGENCY DEPARTMENT CARE AND DISPOSITION

- Volume depletion should be corrected with IV crystalloid infusion. Furosemide 40 to 80 mg IV every 2 hours can then be added.[10]
- Bisphosphonates such as zoledronic acid 4 mg IV over 15 minutes or pamidronate 60 to 90 mg IV over 4 to 24 hours can be initiated in the emergency department.
- Second-line drugs include calcitonin 4 IU/kg SC every 12 hours.
- Hemodialysis provides definitive treatment.[11]

TUMOR LYSIS SYNDROME

EPIDEMIOLOGY

- Tumor lysis syndrome usually occurs within 1 to 3 days after the last radiochemotherapy of hematologic malignancies, especially Burkitt's lymphoma.

PATHOPHYSIOLOGY

- Tumor lysis syndrome refers to a constellation of metabolic abnormalities triggered by the death of neoplastic cells, which releases large quantities of intracellular contents and uric acid into the bloodstream.[9,12]
- High levels of uric acid and phosphate cause sludging and stasis the kidneys, leading to acute renal failure.
- Massive death of tumor cells results in hyperkalemia, hyperuricemia, and hyperphosphatemia.
- Hyperphosphatemia causes deposition of calcium in tissues and secondary hypocalcemia.

CLINICAL FEATURES

- Patients may present with fatigue, lethargy, nausea, vomiting, and cloudy urine.
- Hypocalcemia may cause neuromuscular irritability, muscular spasm, seizure, and altered mentation.
- Acute renal failure exacerbates hyperkalemia, which together with hypocalcemia may contribute to the development of potentially fatal cardiac arrhythmias.

DIAGNOSIS AND DIFFERENTIAL

- An electrolyte panel, including renal function, calcium, phosphate, and uric acid, in the proper clinical context is diagnostic.
- An ECG may show the peaked T waves of hyperkalemia.

EMERGENCY DEPARTMENT CARE AND DISPOSITION

- Hyperkalemia should be treated in the usual fashion with IV calcium, insulin, and bicarbonate, and oral Kayexalate.
- Hyperuricemia is treated by alkalinizing the urine with two ampules of sodium bicarbonate in 1 liter of D_5W, infused to maintain urine pH between 7.1 and 7.5.[12]
- Emergency hemodialysis should be considered in the setting of serum potassium >6.0 mEq/L, uric acid >10.0 mg/dL, phosphate >10 mg/dL, creatinine >10 mg/dL, symptomatic hypocalcemia, or volume overload.[9,12]

ADRENAL CRISIS

EPIDEMIOLOGY

- While 9 to 27% of patients dying from metastatic disease have adrenal metastases, only 20 to 30% of patients with adrenal metastasis develop adrenal insufficiency.[9]

PATHOPHYSIOLOGY

- In primary adrenal insufficiency, the adrenal glands are incapable of producing the mineraloglucocorticoid required for homeostasis.
- Mineralocorticoid (aldosterone) deficiency leads to impaired sodium conservation (hyponatremia) and impaired potassium secretion (hyperkalemia) and proton secretion (acidosis), while glucocorticoid (cortisol) deficiency leads to impaired metabolism of carbohydrate, lipid, protein, and water (hypoglycemia and hypotension).
- In secondary adrenal insufficiency, the hypothalamic-pituitary axis malfunctions. Production of cortisol is impaired due to a low level of adrenocorticotropic hormone, but aldosterone production is still appropriate.
- Long-term glucocorticoid therapy also leads to a depressed level of adrenocorticotropic hormone. Functional adrenal insufficiency similar to secondary adrenal insufficiency can result when long-term glucocorticoid therapy is abruptly withdrawn.

CLINICAL FEATURES

- Patients may complain of fatigue, weakness, nausea, vomiting, and weight loss.
- They may have a history of recent steroid discontinuation.

DIAGNOSIS AND DIFFERENTIAL

- Supportive laboratory tests include hypoglycemia, hyponatremia, and hyperkalemia.
- Septic, cardiogenic, and hypovolemic shock should be considered in the differential diagnosis.

EMERGENCY DEPARTMENT CARE AND DISPOSITION

- Patients in shock should be given IV crystalloid boluses and hydrocortisone 100 to 300 mg IV every 6 to 8 hours while being worked up for other causes of shock.[9]
- If hypoglycemia is present, 50 to 100 mL of D_{50} should be administered.
- A serum cortisol level should be drawn before treatment, if time permits.

SYNDROME OF INAPPROPRIATE SECRETION OF ANTIDIURETIC HORMONE

EPIDEMIOLOGY

- Most cases (60%) of syndrome of inappropriate secretion of antidiuretic hormone (SIADH) is caused by small-cell lung carcinoma, although other primary and metastatic diseases such as brain cancer, pancreatic adenocarcinoma, and carcinoma of the head, neck, and prostate can also be causative.[2]
- SIADH is also caused by chemotherapeutic agents (melphalan, cisplatin, vincristine, vinblastine, and cyclophosphamide), pneumonia, and positive pressure ventilation, among others.

PATHOPHYSIOLOGY

- Antidiuretic hormone (ADH, vasopressin) normally acts on the collecting tubule of the kidneys to increase water absorption during hypovolemia.
- In SIADH, excess ADH is secreted by ectopic tumor cells or through abnormal secretory stimulation of or cytotoxicity of the paraventricular and supraoptic neurons.
- SIADH is a clinical syndrome characterized by hyponatremia, inappropriately concentrated urine

($>$100 mOsm/L), and excessive urine sodium ($>$20 mEq/L) in the face of hypotonic plasma ($<$260 mOsm/L) and euvolemia.[2]

CLINICAL FEATURES

- Clinical presentation is due mainly to hyponatremia, which includes anorexia, nausea, vomiting, headache, altered mentation, and seizure.

DIAGNOSIS AND DIFFERENTIAL

- Hypothyroidism, renal failure, cirrhosis, and adrenal crisis should be excluded.
- Hyponatremia in the proper context should raise the suspicion of SIADH.
- Serum osmolality, urine osmolality, and volume status should be determined before treatment.

EMERGENCY DEPARTMENT CARE AND DISPOSITION

- Mild hyponatremia can be treated with water restriction ($<$500 mL/day).
- Sodium $<$115 mEq/L associated with seizure activity should be treated with 3% normal saline 1 mL/kg/h to raise the sodium concentration by not more than 2 mEq/L/h to avoid central pontine myelinolysis.
- Usually no more than 300 mL of hypertonic saline is required to improve the symptoms of hyponatremic encephalopathy.[9] Patients should be monitored in an intensive care unit.
- Second-line drugs include furosemide 40 mg IV and demeclocycline 300 to 600 mg.

NEUTROPENIC FEVER

EPIDEMIOLOGY

- Infection is frequently the cause of death in cancer patients. In particular, up to 10% of cancer patients die from infection associated with neutropenia.
- Fever, defined as recurrent temperatures $>$38°C or a single temperature $>$38.3°C, in the presence of neutropenia, defined as an absolute neutrophil count $<$500 cells/mL, is a medical emergency.[13]

PATHOPHYSIOLOGY

- Bone marrow transplant and cancer chemotherapy are associated with neutropenia, making cancer patients vulnerable to bacterial infections, especially by the encapsulated types, and fungal infections.
- The use of immunosuppressants leads to lymphopenia and impaired cell-mediated immunity. The normal physical defense barrier is compromised via mucositis and indwelling catheters.

CLINICAL FEATURES

- Febrile neutropenic patients may initially have minimal symptoms and findings, but can succumb rapidly to sepsis and death.
- Typical infectious agents can be viral (cytomegalovirus, herpes simplex virus, varicella-zoster virus), bacterial (*Staphylococcus, Streptococcus,* enterococci, *Haemophilus influenzae, Escherichia coli, Klebsiella, Pseudomonas aeruginosa*), or fungal (*Candida, Aspergillus*).[13]

DIAGNOSIS AND DIFFERENTIAL

- The sites of infection include central venous access catheter (exit site, tunnel, abscess, line sepsis), skin, mouth, sinuses, chest/lung, abdomen (typhlitis, hepatosplenic candidiasis), perianal region (abscess), and central nervous system (meningitis, encephalitis, brain abscess).
- Cultures should be taken from all lumens, skin/line site, urine, sputum, and stool. They should be sent for bacterial, fungal, and viral studies as indicated.
- A chest radiograph may appear normal in neutropenic febrile patients with pneumonia since neutrophils are required for an infiltrate to appear.

EMERGENCY DEPARTMENT CARE AND DISPOSITION

- Resuscitative measures should be initiated for hemodynamically unstable patients.
- Initial empiric antibiotic therapy should include an antipseudomonal agent, such as ceftazidime (2 g IV), cefepime (2 g IV), or imipenem (500 mg IV), and an aminoglycoside.[13,14]
- Vancomycin (1 g IV) is often added to cover methicillin-resistant *Staphylococcus aureus* and penicillin-resistant *Streptococcus pneumoniae.*

HYPERVISCOSITY SYNDROME

PATHOPHYSIOLOGY

- Hyperviscosity syndrome refers to the condition of impaired blood rheology due to abnormal elevations

of paraproteins (eg, Waldenström's macroglobulinemia), pathologic erythrocytosis, or leukocytosis (eg, hematocrit >60%, white blood cell count >100,000 cells/μL).[12]
- The hyperviscosity causes abnormal blood rheology, which manifests medically as sludging, stasis, impaired microcirculation, and tissue hypoperfusion.

CLINICAL FEATURES

- An elevated hematocrit (polycythemia) can be due to primary overproduction of red blood cells by the bone marrow (polycythemia vera) or as a paraneoplastic syndrome associated with renal cell carcinoma and hepatomas, among others.
- At levels >60%, patients can develop symptoms such as headache, fatigue, and blurred vision, and thrombotic complications such as stroke or mesenteric ischemia.
- Acute and chronic leukemias can produce white blood cell counts >100,000/μL.
- Patients also may present with bleeding, abdominal pain, dyspnea, and altered mentation.
- Funduscopic examination may reveal the classic "sausage link" effects.

DIAGNOSIS AND DIFFERENTIAL

- Hyperviscosity syndrome is usually suspected from history and physical examination, aided by findings of rouleaux formation (stacks of red blood cells) on routine smear.
- Serum viscosity may be >4 to 5 (normal of 1.4 to 1.8).
- Protein electrophoresis is diagnostic.

EMERGENCY DEPARTMENT CARE AND DISPOSITION

- Patients who present with hyperviscosity syndrome should undergo a 2-unit phlebotomy and have 2 to 3 L of crystalloid infused.
- Definitive treatments for symptomatic hyperviscosity due to increased serum proteins, leukocytosis, and erythrocytosis include emergency plasmapheresis, leukapheresis, and phlebotomy, respectively, with or without chemotherapy.

NAUSEA AND VOMITING

EPIDEMIOLOGY

- Almost 75% of cancer patients that undergo chemotherapy experience nausea and vomiting.[2]

PATHOPHYSIOLOGY

- Cancer causes nausea and vomiting via infiltration of the gastrointestinal tract with neoplastic cells.
- Chemotherapy causes nausea and vomiting by acting directly on the vomiting center in the medulla.
- Along with radiation therapy, chemotherapy can also cause nausea and vomiting by causing injury to the enterochromaffin cells in the gastrointestinal tract, with the resultant release of serotonin. Subsequent binding of the serotonin receptors in the gastrointestinal tract leads to activation of the chemoreceptor trigger zone (area postrema) in the vomiting center via the vagus nerve to cause nausea and vomiting.[2]

CLINICAL FEATURES

- Cancer patients present with a recent history of chemotherapy and may show signs of dehydration or infection.

DIAGNOSIS AND DIFFERENTIAL

- Increased intracranial pressure, bowel obstruction, infection, or cardiopulmonary disease should be excluded.

EMERGENCY DEPARTMENT CARE AND DISPOSITION

- Nausea and vomiting in cancer patients receiving chemotherapy can be treated with dopamine receptor antagonists (metoclopramide, promethazine), dexamethasone, benzodiazepines (lorazepam), or a histamine antagonist (diphenhydramine).
- Serotonin antagonists (ondansetron, dolasetron, granisetron) are the drugs of choice for nausea and vomiting in cancer patients.
- Besides antiemetics, dehydration and electrolyte abnormalities should be corrected with IV crystalloid and electrolyte replacement.

PAIN CONTROL IN CANCER

EPIDEMIOLOGY

- Pain is highly prevalent in cancer patients. Approximately two thirds of cancer patients experience severe pain and up to 84% of hospice patients report cancer pain.[15]

PATHOPHYSIOLOGY

- Pain is inherently subjective and reflects a collective sensation of pain from pain fibers, modified by the individual's lifelong physical, spiritual, cultural, and personal experience.
- Cancer pain can be broadly categorized into somatic pain (eg, bone pain from metastatic disease), visceral pain (eg, cancer cell–induced injury to the sympathetically innervated organs), and neuropathic pain (eg, infiltration or compression of central or peripheral nerves by cancer cells).[15]

CLINICAL FEATURES

- Different cancer pain syndromes have been recognized. Radiation- and chemotherapy-induced mucositis causes pain due to injury of the mucosa in the upper (mouth) and lower (colorectal) portions of the gastrointestinal tract.
- A number of chemotherapeutic agents (eg, vinca alkaloids) can cause chemotherapy-induced polyneuropathy.
- Radiation can also cause radiation neuropathy, plexopathy, and myelopathy.

DIAGNOSIS AND DIFFERENTIAL

- Acute spinal cord compression, cauda equina syndrome, pathologic fractures, bowel obstruction, infection, and metastatic disease should be excluded in the evaluation.

EMERGENCY DEPARTMENT CARE AND DISPOSITION

- Parenteral narcotic analgesics are initially preferred for all pain syndromes, though recognizing their limited efficacy for neuropathic pain.
- The underlying cause of pain should then be identified and treated.
- Patients with intractable pain or inadequate social support should be admitted to the hospital for pain control.

REFERENCES

1. Eakin R: Bone emergencies, in Johnston PG, Spence RAJ (eds.): *Oncologic Emergencies.* Oxford: Oxford University Press, 2002, p. 175.
2. Talamo G: Pathophysiology of emergency illness due to cancer, in Yeung S, Escalante CP (eds.): *Holland-Frei Oncologic Emergencies.* Hamilton, Ont.: BC Decker, 2002, p. 61.
3. Loblaw DA, Laperriere NJ: Emergency treatment of malignant extradural spinal cord compression: an evidence-based guideline. *J Clin Oncol* 16:1613, 1998.
4. Shannon VR, Ng A: Noninfectious pulmonary emergencies, in Yeung S, Escalante CP (eds.): *Holland-Frei Oncologic Emergencies.* Hamilton, Ont.: BC Decker, 2002, p. 191.
5. Shepherd FA: Malignant pericardial effusion. *Curr Opin Oncol* 9:170, 1997.
6. Wudel LJ Jr, Nesbitt JC: Superior vena cava syndrome. *Curr Treat Options Oncol* 2:77, 2001.
7. Bick RL, Strauss JF, Frenkel EP: Thrombosis and hemorrhage in oncology patients. *Hematol Oncol Clin North Am* 10:875, 1996.
8. Wolfe TR, Hartsell SC: Pulmonary embolism: making sense of the diagnostic evaluation. *Ann Emerg Med* 37:504, 2001.
9. Yeung S, Lazo-Diza G, Gagel RF: Metabolic and endocrine emergencies, in Yeung S, Escalante CP (eds.): *Holland-Frei Oncologic Emergencies.* Hamilton, Ont.: BC Decker, 2002, p. 103.
10. Theriault RL: Hypercalcemia of malignancy: pathophysiology and implications for treatment. *Oncology (Huntingt)* 7:47, 1993.
11. Walls J, Bundred N, Howell A: Hypercalcemia and bone resorption in malignancy. *Clin Orthop* 312:51, 1995.
12. Hussei M, Cullen K:. Metabolic emergencies, in Johnston PG, Spence RAJ (eds.): *Oncologic Emergencies.* Oxford: Oxford University Press, 2002, p. 52.
13. Pizzo PA: Fever in immunocompromised patients. *N Engl J Med* 341:893, 1999.
14. Freifeld AG: Infectious complications in the immunocompromised host. The antimicrobial armamentarium. *Hematol Oncol Clin North Am* 7:813, 1993.
15. Kelly S, Corcoran B: Acute pain emergencies, in Johnston PG, Spence RAJ (eds.): *Oncologic Emergencies.* Oxford: Oxford University Press, 2002, p. 201.

For further reading in *Emergency Medicine: A Comprehensive Study Guide,* 6th ed., see Chap. 225, "Emergency Complications of Malignancy," by Paul Blackburn.

143 HEADACHE AND FACIAL PAIN

Jason Graham

EPIDEMIOLOGY

- Approximately 3.8% of patients presenting to the emergency department have a serious cause of their headache.[1]
- Subarachnoid hemorrhages represent 1% of all non-traumatic headaches.[1]
- Migraine headaches are prevalent in 17% of women and 5% of men.[2]

PATHOPHYSIOLOGY

- As diastolic pressures rises, stretch of the cerebral vasculature may cause headaches. Typically pain will become more severe as the diastolic pressure itself rises.
- Migraine headaches are primarily caused by the response of the brain to a sensory trigger, resulting in a brainstem dysfunction that controls sensory input. Secondary blood vessel disorganization may be responsible for the aura, and finally the headache itself.
- Temporal arteritis is a systemic panarteritis.

CLINICAL FEATURES

SUBARACHNOID HEMORRHAGE

- Patients with subarachnoid hemorrhage (also see Chaps. 144 and 163) most commonly complain of the sudden onset of a severe headache that is located in the occipital or neck region. The headache may be associated with nausea and vomiting.
- The onset of the headache may coincide with activities that elevate the blood pressure, such as exertion, defecation, intercourse, or coughing.
- Fifty percent of patients with subarachnoid hemorrhage will have normal vital signs, normal level of consciousness, and no neck stiffness.

SUBDURAL HEMATOMA

- Subdural hematomas (see Chap. 163) should be suspected in any patient with a remote history of trauma and headache.
- Pain may be localized to the area of trauma or at another site as a result of a contrecoup injury.
- High-risk patients include alcoholics, those taking anticoagulants, and the elderly.

MENINGITIS

- Meningitis (see Chap. 151) should be suspected in any patient presenting with headache, fever, and neck pain. The headache is usually diffuse in location and severity.
- Nuchal rigidity and photophobia may be present.

MIGRAINE HEADACHE

- Migraine headaches are typically of gradual onset and become more severe. Pain is usually unilateral and exacerbated by physical activity, light, or loud noises.
- Aura-free migraine headaches account for approximately 80% of cases.

- Nausea and vomiting are usually associated with the onset of the headache.
- Virtually any neurologic sign or symptom may occur with a migraine headache.
- Any change from the patient's typical migraine should raise the suspicion for other causes of headache.

BRAIN TUMORS

- Patients with brain tumors may describe the headache to be bilateral, unilateral, constant, or intermittent.
- The headache may be worse in the morning, associated with nausea and vomiting, and positional.

HYPERTENSIVE HEADACHE

- Hypertensive headaches will typically become more severe as the diastolic blood pressure rises.
- Care must be taken to consider other causes of hypertension, such as pheochromocytoma, stroke, intracerebral process, pre-eclampsia, or any other cause of life-threatening headache.
- Distinction must be made from a hypertensive emergency, in which there is end-organ damage present.

TENSION HEADACHE

- Tension headaches are usually bilateral, nonpulsatile, and not worsened by physical activity.
- Patients may complain of pain radiating from the neck up to the occiput.

CLUSTER HEADACHE

- Cluster headaches are rare and usually resolve without treatment. They can be of sudden onset, severe, and short acting.
- Headaches usually are unilaterally located in the temple, orbit, or supraorbital region.
- The pain is not exacerbated by movement and patients will typically be pacing or unable to get into a position of comfort.
- Clinical findings associated with cluster headaches include conjunctival injection, lacrimation, nasal congestion, miosis, ptosis, and facial swelling.

OPHTHALMIC DISORDERS

- Ophthalmic disorders, such as glaucoma, iritis, and optic neuritis, may also cause headache.

- Patients may complain of a headache that is localized to the globe, orbit, or retro-orbital region.

TEMPORAL ARTERITIS

- Temporal arteritis is a vasculitis affecting branches of the external carotid artery.
- Women are affected four times more frequently than men and it occurs almost exclusively in patients older than 50 years.
- Headache is the most common complaint in patients with this disorder and is usually localized in the unilateral temple region. The pain is usually described as severe and throbbing.
- Systemic signs and symptoms may be present and include fever, malaise, weight loss, anorexia, diplopia, blurred vision, and polymyalgia.
- Physical examination may reveal tenderness to palpation of the temporal artery.
- Vision loss secondary to ischemic optic neuritis is the most serious complication of temporal arteritis.[3]

DIAGNOSIS AND DIFFERENTIAL

- Tables 143-1 and 143-2 review the primary and secondary causes of headache syndromes and the differential diagnosis of headache, respectively.
- For a patient with a worrisome history or physical examination, computed tomography (CT) of the head without contrast is usually the next step in the work-up.[5]
- The sensitivity of CT for detection of a subarachnoid hemorrhage is approximately 93%.[4]
- The sensitivity may be even higher if the scan is performed within the first 12 hours of hemorrhage; CT sensitivity falls to approximately 80% after 24 hours.
- If subarachnoid hemorrhage is suspected and the head CT is negative, then the clinician must perform a lumbar puncture to screen for xanthochromia in the cerebrospinal fluid (CSF).
- A negative spectrophotometric test for CSF xanthochromia in a patient with greater than 12 hours of headache is nearly 100% sensitive.
- Xanthochromia may remain present for up to 2 weeks following a bleed.
- Persistently bloody CSF from tube 1 to tube 4 should raise the suspicion of subarachnoid hemorrhage regardless of the presence of xanthochromia.
- The diagnosis of temporal arteritis is established by meeting at least three of five criteria: $\geq$50 years of age, new-onset headache, temporal artery tenderness or diminished pulse of the temporal artery, erythrocyte sedimentation rate >50 mm/h, or abnormal temporal artery biopsy.[3]

TABLE 143-1   Primary and Secondary Causes of Headache

Primary Headache Syndromes

Migraine
Tension type
Cluster

Secondary Headache Syndromes

Vascular
   Subarachnoid hemorrhage
   Intraparenchymal hemorrhage
   Subdural or epidural hematoma
   Ischemic (stroke, transient ischemic attack)
   Cavernous sinus thrombosis
   Arteriovenous malformation
   Temporal arteritis
   Carotid or vertebral artery dissection

Central nervous system (CNS) infection
   Meningitis (bacterial, viral, other)
   Encephalitis
   Cerebral abscess

Non-CNS infection
   Focal or systemic
   Sinusitis
   Herpes zoster of face or scalp

Other CNS pathology
   Tumor (benign or malignant)
   Pseudotumor cerebri

Ophthalmic
   Glaucoma
   Iritis
   Optic neuritis

Drug-related and toxic or metabolic
   Nitrates and nitrites
   Chronic analgesic use and abuse
   Hypoxia or high altitude
   Hypercapnia
   Hypoglycemia
   Monosodium glutamate
   Carbon monoxide poisoning
   Alcohol withdrawal

Miscellaneous
   Malignant hypertension
   Pre-eclampsia
   Fever
   Post-lumbar puncture
   Dental (referred)

EMERGENCY DEPARTMENT CARE AND DISPOSITION

- For patients with subarachnoid hemorrhage, rebleeding and vasospasm are the major complications.
- Lowering the systolic blood pressure to 160 mm Hg and/or maintaining a mean arterial pressure of 110 mm Hg is associated with a decreased risk of rebleeding and lowered mortality rate in subarachnoid hemorrhage.
- Nimodipine (60 mg orally every 6 hours) reduces the incidence and severity of vasospasm, and should be administered to all patients with subarachnoid hemorrhage. Neurosurgical consultation is indicated.
- Care of the patient with migraine headache consists of general comfort measures, abortive medications, and prophylactic therapy.
- Abortive medications used in the treatment of the patient with migraine headache include dihydroergotamine mesylate (DHE), sumatriptan, and phenothiazine derivatives. Doses and considerations in the use of these agents are reviewed in Table 143-3.
- Treatment of tension headaches consists of relaxation techniques, nonsteroidal anti-inflammatory drugs (NSAIDs), and other types of pain control.
- Severe tension headaches may be treated with the same medications as migraine headaches.
- Cluster headaches will resolve with the administration of high-flow oxygen in 70% of patients.
- DHE, NSAIDs, and sumatriptan also may be effective for cluster headaches; however, oral medications may be ineffective because of the length of time required for absorption and the short duration of the headache.
- For patients with a hypertensive headache, reduction of blood pressure may be performed with a wide range of medications, including nitroglycerin, nitroprusside, or β-blockers.
- Care should be taken to decrease the mean arterial pressure by no more than 25% over the first hour.
- Patients diagnosed with a subdural hematoma should receive an emergent neurosurgical consultation (see Chap. 163).
- The emergency physician should administer empiric antibiotic therapy to any patient with suspected bacterial meningitis (see Chap. 151). Antibiotic therapy should not be delayed for the lumbar puncture.[5]
- Treatment with prednisone (40 to 60 mg/day) should be initiated immediately upon suspicion of temporal arteritis.[6] Evaluation by an ophthalmologist should be made within 24 hours for definitive diagnosis.
- Reasonable indications for admission to manage pain associated with headache include: (1) migraine lasting for days associated with vomiting and dehydration, (2) chronic headache unresponsive to outpatient therapy, (3) underlying significant medical or surgical pathology, and (4) headache that significantly interferes with activities of daily living.

FACIAL PAIN

TEMPOROMANDIBULAR DISORDER

- Temporomandibular disorder is a painful syndrome involving the temporomandibular joint and the surrounding muscles and ligaments.

TABLE 143-2   Differential Diagnosis of the Patient with Headache

TYPE OF HEADACHE	HISTORY/PHYSICAL FINDINGS
Migraine headache	Young at onset; lasts longer than 60 min; unilateral, pulsating, throbbing; +/− visual aura; nausea and vomiting; precipitated by foods, drugs, alcohol, exercise or orgasm; family history
Cluster headache	Onset in 20s; predominantly male; brief episodes of pain (45–60 min); orbital/retro-orbital pain; periodic and seasonal (spring/autumn); nasal congestion and conjunctival injection/tearing associated
Tension headache	Onset at any age; dull, nagging, persistent pain; progressively worse throughout day
Subarachnoid hemorrhage	Sudden onset; "worst headache ever"; loss of consciousness; meningismus; vomiting; occipital-nuchal location
Hypertensive headache	Throbbing, occipital
Meningitis	Entire head; fever; meningismus
Mass lesions	
Subdural hematoma	Depressed mental status; variable quality headache
Epidural hematoma	History of trauma; consciousness with headache followed by unconsciousness; fracture across groove of middle meningeal artery
Brain tumor	Pain on awakening or with Valsalva; new headache associated with nausea and vomiting
Brain abscess	Findings similar to those of mass lesions; fever
Sinusitis	Stabbing or aching pain, worse with bending or coughing, decreased in supine position
Toxic/metabolic headache	Diffuse; headache remits after removal from offending agent/ environment
Postconcussion headache	History of trauma within hours to days; vertigo, nausea, vomiting, mood alterations, concentration difficulty associated
Pseudotumor cerebri	Obese, young female; irregular menstrual cycles/amenorrhea; papilledema
Acute glaucoma	Nausea, vomiting, orbital pain; edematous/cloudy cornea; mid-position pupil; conjunctival injection; increased intraocular pressure

- Patients often will complain of joint crepitance and pain with chewing, locking of the jaw with opening, and limited jaw movements.
- Treatment of temporomandibular disorder consists of NSAIDs or narcotic analgesics.

TRIGEMINAL NEURALGIA (TIC DOULOUREUX)

- Trigeminal neuralgia is often characterized as a sharp, electric-like pain that is brief and present in the unilateral trigeminal nerve distribution.

TABLE 143-3   Agents Used in the ED Treatment of Migraine Headache

AGENT	ROUTE	CONSIDERATIONS
Ergotamine	inhalation, rectal	Contraindicated in coronary artery disease, hypertension, pregnancy
Chlorpromazine	0.1 mg/kg IV	May cause extrapyramidal effects, excellent antiemetic
Prochlorperazine	10 mg IV	May cause extrapyramidal effects, excellent antiemetic
Metoclopramide	10–20 mg IV	May cause extrapyramidal effects, excellent antiemetic
Dihydroergotamine	0.75–1.0 mg IV over 2 min	Contraindicated in coronary artery disease, hypertension, pregnancy
Sumatriptan	6 mg SC	Contraindicated in coronary artery disease, hypertension, pregnancy
Ketorolac	60 mg IM	Moderately effective

- Paroxysms of pain are integral in the diagnosis and the patient should be completely pain free in the interim. The pain typically lasts only a few seconds.
- The neurologic examination will be normal.
- Initial medical treatment may include carbamazepine, which has been shown to be very effective.

REFERENCES

1. Ramirez-Lassepas M, Espinosa CE, Cicero JJ, et al: Predictors of intracranial pathologic findings in patients who seek emergency care because of headache. *Arch Neurol* 54:1506, 1997.
2. Pryse-Phillips WE, Dodick DW, Edmeads JG, et al: Guidelines for the diagnosis and management of migraines in clinical practice. *Can Med Assoc J* 156:1273, 1997.
3. Hellman DB: Temporal arteritis: A cough, toothache, and tongue infarction. *JAMA* 287:2996, 2002.
4. Sidman R, Connolly E, Lemke T: Subarachnoid hemorrhage diagnosis: Lumbar puncture is still needed when the computed tomography scan is normal. *Acad Emerg Med* 3:16, 1996.
5. American College of Emergency Physicians: Clinical policy for the initial approach to adolescents and adults presenting to the emergency department with a chief complaint of headache. *Ann Emerg Med* 27:821, 1996.
6. Hunder GG: The American College of Rheumatology 1990 criteria for the classification of giant cell arteritis. *Arthritis Rheum* 33:1122, 1990.

For further reading in *Emergency Medicine: A Comprehensive Study Guide*, 6th ed., see Chap. 227, "Headache and Facial Pain," by Christopher J. Denny and Michael J. Schull.

144 STROKE AND TRANSIENT ISCHEMIC ATTACK

J. Stephen Huff

EPIDEMIOLOGY

- Stroke is the third leading cause of death and the leading cause of disability in the U.S.
- Twenty percent of patients with acute stroke will die within 1 year.
- One third of strokes occur in patients younger than 65 years of age.[1]

PATHOPHYSIOLOGY

- The term "stroke" refers to any disease process that disrupts blood flow to a focal region of the brain.
- Injury is rapid from the loss of oxygen and glucose supply to neuronal tissue, and can be delayed by complex secondary mediators of cellular injury.
- Approximately 80% of strokes are ischemic from vascular occlusion; the remainder are caused by intracranial hemorrhage.
- Thrombotic disease is the most common type of ischemic stroke and occurs as a result of narrowing of the vascular lumen, with subsequent platelet adhesion and clot formation.
- About 20% of ischemic strokes are embolic in nature, resulting from intravascular material originating at a proximal source such as the heart (eg, atrial fibrillation), or artery-to-artery emboli subsequently occluding a distal vessel.
- Systemic hypoperfusion is a less-common mechanism of ischemic stroke and may be caused by cardiac failure, leading to a more diffuse injury pattern.
- Hemorrhagic strokes are typically divided into two subtypes: intracerebral (ICH) and nontraumatic subarachnoid (SAH) hemorrhages.
- In ICH, the more common form, bleeding occurs directly into brain parenchyma from small arterioles previously weakened by elevated blood pressure.
- Cerebral vascular amyloidosis is another major cause of ICH, as well as bleeding diathesis due to anticoagulant or thrombolytic use, vascular malformations, and cocaine use.
- SAH involves blood leaking from a cerebral vessel into the subarachnoid space and often into the brain substance. Most nontraumatic SAHs result from berry aneurysm rupture.

CLINICAL FEATURES

- The clinical presentation of stroke is variable and depends upon the area of brain injured and the degree of injury (Table 144-1).
- Transient ischemic attack (TIA) is a neurologic deficit that resolves within 24 hours, although most resolve within minutes.
- In the past, TIAs were not thought to result in permanent tissue injury; however, follow-up studies indicate that more than 60% may be associated with radiologic changes of infarction, even in the absence of clinically detectable neurologic deficit.
- Ten percent of patients with TIAs may have a stroke within 90 days.[2]
- Ischemic stroke involving the anterior cerebral artery typically causes leg weakness greater than arm

TABLE 144-1   Stroke Syndromes

Ischemic stroke syndromes
   Transient ischemic attack: resolves within 24 h (most within 30 min) 5–6% risk of stroke per year
   Dominant hemispheric infarct: contralateral weakness or numbness, contralateral visual field cut, gaze preference, dysarthria, aphasia
   Nondominant hemispheric infarct: contralateral weakness or numbness, visual field cut, constructional apraxia, dysarthria
   Anterior cerebral artery infarct: contralateral weakness or numbness (leg more than arm), dyspraxia, speech perseveration, slow responses
   Middle cerebral artery infarct: most common area involved, contralateral weakness or numbness (arm or face more than leg)
   Posterior cerebral artery infarct: often go unrecognized by patient, minimal motor involvement, light-touch and pinprick sensation significantly affected
   Vertebrobasilar syndrome: dizziness, vertigo, diplopia, dysphagia, ataxia, cranial nerve palsies, bilateral limb weakness, crossed neurologic deficits
   Basilar artery occlusion: quadriplegia, coma, locked-in syndrome
   Cerebellar infarct: "drop attack" associated with vertigo, headache, nausea, vomiting, and/or neck pain, cranial nerve abnormalities
   Lacunar infarct: pure motor or sensory deficits
   Arterial dissection: often associated with severe trauma, headache and neck pain hours to days prior to onset of neurologic symptoms

Hemorrhagic stroke syndromes
   Intracerebral hemorrhage: similar to cerebral infarction with lethargy, headache, nausea, vomiting, significant hypertension
   Cerebellar hemorrhage: dizziness, vomiting, truncal ataxia, inability to walk, rapidly progress to coma, herniation and death
   Subarachnoid hemorrhage: severe headache, vomiting, decreased level of consciousness

weakness, contralateral to the vascular occlusion. Patients may perseverate with speech or motor actions.

- A stroke involving the territory of the middle cerebral artery (MCA) presents with contralateral weakness and numbness, typically with the arm affected more than the leg.
- The face is variably affected. A gaze preference toward the side of the infarct may be present.
- If the dominant hemisphere (left in most patients regardless of handedness) is involved in a MCA stroke, aphasia (receptive, expressive, or both) is often present.
- In MCA stroke, inattention, neglect, or extinction on double-simultaneous stimulation (cortical sensory loss) may help to localize the lesion to the nondominant hemisphere.
- The posterior circulation supplies blood to the brainstem, cerebellum, and visual cortex. Signs and symptoms attributable to a stroke in this distribution may include findings such as dizziness, vertigo, diplopia, dysphagia, ataxia, cranial nerve palsies, or bilateral limb weakness, singly or in combination.
- Occlusion of the basilar artery causes severe quadriplegia, coma, and the locked-in syndrome.
- The hallmark of a brainstem stroke is crossed neurologic deficits (ie, ipsilateral cranial nerve deficits with contralateral motor weakness).

- The lateral medullary syndrome (Wallenberg's syndrome) is a specific posterior stroke syndrome resulting from occlusion of a vertebral artery and/or the posterior inferior cerebellar artery.
- Presenting signs of lateral medullary syndrome include ipsilateral loss of facial pain and temperature sensation with contralateral loss of these senses on the body, and gait or limb ataxia.
- In lateral medullary syndrome, deficits of cranial nerves V, IX, X, or XI ipsilateral to the stroke may be present. Nausea and vomiting may be severe.
- An important subset of posterior circulation strokes is those involving the cerebellum. Early symptoms may include vertigo, headache, inability to walk, or nausea and vomiting. Cranial nerve abnormalities may be present.
- Lacunar infarcts are fragments of the large vessel syndromes, and may be pure motor or sensory deficits. They are caused by infarction of small penetrating arteries and are commonly associated with chronic hypertension.
- Lacunar infarcts are primarily located in the pons, deep white matter, internal capsule, and the basal ganglia.
- ICH may be clinically indistinguishable from cerebral infarction and may present with any of the anatomic syndromes discussed previously. Headache, nausea, and vomiting may precede the neurologic deficit; the patient's condition may quickly deteriorate.
- Bleeding may occur in the putamen, thalamus, pons, or cerebellum (in order of decreasing frequency).
- Patients with SAH may develop focal findings related to location of an aneurysm.
- Patients with SAH typically present with a severe, constant headache, often occipital or nuchal in location. A recent history suggestive of a warning leak, or "sentinel hemorrhage," may be obtained in many patients.
- Vomiting often occurs with the onset of headache and patients may have altered consciousness.
- With SAH, onset of headache is usually sudden, and a careful history may reveal onset with activity associated with elevated blood pressures such as exertion, defecation, intercourse, or coughing.

DIAGNOSIS AND DIFFERENTIAL

- Although strokes are the most common cause of focal neurologic deficits, other causes must be considered in the differential diagnosis (Table 144-2).
- An emergent noncontrast computed tomography (CT) scan of the head is essential to quickly differentiate hemorrhage from ischemia.
- Most acute ischemic strokes will not be visualized by routine CT for at least 6 hours.

TABLE 144-2   Differential Diagnosis of Acute Stroke

Hypoglycemia

Postictal paralysis (Todd's paralysis)

Bell's palsy

Hypertensive encephalopathy

Epidural or subdural hematoma

Brain tumor or abscess

Complicated migraine

Encephalitis

Diabetic ketoacidosis

Hyperosmotic coma

Meningoencephalitis

Wernicke's encephalopathy

Multiple sclerosis

Meniere's disease

Drug toxicity (lithium, phenytoin, carbamazepine)

- Some hypodensity indicating infarction usually appears within 24 to 48 hours.
- CT identifies almost all parenchymal hemorrhages greater than 1 cm in diameter and up to 95% of SAH (if obtained within 12 hours of symptom onset).
- If SAH is still strongly suspected after a nondiagnostic CT scan, lumbar puncture is indicated.

EMERGENCY DEPARTMENT CARE AND DISPOSITION

- Priority should be given to airway management and oxygenation. Patients should be placed on a cardiac monitor and IV access established.
- Dextrose-containing solutions should be avoided except in patients with proven hypoglycemia.
- Only persistent, severe hypertension (systolic blood pressure >220 mm Hg systolic or mean arterial pressure >130 mm Hg) should be treated. Recommended agents include labetalol or enalapril.[3]
- In hypertensive patients being considered for thrombolytic therapy, the use of labetalol is recommended to reduce blood pressure below 185/115 mm Hg. Requirements for more aggressive treatment of hypertension exclude the use of recombinant tissue-type plasminogen activator (rt-PA) in stroke patients.
- Following the use of rt-PA in acute stroke, however, aggressive treatment is warranted to maintain the blood pressure below 185/115 mm Hg.
- The Food and Drug Administration approved the use of IV rt-PA (Activase/Alteplase) in acute ischemic stroke in 1996.[4]
- Thrombolytic therapy in stroke is not recommended when the time of onset cannot be ascertained reliably.

Strokes recognized upon awakening should be timed from when the patient was last known to be without symptoms.
- The use of intra-arterial delivery of thrombolytics remains investigational.
- A review of rt-PA inclusion and exclusion criteria (Table 144-3) should be performed and an emergent noncontrast head CT and neurologic consultation arranged.
- Any hemorrhage on CT excludes the use of rt-PA; detection of a large area of hypodensity may indicate an acute stroke and may suggest that onset was at least several hours previously.
- The total dose of rt-PA is 0.9 mg/kg IV, with a maximum dose of 90 mg; 10% of the dose is administered as a bolus, with the remaining amount infused over 60 minutes.
- No aspirin or heparin should be administered in the initial 24 hours following treatment.
- Intracerebral bleeding should be suspected as the cause of any neurologic worsening until repeat CT imaging is obtained.
- Antiplatelet strategies form the cornerstone for secondary stroke prevention in most stroke and TIA patients.
- Aspirin (50 to 300 mg orally) remains the initial choice in the patient with a first-ever stroke or TIA. Aspirin use, however, will interfere with any subsequent consideration of use of rt-PA.
- Dipyridamole and clopidogrel are other antiplatelet activity agents.
- Although frequently used in the past for stroke treatment, the benefit of unfractionated heparin in any stroke syndrome remains unproven.
- Heparin use may be considered in patients with recent TIAs who are at high risk for stroke. This includes patients with: (1) known high-grade stenosis in the appropriate vascular distribution for the symptoms, (2) a cardioembolic source such as atrial fibrillation or valvular disease (except infective endocarditis), (3) TIAs of increasing frequency (crescendo TIAs), and (4) TIAs despite antiplatelet therapy.
- Early neurosurgical consultation may be needed for patients with cerebellar infarction or hemorrhage.
- Cerebellar swelling with compressions of the brainstem may lead to rapid deterioration. Emergency posterior fossa decompression in selected patients may be life saving.
- Management of blood pressure in ICH remains controversial. Current recommendations are that only severe hypertension (ie, systolic blood pressure >220 mm Hg or diastolic blood pressure >120 mm Hg) be treated.
- When treated, blood pressure should be lowered gradually to prehemorrhage levels using either labetalol or nitroprusside.

TABLE 144-3   Criteria for Use of rt-PA in Acute Ischemic Stroke and Management of Patients Following Use of rt-PA

INCLUSION	EXCLUSION
Age 18 or over	Minor stroke syndromes
Clinical diagnosis of ischemic stroke	Rapidly improving neurologic signs
Well-established time of onset <3 h	Prior intracranial hemorrhage
	Blood glucose <50 or >400 mg/dL
	Seizure at onset of stroke
	Gastrointestinal or genitourinary bleeding within preceding 21 days
	Recent myocardial infarction
	Major surgery within 14 days
	Pretreatment SBP >185 mm Hg or DBP >110 mm Hg
	Previous stroke or head injury within 90 days
	Current use of oral anticoagulants
	Use of heparin within preceding 48 h
	Platelet count 100,000/mL
	Suspected aortic or vascular dissection or LP

MANAGEMENT

Monitor arterial blood pressure during the first 24 h after starting treatment, every 15 min for 2 h after starting infusion, then every 30 min for 6 h, and then every 60 min for 24 h total.

If SBP is 180–230 mm Hg or DBP is 105–120 mm Hg for two or more readings 5–10 min apart:
Give IV labetalol 10 mg over 1–2 min. The dose may be repeated or doubled every 10–20 min up to a total dose of 150 mm Hg
Monitor blood pressure every 15 min during labetalol treatment and observe for hypotension.

If SBP is >230 mm Hg or if DBP is 121–140 mm Hg for two or more readings 5–10 min apart:
Give IV labetalol 10 mg over 1–2 min. The dose may be repeated or doubled every 10–20 min up to a total dose of 150 mm Hg
Monitor blood pressure every 15 min during labetalol treatment and observe for hypotension.
If no satisfactory response, infuse sodium nitroprusside 0.5–10 μg/kg/min; continuous arterial pressure monitor is advised.

If DBP >140 mm Hg for two or more readings 5–10 min apart:
Infuse sodium nitroprusside 0.5–10 μg/kg/min; continuous arterial pressure monitoring is advised.

ABBREVIATIONS: DBP, diastolic blood pressure; IV, intravenous; SBP, systolic blood pressure.

- For patients with evidence of increased intracranial pressure (ICP), head elevation to 30 degrees and mannitol (0.25 to 1.0 g/kg IV) are standard recommendations.
- Neurosurgical consultation for ICP monitoring should be considered in patients with a Glasgow Coma Scale score of <9, and in all patients whose condition is thought to be deteriorating because of elevated ICP.
- In patients with SAH, risk of rebleeding is greatest in the first 24 hours. Rebleeding and vasospasm are the major complications.
- In SAH patients with elevated blood pressures, lowering systolic blood pressure to 160 mm Hg and/or maintaining a mean arterial pressure of 110 mm Hg is associated with lower risk of rebleeding and a decreased mortality rate.
- Nimodipine 60 mg orally every 6 hours, reduces the incidence and severity of vasospasm and should be given to all patients with SAH.
- Phenytoin loading to decrease possible seizures is often recommended.
- Patients with new-onset ischemic strokes or hemorrhages should be admitted for monitoring and obser-

vation even if they are not candidates for interventional therapy.
- Patients with new-onset TIAs should be evaluated for possible cardiac sources of emboli or high-grade stenosis in the carotid arteries.
- Because of the proven efficacy of carotid endarterectomy, patients should be considered for admission unless high-grade stenosis of the carotid artery can be excluded promptly by imaging (ultrasound, magnetic resonance angiography).

REFERENCES

1. American Heart Association: *2002 Heart and Stroke Facts Statistical Update.* Dallas: American Heart Association, 2001.
2. Johnston SC, Gress DR, Browner WS et al: Short-term prognosis after emergency department diagnosis of TIA. *JAMA* 284:2901, 2000.
3. Adams HP Jr, Brott TG, Furlan AJ, et al from the Special Writing Group of the Stroke Council, American Heart Association:

Guidelines for the Management of Patients with Acute Ischemic Stroke: American Heart Association Medical/Scien-
tific Statement 1994. Dallas: American Heart Association,
1994.
4. National Institute of Neurological Disorders and Stroke rt-PA
Stroke Study Group: Tissue plasminogen activator for acute
ischemic stroke. *N Engl J Med* 333:1581, 1995.

For further reading in *Emergency Medicine: A Compre-
hensive Study Guide,* 6th ed., see Chap. 228, "Stroke,
Transient Ischemic Attack, and Other Central Focal
Conditions," by Phillip A. Scott and Caroline A.
Timmerman.

145 ALTERED MENTAL STATUS AND COMA
C. Crawford Mechem

DELIRIUM

EPIDEMIOLOGY

- On admission, 10 to 25% of elderly patients have delirium.[1]

PATHOPHYSIOLOGY

- Delirium always has an organic cause.
- Four pathologic groups encompass most patients: primary intracranial disease, systemic disease secondarily affecting the central nervous system (CNS), exogenous toxins, and drug withdrawal.

CLINICAL FEATURES

- Delirium is a transient disorder characterized by impairment of attention and cognition.
- Delirium is a constellation of signs and symptoms due
to an underlying cause, as opposed to being a distinct
disease entity.
- Delirium may begin abruptly, but by definition lasts
for less than 1 month.[2]
- Attention, perception, thinking, and memory are distorted to varying degrees.
- Alertness is reduced, as manifested by a difficulty
maintaining attention and concentration.
- Activity levels may be increased, decreased, or alternate between the two extremes of agitation and
somnolence.[3]
- Evidence of organic disease such as tachycardia, hypertension, tremor, asterixis, sweating, or emotional
outbursts may be present. Hallucinations, more commonly visual, may also be noted.
- Delirium, dementia, and psychosis have features that
might aid the clinician in distinguishing between
them (Table 145-1).

DIAGNOSIS AND DIFFERENTIAL

- Both historical and physical examination findings are
needed to confirm the diagnosis.
- The acute onset of attention deficits and cognitive
abnormalities with fluctuating severity through the
day and worsening at night is virtually diagnostic of
delirium.
- The differential diagnosis of delirium in the elderly is
listed in Table 145-2.[2]

TABLE 145-1 Features of Delirium, Dementia, and Psychosis

CHARACTERISTIC	DELIRIUM	DEMENTIA	PSYCHOSIS
Onset	Over days	Insidious	Sudden
Course over 24 h	Fluctuating	Stable	Stable
Consciousness	Reduced	Alert	Alert
Attention	Disordered	Normal	May be disordered
Cognition	Disordered	Impaired	May be impaired
Orientation	Impaired	Often impaired	May be impaired
Hallucinations	Visual and/or auditory	Often absent	Usually auditory
Delusions	Transient, poorly organized	Usually absent	Sustained
Movements	Asterixis, tremor may be present	Often absent	Absent

SOURCE: Modified from Lipowski.[2]

TABLE 145-2 Important Medical Causes of Delirium in Elderly Patients

Infection	Pneumonia
	Urinary tract infection
	Meningitis or encephalitis
	Sepsis
Metabolic/toxic	Hypoglycemia
	Alcohol ingestion
	Electrolyte abnormalities
	Hepatic encephalopathy
	Thyroid disorders
	Alcohol or drug withdrawal
Neurologic	Stroke or transient ischemic attack
	Seizure or postictal state
	Subarachnoid hemorrhage
	Intracranial hemorrhage
	Mass CNS lesion
	Subdural hematoma
Cardiopulmonary	Congestive heart failure
	Myocardial infarction
	Pulmonary embolism
	Hypoxia or CO_2 narcosis
Drug-related	Antiemetics
	Antihistamines
	Antiparkinsonian agents
	Antipsychotics
	Antispasmodics
	Muscle relaxants
	Tricyclic antidepressants
	Digoxin
	Sedative-hypnotics
	Narcotic analgesics

EMERGENCY DEPARTMENT CARE AND DISPOSITION

- Treatment is directed at the underlying cause.
- Sedation is often necessary to relieve severe agitation. Haloperidol, 5 to 10 mg orally or parenterally, is a frequent first choice. The dose should be reduced in the elderly.
- Lorazepam, 0.5 to 2 mg orally or parenterally, may be used in conjunction with haloperidol, with the dose dictated by the patient's age and weight.
- Unless a readily reversible cause for the acute mental status change is identified and corrected and there is a return to baseline mental status, most patients should be admitted for further evaluation and treatment.

DEMENTIA

EPIDEMIOLOGY

- Dementia is largely a disease of the elderly. It is estimated that 1% of the U.S. population suffers from dementia at age 60.

PATHOPHYSIOLOGY

- Up to 70% of cases are due to Alzheimer's disease, which is a neurodegenerative disorder of unknown etiology. A reduction in neurons in the cerebral cortex, deposition of amyloid into plaques, and production of neurofibrillary tangles have been noted.
- Vascular dementia accounts for approximately 10 to 20% of cases and is due to cerebrovascular disease with multiple infarctions.

CLINICAL FEATURES

- Dementia is characterized by slowly progressing impairment of cognitive function while alertness remains intact.
- A rapid evolution of symptoms should prompt the emergency physician to search for another process simulating dementia or a comorbidity that may be hastening the progression of dementia.
- Impairment of memory and orientation with preservation of motor function and speech is characteristic of the onset of Alzheimer's disease.
- Short-term memory is more frequently affected, while long-term memory may be preserved.
- The progression of symptoms may include memory loss, difficulty naming objects, forgetting items, loss of reading ability, difficulty in social interactions, disorientation, speech difficulties, anxiety, depression, inability to care for oneself, and personality change.
- Patients with vascular dementia share many of the same symptoms of Alzheimer's disease. However, on physical examination they may have exaggerated or asymmetric reflexes, gait abnormalities, or focal extremity weakness.

DIAGNOSIS AND DIFFERENTIAL

- The history of memory problems is generally one of slow, steady progression. Abrupt changes increase the likelihood of a vascular etiology.
- Physical examination does not determine the diagnosis of dementia but may help to identify associated causes.[3]
- Focal neurologic deficits may suggest vascular dementia or a mass lesion. Increased motor tone, muscle rigidity, or a movement disorder may suggest Parkinson's disease.
- Diagnosis of probable vascular dementia requires signs of cerebrovascular disease. There must be a temporal relationship between stroke and dementia, with dementia developing within 3 months of stroke.[4,5]

TABLE 145-3   Classification of Dementia by Cause

Degenerative
  Alzheimer's disease
  Huntington's disease
  Parkinson's disease, others

Vascular
  Multiple infarcts
  Hypoperfusion (cardiac arrest, profound hypotension, others)
  Subdural hematoma
  Subarachnoid hemorrhage

Infectious
  Meningitis (sequelae of bacterial, fungal, or tubercular)
  Neurosyphilis
  Viral encephalitis (herpes, HIV), Creutzfeldt-Jakob disease

Inflammatory
  Systemic lupus erythematosus
  Demyelinating disease, others

Neoplastic
  Primary tumors and metastatic disease
  Carcinomatous meningitis
  Paraneoplastic syndromes

Traumatic
  Traumatic brain injury
  Subdural hematoma

Toxic
  Alcohol
  Medications (anticholinergics, polypharmacy)

Metabolic
  Vitamin B_{12} or folate deficiency
  Thyroid disease
  Uremia, others

Psychiatric
  Depression

Hydrocephalus
  Normal-pressure hydrocephalus (communicating hydrocephalus)
  Noncommunicating hydrocephalus

SOURCE: Modified from Fleming et al.[3]

- The differential diagnosis of dementia includes delirium and a variety of other disease processes (Table 145-3).

EMERGENCY DEPARTMENT CARE AND DISPOSITION

- Approximately 10 to 20% of patients have a treatable form of dementia, implying that in the majority of cases the underlying process cannot be reversed.
- However, all types of dementia may benefit from environmental or psychosocial interventions.
- Antipsychotic medications have been used to manage psychotic and nonpsychotic behavior among Alzheimer's patients, but are associated with adverse effects. They should therefore be reserved for patients with persistent psychotic features or disruptive or violent behavior.[6]
- Treatment of vascular dementia is limited to management of risk factors, including hypertension.

- Most patients with a new diagnosis of dementia will require admission for further evaluation and management. However, patients with long-standing symptoms, consistent caregivers, and reliable follow-up may be discharged for outpatient evaluation after life-threatening conditions have been excluded.

COMA

EPIDEMIOLOGY

- It is estimated that acute unresponsiveness is present in 0.5 to 1% of emergency department admissions.

PATHOPHYSIOLOGY

- The pathophysiology is affected by the underlying etiology, which may be a systemic disease that affects the CNS secondarily or a primary CNS process. For coma to develop, both cerebral hemispheres or the brainstem must be involved.
- Examples of systemic disease secondarily resulting in coma are hypoxemia and hypoglycemia, in which substrates needed for neuronal function are lacking.
- In primary CNS causes, coma may result from bilateral cortical dysfunction or from localized brainstem pathology.
- Elevated intracranial pressure and associated decreased cerebral perfusion may affect both hemispheres.
- Brainstem disorders include hemorrhage and the uncal herniation syndrome.
- Uncal herniation results from an expanding mass that causes the medial temporal lobe to shift and compress the upper brainstem, resulting in coma. The ipsilateral pupil will become fixed and dilated as a result of third cranial nerve compression. Hemiparesis ipsilateral to the mass may also develop from compression of the descending motor tracts in the opposite cerebral peduncle.

CLINICAL FEATURES

- Coma may be defined as an eyes-closed state with inappropriate responses to environmental stimuli.
- Alertness, self-awareness, language, reasoning, spatial relationship integration, and emotions are all impaired.
- The causes of coma may be divided into two large categories: diffuse CNS dysfunction (toxic-metabolic etiologies) and structural coma.
- Structural coma may be further divided into hemispheric (supratentorial) and posterior fossa coma.

- In most cases of toxic and metabolic causes of coma, physical examination findings will be symmetric without focal deficits, reflecting the diffuse insult to the brain. In general, pupils are small but reactive.
- Coma resulting from lesions of the hemispheres or supratentorial masses often presents with progressive hemiparesis and asymmetry of muscle tone and reflexes.
- Eyes may be conjugately deviated toward the side of the lesion.
- Posterior fossa (or infratentorial) lesions often cause abrupt coma, abnormal extensor posturing, loss of pupillary reflexes, and impaired extraocular movements.

DIAGNOSIS AND DIFFERENTIAL

- History is crucial in determining the etiology of coma. Valuable sources of information may include prehospital personnel, caregivers, family, bystanders, and old medical records.
- An abrupt onset of coma suggests a potentially catastrophic process such as an intracranial hemorrhage.
- A more gradual progression of symptoms may result from a metabolic process or tumor.
- A detailed physical examination may reveal signs of trauma or evidence of a toxidrome.
- Assessment of cranial nerves through pupillary examination and testing of corneal and oculovestibular reflexes may suggest a focal CNS lesion that is potentially treatable with surgery.
- Extensor or flexor posturing are nonspecific, but suggest profound CNS dysfunction.
- CT of the head should be obtained even if the pretest probability is low, because some intracranial processes may be corrected by emergency surgery.
- The differential diagnosis of coma includes generalized disease processes that also affect the brain, as well as primary CNS disorders (Table 145-4).

EMERGENCY DEPARTMENT CARE AND DISPOSITION

- Treatment of coma involves identification of the etiology and initiation of specific therapy.
- Stabilization of airway, ventilation, and circulation is the top priority. Endotracheal intubation may be indicated to protect the airway.
- Readily reversible causes such as hypoglycemia, hypoxia, and opiate overdose should be sought.
- If elevated intracranial pressure is suspected, urgent neurosurgical consultation should be requested. Standard methods should be used to decrease intracranial pressure (see Chap. 163).

TABLE 145-4 Differential Diagnosis of Coma

Coma from causes affecting the brain diffusely
  Encephalopathies
    Hypoxic encephalopathy
    Metabolic encephalopathy
      Hypoglycemia
      Hyperosmolar state (eg, hyperglycemia)
      Electrolyte abnormalities (eg, hyper- or hyponatremia, hypercalcemia)
      Organ system failure
        Hepatic encephalopathy
        Uremia/renal failure
        Endocrine (eg, Addison's, hypothyroid, etc)
        Hypoxia
        CO_2 narcosis
    Hypertensive encephalopathy
  Toxins
  Drug reactions (eg, neuroleptic malignant syndrome)
  Environmental causes—hypothermia, hyperthermia
  Deficiency state—Wernicke's encephalopathy
  Sepsis
Coma from primary CNS disease or trauma
  Direct CNS trauma
  Vascular disease
    Intraparenchymal hemorrhage (hemispheric, basal ganglia, brainstem, cerebellar)
  Subarachnoid hemorrhage
  Infarction
    Hemispheric, brainstem
  CNS infections
  Neoplasms
  Seizures
    Nonconvulsive status epilepticus
    Postictal state

- Patients with readily reversible causes of coma, such as insulin-induced hypoglycemia, may be discharged if treatment is initiated, the patient returns to baseline mental status, the cause of the episode is clear, and the patient has reliable home care and follow-up.
- In all other cases, admission is warranted for further evaluation and treatment.

REFERENCES

1. Rummans TA, Evans JM, Krahn LE et al: Delirium in elderly patients: Evaluation and management. *Mayo Clin Proc* 70: 989, 1995.
2. Lipowski Z: Delirium in the elderly patient. *N Engl J Med* 320:578, 1989.
3. Fleming KC, Adams AC, Petersen RC: Dementia: Diagnosis and evaluation. *Mayo Clin Proc* 70:1093, 1995.
4. Knopman DS, DeKosky ST, Cummings JL et al: Practice parameter: Diagnosis of dementia (an evidence-based review): Report of the Quality Standards Subcommittee of the American Academy of Neurology. *Neurology* 56:1143, 2001.
5. Gold G, Giannakopoulos P, Montes-Paixao C et al: Sensitivity and specificity of newly proposed clinical criteria for possible vascular dementia. *Neurology* 49:690, 1997.

6. Borson S, Raskind MA. Clinical features and pharmacologic treatment of behavioral symptoms of Alzheimer's disease. *Neurology* 48(Suppl 6):S17, 1997.

For further reading in *Emergency Medicine: A Comprehensive Study Guide,* 6th ed., see Chap. 229, "Altered Mental Status and Coma," by J. Stephen Huff.

146 ATAXIA AND GAIT DISTURBANCES

C. Crawford Mechem

PATHOPHYSIOLOGY

- Ataxia is the failure to produce smooth, intentional movements.
- Gait disturbances include ataxia as well as other conditions.
- Ataxia and gait disturbances result from systemic illnesses and conditions affecting the nervous system (Table 146-1).
- Systemic illnesses include intoxication (ethanol, anticonvulsants, sedative-hypnotics, heavy metals) or metabolic conditions (hyponatremia, inborn errors of metabolism). Neurologic causes include peripheral and central nervous system (CNS) pathology.
- Ataxia may be categorized into two types. Motor ataxia is usually due to cerebellar processes. Sensory ataxia results from failure of transmission of proprioceptive information to the CNS, usually from disorders of peripheral nerves, spinal cord, or cerebellar input tracts.

CLINICAL FEATURES

- An abrupt onset of gait disturbance and a severe headache may reflect a catastrophic CNS event requiring immediate intervention.
- In children, any history of musculoskeletal pathology, metabolic disorders, recent immunizations, or viral illnesses including varicella should be elicited.[1]
- The patient should be observed sitting upright, rising to a standing position, walking, and turning.
- Gait abnormalities may be manifested by asking the patient to walk at a normal speed, then on the heels and on the toes, and by tandem toe-to-toe walking.
- A cerebellar or motor ataxic gait is wide based with unsteady, irregular steps.

TABLE 146-1 Common Etiologies of Acute Ataxia and Gait Disturbances

Systemic conditions
  Intoxications with diminished altertness*
    Ethanol
    Sedative-hypnotics
  Intoxications with relatively preserved alertness (diminished alertness
    at higher levels)*
    Phenytoin
    Carbamazepine
    Valproic acid
    Heavy metals—lead, organic mercurials
  Other metabolic disorders
    Hyponatremia*
    Inborn errors of metabolism

Disorders predominantly of the nervous system
  Conditions affecting predominantly one region of the
    central nervous system
    Cerebellum
      Hemorrhage*
      Infarction*
      Degenerative changes
      Abscess*
    Cortex
      Frontal tumor, hemorrhage, or trauma*
      Hydrocephalus
    Subcortical
      Thalamic infarction or hemorrhage*
      Parkinson's disease
    Spinal cord
      Cervical spondylosis
      Posterior column disorders
  Conditions affecting predominantly the peripheral nervous system
    Peripheral neuropathy
    Vestibulopathy

*Conditions that generally require consideration in acute or deteriorating presentations.

- The gait of sensory ataxia involves abrupt movement of the legs and slapping impact of the feet.
- An apraxic gait is one in which the patient has lost the ability to initiate the process of walking despite normal motor function.
- An equine gait is characterized by foot drop due to peroneal muscle weakness.
- A festinating gait is narrow based with small, shuffling steps that become more rapid, common in Parkinson's disease.
- A senile gait is slow with a short stride and wide base, commonly seen in the elderly and in those with neurodegenerative disorders.[2]
- A functional gait is one in which the patient is seemingly unable to walk steadily, though sensory and motor pathways and cerebellar function are intact, and is usually a manifestation of conversion disorder.
- The cerebellum is tested by having the patient perform smooth, voluntary movements and rapidly alternating movements.
- Abnormalities include dysmetria, characterized by inaccurate fine movements.

- Dyssynergia is the breakdown of movements into parts, assessed by finger-to-nose testing.
- Dysdiadochokinesia is characterized by clumsy rapid movements, identified by having the patient pat the thigh with the palm and then the back of the hand in rapidly alternating movements. This should be performed on both sides.
- The heel-to-shin test also assesses cerebellar function. In cerebellar disease, there is an action tremor and the knee is initially overshot. In posterior column disease, there is difficulty locating the knee and the heel weaves from side-to-side or falls off the shin.
- The Romberg test assesses sensation and distinguishes sensory from motor ataxia. The patient stands upright with feet close together, arms outstretched, and eyes open. Inability to maintain a steady posture confirms the presence of ataxia.
- Next, the patient closes the eyes. If the ataxia worsens, the test is positive, suggesting a sensory ataxia. If there is no change with eyes closed (Romberg test negative), a motor ataxia is suggested with possible localization to the cerebellum.
- Sensory examination should include position or vibration testing and sensation to pinprick.[3]
- Nystagmus suggests a cause in the CNS, rather than in the spinal cord or peripheral nerves.

DIAGNOSIS AND DIFFERENTIAL

- The extent of patient evaluation will be dictated by the acuity of symptom onset. Patients with an acute gait disturbance, as well as children, warrant an in-depth initial evaluation.
- Neuroimaging, such as computed tomography or magnetic resonance imaging, is appropriate in the proper clinical setting, as is neurology consultation.
- Ordering of laboratory studies such as electrolytes or a vitamin B_{12} level should be case specific.
- For patients with ataxia, efforts should be directed at determining if it is motor or sensory, and whether the etiology is a systemic illness or nervous system pathology. In the latter case, distinguishing a central versus peripheral etiology is important.

EMERGENCY DEPARTMENT CARE AND DISPOSITION

- Treatment is directed at the suspected etiology.
- Thiamine 100 mg IV should be administered to patients such as alcoholics, who are suspected of having Wernicke's disease, which is suggested by findings of ataxia, altered mental status, and ophthalmoplegia.
- Vitamin B_{12} replacement is appropriate for patients

with suspected deficiency manifesting as posterior column dysfunction.
- Disposition depends on the presumptive diagnosis, likely progression, and consideration of patient safety.
- Patients unable to walk or care for themselves should be admitted.
- In the case of a slowly progressing process with which the patient can be safely cared for at home, referral for further outpatient evaluation may be appropriate once life-threatening processes have been excluded.

REFERENCES

1. Belcher RS: Preeruptive cerebellar ataxia in varicella. *Ann Emerg Med* 27:511, 1996.
2. Waite LM, Broe GA, Creasy H, et al: Neurologic signs, aging, and the neurodegenerative disorders. *Arch Neurol* 53:498, 1996.
3. Diener H-C, Dichgans J: Pathophysiology of cerebellar ataxia. *Mov Disord* 7:95, 1992.

For further reading in *Emergency Medicine: A Comprehensive Study Guide,* 6th ed., see Chap. 230, "Ataxia and Gait Disturbances," by J. Stephen Huff.

147 VERTIGO AND DIZZINESS
Andrew Chang

EPIDEMIOLOGY

- Dizziness is a common (8 million outpatient visits/year) but nonspecific complaint.
- Benign paroxysmal positional vertigo (BPPV) is generally a disease of the elderly unless the patient has a history of head trauma (increased risk for dislodging otoliths out of the utricle and into the semicircular canal).

PATHOPHYSIOLOGY

- There are four general categories of dizziness: vertigo, near-syncope, disequilibrium, and psychogenic dizziness.[1]
- Sensory inputs from three systems (proprioception, visual, and vestibular) gets centrally processed, and the output is either an eye movement or an adjustment in gait and/or posture.
- The sensory conflict theory states that when there is a conflict of information between any two of the three

oyotomo, nausea and emesis occur acutely, although with time habituation occurs.

- The vestibular system (inner ear) is composed of three semicircular canals and otolithic organs (saccule and utricle). This entire system is filled with endolymph.
- The utricle is unique in that it contains calcium particles called otoliths (or otoconia).
- Sudden, unilateral disturbance of the tonic bilateral vestibular input from either a destructive lesion (eg, viral labyrinthitis) or a stimulatory lesion (eg, BPPV) results in vertigo and nystagmus.
- Nystagmus is the rhythmic movement of the eyes that is comprised of a fast and slow component.
- Nystagmus is usually described by the axis of movement (horizontal, vertical, rotatory), and direction is identified with the direction of the fast component.
- The slow phase of nystagmus indicates the injured side of the vestibular system.
- Direction-changing nystagmus (with eye or head position change) suggests a central process or a medication-related effect.
- BPPV results when otoliths inappropriately leave the utricle and enter the semicircular canal (usually the posterior canal, since it is the most dependent of the canals).[2]

CLINICAL FEATURES

VERTIGO

- Vertigo is defined as an illusion of movement and is classically described as "the room is spinning." Other descriptions (such as rocking, tilting, somersaulting, and descending in an elevator) also qualify as vertigo.
- Vertigo is classified as either peripheral or central.
- Peripheral vertigo means peripheral to the brainstem (eg, the eighth cranial nerve and the vestibular apparatus). Although the onset is usually abrupt and intense, the causes of peripheral vertigo are not typically life-threatening.
- Central vertigo indicates dysfunction at the level of the brainstem (vestibular nuclei in the pons and medulla) or cerebellum.
- Table 147-1 reviews the differences between peripheral and central vertigo.
- Central vertigo presents with other neurologic signs and symptoms, whereas peripheral vertigo presents with a nonfocal neurologic exam. However, sudden severe vertigo is observed in cerebellar hemorrhages and strokes and may simulate peripheral vestibular neuritis.[3]
- BPPV is the most common cause of vertigo. It is associated with position change (with a latency of 1 to 5 seconds between movement and symptoms), subsides in less than 1 minute, and fatigues over the course of the day.

TABLE 147-1   Differentiating Factors between Peripheral and Central Causes of Vertigo

	PERIPHERAL	CENTRAL
Onset	Sudden	Gradual
Severity	Intense	Less intense
Pattern	Paroxysmal	Constant
Associated nausea/diaphoresis	Frequent	Infrequent
Fatigue of symptoms and signs	Yes	No
Hearing loss/tinnitus	May occur	Does not occur
CNS symptoms/signs	Absent	Usually present

- The episodic vertigo in BPPV typically resolves spontaneously after days to weeks as the otoliths dissolve (but can be cured immediately at the bedside with the use of the Epley maneuver).
- Patients with BPPV sometimes state that their vertigo is continuous. These patients may be having such frequent attacks that they think their vertigo is continuous, when in fact they are having many discrete episodes of BPPV, each typically lasting less than 1 minute.
- One helpful way to differentiate BPPV from vestibular neuritis and labyrinthitis is to ask whether the patient is experiencing vertigo during the interview. A patient with BPPV should be asymptomatic while providing the history (assuming there is no head movement).

NEAR SYNCOPE

- Near syncope is the feeling that one is going to faint. This is due to global hypoperfusion of the brain.
- Patients often have associated autonomic warning signs, such as pallor, diaphoresis, and nausea.
- Common causes include orthostasis (anemia, hypovolemia, antihypertensive medications), cardiac disease (cardiomyopathy, aortic stenosis, cardiac dysrhythmias), vasovagal episode, and environmental factors (alcohol, high temperature, hyperventilation).
- If the patient is unable to lie down (making it easier for the heart to perfuse the brain), then the patient will convert from near syncope to true syncope.
- If the patient is still unable to lie in a horizontal position, the body will start to make antigravity movements that a lay person may interpret as a seizure.

DISEQUILIBRIUM

- Disequilibrium is a sense of imbalance or unsteadiness while ambulating. Patients may state that they feel like they are going to fall.

- Patients with this type of dizziness are often asymptomatic lying down or sitting, but become symptomatic while standing or walking.
- Common causes include cervical spondylosis (which leads to myelopathy and poor proprioception in the legs), extrapyramidal diseases, and cerebellar diseases.

PSYCHOGENIC DIZZINESS

- Psychogenic dizziness is generally attributed to anxiety states.
- The physical examination in the dizzy patient should include a complete assessment of the auditory, neurologic, and cardiac systems.

DIAGNOSIS AND DIFFERENTIAL

VERTIGO

- The Hallpike test confirms the diagnosis by inducing torsional nystagmus and causing reproduction of symptoms after a short latency (1 to 5 seconds).[4] The symptoms then resolve within 1 minute and become less intense with repeated positioning (the otoliths become scattered throughout the canal and exert less of an effect). Central causes of positional vertigo rarely show these features.
- The head-thrust test is also used to evaluate patients with peripheral vertigo. This is a simple bedside test of the horizontal vestibulo-ocular reflex.
- The head-thrust test is performed by grasping the patient's head and applying a brief, small-amplitude, high acceleration head turn, first to one side and then to the other. The patient fixates on the examiner's nose and the examiner watches for corrective rapid eye movements (saccades) that are a sign of decreased vestibular response. If "catch-up" saccades occur in one direction but not the other, this indicates a peripheral vestibular lesion on that side.[5,6]
- Vestibular neuritis is characterized by the sudden onset of severe, often incapacitating vertigo. Episodes may last for days to weeks. Hearing is not affected.[6]
- A viral etiology is suspected in vestibular neuritis, and patients may have concurrent or recent symptoms of an upper respiratory infection.
- Labyrinthitis, although commonly viral, can also be due to bacterial infection from otitis media, meningitis, and mastoiditis. Hearing loss differentiates this entity from vestibular neuritis.[6]
- Ménière's disease is thought to be caused by distension in the endolymphatic system with occasional ruptures and leakage of fluid from the endolymph into the perilymph.
- Symptoms in Ménière's disease typically last for hours instead of seconds. Roaring tinnitus and a sense of fullness and diminished hearing in the affected ear are typical.
- Since the diagnosis requires multiple episodes of attacks with progressive hearing loss, Ménière's disease cannot be diagnosed on the first presentation of vertigo.
- Perilymphatic fistula at the round or oval window, which is caused by blunt or barotrauma, results in sudden vertigo with sensorineural hearing loss. Insufflation during otoscopy worsens symptoms (Hennebert's sign).
- Trauma, including barotrauma, and infection may cause a perilymph fistula, and symptoms are typically associated with situations resulting in pneumatic fluctuation such as flying, diving, or sneezing.
- Tumors of the eighth cranial nerve and cerebellopontine angle such as meningioma, acoustic neuroma, and acoustic schwannoma also may present as vertigo with hearing loss. These tumors may be associated with ipsilateral facial weakness and impaired corneal reflexes and cerebellar signs.
- Vertigo may occur following closed head injury due to direct labyrinthine trauma or dislodgement of otoliths leading to BPPV. Posttraumatic vertigo may be associated with basilar skull fracture.
- Ototoxicity from a multitude of drugs and chemicals may induce vertigo and hearing loss. Common offenders causing peripheral toxicity include aminoglycosides, cytotoxic agents, quinidine, and quinine-related antimalarial agents.
- Anticonvulsants, antidepressants, neuroleptics, hydrocarbons, alcohol, and phencyclidine may cause centrally mediated vertigo.
- Cerebellar infarction or hemorrhage are potentially devastating causes of central vertigo. Vertigo, nausea, and vomiting may be sudden and severe or mild.
- Truncal ataxia and abnormal gait on Romberg testing are frequently associated with cerebellar infarction or hemorrhage. The nystagmus may change direction with change in direction of the gaze.
- Lateral medullary infarction of the brainstem (Wallenberg's syndrome) causes vertigo along with ipsilateral facial numbness, loss of the corneal reflex, Horner's syndrome, and pharyngeal and laryngeal paralysis. Contralateral loss of pain and temperature sensation in the extremities also occurs.
- Vertebrobasilar insufficiency (VBI) may result in vertigo due to brainstem transient ischemic attacks in patients with the typical risk factors for cerebrovascular disease.
- The vertigo associated with VBI may be sudden in onset and last minutes to hours, but should not last more than 24 hours. Associated focal brainstem signs and syncope are also likely to be present.

- Unlike other causes of central vertigo, VBI may be induced by movement of the head, resulting in decreased vertebral artery blood flow.
- The aura of basilar migraines may include vertigo, visual loss, tinnitus, hearing loss, diplopia, dysarthria, ataxia, and other manifestations of VBI. The aura develops over 5 to 20 minutes and may or may not be followed by the headache.
- Multiple sclerosis can also cause vertigo. Internuclear ophthalmoplegia consisting of defective adduction of one eye and nystagmus of the other abducting eye is a classic finding in multiple sclerosis.

EMERGENCY DEPARTMENT CARE AND DISPOSITION

- With peripheral vertigo, the most effective medications are usually the antihistaminic and antiserotonergic medications. Promethazine, meclizine, and ondansetron are effective in providing symptomatic relief.
- Benzodiazepines prevent the process of vestibular rehabilitation and should be used as second-line agents.
- Scopolamine is a pure anticholinergic medication that works by blocking the conflict signal size.
- Patients with BPPV should be treated with the Epley maneuver (canalith repositioning maneuver). This maneuver is easily performed at the patient's bedside and takes only a few minutes. By moving the otoliths out of the posterior semicircular canal and back into the utricle where they belong, the patient potentially can be cured at the bedside.[7]
- Because of their likely viral etiology, some experts recommend treating vestibular neuritis and labyrinthitis with oral steroids and acyclovir.
- Patients with perilymph fistula, labyrinthitis of suspected bacterial etiology, and Ménière's disease should be referred for follow-up with an ENT specialist.
- Posterior fossa hemorrhage is an emergency for which immediate neurosurgical consultation must be obtained.
- Suspected tumors should have urgent neurosurgical consultation and appropriate imaging studies.

REFERENCES

1. Kroenke K, Lucas CA, Rosenberg ML, et al: Causes of persistent dizziness. A prospective study of 100 patients in ambulatory care. *Ann Intern Med* 117:898, 1992.
2. Parnes LS, McClure JA: Free-floating endolymph particles: a new operative finding during posterior semicircular canal occlusion. *Laryngoscope* 102:988, 1992.
3. Hotson JR, Baloh RW: Acute vestibular syndrome. *N Engl J Med* 339:680, 1998.
4. Furman JM, Cass SP: Benign paroxysmal positional vertigo. *N Engl J Med* 341:1590, 1999.
5. Halmagyi GM, Curthoys IS: A clinical sign of canal paresis. *Arch Neurol* 45:737, 1988.
6. Baloh RW: Vestibular neuritis. *N Engl J Med* 348:1027, 2003.
7. Epley JM: The canalith repositioning procedure: for treatment of benign paroxysmal positional vertigo. *Otolaryngol Head Neck Surg* 107:399, 1992.

For further reading in *Emergency Medicine: A Comprehensive Study Guide*, 6th ed., see Chap. 231, "Vertigo and Dizziness," by Brian Goldman.

148 SEIZURES AND STATUS EPILEPTICUS IN ADULTS
C. Crawford Mechem

EPIDEMIOLOGY

- There are 100,000 new cases of seizures diagnosed in the U.S. each year.
- The overall age-adjusted incidence of seizures worldwide is 30.9 to 56.8 per 100,000, with highest rates among those less than 20 years old followed by those over 60 years.[1]

PATHOPHYSIOLOGY

- A seizure is an episode of abnormal neurologic function caused by inappropriate electrical discharge of brain neurons.
- Epilepsy is a clinical condition in which an individual is subject to recurrent seizures. The term is ordinarily not applied to seizures caused by reversible conditions such as alcohol withdrawal, hypoglycemia, or other metabolic derangements.
- Primary or idiopathic seizures are those without a clear cause.
- Secondary or symptomatic seizures are the result of another identifiable neurologic condition, such as a mass lesion.
- Seizures may be classified in two major groups: generalized and partial (focal) (Table 148-1).
- A subclass of generalized seizures is absence (petit mal) seizures, which classically are seen in school-aged children.

TABLE 148-1 Classification of Seizures

Generalized seizures (consciousness always lost)
   Tonic-clonic seizures (grand mal)
   Absence seizures (petit mal)
  Myoclonic seizures
  Tonic seizures
  Clonic seizures
  Atonic seizures

Partial (focal) seizures
  Simple partial (no alteration of consciousness)
  Complex partial (consciousness impaired)
  Partial seizures (simple or complex) with secondary generalization

Unclassified (due to inadequate information)

- Generalized seizures are believed to be caused by a nearly simultaneous activation of the entire cerebral cortex.
- Partial seizures are due to electrical discharges in a localized, structural lesion of the brain. The discharges may remain local or can spread to nearby regions or the entire cortex (generalized).
- Partial seizures may be either simple, in which consciousness is not affected, or complex, in which consciousness is altered.
- Complex partial seizures are often due to focal discharges in the temporal lobe (termed temporal lobe seizures).
- Eclampsia refers to the combination of seizures, hypertension, edema, and proteinuria in pregnant women beyond 20 weeks' gestation or up to 8 weeks postpartum.
- Status epilepticus has historically been defined as continuous seizure activity lasting for at least 30 minutes, or two or more seizures without intervening return to baseline.[2]
- Nonconvulsive status epilepticus is associated with minimal or imperceptible convulsive activity and is confirmed by electroencephalogram (EEG).

CLINICAL FEATURES

- Generalized seizures begin with abrupt loss of consciousness and loss of postural tone. The patient may then become rigid, with extension of the trunk and extremities.
- Apnea, cyanosis, and urinary incontinence are common with generalized seizures.
- As the rigid (tonic) phase subsides, symmetric rhythmic (clonic) jerking of the trunk and extremities develop. After the attack, the patient is flaccid and unconscious.
- A typical generalized seizure episode lasts from 60 to 90 seconds. Consciousness returns gradually, and postictal confusion may persist for several hours.
- Absence seizures are very brief, usually lasting only a few seconds. Patients suddenly lose consciousness without losing postural tone.
- Patients with absence seizures appear confused or withdrawn, and current activity ceases. They may stare and have twitching of their eyelids. They do not respond to voice or other stimulation, do not exhibit voluntary movement, and are not incontinent.
- Absence seizure attacks end abruptly, and there is no postictal period.
- Simple partial seizures remain localized and consciousness is not affected. The likely location of the initial cortical discharge can be deduced from the clinical features at onset.
- Unilateral tonic or clonic movements limited to one extremity suggest a focus in the motor cortex, while tonic deviation of the head and eyes suggests a frontal lobe focus.
- Visual symptoms often result from an occipital focus, while olfactory or gustatory hallucinations may arise from the medial temporal lobe.
- Such sensory phenomena, or auras, are often the initial symptoms of attacks.
- Complex partial seizures are focal seizures in which consciousness is affected. Because of their effect on thinking and behavior, they are occasionally called psychomotor seizures.
- Symptoms of complex partial seizures may include automatisms, which are typically simple, repetitive purposeless movements such as lip smacking or fiddling with clothing.
- Visceral symptoms, such as a sensation of butterflies rising up from the epigastrium, and olfactory, gustatory, visual, or auditory hallucinations may develop.
- Fear, paranoia, depression, or elation may also be noted with complex partial seizures.

DIAGNOSIS AND DIFFERENTIAL

- The first step in diagnosis is determining if the episode was indeed a true seizure. A careful history should be obtained from the patient and witnesses.
- Important historical information includes the rapidity of onset, presence of a preceding aura, progression of motor activity, whether the activity was local or generalized, and whether the patient became incontinent.
- The duration of the episode and whether there was postictal confusion should also be determined.
- If the patient has a known seizure disorder, the regular pattern of seizures, medications taken and any dosage changes, and the possibility of lack of compliance with the medication regimen should be sought.
- Contributing factors such as sleep deprivation, alcohol withdrawal, infection, and use or cessation of other drugs should be investigated.

TABLE 148-2 Causes of Secondary Seizures

Trauma (recent or remote)*

Intracranial hemorrhage (subdural, epidural, subarachnoid, intraparenchymal)

Structural abnormalities*
  Vascular lesion (aneurysm, arteriovenous malformation)
  Mass lesions (primary or metastatic neoplasms)
  Degenerative diseases
  Congenital abnormalities

Infection (meningitis, encephalitis, abscess)

Metabolic disturbances
  Hypo- or hyperglycemia*
  Hypo- or hypernatremia
  Hyperosmolar states
  Uremia
  Hepatic failure
  Hypocalcemia, hypomagnesemia (rare)

Toxins and drugs (many)
  Cocaine, lidocaine
  Antidepressants
  Theophylline
  Alcohol withdrawal*
  Drug withdrawal

Eclampsia of pregnancy (may occur up to 8 weeks postpartum)

Hypertensive encephalopathy

Anoxic-ischemic injury (cardiac arrest, severe hypoxemia)

*Most common etiologies.

- In patients with first-time seizures, a more detailed history should include any recent or remote head trauma or headaches, current pregnancy or recent delivery; a history of metabolic derangements or hypoxia; systemic illness such as cancer, coagulopathy, or HIV; drug ingestion or withdrawal; and alcohol use (Table 148-2).[3,4]
- The physical examination should include a search for any injuries resulting from the seizure, such as fractures, sprains, strains, posterior shoulder dislocation, tongue lacerations, and aspiration.
- Any localized neurologic deficits should be sought. A transient focal deficit following a focal seizure is referred to as Todd's paralysis, and should resolve within 48 hours.
- In a patient with a known seizure disorder who has had a typical seizure, only a fingerstick serum glucose level and an anticonvulsant level may be needed.
- The therapeutic level of a drug is that level that controls seizures without intolerable side effects, regardless of the normal range provided by the laboratory.
- In patients with a first-time seizure or a change in their established seizure pattern, a noncontrast computed tomography (CT) scan of the head is warranted to investigate for hemorrhage or a structural lesion.[5,6]
- Because many processes such as tumors or vascular anomalies are poorly visualized without contrast, a follow-up contrast CT or magnetic resonance imaging scan may be arranged.

- The differential diagnosis of seizures includes the various causes of syncope, hyperventilation syndrome, migraines, movement disorders, and narcolepsy. Pseudoseizures are psychogenic and may be difficult to distinguish from true seizures.

EMERGENCY DEPARTMENT CARE AND DISPOSITION

- Oxygen should be administered and pulse oximetry initiated. Suction and airway adjuncts must be readily available. IV access should be obtained.
- Endotracheal intubation should be considered for prolonged seizures or if GI decontamination is indicated. If rapid sequence intubation is performed, a short-acting paralytic agent should be used so that ongoing seizure activity can be observed. If longer-acting paralytics are required, electroencephalographic (EEG) monitoring should be initiated.
- IV thiamine and glucose should be given if hypoglycemia is confirmed.
- The anticonvulsants most frequently used are the benzodiazepines (eg, lorazepam), phenytoin, fosphenytoin, and phenobarbital (Fig. 148-1).
- Phenytoin may be administered immediately after benzodiazepines or as a single agent in patients with less frequent seizures.
- Fosphenytoin is a prodrug of phenytoin that has the

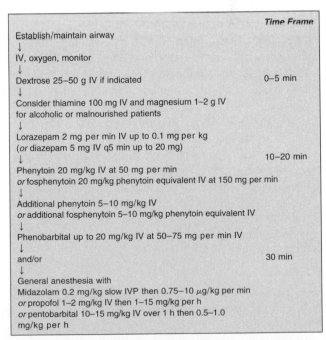

FIG. 148-1. Guidelines for management of status epilepticus. (Adapted from Lowenstein DH, Alldredge BK: Status epilepticus. *N Engl J Med* 338:970, 1998.)

TABLE 148-3 Properties of Commonly Used Anticonvulsant Drugs

DRUG	ORAL DOSE, MG PER DAY*	THERAPEUTIC LEVEL, μg/mL	DAYS TO REACH STEADY STATE†	SERUM HALF-LIFE, h
Phenytoin	300–600 divided tid	10–20	5–10	7–42
Carbamazepine	400–1200 divided tid or qid	6–12	2–4	12–17
Phenobarbital	60–200 qd	10–40	14–21	48–144
Primidone	750–2000 divided tid or qid	5–12	4–7	10–21
Valproic acid	15–60 mg/kg per d divided bid or tid	50–150	2–4	12–18

*Average therapeutic dose. Initiation dosing may be different. Daily dose is individualized. Drug-drug interactions may dramatically change daily doses in patients receiving multiple drugs.
†Indicates time required to establish stable serum levels after any change in dose.

advantages of fewer infusion site reactions, more rapid administration, and intramuscular injection.

- Phenobarbital is a third-line agent in patients who cannot tolerate phenytoin or who do not respond to full doses of benzodiazepines and phenytoin. Respiratory and circulatory depression are common with its use.
- Eclamptic patients should be administered magnesium sulfate 4 to 6 g IV followed by an infusion of 1 to 2 g/h, in addition to the above regimen.[7,8]
- Status epilepticus refractory to the above measures is best controlled by induction of general anesthesia using agents such as midazolam, propofol, or pentobarbital.[9–12]
- Patients with a known seizure disorder who present after their typical seizure may be discharged once they return to baseline and serum anticonvulsant levels are addressed.
- When necessary, IV loading is preferable to the oral route because of the more rapid establishment of a therapeutic level (Table 148-3).
- Patients with a new-onset seizure may be discharged for further outpatient evaluation if they return to baseline and life-threatening conditions have been excluded. Disposition of such patients is ideally made in consultation with a neurologist or primary care physician.
- Indications for admission following a new-onset seizure include persistent altered mental status, central nervous system infection or mass, eclampsia, underlying metabolic derangements not readily corrected in the emergency department, associated head trauma, absence of reliable caretakers at home, and inability to arrange a close follow-up appointment for further evaluation and therapy adjustment.

REFERENCES

1. Hauser WA, Hesdorffer DC: *Epilepsy Frequency, Causes and Consequences.* New York: Demos, 1990, p. 12.

2. Lowenstein DH, Bleck T, Macdonald RL: It's time to revise the definition of status epilepticus. *Epilespia* 40:120, 1999.

3. Holtzman DM, Kaku DA, So YT: New-onset seizures associated with human immunodeficiency virus infection: Causation and clinical features in 100 cases. *Am J Med* 87:173, 1989.

4. Modi G, Modi M, Martinus I, et al: New-onset seizures associated with HIV infection. *Neurology* 55:1558, 2000.

5. American College of Emergency Physicians, American Academy of Neurology, American Association of Neurologic Surgeons, and American Society of Neurology: Practice parameter: Neuroimaging in the emergency patient presenting with seizure (summary statement). *Ann Emerg Med* 28:114, 1996.

6. American College of Emergency Physicians: Clinical policy for the initial approach to patients presenting with a chief complaint of seizure who are not in status epilepticus. *Ann Emerg Med* 29:706, 1997.

7. The Eclampsia Trial Collaborative Group: Which anticonvulsant for women with eclampsia? Evidence from the Collaborative Eclampsia Trial. *Lancet* 345:1455, 1995.

8. Witlin AG, Sibai BM: Magnesium sulfate therapy in preeclampsia and eclampsia. *Obstet Gynecol* 92:883, 1998.

9. Kumar A, Bleck TP: Intravenous midazolam for the treatment of refractory status epilepticus. *Crit Care Med* 20:483, 1992.

10. Parent JM, Lowenstein DH: Treatment of refractory generalized status epilepticus with continuous infusion of midazolam. *Neurology* 44:1837, 1994.

11. Stecker MM, Kramer TH, Raps EC, et al: Treatment of refractory status epilepticus with propofol: clinical and pharmacokinetic findings. *Epilepsia* 39:18, 1998.

12. Prasad A, Worrall BB, Bertram EH, et al: Propofol and midazolam in the treatment of refractory status epilepticus. *Epilepsia* 42:380, 2001.

For further reading in *Emergency Medicine: A Comprehensive Study Guide,* 6th ed., see Chap. 232, "Seizures and Status Epilepticus in Adults," by Christina L. Catlett.

149 ACUTE PERIPHERAL NEUROLOGIC LESIONS

Howard E. Jarvis III

MYOPATHIES

POLYMYOSITIS

- Polymyositis is an inflammatory myopathy characterized by chronic or subacute proximal symmetric weakness.
- Patients may have dysphagia and muscular pain, and a few may progress to respiratory failure.
- Sensation and reflexes are normal except with very severe weakness.
- Laboratory studies may reveal an elevated erythrocyte sedimentation rate, creatine kinase level, and leukocytosis.
- The differential diagnosis includes Lambert-Eaton syndrome, endocrinopathies, toxic myopathies, dermatomyositis, and others.
- Admission is usually warranted to monitor the airway and clinical progression and to complete the evaluation.

DERMATOMYOSITIS

- Dermatomyositis has similar laboratory findings and clinical manifestations as polymyositis, with the addition of a violaceous rash, often on the face and hands.
- Treatment is aimed at immunosuppression.
- Numerous other etiologies of myopathy include environmental (eg, alcohol), occupational, drugs (eg, steroids, azidothymidine, cholesterol-lowering agents), and infection (eg, trichinosis and viral agents).

DISORDERS OF THE NEUROMUSCULAR JUNCTION

- Botulism is caused by *Clostridium botulinum* toxin and occurs in three forms: food-borne, wound, and infantile.
- In the United States, the principal source is improperly prepared or stored food.
- In infantile botulism, organisms arise from ingested spores, often in honey, and produce a systemically absorbed toxin.
- Wound botulism should be considered in patients with a wound or a history of IV drug use and progressive, symmetric descending paralysis.
- Clinical features appear 1 to 2 days following inges-

tion and may be preceded by nausea, vomiting, and diarrhea.
- Early complaints commonly involve the eye or bulbar musculature, and progress to descending weakness and respiratory insufficiency.
- Absent light reflex is a diagnostic clue, and mentation is normal.
- Infants may present with poor suck, listlessness, constipation, regurgitation, and weakness.
- Treatment includes respiratory support, gastrointestinal and wound decontamination, antibiotics (infants only), immune serum (adults and infants), and admission.
- Myasthenia gravis is discussed in Chap. 150.

ACUTE PERIPHERAL NEUROPATHIES

GUILLAIN-BARRÉ SYNDROME

- Guillain-Barré syndrome affects all ages and usually follows a viral illness, especially gastroenteritis. It may be rapidly progressive.
- Although numerous variants exist, extremity weakness, more pronounced initially in the legs, is typical. Bulbar musculature may be involved.
- Respiratory failure and lethal autonomic fluctuations may occur.
- The absence of deep tendon reflexes is classic.
- Cerebrospinal fluid (CSF) analysis typically reveals a high protein level and a normal glucose level and cell count.
- The differential diagnosis includes diphtheria, botulism, lead poisoning, tick paralysis, Lyme disease, spinal cord compression, and porphyria.
- Emergency department (ED) treatment includes respiratory support, admission to a monitored setting, and neurologic consultation.

ACUTE INTERMITTENT PORPHYRIA

- Acute intermittent porphyria is a rare autosomal dominant disorder involving the triad of weakness, psychosis, and abdominal pain. Occasionally they occur together, but each may occur independently.
- Seizures may be seen.
- Certain medications may trigger flares, such as phenytoin, barbiturates, sulfonamides, and estrogen.
- Neurologic findings include weakness and diminished reflexes, particularly in the lower extremities. Sensory abnormalities may occur.
- The differential diagnosis includes causes of pain and lower extremity weakness, such as spinal cord compression (brisk reflexes and up-going toes) and aortic aneurysm or dissection.

- ED treatment includes discontinuation of the offending drug, supportive care, glucose infusions, vitamin B_6, and hematin.

ENTRAPMENT NEUROPATHIES

- Carpal tunnel syndrome is discussed in Chap. 185.
- Other common nerve entrapments include ulnar (which can mimic C8 radiculopathy), deep peroneal (causing foot drop and numbness between the first and second toes), and meralgia paresthetica (entrapment of the lateral cutaneous nerve of the thigh).
- Meralgia paresthetica may follow weight loss and pelvic or gynecologic surgery, and causes lateral thigh numbness.
- These and other entrapments often cause numbness and/or weakness, and require referral to a specialist.

PLEXOPATHIES

BRACHIAL NEURITIS

- Brachial neuritis causes severe shoulder, back, or arm pain followed by weakness in the arm or shoulder girdle, and is bilateral in up to one third of cases.
- Patients have weakness in various distributions of the brachial plexus.
- Sensory deficits are less profound, and reflexes in the involved arm are diminished.
- The differential diagnosis includes multiple radiculopathies, Pancoast tumors, and neoplastic or inflammatory infiltration of the plexus, although a history of pain followed by weakness that plateaus in 1 to 2 weeks makes other diagnoses unlikely.
- A chest radiograph should be ordered to screen for mass lesions involving the plexus.
- ED treatment consists of conservative management, and close neurologic follow-up is indicated.

LUMBAR PLEXOPATHY

- Lumbar plexopathy, or diabetic amyotrophy, presents in diabetics with acute back pain followed within days by ipsilateral progressive leg weakness.
- Decreased strength (and possibly reflexes) in a variety of patterns with relatively symmetric sensation is found.
- Bowel and bladder functions are not affected.
- Plain radiographs and magnetic resonance imaging (MRI) are ultimately needed.
- The differential diagnosis includes cauda equina and conus medullaris syndromes and arteriovenous malformation compression.

- Abdominal computed tomography (CT) scanning aids in excluding aortic aneurysm and psoas muscle masses.
- Patients should be admitted for further evaluation of weakness.

HIV-ASSOCIATED PERIPHERAL NEUROLOGIC DISEASE

- HIV infection and its complications and treatments cause a variety of peripheral nerve disorders.
- The most common, drug-induced and HIV neuropathies, are chronic and do not cause acute symptoms.
- Patients with HIV have a higher rate of mononeuritis multiplex and a myopathy resembling polymyositis.
- In early infection, they are more prone to Guillain-Barré syndrome.
- In the latter stages of AIDS, they may develop cytomegalovirus radiculitis, with acute weakness, primarily lower extremity involvement, and variable bowel or bladder dysfunction.
- Primarily, lower extremity weakness and hyporeflexia, as well as sensory deficits, are seen. Rectal tone may be decreased.
- MRI (indicated to exclude mass lesion) shows swelling and clumping of the cauda equina.
- Admission is required; treatment, which should precede definitive diagnosis, consists of ganciclovir.

OTHER CONDITIONS

MONONEURITIS MULTIPLEX

- Mononeuritis multiplex is caused by a vasculitis and involves multiple deficits in a stepwise fashion, usually involving both sides of the body.
- Mononeuritis multiplex must be differentiated from multiple compression neuropathies, and it requires urgent referral to a neurologist.

BELL'S PALSY

- Bell's palsy causes seventh cranial nerve dysfunction, and patients may complain of facial weakness, articulation problems, difficulty keeping an eye closed, or inability to keep food in the mouth on one side.
- Physical examination findings reveal weakness on one side of the face, including the forehead, and no other focal neurologic findings.
- The differential diagnosis includes stroke, Lyme disease, Guillain-Barré syndrome, parotid tumors, middle ear lesions, cerebellopontine angle tumors, eighth cranial nerve lesions, HIV, and vascular disease.

- The ear should be inspected for ulcerations caused by cranial herpes zoster activation (Ramsay Hunt syndrome) which should be treated with oral acyclovir.
- If muscle strength is retained in the forehead, the lesion is most probably central (ie, in the brainstem or above); this would exclude Bell's palsy, and CT scanning of the head is indicated.
- Treatment of Bell's palsy is controversial, though most neurologists favor a short course of prednisone (50 mg/day for 7 days).[1]
- Steroids are withheld if paresis has been present for more than a week.
- Acyclovir (200 mg five times a day for 10 days) may be beneficial.
- Patients should apply Lacri-Lube in order to prevent corneal drying at night.
- Close follow-up with a neurologist or ENT specialist is indicated.

LYME DISEASE

- Lyme disease is caused by exposure to the tick-borne pathogen *Borrelia burgdorferi*, and prior tick exposure or exposure to areas endemic to deer ticks may be noted.
- In addition to initial arthralgias and fatigue, multiple neurologic manifestations may develop, including seventh cranial nerve palsy.
- Unless there is encephalitis, a rare complication, mental status is normal.
- Peripheral nerves and the nerve root are affected.
- Patients may describe acute or subacute progression of limb weakness and sensory loss, sometimes with radicular pain.
- Selected deep tendon reflexes may be diminished.
- Serum and CSF Lyme antibodies are suggestive of disease. CSF pleocytosis and increased protein with normal glucose are the most common laboratory findings.
- Duration and route of antibiotic administration depends on the severity of clinical findings.

REFERENCES

1. Adour KK, Ruboyianes JM, Von Doersten PG, et al: Bell's palsy treatment with acyclovir and prednisone compared with prednisone alone: A double-blind, randomized controlled trial. *Ann Otol Rhinol Laryngol* 105:371, 1996.

For further reading in *Emergency Medicine: A Comprehensive Study Guide*, 6th ed., see Chap. 233, "Acute Peripheral Neurologic Lesions," by Michael M. Wang.

150 CHRONIC NEUROLOGIC DISORDERS
Mark B. Rogers

AMYOTROPHIC LATERAL SCLEROSIS

EPIDEMIOLOGY

- The typical time of onset for amyotrophic lateral sclerosis (ALS) is over age 50.

PATHOPHYSIOLOGY

- ALS is caused by upper and lower motor neuron degeneration from an unknown etiology, which leads to rapidly progressive muscle wasting and weakness.

CLINICAL FEATURES

- Upper motor neuron dysfunction causes limb spasticity, hyperreflexia, and emotional lability.
- Lower neuron dysfunction causes limb muscle weakness, atrophy, fasciculations, dysarthria, dysphagia, and difficulty in mastication.
- Symptoms are often asymmetric and more prominent in the upper extremities.[1]
- Patients may initially have cervical or back pain consistent with an acute compressive radiculopathy.[2]
- Respiratory difficulty progresses to failure.

DIAGNOSIS AND DIFFERENTIAL

- The diagnosis is clinical and is often previously established.
- Electromyography (EMG) is the most useful test.
- Other illnesses that should be considered include myasthenia gravis, diabetes, dysproteinemia, thyroid dysfunction, vitamin B_{12} deficiency, lead toxicity, vasculitis, and central nervous system (CNS) and spinal cord tumors.

EMERGENCY DEPARTMENT CARE AND DISPOSITION

- Emergency care is required for acute respiratory failure, aspiration pneumonia, choking episodes, or trauma from falls.

- The treatment goal is to optimize pulmonary function through the use of nebulizer treatments, steroids, antibiotics, or endotracheal intubation.[3]
- Patients with impending respiratory failure, pneumonia, inability to handle secretions, and worsening disease process that may require long-term care should be admitted.

MULTIPLE SCLEROSIS

EPIDEMIOLOGY

- Three clinical courses are seen in multiple sclerosis (MS): relapsing and remitting (80% of cases), relapsing and progressive, or chronically progressive.[4]
- Peak age of onset is the third decade of life. Females are two to three times more likely to contract MS than are males.

PATHOPHYSIOLOGY

- Although the etiology of MS is unknown, it involves multifocal areas of CNS demyelination, causing motor, sensory, visual, and cerebellar dysfunction.

CLINICAL FEATURES

- Deficits associated with MS are described as a heaviness, weakness, stiffness, or numbness of an extremity. Lower extremity symptoms are usually more severe.
- Lhermitte's sign is an electric shock–like sensation, a vibration, or dysesthetic pain going down the back into the arms or legs from neck flexion.
- Decreased strength, increased tone, hyperreflexia, clonus, decreased proprioception, and reduced pain and temperature sense may be seen.
- Increases in body temperature, associated with exercise, hot baths, or fever, may worsen symptoms.
- Rarely, acute transverse myelitis may occur. Cerebellar lesions may cause intention tremor or ataxia.
- Brainstem lesions may cause vertigo.
- Cognitive and emotional problems are common (eg, mood disorders or dementia).
- Optic neuritis, usually causing unilateral loss of central vision, is the first presenting symptom in up to 30% of cases and may cause an afferent papillary defect (Marcus Gunn pupil).
- Retrobulbar or extraocular muscle pain usually precedes vision loss. Funduscopy is usually normal, but the disc may appear pale.
- Acute bilateral internuclear ophthalmoplegia (INO), which causes abnormal adduction and horizontal nystagmus, is highly suggestive of MS.

- Dysautonomia causes vesicourethral, gastrointestinal tract, and sexual dysfunction.

DIAGNOSIS AND DIFFERENTIAL

- The diagnosis of MS is clinical and is suggested by two or more episodes, lasting days to weeks, causing dysfunction that implicates different sites in the white matter.[5]
- Magnetic resonance imaging (MRI) of the head may demonstrate various abnormalities, including discrete lesions in the supratentorial white matter or periventricular areas.
- Cerebrospinal fluid (CSF) protein and gamma-globulin levels are often elevated.
- The differential diagnosis includes systemic lupus erythematosus, Lyme disease, neurosyphilis, and HIV disease.

EMERGENCY DEPARTMENT CARE AND DISPOSITION

- Those with severe motor or cerebellar dysfunction may be treated with steroids. A short-term (up to 5 days), high-dose course of pulsed IV methylprednisolone (250 mg IV every 6 hours), followed by oral prednisone tapered over 2 to 3 weeks, may be beneficial.
- Fever must be reduced to minimize symptoms. A careful search for a source of infection should be performed.
- Respiratory infections and distress must be aggressively managed.
- Acute cystitis and pyelonephritis are frequently the sources. Any infection associated with postvoid residuals greater than 100 mL requires intermittent catheterization.
- Admission is required for those at risk for further complications, respiratory compromise, depression with suicidal ideation, and those requiring IV antibiotics or steroids.

MYASTHENIA GRAVIS

EPIDEMIOLOGY

- Peak age of onset for myasthenia gravis (MG) is in the second or third decade of life for females and in the seventh or eighth decade for males.[6]

PATHOPHYSIOLOGY

- Myasthenia gravis (MG) is an autoimmune disease caused by antibody destruction of the acetylcholine receptors at the neuromuscular junction, which results in muscle weakness.

- The thymus is abnormal in 75% of patients and thymectomy resolves or improves symptoms in most patients.[7]

CLINICAL FEATURES

- Most MG patients have generalized weakness, specifically of the proximal extremities, neck extensors, and facial or bulbar muscles. There is usually no deficit in sensory, reflex, and cerebellar function.
- Ptosis and diplopia are the most common symptoms. Symptoms usually worsen as the day progresses or with muscle use (eg, prolonged chewing or reading) and improve with rest.
- Myasthenic crisis is a life-threatening condition involving extreme weakness of the respiratory muscles that may progress to respiratory failure.

DIAGNOSIS AND DIFFERENTIAL

- The diagnosis is confirmed through administration of edrophonium (Tensilon test), electromyogram, and serum testing for acetylcholine receptor antibodies.
- The differential diagnosis includes Lambert-Eaton syndrome, drug-induced disorders (eg, penicillamines, aminoglycosides, and procainamide), ALS, botulism, thyroid disorders, and other CNS disorders (eg, intracranial mass lesions).

EMERGENCY DEPARTMENT CARE AND DISPOSITION

- With myasthenic crisis, supplemental oxygen and aggressive airway management, including endotracheal intubation, should be considered.
- Depolarizing paralytic agents (eg, succinylcholine) and long-acting nondepolarizing agents should be avoided.[8]
- If the Tensilon test is positive, then neostigmine can be administered (0.5 to 2 mg IV or SC, or 15 mg orally), which will be effective within 30 minutes and last for 4 hours.
- Severe MG patients should receive high-dose steroid therapy (mandating a stay in the intensive care unit due to possible increased weakness) and possible plasmapheresis or IV immunoglobulin therapy.
- Several drugs should be used with caution in patients with myasthenia gravis (Table 150-1).
- A neurologist should be consulted for disposition and admission.

LAMBERT-EATON MYASTHENIC SYNDROME

- Lambert-Eaton myasthenic syndrome is an autoimmune disorder that causes fluctuating proximal limb muscle weakness and fatigue.
- Lambert-Eaton syndrome is seen mostly in older men with lung cancer.

TABLE 150-1 Drugs That Should Be Used With Caution in Myasthenia Gravis

Steroids	Neomycin*	Lithium carbonate*	Sotalol	Ecothiopate
ACTD*	Streptomycin*	Amitriptyline	Lidocaine	**Others**
Methylprednisolone*	Kanamycin*	Droperidol	Dilantin	Amantadine
Prednisone*	Gentamicin	Haloperidol	Trimethaphan	Diphenhydramine
	Tobramycin	Imipramine		Emetine
Anticonvulsants	Dihydrostreptomycin*	Paraldehyde	**Local Anesthetic**	Diuretics
Dilantin	Amikacin	Trichlorethanol	Lidocaine*	Muscle relaxants
Ethosuximide	Polymyxin A		Procaine*	CNS depressants
Trimethadione	Polymyxin B	**Antirheumatics**		Respiratory depressants
Paraldehyde	Bacitracin	D-Penicillamine	**Analgesics**	Sedatives
Magnesium sulfate	Sulfonamides	Colchicine	Narcotics	Procaine*
Barbiturates	Viomycin	Chloroquine	Morphine	Tranquilizers
	Colistin		Dilaudid	
Antimalarials	Colistimethate*	**Cardiovascular**	Codeine	**Neuromuscular blocking**
Chloroquine*	Lincomycin	Quinidine*	Pantopon	**agents**
Quinine*	Clindamycin	Procainamide*	Meperidine	Tubocurarine
	Tetracycline	Beta blockers		Pancuronium
IV Fluids	Oxytetracycline	Propranolol	**Endocrine**	Gallamine
Na lactate solution	Rolitetracycline	Oxprenolol	Thyroid replacement*	Dimethyl tubocurarine
		Practolol		Succinylcholine
Antibiotics	**Psychotropics**	Pindolol	**Eyedrops**	Decamethonium
Fluoroquinolones	Chlorpromazine*		Timolol*	
Aminoglycosides				

*Case reports implicate drugs in exacerbations of myasthenia gravis.
SOURCE: This table is a modified version of the table from Adams SL, Matthews J, Grammer LC: Drugs that may exacerbate myasthenia gravis. *Ann Emerg Med* 13:532, 1984, with permission.

- Unlike MG, strength is improved with sustained activity.
- Patients complain of myalgias, stiffness, paresthesias, metallic tastes, and autonomic symptoms (eg, impotence and dry mouth). Eye movements are unaffected.
- Treatment of the underlying neoplasm greatly improves symptoms.
- The EMG is abnormal and serum tests are specific for antibodies to voltage-gated calcium channels.
- Pyridostigmine and immunosuppressive drugs (eg, corticosteroids and azathioprine) may reduce symptom severity.[9]
- Immunoglobulin therapy or plasmapheresis may be necessary.

PARKINSON'S DISEASE

EPIDEMIOLOGY

- The average age of onset for Parkinson's disease is 55 to 60 years of age.[10]

PATHOPHYSIOLOGY

- The etiology of Parkinson's disease is unknown, but patients have reduced dopaminergic receptors in the substantia nigra.

CLINICAL FEATURES

- Parkinson's disease (PD) presents with four classic signs (mnemonic "TRAP"): resting tremor, cogwheel rigidity, akinesia or bradykinesia, and impaired posture and equilibrium.
- Other signs include facial and postural changes, voice and speech abnormalities, depression, and fatigue.
- Initially, most complain of a unilateral resting arm tremor, described as pill rolling, which improves with intentional movement.

DIAGNOSIS AND DIFFERENTIAL

- The diagnosis is clinical and is most often previously established. No laboratory test or neuroimaging study is pathognomonic.
- Parkinsonism can result from street drugs, toxins, neuroleptic drugs, hydrocephalus, head trauma, and other rare neurologic disorders.

EMERGENCY DEPARTMENT CARE AND DISPOSITION

- Parkinson's disease patients may be on medications that increase central dopamine (eg, levodopa, carbidopa, and amantadine), anticholinergics (eg, benztropine), and dopamine receptor agonists (eg, bromocriptine).
- Medication toxicity includes psychiatric or sleep disturbances, cardiac dysrhythmias, orthostatic hypotension, dyskinesias, and dystonia.
- With significant motor or psychiatric disturbances (eg, hallucinations or frank psychosis) or decreased drug efficacy, a "drug holiday" for 1 week should be initiated.

POLIOMYELITIS AND POSTPOLIO SYNDROME

EPIDEMIOLOGY

- Poliomyelitis leads to paralysis in less than 5% of infected patients.[11]

PATHOPHYSIOLOGY

- Poliomyelitis is caused by an enterovirus that causes paralysis via motor neuron destruction and muscle denervation and atrophy.
- In developed countries, transmission is oral to oral; however, transmission is fecal to oral in developing countries.

CLINICAL FEATURES

- Most symptomatic patients have only a mild viral syndrome and no paralysis. Symptoms include fever, malaise, headache, sore throat, and gastrointestinal symptoms.
- Spinal polio results in asymmetric proximal limb weakness and flaccidity, absent tendon reflexes, and fasciculations; sensory deficits are usually not seen. Maximal paralysis occurs within 5 days.
- Other sequelae include bulbar polio (speech and swallowing dysfunction) and encephalitis.
- Postpolio syndrome is the recurrence of motor symptoms after a latent period of several decades.
- Symptoms of postpolio syndrome may include muscle fatigue, joint pain, or weakness of new and previously affected muscle groups.[12] Patients may have new bulbar, respiratory, or sleep difficulties.

DIAGNOSIS AND DIFFERENTIAL

- Polio should be considered in patients with an acute febrile illness, aseptic meningitis, and asymmetric flaccid paralysis.
- CSF may reveal an elevated white blood cell count (mostly neutrophils) and positive cultures for poliovirus.
- Throat and rectal swabs are high yield tests.
- The diagnosis of postpolio syndrome is based on a prior history of paralytic polio with recovery and new symptoms.
- The differential diagnosis includes Guillain-Barré syndrome, peripheral neuropathies (eg, mononucleosis, Lyme disease, and porphyria), abnormal electrolyte levels, toxins, inflammatory myopathies, and other viruses (eg, coxsackievirus, mumps, echovirus, and various enteroviruses).

EMERGENCY DEPARTMENT CARE AND DISPOSITION

- Treatment is supportive.
- Disposition should be made in consultation with a neurologist.

REFERENCES

1. Swash M: Early diagnosis of ALS/MND. *J Neurol Sci* 160: S33, 1998.
2. Sostarko M, Vranjes D, Brinar V, Brzovic Z: Severe progression of ALS/MND after intervertebral discectomy. *J Neurol Sci* 160:S42, 1998.
3. Miller RG, Rosenberg JA, Gelinas DF, et al: Practice parameter: The care of the patient with amyotrophic lateral sclerosis (an evidence-based review): Report of the Quality Standards Subcommittee of the American Academy of Neurology: ALS Parameters Task Force. *Neurology* 52:1311, 1999.
4. Weinshenker BG: Epidemiology of multiple sclerosis. *Neuro Clin* 14:291, 1996.
5. Poser CM, Brinar VV: Diagnostic criteria for multiple sclerosis. *Clin Neurol Neurosurg* 103:1, 2001.
6. Jacobson DL, Gange SJ, Rose NR, Graham NM: Epidemiology and estimated population burden of selected autoimmune diseases in the United States. *Clin Immunol Immunopathol* 84:223, 1997.
7. Gronseth GS, Barohn RJ: Practice parameter: Thymectomy for autoimmune myasthenia gravis (an evidence based review): Report of the Quality Standards Subcommittee of the American Academy of Neurology. *Neurology* 55:7, 2000.
8. Barrons RW: Drug-induced neuromuscular blockade and myasthenia gravis. *Pharmacotherapy* 17:1220, 1997.
9. Pascuzzi RM: Myasthenia gravis and Lambert-Eaton syndrome. *Ther Apher* 6:57, 2002.
10. Tanner CM, Goldman SM: Epidemiology of Parkinson's disease. *Neurol Clin* 14:317, 1996.
11. Jubelt B: Enterovirus and mumps virus infections of the nervous system. *Neurol Clin* 2:187, 1984.
12. Wekre LL, Stanghelle JK, Lobben B, Oyyhaugen S, The Norwegian Polio Study 1994: a nationwide survey of problems in long-standing poliomyelitis. *Spinal Cord* 36:280, 1998.

For further reading in *Emergency Medicine: A Comprehensive Study Guide,* 6th ed., see Chap. 234, "Chronic Neurologic Disorders," by Edward P. Sloan.

151 MENINGITIS, ENCEPHALITIS, AND BRAIN ABSCESS

O. John Ma

MENINGITIS

EPIDEMIOLOGY

- There are approximately 25,000 cases of bacterial meningitis annually in the United States; two thirds of these cases occur in children. The mortality rate is 25% in neonates, 5% in children beyond infancy, and 25% in adults.[1]
- There is an increasing prevalence of ceftriaxone- and penicillin-resistant *Streptococcus pneumoniae* strains in the community.

PATHOPHYSIOLOGY

- Over two thirds of bacterial meningitis cases are caused by S. pneumoniae, *Neisseria meningitidis,* or *Haemophilus influenzae.*
- Infection begins with entrance of bacteria into the subarachnoid space, usually by upper airway inoculation, and is followed by dissemination into the bloodstream and invasion across the blood-brain barrier. Direct inoculation is also possible from infection of parameningeal structures (eg, otitis media, brain abscess, and sinusitis), neurosurgery, and traumatic or congenital communications with the exterior.
- The brain becomes edematous through the following mechanisms. (1) There is reduced cerebrospinal fluid

(CSF) drainage due to interference with flow and absorption by arachnoid granulations; the increased quantity of CSF results in periventricular edema and hydrocephalus. (2) There is disruption of the blood-brain barrier, which allows entry of protein and water. These mechanisms lead to ischemia as intracranial pressure exceeds cerebral perfusion pressure.

CLINICAL FEATURES

- In classic and fulminant cases of bacterial meningitis, the patient presents with fever, headache, stiff neck, photophobia, and altered mental status. Seizures may occur in up to 25% of cases.
- The presenting picture, however, may be more nonspecific, particularly in the very young and elderly. Confusion and fever may be symptoms of meningeal irritation in the elderly.
- It is important to inquire about recent antibiotic use, which may cloud the clinical picture in a less florid case. Other key historical data include living conditions (eg, army barracks, college dormitories), trauma, immunocompetence, immunization status, and recent neurosurgical procedures.
- Physical examination must include assessment for meningeal irritation with resistance to passive neck flexion, Brudzinski's sign (flexion of hips and knees in response to passive neck flexion), and Kernig's sign (contraction of hamstrings in response to knee extension while the hip is flexed).
- The skin should be examined for the purpuric rash characteristic of meningococcemia. Paranasal sinuses should be percussed and ears examined for evidence of primary infection in those sites.
- Focal neurologic deficits, which are present in 25% of cases, should be documented. Fundi should be assessed for papilledema, indicating increased intracranial pressure.

DIAGNOSIS AND DIFFERENTIAL

- When the diagnosis of bacterial meningitis is entertained, performing a lumbar puncture (LP) is mandatory. At a minimum, CSF should be sent for Gram's stain and culture, cell count, protein, and glucose. Typical CSF results for meningeal processes are listed in Table 151-1.
- Additional CSF studies to be considered are latex agglutination or counterimmune electrophoresis for bacterial antigens in potentially partially-treated bacterial cases, India ink or serum cryptococcal antigen in immunocompromised patients, acid-fast stain and culture for mycobacteria in tuberculous meningitis, *Borrelia* antibodies for possible Lyme disease, and viral cultures in suspected viral meningitis.
- Other laboratory tests should include a complete blood count, blood cultures, and partial thromboplastin and prothrombin times, as well as serum glucose, sodium, and creatinine.
- LP can be performed safely if intracranial mass lesions and coagulopathy are unlikely based on clinical grounds. Patients who are immunocompetent, have no history of central nervous system (CNS) disease, have had no recent seizure (<1 week), and have no papilledema or focal neurologic deficits are safe candidates for LP without prior neuroimaging.
- The differential diagnosis includes subarachnoid hemorrhage, meningeal neoplasm, brain abscess, viral encephalitis, cerebral toxoplasmosis, and other infectious meningitides.

EMERGENCY DEPARTMENT CARE AND DISPOSITION

- Upon presentation of the patient with suspected bacterial meningitis, the LP should be performed expeditiously. Empiric antibiotic therapy should be

TABLE 151-1 Typical Spinal Fluid Results for Meningeal Processes

PARAMETER (NORMAL)	BACTERIAL	VIRAL	NEOPLASTIC	FUNGAL
OP (<170 mm CSF)	>300 mm	200 mm	200 mm	300 mm
WBC (<5 mononuclear)	>1000/μL	<1000/μL	<500/μL	<500/μL
% PMNs (0)	>80%	1–50%	1–50%	1–50%
Glucose (>40 mg/dL)	<40 mg/dL	>40 mg/dL	<40 mg/dL	<40 mg/dL
Protein (<50 mg/dL)	>200 mg/dL	<200 mg/dL	>200 mg/dL	>200 mg/dL
Gram's stain (−)	+	−	−	−
Cytology (−)	−	−	+	+

ABBREVIATIONS: OP = opening pressure; PMNs = polymorphonuclear cells; WBC = white blood cells.
SOURCE: From Greenlee JE: Approach to diagnosis of meningitis: Cerebrospinal fluid evaluation. *Infect Dis Clin North Am* 4:583, 1990.

initiated as preparations for LP are made. Antibiotic therapy administered up to 2 hours prior to LP will not decrease the diagnostic sensitivity if CSF bacterial antigen assays are obtained along with CSF cultures.[2,3]

- However, if the patient has focal neurologic deficits or papilledema, a computed tomography (CT) scan of the head should be performed prior to LP in order to determine the possible risks for transtentorial or tonsillar herniation associated with LP. In these cases, empiric antibiotic therapy must be initiated prior to patient transport to the radiology suite for CT scanning. Antibiotic therapy should **always** be initiated in the emergency department (ED) and never be delayed for neuroimaging or LP.
- Empiric treatment for bacterial meningitis is based on the likelihood of certain pathogens and risk factors (Table 151-2).[4,5] For the patient who is severely penicillin-allergic, the combination of chloramphenicol 1 g IV, vancomycin 1 g IV, and rifampin 300 mg PO or IV is recommended.
- Steroid therapy (dexamethasone 10 mg IV 15 minutes prior to antibiotic administration) has proven to be beneficial in adults. Its precise role in the ED, where emergency physicians rarely manage known cases of bacterial meningitis and appropriately administer antibiotics prior to confirmed diagnosis, remains unclear.[6,7]
- Other general management measures are also important. Hypotonic fluids should be avoided. Serum sodium levels should be monitored to detect the syndrome of inappropriate secretion of antidiuretic hormone or cerebral salt wasting. Hyperpyrexia should be treated with acetaminophen. Coagulopathy needs to be corrected using specific replacement therapies.
- Seizures should be treated with benzodiazepines and, if needed, phenytoin loading. Evidence of marked intracranial pressure should be treated with head elevation and mannitol.
- Viral meningitis, without evidence of encephalitis, can be managed on an outpatient basis provided the patient is nontoxic in appearance, can tolerate oral fluids, and has reliable follow-up within 24 hours. However, it remains a diagnosis of exclusion; unless the diagnosis of viral meningitis is obvious, admission is warranted.

ENCEPHALITIS

EPIDEMIOLOGY

- Viral encephalitis is a viral infection of brain parenchyma producing an inflammatory response. It is distinct from, although often coexists with, viral meningitis.
- The incidence of encephalitis is about one tenth that of bacterial meningitis.
- Arboviruses can account for up to 50% of cases during epidemic outbreaks. The four most common arboviral encephalitides in the United States are the La Crosse encephalitis, St. Louis equine encephalitis, western equine encephalitis, and eastern equine encephalitis.[5]
- Herpes simplex virus type 1 (HSV-1) is typically seen in older children and adults as a reactivation disease. Herpes simplex virus type 2 (HSV-2) is seen in neonates as a result of perinatal transmission.

TABLE 151-2 Guidelines for Empiric Treatment of Bacterial Meningitis with No Organisms on Gram's Stain

PATIENT CATEGORY	POTENTIAL PATHOGENS	EMPIRICAL THERAPY
Age		
18–50 years	*Streptococcus pneumoniae, Neisseria meningitidis*	Ceftriaxone 2 g IV q12h plus vancomycin or rifampin if *S. pneumoniae* resistance possible
Older than 50 years	*S. pneumoniae, N. meningitidis, Listeria monocytogenes,* aerobic gram-negative bacilli	Ceftriaxone 2 g IV q12h plus ampicillin 2 g IV q4h plus vancomycin or rifampin if *S. pneumoniae* resistance possible
Special Circumstances		
CSF leak with history of closed head trauma	*S. pneumoniae, Haemophilus influenzae,* group B streptococci	Ceftriaxone 2 g IV q12h
History of recent penetrating head injury, neurosurgery, CSF shunt	*Staphylococcus aureus, Staphylococcus epidermidis,* diphtheroids, aerobic gram-negative bacilli	Vancomycin 25 mg/kg IV load (max infusion rate 500 mg per h), then 19 mg/kg at intervals dictated by Matzke nomogram plus ceftazidime 2 g IV q8h†
Immunocompromised host	*S. pneumoniae, N. meningitidis, L. monocytogenes,* aerobic gram-negative bacilli	Vancomycin 25 mg/kg IV load (max infusion rate 500 mg per h), then 19 mg/kg at intervals dictated by Matzke nomogram plus ampicillin 2 g IV q4h plus ceftazidime 2 g IV q8h†

†Matzke GR, Kovarik JM: Evaluation of the vancomycin-clearance: creatinine-clearance relationship for predicting vancomycin dosage. *Clin Pharm* 4:311, 1985.
SOURCE: From Quagliarello and Scheld,[1] with permission.

PATHOPHYSIOLOGY

- In North America, viruses that cause encephalitis are the arboviruses (including the West Nile virus), herpes simplex virus (HSV), herpes zoster, Epstein-Barr virus, cytomegalovirus (CMV), and rabies.
- The arboviruses are transmitted by mosquitoes and ticks. Rabies is transmitted by the bite of an infected animal. Impaired immune status plays a role in herpes zoster and CMV encephalitis.
- Neurologic dysfunction and damage are caused by disruption of neural cell functions by the virus and by the effects of the host's inflammatory responses. Gray matter is predominantly affected, resulting in cognitive and psychiatric signs, lethargy, and seizures.

CLINICAL FEATURES

- Encephalitis should be considered in patients presenting with any or all of the following features: new psychiatric symptoms, cognitive deficits (aphasia, amnestic syndrome, acute confusional state), seizures, and movement disorders.
- Signs and symptoms of headache, photophobia, fever, and meningeal irritation may be present. Assessment for neurologic findings and cognitive deficits is crucial. Motor and sensory deficits are not typical.
- Encephalitides may show special regional trophism. HSV involves limbic structures of the temporal and frontal lobes, with prominent psychiatric features, memory disturbance, and aphasia. Some arboviruses predominantly affect the basal ganglia, causing chorea-athetosis and parkinsonism. Involvement of the brainstem nuclei leads to hydrophobic choking characteristic of rabies encephalitis.[6]
- Symptoms of West Nile virus infection include fever, headache, muscle weakness, and lymphadenopathy. Most infections are mild and last only a few days. More severe symptoms and signs consist of high fever, neck stiffness, altered mental status, tremors, and seizures. In rare cases (mostly involving the elderly), the infection can lead to encephalitis and death.

DIAGNOSIS AND DIFFERENTIAL

- ED diagnosis can be suggested by findings on CT or magnetic resonance imaging (MRI) and LP. Neuroimaging, particularly MRI, not only excludes other potential lesions such as brain abscess, but may display findings highly suggestive of HSV encephalitis if the medial temporal and inferior frontal gray matter is involved.
- On LP, findings of aseptic meningitis are typical. For the West Nile virus, the most widely used screening test is the IgM enzyme-linked immunosorbent assay (ELISA) test for detecting acute antibody.
- The differential diagnosis includes brain abscess; Lyme disease; subacute subarachnoid hemorrhage; bacterial, tuberculous, fungal, or neoplastic meningitis; bacterial endocarditis; postinfectious encephalomyelitis; toxic or metabolic encephalopathies; and primary psychiatric disorders.

EMERGENCY DEPARTMENT CARE AND DISPOSITION

- The patient suspected of suffering from viral encephalitis should be admitted. Of the viruses causing encephalitis, only HSV has been shown by clinical trial to be responsive to antiviral therapy. The agent of choice is acyclovir 10 mg/kg IV every 8 hours for 14 days.[7]
- Potential complications of encephalitis—seizures, disorders of sodium metabolism, increased intracranial pressure, and systemic consequences of a comatose state—should be managed with standard methods.
- There is no specific treatment for the West Nile virus infection. In more severe cases, intensive supportive therapy is indicated. The primary prevention step is advocating the use of insect repellant containing DEET when people go outdoors during dawn or dusk.

BRAIN ABSCESS

EPIDEMIOLOGY

- The incidence of brain abscess has progressively declined over the past century, reflecting the effect of antibiotics on predisposing conditions such as otitis media.

PATHOPHYSIOLOGY

- A brain abscess is a focal pyogenic infection. It is composed of a central pus-filled cavity, ringed by a layer of granulation tissue and an outer fibrous capsule.
- Three known routes are available for organisms to reach the brain: hematogenously (33%); from contiguous infection of the middle ear, sinus, or teeth (33%); or by direct implantation after neurosurgery or penetrating trauma (10%). The route is unknown in 20% of cases.

CLINICAL FEATURES

- Since patients typically are not acutely toxic, the presenting features of brain abscess are nonspecific. For this reason, the initial diagnosis can be difficult in the ED.
- Presenting signs and symptoms include headache, neck stiffness, fever, vomiting, confusion, or obtundation. The presentation may be dominated by the origin of the infection (eg, ear or sinus pain). Meningeal signs and focal neurologic findings, such as hemiparesis, seizures, and papilledema, are present in less than half the cases.

DIAGNOSIS AND DIFFERENTIAL

- Classically, brain abscess can be diagnosed by a CT scan with contrast of the head , which demonstrates one or several thin, smoothly contoured rings of enhancement surrounding a low-density center, that is in turn surrounded by white matter edema.
- LP is contraindicated when brain abscess is suspected and after the diagnosis has been established. Other routine laboratory studies are usually nonspecific. Blood cultures should be obtained.
- The differential diagnosis includes cerebrovascular disease, meningitis, brain neoplasm, subacute cerebral hemorrhage, and other focal brain infections, such as toxoplasmosis.

EMERGENCY DEPARTMENT CARE AND DISPOSITION

- Decisions on antibiotic therapy for brain abscess should depend on the likely source of the infection. In a suspected otogenic case, initial therapy should consist of a third-generation cephalosporin, such as ceftriaxone or cefotaxime 2 g IV, or trimethoprim-sulfamethoxazole plus chloramphenicol or metronidazole.
- In a suspected sinogenic or odontogenic case, initial therapy should consist of high-dose penicillin 4 million units IV and metronidazole 1 g IV. This antibiotic regimen is also appropriate when a hematogenous source is suspected.

- In a suspected cardiac case, initial therapy should consist of vancomycin 15 mg/kg IV with metronidazole 1 g IV or chloramphenicol.
- When communication with the exterior is suspected, as in penetrating trauma or post–neurosurgical procedure, initial therapy should consist of nafcillin 2 g IV or vancomycin. Ceftazidime 2 g IV should be added if gram-negative aerobes are suspected.
- In cases in which no clear etiology exists, initial empiric therapy should consist of a third-generation cephalosporin and metronidazole.
- Neurosurgical consultation and admission are warranted since many cases will require surgery for diagnosis, bacteriology, and often, definitive treatment.

REFERENCES

1. Quagliarello VJ, Scheld WM: Bacterial meningitis: Pathogenesis, pathophysiology, and progress. *N Engl J Med* 327:864, 1992.
2. Talan DA, Zibulewsky J: Relationship of clinical presentation to time of antibiotics for the emergency department management of suspected bacterial meningitis. *Ann Emerg Med* 22:1733, 1993.
3. Kanegaye JT, Soliemanzadeh P, Bradley JS: Lumbar puncture in pediatric bacterial meningitis: Defining the time interval for recovery of cerebrospinal fluid pathogens after parenteral antibiotic pretreatment. *Pediatrics* 108:1169, 2001.
4. Quagliarello VJ, Scheld WM: Treatment of bacterial meningitis. *N Engl J Med* 336:708, 1997.
5. Choi C: Bacterial meningitis in aging adults. *Clin Infect Dis* 33:1384, 2001.
6. Wald ER, Kaplan SI, Mason EO Jr, et al: Dexamethasone therapy for children with bacterial meningitis. *Pediatrics* 95:21, 1995.
7. de Gans J, van de Beck D: Dexamethasone in adults with bacterial meningitis. *N Engl J Med* 347:1549, 2002.

For further reading in *Emergency Medicine: A Comprehensive Study Guide,* 6th ed., see Chap. 235, "CNS Infections," by Keith E. Loring.

152 OCULAR EMERGENCIES

Steven Go

INFECTIONS

STYE (EXTERNAL HORDEOLUM)

- A stye is an acute infection of an oil gland at the lid margin.
- Emergency department (ED) care of a stye includes warm compresses and erythromycin ointment for 7 to 10 days.

CHALAZION (INTERNAL HORDEOLUM)

- A chalazion is an acute or chronic infection of the meibomian gland.
- ED care is the same as for a stye, plus a 14- to 21-day regimen of doxycycline for refractory cases.
- Persistent chalazia should be referred to an ophthalmologist for incision, curettage, and biopsy.

CONJUNCTIVITIS

- Bacterial conjunctivitis presents with eyelash matting, mucopurulent discharge, and conjunctival inflammation without corneal lesions.
- Bacterial conjunctivitis is treated with topical antibiotic drops (infants: sulfacetamide 10%; adults: trimethoprim-polymyxin B or erythromycin drops).
- Contact lens wears should receive ciprofloxacin, ofloxacin, or tobramycin topical antibiotic coverage for *Pseudomonas*. The worn contact lenses should be discarded and use of new contact lenses should not be resumed until the infection has completely cleared.
- A severe purulent discharge with a hyperacute onset (within 12 to 24 hours) should prompt an emergent consult with an ophthalmologist for an aggressive work-up of possible gonococcal conjunctivitis.
- Viral conjunctivitis presents as a monocular or binocular watery discharge, chemosis, and conjunctival inflammation.
- Viral conjunctivitis is often associated with viral respiratory symptoms and a palpable preauricular node.
- Fluorescein staining may reveal occasional superficial punctate keratitis, but should otherwise be clear.
- Treatment of viral conjunctivitis consists of cool compresses, naphazoline/pheniramine as needed for conjunctival congestion, and ophthalmology follow-up in 7 to 14 days.
- Allergic conjunctivitis presents as a monocular or binocular pruritus, watery discharge, and chemosis with a history of allergies.
- There should be no lesions with fluorescein staining, and preauricular nodes should be absent. Conjunctival papillae are seen on slitlamp exam.
- Treatment of allergic conjunctivitis consists of elimination of the inciting agent, cool compresses, artificial tears, and naphazoline/pheniramine. Diphenhydramine and topical fluorometholone may be helpful in severe cases.

HERPES SIMPLEX VIRUS

- Herpes simplex virus (HSV) infection can involve eyelids, conjunctiva, and cornea. HSV classically causes a dendritic epithelial defect.
- ED care depends on the site of infection: eyelid and conjunctival involvement requires topical antivirals

515

(trifluorothymidine drops or vidarabine ointment) five times daily with topical erythromycin ointment and warm soaks.

- If the cornea is involved, the trifluorothymidine dosage is increased to nine times daily (the vidarabine dosage remains the same).
- If there is anterior chamber involvement, a cycloplegic agent may be used.
- Acyclovir or famciclovir may be considered within the first 3 days of the HSV outbreak.

HERPES ZOSTER OPHTHALMICUS

- Herpes zoster ophthalmicus (HZO) is shingles with a trigeminal distribution, ocular involvement, and frequently, a concurrent iritis.
- A "pseudodendrite" (mucous corneal plaque without epithelial erosion) may be seen.
- ED care includes oral acyclovir therapy and topical erythromycin with warm compresses.
- Oral narcotics and cycloplegic agents are useful for comfort. In the absence of corneal lesions, iritis may be treated with topical steroids and cycloplegics.
- Ophthalmologic consultation is mandatory. Hospitalization and parenteral acyclovir may be required.

PERIORBITAL CELLULITIS (PRESEPTAL CELLULITIS)

- Periorbital cellulitis presents with warm, indurated, and erythematous eyelids, without restriction of ocular motility, proptosis, painful eye movement, or impairment of pupillary function.
- ED care in patients older than 5 years includes oral amoxicillin-clavulanate.
- For toxic-appearing patients, patients with significant comorbidities, or children younger than 5 years old, hospital admission for parenteral ceftriaxone and vancomycin may be required.
- Children younger than 5 years also require a septic work-up because concurrent bacteremia and meningitis may be present.

ORBITAL CELLULITIS (POSTSEPTAL CELLULITIS)

- Orbital cellulitis should be suspected whenever signs and symptoms of periorbital cellulitis presents with fever, toxicity, proptosis, painful ocular motility, or limited ocular excursion.
- Emergent diagnosis with orbital and sinus thin-slice computed tomography (CT) scan without contrast is required. If this study is negative, a CT scan with con-

trast should be done, which may reveal a subperiosteal abscess.
- Ophthalmologic consultation and hospital admission for intravenous cefuroxime are required.

CORNEAL ULCER

- These infections of the corneal stroma present with pain, redness, and photophobia. Etiologies include desiccation, trauma, direct invasion, and contact lens use.
- Slitlamp examination reveals a staining corneal defect with a hazy infiltrate. A hypopyon may be seen.
- ED care includes hourly topical ofloxacin or ciprofloxacin drops.
- Topical cycloplegia helps relieve pain, but patching is contraindicated. An ophthalmologist should evaluate the patient within 24 hours.

TRAUMA

SUBCONJUNCTIVAL HEMORRHAGE

- Disruption of conjunctival blood vessels may occur from trauma, sneezing, gagging, or the Valsalva maneuver, and will resolve spontaneously within 2 weeks.
- When a dense, circumferential bloody chemosis is present, globe rupture must be excluded.

CONJUNCTIVAL ABRASION

- Superficial conjunctival abrasions are treated with erythromycin ointment for 2 or 3 days.
- In the presence of abrasions, an ocular foreign body should be excluded.

CORNEAL ABRASION

- Trauma may cause superficial or deep corneal abrasions that present with tearing, photophobia, blepharospasm, and severe pain, which are relieved by a topical anesthetic.
- Instilled fluorescein will reveal dye uptake at the site of the defect. An ocular foreign body must be excluded.
- ED care includes administration of a cycloplegic (contraindicated in narrow anterior chamber angle patients) and topical tobramycin, erythromycin, or bacitracin/polymyxin.
- Contact lens abrasions are treated with ciprofloxacin, ofloxacin, or tobramycin drops.

- Tetanus status should be updated on all patients with corneal abrasions.
- Recent studies suggest that patching does not facilitate abrasion healing and is also absolutely contraindicated in dirty abrasions and contact lens abrasions.
- Oral analgesics and topical cycloplegics are appropriate; however, topical anesthetics are strictly contraindicated.
- Intraocular foreign bodies should be suspected if a history compatible with penetrating injury is present.
- Ophthalmology follow-up is advised within 24 hours for all corneal abrasions.

CONJUNCTIVAL FOREIGN BODIES

- When a corneal abrasion or a foreign body sensation is present, conjunctival foreign bodies should be sought with lid eversion.
- Foreign bodies may be removed with a moistened sterile swab.

CORNEAL FOREIGN BODIES

- Corneal foreign bodies may be removed with a fine needle tip, eye spud, or eye burr after applying a topical anesthetic. The resultant corneal defect should be treated as a corneal abrasion.
- Deep corneal stoma foreign bodies or those in the central visual axis require ophthalmologic consultation for removal.
- Rust rings may be removed with an eye burr, although emergent removal is not required.
- Residual rust or deep stromal involvement requires ophthalmologic follow-up within 24 hours.

LID LACERATIONS

- Damage to the eye and nasolacrimal system must be excluded in all eyelid and adnexal lacerations.
- Fluorescein instilled into the tear layer that appears in an adjacent laceration confirms injury to the nasolacrimal system.
- Suspected or proven nasolacrimal injuries, lid margin lacerations, levator mechanism lacerations, and all through-and-through lid lacerations require ophthalmology consultation.

BLUNT TRAUMA

- In blunt trauma, the integrity of the globe must be immediately assessed, as well as the visual acuity.

- Signs such as an abnormal anterior chamber depth, an irregular pupil, or blindness indicate a ruptured globe until proven otherwise, and an emergent ophthalmology referral is indicated.
- Traumatic iritis in the absence of a corneal injury can be treated with topical prednisolone acetate and cyclopentolate.
- The care of the blunt trauma eye patient should be discussed with an ophthalmologist, and the patient should follow-up with them within 48 hours even if no significant injuries are initially found.

HYPHEMA

- A hyphema is blood in the anterior chamber, and it can occur spontaneously or following trauma.
- Rebleeding can occur 3 to 5 days following the initial injury and is associated with a high complication rate.
- ED care includes placing the patient upright to allow the blood to settle inferiorly, placement of a protective eye shield, exclusion of a ruptured globe, and dilation of the pupil with atropine.
- After ruptured globe is excluded, intraocular pressure should be measured. If the intraocular pressure is greater than 30 mm Hg, topical timolol is used initially.
- Apraclonidine drops and oral acetazolamide may be necessary if elevated intraocular pressure persists.
- If the intraocular pressure is greater than 24 mm Hg in a sickle cell patient or in a patient with a spontaneous hyphema, topical timolol alone should be used because acetazolamide is contraindicated.
- Mannitol intravenously may be used if initial measures are ineffective.
- In every hyphema, emergent evaluation at the bedside by an ophthalmologist is indicated.

BLOWOUT FRACTURES

- The inferior and medial wall of the orbit may be fractured from blunt trauma.
- Physical examination signs include evidence of inferior rectus entrapment (diplopia on upward gaze), paresthesia of the infraorbital nerve, and subcutaneous emphysema, especially when sneezing or blowing the nose.
- CT of the orbit with thin cuts is the radiographic test of choice to define the lesion.
- ED care includes excluding associated ocular traumatic lesions and administration of cephalexin orally.
- Isolated blowout fractures (with or without entrapment) require referral to an ophthalmologist within 3 to 10 days.

PENETRATING TRAUMA/RUPTURED GLOBE

- Suggestive findings include a severe subconjunctival hemorrhage, shallow or deep anterior chamber compared with the other eye, hyphema, teardrop-shaped pupil, limitation of extraocular motility, extrusion of globe contents, or a significant reduction in visual acuity.
- A penetrating injury should be suspected when the history of a high-speed foreign body or a penetrating injury in proximity of the orbit is present.
- Fluorescein streaming (Seidel's test) is pathognomonic, though it may be absent.
- Once a globe injury is suspected, any further manipulation or examination of the eye must be avoided at all costs.
- ED care includes placing the patient upright and NPO (nothing by mouth), placing a protective metallic eye shield, administration of cephazolin and an antiemetic intravenously, and updating the patient's tetanus status.
- A CT of the orbit with thin cuts is the test of choice to screen for an intraocular foreign body.
- An ophthalmologist should be called immediately if a globe rupture or a penetrating injury is strongly suspected.

CHEMICAL OCULAR INJURY

- Acid and alkali burns are managed in a similar manner. The eye should be immediately flushed at the scene and sterile normal saline or Ringer's lactate irrigation should be continued in the ED immediately upon arrival (even before visual acuities or patient registration) until the pH is normal (7.0).
- Once the pH is normal, the fornices should be swept to remove residual particles and any necrotic conjunctiva. The pH should be rechecked in 10 minutes to ensure that no additional corrosive is leaching out from the tissues.
- Intraocular pressure should be measured.
- A cycloplegic, erythromycin ointment, and narcotic pain medications should be prescribed. Tetanus status should be updated.
- An ophthalmologist should evaluate the patient in the ED if there are signs of a severe injury, such as a pronounced chemosis, conjunctival blanching, corneal edema or opacification, or increased intraocular pressure.

CYANOACRYLATE (SUPER GLUE/CRAZY GLUE) EXPOSURE

- Cyanoacrylate glue easily adheres to the eyelids and corneal surface. Its primary morbidity stems from corneal injuries from the hard particles that form.
- Initial manual removal is facilitated by heavy application of erythromycin ointment, with special care taken not to damage underlying structures.
- After the easily removable pieces are removed, the patient should be discharged with erythromycin ointment to be applied five times a day in order to soften the remaining glue.
- Complete removal of the residual glue can be accomplished by the ophthalmologist at a follow-up visit within 48 hours.

ULTRAVIOLET KERATITIS

- Ultraviolet (UV) keratitis results from excess UV exposure, typically from tanning booths, welding flashes, or prolonged sun exposure.
- Severe pain and photophobia develop 6 to 12 hours after exposure. Conjunctival hyperemia and superficial punctate keratitis are seen.
- ED care is the same as for superficial corneal abrasions.

ACUTE VISUAL REDUCTION OR LOSS

ACUTE ANGLE CLOSURE GLAUCOMA

- Acute angle closure glaucoma presents with eye pain, headache, cloudy vision, colored halos around lights, conjunctival injection, a fixed, mid-dilated pupil, and increased intraocular pressure of 40 to 70 mm Hg (normal range: 10 to 20 mm Hg). Nausea and vomiting is also common.
- Sudden attacks in patients with narrow anterior chamber angles can be precipitated in movie theaters, while reading, and after administration of dilatory agents or inhaled anticholinergics.
- ED care is designed to decrease the intraocular pressure. Immediate medications to administer include timolol, apraclonidine, and prednisolone acetate.
- If intraocular pressure is greater than 50 mm Hg or if vision loss is severe, then acetazolamide 500 mg IV should be considered.
- If intraocular pressure does not decrease and vision does not improve in 1 hour, IV mannitol should be given.
- Pilocarpine 1 to 2% in the affected eye and pilocarpine 0.5% in the contralateral eye may be administered once intraocular pressure is less than 40 mm Hg as long as the patient has a natural lens in place.
- Symptoms of pain and nausea should be treated, and the intraocular pressure monitored hourly. All cases require immediate ophthalmologic consultation.

OPTIC NEURITIS

- Inflammation of the optic nerve can be caused by infection, demyelination, and autoimmune disorders.
- Optic neuritis may present with reduction of vision (often with poor color perception), pain during extraocular movement, visual field cuts, and an afferent pupillary defect.
- Swelling of the optic disc may be seen in anterior optic neuritis.
- Diagnosis can be made with the red desaturation test (after staring at a bright red object with the normal eye only, the object may subsequently appear pink or light red in the affected eye).
- ED care is controversial and the use of IV steroids should be discussed with an ophthalmologist.

CENTRAL RETINAL ARTERY OCCLUSION

- Central retinal artery occlusion may be caused by embolus, thrombosis, giant-cell arteritis, vasculitis, sickle cell disease, and trauma.
- It is often preceded by amaurosis fugax.
- The vision loss is a painless, complete or near complete vision loss, unless only a single arterial branch is affected.
- An afferent pupillary defect is often present and funduscopy classically reveals a pale fundus with narrowed arterioles with segmented flow ("boxcars"), with a bright red macula ("cherry red spot").
- ED care includes ocular massage (digital pressure for 15 seconds, followed by sudden release) and topical timolol or IV acetazolamide. Emergent ophthalmologic consultation is indicated.

CENTRAL RETINAL VEIN OCCLUSION

- Thrombosis of the central retinal vein causes painless, rapid monocular vision loss.
- Funduscopy classically reveals diffuse retinal hemorrhages, cotton wool spots, and optic disc edema ("blood-and-thunder"). The contralateral optic nerve and fundus are usually normal.
- Predisposing drugs (eg, oral contraceptives, diuretics) should be discontinued
- ED care may include aspirin 60 to 325 mg daily and all patients should be referred to an ophthalmologist within 24 hours.

GIANT CELL ARTERITIS (TEMPORAL ARTERITIS)

- Giant cell arteritis is a systemic vasculitis that can cause ischemic optic neuropathy. Patients are usually over 50 years of age, female, and often have polymyalgia rheumatica.
- Symptoms and signs include headache, jaw claudication, myalgias, fatigue, fever, anorexia, temporal artery tenderness, and often neurologic findings (including transient ischemic attack [TIA] and stroke).
- An afferent pupillary defect is often present.
- C-reactive protein and erythrocyte sedimentation rate are usually elevated (70 to 110 seconds).
- ED care includes IV steroids and ophthalmologic consultation.

BIBLIOGRAPHY

Chang B, Cullom R: *The Wills Eye Manual: Office and Emergency Room Diagnosis and Treatment of Eye Disease,* 2nd ed. Philadelphia: Lippincott, 1994.

Kanski J: *Clinical Ophthalmology: A Systematic Approach,* 3rd ed. London: Butterworth-Heinemann, 1994.

Kline L: Optic Nerve Disorders: Ophthalmology Monographs, no. 10. San Francisco: American Academy of Ophthalmology, 1996.

Spalton D, Hitchings R, Hunter P: *Atlas of Clinical Ophthalmology,* 2nd ed. London: Mosby-Year Book Europe, 1994.

Trobe J: *The Physician's Guide to Eye Care.* San Francisco: American Academy of Ophthalmology, 1993.

Vaughan D, Asbury T, Riordan-Eva P: *General Ophthalmology,* 14th ed. Norwalk, CT: Appleton & Lange, 1995.

Weingeist T, Liesegang T, Slamovits T: Basic and Clinical Science Course, 1997-1998. San Francisco: American Academy of Ophthalmology, 1997.

Wright K: *Textbook of Ophthalmology.* Baltimore: Williams & Wilkins, 1997.

For further reading in *Emergency Medicine: A Comprehensive Study Guide,* 6th ed., see Chap. 238, "Ocular Emergencies," by John D. Mitchell.

153 FACE AND JAW EMERGENCIES

Robert J. French

FACIAL INFECTIONS

IMPETIGO

- Impetigo is a superficial epidermal infection.
- Impetigo may occur after minor skin trauma on exposed body surfaces such as the face and extremities.[1] In the majority of cases, it develops on apparently uninjured skin.[2]

- There are two different presentations of impetigo: bullous and nonbullous.
- Bullous impetigo is caused by *Staphylococcus aureus*. It presents as a vesicle that rapidly enlarges to form a bulla (2 to 5 cm) that collapses, leaving a honey-colored central crust.[2]
- Nonbullous impetigo is caused by *Streptococcus pyogenes* and *S. aureus*. This form presents as a vesicle that develops into a pustule, and eventually forms the characteristic honey-colored crust.
- Symptoms of mild itching are present, but systemic symptoms are infrequent.[1]
- Glomerulonephritis may follow streptococcal impetigo with an overall incidence of 2 to 5%.[1] Antibiotic treatment does not prevent glomerulonephritis.[1]
- Mupirocin ointment 2% applied topically tid is the treatment of choice for localized infections.
- A 7- to 10-day course of oral antibiotics is indicated for more diffuse infections. Oral antibiotic regimens include dicloxacillin, cephalexin, or amoxicillin-clavulanate.
- Clindamycin or azithromycin are appropriate alternatives for individuals with a penicillin allergy.

ERYSIPELAS

- Erysipelas most often occurs in the very young and older adults aged 50 to 60 years.[3]
- Erysipelas is a superficial cellulitis, usually limited to the epidermis and dermis, with prominent lymphatic involvement.
- Erysipelas is almost always due to *S. pyogenes* and rarely *S. aureus.*
- The face, ears, and lower legs are common sites of infection.
- Erysipelas is painful and presents as a fiery red, edematous, indurated lesion with a sharply demarcated palpable border.
- Streptococcal bacteremia occurs in 5% of patients.
- Mild early cases of erysipelas secondary to *S. pyogenes* can be treated orally with penicillin V.
- When *S. aureus* cannot be excluded, oral dicloxacillin is indicated.
- For severe cases of facial erysipelas, IV nafcillin or oxacillin is appropriate.
- Diabetic patients may require broader coverage with ampicillin-sulbactam, amoxicillin-clavulanate, or a second- or third-generation cephalosporin.
- In penicillin-allergic patients, clindamycin, erythromycin, azithromycin, clarithromycin, gatifloxacin, or moxifloxacin can be prescribed.

CELLULITIS

- Cellulitis is a painful, acute, spreading infection of the skin that extends deeper than erysipelas and involves the subcutaneous tissue. In contrast to erysipelas, the borders are not elevated and are less clearly defined.[1]
- Cellulitis commonly occurs secondary to violation of the skin barrier.
- If there is no obvious portal of entry, then contiguous spread from deep space infection or lymphatic/hematogenous seeding should be considered.[2]
- The pathogen usually is *S. pyogenes* or *S. aureus*. In children (and rarely in adults), *Haemophilus influenzae* and *Streptococcus pneumoniae,* as well as anaerobic and oral commensals, may play a role in facial cellulitis.[4]
- In streptococcal cellulitis, the skin is red, progression is rapid, and toxicity is more common.
- Staphylococcal skin infections are red, may blister, progress more indolently, and form an abscess more commonly.
- In children with *H. influenzae* cellulitis, the skin often has a violaceous tinge, and there is an absence of integument violation.
- In *H. influenzae* facial cellulitis should be suspected in children, particularly if there is no identifiable portal of entry. The infection is believed to result from either local mouth trauma or spread from otitis media.[2]
- These patients appear acutely ill and have a high fever, white blood cell count >15,000/μL, and up to 90% positive blood cultures.
- In adults, *H. influenzae* facial cellulitis is often preceded by pharyngitis and fever.
- Empiric antibiotic treatment should begin early and provide coverage for both *S. pyogenes* and *S. aureus*. These include cefazolin, cephalexin, and dicloxacillin.
- If *Haemophilus influenzae* is clinically suspected, appropriate agents are ampicillin-sulbactam, amoxicillin-clavulanate, or a second- or third-generation cephalosporin.
- Patients with a penicillin allergy can be treated with clindamycin, erythromycin, azithromycin, clarithromycin, gatifloxacin, or moxifloxacin.
- Patients with severe infections or signs of toxicity should be admitted.
- Immunocompromised patients should be treated aggressively and have a lower threshold for admission.

SALIVARY GLAND DISORDERS

VIRAL PAROTITIS

- Mumps, a paramyxovirus, is the most common cause of viral parotitis in children under age 15 years.
- Other viral etiologies include influenza, parainfluenza, coxsackieviruses, echoviruses, lymphocytic choriomeningitis, and HIV.[5]
- The virus is spread by airborne droplets.
- Symptoms begin after an incubation period of 2 to 3

weeks and consist of fever, malaise, headache, myalgias, arthralgias, and anorexia.

- Prodromal symptoms continue for 3 to 5 days and are followed by parotid gland enlargement.
- Bilateral parotid enlargement occurs in 75% of cases and lasts up to 5 days. The gland is tense and painful, but erythema and warmth are absent.[5]
- There is no discharge from the parotid duct. Diagnosis is clinical.
- Treatment is supportive and consists of analgesics and antipyretics.
- The patient is contagious for 9 days after the onset of parotid gland swelling.
- Epididymo-orchitis is the most common extra–salivary gland involvement in postpubertal males, affecting 20 to 30% of patients. It can precede or follow parotitis.
- Epididymo-orchitis may present as the sole manifestation of mumps.
- Oophoritis occurs in only 5% of females.
- Vaccination has reduced the incidence of mumps substantially.[5,6]

SUPPURATIVE PAROTITIS

- Suppurative parotitis is a potentially fatal bacterial infection that occurs in patients with diminished salivary flow.
- Bilateral parotid gland involvement is found in 25% of cases.[5]
- Retrograde transmission of bacteria leads to infection.
- Factors and conditions that lead to decreased salivary flow include recent anesthesia, dehydration, prematurity, advanced age, sialolithiasis, medications (eg, diuretics, β-blockers, antihistamines, phenothiazines, tricyclic antidepressants), and certain disorders (eg, diabetes, HIV, hypothyroidism, Sjögren's syndrome).[5]
- Suppurative parotitis is usually caused by *S. aureus* and less often by *Streptococcus pneumoniae, S. pyogenes,* and *Haemophilus influenzae.*[6] Anaerobes such as *Bacteroides* species, *Peptostreptococci,* and *Fusobacterium* are found in 43% of isolates.[7]
- Symptoms progress rapidly and consist of fever, trismus, and severe pain over the parotid gland.
- Physical examination reveals induration, erythema, and tenderness to palpation over the cheek and angle of the mandible.
- In contrast to mumps, pus may be expressed from the parotid duct.
- Treatment consists of hydration, local massage, heat, sialogogues (eg, lemon drops, orange juice), and either β-lactamase- or penicillinase-resistant antibiotics. Amoxicillin-clavulanate or ampicillin-sulbactam contains β-lactamase inhibitors.[5]

- Dicloxacillin, oxacillin, and second-generation cephalosporins are penicillinase resistant.
- Some authors recommend adding metronidazole to enhance anaerobic coverage.[5]
- In penicillin-allergic patients, clindamycin or a combination of cephalexin and metronidazole should be used.
- ENT consultation is required in severe cases or treatment failures.

SIALOLITHIASIS

- Eighty percent of salivary calculi (sialoliths) occur in the submandibular duct and most of the remainder in the parotid duct.
- Sialoliths are more common in the submandibular duct because of the viscous secretions and uphill course.[8]
- Patients present with unilateral pain, swelling, and tenderness of the involved gland. The stone may be palpable and the gland will be firm.
- Submandibular calculi are usually radiopaque and can be visualized on intraoral radiographs.
- Sialolithiasis is often difficult to distinguish from suppurative sialoadenitis, and at times the two may coexist.
- Treatment initially consists of analgesics, massage, and sialogogues.[8] If concurrent infection is suspected, treatment with antibiotics is indicated.
- Palpable stones can be milked from the duct.
- Persistently retained calculi can be removed electively by an otolaryngologist via dilatation or incision of the ductal orifice.

MASTICATOR SPACE ABSCESS

- The masticator space consists of four contiguous potential spaces bounded by the muscles of mastication. These spaces include the masseteric, pterygomandibular, superficial temporal, and deep temporal spaces.[9]
- Infection in these spaces, commonly associated with an odontogenic source, are polymicrobial. Typical organisms include species of *Streptococcus, Peptostreptococcus, Bacteroides, Prevotella, Porphyromonas, Fusobacterium, Actinomyces, Veillonella,* and anaerobic spirochetes.[9]
- Abscesses in these spaces result in swelling over the buccal, submandibular, or sublingual areas.
- Signs and symptoms depend partly on the abscess location and include fever, facial swelling, pain, erythema, fever, and trismus.
- Contrast-enhanced CT can help differentiate cellulitis from abscess, and if an abscess is present, its extent can be detailed.
- Since these spaces ultimately communicate with the

tissue planes that extend into the mediastinum, early treatment is imperative.

- Well-appearing patients with minimal symptoms and no palpable abscess are candidates for outpatient treatment. Therapy includes analgesics and oral antibiotics (clindamycin or amoxicillin-clavulanate) for 10 to 14 days.
- Patients with significant trismus, potential airway compromise, palpable abscess, diffuse cellulitis, or sepsis should be admitted.
- IV clindamycin is recommended. Alternative agents include ampicillin-sulbactam, cefoxitin, or combination therapy with penicillin and metronidazole.
- In severe cases, emergent ENT consultation is needed for operative drainage.

MANDIBLE DISORDERS

TEMPOROMANDIBULAR JOINT DYSFUNCTION

- The temporomandibular joint (TMJ) combines a hinge and gliding movement. Anatomic internal derangement or systemic disease can cause dysfunction of this joint.
- Patients present with unilateral dull pain in the region of the TMJ or localized over one of the muscles of mastication. The pain worsens over the course of the day and in severe cases can cause trismus.
- Physical examination findings include reduced mandible range with a <35 mm maximum interincisor distance.
- Tenderness to palpation over the condylar head may be present when opening and closing the mouth.
- Treatment consists of warm compresses, soft diet, analgesics, and muscle relaxants. Patients should be referred to a dental specialist for evaluation and consideration for occlusal splint therapy.

MANDIBLE DISLOCATION

- The mandible can be dislocated in an anterior, posterior, lateral, or superior direction.
- Anterior dislocation is most common.
- Patients with acute mandible dislocations present with severe pain, difficulty swallowing, and malocclusion.
- In anterior dislocations, pain is localized anterior to the tragus and a history of extreme mouth opening is typical.
- All other mandibular dislocations require significant trauma.
- The diagnosis of a nontraumatic anterior dislocation is made clinically.
- In other dislocations or if there is a history of trauma, radiographs are needed.

- Reduction may be attempted in closed anterior dislocations without fracture.
- Patients with open or nonreducible dislocations, associated fractures, or nerve injury should be emergently referred to an oral maxillofacial surgeon.
- After successful reduction, patients are placed on a soft diet and instructed not to open their mouths more than 2 cm for 2 weeks.[10]

REFERENCES

1. Rhody C: Bacterial infections of the skin. *Prim Care Clin Office Pract* 27:459, 2000.
2. Habif TP: *Clinical Dermatology,* 3rd ed. St. Louis: Mosby-Year Book, 1996, p. 378.
3. Jorup-Ronstrom C: Epidemiological, bacteriological and complicating features of erysipelas. *Scand J Infect Dis* 18:519, 1986.
4. Dodson TB, Leonard KB: Oral-facial emergencies: Special considerations for the pediatric emergency patient. *Emerg Med Clin North Am* 18:539, 2000.
5. McQuone SJ: Acute viral and bacterial infections of the salivary glands. *Otolaryngol Clin North Am* 32:793, 1999.
6. Gold E: Almost extinct diseases: Measles, mumps, rubella and pertussis. *Pediatr Rev* 17:120, 1996.
7. Brook I: Aerobic and anaerobic microbiology of acute suppurative parotitis. *Laryngoscope* 101:170, 1991.
8. Williams MF: Sialolithiasis. *Otolaryngol Clin North Am* 32: 819, 1999.
9. Flynn TR: The swollen face. *Emerg Med Clin North Am* 18: 481, 2000.
10. Undt G, Kerner C: Treatment of recurrent mandibular dislocation. *Int J Oral Maxillofac Surg* 26:92, 1997.

For further reading in *Emergency Medicine: A Comprehensive Study Guide,* 6th ed., see Chap. 240, "Face and Jaw Emergencies," by Robert Haddon and W. Franklin Peacock IV.

154   EAR AND NOSE EMERGENCIES
Jeffrey N. Glaspy

OTOLOGIC EMERGENCIES

OTITIS EXTERNA

PATHOPHYSIOLOGY

- The most common organisms implicated in otitis externa (OE) are *Pseudomonas aeruginosa* and *Staphy-*

lococcus aureus [1] *Bacteroides* species and polymicrobial infection may account for a significant number of cases.

- Otomycosis (fungal OE) accounts for approximately 10% of cases, especially in tropical climates.
- *Aspergillus* and *Candida* are the most common fungal pathogens.
- Risk factors for development of OE include swimming, trauma of the external auditory canal (EAC), and any process that elevates the pH of the EAC.

CLINICAL FEATURES

- OE is characterized by pruritus, pain, and tenderness of the external ear.
- Erythema and edema of the EAC may also be present and may cause hearing loss of the involved ear. Clear or purulent otorrhea may be present.
- Pain is elicited with movement of the pinna or tragus.

EMERGENCY DEPARTMENT CARE AND DISPOSITION

- The treatment of OE includes analgesics, cleansing of the EAC, acidifying agents, topical antimicrobials, and occasionally topical steroid preparations.
- Floxin otic, Cortisporin otic suspension, and CiproHC otic are commonly used to treat OE.
- If significant swelling of the EAC is present, a wick or piece of gauze may be inserted into the EAC to allow passage of topical medications.

MALIGNANT OTITIS EXTERNA

- Malignant otitis externa is a potentially life-threatening infection of the EAC with variable extension to the base of the skull.
- *Pseudomonas aeruginosa* is the most common causative organism.
- Elderly patients, diabetics, and HIV patients are most commonly affected.
- Computed tomography (CT) imaging is necessary to determine the extent and stage of the disease. Emergent otolaryngologic (ENT) consultation, IV aminoglycoside and antipseudomonal penicillin, cephalosporin, or fluoroquinolone therapy, and admission to the hospital are mandatory.

OTITIS MEDIA

PATHOPHYSIOLOGY

- The incidence and prevalence of otitis media (OM) peak in the preschool years and decline with advancing age.
- The most common bacterial pathogens in acute OM are *Streptococcus pneumoniae, Haemophilus influenzae,* and *Moraxella catarrhalis.*

- The predominant organisms involved in chronic OM are *Staphylococcus aureus, Pseudomonas aeruginosa,* and anaerobic bacteria.

CLINICAL FEATURES

- Patients with OM present with otalgia with or without fever; occasionally hearing loss and otorrhea are present.
- The tympanic membrane (TM) may be retracted or bulging and will have impaired mobility on pneumatic otoscopy. Loss of TM mobility on insufflation is considered the most sensitive sign of OM.
- The TM may appear red as a result of inflammation, or may be yellow or white due to middle ear secretions.
- Complications of OM include TM perforation, conductive hearing loss, acute serous labyrinthitis, facial nerve paralysis, acute mastoiditis, lateral sinus thrombosis, cholesteatoma, and central nervous system infections.

EMERGENCY DEPARTMENT CARE AND DISPOSITION

- A 10-day course of amoxicillin is the preferred initial treatment for OM. Alternative agents include trimethoprim-sulfamethoxazole, azithromycin, or cefuroxime.
- Cefuroxime or amoxicillin-clavulanate may be given for OM unresponsive to first-line therapy after 72 hours.
- TM perforation and conductive hearing loss are most often self-limiting and often require no specific intervention.

BULLOUS MYRINGITIS

- Bullous myringitis is a painful condition of the ear characterized by bulla on the TM and deep EAC.
- Numerous pathogens have been reported in the etiology, including viruses, *Mycoplasma pneumoniae,* and *Chlamydia psittaci.*
- The diagnosis is made by clinical examination.
- The treatment consists of pain control, warm compresses, and oral antibiotics if an associated middle ear effusion is present.

MASTOIDITIS

- Acute mastoiditis occurs as infection spreads from the middle ear to the mastoid air cells.
- Patients present with otalgia, fever, and postauricular erythema, swelling, and tenderness.
- Protrusion of the auricle with obliteration of the postauricular crease may be present.
- CT scan will delineate the extent of bony involvement.

- Emergent ENT consultation, IV cefuroxime, and admission to the hospital are necessary. Surgical drainage ultimately may be required.

LATERAL SINUS THROMBOSIS

- This condition arises from extension of infection and inflammation into the lateral and sigmoid sinuses.
- Headache is common and papilledema, sixth nerve palsy, and vertigo may be present.
- Diagnosis may be made with CT scan, although magnetic resonance imaging or angiography may be necessary.
- Therapy consists of emergent ENT consultation, combination of IV nafcillin, ceftriaxone, and metronidazole therapy, and hospital admission.

TRAUMA TO THE EAR

- Lacerations to the ear should be copiously irrigated and any injury to the perichondrium should be closed with 5-0 or 6-0 absorbable suture.
- ENT or plastic surgery should be consulted for significant injuries, especially in avulsion injuries with tissue loss.
- A hematoma can develop from any type of trauma to the ear.
- Improper treatment of ear hematomas can result in stimulation of the perichondrium and development of asymmetric cartilage formation. The resultant deformed auricle has been termed cauliflower ear.
- Immediate incision and drainage of the hematoma with a compressive dressing is necessary to prevent reaccumulation of the hematoma.
- Thermal injury to the auricle may be caused by excessive heat or cold.
- Superficial injury of either type is treated with cleansing, topical non–sulfa containing antibiotic ointment and a light dressing.
- Frostbite is treated with rapid rewarming using saline-soaked gauze at 38° to 40°C.
- The rewarming process will be quite painful and may necessitate analgesics or conscious sedation.
- Any second- or third-degree burn requires immediate ENT or burn center consultation.

TYMPANIC MEMBRANE PERFORATIONS

- Tympanic membrane perforation may result from blunt or penetrating trauma, noise, barotrauma, infection, or lightning. Patients may complain of pain, bleeding, or decreased hearing.

- Ninety percent will heal without intervention. Antibiotics are not indicated unless a coexistent infection is present.

OTALGIA

- Primary otalgia, caused by auricular and periauricular disease, may occur from trauma, infection, foreign body, cerumen impaction, cholesteatoma, and neoplasm.
- Referred otalgia may occur with dental disease, oropharyngeal and retropharyngeal processes, nasal cavity pathology, and disorders of the throat and neck.
- The sensory distribution of the ear is from: (1) the mandibular division of the trigeminal nerve (supplying the auricle, tragus, external auditory canal and external surface of the TM), (2) the facial nerve (supplying the external auditory canal and posterior auricle), and (3) the glossopharyngeal nerve and the auricular branch of the vagus nerve (supplying the middle ear structures).

TINNITUS

- Tinnitus is the perception of sound without external stimuli. It may be constant, pulsatile, high- or low-pitched, hissing, clicking, or ringing in nature.
- Causes of tinnitus include sensorineural hearing loss, hypertension, conductive hearing loss, head trauma, medications (aspirin, nonsteroidal anti-inflammatory drugs [NSAIDS], aminoglycosides, loop diruetics, and chemotherapeutics), temporomandibular joint disorders, depression, acoustic neuromas, multiple sclerosis, benign intracranial hypertension, Ménière's disease, Cogan's syndrome, arteriovenous malformations, arterial bruits, enlarged eustachian tube, palato-myoclonus, and stapedial muscle spasm.
- Pharmacologic treatment with antidepressant medications may alleviate tinnitus in which no correctable cause can be found.

HEARING LOSS

- Causes of sudden hearing loss include idiopathic (most common), infectious (mumps, Epstein-Barr virus, herpes, CMV, syphilis, and labyrinthitis), vascular/hematologic (leukemia, sickle cell disease, polycythemia, Berger's disease, and cerebral aneurysm), metabolic (diabetes, hyperlipidemia), rheumatologic (temporal arteritis, Wegener's granulomatosis), conductive causes (otitis externa, otitis media, ruptured tympanic membrane, neoplasm, osteonecrosis), Ménière's disease, Cogan's syndrome, acoustic neuroma, cochlear rupture, and ototoxic medications.

- Indictors of poor prognosis include severe hearing loss on presentation and the presence of vertigo.
- If the cause is not readily determined by history and physical examination, otolaryngologic consultation is necessary.

NASAL EMERGENCIES

EPISTAXIS

- Anterior epistaxis accounts for about 90% of all nosebleeds, with the majority originating from Kiesselbach's plexus.
- Posterior epistaxis originates from branches of the sphenopalatine artery and is more common in elderly patients.
- Posterior epistaxis is suspected when an anterior source of bleeding is not identified, bleeding occurs from both nostrils, or when blood is seen draining into the posterior pharynx after anterior sources have been controlled.
- Treatment options for anterior epistaxis include direct pressure, vasoconstrictive agents (Neo-Synephrine, cocaine), silver nitrate cautery, and anterior nasal packing.
- Treatment options for posterior epistaxis include dehydrated sponge packing, balloon tamponade devices, or arterial ligation or embolization.
- All patients with nasal packing require antibiotic prophylaxis with antistaphylococcal agents to prevent sinusitis and toxic shock syndrome.

NASAL FRACTURES

- Nasal fractures are a clinical diagnosis suggested by the injury mechanism, swelling, tenderness, crepitance, gross deformity, and periorbital ecchymosis.
- Intermittent ice application, analgesics, and over-the-counter decongestants are the normal treatment.
- Follow-up in 2 to 5 days for re-examination and possible fracture reduction is prudent.
- The nose should be examined for a septal hematoma, which is a collection of blood beneath the perichondrium of the nasal septum. They appear as bluish, fluid-filled sacs (or grape-like clusters) on the nasal septum.
- If left untreated, a septal hematoma may result in abscess formation or necrosis of the nasal septum.
- Treatment of septal hematoma is local incision and drainage with subsequent placement of an anterior nasal pack.
- A fracture of the cribriform plate may violate the sub-

arachnoid space and cause cerebrospinal fluid rhinorrhea. Symptoms may be delayed for several weeks.
- If a cribriform plate injury is suspected, a CT scan and immediate neurosurgical consultation should be obtained.

NASAL FOREIGN BODIES

- Nasal foreign bodies should be suspected in patients with unilateral nasal obstruction, foul rhinorrhea, or persistent unilateral epistaxis.
- After topical vasoconstrictors and anesthetic agents have been used, the foreign body should be removed under direct visualization.
- Tools for removal include forceps, suction catheters, hooked probes, and balloon-tipped catheters.
- For pediatric patients, one technique is to apply positive pressure via a puff of air blown into the patient's mouth with a finger occluding the unobstructed nostril.

SINUSITIS

PATHOPHYSIOLOGY
- Viral upper respiratory infections and allergic rhinitis are the most common precipitating factors.[2]
- The most common pathogens associated with acute bacterial sinusitis are *Streptococcus pneumoniae, Haemophilus influenzae,* and *Moraxella catarrhalis.*[3]

CLINICAL FEATURES
- Maxillary sinusitis presents with pain in the infraorbital area, whereas frontal sinusitis causes pain in the supraorbital and lower forehead region.
- Ethmoidal sinusitis, which is especially serious in children because of its tendency to spread to the central nervous system, often produces a dull, aching sensation in the retro-orbital area.
- Sphenoidal sinusitis is uncommon and has vague signs and symptoms.
- The diagnosis of sinusitis is often clinical.
- Radiographs may show sinus opacification, air-fluid levels, or mucosal thickening of at least 6 mm, but they are generally not required in the ED.

EMERGENCY DEPARTMENT CARE AND DISPOSITION
- Treatment includes nasal decongestant sprays, such as oxymetazoline or phenylephrine, for no longer than 3 days.
- Antibiotic choices for 14- to 21-day regimens include ampicillin, trimethoprim-sulfamethoxazole, clarithromycin, second-generation cephalosporins, and amoxicillin-clavulanate.

• Complications of sinusitis include osteomyelitis, meningitis, intracranial abscess, Pott's puffy tumor, periorbital cellulitis, orbital cellulitis, and cavernous sinus thrombosis.

REFERENCES

1. Selesnick SH: Otitis externa: Management of the recalcitrant case. *Am J Otolaryngol* 15:408, 1994.
2. Hickner JM, Bartlett JG, Besser RE, et al: Principles of appropriate antibiotic use for acute rhinosinusitis in adults. *Ann Intern Med* 134:498, 2001.
3. Kaiser L, Morabia A, Stalder H, et al: Role of nasopharyngeal culture in antibiotic prescription for patients with common cold or acute sinusitis. *Eur J Clin Microbiol Infect Dis* 20:445, 2001.

For further reading in *Emergency Medicine: A Comprehensive Study Guide,* 6th ed., see Chap. 239, "Common Disorders of the External, Middle, and Inner Ear," by Anne Tintinalli and Michael Lucchesi; and Chap. 241, "Nasal Emergencies and Sinusitis," by Thomas A. Waters and W. Frank Peacock IV.

155 ORAL AND DENTAL EMERGENCIES

Steven Go

OROFACIAL PAIN

• Eruption of the primary teeth in infants and children may be associated with pain, irritability, and drooling.
• The most common cause of toothache is periapical pathology.
• Fluctuant oral abscesses require local incision and drainage, oral antibiotics effective against mouth flora, oral analgesia, warm saline rinses, and close follow-up.
• Odontogenic infections can spread readily to the facial spaces.
• Ludwig's angina is a cellulitis involving the submandibular spaces and the sublingual space that can spread to the neck and mediastinum, causing airway compromise, overwhelming infection, and death.
• If dental infections spread to the infraorbital space, a cavernous sinus thrombosis may result, which may present with limitation of lateral gaze, meningeal signs, sepsis, and coma.

• Treatment of Ludwig's angina and cavernous sinus thrombosis includes intravenous broad-spectrum antibiotics, such as ampicillin-sulbactam, and emergent oral and maxillofacial surgical consultation for consideration of surgical intervention.
• Periosteitis causes pain within 24 to 48 hours of a tooth extraction; it responds well to analgesics.
• Postextraction alveolar osteitis ("dry socket") occurs when the clot from the socket is displaced, typically on postoperative day 2 or 3. It presents with severe pain with foul odor and taste.
• Treatment of postextraction alveolar osteitis consists of saline irrigation and packing of the socket with eugenol-impregnated gauze.
• Acute necrotizing ulcerative gingivitis (ANUG or "trench mouth") is the only periodontal disease in which bacteria invade non-necrotic tissue.
• ANUG presents with pain, ulcerated or "punched out" interdental papillae, gingival bleeding, fever, malaise, and fetid breath. It occurs mainly in patients with lowered resistance due to HIV, malnourishment, and stress.
• Treatment of ANUG consists of oral metronidazole and chlorhexidine mouth rinses.[1]

SOFT TISSUE LESIONS OF THE ORAL CAVITY

• Oral candidiasis lesions consist of removable white, curd-like plaques on an erythematous mucosal base. Risk factors include extremes of age, immunocompromised states, use of intraoral prosthetic devices, concurrent antibiotic use, and malnutrition.
• Treatment of oral candidiasis is with oral antifungal agents such as clotrimazole troches or nystatin oral suspension.
• Aphthous stomatitis is a common pattern of mucosal ulceration triggered by cell-mediated immunity. The painful lesions typically resolve when treated with topical steroids.
• Herpes gingivostomatitis causes painful ulcerations of the gingiva and mucosal surfaces. Fever, lymphadenopathy, and tingling often precede the eruption of numerous vesicles, which then rupture and form ulcerative lesions.
• If acyclovir or valacyclovir is initiated during the prodromal phrase of herpes gingivostomatitis, the clinical duration and severity may be attenuated.
• Herpangina and hand, foot, and mouth disease (HFMD) are both caused by infection with coxsackievirus A species.
• Herpangina presents with high fever, sore throat, headache, and malaise, followed by eruption of oral vesicles, which rupture to form painful, shallow

ulcers on the soft palate, uvula, and tonsillar pillars. Unlike herpes infection, the buccal mucosa, tongue, and gingiva are spared.

- HFMD causes vesicles to initially form on the soft palate, gingiva, tongue, and buccal mucosa. The vesicles then rupture, leaving painful ulcers surrounded by red halos. Lesions may also appear on the buttocks, palms, and soles.
- Treatment of herpangina and HFMD is supportive and consists of hydration and acetaminophen or ibuprofen.

LESIONS OF THE TONGUE

- Erythema migrans ("geographic tongue" or "migratory glossitis") is a common benign finding marked by multiple circumscribed zones of erythema found predominantly on the tip and lateral borders of the tongue. The lesions wax and wane with stress and menstrual cycle.
- Symptomatic lesions of erythema migrans respond to topical fluocinonide gel applied several times daily.[2]
- Strawberry tongue appears as red spots on a white-coated background. It is associated with Kawasaki's disease and also with streptococcal infection. If it is due to the latter, it responds to antibiotics effective against group A streptococci.
- Black hairy tongue is a brown discoloration of unknown etiology that affects the dorsum of the tongue.
- Treatment of black hairy tongue consists of frequent tongue brushing and avoidance of tobacco, strong mouthwashes, and antibiotics. Symptomatic resolution is usually spontaneous.[3]

OROFACIAL TRAUMA

DENTAL FRACTURES

- In dentoalveolar trauma, a search for associated injuries should be undertaken and the patient should be warned of the possibility of occult damage to the neurovascular bundle, with subsequent pulp necrosis or root resorption.
- Ellis class 1 fractures involve only the enamel of the tooth. These injuries may be smoothed with an emery board or referred to a dentist for cosmetic repair.[4-6]
- Ellis class 2 fractures (70% of tooth fractures) involve the creamy yellow dentin underneath the white enamel. The patient complains of air and temperature sensitivity.
- To decrease the chances of contamination in Ellis class 2 fractures, the exposed dentin must be thoroughly dried and promptly covered with a temporary dental dressing such as zinc oxide/eugenol paste.

- In patients under the age of 12, the protective dentinal layer is thin. A visible blush of pulp under this thin dentinal layer thus indicates that the pulp is at risk, and should be treated like an Ellis class 3 fracture.[4-6]
- Ellis class 3 fractures are tooth-threatening fractures that involve the pulp and can be identified by a red blush of the dentin or a visible drop of blood after wiping the tooth.
- Ideally, a dentist should evaluate the patient with an Ellis class 3 fracture immediately. If a dentist is not immediately available, the tooth may be temporarily covered with a dental dressing such as zinc oxide/eugenol paste until the patient is seen within 24 hours.
- Oral analgesics may be needed, but topical anesthetics are contraindicated. The use of prophylactic antibiotics is controversial.[4-6]

CONCUSSIONS, LUXATIONS, AND AVULSIONS

- Concussion injuries involve tenderness to percussion with no mobility.
- Dental trauma with tenderness to percussion and mobility without evidence of dislodgment is called subluxation, which has a higher incidence of future pulp necrosis.
- Management of concussion injuries and subluxation includes nonsteroidal anti-inflammatory drugs (NSAIDs), soft diet, and referral to a dentist.
- Extrusive luxation occurs when a tooth is partially avulsed from alveolar bone. Treatment involves gentle repositioning of the tooth to its original location and splinting with zinc oxide periodontal dressing.
- When the tooth is laterally displaced with a fracture of the alveolar bone, the condition is called lateral luxation.
- Although manual relocation is possible, the treatment of lateral luxation is best done in consultation with a dentist in the emergency department (ED), especially if the alveolar fracture is significant.
- An intrusive luxation occurs when the tooth is forced below the gingiva and often has a poor outcome. Treatment is similar to that of subluxations.
- Dental avulsion is a dental emergency in which a tooth has been completely removed from the socket.
- Primary teeth in children should not be replaced because of potential damage to the permanent teeth.
- Permanent teeth that have been avulsed for less than 3 hours must be immediately reimplanted in an attempt to save the periodontal ligament fibers.
- If reimplantation at the scene is not possible due to risk of aspiration, the tooth should be rinsed and placed in a nutrient solution, such as Hank's solution,

sterile saline, or milk, and the tooth transported immediately with the patient to the ED.

- Upon arrival in the ED, the socket can be gently irrigated with sterile normal saline prior to reimplantation if the root is still moist. If the root of the tooth has been dry for longer than 20 minutes, it may be soaked in various solutions prior to implantation in attempt to improve outcome.
- A dentist should evaluate the patient as soon as possible to stabilize the tooth, but reimplantation should not be delayed while awaiting the arrival of the specialist.
- If a patient arrives with an empty socket and the tooth cannot be located, adjacent tissue should be searched. Radiographs may be necessary to exclude displaced or aspirated teeth.[7,8]

ORAL SOFT TISSUE TRAUMA

- Stabilization of dental injuries and an aggressive search for retained foreign bodies should take place before repair of lacerations.
- Most intraoral mucosal lacerations will heal by themselves; however, they should be repaired if they are gaping or if flaps are present. Treatment consists of achieving good anesthesia, débridement, irrigation, and closure with 5-0 absorbable sutures.[9]
- The repair of through and through lacerations is controversial. Some advocate first repairing the intraoral laceration, then irrigating the wound before finally closing the external laceration, using both superficial and deep sutures if necessary. Others advocate leaving the intraoral lacerations open.
- Tongue lacerations that gape widely, actively bleed, are flap-shaped, or involve muscle should be closed. Lacerations may be repaired with 4-0 absorbable sutures. Extensive lesions or those in uncooperative patients may require operative repair.
- Lip lacerations are potentially complex because of the possible involvement of the vermilion border (the transition between lip tissue and the skin of the face), which must be aligned precisely with 6-0 nonabsorbable sutures to avoid a noticeable cosmetic defect.
- Violated deep muscle layers and intraoral lesions must be closed as well. Prophylactic penicillin VK or clindamycin should be prescribed.[9]
- A cosmetic surgeon should be consulted to repair extensive lip lacerations.
- Laceration of the maxillary labial frenulum does not usually require repair.
- The lingual frenulum is very vascular and usually should be repaired with 4-0 absorbable sutures.

ORAL HEMORRHAGE

POSTOPERATIVE BLEEDING

- Bleeding following dental extraction is usually controlled by direct pressure for 20 minutes applied by biting on gauze.
- If bleeding persists, packing the socket may be effective. Sutures may be used to hold these packing agents in place.
- Failure of the above measures warrants a screening coagulation profile and consultation with an oral surgeon.

REFERENCES

1. Horning GM: Necrotizing gingivostomatitis: NUG to noma. *Compend Contin Educ Dent* 17:951, 1996.
2. Espelid M, Bang G, Johannessen AC, et al: Geographic stomatitis: Report of 6 cases. *J Oral Pathol Med* 20:425, 1991.
3. Sarti GM, Haddi RI, Schaffer D, et al: Black hairy tongue. *Am Fam Phys* 41:1751, 1990.
4. Antrim DD: Treatment of endodontic urgent care cases. *Dent Clin North Am* 30:549, 1986.
5. Dumsha TC: Luxation injuries. *Dent Clin North Am* 39:79, 1995.
6. Rauschenberger CR, Hovland EJ: Clinical management of crown fractures. *Dent Clin North Am* 39:25, 1995.
7. Trope M: Clinical management of the avulsed tooth. *Dent Clin North Am* 39:93, 1995.
8. Blomlof L: Milk and saliva as possible storage media for traumatically exarticulated teeth prior to reimplantation. *Swed Dent J* 8:1, 1981.
9. Trott T: *Wounds and Lacerations: Emergency Care and Closure,* 2nd ed. St. Louis: Mosby, 1997.

For further reading in *Emergency Medicine: A Comprehensive Study Guide,* 6th ed., see Chap. 242, "Oral and Dental Emergencies," by Ronald W. Beaudreau.

156 NECK AND UPPER AIRWAY DISORDERS

Robert J. French

PHARYNGITIS/TONSILLITIS

PATHOPHYSIOLOGY

- Pharyngotonsillitis in adults is often due to an infectious etiology, most commonly viral. Other infectious causes include bacteria, fungi, and parasites.

- Transmission of most cases of pharyngitis is via person-to-person contact with droplets of saliva. In temperate climates the incidence is higher in winter and early spring.[1]

CLINICAL FEATURES

- Group A β-hemolytic streptococci (GABHS) cause up to 15% of acute pharyngitis cases, typically with sudden onset of sore throat, painful swallowing, chills, and fever.
- Other bacterial causes of pharyngitis include group C and G streptococci, *Haemophilus influenzae*, *Mycoplasma pneumoniae*, *Chlamydia pneumoniae*, *Neisseria gonorrhoeae*, and *Corynebacterium diphtheriae*.
- Clinical criteria for GABHS pharyngitis include: (1) tonsillar exudate, (2) tender anterior cervical adenopathy, (3) history of fever, and (4) absence of cough.[2,3]

DIAGNOSIS AND DIFFERENTIAL

- Most rapid streptococcal antigen detection tests report sensitivities of 80 to 90% with specificities >95%.[2]

EMERGENCY DEPARTMENT CARE AND DISPOSITION

- Penicillin remains the antibiotic of choice for treatment of GABHS pharyngotonsillitis.[2]
- In penicillin-allergic patients, a 10-day course of erythromycin is the recommended alternative. Oral cephalosporins and clindamycin are additional alternative agents for GABHS pharyngitis.
- Treatment with antibiotics is recommended in patients with GABHS, to help prevent both suppurative and nonsuppurative poststreptococcal sequelae.
- Suppurative complications include cervical lymphadenitis, peritonsillar abscess, retropharyngeal abscess, sinusitis, and otitis media.[2]
- Virulent strains of GABHS are associated with acute rheumatic fever and poststreptococcal glomerulonephritis. Treatment with appropriate antibiotics, resulting in eradication of GABHS infection, can help prevent acute rheumatic fever.[2]
- Antibiotic treatment of GABHS does not prevent poststreptococcal glomerulonephritis.[2]
- Dexamethasone may be used in patients with severe symptoms.[4]

PERITONSILLAR ABSCESS

PATHOPHYSIOLOGY

- Peritonsillar abscess (PTA) is the most frequent deep-space infection of the head and neck. It is caused by a collection of purulent material between the palatine tonsil capsule and the superior constrictor and palatopharyngeus muscle.[5]
- Although GABHS is the most common cause of PTA, mixed aerobic/anaerobic bacteria are often present.[5]

CLINICAL FEATURES

- Symptoms of PTA include fever, malaise, sore throat, odynophagia, dysphagia, "hot potato voice," sore throat, otalgia, and varying degrees of trismus.
- Signs include unilateral tonsillar enlargement with inferomedial displacement, palatal and uvula edema, contralateral deflection of the uvula, tender ipsilateral anterior lymphadenopathy, drooling, and dehydration.

DIAGNOSIS AND DIFFERENTIAL

- The differential diagnosis includes tonsillitis, peritonsillar cellulitis, infectious mononucleosis, retropharyngeal abscess, tumor, and internal carotid artery aneurysm.[5]
- Digital or cotton-tipped applicator palpation for fluctuance may help differentiate PTA from cellulitis. Trismus is uncommon in peritonsillar cellulitis.

EMERGENCY DEPARTMENT CARE AND DISPOSITION

- Aspiration of purulent material with an 18- or 20-gauge needle is both diagnostic and therapeutic for PTA and will effectively treat 85% of these patients.[5]
- Care must be taken to avoid puncture of the internal carotid artery that is located 2.5 cm behind and lateral to the tonsil.[6]
- Emergency department intraoral bedside ultrasound can aid in detection and guidance of needle aspiration.[7]
- Following needle aspiration, antibiotic therapy is recommended to eradicate offending organisms. Penicillin is the treatment of choice. In penicillin-allergic patients, clindamycin is recommended.
- Broader-spectrum agents, such as amoxicillin-clavulanate or cefuroxime plus metronidazole, can be used if there is inadequate clinical improvement.
- Complications of PTA include airway obstruction, aspiration of ruptured abscess contents, septicemia, retropharyngeal abscess, and mediastinitis.

RETROPHARYNGEAL ABSCESS

PATHOPHYSIOLOGY

- Retropharyngeal abscess is most common in children less than 5 years old, but it can also occur in adults.
- Due to anatomic and pathophysiologic differences, retropharyngeal abscess in children is typically more localized than in adults.[8]
- In adults, retropharyngeal abscess is caused by direct extension of purulent material from an adjacent site or abscess formation following retropharyngeal cellulitis. Other causes include foreign body (eg, fish bone) penetration, vertebral osteomyelitis or diskitis, and hematogenous spread from distant sites.[9]
- The most common aerobic species are *Streptococcus viridans* and *Streptococcus pyogenes*. *Bacteroides* and *Peptostreptococcus* are the most commonly isolated anaerobes.[10]

CLINICAL FEATURES

- Patients present with fever, sore throat, odynophagia, dysphagia, neck stiffness, neck pain, muffled voice, stridor, and respiratory distress.
- These patients gravitate toward a supine position with the neck in slight extension to minimize compression of the upper airway. Sitting them up can increase their dyspnea.[11]
- Physical examination may reveal tender cervical lymphadenopathy, neck swelling, torticollis, pharyngeal erythema, and edema.

DIAGNOSIS AND DIFFERENTIAL

- The lateral soft tissue neck radiograph may demonstrate thickening in the prevertebral space.
- A contrast-enhanced computed tomography (CT) scan of the neck can help differentiate cellulitis from abscess and help define the extent of the infection.
- Differential diagnosis includes retropharyngeal space tumor, foreign body, aneurysm, hematoma, edema, and lymphadenopathy.

EMERGENCY DEPARTMENT CARE AND DISPOSITION

- Emergency department treatment consists of airway management, parenteral antibiotics, and urgent ENT consultation for operative drainage.
- First-line treatment options for adults include clindamycin or penicillin G plus metronidazole. Ampicillin-sulbactam is an appropriate alternative.[12]

PARAPHARYNGEAL ABSCESS

PATHOPHYSIOLOGY

- Parapharyngeal abscess occurs secondary to odontogenic and pharyngotonsillar infections or as a result of direct extension from an adjacent deep neck abscess. This space is shaped like an inverted pyramid and extends from the base of the skull to the hyoid.
- The styloid process arbitrarily divides this space into anterior and posterior compartments.[15]

CLINICAL FEATURES

- Patients with anterior space infection will present with trismus along with bulging of the lateral pharyngeal wall.
- Posterior space infections are more ominous and can result in palsies of cranial nerves IX through XII, Horner's syndrome, internal jugular vein thrombosis, and carotid artery rupture and/or pseudoaneurysm formation.[16]

DIAGNOSIS AND DIFFERENTIAL

- The lateral soft tissue neck radiograph is less sensitive in detection of parapharyngeal abscess compared with retropharyngeal space infections.
- Contrast-enhanced neck CT can accurately diagnose and delineate the extent of the parapharyngeal abscess. Doppler ultrasound or angiography may be required if vascular encroachment is a concern.[15]

EMERGENCY DEPARTMENT CARE AND DISPOSITION

- The management and treatment are similar to that followed for retropharyngeal space infections.

EPIGLOTTITIS

CLINICAL FEATURES

- Epiglottitis can lead to rapid, unpredictable airway obstruction. Once a disease primarily of childhood, it is now most often seen in adults with a mean age of 46 years.[13]
- Supraglottic inflammatory changes are most commonly secondary to *Haemophilus influenzae* type b infection.[14]
- Adults present with a 1- to 2-day history of worsening dysphagia, odynophagia, and dysphonia.

- The throat pain is disproportionate to clinical examination findings. Other signs include anxiety, fever, tachycardia, cervical adenopathy, and pain with gentle palpation of the trachea or larynx.
- Clinical indicators of imminent airway obstruction include dyspnea, drooling, aphonia, and stridor.

DIAGNOSIS AND DIFFERENTIAL

- All diagnostic procedures should be deferred in the unstable patient and attention focused on airway patency.
- Lateral soft-tissue neck radiographs may show an edematous epiglottis ("thumbprint sign") with loss of the vallecula and ballooning of the hypopharynx.[15]
- Direct fiberoptic laryngoscopy classically reveals a cherry red epiglottis.
- Differential diagnosis includes pharyngitis, infectious mononucleosis, croup, deep space neck abscess, diphtheria, pertussis, laryngeal trauma, foreign body aspiration, and laryngospasm.

EMERGENCY DEPARTMENT CARE AND DISPOSITION

- Patients with suspected epiglottitis require emergent otolaryngology consultation, and the emergency physician must be prepared to establish a definitive airway.
- Initial airway management consists of supplemental humidified oxygen and comfortable patient positioning. Heliox can be given as a temporizing measure.
- The stable pediatric patient preferably should have the definitive airway established in the operating room.
- Stable adults are often managed without intubation. If airway intervention is needed and the clinical situation permits, awake nasotracheal fiberoptic intubation is the preferred method.
- Orotracheal intubation can be attempted but will be difficult secondary to anatomic distortion. If intubation is unsuccessful, patients under 8 years of age may require needle cricothyroidotomy and those older than 8 years may require surgical cricothyroidotomy.
- Intravenous cefuroxime is the recommended first-line treatment. Cefotaxime, ceftriaxone, or ampicillin-sulbactam are acceptable alternatives.

ODONTOGENIC ABSCESS

PATHOPHYSIOLOGY

- Suppurative odontogenic infections are polymicrobial, consisting of *Streptococcus* species and oral anaerobes. Untreated, they can erode cortical bone and spread into soft tissue.
- Ludwig's angina is an odontogenic infection of the submandibular, sublingual, and submandibular spaces.
- Dental disease is the most common cause of Ludwig's angina. A history of an infected or extracted tooth is usually obtained, typically the lower second or third molars.[16]
- Other causes of Ludwig's angina include fractured mandible, floor of the mouth foreign body or laceration, and tongue piercing.

CLINICAL FEATURES

- Patients with Ludwig's angina present with edema of the upper midline neck, dysphagia, trismus, and marked edema of the floor of the mouth.
- The tongue can rapidly become elevated and displaced posteriorly, leading to airway compromise.[16] Anxiety, drooling, and stridor suggest impending airway collapse.
- Sublingual and submandibular abscesses may extend into deep neck spaces, including the prevertebral, parapharyngeal, and retropharyngeal spaces.
- Physical examination findings in Ludwig's angina are bilateral submandibular swelling and elevation or protrusion of the tongue. A tense, brawny edema may develop in the anterior neck between the hyoid bone and the genu of the mandible.

DIAGNOSIS AND DIFFERENTIAL

- A contrast-enhanced CT scan should be used to diagnose the location of the deep neck space abscess.

EMERGENCY DEPARTMENT CARE AND DISPOSITION

- Endotracheal intubation may be difficult due to anatomic distortion, trismus, and decreased submandibular compliance.[17] Therefore, fiberoptic nasotracheal intubation is the preferred method of airway control. If unsuccessful, emergent surgical cricothyroidotomy or tracheostomy is indicated.
- Treatment of odontogenic abscesses includes operative drainage and intravenous antibiotics. Emergent otolaryngologic consultation is warranted.
- First-line parenteral antibiotic therapy in adults is: (1) clindamycin or (2) penicillin G plus metronidazole. Alternative agents include cefoxitin or ampicillin-sulbactam.[12]

ACUTE AIRWAY OBSTRUCTION

CLINICAL FEATURES

- Foreign bodies can cause partial or complete airway obstruction. Size, shape, and location of the foreign body dictate symptoms.[18]
- Lodging at the laryngeal inlet or subglottic region (upper airway) can cause acute airway obstruction with choking crisis, stridor, and subsequent respiratory arrest.[19]
- Foreign bodies that are distal to the trachea (lower airway) are less likely to cause acute obstructive symptoms, but may present instead with cough, wheezing, dyspnea, or pneumonia.

DIAGNOSIS AND DIFFERENTIAL

- Differential diagnosis includes epiglottitis, retropharyngeal or parapharyngeal abscess, Ludwig's angina, anaphylaxis, angioedema, extrinsic compression from esophageal bolus, and neoplasm.

EMERGENCY DEPARTMENT CARE AND DISPOSITION

- In the stable patient, foreign body detection can be aided by direct inspection of the oropharynx with indirect or direct laryngoscopy or fiberoptic nasopharyngoscopy.
- In the patient with critical upper airway obstruction, an expeditious attempt at removal with Magill forceps under direct laryngoscopy is indicated.
- If the foreign body is visualized but cannot be removed, a surgical airway may be required.
- If the foreign body is not visualized and the patient is unstable, endotracheal intubation should be performed.
- The endotracheal tube should be passed distal to the carina, forcing the foreign body into the right (usually) or left mainstem bronchus. The endotracheal tube is then pulled back and secured at its normal position.
- Ventilation of the unobstructed lung is achieved while preparation is made for emergent bronchoscopy.

ANGIOEDEMA OF THE UPPER AIRWAY

PATHOPHYSIOLOGY

- Causes of angioedema include (1) C1-esterase inhibitor deficiency, (2) IgE-mediated type 1 allergic reaction, (3) adverse reaction to angiotensin-converting enzyme (ACE) inhibitor therapy, and (4) idiopathic reaction.

- The incidence of ACE inhibitor–related angioedema is 0.1 to 0.2%.[20]
- Sixty percent of these cases occur within 1 week of starting the drug, but ACE inhibitor–related angioedema can occur months to years after initiation of treatment.[20]

CLINICAL FEATURES

- Angioedema of the upper airway can progress rapidly and lead to airway obstruction.
- Patients with airway involvement can present with "throat tightness," dyspnea, cough, hoarseness, and stridor.

EMERGENCY DEPARTMENT CARE AND DISPOSITION

- In adults, 0.3 mL (0.3 mg) of epinephrine 1:1000 is administered subcutaneously. This can be repeated every 15 to 20 minutes as needed.
- Additional medications that should be administered include diphenhydramine, methylprednisolone, and a histamine antagonist.
- Fiberoptic nasopharyngoscopy is used to assess possible laryngeal edema.
- Patients with laryngeal edema, potential for airway compromise, and/or worsening symptoms despite maximal therapy require admission.

LARYNGEAL TRAUMA

CLINICAL FEATURES

- Laryngeal injuries may result from blunt or penetrating trauma.
- Patients may present with hoarseness, dyspnea, dysphagia, stridor, hemoptysis, and aphonia.
- Pain with tongue movement implies an injury to the epiglottis, hyoid bone, or larynx.
- Physical examination may reveal anterior neck tenderness, laryngeal swelling, tracheal displacement, or subcutaneous emphysema.
- Asphyxia, secondary to laryngotracheal separation, can occur at the scene in patients with high-impact mechanisms.
- Minor laryngeal injuries may progress, due to edema and expanding hematomas, and close observation is needed.
- A high level of suspicion for cervical spine injury is appropriate.

EMERGENCY DEPARTMENT CARE AND DISPOSITION

- Emergent otolaryngologic consultation is warranted.
- In stable patients, bedside nasopharyngoscopy can evaluate airway integrity. This can be followed by spiral neck CT to delineate the extent of the injury.
- In unstable patients with massive laryngeal trauma, immediate tracheostomy should be performed. If this cannot be performed, endotracheal intubation or fiberoptic intubation should be attempted.

REFERENCES

1. Bisno AL: Acute pharyngitis. *N Engl J Med* 344:205, 2001.
2. Bisno AL, Gerber MA: Practice guidelines for the diagnosis and management of group A streptococcal pharyngitis. *Clin Infect Dis* 35:125, 2002.
3. Centor RM, Witherspoon JM: The diagnosis of pharyngitis in the emergency room. *Med Decision Making* 1:239, 1981.
4. Wei JL: Efficacy of single-dose dexamethasone as adjuvant therapy for acute pharyngitis. *Laryngoscope* 112:87, 2002.
5. Steyer TE: Peritonsillar abscess: Diagnosis and treatment. *Am Fam Phys* 65:93, 2002.
6. Roberts JR, Hedges JR (eds.): *Clinical Procedures in Emergency Medicine,* 3rd ed. Philadelphia: WB Saunders, 1998, p. 1122.
7. Blaivas M, Theodoro D, Duggal S: Ultrasound-guided drainage of a peritonsillar abscess by the emergency physician. *Am J Emerg Med* 21:155, 2003.
8. Goldenberg D: Retropharyngeal abscess: a clinical review. *J Laryngol Otol* 111:546, 1997.
9. Kirse DJ, Roberson DW: Surgical management of retropharyngeal space infections in children. *Layrngoscope* 111: 1413, 2001.
10. Asmar BI: Bacteriology of retropharyngeal abscess in children. *Pediatr Infect Dis J* 9:595, 1990.
11. Hamer R: Retropharyngeal abscess: a clinical review. *J Laryngol Otol* 111:549, 1982.
12. Gilbert D: *The Sanford Guide to Antimicrobial Therapy,* 33rd ed. 2003, p. 32.
13. Senior BA: Changing patterns in pediatric supraglottitis: A multi-institutional review, 1980 to 1992. *Laryngoscope* 104:1314, 1994.
14. Nakamura H: Acute epiglottitis: A review of 80 patients. *J Laryngol Otol* 115:31, 2001.
15. Bansal A: Otolaryngologic critical care. *Crit Care Clin* 19: 55, 2003.
16. Flynn RT: Oral-facial emergencies : The swollen face. *Emerg Med Clin North Am* 18:481, 2000.
17. Stackhouse RA: Fiberoptic airway management. *Anesthesiol Clin North Am* 20:933, 2002.
18. National Safety Council: *Accident Facts,* 1998 edition. Itasca, IL: National Safety Council 1998, p. 21.
19. Baharloo F: Tracheobronchial foreign bodies. *Chest* 115: 1357, 1999.
20. Vleeming W: ACE inhibitor-induced angioedema: Incidence, prevention and management. *Drug Safety* 18:171, 1998.

For further reading in *Emergency Medicine: A Comprehensive Study Guide,* 6th ed., see Chap. 243, "Infections and Disorders of the Neck and Upper Airway," by Carol G. Shores.

Section 19
DISORDERS OF THE SKIN

157 DERMATOLOGIC EMERGENCIES

Michael Blaivas

EXFOLIATIVE DERMATITIS

EPIDEMIOLOGY

- Males are affected twice as often as females, and most patients are over the age of 40.

PATHOPHYSIOLOGY

- Exfoliative dermatitis, a cutaneous reaction to a drug, chemical, or underlying systemic disease state, occurs when most or all of the skin is involved with a scaling erythema, leading subsequently to exfoliation.
- The underlying mechanism is largely unknown.
- Etiologies responsible for exfoliative dermatitis include (in decreasing order of incidence) generalized flares of pre-existing skin disease (eg, psoriasis, atopic and seborrheic dermatitides, lichen planus, pemphigus foliaceus, etc), contact dermatitis, malignancy, and medications or chemicals.

CLINICAL FEATURES

- Patients may present with either acute, acute on chronic, or chronic disease.
- The acute onset form is encountered most often in cases involving medications, contact allergens, or malignancy, while the chronic variety usually is related to an underlying cutaneous disease.

- Patients may complain of pain, pruritus, tightening of the skin, a chilling sensation of the skin, fever, nausea, vomiting, weight loss, and fatigue.
- The physical examination may show generalized warmth and erythroderma, scaling with desiccation, and exfoliation of the skin, as well as fever and other signs of systemic toxicity.
- The process usually begins on the face and upper trunk with progression to other skin surfaces.
- Chronic findings include dystrophic nails, thinning of body hair, alopecia, and hypo- or hyperpigmentation.
- Acute complicating factors include fluid and electrolyte losses, secondary infection, and excessive heat loss with hypothermia.
- High-output congestive heart failure (CHF) may be noted due to extensive cutaneous vasodilation in poorly compensated individuals.

DIAGNOSIS AND DIFFERENTIAL

- Diffuse erythema with desiccation or exfoliation must be considered exfoliative dermatitis until proven otherwise.
- Diagnosis of exfoliative dermatitis is confirmed by skin biopsy.
- The differential diagnosis includes acute generalized exanthematous pustulosis, toxic epidermal necrolysis, primary blistering disorders, Kawasaki's disease, and the toxic-infectious erythemas.

EMERGENCY DEPARTMENT CARE AND DISPOSITION

- Management should focus on airway, breathing, and circulation support, with appropriate correction of any life-threatening abnormality.

- After resuscitation has been completed, treatment of secondary infection, correction of electrolyte disorders, control of body temperature, and management of CHF are clinical issues to address.
- Dermatologic treatment includes oral antihistamines, systemic corticosteroids, oatmeal baths, and bland lotions.
- For patients with a new presentation or a significant recurrence of exfoliative dermatitis, admission with dermatologic consultation is advised.
- For patients with chronic disease with mild recurrence who are not systemically ill, outpatient treatment with prompt dermatologic follow-up is reasonable.

ERYTHEMA MULTIFORME

EPIDEMIOLOGY

- The highest incidence affects young adults (20 to 40 years of age), with males affected twice as often as females.

PATHOPHYSIOLOGY

- Erythema multiforme (EM) is an acute inflammatory skin disease that ranges from a mild papular eruption (EM minor) to a severe vesiculobullous form with mucous membrane involvement and systemic toxicity (Stevens-Johnson syndrome).
- EM is usually due to infection, drugs (antibiotics and anticonvulsants), malignancy, rheumatologic disorders, or pregnancy.
- No cause is found in 50% of cases.

CLINICAL FEATURES

- Symptoms include malaise, arthralgias, myalgias, fever, diffuse pruritus, and a generalized burning sensation that may be noted days prior to skin abnormalities.
- Signs noted on examination primarily involve the skin and mucosal surfaces, including erythematous papules (which appear first) and maculopapules, target lesion (evolves in 24 to 48 hours), urticarial plaques, vesicles, bullae, vesiculobullous lesions, and mucosal (oral, conjunctival, respiratory, and genitourinary) erosions.
- The target lesion is highly characteristic of EM. The erythematous papules appear symmetrically on the dorsum of the hands and feet, and the extensor surfaces of the extremities.
- Ocular involvement occurs in 10% of patients with

EM minor and in 75% of patients with Stevens-Johnson syndrome.
- Patients are at risk for significant fluid and electrolyte deficiencies as well as secondary infection.
- Recurrence is noted, especially involving cases in which infection or medication is involved.

DIAGNOSIS AND DIFFERENTIAL

- The diagnosis of EM is based on the simultaneous presence of lesions with multiple morphologies at times with mucous membrane involvement.
- The differential diagnosis includes herpetic infections, vasculitis, toxic epidermal necrolysis, primary blistering disorders, Kawasaki's disease, and toxic-infectious erythemas.

EMERGENCY DEPARTMENT CARE AND DISPOSITION

- Patients with localized papular disease without systemic manifestations and mucous membrane involvement may be managed on an outpatient basis with dermatologic consultation. Topical steroids to non-eroded skin as well as oral analgesics and antihistamines are recommended.
- For patients with extensive disease or systemic toxicity, inpatient therapy in a critical care setting with immediate dermatologic consultation is advised.
- In addition to intensive management of potential fluid, electrolyte, infectious, nutritional, and thermoregulatory issues, parenteral analgesics and antihistamines are required.
- Systemic steroids are recommended by some authorities. Diphenhydramine and lidocaine rinses are useful for painful oral lesions; cool Burrow's solution compresses are applied to blistered regions.

TOXIC EPIDERMAL NECROLYSIS

PATHOPHYSIOLOGY

- Toxic epidermal necrolysis (TEN) is an explosive dermatosis characterized by tender erythema, bullae formation, and subsequent exfoliation.
- The most common cause of TEN is medications; other etiologies include chemicals, infections (eg, HIV), malignancy, or immunologic factors.
- Sulfa-based drugs, penicillin, anticonvulsants, and nonsteroidal anti-inflammatory drugs (NSAIDs) are the most frequent medication triggers for TEN.

CLINICAL FEATURES

- Patients may complain of malaise, anorexia, myalgias, arthralgias, fever, painful skin, and symptoms of upper respiratory infection. These symptoms may be present for 1 to 2 weeks prior to the development of skin abnormalities.
- Physical examination findings include a warm and tender erythema, flaccid bullae, positive Nikolsky's sign, erosions with exfoliation, mucous membrane (oral, conjunctival, respiratory, and genitourinary) lesions, and systemic toxicity.
- Nikolsky's sign is positive when the superficial layers of skin slip free from the lower layers with a slight rubbing pressure; large areas of the skin will blister and peel away, leaving wet, red, painful areas.
- Infection, hypovolemia, and electrolyte disorders are typical causes of death, an end result in as many as 30% of cases.
- Predictors of poor prognosis include advanced age, extensive disease, leukopenia, azotemia, and thrombocytopenia.

DIAGNOSIS AND DIFFERENTIAL

- Diagnosis of TEN is confirmed by skin biopsy.
- The differential diagnosis includes toxic-infectious erythemas, exfoliative drug eruptions, primary blistering disorders, Kawasaki's disease, and Stevens-Johnson syndrome.

EMERGENCY DEPARTMENT CARE AND DISPOSITION

- Patients with TEN are best cared for in a critical care setting such as a burn unit.
- Attention to adequate cardiorespiratory function is essential; correction of fluid, electrolyte, and infectious complications are early treatment considerations.
- Immediate dermatologic consultation is required.

TOXIC INFECTIOUS ERYTHEMAS

PATHOPHYSIOLOGY

- Toxic infectious erythemas include toxic shock syndrome (TSS), streptococcal toxic shock syndrome (STSS), and staphylococcal scalded-skin syndrome (SSSS).
- TSS is a multisystem illness presenting with fever, shock, and erythroderma followed by desquamation associated with toxigenic *Staphylococcus aureus*.

- The causative agent of STSS is *Streptococcus pyogenes* (group A strep).
- SSSS is divided into three stages: (1) initial and erythroderma, (2) exfoliative, and (3) desquamation and recovery.
- In SSSS, exotoxins released by bacteria cause acantholysis and intraepidermal cleavage of the skin.
- SSSS occurs primarily in infants, young children, and the immunocompromised.

CLINICAL FEATURES

- The manifestations of TSS range from a mild, trivial disease to a rapidly progressive, potentially fatal, multisystem illness.
- The dermatologic hallmark of TSS is a nonpruritic, blanching macular erythroderma.
- The clinical presentation of STSS is similar to that of TSS; in fact, similar criteria may be used for the diagnosis.
- STSS presents with fever, hypotension, and skin infections.
- The majority of cases of STSS are associated with soft tissue infections; cellulitis, myositis, and fasciitis were the most common presenting diagnoses.
- In SSSS, there is a sudden appearance of a tender, diffuse erythroderma. The involved skin may have a sandpaper texture similar to the rash of scarlet fever.
- The exfoliative stage of SSSS begins on the second day of the illness with a wrinkling and peeling of the previously erythematous skin; Nikolsky's sign is found. Large, flaccid, fluid-filled bullae and vesicles then appear. These lesions easily rupture and are shed in large sheets; the underlying tissue resembles scalded skin and rapidly desiccates.
- During the exfoliative phase of SSSS, the patient is often febrile and irritable. After 3 to 5 days of illness, the involved skin desquamates, leaving normal skin in 7 to 10 days.

DIAGNOSIS AND DIFFERENTIAL

- The diagnosis of TSS requires the presence of all four major criteria and three or more indications of multisystem involvement.

MAJOR CRITERIA
1. Fever: temperature >102°F
2. Rash: erythroderma (localized or diffuse) followed by peripheral desquamation
3. Mucous membranes: hyperemia of oral and vaginal mucosa and of conjunctiva
4. Hypotension: history of dizziness, orthostatic changes, or hypotension

MULTISYSTEM MANIFESTATIONS

1. Central nervous system: altered mentation without focal neurologic signs
2. Cardiovascular: distributive shock, heart failure, dysrhythmias
3. Pulmonary: acute respiratory distress syndrome (ARDS)
4. Gastrointestinal: vomiting and diarrhea
5. Hepatic: elevations in bilirubin, alkaline phosphatase, and the transaminases
6. Renal: blood urea nitrogen (BUN) and/or creatinine elevations, abnormal urinary sediment, oliguria
7. Hematologic: thrombocytopenia or thrombocytosis, anemia, leukopenia or leukocytosis
8. Musculoskeletal: myalgias, arthralgias, rhabdomyolysis
9. Metabolic: hypocalcemia, hypophosphatemia
10. Absence of other etiologic agent

- For TSS and STSS, fever and hypotension with associated erythroderma should suggest the diagnosis.
- Infants and toddlers with fever and diffuse erythroderma suggest SSSS.

EMERGENCY DEPARTMENT CARE AND DISPOSITION

- Management of patients with TSS and STSS is dictated by the severity of their illness. If the patient presents in extremis, airway control, ventilatory status, and hemodynamic status should be addressed emergently.
- Patients must be checked for evidence of organ system dysfunction. The vast majority of patients with TSS require hospital admission; the patient who is critically ill is best managed in the intensive care setting.
- Management of the patient with SSSS includes fluid resuscitation and correction of electrolyte abnormalities, as well as identification and treatment of the source of the toxigenic *Staphylococcus* with the appropriate antistaphylococcal antibiotic, preferably a penicillinase-resistant penicillin.
- The newborn may be treated with topical sulfadiazine or its equivalent.
- Corticosteroids are not recommended.

BULLOUS DISEASES

PATHOPHYSIOLOGY

- Pemphigus vulgaris (PV) is a generalized mucocutaneous autoimmune blistering eruption characterized by intraepidermal acantholytic blistering.

- Bullous pemphigoid (BP) is a generalized mucocutaneous blistering disease of the elderly, with an average age of 70 years at the time of initial diagnosis.

CLINICAL FEATURES

- The primary lesions of PV are vesicles or bullae that vary in diameter from less than 1 cm to several centimeters, commonly first affecting the head, trunk, and mucous membranes.
- The blisters are usually clear and tense, originating from normal skin or atop an erythematous or urticarial plaque. Within 2 to 3 days, the bullae become turbid and flaccid with rupture soon following, producing painful, denuded areas. These erosions are slow to heal and prone to secondary infection.
- Nikolsky's sign is positive in PV and absent in other autoimmune blistering diseases. Mucous membranes are affected in 95% of PV patients.
- BP is characterized by tense blisters (up to 10 cm in diameter) arising from either normal skin or from erythematous or urticarial plaques. Frequent sites of involvement include intertriginous and flexural areas. Ulceration with tissue loss follows blister formation.
- Lesions of the oral cavity occur in BP in 40% of cases, but with less consistency and severity than in PV.

DIAGNOSIS AND DIFFERENTIAL

- Diagnosis is suspected with the appearance of the blistering lesions and confirmed by skin biopsy and immunofluorescence testing.
- The differential diagnosis of PV and BP includes all of those diseases that can present with primary skin blistering, including TEN, EM, other autoimmune blistering diseases, burns, severe contact dermatitis, bullous diabeticorum, and friction blisters.

EMERGENCY DEPARTMENT CARE AND DISPOSITION

- Patients with PV should be hospitalized with early dermatologic consultation; high-dose parenteral steroids and other therapies are best administered to the elderly in the hospital.
- Blisters or eroded skin should be treated as burns with silver sulfadiazine cream or antibiotic ointments with clean dressings. Pain originating from oral lesions may be partially relieved with soothing mouthwashes (1:1 mixture of diphenhydramine elixir with Mylanta) or with viscous lidocaine.

- Close observation and rapid treatment with appropriate antibiotics for superficial infection is imperative.
- BP is also managed by systemic steroids.

MENINGOCOCCEMIA

PATHOPHYSIOLOGY

- Meningococcemia is a potentially fatal infectious illness caused by *Neisseria meningitidis.*
- It has a wide clinical spectrum, including pharyngitis, meningitis, and bacteremia.
- Illness typically affects patients under 20 years of age. Epidemics are seen with very virulent strains.

CLINICAL FEATURES

- Infection develops 2 to 10 days after exposure and presents with severe headache, fever, altered mental status, nausea, vomiting, myalgias, arthralgias, and neck stiffness.
- Dermatologic manifestations include petechiae, urticaria, hemorrhagic vesicles, and macules.
- Fulminant disease is seen in less than 5% of patients.

DIAGNOSIS AND DIFFERENTIAL

- Diagnosis relies on clinical suspicion based on presentation of an ill-appearing patient with petechial rash and associated symptoms.
- Cerebrospinal fluid cultures may be positive.
- The differential diagnosis includes Rocky Mountain spotted fever, TSS, gonococcemia, bacterial endocarditis, vasculitis, viral and bacterial infection, and disseminated intravascular coagulation.

EMERGENCY DEPARTMENT CARE AND DISPOSITION

- Ceftriaxone 2 g IV and vancomycin 1 g IV should be administered empirically as soon as the disease is suspected.
- Hospital admission is necessary.

DISSEMINATED GONOCOCCAL INFECTION

PATHOPHYSIOLOGY

- Two percent of patients with mucosal lesions develop disseminated disease.

- Up 75% of those diagnosed with disseminated gonococcal infection are in late pregnancy, immediate post-partum period, or within 1 week of onset of menses.

CLINICAL FEATURES

- Fever, arthralgias, and multiple papular, vesicular, or pustular skin lesions are noted.
- Rash develops on dorsal aspects of ankles and feet.
- Lesions are initially small red papules or maculopapules; they either resolve or evolve into vesicles with purulent fluid and central necrosis.

DIAGNOSIS AND DIFFERENTIAL

- Diagnosis is made in sexually active persons with tenosynovitis, arthralgias, and appropriate dermatologic symptoms.
- Gram's stain of lesion fluid may show *Neisseria gonorrhoeae.* Blood cultures may be positive.

EMERGENCY DEPARTMENT CARE AND DISPOSITION

- Parenteral ceftriaxone or ciprofloxacin should be administered for 7 days.

BIBLIOGRAPHY

Freedman JD, Beer DJ: Expanding perspectives on the toxic shock syndrome. *Adv Intern Med* 36:363, 1991.

Hoge CW, Schwartz B, Talkington DF, et al: National Centers for Disease Control and Prevention: The changing epidemiology of invasive group A streptococcal infections and the emergence of streptococcal toxic shock-like syndrome: A retrospective population-based study. *JAMA* 269:384, 1993.

Pauquet P, Pierard GE: Erythema multiforme and toxic epidermal necrolysis: A comparative study. *Am J Dermatopathol* 19:127, 1997.

Roujeau JC, Kelly JP, Naldi L, et al: Medication use and the risk of Stevens-Johnson syndrome or toxic epidermal necrolysis. *N Engl J Med* 333:1600, 1995.

Rzany B, Hering O, Mockenhaupt M, et al: Histopathological and epidemiological characteristics of Stevens-Johnson syndrome and toxic epidermal necrolysis. *Br J Dermatol* 135:6, 1996.

Seidenbaum M, David M, Sandbank M: The course and prognosis of pemphigus: A review of 115 patients. *Int J Dermatol* 27:580, 1988.

Wong KS, Wong SM, Tham SM, et al: Generalized exfoliative dermatitis: a clinical study of 108 patients. *Ann Acad Med* 17:520, 1988.

For further reading in *Emergency Medicine: A Compre-hensive Study Guide,* 6th ed., see Chap. 246, "Serious Generalized Skin Disorders," by William J. Brady, Andrew D. Perron, and Daniel J. DeBehnke.

158 OTHER DERMATOLOGIC DISORDERS

Michael Blaivas

PHOTOSENSITIVITY

CLINICAL FEATURES

- Patients with sunburn have an inflammatory response to ultraviolet radiation and may present with minimal discomfort or extreme pain with extensive blistering.
- A tender, warm erythema is seen in sun-exposed areas. Vesiculation may occur, representing a second-degree burn injury.
- Exogenous photosensitivity results from either the topical application or the ingestion of an agent that increases the skin's sensitivity to ultraviolet light.
- Furocoumarins—lime juice, various fragrances, figs, celery, and parsnips—when topically applied are the most common group of agents causing photoeruptions. Other topical photosensitizers include PABA esters and topical psoralens.
- The exogenous photoeruption is similar to a severe sunburn reaction, often with blistering.

DIAGNOSIS AND DIFFERENTIAL

- Sunburn should be suspected in a patient who has frequented the outdoors with significant ultraviolet light exposure.
- The diagnosis of exogenous photosensitivity is based on identifying the offending agent.
- A linear appearance to the rash suggests an externally applied substance.

EMERGENCY DEPARTMENT CARE AND DISPOSITION

- Sunburns are treated symptomatically with tepid baths, oral analgesics, and burn wound care, including topical antibiotics to blistered areas.

- Initial management of exogenous photosensitivity is similar to the sunburn reaction, including the avoidance of the sun until the eruption has cleared. Any causative agent should be discontinued if possible.

CONTACT DERMATITIS

CLINICAL FEATURES

- Contact dermatitis may be a primary irritant reaction or an allergic-mediated event.
- Agents capable of causing an aerosolized reaction include rhus (poison ivy and oak) when the plant has been burned.
- Allergic contact dermatitis resulting from an aerosolized allergen presents with erythema or scaling, at times accompanied by blistering. The involvement is diffuse with upper and lower eyelids affected.

DIAGNOSIS AND DIFFERENTIAL

- Direct application of the allergen produces similar finding on the most sensitive skin areas, such as the eyelids.

EMERGENCY DEPARTMENT CARE AND DISPOSITION

- Corticosteroids (topical or oral, depending on the severity) are often required. Only low-potency topical corticosteroids (hydrocortisone 2.5%) should be used on the face; cream or ointment should be used initially.
- Extensive and severe periocular involvement requires oral prednisone.
- Oral antihistamines are also useful in reducing pruritus.

ALOPECIA

CLINICAL FEATURES

- The causative syndromes of hair loss include the non-scarring (secondary syphilis, alopecia areata, contact dermatitis, thyroid disorders, medication-related) and scarring (tinea capitis, zoster infection, discoid lupus, sarcoidosis, scleroderma, malignancy) syndromes.
- Tinea capitis is a dermatophyte infection of the scalp that is most commonly seen in children. Areas of alopecia with broken hair shafts and peripheral scaling are noted; the alopecia is patchy and usually nonscarring.

- Alopecia areata presents with a patchy alopecia. Loose round patches of hair are lost, leaving behind normal scalp that lacks scaling or scarring. Any hair-bearing area may be affected, but the scalp is the most common site of involvement.
- Alopecia areata usually resolves spontaneously within 2 to 6 months, particularly if the initial involvement is mild. Extensive disease is less likely to resolve.
- Telogen effluvium is hair loss resulting from major stressors such as pregnancy, major surgery, or illness. Occurrence is delayed by 2 to 3 months after the stressor and recovery is spontaneous.

DIAGNOSIS AND DIFFERENTIAL

- Diagnosis of tinea capitis is based on a potassium hydroxide (KOH) preparation or positive fungal culture.
- Diagnosis of alopecia areata is based on clinical examination.

EMERGENCY DEPARTMENT CARE AND DISPOSITION

- Griseofulvin is the first-line agent for tinea capitis; topical treatment alone is not effective. The patient should be re-evaluated after 6 weeks of treatment.
- Ketoconazole shampoo is recommended in addition to griseofulvin.
- No specific emergency department–based therapy is available for alopecia areata. If the disease is extensive or rapidly progressive, dermatology referral is recommended.

TINEA INFECTIONS

CLINICAL FEATURES

- Tinea pedis is a fungal infection of the feet, also known as athlete's foot.
- Tinea manuum, a dermatophyte infection of the hand, is often unilateral and frequently associated with tinea pedis.
- The most common form of tinea pedis is the interdigital presentation, manifested by maceration and scaling in the web spaces between the toes. Ulcerations may be present in severe cases with secondary infection.
- The second type of tinea pedis is characterized by chronic, dry scaling with minimal inflammation on the palmar or plantar surfaces. It often extends to the medial and lateral aspects of the feet, but not the dorsal surface. Maceration between the toes is common.

- The third type of fungal infection presents as an acute, painful, pruritic vesicular eruption on the palms or soles. Erythema is a prominent feature, while the nails and web spaces are usually spared.
- Tinea cruris, a fungal infection of the groin commonly called jock itch, is very common in males. Erythema with a peripheral annular, scaly edge is seen. The rash extends onto the inner thighs and the buttocks and spares the penis and scrotum—a feature which is important in distinguishing tinea cruris from other eruptions in the groin.

DIAGNOSIS AND DIFFERENTIAL

- Identification of fungal elements on a KOH preparation or with fungal culture may be required if the diagnosis is uncertain. Typically, the diagnosis is made clinically.

EMERGENCY DEPARTMENT CARE AND DISPOSITION

- Nonbullous tinea pedis and tinea manuum can be treated with topical antifungal agents, such as clotrimazole, miconazole, ketoconazole, or econazole.
- Nail infections also should be treated with oral antifungal agents (itraconazole, fluconazole, or terbinafine) as well.
- Bullous tinea pedis often does not respond to topical treatment; oral antifungal treatment is necessary.
- Treatment of tinea cruris is with antifungal creams such as clotrimazole, ketoconazole, or econazole. Antifungal powders should be used on a daily basis to prevent recurrences.

CANDIDA INTERTRIGO

- Candidal infections of the skin favor moist, occluded areas of the body.
- Superficial candidal infections are commonly seen in the diaper area, the vulva and groin of women, the glans penis (balanitis) in uncircumcised males, and the inframammary and pannus folds of obese patients.
- Antibiotic therapy, systemic corticosteroid therapy, urinary or fecal incontinence, immunocompromised states, and obesity are predisposing factors.
- The typical presentation of candida intertrigo is erythema and maceration with surrounding small erythematous papules or pustules. The satellite pustules are a characteristic finding in differentiating between candida intertrigo and other inflammatory disorders affecting the skin folds.

- KOH preparation of the pustules may demonstrate short hyphae and spores.
- Topical antifungals such as clotrimazole, ketoconazole, or econazole should be applied.
- Hydrocortisone 1% cream can provide symptomatic relief.

PSORIASIS

- Psoriasis vulgaris presents with erythema, scales, and fissures as discrete plaques located on palms and soles.
- In pustular psoriasis erythema, some scaling and numerous pustules are seen on the palms and soles.
- The diagnosis is usually made clinically. Biopsy may be helpful.
- Hand and foot dermatitis, lichen simplex chronicus, and Reiter's syndrome are in the differential diagnosis for vulgaris.
- Topical corticosteroids, tar preparations, and lubrication are beneficial.

HUMAN SCABIES

CLINICAL FEATURES

- Human scabies is an infestation of the skin by *Sarcoptes scabiei*. Scabies is transmitted by close physical contact or linens and clothing.
- Scabetic mites burrow into the stratum corneum. The time from infestation to clinical symptoms is 3 to 4 weeks.
- The eruptions are very pruritic. Hands, feet, elbows, knees, umbilicus, groin, and genitals may be involved.
- Excoriations and pruritic papules may be the only visible clues.
- In crusted scabies, hyperkeratosis develops on the hands and feet, with nails frequently affected.

DIAGNOSIS AND DIFFERENTIAL

- Diagnosis is based on high clinical suspicion and positive scabies preparation.

EMERGENCY DEPARTMENT CARE AND DISPOSITION

- Topical scabicides are applied from the neck down to the feet. Permethrin 5% cream and lindane 1% lotion are equally effective.

- Lindane is neurotoxic in infants, children, and pregnant women.
- Oral antihistamines and topical corticosteroids help relieve symptoms.

PEDICULOSIS

CLINICAL FEATURES

- Pediculosis capitis is an infestation of the hair and scalp with the mite *Pediculus capitis,* and occurs most commonly in school-aged children.
- The louse is spread via close personal contact, clothing, and bed linens. Itching can be mild or intense.
- Excoriation may be seen in the posterior neck and occiput.
- *Pediculus corporis* (body lice) is less commonly seen. It typically occurs in overcrowded conditions with poor hygiene.
- Bites are typically not felt by individuals, but red urticarial papules are left. Areas not covered by clothing are typically spared.
- *Pthirus pubis* is pubic lice and is sexually transmitted.

DIAGNOSIS AND DIFFERENTIAL

- Diagnosis of pediculosis capitis is made by visualization of lice and nits (eggs firmly attached to hair shafts) on physical examination.

EMERGENCY DEPARTMENT CARE AND DISPOSITION

- Permethrin 1% rinse is first-line therapy for head, body, and pubic lice. It should be applied to the scalp for 10 minutes.
- Fifty percent vinegar solution rinse followed by combing can remove nits.

HERPES ZOSTER INFECTION

CLINICAL FEATURES

- Herpes zoster results from activation of latent varicella zoster virus.
- Pain or dysesthesia precedes the eruption by 3 to 5 days.
- Eruptions can occur anywhere on the body, but commonly involve thoracic dermatomes.
- Erythematous papules progress to clusters of vesicles with an erythematous base.

- In 10% of cases, branches of the trigeminal nerve are involved.
- Lesions involving the nose should lead to significant concern for ophthalmic involvement and development of keratitis, which can lead to blindness.

DIAGNOSIS AND DIFFERENTIAL

- A Tzanck prep and viral culture can confirm a diagnosis typically made on history and physical examination.
- The differential diagnosis includes herpes simplex, impetigo, and contact dermatitis.

EMERGENCY DEPARTMENT CARE AND DISPOSITION

- Antivirals such as acyclovir or valacyclovir are beneficial if administered within 72 hours after the eruption of the lesions.

- Domeboro's solution compresses provide symptomatic treatment.

BIBLIOGRAPHY

Epstein E: Hand dermatitis: practical management and current concepts. *J Am Acad Dermatol* 10:395, 1984.

Guitart J, Woodley D: Intertrigo: a practical approach. *Compr Ther* 28:402, 1994.

Omura EF, Rye B: Dermatologic disorders of the foot. *Clin Sports Med* 13:825, 1994.

For further reading in *Emergency Medicine: A Comprehensive Study Guide,* 6th ed., see Chap. 247, "Disorders of the Face and Scalp," Chap. 248, "Disorders of the Hands, Feet, and Extremities," and Chap. 250, "Infestations," all by Dean Morrell and Lisa May.

159 INITIAL APPROACH TO THE TRAUMA PATIENT

J. Christian Fox

EPIDEMIOLOGY

- Trauma results in the deaths of 150,000 Americans each year and is the fourth leading cause of death.
- Deaths due to traumatic injuries is the most common cause of death in patients younger than 45 years.[1]
- Trauma causes more deaths among children and adolescents (ages 1 to 19) than all other diseases combined.[2]

CLINICAL FEATURES

- Trauma patients who present with obviously abnormal vital signs must prompt a thorough search for the specific underlying injuries.
- Nonspecific signs such as tachycardia, tachypnea, or mild alterations in consciousness must similarly be presumed to signify serious injury until proven otherwise, and these aggressively evaluated and treated.
- Without signs of significant trauma, the mechanism of injury may suggest potential problems and these also should be pursued diligently.

DIAGNOSIS AND DIFFERENTIAL

- The history should be obtained from the patient, witnesses, or paramedics, and include mechanism of injury, sites of injury, blood loss at the scene, degree of damage to any vehicles, and descriptions of weapons used.
- Past medical history, medications, and illicit drug and alcohol use need to be extracted to help understand the patient's physiologic response to injury.
- The primary survey (ABCDE), including the assessment of a complete set of vital signs, is characterized by the orderly identification and concomitant treatment of the most life-threatening injuries.
- Airway patency and breathing are assessed by means of examination for gag reflex, pooling of secretions, airway obstruction, tracheal deviation, presence and quality of breath sounds, flail chest, crepitation, sucking chest wounds, and fractures of the sternum.
- Ensuring cervical spine immobilization in the appropriate clinical setting is a key component during the airway assessment.
- Problems such as tension pneumothorax, pneumothorax, hemothorax, and malpositioned endotracheal tube should be remedied before proceeding any further.
- Circulatory status is evaluated via vital signs and cardiac monitoring. Sites of obvious bleeding, indications of shock, and signs of cardiac tamponade (Beck's triad of hypotension, jugular venous distention, and muffled heart sounds) are identified.
- The primary survey concludes with a brief neurologic examination for disability using the Glasgow Coma Scale, pupil size and reactivity, and motor function assessment.
- The patient is then completely exposed in order to identify other injuries.
- The secondary survey is a rapid but thorough head-to-toe examination to identify all injuries and to set priorities for care. Resuscitation and frequent monitoring of vital signs continue throughout this process.
- Evidence of significant head injury (eg, skull and facial fractures) is sought and the pupils rechecked. The

neck, chest, and abdominal examinations are completed and the stability of the pelvis assessed.

- Radiographs of the cervical spine, chest, and pelvis are obtained, as appropriate for the scenario.
- A gastric tube should be inserted (orally in the setting of facial fractures) to decompress the stomach and assess for hemorrhage.
- The genitourinary system is evaluated by external inspection and rectal examination; a urethrogram should be ordered if urethral injury (blood at the meatus or the finding of a displaced prostate) is suspected. Otherwise, a Foley catheter is placed and the urine should be checked for blood. A pregnancy test should be ordered for female patients of childbearing age.
- Vaginal blood on a bimanual exam is an indication for a speculum examination.
- Extremities should be checked for soft tissue injury, fractures, and pulses.
- A more thorough neurologic examination is completed, carefully checking motor and sensory function.
- After the secondary survey, laboratory studies and additional radiographic studies, such as cystogram, intravenous pyelogram, aortogram, or computed tomography (CT) scans, should be considered.
- In patients who are too hemodynamically unstable for CT scan, the focused assessment with sonography for trauma (FAST) examination is used for the rapid bedside identification of free intraperitoneal fluid, hemothorax, and hemopericardium.[3]
- Diagnostic peritoneal lavage (DPL) is an alternative method of identifying intraperitoneal blood in lieu of a FAST exam.[4]

EMERGENCY DEPARTMENT CARE AND DISPOSITION

- Airway patency should be confirmed at the outset of the primary survey.
- A chin lift may initially help in opening the airway; suctioning may remove foreign material, blood, loose tissue, or avulsed teeth.
- Endotracheal intubation via a rapid sequence technique is indicated for patients with altered mental status, including severe agitation, or those who for any reason are unable to maintain a patent airway on their own.
- Patients with evidence of intracranial injury on examination may benefit from endotracheal intubation for airway protection.
- In cases of extensive facial trauma or when endotracheal intubation is not possible, cricothyrotomy or another advanced airway technique may be employed to secure the airway.
- Patients should be administered 100% oxygen via mask or endotracheal tube.

- Suspected tension pneumothorax is treated immediately with needle decompression followed by tube thoracostomy.
- For large hemothoraces, consideration may be given to autotransfusion and immediate operative exploration for initial chest tube output of >1500 mL of blood.
- The presence of a flail chest may mandate endotracheal intubation to ventilate patients adequately.
- Sucking chest wounds require placement of an occlusive dressing followed by chest tube placement.
- If the patient is hypotensive, then 2 L of warm crystalloid should be administered to treat shock. This may be followed by administering O-negative or type-specific blood as required.[5]
- Severe external hemorrhage should be managed with compression at the bleeding site.
- Bleeding from scalp lacerations should be controlled with Raney clips.
- Tamponade of severe epistaxis may be achieved with balloon compression devices.
- Reduction of fractures may prevent distal neurovascular compromise; all fractures should be splinted.
- Open fractures should be treated with cephalexin 2 g IV, with consideration given to additional antibiotic coverage for particularly contaminated injuries.
- Patients with pelvic fractures and signs of persistent hemorrhage may benefit from pelvic arteriography and embolization.
- Tetanus prophylaxis must be assured; an antibiotic such as cefotetan 2 g IV is indicated for possible ruptured abdominal viscus and vaginal or rectal lacerations.
- Intravenous mannitol 0.25 to 1.0 g/kg should be considered for acute neurologic deterioration.

REFERENCES

1. Committee on Injury Prevention and Control Division of Health Promotion and Disease Prevention, Bonnie RJ, Fulco CE, Liverman CT (eds.): *Reducing the Burden of Injury. Advancing Prevention and Treatment.* Washington: National Academy Press, 1999.
2. Baker SP: *The Injury Fact Book,* 2nd ed. New York: Oxford Press, 1992.
3. Ma OJ, Mateer JR, Ogata M, et al: Prospective analysis of rapid trauma ultrasound examination performed by emergency physicians. *J Trauma* 38:879, 1995.
4. McKenney GS, Oshsner MG, Schmidt JA, et al: Can ultrasound replace diagnostic peritoneal lavage in the assessment of blunt trauma? *J Trauma* 37:439, 1994.
5. Bickell WH, Wall MJ, Pepe PE, et al: Immediate versus delayed fluid resuscitation for hypotensive patients with penetrating torso injuries. *N Engl J Med* 331:1105, 1997.

For further reading in *Emergency Medicine: A Comprehensive Study Guide,* 6th ed., see Chap. 251, "Initial Approach to Trauma," by Edward E. Cornwell III.

160 PEDIATRIC TRAUMA

Charles J. Havel, Jr.

EPIDEMIOLOGY

- Trauma is the most common cause of death and disability in children 1 year of age and older; motor vehicle crash is the leading mechanism of injury in these children.[1]
- Head injury is the most frequent cause of death.[1]
- Homicide accounts for up to 25% of pediatric trauma deaths.[2]

PATHOPHYSIOLOGY

- As obligate nose breathers, infants less than 6 months of age with facial trauma or bleeding into the nasopharynx will evidence significant respiratory distress.
- In children, the primary cardiovascular response to hemorrhage is not increased stroke volume (as in adults) but an increase in heart rate.
- Age-dependent developmental differences in children demand adaptation of the traditional Glasgow coma score.
- The ratio of surface area to mass is greater in children than in adults.

CLINICAL FEATURES

- Tachypnea and accessory muscle use are early signs of dyspnea in children. Nasal flaring, grunting, and retractions are also signs of respiratory distress.
- Tachycardia is the most sensitive and earliest sign of volume loss in pediatric trauma patients. Hypotension is a late and therefore ominous finding.
- Other important signs of significant blood loss are increased capillary refill time, decreased degree of responsiveness, decreased urine output, narrowed pulse pressure, and decreased skin temperature.
- The signs of neurologic injury in children tend to be subtle and nonspecific. Manifestations of spinal cord injury may occur on a delayed basis.
- Children with major injuries are at significant risk for hypothermia.

DIAGNOSIS AND DIFFERENTIAL

- Simple scalp injuries, particularly in younger children, may result in significant blood loss due to the high degree of vascularity of the scalp.
- Liberal use of noncontrast computed tomography (CT) imaging is warranted in pediatric head trauma. Specific indications include significant loss of consciousness, alteration in mental status or seizure, deteriorating neurologic status, neurologic deficit, suspicion of skull fracture, and persistent vomiting.
- The increased flexibility of the spine in children is responsible for the clinical entity of spinal cord injury without radiographic abnormality (SCIWORA). A high degree of clinical suspicion and subsequent neurosurgical consultation and/or magnetic resonance imaging is warranted in these cases.
- A flexible spine also results in a decreased incidence of spinal fracture in children.[3] Nonetheless, "clearing" the spine in pediatric patients by physical examination alone and without radiographs, especially the cervical spine, is somewhat controversial. Applying criteria such as those utilized in the NEXUS trial can be difficult, particularly in the very young.
- In blunt chest trauma, considerable force may be transmitted to intrathoracic structures, causing serious injury with a paucity of external signs.
- Radiographic identification of any rib fracture carries great significance as a sensitive indicator of underlying lung injury, even if early imaging is otherwise unremarkable.
- The physical examination in children has been shown to be unreliable in determining the severity of injury in up to 45% of pediatric trauma patients.
- CT imaging is indicated in patients with a suspicious mechanism of injury, those who are symptomatic, or those with elevations of liver enzymes, amylase, lipase, and/or greater than 20 red blood cells per high power field on urinalysis.
- Identification of a pelvic fracture, particularly an anterior ring fracture, should prompt investigation for associated urethral or bladder injury.
- In the case of thermal injuries, careful documentation of the depth and extent of injury must be performed, recognizing that the Rule of Nines may be inaccurate in estimating burn surface area in children.
- Carbon monoxide levels should be obtained in patients with thermal injuries sustained in closed spaces.
- Nonaccidental trauma (child abuse) should be suspected when evaluating pediatric trauma patients, especially when the described mechanism of injury is inconsistent with the injuries sustained.
- Other markers for child abuse include the presence of retinal hemorrhages, specific pattern injuries, unexplained bruising, or skeletal fractures in various stages of healing.

EMERGENCY DEPARTMENT CARE AND DISPOSITION

- A complete and organized primary and secondary survey should be completed for all pediatric patients with significant mechanism of injury. Many problems are managed in a similar fashion to that used in adult patients.
- All patients should initially be administered 100% oxygen. Suctioning, jaw thrust, or chin lift maneuvers, and placement of either a nasal or an oral airway are airway maneuvers to be considered.
- In patients requiring tracheal intubation, orotracheal intubation is the route of choice. Choosing an appropriate endotracheal tube size is conveniently done by using the following formula: internal diameter (in mm) = (16 + age of patient in years)/4. In patients younger than 8 years old, an uncuffed endotracheal tube is generally placed.
- Rapid sequence intubation using pretreatment with 100% oxygen, intravenous lidocaine at 1.0 mg/kg, intravenous atropine at 0.02 mg/kg (minimum dose 0.1 mg, maximum dose 1.0 mg), and appropriate sedation and pharmacologic paralysis is indicated for patients with head injuries or those who are uncontrollably combative.
- Securing an airway in the setting of severe facial trauma if tracheal intubation cannot be established is best achieved by transtracheal catheter ventilation.
- Early employment of intraosseous cannulation, particularly in young children and infants, should be considered if intravenous access cannot be promptly established.
- Resuscitative fluids should be administered in 20-mL/kg boluses of isotonic crystalloid. If there is no improvement or deterioration occurs after an initial response, 10-mL/kg boluses of packed red blood cells should be infused.
- Burn patients should be resuscitated according to a standard burn formula, such as the Parkland formula.
- Neurologic injuries present special challenges given the high anxiety levels in pediatric patients. Sedation/analgesia with morphine sulfate and midazolam, each at 0.05 to 0.1 mg/kg IV (or similar agents at corresponding dosages), is appropriate after completion of the neurologic examination and may be required to facilitate advanced imaging.
- Aggressive treatment of hypoxia and hypotension accompanying severe head injury is critical. Patients should be tracheally intubated, the head of the bed elevated to 30 degrees, and the head and neck positioned at neutral.
- Mannitol at 0.25 to 1.0 g/kg and furosemide at 1.0 mg/kg IV can be used to treat cerebral edema. Hyperventilation should be reserved for those patients with clear signs of impending herniation.
- Posttraumatic seizures are more common in children than adults. Prophylaxis with fosphenytoin 18 mg/kg (phenytoin equivalents) should be considered.
- Spinal immobilization must be achieved in infants and younger children with allowance for their relatively larger head by placement of padding behind the shoulders.
- For neurologic deficit attributable to closed spinal cord injury, steroids should be administered within 8 hours. Dosing consists of a bolus of methylprednisolone 30 mg/kg IV over 15 minutes followed 45 minutes later by an IV infusion at 5.4 mg/kg/h for 48 hours.
- Children with any of the following injuries should be hospitalized: skull fractures or evidence of intracranial injury on CT scan, spinal trauma, significant chest trauma, abdominal trauma with internal organ injury, or significant burns. Referral to a pediatric trauma center should be considered for these patients.
- Social service consultation and reporting to child protective services are indicated if there is any suspicion of nonaccidental trauma.

REFERENCES

1. Rhodes M, Smith S, Boorse D: Pediatric trauma patients in an "adult" trauma center. *J Trauma* 35:384, 1993.
2. Fingerhut LA, Warner M: *Injury Chartbook, Health, United States, 1996-97.* Hyattsville, MD: National Center for Health Statistics, 1997, p. 38.
3. Hadley MN, Zabramski JM, Browner CM, et al: Pediatric spinal trauma: Review of 122 cases of spinal cord and vertebral column injuries. *J Neurosurg* 68:18, 1998.

For further reading in *Emergency Medicine: A Comprehensive Study Guide,* 6th ed., see Chap. 252, "Pediatric Trauma," by William E. Hauda II.

161 GERIATRIC TRAUMA
O. John Ma

EPIDEMIOLOGY

- While persons over 65 years of age represent 12% of the population, they account for 36% of all ambulance transports, 25% of hospitalizations, and 25% of total trauma costs.[1]

- Approximately 28% of deaths due to accidental causes involve persons 65 years and older. The elderly have the highest population-based mortality rate of any age group.[1]

PATHOPHYSIOLOGY

- Chronologic age is the actual number of years the individual has lived. Physiologic age describes the actual functional capacity of the patient's organ systems in a physiologic sense.
- Comorbid disease states such as diabetes mellitus, coronary artery disease, renal disease, arthritis, and pulmonary disease can decrease the physiologic reserve of certain patients, which makes it more difficult for them to recover from a traumatic injury.[2]
- Physiologic reserve describes the various levels of functioning of the patient's organ systems that allow them to compensate for traumatic derangement.[1]
- Falls are the most common cause of injury in patients over 65 years of age.[3,4] Falls are reported as the underlying cause of 9500 deaths each year in patients over the age of 65 years. In the >85-year-old age group, 20% of fatal falls occur in nursing homes.[5]
- Motor vehicle crashes rank as the second leading mechanism of injury that brings elderly patients to trauma centers in the United States, and are the most common mechanism for fatal incidents in elderly persons through 80 years of age.[1]
- The elderly constitute between 13 and 20% of admissions to burn units, but have the highest case fatality rate of any age group.

CLINICAL FEATURES

- Following injury, older patients have higher admission rates, longer hospital stays, increased long-term morbidity, and higher mortality rates despite lower injury severity.[6]
- The clinician should not be lulled into a false sense of security by "normal" vital signs. In one study of 15 patients initially considered to be hemodynamically "stable," eight had cardiac outputs less than 3.5 L/min and none had an adequate response to volume loading. Of seven patients with a normal cardiac output, five had inadequate oxygen delivery.[7]
- There is progressive stiffening of the myocardium with age that results in a decreased effectiveness of the pumping mechanism. A normal tachycardic response to pain, hypovolemia, or anxiety may be absent or blunted in the elderly trauma patient.[8] Medications such as β-blockers may mask tachycardia and hinder the evaluation of the elderly patient.

- Elderly persons suffer a much lower incidence of epidural hematomas than the general population; however, there is a higher incidence of subdural hematomas. As the brain mass decreases with advancing age, there is greater stretching and tension of the bridging veins that pass from the brain to the dural sinuses.[9]
- The incidence of cervical spine injury has been found to be twice as great in geriatric patients as in a younger cohort of blunt trauma patients. Odontoid fractures were particularly common in geriatric patients, accounting for 20% of geriatric cervical spine fractures compared with 5% of nongeriatric fractures.[10]
- Severe thoracic injuries such as hemopneumothorax, pulmonary contusion, flail chest, and cardiac contusion, can quickly lead to decompensation in elderly individuals whose baseline oxygenation status may already be diminished.
- Reduction in pulmonary compliance, total lung surface area, and mucociliary clearance of foreign material and bacteria result in an increased risk for elderly patients to develop nosocomial gram-negative pneumonia.[8]
- Hip fracture is the single most common diagnosis that leads to hospitalization in all age groups in the United States.
- Hip fractures occur primarily in four areas: intertrochanteric, transcervical, subcapital, and subtrochanteric. Intertrochanteric fractures are the most common, followed by transcervical fractures.[8] Emergency physicians must be aware that pelvic and long bone fractures are frequently the sole etiology for hypovolemia in elderly patients.
- The incidence of humeral head and surgical neck fractures in elderly patients is increased by falls on the outstretched hand or elbow.

DIAGNOSIS AND DIFFERENTIAL

- For older patients, the adhesions associated with previous abdominal surgical procedures may increase the risk of performing diagnostic peritoneal lavage.[1]
- For CT scanning, it is important to ensure adequate hydration and baseline assessment of renal function prior to the contrast load for the CT scan. Some patients may be volume depleted due to medications such as diuretics. This hypovolemia coupled with contrast administration may exacerbate any underlying renal pathology.[1]
- For unstable patients, and especially those with multiple scars on the abdominal wall from previous procedures, the focused assessment with sonography for trauma (FAST) examination is the ideal diagnostic study to detect free intraperitoneal fluid.

EMERGENCY DEPARTMENT CARE AND DISPOSITION

- Prompt tracheal intubation and use of mechanical ventilation should be considered in patients with more severe injuries, respiratory rates greater than 40 breaths per minute, or when the Pa_{O_2} is <60 mm Hg or the Pa_{CO_2} is >50 mm Hg.[11]
- Early invasive monitoring has been advocated to help physicians assess hemodynamic status in the elderly. One study demonstrated that by reducing the time to invasive monitoring in elderly trauma patients from 5.5 hours to 2.2 hours, and thus recognizing and appropriately treating occult shock, the survival rate of their patients increased from 7 to 53%. Survival was improved because of enhanced oxygen delivery through the use of adequate volume loading and inotropic support.[7]
- During the initial resuscitative phase, crystalloid, while the primary option, should be administered judiciously since elderly patients with diminished cardiac compliance are more susceptible to volume overload. Strong consideration should be made for early and more liberal use of packed red blood cell transfusion.
- Among geriatric trauma patients who are hospitalized, the mortality rate has been reported to be between 15 and 30%. These figures far exceed the mortality rate of 4 to 8% found in younger patients.[1] In general, multiple organ failure and sepsis cause more deaths in elderly patients than in younger trauma victims.[12]
- Several markers for poor outcome in elderly trauma patients have been determined. Age greater than 75 years, Glasgow Coma Scale score ≤7, presence of shock upon admission, severe head injury, and the development of sepsis are associated with worse outcome and higher mortality figures.[13]
- One study demonstrated that immediately after discharge, one third of trauma survivors return to independent living, one third return to dependent status but living at home, and one third require nursing home facilities. Altogether, at long term follow-up 89% returned home after trauma and 57% returned to independent living.[14]

REFERENCES

1. Schwab CW, Kauder DR: Trauma in the geriatric patient. *Arch Surg* 127:701, 1992.
2. Morris JA, MacKenzie EJ, Edelstein SL: The effect of pre-existing conditions on mortality in trauma patients. *JAMA* 263:1942, 1990.
3. Osler T, Hales K, Baack B, et al: Trauma in the elderly. *Am J Surg* 156:537, 1988.
4. Smith DP, Enderson BL, Maull KI: Trauma in the elderly: Determinants of outcome. *South Med J* 83:171, 1990.
5. Tinetti ME, Speechley M: Prevention of falls among the elderly. *N Engl J Med* 320:1055, 1989.
6. Finelli FC, Johnsson J, Champion HR, et al: A case control study for major trauma in geriatric patients. *J Trauma* 29:541, 1989.
7. Scalea TM, Simon HM, Duncan AO, et al: Geriatric blunt trauma: Improved survival with early invasive monitoring. *J Trauma* 30:129, 1990.
8. Demarest GB, Osler TM, Clevenger FW: Injuries in the elderly: evaluation and initial response. *Geriatrics* 45:36, 1990.
9. Kirkpatrick JB, Pearson J: Fatal cerebral injury in the elderly. *J Am Geriatr Soc* 26:489, 1978.
10. Touger M, Gennis P, Nathanson N, et al: Validity of a decision rule to reduce cervical spine radiography in elderly patients with blunt trauma. *Ann Emerg Med* 40:287, 2002.
11. Allen JE, Schwab CW: Blunt chest trauma in the elderly. *Am Surg* 51:697, 1985.
12. Horst HM, Obeid FN, Sorensen VJ, et al: Factors influencing survival of elderly trauma patients. *Crit Care Med* 14:681, 1986.
13. van Aalst JA, Morris JA, Yates HK, et al: Severely injured geriatric patients return to independent living: A study of factors influencing function and independence. *J Trauma* 31:1096, 1991.
14. DeMaria EJ, Kenney PR, Merriam MA, et al: Survival after trauma in geriatric patients. *Ann Surg* 206:738, 1987.

For further reading in *Emergency Medicine: A Comprehensive Study Guide*, 6th ed., see Chap. 253, "Geriatric Trauma," by O. John Ma and Stephen W. Meldon.

162 TRAUMA IN PREGNANCY

C. Crawford Mechem

EPIDEMIOLOGY

- Trauma is the leading cause of nonobstetric morbidity and mortality in pregnant women.
- Significant trauma complicates 6 to 8% of all pregnancies.[1] The maternal trauma mortality rate does not differ from that of nonpregnant women.[2]
- A positive toxicology screen has been noted in 16% of cases.[3]

PATHOPHYSIOLOGY

- Motor vehicle crash is the most common mechanism of blunt abdominal trauma in pregnant patients; this is followed by falls and direct assault.[1,4]

- Gunshot wounds are the most common form of penetrating abdominal trauma in pregnancy. Fetal mortality rate may be as high as 70% in these cases.
- Up to 5% of patients with minor abdominal trauma may experience placental abruption.
- A significant percentage of trauma in pregnancy results from interpersonal violence, which in many cases was committed by a husband or boyfriend.[5,6]
- Physiologic changes of pregnancy make determination of injury severity problematic.
- Heart rate increases 10 to 20 beats per minute in the second trimester, while systolic and diastolic blood pressures drop 10 to 15 mm Hg.
- Blood volume increases up to 45%. Red cell mass increases to a lesser extent, leading to a physiologic anemia of pregnancy.
- Tachycardia, hypotension, or anemia may be due to blood loss or normal physiologic changes.
- Due to the hypervolemic state, a patient may lose 30 to 35% of her blood volume before manifesting signs of shock.[1]
- Pulmonary changes in pregnancy include elevation of the diaphragm and decreases in residual volume and function residual capacity.
- Tidal volume increases, resulting in hyperventilation with associated respiratory alkalosis. Renal compensation causes the serum pH to remain unchanged.

CLINICAL FEATURES

- After 12 weeks' gestation, the enlarging uterus emerges from the pelvis, and by 20 weeks reaches the level of the umbilicus. Its blood flow increases, making severe maternal hemorrhage from uterine trauma more likely.
- The uterus can also compress the inferior vena cava when the patient is supine, leading to the "supine hypotension syndrome."
- As pregnancy progresses, the small intestines are pushed cephalad, increasing their likelihood of injury in penetrating trauma to the upper abdomen.[4]
- Decreased intestinal motility is associated with gastroesophageal reflux, predisposing the patient to vomiting and aspiration.
- The bladder moves into the abdomen in the third trimester, increasing its susceptibility to injury.
- Splenic injury remains the most common cause of abdominal hemorrhage in the pregnant trauma patient.
- Fetal injuries are more likely to be seen in the third trimester, often associated with pelvic fractures or penetrating trauma.
- Uterine rupture is rare, but is associated with a fetal mortality rate of close to 100%.[4,7]
- More common complications of trauma include preterm labor and abruptio placentae.

- Second only to maternal death, abruptio placentae is the most common cause of fetal death.[4] It presents with abdominal pain, vaginal bleeding, uterine contractions, and signs of disseminated intravascular coagulation.[6,8]
- Fetal-maternal hemorrhage occurs in over 30% of cases of significant trauma and may result in Rh-isoimmunization of Rh-negative women.[4]

DIAGNOSIS AND DIFFERENTIAL

- Since maternal stability and survival offer the best chance for fetal well-being, no critical interventions or diagnostic procedures should be withheld out of concern for potential adverse effects on the fetus.
- In addition to the standard trauma evaluation, special attention should be directed to the gravid abdomen, looking for evidence of injury, tenderness, or uterine contractions.
- If abdominal or pelvic trauma is suspected, a sterile pelvic examination is indicated, looking for genital trauma, vaginal bleeding, or ruptured amniotic membranes.
- Fluid with a pH of 7 in the vaginal canal suggests amniotic rupture, as does a branch-like pattern, or "ferning," on drying of vaginal fluid on a microscope slide.
- Shielding the uterus when possible and limiting radiographs to those that will significantly impact the patient's care are prudent measures.
- Adverse fetal effects from radiation are negligible with doses less than 10 rad, which is an exposure far greater than that received from most trauma radiographs.
- Abdominal and pelvic computed tomography (CT) scanning, pelvic angiography, and pelvic fluoroscopy result in the highest doses of radiation.
- In the case of CT, exposure may be decreased by reducing the number of cuts obtained.[9]
- Bedside ultrasonography is a highly sensitive and specific radiation-free alternative for imaging the abdomen. In addition to evaluating fetal heart rate, ultrasonography can also assess gestational age, fetal activity or demise, placental location, and amniotic fluid volume.[10]
- Magnetic resonance imaging (MRI) and ventilation-perfusion scanning have not been associated with adverse fetal outcome.
- Diagnostic peritoneal lavage remains a valid modality for evaluating the pregnant abdominal trauma patient. An open supraumbilical technique should be used.[1,4]
- Auscultation of fetal heart tones for determining fetal viability and identifying fetal distress should be performed early in the evaluation.
- A normal fetal heart rate is in the range of 120 to 160 beats per minute.
- Fetal bradycardia is most likely from hypoxia due to

maternal hypotension, respiratory compromise, or placental abruption.

- Fetal tachycardia is most likely due to hypoxia or hypovolemia.

- Absence of fetal heart tones in the setting of trauma precludes fetal viability.

- In the setting of blunt abdominal trauma, external fetal monitoring is indicated for all patients beyond 20 weeks' gestation and is more predictive than ultrasound for abruptio placentae. Four hours is the recommended initial period of monitoring, extended up to 24 hours in case of documented uterine irritability.

- Beyond the viable gestational age of 23 weeks, fetal tachycardia, lack of beat-to-beat or long-term variability, or late decelerations on tocodynamometry are diagnostic of fetal distress and may be indications for emergent cesarean section.

EMERGENCY DEPARTMENT CARE AND DISPOSITION

- As is the case in all trauma patients, initial priorities remain the ABCs of resuscitation directed at the mother. Care should be coordinated with surgical and obstetric consultants.

- All pregnant trauma patients should receive supplemental oxygen.

- Large-bore, peripheral IV lines with crystalloid infusions should be initiated.

- For patients beyond 20 weeks' gestation who must remain supine, a wedge may be placed under the right hip, tilting the patient 30 degrees to the left, thus reducing the likelihood of supine hypotension syndrome. Otherwise, the patient should be kept in a left lateral decubitus position whenever possible.

- Early gastric intubation should be performed to reduce the risk of aspiration.

- Vasopressors can have deleterious effects on uterine perfusion and should be avoided.

- Tetanus prophylaxis is not contraindicated in pregnancy and should be administered when indicated.

- D immune globulin, 300 μg IM, should be administered to all unsensitized D-negative pregnant patients following abdominal trauma.[4]

- Tocolytics have a variety of side effects, including fetal and maternal tachycardia. They should only be administered in consultation with an obstetrician.

- Indications for emergent laparotomy in the pregnant patient remain the same as in the nonpregnant patient.

- Emergent cesarean section has been associated with a 75% fetal survival rate when the gestational age is at or greater than 26 weeks, fetal heart tones are present on admission, and the procedure is performed at the earliest sign of fetal distress.[11]

- Perimortem cesarean section has also been associated with favorable fetal outcomes. It should be considered only after optimal resuscitation efforts have been initiated in patients beyond 23 weeks of pregnancy. Improved outcomes are associated with delivery within 5 minutes of maternal death.[12,13]

- The decision to admit or discharge a pregnant trauma patient is based on the nature and severity of the presenting injuries and is often made after consultation with surgical and obstetric consultants.

- Patients who display evidence of fetal distress or increased uterine irritability during initial observation should be admitted.

- Patients who are discharged should be instructed to seek medical attention immediately if they develop abdominal pain or cramps, vaginal bleeding, leakage of fluid, or perception of decreased fetal activity.

REFERENCES

1. Scorpio RJ, Esposito TJ, Smith LG, et al: Blunt trauma during pregnancy: Factors affecting fetal outcome. *J Trauma* 32: 213, 1992.
2. Esposito TJ, Gens DR, Smith LG, et al: Trauma during pregnancy: A review of 79 cases. *Arch Surg* 126:1073, 1991.
3. Esposito TJ, Gens DR, Smith LG, et al: Evaluation of blunt trauma occurring during pregnancy. *J Trauma* 29:1628, 1989.
4. Obstetric aspects of trauma. *Am Coll Obstet Gynecol Educ Bull* 22:251, 1998.
5. Gazmararian JA, Lazorick S, Spitz AM, et al: Prevalence of violence against pregnant women. *JAMA* 275:1915, 1996.
6. Poole GV, Martin JN, Perry KG Jr, et al: Trauma in pregnancy: The role of interpersonal violence. *Am J Obstet Gynecol* 174:1873, 1996.
7. Astarita DC, Feldman B: Seat belt placement resulting in uterine rupture. *J Trauma* 42:738, 1997.
8. Ali J, Yeo A, Gana TJ, et al: Predictors of fetal mortality in pregnant trauma patients. *J Trauma* 42:782, 1997.
9. Goldman SM, Wagner LK: Radiologic management of abdominal trauma in pregnancy. *Am J Radiol* 166:763, 1996.
10. Ma OJ, Mateer JR, DeBehnke DJ: Use of ultrasonography for the evaluation of pregnant trauma patients. *J Trauma* 40: 665, 1996.
11. Morris JA, Rosenbower TJ, Jurkovich GJ, et al: Infant survival after cesarean section for trauma. *Ann Surg* 223:481, 1996.
12. Katz VL, Dotters DJ, Droegemueller W: Perimortem cesarean delivery. *Obstet Gynecol* 68:571, 1986.
13. Kupas DF, Harter SC, Vosk A: Out-of-hospital perimortem cesarean section. *Prehosp Emerg Care* 2:206, 1997.

For further reading in *Emergency Medicine: A Comprehensive Study Guide,* 6th ed., see Chap. 254, "Trauma in Pregnancy," by Nelson Tang and Drew White.

163 HEAD INJURY

O. John Ma

EPIDEMIOLOGY

- Approximately 1.5 million people per year sustain a nonfatal traumatic brain injury (TBI). TBI accounts for approximately one third of all trauma-related deaths in persons younger than 45 years of age.[1]
- Young men, elderly individuals, children, and alcoholics are at greater risk for TBI.

PATHOPHYSIOLOGY

- Direct injury is caused immediately by the forces of an object striking the head or by penetrating injury.
- Indirect injuries are from acceleration/deceleration forces that result in the movement of the brain inside the skull.
- Secondary brain injury occurs from potentially treatable factors such as intracranial hemorrhage and masses, cerebral edema, ischemia, hypoxia (Po_2 <60 mm Hg), hypotension (systolic blood pressure <90 mm Hg), anemia (hematocrit <30%), and increased intracranial pressure (ICP).[2]
- Cerebral perfusion pressure (CPP) is the difference between the mean arterial pressure (MAP) and the ICP. Elevation of the ICP and/or hypotension results in a depressed CPP and leads to further brain injury.

- Rapid rises in the ICP can lead to the "Cushing reflex," characterized by hypertension, bradycardia, and respiratory irregularities. The Cushing reflex is seen uncommonly and usually occurs in children.

CLINICAL FEATURES

- Mild TBI involves patients with a Glasgow Coma Scale score (GCS, see Table 163-1) ≥14. Patients may be asymptomatic with only a history of head trauma, or may be confused and amnestic of the event. They may have experienced brief loss of consciousness and complain of a diffuse headache, nausea, and vomiting.
- Mild TBI patients at high risk include those with a skull fracture, large subgaleal swelling, focal neurologic findings, coagulopathy, age >60 years, or drug/alcohol intoxication.[3]
- Moderate TBI (GCS 9 to 13) accounts for approximately 10% of all patients with head injuries. Overall, 40% of moderate TBI patients have a positive computed tomography (CT) scan and 8% require neurosurgical intervention. Roughly 10% of these patients will deteriorate and progress to severe TBI.[4]
- Severe TBI (GCS <9) accounts for approximately 10% of head injury patients. The mortality of severe TBI approaches 40%. The immediate clinical priority in these patients is to prevent secondary brain injury, identify other life-threatening injuries, and identify treatable neurosurgical conditions.
- Out-of-hospital medical personnel often may provide

TABLE 163-1 The Glasgow Coma Scale for All Age Groups

	4 YEARS TO ADULT	CHILD <4 YEARS	INFANT
Eye Opening			
4	Spontaneous	Spontaneous	Spontaneous
3	To speech	To speech	To speech
2	To pain	To pain	To pain
1	No response	No response	No response
Verbal Response			
5	Alert and oriented	Oriented, social, speaks, interacts	Coos, babbles
4	Disoriented conversation	Confused speech, disoriented, consolable, aware	Irritable cry
3	Speaking but nonsensical	Inappropriate words, inconsolable, unaware	Cries to pain
2	Moans or unintelligible sounds	Incomprehensible, agitated, restless, unaware	Moans to pain
1	No response	No response	No response
Motor Response			
6	Follows commands	Normal, spontaneous movements	Normal, spontaneous moves
5	Localizes pain	Localizes pain	Withdraws to touch
4	Movement or withdrawal to pain	Withdraws to pain	Withdraws to pain
3	Decorticate flexion	Decorticate flexion	Decorticate flexion
2	Decerebrate extension	Decerebrate extension	Decerebrate extension
1	No response	No response	No response
3–15			

GCS reporting should be modified for intubated and paralyzed patients.

- critical parts of the history, including mechanism and time of injury, presence and length of unconsciousness, initial mental status, seizure activity, vomiting, verbalization, and movement of extremities.
- Clinically important features of the neurologic examination that should be addressed include assessing the mental status and GCS; pupils for size, reactivity, and anisocoria; cranial nerve function; motor, sensory, and brainstem function; deep tendon reflexes; and noting any development of decorticate or decerebrate posturing.
- Isolated linear nondepressed fractures with an intact scalp are common and do not require treatment. However, life-threatening intracranial hemorrhage may result if the fracture causes disruption of the middle meningeal artery or a major dural sinus. Depressed skull fractures are classified as open or closed, depending on the integrity of the overlying scalp.
- Although basilar skull fractures can occur at any point in the base of the skull, the typical location is in the petrous portion of the temporal bone. Findings associated with a basilar skull fracture include hemotympanum, cerebrospinal fluid (CSF) otorrhea or rhinorrhea, periorbital ecchymosis ("raccoon eyes"), and retroauricular ecchymosis (Battle's sign).
- Brain concussion is a diffuse head injury usually associated with transient loss of consciousness that occurs immediately following a nonpenetrating blunt impact to the head. It generally occurs when the head, while moving, strikes or is struck by an object. The duration of unconsciousness is typically brief (seconds to minutes).
- Symptoms of amnesia and confusion are clinical hallmarks of concussion. Complete recovery is typical, although persistent headache and problems with memory, anxiety, insomnia, and dizziness can continue in some patients for weeks after the injury.
- Common locations for brain contusions are the frontal poles, the subfrontal cortex, and the anterior temporal lobes. Contusions may occur directly under the site of impact or on the contralateral side (contrecoup lesion).
- The contused area is usually hemorrhagic with surrounding edema, and occasionally associated with subarachnoid hemorrhage. Neurologic dysfunction may be profound and prolonged, with patients demonstrating mental confusion, obtundation, or coma. Focal neurologic deficits are usually present.
- Combination of parenchymal hemorrhage and contusion can produce an expanding mass lesion. When present in the anterior temporal lobe, uncal herniation can occur without a diffuse increase in ICP.
- Traumatic subarachnoid hemorrhage results from the disruption of subarachnoid vessels and presents with blood in the CSF. Patients may complain of diffuse headache, nausea, or photophobia.

- Traumatic subarachnoid hemorrhage may be the most common CT abnormality in patients with moderate or severe TBI. Some cases may be missed if the CT scan is obtained less than 6 hours after injury.[5]
- An epidural hematoma results from an acute collection of blood between the inner table of the skull and dura. Approximately 80% of the time it is associated with a skull fracture that lacerates a meningeal artery, most commonly the middle meningeal artery. Underlying injury to the brain may not necessarily be severe.
- In the classic scenario (20% of cases) of epidural hematoma, the patient experiences loss of consciousness after a head injury. The patient may present to the emergency department (ED) with clear mentation, signifying the "lucid interval," and then begin to develop mental status deterioration in the ED. A fixed and dilated pupil on the side of the lesion with contralateral hemiparesis are classic late findings. The high pressure arterial bleeding of an epidural hematoma can lead to herniation within hours of injury.
- A subdural hematoma (SDH), which is a collection of venous blood between the dura mater and the arachnoid, results from tears of the bridging veins that extend from the subarachnoid space to the dural venous sinuses. A common mechanism is sudden acceleration-deceleration. Patients with brain atrophy, such as alcoholics or the elderly, are more susceptible to a subdural hematoma.
- In acute SDH, patients present within 14 days of the injury, and most become symptomatic within 24 hours of injury.
- After 2 weeks, patients are defined as having a chronic SDH. Symptoms may range from a headache to lethargy or coma. It is important to distinguish between acute and chronic subdural hematomas by history, physical examination, and CT scan.
- Diffusely or focally increased ICP can result in herniation of the brain at several locations.
- Transtentorial (uncal) herniation occurs when a SDH or temporal lobe mass forces the ipsilateral uncus of the temporal lobe through the tentorial hiatus into the space between the cerebral peduncle and the tentorium. This results in compression of the oculomotor nerve and parasympathetic paralysis of the ipsilateral pupil, causing it to become fixed and dilated. The cerebral peduncle is simultaneously compressed, resulting in contralateral hemiparesis. The increased ICP and brainstem compression result in progressive deterioration in the level of consciousness.
- Occasionally, in transtentorial herniation, the contralateral cerebral peduncle is forced against the free edge of the tentorium on the opposite side, resulting in paralysis ipsilateral to the lesion—a false localizing sign. The posterior cerebral artery can be compressed

against the free edge of the tentorium, resulting in infarction of the occipital lobe. If the herniation continues untreated, there is progressive brainstem deterioration leading to hyperventilation, decerebration, and then to apnea and death.

- Cerebellotonsillar herniation through the foramen magnum occurs much less frequently. Resultant medullary compression causes bradycardia, respiratory arrest, and death.
- Cingulate or subfalcial herniation occurs when one cerebral hemisphere is displaced underneath the falx cerebri into the opposite supratentorial space. This is rarely clinically diagnosed.
- Gunshot wounds and penetrating sharp objects can result in penetrating injury to the brain. The degree of neurologic injury will depend on the energy of the missile, whether the trajectory involves a single or multiple lobes or hemispheres of the brain, the amount of scatter of bone and metallic fragments, and whether a mass lesion is present.

DIAGNOSIS AND DIFFERENTIAL

- Approximately 4% of patients suffering a severe TBI will have an associated cervical spine fracture. Cervical spine radiographs should be obtained on all trauma patients who present with altered mental status, neck pain, intoxication, neurologic deficit, or severe distracting injury.
- All patients with a GCS of 14 or less should undergo an emergent head CT scan without contrast after stabilization.
- Patients with a GCS of 15 should undergo a CT scan if they experienced loss of consciousness, nausea or vomiting, posttraumatic seizure, amnesia, continued diffuse headache, a history of coagulopathy, or intoxication without significant improvement after a period of observation.
- Other indications for CT scan include clinical neurologic deterioration during observation, presence of distracting injuries, persistent focal neurologic or mental status deficit, and skull fractures in the vicinity of the middle meningeal artery or major venous sinuses.
- Routine skull radiographs are not indicated. Anteroposterior and lateral skull radiographs may be obtained for penetrating wounds of the skull or for suspected depressed skull fracture.
- Skull radiographs may help localize the position of a foreign body within the cranium and may determine the amount of bony depression. If a CT scan of the head will be obtained, bone windows can be obtained, eliminating the need for skull films.
- Laboratory work for significant head injury patients should include type and cross-matching, complete blood count, electrolytes, glucose, arterial blood gas analysis, directed toxicologic studies, prothrombin time (PT), partial thromboplastin time (PTT), platelets, and disseminated intravascular coagulation (DIC) panel.

EMERGENCY DEPARTMENT CARE AND DISPOSITION

- Standard protocols for evaluation and stabilization of trauma patients should be initiated. A careful search for other significant injuries should be made since up to 60% of patients with severe TBI have associated major injuries.
- The patient should be administered 100% oxygen, and cardiac monitoring and two IV lines should be secured.
- For patients with severe TBI, endotracheal intubation (via rapid sequence intubation) to protect the airway and prevent hypoxemia is the top priority. When properly performed, rapid sequence intubation assists in preventing increased ICP and has a low complication rate. When performing rapid sequence intubation, it is imperative to provide adequate cervical spine immobilization and use an adequate sedation/induction agent
- Since hypotension can lead to depressed cerebral perfusion pressure, restoration of an adequate blood pressure is vital. Resuscitation with IV crystalloid fluid to a MAP of 90 mm Hg is indicated; if hypertensive, a 25 to 30% reduction in MAP should be achieved.[3]
- Once an adequate blood pressure is maintained, IV fluids should be administered cautiously to prevent cerebral edema. Hypotonic and glucose-containing solutions should be avoided.
- Once a head CT scan demonstrating intracranial injury has been identified, immediate neurosurgical consultation is indicated. Patients with new neurologic deficits from an acute epidural or subdural hematoma require emergent neurosurgical consultation for definitive operative care.
- All patients who demonstrate signs of increased ICP should have the head of their bed elevated 30 degrees (provided that the patient is not hypotensive), adequate volume resuscitation to a MAP of 90 mm Hg, and maintenance of adequate arterial oxygenation. After these steps, mannitol, 0.25 to 1.0 g/kg IV bolus, should be administered.
- Hyperventilation is no longer recommended as a prophylactic intervention to lower ICP because of its potential to cause cerebral ischemia. Hyperventilation should be reserved as a last resort for decreasing ICP; if used, it should be implemented as a temporary

measure and the P_{CO_2} monitored closely to maintain the range of 30 to 35 mm Hg.[6]

- When all other methods to control the ICP have failed, patients with signs of impending brain herniation may need emergency decompression by trephination (burr holes). CT scanning prior to attempting trephination is recommended to localize the lesion and direct the decompression site.
- For posttraumatic seizures, prophylactic anticonvulsants should be administered in consultation with the neurosurgeon. Seizures should be treated with benzodiazepines, such as lorazepam, and fosphenytoin at a loading dose of 18 to 20 mg/kg IV.
- Patients with a basilar skull fracture or penetrating injuries (gunshot wound or stab wound) should be admitted to the neurosurgical service and started on prophylactic antibiotic therapy (eg, ceftriaxone 1 g every 12 hours).[7]
- The use of nimodipine (2 mg/h) in patients with traumatic subarachnoid hemorrhage reduces the likelihood of death or severe disability by 55%.[8]
- Patients with an initial GCS of 15 that is maintained during the observation period, normal serial neurologic examinations, and a normal CT scan may be discharged home.
- Those with a positive CT scan require neurosurgical consultation and admission.
- Patients with an initial GCS of 14 and a normal CT scan should be observed in the ED for at least 6 hours. If their GCS improves to 15 and they remain completely neurologically intact, they can be discharged home.
- All patients who experience a head injury should be discharged home with a reliable companion who can observe the patient for at least 24 hours, carry out appropriate discharge instructions, and follow the head injury sheet instructions.

REFERENCES

1. Thurman DJ, Alverson C, Dunn KA, et al: Traumatic brain injury in the United States: A public health perspective. *J Head Trauma Rehabil* 14:602, 1999.
2. Chestnut RM, Marshall LF, Klauber MR, et al: The role of secondary brain injury: Determining outcome from severe head injury. *J Trauma* 34:216, 1993.
3. Servadei F, Teasdale G, Merry G, et al: Neurotraumatology Committee of the World Federation of Neurosurgical Societies: Defining acute mild head injury in adults. *J Neurotrauma* 18:657, 2001.
4. Stein SC, Ross SE: Moderate head injury: A guide to initial management. *J Neurosurg* 77:562, 1992.
5. Servadei F, Murray GD, Teasdale G, et al: Traumatic subarachnoid hemorrhage: Demographic and clinical study of 750 patients from the European brain injury consortium survey of head injuries. *Neurosurgery* 50:261, 2002.
6. Bullock RM: Management and prognosis of severe traumatic brain injury, part 1. *J Neurotrauma* 17:451, 2000.
7. Friedman JA, Ebersold MJ, Quast LM: Post-traumatic cerebrospinal fluid leakage. *World J Surg* 25:1062, 2001.
8. Harders A, Kakarieka A, Braakman R: Traumatic subarachnoid hemorrhage and its treatment with nimodipine. *J Neurosurg* 85:82, 1996.

For further reading in *Emergency Medicine: A Comprehensive Study Guide,* 6th ed., see Chap. 255, "Head Injury," by Thomas D. Kirsch and Christopher A. Lipinski.

164 SPINE AND SPINAL CORD INJURIES

Jeffrey N. Glaspy

EPIDEMIOLOGY

- The incidence of spinal cord injuries (SCIs) has been estimated at 30 cases per million population at risk. There is a male-to-female predominance of 4 to 1.
- Ninety percent of SCIs are related to motor vehicle crashes.
- The cervical spine is the most often injured segment of the spine.

PATHOPHYSIOLOGY

- Three main vertebral columns provide stability to the spine.[1]
- The anterior column is made up of the anterior wall of the vertebral body, the anterior annulus, and the anterior longitudinal ligament.
- The middle column consists of the posterior wall of the vertebral body, the posterior annulus fibrosus, and the posterior longitudinal ligament.
- The posterior column includes the bony complex of the posterior vertebral arch and the posterior ligamentous complex.
- For a thoracolumbar injury to be considered unstable, disruption of two or more of these columns must be present.
- While compression fracture of 25% is considered unstable in the cervical region,[2] thoracic or lumbar vertebral body compression of more than 50% is generally considered unstable.

CLINICAL FEATURES

- Damage to the spinal cord results in two phases of injury. Initially, a direct mechanical injury may result in hemorrhage, edema, and ischemia. Within hours, a secondary tissue degeneration phase begins with release of membrane-destabilizing enzymes and inflammatory mediators, which induces lipid peroxidation and hydrolysis.
- There are three main spinal cord tracts. The corticospinal tract fibers decussate in the lower medulla and descend through the lateral aspect of the spinal cord. Damage to the corticospinal tract (upper motor neurons) results in ipsilateral muscle weakness, spasticity, increased deep tendon reflexes, and Babinski's sign.
- The other two main spinal cord tracts, the spinothalamic and dorsal columns, are ascending pathways that transmit sensory information.
- The spinothalamic tracts transmit pain and temperature sensation and decussate shortly after entering the vertebral column. Injury to the spinothalamic tract causes contralateral loss of pain and temperature sensation.
- The dorsal (or posterior) columns transmit vibration and proprioception sensation. The neurons in this tract do not synapse until they reach the medulla, where they then decussate. Injury to a dorsal column will cause ipsilateral loss of vibration and proprioception sensation.
- Light touch is transmitted through both the spinothalamic and dorsal tracts. Light touch is not lost unless there is damage to both of these tracts.
- SCIs are either complete or incomplete lesions.
- The severity of injury determines the prognosis for recovery of function. Lesions cannot be deemed complete until spinal shock has resolved, which usually occurs over a 24- to 48-hour period.
- Not all patients with SCI have neurologic deficits on initial presentation. Many unstable spinal fractures may present without spinal cord or nerve root trauma.
- Symptomatic patients may complain of paresthesias, dysesthesias, weakness, or other sensory disturbances with or without specific physical examination findings. More severely injured patients may have an obvious neurologic deficit on physical examination.
- Patients may present with spinal shock, in which hypotension and bradycardia are commonly seen.
- Although hypotension in spinal shock is due to a transection of sympathetic tone, hypovolemic shock must be considered the cause of the hypotension until proven otherwise.
- Patients with spinal shock generally have pink, warm extremities and adequate urine output.
- Other signs of autonomic dysfunction may accompany spinal shock, such as gastrointestinal ileus, urinary retention, fecal incontinence, priapism, and loss of the normal ability to regulate body temperature.

DIAGNOSIS AND DIFFERENTIAL

- The mechanism of injury is useful in determining the most likely spine or spinal cord injuries (Table 164-1).
- Any neurologic complaints, even if transitory, must raise suspicion for a SCI. Palpation of the entire spine will identify any potential areas for spinal injury.
- A complete neurologic examination should include motor strength and tone (corticospinal tract), pain and temperature sensation (spinothalamic tract), proprioception and vibration sensation (dorsal columns), and reflexes.
- A rectal examination and bulbocavernosus reflex test should be performed. Preservation of rectal tone or reflexes indicates an incomplete spinal cord lesion.
- NEXUS criteria for cervical spine radiography are summarized in Table 164-2.[3]
- For the cervical spine, a minimum of three radiographic views (lateral, odontoid, and anteroposterior) are necessary. These views will identify most

TABLE 164-1 Cervical Spine Injuries: Mechanism of Injury

Flexion
 Anterior subluxation (hyperflexion sprain)
 Bilateral interfacetal dislocation
 Simple wedge (compression) fracture
 Clay-shoveler's (coal-shoveler's) fracture
 Flexion teardrop fracture

Flexion–rotation
 Unilateral interfacetal dislocation

Pillar fracture
 Fracture or separation (pedicolaminar fracture)

Vertical compression
 Jefferson burst fracture of atlas
 Burst (bursting, dispersion, axial-loading) fracture

Hyperextension
 Hyperextension dislocation
 Avulsion fracture of anterior arch of atlas
 Extension teardrop fracture
 Fracture of posterior arch of atlas
 Laminar fracture
 Traumatic spondylolisthesis ("hangman's" fracture)

Lateral flexion
 Uncinate process fracture

Injuries caused by diverse or poorly understood mechanisms
 Occipitoatlantal dissociation
 Occipital condylar fractures
 Dens fractures

SOURCE: Harris J: Spine, including soft tissue of the pharynx and neck, in Harris J, Harris W (eds): *The Radiology of Emergency Medicine,* 4th ed. Baltimore, Lippincott Williams & Wilkins, 2000, p. 137.

TABLE 164-2 NEXUS Criteria for Cervical Spine Radiography

According to NEXUS low-risk criteria, cervical spine radiography can be omitted for trauma patients only if they exhibit *all* of the following criteria:

No posterior midline cervical spine tenderness

No evidence of intoxication

Normal level of alertness

No focal neurologic deficit

No painful distracting injuries

bony injuries; they cannot, however, exclude ligamentous or occult bony injuries.

- Since occult fractures and ligamentous injuries may be missed on plain radiographs, clinical clearance of the cervical spine must be performed after a negative cervical spine series. Patients with painful distracting injuries, altered mental status, or intoxication should not undergo clinical clearance of the cervical spine.

- The characteristics and stability of common cervical spine fractures are summarized in Table 164-3.
- A Jefferson fracture is a burst fracture of C1 and usually occurs with an axial load injury. On the odontoid view the lateral masses of C1 will be displaced. If the displacement of the lateral masses on each side added together is greater than 7 mm, rupture of the transverse ligament is likely.
- Type I fractures of the odontoid include avulsions of the tip of the odontoid and are considered stable fractures.
- Type II fractures of the odontoid occur at the junction of the odontoid and the body of C2 and are the most common odontoid fracture.
- Type III fractures of the odontoid occur through the superior portion of C2 at the base of the dens.
- A hangman's fracture is located in the pedicles of C2, with anterior displacement of C2 on C3. These are caused by hyperextension injuries and are unstable fractures.

TABLE 164-3 Characteristics of Common Cervical Spine Fractures and Injuries, Arranged in Descending Order from the Most Unstable Fractures to the Least Unstable

TYPE OF FRACTURE	MECHANISM	OTHER FACTS	STABILITY
Occipitoatlantal dislocation	Skull is displaced from the cervical spine	Frequently results in death	Most unstable
Transverse ligament disruption	Diverse mechanism, possibly a blow to the occiput	Identified by examination of predental space (>3 mm)	Highly unstable
Odontoid fracture	Diverse mechanism	Classified as type I, II, or III	Depends on type of fracture
Flexion teardrop	Extreme flexion	Complete disruption of all ligamentous structures at the level of injury	Unstable
Bilateral facet dislocation	Hyperflexion	Disruption of all ligamentous structures occurs	Unstable
Burst fracture	Direct axial load	Fracture fragments may displace into spinal cord	Unstable
Hyperextension dislocation	Hyperextension	Complete tear of anterior longitudinal ligament and intervertebral disk, with disruption of posterior ligamentous complex	Unstable
Hangman's fracture (traumatic spondylolisthesis of the axis	Hyperextension	Located in pedicles of C2, with C2 displacing anteriorly on C3	Unstable
Extension teardrop	Hyperextension	Anterior longitudinal ligament avulses inferior portion of anterior vertebral body	Unstable in extension
Jefferson's fracture (burst fracture of C1)	Axial load	Lateral masses of C1 are displaced on odontoid view	Likely unstable
Unilateral facet dislocation	Flexion and rotation	Anteroposterior view will reveal the rotation	Mechanically stable unless associated with fracture
Anterior subluxation (a.k.a. hyperflexion sprain)	Hyperflexion	Failure of posterior ligamentous structures	Potentially unstable
Simpe wedge fracture	Hyperflexion	Posterior ligaments may be disrupted	Unstable if posterior element disruption occurs
Pillar fracture	Extension and rotation	Impaction of a superior vertebrae on the inferior articular mass occurs	Stable
Spinous process fracture	Hyperflexion	Intense flexion against contracted posterior erector spinal muscles	Isolated fractures are stable

- Hyperflexion injuries include anterior subluxation, clay-shoveler's fracture, simple wedge fractures, flexion teardrop fracture, and bilateral interfacetal dislocation.
- Unilateral facet dislocations result from flexion and rotation injuries.
- Extension and rotation injuries include pillar fractures and pedicolaminar fractures.
- Burst fractures result from vertical compression injuries and are unstable fractures.
- Hyperextension injuries include hyperextension dislocations, extension teardrop fractures, and laminar fractures.
- Uncinate process fractures result from lateral flexion injuries.
- Flexion and extension views may indicate ligamentous injury. A step-off of 3.7 mm or an angulation of greater than 11 degrees indicates cervical instability.[4]
- Ten percent of patients with spine fracture in one segment will have a second fracture in another. Therefore, determination of spinal column injury at one level mandates radiographic evaluation of the entire spine.
- The thoracolumbar spine is the second most commonly injured area of the spine. This is due to the high degree of mobility associated with this area.
- A Chance fracture is most often a fracture of L1, and occurs from flexion injury, often in passengers involved in motor vehicle crashes who are wearing only lap seat belts.
- Computed tomography (CT) scans are indicated for all patients with fractures or dislocations that can be seen on plain films.
- CT scan, especially with 3-D reconstructions, can define the anatomy of the fracture and reveal the extent of spinal canal impingement by bone fragments.

- Magnetic resonance imaging (MRI) offers better determination of neurologic, ligamentous, muscular, and soft tissue anatomy and injury. MRI is indicated in patients with neurologic findings without a clear explanation following plain films and/or CT scan.
- The difference between complete and incomplete lesions is crucial; prognosis for complete lesions is poor, while patients with incomplete lesions can be expected to have at least some degree of improvement.
- The characteristics of some of the more common spinal cord syndromes are listed in Table 164-4.
- Spinal cord injury without radiographic abnormality (SCIWORA) is an entity that is most commonly seen in the pediatric population.[5]
- Spine or SCI in children should raise a suspicion for child abuse.

EMERGENCY DEPARTMENT CARE AND DISPOSITION

- Airway assessment and management with in-line cervical immobilization is the first and most pressing treatment in the emergency department.
- For patients with cervical spine injury (especially for injuries of C5 and above) a low threshold for endotracheal intubation should be maintained. Diaphragmatic weakness or paralysis can lead to hypoventilation or hypoxemia.
- The patient should be placed on high-flow oxygen and have two large-bore IVs established.
- Fluid resuscitation facilitates spinal cord resuscitation; obvious bleeding must be controlled and a rapid assessment of other life-threatening injuries must ensue.

TABLE 164-4 Spinal Cord Syndromes

SYNDROME	ETIOLOGY	SYMPTOMS	PROGNOSIS
Anterior cord	Direct anterior cord compression; Flexion of cervical spine; Thrombosis of anterior spinal artery	Complete paralysis below the lesion with loss of pain and temperature sensation; Preservation of proprioception and vibratory function	Poor
Central cord	Hyperextension injuries; Disruption of blood flow to the spinal cord; Cervical spinal stenosis	Quadriparesis—greater in the upper extremities than the lower extremities; some loss of pain and temperature sensation, also greater in the upper extremities	Good
Brown-Séquard	Transverse hemisection of the spinal cord; Unilateral cord compression	Ipsilateral spastic paresis, loss of proprioception and vibratory sensation and contralateral loss of pain and temperature sensation	Good
Cauda equina	Peripheral nerve injury	Variable motor and sensory loss in the lower extremities, sciatica, bowel/bladder dysfunction and "saddle anesthesia"	Good
Spinal shock	Partial or complete injury, usually at the T6 level and above	Areflexia, loss of sensation, and flaccid paralysis below the level of the lesion; a flaccid bladder and loss of rectal tone; bradycardia and hypotension	Complete lesions have a poor prognosis; Incomplete lesions have some degree of recovery

- Patients should be log rolled (while maintaining in-line spinal immobilization that prevents secondary injury to the spine and preserves residual spinal cord function) to identify any obvious fractures or associated injuries.
- Patients should be removed from hard backboards to prevent skin breakdown and pressure sores.
- Spinal shock should be treated with oxygen, IV fluids, and vasopressors, such as norepinephrine or dopamine, as necessary.
- For blunt trauma patients who have sustained a SCI with neurologic deficits, methylprednisolone should be administered if the patient presents within 8 hours of injury. The dose is 30 mg/kg IV over 15 minutes, followed by 45 minutes with no medication, and then 5.4 mg/kg/h for 23 hours.
- Methylprednisolone therapy has not been proven to be beneficial in penetrating spinal cord injury.
- Penetrating spinal injuries should receive empiric antibiotics in the emergency department. Patients with progressive neurologic deterioration require operative intervention. Most injuries that do not progress are treated nonoperatively.
- Any patient with a significant injury to the spine or spinal cord or any patient with significant associated injury should be admitted to the hospital.

REFERENCES

1. Denis F: The three column spine and its significance in the classification of acute thoracolumbar spinal injuries. *Spine* 8: 817, 1983.
2. Mazur JM, Stauffer ED: Unrecognized spinal instability associated with seemingly "simple" cervical compression fractures. *Spine* 8:687, 1983.
3. Hoffman JR, Mower WR, Wolfson AB, et al: Validity of a set of clinical criteria to rule out injury to the cervical spine in patients with blunt trauma. *N Engl J Med* 343:94, 2000.
4. Panjabi MM, Tech D, White AA: Basic biomechanics of the spine. *Neurosurgery* 7:76, 1980.
5. Gupta SK, Khosla RK, Sharma BS, et al: Spinal cord injury without radiographic abnormality in adults. *Spinal Cord* 38: 129, 2000.

For further reading in *Emergency Medicine: A Comprehensive Study Guide,* 6th ed., see Chap. 256, "Spinal Cord Injuries," by Bonny J. Baron and Thomas M. Scalea; and Chap. 272, "Injuries to the Spine," by James L. Larson, Jr.

165 MAXILLOFACIAL TRAUMA

C. Crawford Mechem

CLINICAL FEATURES AND DIAGNOSIS

- In patients who have sustained maxillofacial trauma, important points that should be obtained in the history include mechanism of injury, loss of consciousness, facial paresthesias, malocclusion, and visual changes such as diplopia.[1]
- Monocular diplopia suggests lens dislocation or corneal or retinal injury, while binocular diplopia implies dysfunction of the extraocular muscles or nerves.
- The physical examination should begin with a close inspection of the face, evaluating for elongation or asymmetry. The muscles of facial expression should be assessed.
- Ecchymoses around the eyes (raccoon's eyes) or over the mastoids (Battle's sign) suggest basilar skull fracture.
- A posttraumatic Bell's palsy may be the result of a temporal bone fracture.
- Subcutaneous air is pathognomonic for a sinus or nasal fracture.
- Simultaneous palpation of the zygomatic arches will reveal any asymmetry.
- Facial stability is assessed by grasping the maxillary arch with the mouth open. LeFort fractures are diagnosed by rocking the maxillary arch while feeling the central face for movement with the opposite hand (Fig. 165-1).
- In LeFort I, a transverse fracture separates the body of the maxilla from the lower portion of the pterygoid plate and nasal septum. With stress on the maxilla, only the hard palate and upper teeth move.
- A pyramidal fracture of the central maxilla and the palate defines a LeFort II. Facial tugging moves the nose but not the eyes.
- LeFort III, or cranial-facial disjunction, occurs when the facial skeleton separates from the skull. The entire face shifts with tugging.
- A LeFort IV fracture includes the frontal bone as well as the midface.
- A sensory examination of the face should be performed. Anesthesia may be seen due to nerve contusion or bony fracture.
- Damage to the infraorbital nerve, often from a blowout or orbital rim fracture, may result in anesthesia of the ipsilateral upper lip, nasal mucosa at the vestibule, lower eyelid, and maxillary teeth.
- Lower lip and lower tooth anesthesia may occur with mandible fractures.

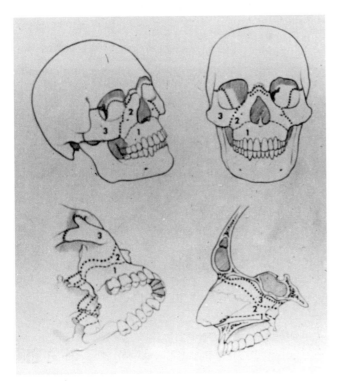

FIG. 165-1. Schematic of midfacial fracture lines. (Reproduced with permission from Dingman RO, Natvig P: *Surgery of Facial Fractures.* Philadelphia: Saunders, 1964, p. 248.)

- If the patient is unable to see the Snellen eye chart, the ability to count fingers or perceive light should be documented.
- The pupils should be examined for reactivity, alignment, and shape. A teardrop shape may suggest globe rupture or penetration.
- A swinging light test is performed to check for a Marcus Gunn pupil, which initially dilates (rather than constricts) when first illuminated, indicating damage to the retina or optic nerve.
- The eyes are checked for hyphema, preferably with the patient in a seated position. The presence of subconjunctival hemorrhage or eyelid trauma should be noted.
- Penetrating trauma to the medial third of the lids may cause damage to the lacrimal apparatus.
- Diplopia, especially on upward gaze, may be due to fractures of the zygomatic arch or orbital floor.
- Pain with extraocular motions may suggest an occult orbital fracture.
- The distance between the medial canthi, normally 35 to 40 mm, should be measured. Widening, or telecanthus, suggests serious nasoethmoidal-orbital complex trauma, as does medial canthus tenderness.
- Widening of the distance between the pupils, or hypertelorism, results from orbital dislocation and is often associated with blindness.

- The nose should be examined for deformity, crepitus, or subcutaneous air. Septal hematoma may be observed, appearing as a bluish, bulging mass on a widened septum.
- Cerebrospinal fluid (CSF) rhinorrhea is suggested by clear nasal drainage mixed with blood that forms a double ring, or halo sign, when dropped on a paper towel or bed sheet.
- The ears should be examined for subperichondral hematoma and the canals inspected for lacerations, CSF leak, hemotympanum, or tympanic membrane rupture.
- The mouth should be inspected for lacerations, malocclusion, tooth trauma, or lip or gingival anesthesia, often due to fracture-induced nerve injury.
- To assess for mandibular fracture, the physician may have the patient bite down on a tongue blade, then twist it in an attempt to break it. Patients with a mandible fracture will open their mouth, whereas those with an intact mandible will break the tongue blade.[2]
- The choice and timing of radiographs depends on the stability of the patient. Associated head, chest, and abdominal injuries take precedence.
- Plain films are excellent as screening studies. Facial computed tomography (CT) imaging is frequently required to make the definitive diagnosis and guide surgical management.

EMERGENCY DEPARTMENT CARE AND DISPOSITION

- Initial management should focus on airway control. A chin lift or jaw thrust without neck extension often restores airway patency.
- In severe mandible fractures, loss of bony support may result in posterior displacement of the tongue. To prevent airway obstruction, the tongue should be pulled forward with a gauze pad, towel clips, or a suture passed through the tip.
- When endotracheal intubation is required, the oral route is preferred because of concern for nasocranial intubation or severe epistaxis with the nasal route.
- Rapid sequence intubation carries the risk of inability to ventilate the patient if intubation is unsuccessful.
- Alternative strategies include awake intubation or use of sedatives, such as benzodiazepines or ketamine, at doses that minimize respiratory depression.
- If patients are administered paralytic agents, equipment for emergent cricothyroidotomy should be at the bedside and the neck prepped.
- The laryngeal mask airway may be used as a bridge to intubation or surgical airway, provided that the hypopharynx remains intact.

- Hemorrhage may be controlled with direct pressure. Blind clamping should be avoided because of the risk of damaging the facial nerve or parotid duct.
- Pharyngeal bleeding may require packing around a cuffed endotracheal tube.
- In LeFort fractures, bleeding may be controlled by manually realigning the fragments.
- Severe epistaxis requires direct pressure or nasal packing. In massive nasopharyngeal bleeding, passing a Foley catheter along the floor of the nose and inflating the balloon may be life-saving.

CARE OF SPECIFIC FACIAL FRACTURES

FRONTAL SINUS/FRONTAL BONE FRACTURES

- These injuries usually result from blunt trauma to the frontal bone and are frequently associated with intracranial injury.
- Young children have a high incidence of frontal bone injuries due to its prominence.
- Late complications include cranial empyema and mucopyocele. Consultation with an ear, nose, and throat (ENT) specialist or neurosurgeon may be warranted.
- Antibiotics covering sinus pathogens should be administered. These include first-generation cephalosporins, amoxicillin-clavulanate, or trimethoprim-sulfamethoxazole.
- Depressed fractures or posterior wall involvement warrants admission for IV antibiotics.
- Patients with isolated fractures of the anterior wall may be treated on an outpatient basis.

NASOETHMOIDAL-ORBITAL INJURIES

- These fractures usually result from trauma to the bridge of the nose or medial orbital wall.
- If the medial canthus is tender, evidence of CSF rhinorrhea should be sought. When CSF rhinorrhea is present, a CT of facial bones should be ordered.
- If a nasoethmoidal-orbital fracture is noted, a maxillofacial surgeon should be consulted.
- Blowout fractures are the most common orbital fracture and occur when a blunt object strikes the globe, causing rupture of the orbital floor. Suggestive physical examination findings include enophthalmos, infraorbital anesthesia, diplopia on upward gaze, and a step-off deformity on palpation of the infraorbital rim.
- If a blowout fracture is diagnosed clinically or with plain films, a CT scan should be obtained to determine the surface area of the broken floor.

- Indications for surgery include enophthalmos or persistent diplopia.[3,4]
- Antibiotics covering sinus pathogens are often recommended for patients with subcutaneous emphysema.
- The patient also should be advised to minimize nose blowing to prevent accumulation of subcutaneous air.
- The oculomotor and ophthalmic divisions of the trigeminal nerve course through the superior orbital fissure. An orbital fracture involving this canal leads to the superior orbital fissure syndrome, characterized by paralysis of extraocular motions, ptosis, and periorbital anesthesia.
- When the orbital apex is involved, the patient may develop these symptoms and blindness. The swinging light test and visual acuity determination are crucial in making this diagnosis. Patients with this syndrome require emergent ophthalmologic consultation.

NASAL FRACTURES

- Cosmesis and the ability to breathe are usually the main concerns in patients with nasal fractures.
- A septal hematoma is treated by local anesthesia with benzocaine or cocaine, followed by incision of the inferior border with a no. 11 blade, which will allow it to drain. Packing the nose will prevent reaccumulation.
- All other patients with suspected nasal fracture should be referred for re-evaluation by an ENT specialist in 5 to 7 days.

ZYGOMATIC FRACTURES

- Zygoma fractures occur in two major patterns: tripod fractures and isolated zygomatic arch fractures.
- Tripod fractures involve the infraorbital rim, diastasis of the zygomaticofrontal suture, and disruption of the zygomaticotemporal junction at the arch.
- Plain films are usually adequate to diagnose isolated zygomatic arch fractures, whereas a facial CT is warranted if a tripod fracture is suspected.
- Tripod fractures require admission for open reduction and internal fixation.
- Patients with isolated fractures of the zygomatic arch can have elective outpatient repair.

MAXILLARY FRACTURES

- These are high-energy fractures and are often seen in victims of multisystem trauma. Patients frequently require endotracheal intubation for airway control.

- Visual acuity should be tested, especially with LeFort III fractures, where the incidence of blindness is high.
- A CT scan of the face can be obtained in conjunction with neuroimaging.
- Patients with complex fractures require admission for open reduction and internal fixation.

MANDIBULAR FRACTURES AND TEMPOROMANDIBULAR DISLOCATION

- Patients with open fractures require admission and IV antibiotics. Penicillin, clindamycin, or a first-generation cephalosporin is recommended.
- Many patients with closed fractures may be managed on an outpatient basis. A Barton bandage, an elastic bandage wrapped around the jaw and head, may be worn for comfort.
- To reduce a temporomandibular dislocation, the physician stands behind the seated patient and presses downward and backward on the posterior molars or the mandibular ridge using thumbs wrapped in gauze. A Barton bandage is applied and the patient is discharged on a liquid diet with close follow-up.

REFERENCES

1. Major MS, Macgregor A, Bumpous JM: Patterns of maxillofacial injuries as a function of automobile restraint use. *Laryngoscope* 110:608, 2000.
2. Alonso LL, Purcell TB: Accuracy of the tongue blade test in patients with suspected mandibular fracture. *J Emerg Med* 13: 297, 1995.
3. Bhattacharya J, Moseley IF, Fells P: The role of plain radiography in the management of suspected orbital blow-out fractures. *Br J Radiol* 70:29, 1997.
4. Courtney DJ, Thomas S, Whitfield PH: Isolated orbital blowout fractures: Survey and review. *Br J Oral Maxillofac Surg* 38:496, 2000.

For further reading in *Emergency Medicine: A Comprehensive Study Guide,* 6th ed., see Chap. 257, "Maxillofacial Trauma," by Nael Hasan and Stephen A. Colucciello.

166 NECK TRAUMA

Walter N. Simmons

EPIDEMIOLOGY

- Multiple injuries are sustained 44 to 52% of the time with penetrating neck trauma.[1–5]

PATHOPHYSIOLOGY

- The neck contains a high concentration of vascular, aerodigestive, and spinal structures in a relatively confined space.
- The Roon and Christensen anatomic classification divides the neck into three zones (Table 166-1).[2]
- The at-risk structures located in zone I are the vertebral and proximal carotid arteries, major thoracic vessels, superior mediastinum, lungs, esophagus, trachea, thoracic duct, and spinal cord.
- The at-risk structures located in zone II are the carotid and vertebral arteries, jugular vein, esophagus, trachea, larynx, and the spinal cord.
- The at-risk structures located in zone III are the distal carotid and vertebral arteries, pharynx, and the spinal cord.
- The platysma is the most superficial structure beneath the skin and serves as an important planar landmark in evaluating penetrating neck injuries. Injuries that violate the platysma require more aggressive evaluation.
- Beneath the platysma is the deep cervical fascia and the fascial compartments that support the muscles, vessels, and viscera of the neck.
- The tight fascial compartments offer a tamponade effect, which helps limit potential for external bleeding from vascular injuries. However, bleeding within this confined space can result in extrinsic compression and airway compromise.

CLINICAL FEATURES

- Blunt and penetrating laryngeal or pharyngeal trauma can cause dysphonia, stridor, hemoptysis, hematemesis, dysphagia, neck emphysema, and dyspnea progressing to respiratory arrest.

TABLE 166-1   Zones of the Neck

Zone I	Base of the neck to the cricoid cartilage
Zone II	Cricoid cartilage to the angle of the mandible
Zone III	Angle of the mandible to the base of the skull

TABLE 166-2 Signs and Symptoms of Neck Injury

HARD SIGNS	SOFT SIGNS
Hypotension in emergency department	Hypotension in field
Active arterial bleeding	History of arterial bleeding
Diminished carotid pulse	Tracheal deviation
Expanding hematoma	Nonexpanding large hematoma
Thrill/bruit	Apical capping on chest radiograph
Lateralizing signs	Stridor
Hemothorax >1000 mL	Hoarseness
Air or bubbling in wound	Vocal cord paralysis
Hemoptysis	Subcutaneous emphysema
Hematemesis	Seventh cranial nerve injury
	Unexplained bradycardia (without CNS injury)

- It is not uncommon for an expanding hematoma in the neck to cause significant mass effect that leads to airway compromise.
- Patients may present with signs of shock (diaphoresis, tachycardia, and hypotension) after experiencing significant blood loss.
- Neurologic injury demonstrated by subjective complaints of pain and paresthesias, or more objective findings of hemiplegia, quadriplegia, and coma may be observed.
- Significant esophageal injury may initially be associated with complaints of dysphagia and hematemesis.
- All symptoms and signs associated with neck trauma require diagnostic evaluation, but hard signs are more often associated with significant injury (Table 166-2).
- Strangulation may cause the formation of petechiae of the skin above the site of injury or in the subconjunctivae.[6–9]

DIAGNOSIS AND DIFFERENTIAL

- All patients with neck trauma should be quickly evaluated for hemodynamic stability, obvious aerodigestive injury, and violation of the platysma muscle.
- Probing of neck wounds in the emergency department is not indicated; full exploration should occur in the operating room where the capacity for proximal and distal vascular control is optimal.
- Plain radiographs can identify cervical spine injury, the presence of any penetrating foreign body, air in the soft tissues, and soft tissue swelling.
- A chest radiograph is warranted for any suspected thoracic cavity penetration.
- Additional diagnostic procedures to be considered, in conjunction with surgical consultation, include ar-

teriography or duplex sonography for suspected arterial injury, computed tomography (CT) scanning of the larynx or cervical spine, endoscopy of the airway and esophagus, or contrast studies of the esophagus.

- Stable patients with zone I injuries should undergo angiography, esophagram, and/or esophagoscopy.
- Patients with zone III injuries should undergo angiography.
- Controversy surrounds the management of stable patients with zone II injuries. They may undergo immediate surgical exploration or be evaluated with angiography, esophagram, and/or esophagoscopy.
- Patients with any symptoms suggestive of laryngotracheal injury require laryngoscopy and bronchoscopy.
- Helical CT scanning may be useful in stable patients to visualize the trajectory of penetrating injuries and their proximity to vital structures.
- Vascular injury is most common with penetrating trauma, although major vessel injury can occur due to blunt trauma and may simulate an acute stroke.
- Neurologic injuries include generalized brain ischemia (seen primarily with strangulation), spinal cord trauma, nerve root damage, and peripheral nerve damage.
- Cervical spine injury initially may present without neurologic deficit, but the spine can be cleared clinically in selected blunt trauma and gunshot wound victims.
- Gastrointestinal injuries are often occult and generally require evaluation by endoscopy or contrast radiography.

EMERGENCY DEPARTMENT CARE AND DISPOSITION

- Standard trauma protocols for evaluation and stabilization of trauma patients should be initiated (see Chap. 159). High-flow oxygen, cardiac and respiratory monitoring, and IV access should be quickly established.
- Any patient with acute respiratory distress, airway compromise from blood secretions, evidence of expanding hematoma on the neck, massive subcutaneous emphysema, tracheal shift, impending respiratory arrest, or severe alteration in mental status necessitates the establishment of a definitive airway. Endotracheal intubation is indicated for these patients.
- In cases where oral or nasal intubation is not possible or is contraindicated, cricothyrotomy or transtracheal jet insufflation should be performed.
- The cervical spine should be immobilized and assessed, as clinically appropriate.
- Injuries in proximity to the base of the neck predispose patients to simultaneous injury to the chest. The

chest must also be assessed for injuries such as pneumothorax and hemothorax, which are primarily seen in penetrating trauma.

- Direct pressure can often control active hemorrhage.
- Blind clamping of blood vessels is contraindicated due to the complex vital anatomy compressed into a relatively small space and the danger of causing further injury with a misguided surgical instrument.
- Fluid resuscitation should begin with crystalloid followed by blood products if needed.
- Minor penetrating wounds that do not violate the platysma muscle require standard meticulous wound care and closure. These patients should be observed for several hours in the emergency department. If asymptomatic and hemodynamically stable after 4 to 6 hours, these patients may be discharged home with close follow-up.
- Wounds that violate the platysma muscle mandate surgical consultation. These patients should be admitted for surgical exploration or for further diagnostic evaluation of any significant deep structure injury.
- Patients with blunt neck trauma initially may present with subtle signs of injury and may develop significant symptoms on a delayed basis, particularly those with a strangulation mechanism. After a period of observation, asymptomatic patients may be discharged with close follow-up, although a low threshold for admission should be maintained.
- Hoarseness, dysphagia, and dyspnea are indications for more extensive evaluation in patients with blunt neck trauma.[10]

REFERENCES

1. Irish JC, Hekkenberg R, Gullane PJ, et al: Penetrating and blunt neck trauma: 10 year review of a Canadian experience. *Can J Surg* 40:33, 1997.
2. Roon AJ, Christensen N: Evaluation and treatment of penetrating cervical injuries. *J Trauma* 19:391, 1979.
3. Shearer VE, Giescke AH: Airway management for patients with penetrating neck trauma: A retrospective study. *Anesth Analg* 77:1135, 1993.
4. Baron BJ, Sinert RH, Kohl L, et al: The value of physical examination in penetrating neck trauma. *Acad Emerg Med* 4:347, 1997.
5. Sclafani SJA, Cavaliere G, Atweh N, et al: The role of angiography in penetrating neck trauma. *J Trauma* 31:557, 1991.
6. Fuhrman GM, Stieg FH, Buerk CA: Blunt laryngeal trauma: Classification ad management protocol. *J Trauma* 30:87, 1990.
7. Li MS, Smith BM, Espinosa J, et al: Nonpenetrating trauma to the carotid artery. Seven cases and a literature review. *J Trauma* 36:265, 1994.
8. Watridge CB, Muhlbauer MS, Lowery RD: Traumatic carotid artery dissection: Diagnosis and treatment. *J Neurosurg* 71:854, 1989.
9. Fabian TC, Patton JH, Croce MA, et al: Blunt carotid injury, importance of early diagnosis and anticoagulant therapy. *Ann Surg* 223:513, 1996.
10. Iserson KV: Strangulation: A review of ligature, manual, and postural neck compression injuries. *Ann Emerg Med* 13:179, 1984.

For further reading in *Emergency Medicine: A Comprehensive Study Guide,* 6th ed., see Chap. 258, "Penetrating and Blunt Neck Trauma," by Bonny J. Baron.

167 CARDIOTHORACIC TRAUMA
Jeffrey N. Glaspy

EPIDEMIOLOGY

- Thoracic trauma accounts for 25% of civilian trauma deaths.
- Mortality is less than 5% for isolated chest trauma, but rises to 33% for severe multisystem injuries.

PATHOPHYSIOLOGY

- Penetrating injuries to the thorax frequently result in pneumothorax or hemothorax. Hemothorax accompanies pneumothorax in 75% of cases.
- Blunt trauma causes injury by several mechanisms: compression (organ rupture), direct trauma (fractures, soft tissue injuries), and acceleration/deceleration forces (vessel shear and tear).
- Massive hemothorax causes life-threatening conditions by three mechanisms: (1) hypovolemia (1500 mL of blood is considered massive hemothorax in adults), (2) hypoxia (from lung collapse), and (3) increased intrathoracic pressure (leading to vena cava collapse and compression of the pulmonary parenchyma).

GENERAL PRINCIPLES AND CONDITIONS

- All patients should be assessed with initial consideration for airway, breathing, and circulation. Cervical spine immobilization should be maintained via in-line stabilization until a spinal injury can be safely and completely excluded.

- In all cases of significant respiratory distress, the airway should be secured and adequate oxygenation and ventilation provided.
- Indications for endotracheal intubation include need to protect airway patency, need to optimize oxygenation or ventilation, and planned procedures necessitating intubation (general anesthesia, bronchoscopy).
- The patient's breathing and oxygenation should be rapidly assessed. High-flow oxygen may help prevent secondary injury from hypoxia.
- Tracheal position and breath sounds should be examined.
- The presence of bowel sounds in the chest should suggest the possibility of a diaphragmatic injury.
- Inequality of breath sounds may suggest a pneumothorax, hemothorax, or an improperly placed endotracheal tube.
- It is essential to immediately recognize tension pneumothorax, cardiac tamponade, flail chest, open pneumothorax, and massive hemothorax.
- Any associated hemorrhage must be controlled and any associated injuries must be stabilized.
- Strong consideration must be given to associated abdominal and pelvic injuries.
- If subclavian venous cannulation is required, it should be placed on the side of the injury.
- In patients with cardiac arrest due to chest trauma, external cardiac compression is of no value and may be harmful secondary to additional trauma to thoracic and abdominal organs or vessels.
- If cardiac compression is deemed potentially beneficial, emergency department (ED) thoracotomy and internal cardiac compression are warranted.

CHEST WALL INJURIES

CLINICAL FEATURES AND DIAGNOSIS

- Small open chest wounds (sucking chest wounds) can act as one-way valves, allowing air to enter during inspiration, but none to exit during expiration. This will result in an expanding pneumothorax.
- Small open chest wounds should be covered immediately by a sterile petroleum gauze dressing, and a chest tube should be placed at a separate site to relieve the pneumothorax.
- Injuries with large amounts of chest wall tissue loss will require mechanical ventilation and surgical repair.
- Patients with subcutaneous emphysema should be presumed to have a pneumothorax, even if the initial chest radiograph does not reveal a pneumothorax.
- If severe subcutaneous emphysema is palpated, then a major bronchial injury should be suspected.

- Clavicular fractures occasionally may injure the subclavian vein, producing a large hematoma or venous thrombosis.
- Rib fractures should be assumed to be present in any patient with localized tenderness over one or more ribs after chest trauma. Up to 50% of rib fractures may not be apparent on initial chest radiographs.
- Fractures of the first or second ribs suggest high-force injuries and are frequently associated with other significant thoracic injuries.
- Flail chest refers to segmental fractures (ie, fractures in two or more locations on the same rib) in three or more adjacent ribs.
- Flail chest is characterized by paradoxical inward movement of the involved portion of the chest wall during spontaneous inspiration and outward movement during expiration.
- Sternal fractures should alert the physician to possible underlying injuries, especially to the heart or great vessels.

EMERGENCY DEPARTMENT CARE AND DISPOSITION

- Bleeding from chest wall injuries is best controlled by direct pressure. Probing of these wounds is not recommended in the ED.
- If significant subcutaneous emphysema is noted, then a pneumothorax should be presumed to be present, and a chest tube should be inserted, especially if endotracheal intubation is imminent.
- For rib fractures, adequate analgesia (with narcotic analgesics) and pulmonary toilet are the mainstays of treatment.
- Patients with multiple rib fractures should be admitted for 24 to 48 hours if they cannot cough and clear secretions, are elderly, or have pre-existing pulmonary disease.
- Intercostal nerve blocks, intrapleural administration of anesthetics, and epidural analgesia should be considered in patients with intractable pain.
- The preferred treatment of flail chest injuries is analgesia to allow the patient to fully expand the underlying lung, with a goal of improving ventilation and pulmonary toilet.
- Indications for ventilatory support include three or more associated injuries, severe head trauma, comorbid pulmonary disease, fracture of eight or more ribs, or age greater than 65 years. Surgical repair of flail chest is controversial.[1,2]
- Patients with sternal fractures should have a screening electrocardiogram (ECG) for blunt myocardial injury. If the patient's vital signs and ECG are normal, then a repeat ECG should be obtained in 6 hours.[3] If the re-

peat ECG is normal, no further work-up for blunt myocardial injury is required.

LUNG INJURIES

CLINICAL FEATURES AND DIAGNOSIS

- The diagnosis of a tension pneumothorax should be made on physical examination and not by chest radiograph.
- Signs and symptoms of a tension pneumothorax include dyspnea, hypoperfusion, distended neck veins, decreased or absent breath sounds on the affected side, hyperresonant percussion on the affected side, and deviation of the trachea away from the affected side.
- Tension pneumothorax needs to be recognized and treated immediately.
- Pulmonary contusions are defined as direct damage to the lung resulting in both hemorrhage and edema in the absence of a pulmonary laceration.
- Two sources of injury occur in pulmonary contusion. The first is the direct tissue injury and the second results from fluid administration during resuscitation.
- The radiographic diagnosis of pulmonary contusion may be delayed for up to 6 hours.
- Hemothorax should be considered in any trauma patient with unilateral decreased breath sounds.
- Volumes of blood as low as 200 to 300 mL are usually visualized on an upright chest radiograph. However, volumes in excess of 1 L may be missed on a supine chest radiograph.
- If a pneumothorax is suspected but not seen on the initial chest radiograph, an expiratory chest film may facilitate diagnosis.
- Subcutaneous emphysema in the neck or the presence of a crunching sound (Hamman's sign) over the heart during systole suggests the presence of pneumomediastinum.
- Although readily seen on computed tomography (CT) imaging, pneumomediastinum may be missed on chest radiograph.
- It is essential to evaluate for associated injury to the larynx, trachea, major bronchi, pharynx, or esophagus.

EMERGENCY DEPARTMENT CARE AND DISPOSITION

- When a tension pneumothorax is suspected, immediate needle thoracostomy with a 14-gauge IV catheter in the second intercostal space, midclavicular line is mandatory.
- Needle thoracostomy converts a tension pneumothorax into an open pneumothorax, and often significantly improves the patient's clinical condition. Subsequent placement of a chest tube is required.
- The treatment of pulmonary contusions includes maintenance of adequate ventilation, pain control, and adequate pulmonary toilet.
- Patients with pulmonary contusion who have more than 25% of total lung involvement frequently require mechanical ventilation. Mechanical ventilation with the use of positive end-expiratory pressure may be required, even if less than 25% of the lung volume is involved.
- If a hemothorax or non–tension pneumothorax is suspected in a patient with severe respiratory distress, a chest tube should be inserted prior to obtaining a chest radiograph.
- Tube thoracostomy with a 36 or 40 F chest tube is the mainstay of treatment of a hemothorax.
- Ongoing assessment of blood loss from the chest tube is essential.
- Indications for thoracotomy include: initial drainage of 1500 mL of blood from the chest tube, drainage of 100 mL of blood per hour for six or more hours, persistent air leakage or failure of the lung to completely re-expand after tube thoracostomy, or clinical judgment of the thoracic surgeon in the face of a hemodynamically unstable patient.
- Chest tube drainage of occult pneumothorax (one seen on CT scan but not on plain film) is not required unless the patient requires mechanical ventilation.
- A chest radiograph should be obtained in all patients after insertion of a chest tube.
- Small pneumothoraces that have not expanded on serial chest radiographs taken 6 to 12 hours apart do not usually require chest tube insertion; however, admission for serial examination is recommended.

TRACHEOBRONCHIAL INJURIES

- Most injuries to major bronchi are due to deceleration shearing forces on mobile bronchi from the more fixed proximal structures, although compression against vertebral bodies or forced expiration against a closed glottis may also damage bronchi.
- Dyspnea, hemoptysis, subcutaneous emphysema, Hamman's sign, and sternal tenderness are the most common presenting signs and symptoms, although approximately 10% are asymptomatic.
- On chest radiograph, a large pneumothorax, pneumomediastinum, deep cervical emphysema, or endotracheal tube balloon that appears round, all suggest tracheobronchial injury.
- Most tracheobronchial injuries occur within 2 cm of the carina or at the origin of lobar bronchi.
- Management includes assuring adequate ventilation

and referral for immediate bronchoscopy to evaluate and treat the injury.

- Injuries of the cervical trachea usually occur at the junction of the trachea and cricoid cartilage and are caused by direct trauma.
- Inspiratory stridor is common and indicates a 70 to 80% obstruction.
- Orotracheal intubation, preferably over a bronchoscope, should be attempted.
- If gentle intubation is not possible, a formal tracheostomy should be performed.

DIAPHRAGMATIC INJURIES

- The majority of diaphragmatic injuries are caused by penetrating trauma.
- The incidence of left- versus right-sided diaphragmatic injuries may be equal, although left-sided injuries are more commonly diagnosed, as right-sided lesions may be masked due to the liver blocking herniation of abdominal contents.[4]
- Evidence of intrathoracic injury from a penetrating abdominal wound should alert the physician to the likely possibility of diaphragmatic disruption.
- With blunt trauma, any abnormality of the diaphragm or lower lung fields on chest radiograph should arouse suspicion for diaphragmatic tear.
- CT scan and upper gastrointestinal series may diagnose less obvious diaphragmatic injuries. However, many of these injuries are only diagnosed on laparotomy or thoracotomy.
- The treatment of these injuries is surgical repair of the diaphragm.

PENETRATING INJURIES TO THE HEART

CLINICAL FEATURES AND DIAGNOSIS

- Both blunt and penetrating cardiac injuries have the potential to cause cardiac tamponade.
- The presentation of cardiac tamponade includes Beck's triad of hypotension, distended neck veins, and muffled heart tones.
- Other causes of Beck's triad include tension pneumothorax, myocardial dysfunction, and systemic air embolism.
- A hypotensive patient with penetrating chest injury anywhere near the heart should be considered to have sustained a cardiac injury until proven otherwise.
- Penetrating wounds to the heart are usually rapidly fatal, with fewer than 25% reaching the hospital alive.
- Factors affecting survival include the weapon used,

the size of myocardial injury, the chamber injured, coronary artery damage, the presence of tamponade, associated injuries, and the time taken to reach the hospital.

- Chest radiographs are rarely helpful in diagnosing acute cardiac injury, and changes on ECG are usually nonspecific.
- Bedside ultrasonography and transesophageal echocardiography (TEE) are rapid and sensitive modalities for diagnosing pericardial effusion and tamponade.
- Pericardiocentesis has limited value in the evaluation of patients with possible cardiac injury due to a high incidence of false-positive and false-negative aspirates.[5]
- Pericardiocentesis should be reserved for patients in extremis, when the possibility of tamponade must be excluded in a matter of seconds.
- In the hemodynamically stable patient, when echocardiography is not available, a subxiphoid pericardial window can be performed in the operating room under general anesthesia.

EMERGENCY DEPARTMENT CARE AND DISPOSITION

- The initial management of patients with penetrating cardiac injury includes airway, breathing, and circulation.
- Two large-bore IV catheters should be placed, with one catheter in a leg vein in the event that the superior vena cava or one of its major branches is injured.
- Patients in shock who do not respond to adequate fluid resuscitation and who are suspected of having a cardiac injury should undergo emergent thoracotomy.
- The immediate treatment of cardiac tamponade is pericardiocentesis, with subsequent surgical repair.
- An initial fluid bolus should be given to increase filling pressure in the right atrium; however, this effect is transitory and decompression of the tamponade by pericardiocentesis or surgery will be needed.
- A patient with penetrating thoracic trauma who loses vital signs just prior to hospital arrival may require emergent ED thoracotomy to assess for and treat pericardial or cardiac wall injury.

BLUNT INJURIES TO THE HEART

CLINICAL FEATURES AND DIAGNOSIS

- The most common mechanism of injury causing blunt cardiac trauma is a deceleration injury, such as that seen in motor vehicle crashes (even at speeds less than 20 mph); other causes include falls, direct blows

to the chest, crush injuries, blast injuries, and athletic trauma.
- Blunt cardiac trauma may result in rupture of an outer chamber wall, septal rupture, valvular injuries (with the aortic valve being the most commonly injured), direct myocardial injury (contusion), laceration or thrombosis of coronary arteries, and pericardial injury.
- A history of moderate to severe chest or upper abdominal injury, even without abnormalities on physical examination, should raise the suspicion of cardiac injury.
- Blunt myocardial injury is a term used to include myocardial contusion and myocardial concussion.
- The areas most commonly affected by blunt myocardial injury include the anterior right ventricular wall, the anterior interventricular septum, and the anterior-apical left ventricle.
- The most common clinical features of blunt myocardial injury include tachycardia out of proportion to blood loss, arrhythmias (especially premature ventricular contractions and atrial fibrillation), and conduction defects.
- Screening tests, such as ECG and cardiac isoenzymes, usually do not accurately indicate the severity of blunt myocardial injury, nor are they predictive of major morbidity or mortality.
- Chest radiography has its greatest value in the recognition of associated injuries.
- A normal cardiac troponin I in a patient without other clinical findings is reasonably predictive of absence of serious blunt myocardial injury.[6]
- Echocardiography is best reserved for patients who demonstrate cardiac dysrhythmias or dysfunction.

EMERGENCY DEPARTMENT CARE AND DISPOSITION

- Patients with blunt myocardial injury occasionally may require treatment for heart failure or rhythm and conduction disturbances.
- Patients should be treated with supplemental oxygen and given analgesics as needed.
- Nitrates should be avoided unless the patient has pre-existing coronary artery disease.
- IV fluids and inotropic agents (dopamine or dobutamine) may be used for hypotension once cardiac tamponade has been excluded.
- For patients with blunt myocardial injury, an initial ECG may identify dysrhythmias or injury patterns.
- If the initial ECG is normal, then continuous cardiac monitoring should be performed for 4 to 6 hours. If there are no identified dysrhythmias and the patient is otherwise uninjured, then the patient may be discharged home.[7]

- If the ECG is abnormal and the patient is hemodynamically stable, then the patient should be admitted to a monitored setting with repeat ECG in 12 to 24 hours.
- Upon discharge from the hospital, patients with blunt myocardial injury should have close follow-up to evaluate for posttraumatic pericarditis, ventricular septal defect, valvular defects, and ventricular aneurysms.

PERICARDIAL INFLAMMATION SYNDROME

- Although the cause of this syndrome is unclear, pericardial inflammation syndrome should be suspected in patients who develop chest pain, fever, and pleural or pericardial effusions 2 to 4 weeks after cardiac trauma or surgery.
- A friction rub may be present and ECG may show ST-segment changes consistent with pericarditis.
- Treatment is primarily symptomatic with nonsteroidal anti-inflammatory agents as first-line therapy. Occasionally glucocorticoids may be required.

PENETRATING TRAUMA TO THE GREAT VESSELS

CLINICAL FEATURES AND DIAGNOSIS

- Simple lacerations of the great vessels may cause exsanguination, tamponade, hemothorax, air embolism, and development of an arteriovenous (AV) fistula or false aneurysm.
- The size of the knife, its length, and the angle of penetration may suggest the vessels or organs most likely to be injured.
- Projectile missile wounds may enter a major vessel and embolize to distant locations.
- Assessment of bilateral upper extremity pulses should be noted, and the entire chest should be auscultated for bruits, which may represent a false aneurysm or AV fistula.
- On chest radiograph, widening of the upper mediastinum may indicate injury to the brachiocephalic vessels.
- A fuzzy image of a foreign body on radiograph may indicate motion artifact caused by a foreign body located within or adjacent to pulsatile vascular structures.
- In stable patients, CT scan can localize hematomas adjacent to major vascular structures. The use of contrast helps further evaluate these structures and may demonstrate a vascular defect or false aneurysm.
- A preoperative arteriogram will help visualize the arch of the aorta and its major branches.

EMERGENCY DEPARTMENT CARE AND DISPOSITION

- A patient with no signs of life in the field requires no further resuscitative efforts; however, if the patient lost vital signs immediately prior to hospital arrival, then ED thoracotomy is indicated.
- Early endotracheal intubation should be performed in patients with penetrating injuries to the thoracic inlet. This approach avoids problems with expanding hematomas that may occlude the airway.
- In patients with severe shock (systolic blood pressure <60 mm Hg), immediate surgery is indicated.
- With mild to moderate shock (systolic blood pressure of 60 to 90 mm Hg), infusion of 2 to 3 liters of crystalloid should be rapidly administered while the need for emergent surgery is evaluated.

BLUNT TRAUMA TO THE GREAT VESSELS

CLINICAL FEATURES AND DIAGNOSIS

- About 80 to 90% of patients with blunt trauma to the thoracic great vessels (especially the aorta) die at the scene, and 50% of the remaining patients die within 24 hours if not treated promptly.
- Pre-existing vascular disease (atherosclerosis or medial necrosis) does not appear to predispose patients to traumatic aortic rupture.
- Approximately 90% of patients with blunt aortic injuries who reach the hospital alive have their aortic injury in the isthmus, between the left subclavian artery and the ligamentum arteriosum.
- Other common sites of injury are the innominate or left subclavian artery at their origins or a subclavian artery over the first rib.
- Most patients will initially be asymptomatic after an aortic injury. Therefore this injury should be suspected in anyone with a sudden, severe deceleration or a high-speed impact from the side.
- About one third of patients with blunt trauma to the aorta have no external evidence of thoracic injury.
- Physical examination findings that suggest aortic injury include an acute onset of upper extremity hypertension, difference in pulse amplitude in the upper and lower extremities, and the presence of a harsh systolic murmur over the precordium or interscapular area.
- Up to one third of patients with traumatic rupture of the aorta will present with a normal chest radiograph initially.
- Radiographic abnormalities associated with traumatic aortic rupture include superior mediastinal widening, deviation of the esophagus and/or trachea at T4, ob-

scuration of the aortic knob and/or descending aorta, displacement of the left mainstem bronchus more than 40 degrees below horizontal, widening of the paratracheal stripe, displacement of the paraspinal lines, obscuration of the medial aspects of the left upper lobe, the presence of apical cap, and fracture of the first or second rib.

- TEE is a highly sensitive diagnostic modality for evaluating traumatic aortic rupture. It can also be performed on hemodynamically unstable patients in the ED.
- Newer generation helical CT scans offer a rapid diagnostic modality for traumatic aortic injury; however, angiography remains the gold standard.
- Very few patients with injury to the ascending aorta survive long enough for the diagnosis to be established and the repair to be completed.
- If there is an associated valvular injury, a murmur of aortic insufficiency may be heard.
- Injuries to the descending aorta are uncommon. Descending aortic injuries present with paraplegia, mesenteric ischemia, anuria, or lower extremity ischemia.
- Blunt injuries to the innominate artery are second in frequency only to rupture of the aorta at the isthmus in patients reaching the hospital alive.
- Blunt injuries to the innominate artery are associated with rib fractures, flail chest, hemopneumothorax, fractured extremities, head injuries, facial fractures, and abdominal injuries. Diminished right radial or brachial pulse is found in 50% of patients.
- Chest radiographic findings in injuries to the innominate artery are similar to those for traumatic aortic disruption.
- CT angiography is widely used as an initial screening tool, but aortography is generally required to make the diagnosis of innominate artery injury.
- Subclavian artery injuries are most often caused by fractures to the first rib or clavicle. Absence of a radial pulse on the affected side is the most important sign.
- A pulsatile mass or bruit at the base of the neck is suggestive of injury to the subclavian artery. Associated injury to the brachial plexus occurs in 60% of patients. Horner's syndrome often indicates avulsion of nerve roots from the spinal cord.
- In subclavian artery injuries, the chest radiograph may show a widened superior mediastinum without obscuration of the aortic knob.

EMERGENCY DEPARTMENT CARE AND DISPOSITION

- Patients with traumatic aortic injury should not be allowed to develop a systolic blood pressure over 120 mm Hg or to perform a Valsalva maneuver.

- Fluid administration should be monitored carefully and administration of sedatives, vasodilators, analgesics, and β-blockers may be required to reduce the systolic blood pressure.
- A nasogastric tube should be inserted cautiously to avoid patient gagging or coughing.
- Although surgical repair is the accepted standard of care, aggressive medical control of blood pressure with delayed repair and prolonged observation may be alternatives to patients at high risk for surgery.
- Endovascular stenting may provide a less invasive approach to surgical repair.

ESOPHAGEAL AND THORACIC DUCT INJURIES

- Injury to the thoracic esophagus is rare.
- If suspected, a swallow study with water-soluble contrast should be obtained. If this study is negative, then a follow-up barium swallow is recommended.
- Flexible esophagoscopy is another diagnostic study that may be considered.
- Immediate esophageal repair is the treatment of choice.
- If repair is delayed beyond 24 hours, local edema and tissue necrosis make repair unlikely.
- Mortality for esophageal injury is 5 to 25% if repaired within 12 hours, and 25 to 66% if treated after 24 hours.
- Most injuries to the thoracic duct result in chylothorax on the right side. Tube thoracostomy is the treatment of choice.

REFERENCES

1. Galan G, Penalver JC, Paris E, et al: Blunt chest injuries in 1696 patients. *Eur J Cardiothorac Surg* 6:284, 1992.
2. Tanaka H, Yukioka T, Yamaguti Y, et al: Surgical stabilization or internal pneumatic stabilization? A prospective randomized study of management of severe flail chest patients. *J Trauma-Injury Infect Crit Care* 52:727, 2002.
3. Chiu WC, D'amelio LF, Hammond JS: Sternal fractures in blunt chest trauma: A practical algorithm for management. *Am J Emerg Med* 15:252, 1997.
4. Brown GL, Richardson JD: Traumatic diaphragmatic hernia. *Ann Thorac Surg* 39:172, 1985.
5. Demetriades D, Breckon V, Breckon C, et al: Antibiotic prophylaxis in penetrating injuries of the chest. *Ann Roy Coll Surg Engl* 73:348, 1991.
6. Bertinchant JP, Polge A, Mohty D, et al: Evaluation of incidence, clinical significance, and prognostic value of circulating cardiac troponin I and T elevation in hemodynamically stable patients with suspected myocardial contusion after blunt chest trauma. *J Trauma* 48:924, 2000.
7. Foil MB, Mackersie RC, Furst SR, et al: The symptomatic patient with suspected myocardial contusion. *Am J Surg* 160: 638, 1990.

For further reading in *Emergency Medicine: A Comprehensive Study Guide,* 6th ed., see Chap. 259, "Thoracic Trauma," by Timothy G. Buchman, Bruce L. Hall, William M. Bowling, and Gabor D. Kelen.

168 ABDOMINAL TRAUMA

O. John Ma

EPIDEMIOLOGY

- The most common cause of death and disability from nonintentional injury is the motor vehicle crash. Falls are the second leading cause of accidental death in the United States.

PATHOPHYSIOLOGY

- The injury pattern of blunt abdominal trauma is often diffuse. Blunt injuries involve a compression or crushing mechanism by direct energy transmission. If the compressive, shearing, or stretching forces exceed the tolerance limits of the organ tissue, then tissue disruption occurs.
- Injury also can result from movement of organs within the body. Some organs are rigidly fixed, whereas others are mobile. Typical examples in the abdomen include mesenteric or small bowel injuries, particularly at the ligament of Treitz or at the junction of the distal small bowel and right colon.
- Falls from a height produce solid organ injuries less commonly and hollow visceral injuries more commonly.[1] Retroperitoneal injuries associated with significant blood loss occur from falls because force is transmitted up the axial skeleton.
- Gunshot wounds may injure the victim by having the bullet directly injure the organ or secondarily from missiles such as bone and bullet fragments or from energy transmission from the bullet.

CLINICAL FEATURES

SOLID VISCERAL INJURIES

- Injury to the solid organs causes morbidity and mortality, primarily as a result of acute blood loss.
- The spleen is the most frequently injured organ in blunt abdominal trauma and is commonly associated with other intra-abdominal injuries. Kehr's sign, representing referred left shoulder pain, is a classic finding in splenic rupture. Lower left rib fractures should heighten clinical suspicion for splenic injury.
- The liver also is commonly injured in both blunt and penetrating injuries.
- Tachycardia, hypotension, and acute abdominal tenderness are the primary physical examination findings.
- Some patients with solid organ injury occasionally may present with minimal symptoms and nonspecific findings on physical examination. This is commonly associated with younger patients and those with distracting injuries, head injury, or intoxication.[2]
- A single physical examination is insensitive for diagnosing abdominal injuries. Serial physical examinations on an awake, alert, and reliable patient are important for identifying intra-abdominal injuries.

HOLLOW VISCERAL INJURIES

- These injuries produce symptoms by the combination of blood loss and peritoneal contamination. Perforation of the stomach, small bowel, or colon is accompanied by blood loss from a concomitant mesenteric injury.
- Gastrointestinal contamination will produce peritoneal signs over a period of time. Patients with head injury, distracting injuries, or intoxication may not exhibit peritoneal signs initially.
- Small bowel and colon injuries are most frequently the result of penetrating trauma. However, a deceleration injury can cause a bucket-handle tear of the mesentery or a blowout injury of the antimesenteric border.
- Suppurative peritonitis may develop from small bowel and colonic injuries. Inflammation may take 6 to 8 hours to develop.

RETROPERITONEAL INJURIES

- Duodenal injuries are most often associated with high-speed vertical or horizontal decelerating trauma. Duodenal injuries may range in severity from an intramural hematoma to an extensive crush or laceration.
- Clinical signs of duodenal injury are often slow to develop. Patients may present with abdominal pain, fever, nausea, and vomiting, although these may take hours to become clinically obvious.
- Duodenal ruptures are usually contained within the retroperitoneum.
- Pancreatic injury often accompanies rapid deceleration injury or a severe crush injury. The classic case is a blow to the midepigastrium from a steering wheel or the handlebar of a bicycle.
- Leakage of activated enzymes from the pancreas can produce retroperitoneal autodigestion, which may become superinfected with bacteria and produce a retroperitoneal abscess.

DIAPHRAGMATIC INJURIES

- Presentation of diaphragm injuries is often insidious. Only occasionally is the diagnosis obvious when bowel sounds can be auscultated in the thoracic cavity.
- On chest radiograph, herniation of abdominal contents into the thoracic cavity or a nasogastric tube coiled in the thorax confirms the diagnosis. In most cases, however, the only finding on chest radiograph is blurring of the diaphragm or an effusion.
- This injury is diagnosed most often on the left.

DIAGNOSIS AND DIFFERENTIAL

PLAIN RADIOGRAPHS

- A chest radiograph is helpful in evaluating for herniated abdominal contents in the thoracic cavity and for evidence of free air under the diaphragm.
- An AP pelvis radiograph is important for identifying pelvic fractures, which can produce significant blood loss and be associated with intra-abdominal visceral injury.
- For blunt abdominal trauma, routine use of plain abdominal radiographs is not a cost-effective and prudent method for evaluating the trauma patient.

DIAGNOSTIC PERITONEAL LAVAGE

- Diagnostic peritoneal lavage (DPL) remains an excellent screening test for evaluating abdominal trauma. Its advantages include its sensitivity, availability, the relative speed with which it can be performed, and low complication rate (1%).
- Disadvantages include the potential for iatrogenic injury, its misapplication for evaluation of retroperitoneal injuries, and its lack of specificity. Laparotomy

based solely on a positive DPL results in a nontherapeutic laparotomy approximately 30% of the time.[3]

- For blunt trauma, indications for DPL include: (1) patients who are too hemodynamically unstable to leave the emergency department for computed tomography (CT) scanning, and (2) unexplained hypotension in patients with an equivocal physical examination.
- In penetrating trauma, DPL should be performed when it is not clear that exploratory laparotomy should be performed. DPL is useful in evaluating patients sustaining stab wounds where local wound exploration indicates that the superficial muscle fascia has been violated. Also, it may be useful in confirming a negative physical examination when tangential or lower chest wounds are involved.
- In blunt abdominal trauma, the DPL is considered positive if more than 10 mL of gross blood is aspirated immediately, the red blood cell count is >100,000 cells/µL, the white blood cell count is >500 cells/µL, bile is present, or if vegetable matter is present.
- The only absolute contraindication to DPL is when surgical management is clearly indicated, in which case the DPL would delay patient transport to the operating room.
- Relative contraindications include patients with advanced hepatic dysfunction, severe coagulopathies, previous abdominal surgeries, or a gravid uterus.

ULTRASONOGRAPHY

- The focused assessment with sonography for trauma (FAST) examination, like DPL, is an accurate screening tool for abdominal trauma. The underlying premise behind the use of the FAST examination is that clinically significant injuries will be associated with the presence of free fluid accumulating in dependent areas.
- Advantages of the FAST examination are that it is accurate, rapid, noninvasive, repeatable, portable, and involves no contrast material or radiation exposure to the patient. There is limited risk for patients who are pregnant, coagulopathic, or have had previous abdominal surgery.[4]
- One major advantage of the FAST examination is the ability to also evaluate for free pericardial and pleural fluid.
- Disadvantages include the inability to determine the exact etiology of the free intraperitoneal fluid and the operator-dependent nature of the examination. The FAST examination also cannot evaluate the retroperitoneum as well as CT.[4]
- Other disadvantages of the FAST examination are the difficulty in interpreting the views in patients who are

obese or have subcutaneous air or excessive bowel gas, and the inability to distinguish intraperitoneal hemorrhage from ascites.[4]

COMPUTED TOMOGRAPHY

- Abdominal CT scanning has a greater specificity than DPL and ultrasonography, thus making it the initial diagnostic test of choice at most trauma centers. Oral and IV contrast material should be given to provide optimal resolution.
- Advantages of CT scan include its ability to precisely locate intra-abdominal lesions preoperatively, to evaluate the retroperitoneum, to identify injuries that may be managed nonoperatively, and its noninvasiveness.
- The disadvantages of CT scanning are its expense, the time required to perform the study, the need to transport the trauma patient to the radiology suite, and the need for contrast materials.

EMERGENCY DEPARTMENT CARE AND DISPOSITION

- Patients should be administered 100% oxygen and have cardiac monitoring and two large-bore IV lines secured.
- For hypotensive abdominal trauma patients, resuscitation with IV crystalloid fluid is indicated. Transfusion with O-negative or type-specific packed red blood cells should be considered in addition to crystalloid resuscitation.
- Laboratory work for patients with abdominal trauma should be based on the mechanism of injury (blunt versus penetrating). It may include type and crossmatching, complete blood count, electrolytes, arterial blood gas, directed toxicologic studies, prothrombin time (PT), partial thromboplastin time (PTT), hepatic enzymes, and lipase.
- Table 168-1 lists the indications for exploratory laparotomy. When a patient presents to the emergency department with an obvious high-velocity gunshot wound to the abdomen, DPL or the FAST examination should not be performed as they will only delay transport of the patient to the operating room.
- If organ evisceration is present, it should be covered with a moist, sterile dressing prior to surgery.
- For an equivocal stab wound to the abdomen, surgical consultation for local wound exploration is indicated. If the wound exploration demonstrates no violation of the anterior fascia, the patient can be discharged home safely.
- For the hemodynamically stable blunt trauma patient with a positive FAST examination, further evaluation with CT scan may be warranted prior to admission.

TABLE 168-1   Indications for Laparotomy

	BLUNT		PENETRATING
Absolute	Anterior abdominal injury and hypotension Abdominal wall disruption Peritonitis Free air on chest x-ray CT-diagnosed injury requiring surgery (eg, pancreatic transaction, duodenal rupture)	Absolute	Injury to abdomen, back, and flank with hypotension Abdominal tenderness Gastrointestinal evisceration Positive DPL High suspicion for transabdominal trajectory (GSW) CT-diagnosed injury requiring surgery (eg, ureter or pancreas)
Relative	Positive DPL or FAST in stable patient Solid visceral injury in stable patient Hemoperitoneum on CT without clear source	Relative	Positive local wound exploration (SW)

ABBREVIATIONS: CT = computed tomography; DPL = diagnostic peritoneal lavage; FAST = focused assessment with sonography for trauma; GSW = gunshot wound; SW = stab wound.

REFERENCES

1. Scalea TM, Goldstein AS, Phillips TF, et al: An analysis of 161 falls from a height. *J Trauma* 26:706, 1986.
2. Scalea TM, Holman M, Fourtes M, et al: Central venous blood oxygen saturation: an early, accurate measurement of volume during hemorrhage. *J Trauma* 28:725, 1988.
3. Goldstein AS, Scalfani S, Kupterstein NH, et al: The diagnostic superiority of computed tomography. *J Trauma* 25:939, 1985.
4. Ma OJ, Mateer JR, Ogata M, et al: Prospective analysis of a rapid trauma ultrasound examination performed by emergency physicians. *J Trauma* 38:879, 1995.

For further reading in *Emergency Medicine: A Comprehensive Study Guide,* 6th ed., see Chap. 260, "Abdominal Injuries," by Thomas M. Scalea and Sharon A. Boswell.

169   FLANK AND BUTTOCK TRAUMA

Robert A. Schwab

EPIDEMIOLOGY

- Penetrating trauma to the flank and buttock, while not as common as penetrating injuries to other areas of the trunk, are nevertheless important, as they present diagnostic challenges based on the potential for retroperitoneal injuries.

- The emergency department evaluation and management, consisting of appropriate resuscitation followed by diagnostic and therapeutic interventions used to determine whether operative or nonoperative management is undertaken, is critical to optimizing outcomes in these patients.

PENETRATING TRAUMA TO THE FLANK

PATHOPHYSIOLOGY

- The common pathophysiology of these injuries is related to blood loss with or without frank hemorrhagic shock. Infection due to violation of skin integrity or penetration of hollow or solid organs may occur. Vascular disruptions may produce ischemia distal to the injury. Leakage of bodily fluids such as bile or urine into the peritoneal or retroperitoneal space may produce tissue irritation or sterile abscesses.
- Any intraperitoneal or retroperitoneal structure may be injured; missile pathways are unpredictable and the appearance of stab wound pathways can be misleading.

CLINICAL FEATURES

- The organs most commonly injured by penetrating trauma to the flank include the liver, kidney, colon, duodenum, and pancreas.
- Key historical features include the mechanism of injury and type of weapon; time since injury; postinjury symptoms, particularly hematemesis; and general medical history.

- Physical examination should begin with inspection for evidence of exsanguinating hemorrhage, evisceration, or frank peritoneal signs. Perfusion of the lower extremities should be assessed. Digital rectal examination can identify occult bowel injuries if intraluminal bleeding is significant. Auscultation of the lung fields may help identify thoracic or diaphragmatic injuries.

DIAGNOSIS AND DIFFERENTIAL

- Wound exploration is of limited utility and should be reserved for patients who are stable and whose history and physical examination suggest very low probability of deep penetration.
- Following resuscitation, expeditious determination of the need for immediate operative intervention is the next priority. Unstable patients with signs of peritoneal irritation or with evidence of free intraperitoneal fluid by bedside ultrasonography or diagnostic peritoneal lavage should undergo laparotomy without delay. Other indications include evisceration, gross blood on rectal examination, and gunshot wound with a transpelvic or transperitoneal pathway.
- Computed tomography (CT) is the diagnostic study of choice in stable patients due to its ability to evaluate retroperitoneal as well as intraperitoneal structures. The diagnostic accuracy of triple-contrast CT scanning is approximately 98%.[1] The presence of bowel wall edema may indicate bowel perforation, even when contrast leak is not visible.[2]
- An upright chest radiograph should be obtained to evaluate possible thoracic involvement and to detect free intraperitoneal air. Plain abdominal or pelvic films can assist in determining missile pathway and detect fractures.

EMERGENCY DEPARTMENT CARE AND DISPOSITION

- Standard resuscitation principles apply. Patients should receive two large-bore IV lines, supplemental oxygen, cardiac monitoring, and nasogastric tube insertion. A urinary catheter should be placed unless there is high suspicion of urethral injury. Surgical consultation should be obtained immediately.
- Prophylactic broad-spectrum antibiotics (eg, piperacillin-tazobactam 3.375 g IV) should be administered to patients with evidence of intraperitoneal injury or strong suspicion of extraperitoneal bowel injury.
- If no immediate indication for laparotomy is found, CT should be utilized to determine the need for operation and to detect occult injuries. Free intraperitoneal air or major organ, vessel, or nerve injury identified by imaging may require operation, but fewer nontherapeutic laparotomies and good outcomes with decreased morbidity are achieved through the use of early CT scanning.[3]
- All patients should be admitted for observation with the exception of those sustaining very superficial stab wounds whose diagnostic evaluation reveals no significant injury.

PENETRATING BUTTOCK INJURIES

PATHOPHYSIOLOGY

- The same principles apply as for flank trauma; blood loss, infection, vascular disruption with distal ischemia, fractures, and sterile abscesses can contribute to morbidity and mortality from these injuries.
- Gunshot wounds have much higher potential for injury, because the thick gluteal musculature protects against deep penetration from most stab wounds. Operative intervention is rarely required for stab wounds to the buttock.

CLINICAL FEATURES

- Injuries to the gastrointestinal and genitourinary tracts are of greatest concern for this mechanism of trauma, but injuries to pelvic bony and vascular structures (internal iliac or gluteal vessels) can lead to significant morbidity, as can injuries to major nerves (sciatic and femoral nerves).
- Key historical features include the mechanism of injury and type of weapon; time since injury; postinjury symptoms, particularly hematuria or hematochezia; and general medical history.
- Physical examination should be directed toward detection of evisceration, exsanguinating hemorrhage, or peritonitis first, followed by careful assessment for genitourinary or rectal injuries.
- Inspection of the urethral meatus and genitalia followed by digital rectal examination is mandatory. Genitourinary trauma can present with hematuria and scrotal or penile hematomas.
- Pelvic stability should be assessed by palpation and distal extremity perfusion should be ensured.

DIAGNOSIS AND DIFFERENTIAL

- Wound exploration is of limited utility and should be reserved for patients who are stable and whose history and physical examination suggest very low probability of deep penetration.

- Following resuscitation, expeditious determination of the need for immediate operative intervention is the next priority. Indications for operative intervention include signs of peritonitis, gross hematuria, gross blood on rectal examination, gunshot entrance wound above the level of the greater trochanter, and a transpelvic missile pathway.[4]
- Proctosigmoidoscopy should be performed if the missile pathway suggests possible rectal injury.
- Cystourethrography should be performed in patients with hematuria or when there is strong suspicion of genitourinary tract injury.
- CT scanning with intravenous and rectal contrast and clamping of the urinary catheter can provide a comprehensive diagnostic evaluation of key structures. CT scanning may also demonstrate pelvic fractures and intrapelvic hematomas.
- Arteriography is indicated when there is a distal pulse deficit or perivascular hematoma on CT scan.
- Plain abdominal or pelvic films can assist in determining missile pathway and detecting fractures.

EMERGENCY DEPARTMENT CARE AND DISPOSITION

- Standard resuscitation principles apply. Patients should receive two large-bore IV lines, supplemental oxygen, cardiac monitoring, and nasogastric tube insertion. A urinary catheter should be inserted after careful evaluation for urethral injury. Surgical consultation should be obtained immediately.
- Prophylactic broad-spectrum antibiotics (eg, piperacillin-tazobactam 3.375 g IV) should be administered to patients with evidence of intraperitoneal injury or strong suspicion of extraperitoneal bowel injury.
- If no immediate indication for laparotomy is found, CT should be utilized to determine the need for operation and to detect occult injuries.
- All patients should be admitted for observation with the exception of those sustaining very superficial stab wounds whose diagnostic evaluation reveals no significant injury.

REFERENCES

1. Albrecht RM, Virgil A, Schermer CR, et al: Stab wounds to the back/flank in hemodynamically stable patients: Evaluation using triple-contrast computed tomography. *Am Surg* 65:683, 1999.
2. Himmelman RG, Martin M, Gilkey S, et al: Triple-contrast CT scans in penetrating back and flank trauma. *J Trauma* 31:852, 1991.
3. Boyle EM Jr, Maier RV, Slaazar JD, et al: Diagnosis of injuries after stab wounds to the back and flank. *J Trauma* 42:260, 1997.
4. DiGiacomo JC, Schwab CW, Rotondo MF, et al: Gluteal gunshot wounds: Who warrants exploration? *J Trauma* 37:622, 1994.

For further reading in *Emergency Medicine: A Comprehensive Study Guide,* 6th ed., see Chap. 261, "Penetrating Trauma to the Flank and Buttock," by Alasdair K. T. Conn.

170　GENITOURINARY TRAUMA

C. Crawford Mechem

EPIDEMIOLOGY

- Injuries to the genitourinary system occur in 2 to 5% of adult trauma patients, usually in the setting of blunt trauma.
- Approximately 80% of genitourinary injuries involve the kidney and 10% involve the bladder.
- Approximately 10% of children with blunt abdominal trauma have genitourinary system involvement.

CLINICAL FEATURES

- The history and physical examination should raise suspicion for genitourinary injuries.
- Patients with any abdominal trauma, including penetrating trauma in the vicinity of genitourinary structures, are at risk.
- High-velocity deceleration predisposes to renal pedicle injuries, including lacerations and thromboses of the renal artery and vein.
- Fractures of the lower ribs or lower thoracic or lumbar vertebrae are often associated with renal or ureteral injuries, while pelvic fractures and straddle injuries are associated with urethral or bladder trauma.
- Flank ecchymoses, tenderness, or masses suggest renal injuries.
- The perineum should be inspected for blood or lacerations, which may denote an open pelvic fracture.
- The presence of a penile, scrotal, or perineal hematoma or blood at the penile meatus suggests urethral injury.

- If blood at the meatus is present, then no attempt at inserting a urethral catheter should be made due to the concern for converting a partial urethral laceration into a complete transection.
- A rectal examination should be performed, assessing sphincter tone, checking for blood, and determining the position of the prostate.
- A high-riding prostate or one that feels boggy suggests injury to the membranous urethra.
- In men, the scrotum should be examined for ecchymoses, lacerations, or testicular disruption.
- In women, the vaginal introitus should be inspected for lacerations and hematomas, which are often associated with pelvic fractures. If there is evidence of injury in this area, or if injury is suspected, a bimanual examination should be performed. If blood is present, a speculum examination is warranted to check for vaginal lacerations.

DIAGNOSIS AND DIFFERENTIAL

- Microscopic hematuria is defined as more than 5 red blood cells (RBCs) per high-power field (hpf). This is based on a 10-mL urine specimen centrifuged for 5 min at 2000 rpm.[1]
- Generally, blood at the urethral meatus should be excluded and the urine evaluated for hematuria before passage of a urinary catheter is considered.
- If placement of a catheter is urgent and injury to the urethra has not been excluded, then the suprapubic approach may be used.
- Analysis of the first-voided urine may help localize the injury. Initial hematuria suggests injury to the urethra or prostate, while terminal hematuria is associated with bladder neck trauma.
- Continuous hematuria is often due to injury to the bladder, ureter, or kidney.
- In blunt trauma, the degree of hematuria does not correlate with severity of injury.
- In hemodynamically stable patients, isolated microscopic hematuria rarely represents significant injury. Exceptions to this include associated transient hypotension, a rapid deceleration mechanism that may cause renal pedicle or vascular injury, or pediatric cases.
- In stable children, injury is unlikely if the urine contains less than 50 RBCs/hpf.[2]
- The choice of imaging study will be dictated by the hemodynamic status of the patient and suspicion for associated injuries (Table 170-1).
- Blunt trauma patients who have sustained injury from a rapid deceleration mechanism, demonstrated hemodynamic instability, revealed gross hematuria, or demonstrated microscopic hematuria along with associated injuries should undergo abdominal computed

TABLE 170-1 Selection of Diagnostic Imaging for Suspected Renal System Injury

IMAGING STUDY	SUSPECTED INJURY
Retrograde urethrogram or cystogram	Urethral injury
CT (with IV contrast)	Renal injury (staging) Ureteral injury
Cystogram, plain film (retrograde)	Bladder injury
CT cystogram (retrograde)	Bladder injury
"One-shot" IVP	Unstable patients taken to operating room
IVP	Alternative to CT in unstable patients Ureteral injury
Angiogram or venogram	Pedicle injuries, venous disruption
Retrograde pyelogram	Renal pelvis disruption

ABBREVIATIONS: CT = computed tomography; IVP = intravenous pyelogram.

tomography (CT) imaging. This modality has the advantage of simultaneously imaging other organs.
- CT should only be performed on hemodynamically stable patients. Patients who are unstable should undergo a one-shot intravenous pyelogram (IVP), either in the emergency department or operating room.
- If the patient's systolic blood pressure is 70 mm Hg or less, dye-induced nephrotoxicity may result.
- An IVP can also be used in stable patients if CT is unavailable, but the resolution may be poor.
- IVP remains the mainstay for diagnosing ureteral injuries, which is identified by extravasation of contrast dye.[3]
- In many centers, spiral CT scanners are also being used for this purpose and have the advantage of visualizing the entire retroperitoneal space.
- In penetrating trauma, there is no correlation between degree of hematuria and severity of injury. Therefore penetrating trauma patients with the potential for genitourinary injury should be imaged by CT or IVP, depending on their hemodynamic stability, prior to exploratory laparotomy.[4]
- Cystography is commonly used to diagnose suspected bladder injuries. It is performed by instilling contrast media retrograde into the bladder and looking for extravasation, preferably under fluoroscopy.
- Urethral injuries are investigated by retrograde cystography. An unlubricated urinary catheter is passed 2 to 3 cm into the distal urethra, the balloon inflated with 1 to 3 mL of water, and 20 to 30 mL of contrast material is injected. An oblique film is obtained to evaluate for extravasation.
- Urethral injuries should not be investigated in the case of pelvic trauma until it is certain that pelvic angiography or embolization is not required.

EMERGENCY DEPARTMENT CARE AND DISPOSITION

- Standard protocols for evaluation and stabilization of trauma patients should be initiated (see Chap. 159). Emphasis should be placed on identifying life-threatening injuries.
- Patients with isolated microscopic hematuria and no other injuries may be discharged with repeat urinalysis in 1 to 2 weeks.

MANAGEMENT OF SPECIFIC INJURIES

KIDNEY

- Contusions account for more than 90% of renal injuries, with renal lacerations, pedicle injuries, and shattered kidneys making up the rest.
- Renal contusions and lacerations not involving the collecting system are usually managed nonoperatively. In the absence of other injuries, these patients may be discharged with repeat urinalysis in 1 to 2 weeks.
- Patients with pedicle injuries or lacerations involving the collecting system should be admitted. Many of these patients have associated injuries requiring surgical repair.
- In the case of isolated renal injury, patients may be managed nonoperatively with frequent reassessment. They should be put at bed rest, kept well hydrated, and have frequent hematocrit determinations and urinalyses to assess the degree of hematuria.
- Patients with shattered kidneys require operative repair, as do patients with uncontrolled renal hemorrhage, multiple kidney lacerations, renal vascular injuries, a pulsatile or expanding hematoma on abdominal exploration, or penetrating injuries.

URETER

- Ureteral injuries are the rarest of the genitourinary injuries and usually result from penetrating trauma.
- If the ureter is completely transected, hematuria may be absent.[5]
- Ureter injuries should be managed operatively.

BLADDER

- Bladder contusions are treated expectantly.
- Incomplete bladder lacerations may be managed by catheter placement and observation.
- Bladder rupture is either intra- or extraperitoneal.

- Intraperitoneal rupture usually results from a burst injury of a full bladder and is managed operatively.
- Extraperitoneal rupture is often associated with a pelvic ring fracture.
- Symptoms of extraperitoneal rupture include abdominal pain and tenderness, hematuria, and inability to void. Management involves urethral catheter drainage alone.
- Penetrating bladder injuries are managed operatively.

URETHRA

- Urethral injuries in males involve the posterior (prostatomembranous) urethra and the anterior (bulbous and penile) urethra.
- Posterior injuries are associated with pelvic fractures. Anterior injuries result from direct trauma or instrumentation.
- In females, urethral injuries are often associated with pelvic fractures and commonly present with vaginal bleeding.
- Anterior contusions are managed conservatively, with or without a urethral catheter.
- Partial anterior urethral lacerations are managed with an indwelling catheter or with suprapubic cystotomy.
- Complete lacerations are repaired with end-to-end anastomosis.
- Partial lacerations of the posterior urethra are managed with urethral or suprapubic drainage.
- Complete lacerations are managed either surgically or with suprapubic drainage alone.

TESTICLES AND SCROTUM

- Blunt testicular injuries consist of contusions or rupture.
- Testicular ultrasound can help to determine the type and extent of injury.
- Contusions may be managed conservatively with nonsteroidal anti-inflammatory drugs, ice, elevation, scrotal support, and urologic follow-up.
- Testicular rupture or penetrating trauma requires operative repair to improve outcome.
- Scrotal skin avulsion is managed by housing the testicle in the remaining scrotal skin, which will usually return to normal size in several months.

PENIS

- Injuries range from small contusions to degloving injuries or amputations.
- Lacerations and amputations require operative débridement and reconstruction or reimplantation.

- A fractured penis, due to traumatic rupture of the corpus cavernosum, is managed by immediate surgical drainage of blood clot and repair of the torn tunica albuginea and any associated urethral injuries.
- Penile skin avulsion is managed with split-thickness skin grafting after débridement.
- Zipper injury to the penis results when the penile skin is trapped in the trouser zipper. Mineral oil and lidocaine infiltration are useful in freeing the penile skin from the zipper. Wire-cutting or bone-cutting pliers are used to cut the median bar (diamond) of the zipper, causing the zipper to fall apart.
- Contusions to the perineum or penis are treated conservatively with cold packs, rest, and elevation.
- If the patient is unable to void, catheter drainage may be required.

REFERENCES

1. Ahn JH, Morey AF, McAninch JW: Workup and management of traumatic hematuria. *Emerg Med Clin North Am* 16:145, 1998.
2. Morey AF, Bruce JE, McAninch JW: Efficacy of radiographic imaging in pediatric blunt renal trauma. *J Urol* 156:2014, 1996.
3. Brandes SB, Chelsky MJ, Buckman RF, et al: Ureteral injuries from penetrating trauma. *J Trauma* 36:745, 1994.
4. Medina D, Lavery R, Ross SE, et al: Ureteral trauma: Preoperative studies neither predict injury nor prevent missed injury. *J Am Coll Surg* 186:641, 1998.
5. Morey AF, McAninch JW, et al: Single-shot intraoperative excretory urography for the immediate evaluation of renal trauma. *J Urol* 161:1091, 1999.

For further reading in *Emergency Medicine: A Comprehensive Study Guide*, 6th ed., see Chap. 262, "Genitourinary Trauma," by Frederick Levy and Gabor D. Kelen.

171 PENETRATING TRAUMA TO THE EXTREMITIES
C. Crawford Mechem

EPIDEMIOLOGY

- Of patients presenting with gunshot wounds, 20 to 40% have extremity involvement.
- Penetrating trauma accounts for up to 82% of all vascular injuries to the extremities.
- Gunshot and shotgun wounds account for nearly 65% of penetrating vascular extremity injuries and stab wounds account for approximately 15%.[1]

PATHOPHYSIOLOGY

- Tissue damage caused by a bullet depends on the projectile's velocity, mass, shape, construction, composition, angle of impact, and flight characteristics in tissue. The type of tissue impacted and the size of the temporary cavity produced by the bullet are important factors.
- Tissue damage is usually proportional to the amount of fracture comminution and displacement, blood loss within the limb, and nerve or vascular injury.[2]

CLINICAL FEATURES

- After the primary trauma evaluation and resuscitation are complete, a careful history should be obtained, including the type of weapon used.
- A thorough physical examination should be performed to determine the presence of extremity injuries warranting immediate operative repair.
- The size and shape of wounds or soft tissue injuries should be noted and any obvious bony deformity carefully examined.
- The extremity should be checked for evidence of compartment syndrome.
- Wounds near or overlying joints should be assessed for penetration of the joint capsule.
- Vascular integrity of the affected extremity should be evaluated by assessing distal pulses, which can be compared to the unaffected side. The color, temperature, and capillary refill of the involved extremity may be indicators of subtle vascular injury.
- The presence of "hard signs" of arterial injury include absent or diminished distal pulses, obvious arterial bleeding, large expanding or pulsatile hematoma, audible bruit, palpable thrill, or distal ischemia.
- Distal ischemia is suggested by pain, pallor, paralysis, paresthesias, and coolness.
- "Soft signs" of arterial injury are the presence of a small and stable hematoma, injury to an anatomically related nerve, unexplained hypotension, history of hemorrhage no longer present, proximity of injury to major vessels, or a complex fracture.[3]
- A final component of the clinical assessment of the injured extremity is a careful neuromuscular examination, investigating for evidence of motor or sensory deficits.

DIAGNOSIS AND DIFFERENTIAL

- Diagnostic tests that can assist the emergency physician in evaluating penetrating extremity wounds include ankle-brachial indices (ABI) and radiologic studies.
- Measurement of ABI objectively verifies diminished extremity pulses noted on physical examination.
- Doppler devices are used to measure ABI with a diagnostic accuracy of up to 95%. The sensitivity and specificity vary, depending on whether an abnormal ratio is set at 0.9 or 1.0.[4,5]
- ABI do not reliably detect nonocclusive arterial injuries, such as intimal flaps and pseudoaneurysms.
- ABI are performed by placing the patient in a supine position and measuring the systolic blood pressure in all four extremities.
- To measure an ankle systolic pressure, a standard adult blood pressure cuff is wrapped around the ankle just above the malleoli.
- The cuff is inflated to approximately 30 mm Hg above the systolic pressure and the Doppler flowmeter is used to detect the systolic pressure over the anterior tibial artery just distal to the blood pressure cuff as it is slowly deflated.
- The systolic blood pressure is also measured in both upper extremities using the Doppler device.
- The ABI measurement is then calculated by dividing the ankle systolic pressure by the greater of the two upper extremity pressures.
- An ABI measurement greater than 1.0 is normal.
- An ABI measurement of 0.5 to 0.9 is indicative of injury to a single artery segment, whereas an ABI measurement less than 0.5 indicates severe arterial injury or injury to multiple arterial segments.
- A difference of greater than 20 mm Hg between upper extremity systolic pressures indicates upper extremity arterial injury.
- Underlying medical conditions, such as pre-existing peripheral vascular disease or severe hypothermia, can affect the accuracy of ABI measurement.
- Plain radiographs, including anteroposterior and lateral views, of the involved extremity should be obtained when fractures or retained foreign bodies are a possibility.
- The joints above and below the injury should be included.
- In cases of shotgun wounds, the extremity distal to the wound should be imaged because of the risk of embolized shot pellets.
- Computed tomography may be required to detect fractures and to determine if intra-articular fractures, fragments, or foreign bodies are present.
- Arteriography can be used to delineate the extent, nature, and location of vascular injuries in special situations such as shotgun wounds, multiple or severe fractures, chronic vascular disease, thoracic outlet wounds, or extensive soft tissue injury. It has become the gold standard in the evaluation of patients with wounds in proximity to major neurovascular bundles.[4,6–8]
- Duplex ultrasonography has a diagnostic accuracy of 96 to 98%; it is rapid, safe, and can image extremity vessels with as much resolution as contrast angiography.[1,3,9]

EMERGENCY DEPARTMENT CARE AND DISPOSITION

- The general principles of wound management and tetanus prophylaxis apply.
- There is no proven role for prophylactic antibiotics unless the wound is contaminated or the patient has an underlying immunocompromising condition.
- Venous bleeding can in most cases be controlled by direct pressure.[10]
- While present in fewer than 6% of cases, hard signs of arterial injury require surgical evaluation and either arteriography or immediate exploration in the operating room.
- Soft signs of vascular injury require inpatient observation.
- Wound exploration in the emergency department is reserved for those patients with suspected foreign bodies in the wound, ligamentous involvement, or for control of minor venous bleeding.
- Patients with evidence of compartment syndrome, nerve injuries, or orthopedic injuries should be evaluated by the appropriate surgical subspecialist.
- Patients with no signs of vascular, bony, or nerve injury; minimal soft tissue defect; and no signs of developing compartment syndrome over a 3- to 12-hour period of observation can be discharged home.

REFERENCES

1. Frykberg ER: Advances in the diagnosis and treatment of extremity vascular trauma. *Surg Clin North Am* 75:207, 1995.
2. Fackler ML: Gunshot wound review. *Ann Emerg Med* 28: 194, 1996.
3. Modrall JG, Weaver FA, Yellin AE: Diagnosis and management of penetrating vascular trauma and the injured extremity. *Emerg Med Clin North Am* 16:129, 1998.
4. Gates JD: Penetrating wounds of the extremities: Methods of identifying arterial injury. *Orthopedics* 10:2, 1994.
5. Nassoura ZE, Ivatury RR, Simon RJ, et al: A reassessment of Doppler pressure indices in the detection of arterial lesions

in proximity to penetrating injuries of the extremities: A prospective study. *Am J Emerg Med* 14:151, 1996.

6. Dennis JW, Frykberg ER, Crump JM, et al: New perspectives on the management of penetrating trauma in proximity to major limb arteries. *J Vasc Surg* 11:84, 1990.

7. Dennis JW, Frykberg ER, Veldenz HC, et al: Validation of nonoperative management of occult vascular injuries and accuracy of physical examination alone in penetrating extremity trauma: 5- to 10-year follow-up. *J Trauma* 44:243, 1998.

8. Feliciano DV, Herskowitz K, O'Gorman RB, et al: Management of vascular injuries in the lower extremities. *J Trauma* 28:319, 1988.

9. Bergstien J, Blair J, Edwards J, et al: Pitfalls in the use of color-flow duplex ultrasound for screening of suspected arterial injuries in penetrating extremities. *J Trauma* 33:395, 1992.

10. Yelon JA: Venous injuries of the lower extremities and pelvis: Repair versus ligation. *J Trauma* 33:532, 1992.

For further reading in *Emergency Medicine: A Comprehensive Study Guide,* 6th ed., see Chap. 263, "Penetrating Trauma to the Extremities," by Alan M. Kumar and Richard D. Zane.

172 INITIAL EVALUATION AND MANAGEMENT OF ORTHOPEDIC INJURIES

Michael P. Kefer

PATHOPHYSIOLOGY

- Bone fracture results in severing of the microscopic vessels crossing the fracture line, which cuts off the blood supply to the involved fracture edges.[1] Callus formation ensues and becomes progressively more mineralized.
- Necrotic edges of the fracture are gradually resorbed by osteoclasts. This explains why some occult fractures are not immediately detected on radiographs, but then appear several days later after this resorption process is well established.
- Remodeling deposits new bone along the lines of stress. This process often lasts years.

CLINICAL FEATURES

- Knowing the precise mechanism of injury or listening carefully to the patient's symptoms is important in diagnosing fracture or dislocation.
- Pain may be referred to an area distant from the injury (eg, hip injury presenting as knee pain).
- The physical examination includes: (1) inspection for deformity, edema, or discoloration; (2) assessment of active and passive range of motion of joints proximal and distal to the injury; (3) palpation for tenderness or deformity; and (4) assessment of neurovascular status distal to the injury.

- Careful palpation can prevent missing a crucial diagnosis due to referred pain.
- The neurovascular status should be documented early, before performing reduction maneuvers.
- Radiologic evaluation is based on the history and physical examination, not simply on where the patient reports pain.
- Radiographs of all long bone fractures should include the joints proximal and distal to the fracture to evaluate for coexistent injury.
- A negative radiograph does not exclude a fracture. This commonly occurs with scaphoid, radial head, or metatarsal shaft fractures.
- The emergency department diagnosis is often clinical and is not confirmed until 7 to 10 days after the injury, when enough bone resorption has occurred at the fracture site to detect a lucency on the radiograph.
- An accurate description of the fracture to the orthopedic consultant is crucial and should include the following details:[2]
  - Closed versus open: describes whether the skin overlying the fracture is intact (closed) or not (open).
  - Location: midshaft, junction of proximal and middle or middle and distal third, or distance from bone end. Intra-articular involvement with disruption of the joint surface may require surgery. Anatomic bony reference points should be used when applicable (eg, humerus fracture just above the condyles is described as supracondylar as opposed to distal humerus).
  - Orientation of fracture line: transverse, spiral, oblique, comminuted (shattered), and segmental (single large segment of free-floating bone).
  - Displacement: the amount and direction the distal fragment is offset in relation to the proximal fragment.
  - Separation: the degree two fragments have been pulled apart. Unlike displacement, alignment is maintained.

- Shortening: reduction in bone length due to impaction or overriding fragments.
- Angulation: angle formed by the fracture segments. Describe the degree and direction of deviation of the distal fragment.
- Rotational deformity: degree the distal fragment is twisted on the axis of the normal bone. It is usually detected by physical examination and not seen on the radiograph.
- Fractures combined with dislocation or subluxation: associated disruption of proper joint alignment should be described as fracture-dislocation or fracture-subluxation to clearly communicate the more serious nature of the injury.
- Complications resulting from neurovascular deficit may be immediate or delayed.
- Fat embolus may result from fracture of large bones such as the femur.
- Compartment syndrome that presents with the five classic signs of pain, pallor, paresthesias, pulselessness, and paralysis that is well advanced.
- Long-term complications of fracture include malunion, nonunion, avascular necrosis, arthritis, and osteomyelitis.

EMERGENCY DEPARTMENT CARE AND DISPOSITION

- Swelling should be controlled with application of cold packs and elevation.
- Analgesics should be administered on a timely basis.
- Prompt reduction of fracture deformity with steady, longitudinal traction is indicated to: (1) alleviate pain; (2) relieve tension on associated neurovascular structures; (3) minimize the risk of converting a closed fracture to an open fracture when a sharp, bony fragment tents overlying skin; and (4) restore circulation to a pulseless distal extremity. Distal vascular compromise is the most time-critical.
- Open fractures are treated immediately with prophylactic antibiotics to prevent osteomyelitis.[3,4]
- A common regimen is a first-generation cephalosporin and an aminoglycoside. Irrigation and débridement in the operating room may be indicated.[5]
- The fracture or relocated joint should be immobilized. Fiberglass or plaster splinting material is commonly used.
- The chemical reaction that causes the material to set is an exothermic reaction that begins upon contact with water. The amount of heat liberated is directly proportional to the setting process, which in turn is directly proportional to the temperature of the water.
- Severe burns can result from the splinting material, as the peak temperature to the skin is the sum of the water temperature plus the heat released by the exothermic reaction.
- Splints for midshaft fractures should be long enough to immobilize the joint above and below the fracture.
- Crutches should be prescribed for the patient who has a lower extremity injury that requires prevention of bearing weight.
- The pressure of the crutch pads is borne by the sides of the thorax, not the axilla, to avoid injury to the brachial plexus.

REFERENCES

1. Buckwalter JA, Einhorn TA, Marsh JL: Bone and joint healing, in Bucholz RW, Heckman JD (eds): *Rockwood and Green's Fractures in Adults,* Vol. 1, 5th ed. Philadelphia: Lippincott Williams & Wilkins, 2001, p. 245.
2. Schultz RJ: *The Language of Fractures.* Baltimore: Williams & Wilkins, 1972, p. 32.
3. Braun R, Enzler MA, Rittman WW: A double-blind clinical trial of prophylactic cloxacillin in open fractures. *J Orthop Trauma* 1:12, 1987.
4. Worlock P, Slack R, Harvey L, Mawhinney R: The prevention of infection in open fractures: An experimental study of the effects of antibiotic therapy. *J Bone Joint Surg* 70A:1341, 1988.
5. Olson SA, Finkeheier CG, Moehring HD: Open fractures, in Bucholz RW, Heckman JD (eds): *Rockwood and Green's Fractures in Adults,* Vol. 1, 5th ed. Philadelphia: Lippincott Williams & Wilkins, 2001, p. 285.

For further reading in *Emergency Medicine: A Comprehensive Study Guide,* 6th ed., see Chap. 267, "Initial Evaluation and Management of Orthopedic Injuries," by Jeffrey S. Menkes.

173   HAND AND WRIST INJURIES

Michael P. Kefer

ANATOMY AND EXAMINATION

- There are 27 bones in the hand: 14 phalanges, 5 metacarpals, and 8 carpals. The wrist consists of the area from the distal radius to the carpometacarpal joints.
- The intrinsic muscles of the hand are those that originate and insert within the hand. These are the thenar and hypothenar muscle groups, adductor pollicis, the interossei, and the lumbricals.

- Thenar muscles abduct, oppose, and flex the thumb and are innervated by the median nerve.
- Hypothenar muscles abduct, oppose, and flex the little finger and are innervated by the ulnar nerve.
- The adductor pollicis adducts the thumb and is innervated by the ulnar nerve.
- Interosseous muscles adduct and abduct the fingers from the midline and are innervated by the ulnar nerve.
- Lumbricals provide flexion and extension function to the digits. The two radial lumbricals are innervated by the median nerve. The two ulnar lumbricals are innervated by the ulnar nerve.
- The flexor digitorum superficialis inserts into the middle phalanges and flexes all the joints it crosses. Function is tested when the patient flexes the proximal interphalangeal (PIP) joint while the other fingers are held in extension.
- The flexor digitorum profundus inserts at the base of the distal phalanges and flexes the distal interphalangeal (DIP) joint as well as all the other joints flexed by the flexor digitorum superficialis. Function is tested when the patient flexes the DIP joint while the PIP and metacarpal phalangeal (MCP) joints are held in extension.
- The extensor digitorum extends all the digits. Function is tested by having the patient hold the hand in the "stop traffic" position. This also tests radial nerve motor function.
- The radial nerve provides sensation to the dorsal radial aspect of the hand. None of the intrinsic muscles of the hand are innervated by the radial nerve.
- The ulnar nerve provides sensation to the fifth and ulnar half of the fourth digit, and motor function to the intrinsic hand muscles.
- The median nerve provides sensation to the first, second, third, and radial half of the fourth digit, and motor function to the intrinsic hand muscles.

HAND INJURIES

TENDON INJURIES

- Knowing the position of the hand at the time of injury predicts where along its course a tendon is injured.
- Extensor tendon repair can often be performed by the emergency physician.
- Flexor tendon repair should be performed by the hand surgeon.
- It is common for the emergency care of tendon lacerations to consist of closing the skin and splinting until definitive repair by the hand surgeon, which can occur up to 4 weeks later.

MALLET FINGER

- This results from rupture of the extensor tendon at the base of the distal phalanx.
- When associated with an avulsion fracture involving less than one third of the DIP joint surface, treatment consists of splinting the finger in extension for 6 weeks.
- When more than one third of the joint surface is involved, internal fixation is recommended.

BOUTONNIÈRE DEFORMITY

- This results from an injury at the dorsal surface of the PIP joint that disrupts the extensor hood apparatus.
- Lateral bands of the extensor mechanism become flexors of the PIP joint and hyperextensors of the DIP joint.
- An extensor hood injury is easily missed on emergency department (ED) presentation.
- Treatment consists of splinting the PIP joint in extension and referral to an orthopedist.

GAMEKEEPER'S THUMB

- This injury results from forced radial abduction at the MCP joint with injury to the ulnar collateral ligament of the thumb. This is the most critical of the collateral ligament injuries because it affects pincer function.
- A complete tear is diagnosed when abduction stress causes more than 40 degrees of radial angulation.
- Treatment consists of a thumb spica splint and referral for surgical repair.

DISTAL INTERPHALANGEAL JOINT DISLOCATIONS

- These injuries are uncommon because of the firm attachment of skin and fibrous tissue to underlying bone.
- Dislocations are usually dorsal.
- Reduction is performed under digital-block anesthesia. The dislocated phalanx is distracted, slightly hyperextended, then repositioned.
- Inability to reduce the joint may be from an entrapped volar plate, profundus tendon, or avulsion fracture.

PROXIMAL INTERPHALANGEAL JOINT DISLOCATIONS

- Dorsal dislocation results from rupture of the volar plate.

- Reduction is the same method as described for DIP joint dislocations.
- An irreducible joint from an entrapped volar plate may require surgical reduction.
- Lateral dislocation results from rupture of the collateral ligaments.
- Dorsal and lateral reduced injuries should be splinted at 30 degrees flexion and referred.
- Volar dislocation is rare.

METACARPOPHALANGEAL JOINT DISLOCATIONS

- These are usually dorsal dislocations that require surgical reduction due to volar plate entrapment.
- Closed reduction is attempted with the wrist flexed and pressure applied to the proximal phalanx in a distal and volar direction.
- The joint should be splinted in flexion.

DISTAL PHALANX FRACTURES

- A tuft fracture is the most common injury. If associated with subungual hematoma, drainage is recommended.
- Transverse fractures with displacement are always associated with nail bed laceration, which may require repair.
- Avulsion fracture of the base results in a mallet finger.
- If less than one third of the articular surface is involved, a dorsal extension splint should be applied.
- If more than one third of the articular surface is involved, then internal fixation is recommended.

MIDDLE AND PROXIMAL PHALANX FRACTURES

- This diagnosis is often suspected if the fingertips of the closed hand do not point to the same spot on the wrist and the plane of the nail bed of the involved digit is not aligned with the others.
- Treatment of nondisplaced fractures is a gutter splint in the position of function and referral.
- Treatment of displaced fractures usually requires surgical intervention.
- Rotational malalignment is a common problem and requires correction.

METACARPAL FRACTURES

- A fourth or fifth metacarpal neck fracture, the boxer's fracture, is the most common metacarpal fracture.

Angulation of 20 degrees in the ring finger and 40 degrees in the fifth finger can be tolerated, but ideally angulation greater than 20 degrees should be reduced.
- Second and third metacarpal fractures causing angulation greater than 15 degrees should be reduced. Treatment consists of a gutter splint with the wrist extended 20 degrees and the MCP joint flexed 90 degrees and referral.
- First metacarpal base fractures with intra-articular involvement (Bennett and Rolando fractures) should be immobilized in a thumb spica splint and referred for surgical repair.

COMPARTMENT SYNDROME

- Crush injuries to the hand are especially at risk for compartment syndrome.
- Patients will complain of pain that is out of proportion to the physical examination findings.
- Examination reveals the hand at a resting position is extended at the MCP joint and slightly flexed at the PIP joint. This is associated with pain with passive stretch of the involved compartment and tense edema.
- This condition is a surgical emergency.

HIGH PRESSURE INJECTION INJURY

- This injury occurs when substances under high pressure, such as grease, paint, or hydraulic fluid, are injected into the hand.
- Oil-based paint causes the most severe tissue reaction and can result in ischemia, leading to amputation.
- Radiographs of the hand and forearm are indicated to evaluate for radiopaque substances and subcutaneous air.
- This is a surgical emergency.

WRIST INJURIES

SCAPHOLUNATE DISSOCIATION

- The patient with scapholunate dissociation presents with wrist tenderness that may be localized to the scapholunate joint.
- The radiograph demonstrates a space between the scaphoid and lunate that is more than 3 mm.
- Early referral for ligamentous repair is indicated.

LUNATE AND PERILUNATE DISLOCATION

- The most common carpal bone dislocations are lunate and perilunate.

- In both injuries, a lateral wrist radiograph reveals the dislocation, as the normal alignment of the radius-lunate-capitate (the "3 C's" sign) is lost.
- With a lunate dislocation, the lunate dislocates anterior to the radius, but the remainder of the carpus aligns with the radius.
- On posteroanterior (PA) radiograph, the lunate has a triangular shape, which is the pathognomonic "piece of pie" sign. Lateral radiograph reveals the lunate to be displaced and tilted palmarly ("spilled teacup sign").
- With a perilunate dislocation, the lunate remains aligned with the radius, but the remainder of the carpus is dislocated, usually dorsal to the lunate.
- There is usually concomitant fracture of the scaphoid and the proximal portion of the scaphoid remains with the lunate while the distal portion dislocates with the carpus.
- Prompt referral for closed reduction or surgical repair is indicated.

SCAPHOID FRACTURE

- This is the most common carpal fracture.
- The patient is tender in the anatomic snuffbox.
- The wrist radiograph is commonly negative, so the diagnosis is based on physical examination findings.
- Treatment of the patient with snuffbox tenderness is thumb spica splint and referral.
- Without proper treatment, there is risk of avascular necrosis of the scaphoid bone.

TRIQUETRUM FRACTURE

- This is either a dorsal avulsion or body fracture.
- There is tenderness dorsally, just distal to the ulnar styloid.
- The wrist radiograph is often negative, so diagnosis is based on physical examination findings.
- Treatment consists of a volar splint and referral.

LUNATE FRACTURE

- This is the most important of the carpal fractures since it occupies two thirds of the articular surface of the radius. There is risk of avascular necrosis.
- Tenderness is present over the lunate fossa (distal to the rim of the radius at the base of the third metacarpal).
- Wrist radiograph is commonly negative, so diagnosis is based on physical examination findings.
- Treatment consists of a thumb spica splint and referral.

TRAPEZIUM FRACTURE

- Trapezium fracture results in painful thumb movement.
- Tenderness is present at the apex of the anatomic snuffbox and base of the thenar eminence.
- Treatment consists of a thumb spica splint and referral.

PISIFORM FRACTURE

- The pisiform is a sesamoid bone within the flexor carpi ulnaris tendon.
- There is tenderness at its bony prominence at the base of the hypothenar eminence.
- Treatment consists of a volar splint at 30 degrees flexion with ulnar deviation to relieve tension on the tendon and referral.

HAMATE FRACTURE

- Hamate fracture most commonly involves the hook, which is palpable in the soft tissue of the radial aspect of the hypothenar eminence.
- Treatment consists of a volar splint and referral.

CAPITATE FRACTURE

- Isolated capitate fracture is rare. It is usually associated with scaphoid fracture.
- The capitate is also at risk of avascular necrosis.
- Treatment consists of a thumb spica splint and referral.

TRAPEZOID FRACTURE

- Trapezoid fracture is extremely rare and difficult to see on radiographs.
- Treatment consists of a thumb spica splint and referral.

RADIAL STYLOID FRACTURE

- The major carpal ligaments on the radial side of the wrist insert on the radial styloid.
- Fracture of the radial styloid can produce carpal instability and is associated with scapholunate dissociation.
- Early orthopedic referral is indicated.

ULNAR STYLOID FRACTURE

- Ulnar styloid fracture may result in radial ulnar joint instability.

- Treatment consists of an ulnar gutter splint with the wrist in the neutral position and ulnar deviation.

COLLES' AND SMITH'S FRACTURES

- These fractures involve the distal radius at the metaphysis.
- With a Colles' fracture, the distal radius is displaced dorsally, causing a dinner-fork deformity.
- With a Smith's fracture, the distal radius is displaced volarly, causing a garden-spade deformity.
- Treatment is hematoma block, placement of the hand in a finger trap, and closed reduction.

BIBLIOGRAPHY

Belliappa PP, Scheker LR: Functional anatomy of the hand. *Emerg Med Clin North Am* 11:557, 1993.

Gupta A, Kleinerl HE: Evaluating the injured hand. *Hand Clin* 9:195, 1993.

Ritchie JV, Munter DW: Emergency department evaluation and treatment of wrist injuries. *Emerg Med Clin North Am* 17:823, 1999.

Schnall SB, Mirzayan R: High pressure injection injuries to the hand. *Hand Clin* 15:245, 1999.

Sherman GM, Seitz WH: Fractures and dislocations of the wrist. *Curr Opinion Orthop* 10:237, 1999.

Weeks PM: Hand injuries. *Curr Prob Surg* 30:725, 1993.

For further reading in *Emergency Medicine: A Comprehensive Study Guide*, 6th ed., see Chap. 268, "Injuries to the Hand and Digits," by Robert L. Muelleman and Michael C. Wadman; and Chap. 269, "Wrist Injuries," by Dennis T. Uehara, Dean Wolanyk, and Robert H. Escarza.

174 ELBOW AND FOREARM INJURIES

Sandra L. Najarian

ELBOW DISLOCATIONS

CLINICAL FEATURES

- Most elbow dislocations are posterior and result from a fall on an outstretched hand.

- On examination, the patient usually holds the elbow in 45 degrees of flexion. The olecranon is directed posteriorly and is often obscured by significant swelling.
- Neurovascular injury occurs in 8 to 21% of cases; the ulnar nerve and brachial artery are the most frequently injured structures.
- Absence of a radial pulse before reduction, an open dislocation, and other systemic injuries are often associated with arterial injury.[1,2]

DIAGNOSIS AND DIFFERENTIAL

- Radiographs of the elbow confirm the diagnosis. On the lateral view the ulna and radius are displaced posteriorly.
- On the anteroposterior (AP) view, the ulna and radius may be displaced medially or laterally, but maintain their normal relationship to each other.

EMERGENCY DEPARTMENT CARE AND DISPOSITION

- After adequate sedation, closed reduction of the elbow dislocation is accomplished by gentle traction on the wrist and forearm while an assistant applies countertraction on the upper arm.
- Any medial or lateral displacement is corrected with the other hand. Distal traction is applied to the wrist while downward pressure is applied to the proximal forearm to help disengage the coronoid process from the olecranon fossa.
- Neurovascular status must be reassessed after reduction and a period of observation. Postreduction films should be obtained.
- A long arm posterior splint is used to immobilize the elbow in 90 degrees of flexion.
- The risk of subsequent edema is significant, and cylindrical casts should not be placed.
- Close orthopedic follow-up must be arranged. Patients with instability in extension, neurovascular compromise, or open dislocations require immediate orthopedic consultation.

ELBOW FRACTURES

PATHOPHYSIOLOGY

- The most common fracture of the elbow is a radial head fracture, which usually results from a fall on an outstretched hand.
- Intercondylar fractures result from a force directed against the elbow and occur most commonly in adults.

- Supracondylar fractures are extra-articular fractures that occur most commonly in children.
- Ninety-five percent of supracondylar fractures are extra-articular, resulting from an extension force.
- Olecranon fractures often result from direct trauma.

CLINICAL FEATURES

- Radial head fractures produce lateral elbow pain and tenderness, and an inability to fully extend the elbow.
- Patients with intercondylar and supracondylar fractures will have significant swelling and tenderness and limited range of motion.
- Supracondylar fractures may resemble a posterior elbow dislocation because the olecranon is prominent posteriorly. Evaluation of neurovascular compromise is essential since neurovascular injuries are common with supracondylar fractures.
- The anterior interosseus nerve, a motor branch of the median nerve, is most prone to injury with supracondylar fractures. Anterior interosseus nerve function is demonstrated by flexion of the index finger distal interphalangeal joint and thumb interphalangeal joint.
- The most serious complication of supracondylar fractures is Volkmann's ischemic contracture, which manifests as muscle and nerve necrosis resulting from edema that reduces arterial and venous flow through the volar compartment of the forearm.
- Pain with passive extension of the fingers, forearm tenderness, and refusal to open the hand are signs of impending Volkmann's ischemia.
- Acute vascular injuries are usually secondary to transient vasospasm, which results in a decreased or absent radial pulse.
- Olecranon fractures result in localized swelling and tenderness and limited mobility.
- With olecranon fractures, triceps function is often weak. The ulnar nerve is the most commonly injured nerve with this injury.

DIAGNOSIS AND DIFFERENTIAL

- Radial head fractures may not present with a visible fracture line. A posterior fat pad sign may be the only evidence of injury.
- Careful inspection for a fracture line separating the condyles and the humerus signifies an intercondylar fracture.
- In supracondylar fractures, the AP radiograph shows a transverse fracture line, and the lateral view reveals an oblique fracture line and displacement of the distal fragment proximally and posteriorly.
- In supracondylar fractures, a posterior and anterior fat pad sign may also be seen on the lateral view.[3]

- In olecranon fractures, it is important to note any displacement (>2 mm).

EMERGENCY DEPARTMENT CARE AND DISPOSITION

- Immobilization in a splint and orthopedic referral are appropriate for nondisplaced fractures.
- Minimally displaced radial head fractures may be treated with a sling and early range of motion.
- Immediate orthopedic consultation is warranted for all displaced fractures, open fractures, and evidence of neurovascular compromise.
- Patients with supracondylar fractures warrant orthopedic consultation and admission for observation of neurovascular status.
- Supracondylar fractures are often treated with closed reduction and percutaneous pinning.
- Displaced intercondylar fractures and olecranon fractures often require open reduction and internal fixation.
- Nondisplaced olecranon fractures (less than 2 mm in both flexion and extension) are treated with immobilization; all others are treated surgically.

EPICONDYLE FRACTURES

- Lateral epicondyle fractures are rare because the anatomic position of the condyle reduces the exposure of the epicondyle to direct trauma.
- Lateral condyle fractures occur in children and are more common than medial condyle fractures.
- Isolated medial epicondyle fractures are extra-articular and occur most commonly in children and adolescents. Direct trauma, posterior elbow dislocation, or repeated valgus stress such as throwing a baseball (little league elbow), are mechanisms for injury.
- Patients will present with medial elbow pain and demonstrate tenderness with pronation and with forearm and wrist flexion.
- Medial epicondylar fractures may be associated with ulnar nerve injury.
- Nondisplaced and minimally displaced fractures (less than 2 mm) are treated with long arm splint immobilization. Displaced fractures require orthopedic referral for open reduction and internal fixation.

FOREARM FRACTURES

PATHOPHYSIOLOGY

- Fractures of the ulna and radius usually occur from significant trauma, such as a motor vehicle crash or a fall from height.

- Isolated fractures of the ulna usually occur from a direct blow to the forearm.
- Radius fractures usually result from direct trauma or from a fall on an outstretched hand.

CLINICAL FEATURES

- Isolated ulna or radius fractures present with localized swelling and tenderness over the fracture site.
- Examination of both bone fractures reveals swelling, tenderness, and deformity of the forearm. Open fractures of the forearm are common.
- Nerve function must be carefully assessed. Evaluating radial nerve function is accomplished by having the patient extend both the wrist and fingers against resistance and by testing sensation over the dorsum of the thumb-index finger web space.
- Abducting the thumb against resistance (recurrent branch of the median nerve) and intact sensation on the radial side of the palm indicate intact median nerve function.
- The ability to abduct the index finger against resistance and the presence of intact sensation over the distal tip of the little finger indicate proper ulnar nerve function.
- Monteggia's fracture-dislocation, a fracture of the proximal ulna shaft with a radial head dislocation, presents with significant pain and swelling over the elbow.
- Paralysis of the posterior interosseus nerve (deep branch of the radial nerve) is a potential complication of Monteggia's fracture.
- Galeazzi's fracture-dislocation, a fracture of the distal radius with an associated distal radioulnar joint dislocation, causes localized swelling and tenderness over the distal radius and wrist.

DIAGNOSIS AND DIFFERENTIAL

- The amount of displacement, angulation, and shortening needs to be evaluated.
- Any rotational angulation should be noted. A sudden change in the width of a bone or a change in the normal orientation of various bony prominences suggests rotational deformity.
- Isolated ulna fractures are considered displaced if there is greater than 10 degrees angulation or more than 50% displacement.
- The radial head dislocation in a Monteggia's fracture can be subtle.[4] Normally, the radial head aligns with the capitellum in all radiographic views of the elbow. The radial head dislocation is in the same direction as the apex of the ulnar fracture.

- In Galeazzi's fracture, the distal radioulnar joint dislocation may be difficult to identify. An increase in the distal radioulnar joint space may be seen on the AP view; on the lateral view, the ulna is displaced dorsally.

EMERGENCY DEPARTMENT CARE AND DISPOSITION

- Nondisplaced isolated fractures may be immobilized in a long arm cast and given close orthopedic referral.
- Displaced ulnar fractures with angulation greater than 10 degrees or displacement of more than 50% require open reduction and internal fixation.
- Closed reduction is often adequate for both bone fractures in children.
- Open reduction and internal fixation is usually required for displaced fractures in adults, and Monteggia's and Galeazzi's fracture-dislocations.

BICEP AND TRICEP RUPTURES

CLINICAL FEATURES

- Rupture of the proximal long head of the biceps is the most common type, and usually occurs after a sudden or prolonged contraction against resistance. Patients often describe a snap or pop and complain of pain in the anterior shoulder.
- Swelling, tenderness, and crepitus over the bicipital groove can be seen on examination in biceps ruptures. The distally retracted biceps will appear as a ball in the middle of the arm when the elbow is flexed.
- In biceps ruptures, there is minimal loss of strength in elbow flexion because of the function of the brachialis and supinators.
- Distal biceps injuries are rare.[5,6] Weakness in flexion and supination of the forearm is more apparent than in proximal ruptures.
- Triceps ruptures almost always occur distally as a result of a direct blow to the olecranon or a fall on an outstretched hand, causing a forceful flexion of the extended forearm.
- An associated olecranon avulsion fracture is common.
- On examination with triceps ruptures, swelling and tenderness is noted proximal to the olecranon. Extension of the forearm is weak.
- Triceps function can be assessed using a modified Thompson's test. With the arm supported, the elbow flexed at 90 degrees, and the forearm hanging in a relaxed position, squeezing the triceps should produce extension of the forearm. This is absent in a complete triceps rupture.

DIAGNOSIS AND DIFFERENTIAL

- Diagnosis is clinical.
- Radiographs should be obtained to exclude an associated olecranon avulsion fracture.

EMERGENCY DEPARTMENT CARE AND DISPOSITION

- Treatment includes sling, ice, analgesia, and orthopedic referral for definitive management.
- Surgical repair is indicated for young, active individuals with complete ruptures.

REFERENCES

1. Cohen MS, Hastings H: Acute elbow dislocation: evaluation and management. *J Am Acad Orthop Surg* 6:15, 1998.
2. Hildebrand KA, Patterson SD, King GJ: Acute elbow dislocations: Simple and complex. *Orthop Clin North Am* 30:63, 1999.
3. Villarin LA, Belk KE, Freid R: Emergency department evaluation and treatment of elbow and forearm injuries. *Emerg Med Clin North Am* 17:843, 1999.
4. Perron AD: Orthopedic pitfalls in the ED: Galeazzi and Monteggia fracture-dislocation. *Am J Emerg Med* 19:225, 2001.
5. Baker BE, Bierwagen D: Rupture of the distal tendon of the biceps brachii. *J Bone Joint Surg* 67:414, 1985.
6. Bernstein AD, Breslow MJ, Jazrawi LM: Distal biceps tendon ruptures: A historical perspective and current concepts. *Am J Orthop* 30:193, 2001.

For further reading in *Emergency Medicine: A Comprehensive Study Guide,* 6th ed., see Chap. 270, "Injuries to the Elbow and Forearm," by Arthur F. Proust, Jason H. Bredenkamp, and Dennis T. Uehara.

175 SHOULDER AND HUMERUS INJURIES

Robert J. French

STERNOCLAVICULAR JOINT INJURIES

CLINICAL FEATURES

- The sternoclavicular joint is the most frequently moved nonaxial joint of the body since virtually all movements of the upper extremity are transferred proximally to this joint.
- Sternoclavicular injury results from direct trauma to the joint or forceful rolling of the shoulder forward or backward.
- Sternoclavicular sprains cause localized pain and swelling.
- The sternoclavicular joint is the least commonly dislocated major joint in the body.
- Anterior dislocations are more common than posterior dislocations.[1]
- Posterior dislocations are more ominous due to potential injury to mediastinal contents.
- Patients with sternoclavicular dislocations experience severe pain that is exacerbated by movement or lying supine.
- Anterior dislocations can be diagnosed clinically by visual and palpable prominence of the medial clavicular head.
- In posterior dislocations, the medial clavicular head is less visible and nonpalpable. The expected medial clavicle depression may be obscured by local edema, resulting in a missed or delayed diagnosis.
- Patients with posterior dislocations may present with hoarseness, dysphagia, dyspnea, upper extremity paresthesias, and weakness.

DIAGNOSIS AND DIFFERENTIAL

- Plain radiographs cannot reliably differentiate sprains from dislocations.
- Computed tomography (CT) imaging can accurately diagnose sternoclavicular joint dislocations.

EMERGENCY DEPARTMENT CARE AND DISPOSITION

- Treatment of sternoclavicular sprains consists of ice, analgesics, and an arm sling.
- After closed reduction of an anterior sternoclavicular dislocation, the patient should be placed in a figure-of-eight clavicle splint. These reductions often prove to be unstable.
- For nonreducible anterior dislocations and all posterior dislocations, urgent orthopedic consultation is required.

CLAVICLE FRACTURES

CLINICAL FEATURES

- Clavicle fractures account for almost one-half of significant shoulder girdle injuries and are the most common fracture in children.

- The most common mechanism is a direct blow to the shoulder that causes buckling of the clavicle.
- Patients typically present with pain, swelling, deformity, and localized tenderness.
- Although rare, injuries to the lung and neurovascular bundle can occur.
- Routine clavicle views reveal 80% of fractures in the middle third of the clavicle, 15% in the distal third, and 5% in the medial third.

EMERGENCY DEPARTMENT CARE AND DISPOSITION

- Treatment consists of analgesics and immobilization, preferably by sling, for 4 to 8 weeks.
- Orthopedic consultation is needed for open fractures, neurovascular compromise, skin tenting, or interposition of soft tissue.
- The nonunion rate varies from 0.1 to 15%.[2] Factors associated with nonunion are marked initial displacement and shortening.[3] Early orthopedic follow-up is required.

ACROMIOCLAVICULAR JOINT INJURIES

CLINICAL FEATURES

- Injury to the acromioclavicular joint occurs most commonly in young men secondary to sport-related activities.
- The mechanism of injury is usually direct trauma to the point of the shoulder with the arm adducted.
- Patients typically present with tenderness and deformity at the acromioclavicular joint.

DIAGNOSIS AND DIFFERENTIAL

- These injuries are classified as types I through VI based on severity of injury to the acromioclavicular and coracoclavicular ligaments.[4]
- An acromioclavicular ligament sprain or partial tear is a type I injury and radiographs will be normal.
- Type II injuries, associated with disruption of the acromioclavicular ligament, result in 25 to 50% elevation of the clavicle above the acromial process.
- Type III injuries, characterized by complete disruption of the acromioclavicular and coracoclavicular ligaments, reveal 100% superior displacement of the clavicle and coracoclavicular space widening.
- Types III through VI represent complete acromioclavicular and coracoclavicular ligament disruption with varied orientations of the displaced clavicle.

- In type I and type II injuries, the coracoclavicular distance is 1.1 to 1.3 cm. A coracoclavicular gap differential of more than 5 mm between the injured and uninjured shoulders is diagnostic of a type III injury.

EMERGENCY DEPARTMENT CARE AND DISPOSITION

- Treatment of type I and type II injuries consists of rest, ice, analgesics, and immobilization for 1 to 3 weeks. Once pain-free, the patient can begin range-of-motion and strengthening exercises.
- Treatment of type III injuries is controversial, with proponents for conservative or operative management. The recent trend favors conservative management, as in type I and II injuries.[5]
- More severe injuries, types IV through VI, are generally managed operatively.

GLENOHUMERAL JOINT DISLOCATION

CLINICAL FEATURES

- Dislocation of the glenohumeral joint is the most common major joint dislocation.
- The glenohumeral joint can dislocate anteriorly, posteriorly, inferiorly, and superiorly. Anterior dislocations account for 95 to 97% of all dislocations.
- Posterior dislocations account for 2%. Inferior dislocations (luxatio erecta) are extremely rare, accounting for 0.5% of glenohumeral joint dislocations.
- The most common mechanism for anterior dislocation is an indirect force levered on the joint capsule from a combination of abduction, extension, and external rotation.
- Posterior dislocations occur in patients with convulsive seizures, anterior blows to the shoulder, and falls on an outstretched hand.
- The mechanism for inferior dislocation is either forceful hyperabduction or inferior directed axial load on the abducted shoulder.
- In anterior dislocations, the patient typically is in severe pain and holds the arm in slight abduction and external rotation. The shoulder has a "squared off" and shortened appearance.
- In posterior dislocations, the arm is held across the chest in adduction and internal rotation. The anterior shoulder appears flat with a prominent coracoid process, while the posterior aspect appears full, and external rotation is blocked.
- In inferior dislocations, the patient presents with the arm locked overhead.

- The axillary nerve is the most common neurovascular structure injured in anterior dislocations and can be assessed by pinprick sensation over the skin of the lateral shoulder.

DIAGNOSIS AND DIFFERENTIAL

- Anteroposterior (AP) and lateral scapular "Y" or axillary views should be obtained.[6,7]
- Although associated fractures can be radiographically identified in up to half of patients with glenohumeral dislocation, most of these fractures are compression fractures of the humeral head (Hill-Sachs lesion) that require no additional treatment.[8]
- Other associated injuries include anterior glenoid rim fractures (Bankard lesion), greater tuberosity avulsion fractures, and rotator cuff tears.
- In posterior dislocations, AP radiographs in posterior glenohumeral dislocations show a loss of the elliptical half-moon shape overlap seen on normal films. The humeral head takes on a "light bulb" or "drumstick" appearance due to its internally rotated configuration.

EMERGENCY DEPARTMENT CARE AND DISPOSITION

- Multiple techniques have been described to reduce anterior glenohumeral dislocations.
- Modified Hippocratic technique: This method uses traction-countertraction. The patient is supine with the arm abducted and flexed 90 degrees. The physician gradually applies traction while the assistant provides countertraction. Gentle internal and external rotation may aid reduction.
- Stimson technique: The patient is placed prone on a gurney with the dislocated extremity hanging over the side and a 10-pound weight attached at the wrist. Reduction occurs in 20 to 30 minutes if complete muscle relaxation is achieved.
- Milch technique: With the patient supine, the physician slowly abducts and externally rotates the arm to the overhead position. With the elbow fully extended, gentle traction is applied. If reduction is not achieved, the humeral head can be manipulated into the glenoid fossa with the physician's free hand.
- Scapular manipulation technique: The first step is to apply traction to the arm held in 90 degrees of forward flexion. This can be accomplished in the prone position using the Stimson technique or in a seated position with an assistant applying traction.[9,10] The arm should be positioned in slight external rotation. The scapular tip is then pushed as far medially as possible while stabilizing the superior aspect of the scapula with the other hand.[11] A small amount of dorsal displacement of the scapula tip is recommended.

- External rotation technique: The patient is supine with the arm adducted to the side. The elbow is flexed to 90 degrees and the arm is slowly and gently externally rotated. No traction is applied. Reduction is subtle and usually occurs prior to reaching the coronal plane.
- Aronen technique. This technique is most useful when reduction is easy to achieve, as in recurrent dislocations or immediately after injury, before muscle spasm and swelling have occurred. In this technique, the patient is seated with the ipsilateral leg and knee in flexion. The patient is instructed to clasp his or her hands around the ipsilateral knee and then relax the shoulder muscles, allowing the weight of the lower limb to provide gentle in-line traction. Countertraction is applied by the patient's upper body weight and his or her own paraspinous muscles.[12,13]
- After reduction, a shoulder immobilizer or a sling and swath should be applied and orthopedic follow-up arranged.
- The shoulder should be immobilized for 3 to 6 weeks in younger patients and 1 or 2 weeks in older patients (age >40 years).[13]
- In posterior dislocations, reduction is performed in the supine patient by applying axial traction along the long axis of the humerus, anteriorly directed pressure on the posterior humeral head, and a small amount of external rotation.
- For inferior dislocations, reduction consists of traction in an upward and outward direction in line with the humerus.

SCAPULA INJURIES

CLINICAL FEATURES

- Fractures of the scapula are a rare occurrence, accounting for less than 1% of all fractures.[14]
- Due to the excessive forces needed to fracture this protected bone, associated injuries of the ipsilateral lung, thoracic cage, and shoulder girdle are a major concern.[15]
- Patients will present with localized tenderness over the scapula and the arm held in adduction.

EMERGENCY DEPARTMENT CARE AND DISPOSITION

- A thorough investigation for associated intrathoracic injuries is mandated. Careful consideration should be made for admission of patients with scapula fracture for observation.

- The fracture is managed nonoperatively with a sling for immobilization, ice, analgesics, and early range-of-motion exercises.
- Surgical intervention may be warranted for displaced glenoid articular fractures, angulated glenoid neck fractures, and certain acromion or coracoid fractures.

HUMERUS FRACTURES

CLINICAL FEATURES

- Fractures of the proximal humerus are a relatively common injury, and are typically seen in elderly patients with osteoporosis after a fall on an outstretched hand.
- Humeral shaft fractures occur most commonly in young men and osteoporotic women after direct or indirect trauma to the humeral shaft.
- Patients with proximal humerus and humeral shaft fractures present with localized pain, swelling, tenderness, ecchymosis, and crepitus.
- In proximal humerus fractures, a thorough neurovascular examination can identify injuries of the axillary nerve, axillary artery, or brachial plexus.
- Shortening of the upper extremity may be noted in displaced humeral shaft fractures.
- In humeral shaft fractures, a careful neurovascular exam may reveal injuries to the brachial artery or vein, or the radial, ulnar, or median nerves.
- The most commonly injured nerves in proximal humerus fractures and humeral shaft fractures are the axillary nerve and the radial nerve, respectively.

EMERGENCY DEPARTMENT CARE AND DISPOSITION

- Treatment consists of analgesics, immobilization, and orthopedic referral for simple fractures. Immobilization can be achieved with a sling and swath or a shoulder immobilizer.
- Urgent orthopedic consultation is indicated for multipart proximal humerus fractures, significantly displaced or angulated shaft fractures, open fractures, or any fracture with neurovascular compromise.

REFERENCES

1. Yeh GL, Williams GR: Conservative management of sternoclavicular injuries. *Orthop Clin North Am* 31:189, 2000.
2. Chu CM, Wang SJ, Lin LC: Fixation of mid-third clavicular fractures with Knowles pins: 78 patients followed for 2-7 years. *Acta Orthop Scand* 73:134, 2002.
3. Wick M, Mueller EJ, et al: Midshaft fractures of the clavicle with a shortening of more than 2 cm. Predisposes to nonunion. *Arch Orthop Trauma Surg* 121:2072, 2001.
4. Clarke HD, McCann PD: Acromioclavicular joint injuries. *Orthop Clin North Am* 31:177, 2000.
5. Bradley JP, Hussein E: Decision making: operative versus nonoperative treatment of acromioclavicular joint injuries. *Clin Sports Med* 22:277, 2003.
6. Hendey GW, Kinlaw K: Clinically significant abnormalities in postreduction radiographs after anterior shoulder dislocation. *Ann Emerg Med* 28:399, 1996.
7. Shuster M, Abu-Laban RB, Boyd J: Prereduction radiographs in clinically evident anterior shoulder dislocation. *Am J Emerg Med* 17:653, 1999.
8. Cleeman E, Flatow EL: Shoulder dislocation in the young patient. *Orthop Clin North Am* 31:217, 2000.
9. Anderson D, Zvirbulis R, Ciullo J: Scapular manipulation for reduction of anterior shoulder dislocations. *Clin Orthop Rel Res* 164:181, 1982.
10. McNamara RM: Reduction of anterior shoulder dislocations by scapular manipulation. *Ann Emerg Med* 22:1140, 1993.
11. Kothari RU, Dronen SC: The scapular manipulation technique for the reduction of acute anterior shoulder dislocations. *J Emerg Med* 8:625, 1990.
12. Garrik JG, Webb DR: *Sports Injuries: Diagnosis and Management,* 1st ed. Philadelphia: Saunders,1990, p. 61.
13. Wen DY: Current concepts in the treatment of anterior shoulder dislocations. *Am J Emerg Med* 17:410, 1999.
14. McGinnis M, Denton JR: Fractures of the scapula: a retrospective study of 40 fractured scapulae. *J Trauma* 29:1488, 1989.
15. Ada JR, Miller ME: Scapular fractures: analysis of 113 cases. *Clin Orthop* 269:174, 1991.

For further reading in *Emergency Medicine: A Comprehensive Study Guide,* 6th ed., see Chap. 271, "Injuries to the Shoulder Complex and Humerus," by Dennis T. Uehara and John P. Rudzinski.

176 PELVIS, HIP, AND FEMUR INJURIES

E. Parker Hays, Jr.

PELVIS FRACTURES

EPIDEMIOLOGY

- Pelvic fractures are associated with high morbidity and mortality rates because of the immense forces needed to fracture the bony pelvis; concomitant abdominal, chest, and head injuries; and the potential of severe hemorrhage.

- Most pelvic fractures are the result of motor vehicle passenger or pedestrian accidents or falls in the elderly.

CLINICAL FEATURES

- Pelvic fractures should be suspected whenever there is trauma to the torso or a fall from a height.
- Pain, crepitus, or instability on palpation of the pelvis suggests a fracture.
- Perianal edema, pelvic edema, ecchymoses, lacerations, deformities, and hematomas over the inguinal ligament or the scrotum (Destot's sign) suggest pelvic fracture.
- The fracture line may be palpated on rectal examination (Earle's sign).
- Hypotension may be secondary to abdominal or thoracic injuries, or blood loss from disrupted pelvic bones or vessels.

DIAGNOSIS AND DIFFERENTIAL

- On radiograph, the anteroposterior (AP) pelvic radiograph is the most useful view. Additional views include oblique hemi-pelvis, inlet (to evaluate AP displacement), and outlet views (to evaluate superior-inferior displacement).
- Computed tomography (CT) is superior to plain radiographs in assessing the posterior arch, the acetabulum, and for associated hemorrhage.[1]

- Many classifications for pelvic fractures exist. The Young system is helpful, as its classifications are based on the mechanism and directional forces, and it may predict the likelihood of severe hemorrhage (Table 176-1).[2]
- Four main patterns (suggested by the alignment of pubic rami fractures, pubic symphysis diastasis, and sacroiliac joint displacement) are described in the Young system: (1) lateral compression (LC) may result from a side-impact motor vehicle crash, and has a mortality rate approaching 13%; (2) anteroposterior compression (APC) classically resulting from a head-on motor vehicle crash, with a mortality rate approaching 25%; (3) vertical shear (VS) usually results from a fall or jump from a height, with a mortality rate approaching 25%; and (4) combination mechanisms (CM), with LC/VS being the most common.[3,4]

EMERGENCY DEPARTMENT CARE AND DISPOSITION

- Standard protocols for evaluation and stabilization of trauma patients should be initiated. Patients should receive supplemental oxygen, cardiac monitoring, and two IV lines.
- Blood should be sent for type and cross-matching. Since hemorrhage is the cause of death in 50% of pelvic fractures, early use of blood products is indicated.[2]
- Unstable pelvic fractures may be wrapped in a bed sheet that is tensioned circumferentially to reduce pelvic volume and stem hemorrhage.
- Orthopedics should be consulted expeditiously to consider external fixation, especially if there is evidence of

TABLE 176-1   **Injury Classification Keys According to the Young System**

CATEGORY	DISTINGUISHING CHARACTERISTICS [SEVERE HEMORRHAGE INCIDENCE (%)]

LC	Transverse fracture of pubic rami, ipsilateral or contralateral to posterior injury:
	  I: Sacral compression on side of impact
	  II: Crescent (iliac wing) fracture on side of impact (36%)
	  III: LC-1 or LC-2 injury on side of impact; contralateral open-book (APC) injury (60%)

APC	Symphyseal diastasis and/or longitudinal rami fractures:
	  I: Slight widening of public symphysis and/or anterior SI joint; stretched but intact anterior SI, sacrotuberous, and sacrospinous ligaments; intact posterior SI ligaments
	  II: Widened anterior SI joint; disrupted anterior SI, sacrotuberous, and sacrospinous ligaments; intact posterior SI ligaments (28%)
	  III: Complete SI joint disruption with lateral displacement; disrupted anterior SI, sacrotuberous, and sacrospinous ligaments; disrupted posterior SI ligaments (53%)

VS	Symphyseal diastasis or vertical displacement anteriorly and posteriorly, usually through the SI joint, occasionally through the iliac wing and/or sacrum (75%)
CM	Combination of other injury patterns, LC/VS being the most common (58%)

ABBREVIATIONS: APC = anterior-posterior compression; CM = combination mechanisms; LC = lateral compression; SI = sacroiliac; VS = vertical shear.

continued blood loss with disruption of the posterior elements.
- Angiography for embolization of pelvic vessels is indicated in 2% of pelvic fractures and approaches 100% efficacy.[5] Younger age and shorter time to embolization are associated with improved survival.
- Intra-abdominal solid organ injuries and other sources of blood loss should be considered. If diagnostic peritoneal lavage is performed, a supraumbilical approach should be taken to avoid disruption of a pelvic hematoma.
- Rectal examination (and bimanual pelvic examination for women) should be performed for rectal and gynecologic injuries. Rectal injuries are treated with irrigation, diverting colostomy, and IV antibiotics.
- If blood is found on initial pelvic examination, a speculum examination should be performed to evaluate for vaginal lacerations (which may occur with anterior pelvic fractures). Vaginal lacerations mandate operative débridement, irrigation, and IV antibiotics.

STABLE PELVIC AVULSION AND SINGLE BONE FRACTURES

- Table 176-2 reviews the clinical findings of pelvic avulsion and single bone fractures.

- Avulsion fractures include anterior superior iliac spine (ASIS), anterior inferior iliac spine (AIIS), and the ischial tuberosity, any of which may be avulsed during forceful muscular contraction of attached muscles.
- Avulsion fractures present with localized pain that is worsened with contraction of the involved muscles.
- Treatment of avulsion fractures is conservative with rest in a position of comfort and use of crutches with partial weight bearing followed by full weight bearing.[6]
- Fracture of a single ischial bone or pubic ramus can occur in the elderly from a fall with direct trauma.
- If no other injuries are present, fractures of a single ischial bone or pubic ramus are stable (do not compromise pelvic ring integrity) and are treated with analgesia, rest, crutches if necessary, and primary physician or orthopedic follow-up in 1 to 2 weeks.
- Iliac wing (Duverney) fractures present with pain and swelling over the iliac wing. Intra-abdominal injuries may coexist.[7]
- Sacral fractures occur from large AP traumatic forces. They may be difficult to diagnose on radiograph. Neurologic injury does not occur with fractures below S4. Sacral root injuries may be present in up to one third of sacral fractures.

TABLE 176-2 Pelvic Avulsion and Single Bone Fractures

FRACTURE	MECHANISM OF INJURY	CLINICAL FINDINGS/ ASSOCIATED INJURIES
Iliac wing (Duverney) fracture	Direct trauma, usually lateral to medial	Swelling, tenderness over iliac wing; abdominal pain; ileus; acetabular fractures; serious injury infrequent
Single ramus of pubis or ischium	Fall or direct trauma in elderly; exercise-induced stress fracture in young or in pregnant women	Local pain and tenderness; inability to ambulate; rectal injury
Ischium body	Violent, external trauma or from fall in sitting position; least common fracture	Local pain and tenderness; pain with hamstring movement; rectal injury
Sacral fracture	Transverse fractures from direct AP trauma; upper transverse fractures from fall in flexed position	Pain on rectal exam; sacral root injury with upper transverse fractures
Coccyx fracture	Fall in sitting position; more common in women	Pain, tenderness over sacral region; pain on compression during rectal exam
Anterior superior iliac spine (ASIS)	Forceful sartorius muscle contraction (eg, adolescent sprinters)	Pain with hip flexion and abduction
Anterior inferior iliac spine (AIIS)	Forceful rectus femoris muscle contraction (eg, adolescent soccer players)	Pain in groin; pain with hip flexion
Ischial tuberosity	Forceful contraction of hamstrings	Pain with sitting or flexing the thigh

ABBREVIATION: AP = anteroposterior.

ACETABULAR FRACTURES

- Acetabular fractures account for 20% of pelvic injuries and usually occur secondary to a motor vehicle crash.[8]
- The four anatomic sites of fracture—posterior, ilioischial column, transverse, and iliopubic column—are all associated with hip dislocations.[9]
- The most common complication is a sciatic nerve injury, especially with posterior column fracture.
- Early orthopedic consultation and hospital admission are indicated for patients with acetabular fractures.

HIP AND FEMUR INJURIES

HIP FRACTURES

- The incidence of hip fractures in the United States is 80 per 100,000.[10] The incidence increases with age and doubles for each decade after 50. It is three to four times higher in women than in men.
- The affected leg is classically shortened and externally rotated. The position of the extremity, ecchymoses, deformity, and range of motion should be evaluated.
- Complications of hip fractures include infection, venous thromboembolism, avascular necrosis, and nonunion.
- AP, lateral, and frog-leg views will evaluate the femur and acetabulum. Hip fractures are classified as intracapsular (femoral head and neck) or extracapsular (intertrochanteric and subtrochanteric).
- Intracapsular fractures may compromise blood supply to the femoral head and lead to avascular necrosis.
- Isolated femoral head fractures are most commonly associated with hip dislocations.
- Femoral neck fractures are common in elderly patients with osteoporosis. The leg is shortened, abducted and held in external rotation.
- Significant complications of femoral neck fractures include infection, thromboembolism, nonunion, and avascular necrosis.[11]
- Nondisplaced neck fractures are treated with pin fixation. Displaced fractures are treated with open reduction or prosthesis placement.
- Stress fracture of the femur should be suspected if there is significant pain without radiographic abnormality. Radiographs should reveal a fracture, but a bone scan is more sensitive for subtle fractures.
- Stress fractures are treated conservatively with a bone scan in 1 to 2 days or follow-up radiograph in 10 to 14 days.
- Intertrochanteric fractures generally occur in the elderly after a fall or a motor vehicle crash. The extremity is markedly externally rotated and shortened.

- Intertrochanteric fractures are classified as stable or unstable. Stable fractures are those in which the medial cortices of the femoral neck and the femoral fragments abut. Buck's traction may be applied until surgical fixation is performed. Overall mortality is 10 to 30%.
- Subtrochanteric fractures may be seen in elderly osteoporotic patients and young patients after major trauma. Symptoms include pain, deformity, and swelling.
- Patients with subtrochanteric fractures may present hypotensive secondary to blood loss into the soft tissue of the thigh. Immobilization with a traction apparatus is recommended, with eventual open reduction and internal fixation.[12]
- Greater trochanter fractures may occur in adults (true fracture) or children (avulsion of the apophysis). Pain is present on abduction and extension of the leg.
- Treatment of greater trochanter fractures is controversial, and may include conservative treatment or operative fixation (based on patient age and displacement of fragment).
- Lesser trochanter avulsions are most common in young athletes after avulsion secondary to a forceful contraction of the iliopsoas muscle. There is pain during flexion and internal rotation. If there is more than 2 cm of displacement, operative fixation with screws is recommended.
- Following trauma, significant hip pain with weight bearing, even in the presence of normal plain radiographs, suggests the possibility of an occult fracture, especially of the femoral neck or the acetabulum.
- If an occult fracture is suspected, close follow-up is needed for CT scan or magnetic resonance imaging (MRI). MRI is reliable in detecting occult fractures within 24 hours of injury.[13,14]

HIP DISLOCATIONS

- Hip dislocations are most often the result of massive forces during trauma. Ninety percent are posterior and ten percent are anterior.
- Both types should be treated with early closed reduction (<6 hours) in order to decrease the incidence of avascular necrosis.
- Posterior dislocations, which occur when a posterior force is applied to the flexed knee, may coexist with acetabular fractures. The leg is foreshortened, internally rotated and adducted. AP, lateral, and oblique views will evaluate the status of the acetabulum and the femoral head.
- Treatment of posterior dislocations includes early closed reduction using the Allis maneuver (hip flexion to 90°, then internal and external rotation) or the

Stimson maneuver (patient prone, with the leg hanging over the edge of the stretcher, and application of gentle traction).

- Anterior dislocations occur during forced abduction. The leg is held in abduction and external rotation.
- Treatment of anterior dislocations includes early closed reduction with strong, in-line traction, and flexing and internally rotating the leg with abduction once the femoral head clears the acetabulum.

FEMORAL SHAFT FRACTURES

- Femoral shaft fractures typically occur in active patients from industrial accidents, motor vehicle crashes, and gunshot wounds.[15]
- Spiral midshaft femur fractures can occur in toddlers who are running and trip in a twisting fashion. Midshaft femur fractures in children can be a result of neglect or abuse.
- Since the femur has a rich vascular supply and is surrounded by soft tissue, it can accommodate 1 liter or more of blood, potentially contributing to hypotension and shock after a fracture.
- Open fractures should be grossly decontaminated and IV cephalosporin administered.
- Distal neurovascular function should be thoroughly evaluated as sciatic nerve injury can occur. Diagnosis is confirmed radiographically.
- Treatment involves immediate immobilization with Hare or Sager traction (relatively contraindicated in open fractures and sciatic nerve injury) or a Thomas splint.
- Definitive repair is by operative fixation, or traction in children.
- Open femur fractures require early orthopedic consultation for copious irrigation and débridement in the operating room.[16]

REFERENCES

1. Yang AP, Iannacone WM: External fixation for pelvic ring disruptions. *Orthop Clin North Am* 28:331, 1997.
2. Cryer HM, Miller FB, Evers BM, Rouben LR: Pelvic fracture classification: Correlation with hemorrhage. *J Trauma* 28:973, 1988.
3. Young JWR, Burgess AR: *Radiologic Management of Pelvic Ring Fracture: Systematic Radiologic Diagnosis.* Baltimore: Urban & Schwarzenberg, 1987, p. 134.
4. Dalal SA, Burgess AR, Siegel JH, et al: Pelvic fracture in multiple trauma: Classification by mechanism is key to problem of organ injury, resuscitation requirements and outcome. *J Trauma* 29:981, 1989.
5. Agolini SF, Shah K, Jaffe J, et al: Arterial embolization is a rapid and effective technique for controlling pelvic fracture hemorrhage. *J Trauma* 43:395, 1997.
6. Gruen GS, Leit ME, Gruen RJ, et al: Functional outcome of patients with unstable pelvic ring fractures stabilized with open reduction and internal fixation. *J Trauma* 39:838, 1995.
7. Burgess AR, Jones AL: Fractures of the pelvic ring, in Rockwood CA Jr, Green DP, Bucholz RW, Heckman JD (eds.): *Fractures in Adults,* 4th ed. Philadelphia: JB Lippincott, 1996, p. 1575.
8. Tile M: Fractures of the acetabulum, in Rockwood CA Jr, Green DP, Bucholz RW, Heckman JD (eds.): *Fractures in Adults,* 4th ed. Philadelphia: JB Lippincott, 1996, p. 1617.
9. Perry DC, DeLong W: Acetabular fractures. *Orthop Clin North Am* 28:405, 1997.
10. Zuckerman JD: Hip fracture. *N Engl J Med* 334:1519, 1996.
11. Shah AK, Eissler J, Radomisli T: Algorithms for the treatment of femoral neck fractures. *Clin Orthop* 399:28, 2002.
12. Lyons AR: Clinical outcomes and treatment of hip fractures. *Am J Med* 103:51S, 1997.
13. Alba E, Youngberg R: Occult fractures of the femoral neck. *Am J Emerg Med* 10:64, 1992.
14. Pandey R, McNally E, Ali A, Bulstrode C: The role of MRI in the diagnosis of occult hip fractures. *Injury* 29:61, 1998.
15. Bucholz RW, Brumback RJ: Fractures of the shaft of the femur, in Rockwood CA Jr, Green DP, Bucholz RW, Heckman JD (eds.): *Fractures in Adults,* 4th ed. Philadelphia: JB Lippincott, 1996, p. 1827.
16. Bucholz RW, Jones A: Current concepts review: Fractures of the shaft of the femur. *J Bone Joint Surg* 73A:1561, 1991.

For further reading in *Emergency Medicine: A Comprehensive Study Guide,* 6th ed., see Chap. 273, "Trauma to the Pelvis, Hip and Femur," by Mark T. Steele and Stefanie R. Ellison.

177 KNEE AND LEG INJURIES

Jeffrey N. Glaspy

RADIOGRAPHIC EVALUATION OF KNEE INJURIES

- The Ottawa Knee Rules and the Pittsburgh Knee Rules provide a rapid means for determining which patients require radiographic evaluation of the knee.[1,2] Each of the decision rules has equal sensitivity, but the Pittsburgh Knee Rules are more specific than the Ottawa Knee Rules, and they are also applicable to children as well as adults.
- According to the Pittsburgh Knee Rules, radiographic evaluation is recommended if the patient sustained a

blunt traumatic mechanism and is: (1) less than 12 years of age or older than 50 years of age, or (2) unable to walk four weight-bearing steps in the emergency department (ED).[2]

- Fat-fluid levels seen on a lateral radiographic view is suggestive of an intra-articular fracture.[3]
- If a patellar injury is suspected, a sunrise view should be ordered. This is the most useful view for detecting nondisplaced vertical or marginal fractures of the patella.

FRACTURES

PATELLAR FRACTURES

- Patella fractures occur from direct trauma or from forceful contraction of the quadriceps tendon.
- The fractures may be a transverse (most common), comminuted, or avulsion type.
- Physical examination reveals tenderness, swelling, effusion, and often a palpable defect of the patella. The extensor mechanism of the knee should be evaluated.
- Nondisplaced patellar fractures with intact extensor mechanisms are treated with knee immobilization, ice, analgesics, elevation, and referral for casting.
- Fractures that are displaced more than 3 mm or are associated with disruption of the extensor mechanism require early orthopedic referral for operative repair
- All open fractures of the patella need operative repair and antistaphylococcal antibiotic therapy.

FEMORAL CONDYLE FRACTURES

- Femoral condyle fractures usually result from direct trauma with an axial load or from a blow to the distal femur.
- Supracondylar, intercondylar, condylar, and distal femoral epiphyseal fractures may be seen.
- Signs and symptoms include pain, swelling, deformity, rotation, shortening, and inability to ambulate.
- Associated injuries should be identified and include popliteal artery injury, ipsilateral hip dislocation or fracture, quadriceps mechanism injury, and neurologic injury, especially the deep perineal nerve.
- Orthopedic consultation is required as most fractures will require operative repair.

TIBIAL SPINE AND TUBEROSITY FRACTURES

- Tibial spine fractures are caused by direct anterior or posterior force against the flexed proximal tibia.
- Anterior spine fracture is about tenfold more common than posterior spine fracture.

- Physical examination reveals tenderness, swelling, inability to extend the knee, and a positive Lachman's sign.
- Nondisplaced fractures are treated with knee immobilization in full extension. Displaced fractures require operative repair.
- Avulsion of the tibial tubercle may occur with a sudden force to the flexed knee with the quadriceps muscle contracted. The treatment includes knee immobilization and orthopedic referral.

TIBIAL PLATEAU FRACTURES

- Tibial plateau fractures result from varus or valgus forces combined with axial loading. The lateral plateau is more commonly fractured.
- Symptoms include pain, swelling of the knee, and decreased range of motion.
- Radiographic evaluation may reveal a fracture or only a lipohemarthrosis.
- Computed tomography (CT) may be helpful in evaluating the fracture.
- Ligamentous instability is common and occurs in about one third of cases.
- Early orthopedic consultation is necessary due to the need for precise reconstruction of the articular surface.

TIBIAL FRACTURES

- Fractures to the tibia may result from direct trauma or rotational or torsional stress.
- Patients present with pain, swelling, and crepitance.
- A complete neurovascular evaluation is essential, as is a search for possible compartment syndrome.
- Radiographs of the tibia, ankle, and knee are required to exclude associated fractures.
- Most tibial fractures require emergent orthopedic consultation. Indications for emergent operative repair include open fractures, vascular compromise, or compartment syndrome.

FIBULAR FRACTURES

- Fibular fractures most commonly involve the distal fibula at the ankle. Isolated shaft fractures usually occur from direct trauma.
- Proximal fibular fractures may result from external rotation injuries, whereas distal fibular fractures may result from internal rotation injuries.
- Patients with isolated fibular fracture may be able to bear weight.
- Treatment includes splinting, ice, elevation, and no

weight bearing pending follow-up with an orthopedic specialist or primary care physician.

LIGAMENTOUS INJURIES

- Anterior cruciate ligament (ACL) injuries often result from a deceleration, hyperextension, or internal rotation of the tibia on the femur. Patients will often report hearing a "pop" and develop marked swelling minutes to hours after the injury.
- Lachman's test is the most sensitive test for ACL injuries.[4] Other tests include the anterior drawer test and the lateral pivot shift test.
- Isolated posterior cruciate ligament (PCL) injuries are rare. The mechanism of injury is usually an anterior to posterior force applied to the tibia or lower leg.
- Injuries to the PCL ligament are detected by the posterior drawer test.
- Injuries to the medial collateral ligament and medial capsular structures can be determined by abduction (or valgus) stress testing with the knee in 30 degrees of flexion. If instability exists in flexion, the test should be repeated in full extension (if possible).
- Medial instability in full extension indicates a severe lesion involving the cruciate ligaments and posterior capsule.
- Injuries to the lateral collateral ligament and the lateral capsule are detected by adduction (or varus) stress testing with the knee in 30 degrees of flexion. If instability exists in flexion, the test should be repeated in full extension (if possible).
- Lateral instability in full extension indicates a severe lesion involving the cruciate ligaments and the posterolateral corner of the capsule. Perineal nerve injuries may be associated with lateral injuries.
- Although most ligamentous injuries present with hemarthrosis, serious ligamentous injuries may present with minimal pain and no hemarthrosis due to disruption of the capsule.
- Treatment of most ligamentous injuries consists of knee immobilization, ice, elevation, analgesics, and referral to an orthopedist.
- For severe ligamentous injuries with an unstable knee, immediate orthopedic consultation may be prudent to plan for operative intervention.

MENISCAL INJURIES

- Cutting, squatting, or twisting maneuvers may cause injury to a meniscus.
- The medial meniscus is more often injured than the lateral meniscus.
- Symptoms of meniscal injuries include painful locking of the knee, a popping or clicking sensation, or a sensation of the knee giving out.

- McMurray's test and other tests for meniscal injuries are not sensitive.
- Definitive diagnosis can be made by outpatient magnetic resonance imaging (MRI) or arthroscopy.
- Treatment of meniscal injuries includes knee immobilization, analgesics, ice, elevation, and orthopedic referral.

DISLOCATIONS

KNEE DISLOCATION

- Knee dislocations result from various large force mechanisms and are associated with tremendous ligamentous and capsular injuries.
- Posterior knee dislocations are most common, although anterior, medial, lateral, rotational, or combined injuries may occur. Because of instability, reduction often occurs spontaneously.
- A knee that is severely unstable in multiple directions is suspicious for a spontaneously reduced knee dislocation.
- There is a high incidence of associated popliteal artery and peroneal nerve injury. Determining pre- and postreduction neurovascular status is essential.
- Radiographs should be obtained to exclude associated fractures.
- Early reduction of the dislocation is essential.
- Any patient with absent or diminished pulse, foot ischemia, or bruit requires emergent arteriography or vascular surgery consultation for surgical exploration.
- All patients should be admitted for serial vascular examinations.

PATELLA DISLOCATION

- Patella dislocation usually results from a twisting injury on an extended knee.
- Associated tearing of the medial joint capsule may occur.
- Reduction is accomplished following conscious sedation by flexing the hip, hyperextending the knee, and sliding the patella back into place. Knee immobilization and orthopedic or primary care follow-up is necessary.

TENDON INJURIES

PATELLAR TENDON RUPTURE

- Patellar tendon rupture is more common in patients younger than 40 years old with a history of patellar tendinitis or steroid injections.
- This injury often occurs after forceful contraction of the quadriceps muscle.

- On physical examination, patients will have a defect inferior to the patella and an inability to extend the knee.
- On lateral radiograph a high or low riding patella may be seen.
- Treatment consists of knee immobilization and orthopedic consultation for operative repair.

QUADRICEPS TENDON RUPTURE

- Quadriceps tendon rupture is most common in individuals over 40 years of age after sudden contraction of the quadriceps muscle (landing after a jump).
- Symptoms include sharp pain at the proximal knee with ambulation.
- If the tear is complete the patient may be unable to extend the flexed knee.
- There may be a palpable defect, with tenderness and swelling at the suprapatellar region with distal migration of the patella.
- Radiographs are useful in excluding a patellar or femoral avulsion fracture.
- Treatment consists of knee immobilization and orthopedic consultation for possible operative repair.

ACHILLES TENDON RUPTURE

- Rupture of the Achilles tendon occurs with forceful plantar flexion of the foot.
- Risk factors include rheumatoid arthritis, lupus, quinolone antibiotics, previous steroid injections of the Achilles, and poor athletic conditioning.
- The diagnosis is made clinically with a positive Thompson's test (no plantar flexion of the foot with squeezing of the calf) and inability to toe walk.
- Treatment includes splinting in plantar flexion, no weight bearing, analgesics, elevation, and referral to an orthopedist for possible surgical repair.

OVERUSE INJURIES

PATELLAR TENDINITIS

- This condition, known as "jumper's knee," presents with pain over the patellar tendon that is exacerbated when running up hills or standing from a sitting position.
- Treatment consists of ice, nonsteroidal anti-inflammatory drugs (NSAIDs), and quadriceps strengthening exercises.

CHONDROMALACIA PATELLAE

- This condition is caused by patellofemoral malalignment, which places lateral stress on the articular cartilage.

- It is most common in young, active women and presents with anterior knee pain that worsens with stair climbing or rising from a sitting position.
- Diagnosis is assisted using the patellar compression test and the apprehension test.
- Treatment includes rest, NSAIDs, and quadriceps strengthening exercises.

REFERENCES

1. Stiell IG, Wells GA, Hoag RH, et al: Implementation of the Ottawa Knee Rules for the use of radiography in acute knee injuries. *JAMA* 278:2075, 1997.
2. Seaberg DC, Yealy DM, Lukens T, et al: Multicenter comparison of two clinical decision rules for the use of radiography in acute, high-risk knee injuries. *Ann Emerg Med* 32:8, 1998.
3. Lugo-Olivieri CH, Scott WW Jr, Zehovni EA: Fluid-fluid levels in injured knees: Do they always represent lipohemarthrosis? *Radiology* 198:499, 1996.
4. Solomon DH, Simel DL, Bates DW, et al: Does this patient have a torn meniscus or ligament of the knee? Value of the physical examination. *JAMA* 286:1610, 2001.

For further reading in *Emergency Medicine: A Comprehensive Study Guide,* 6th ed., see Chap. 274, "Knee Injuries," by Mark T. Steele and Jeffrey N. Glaspy; and Chap. 275, "Leg Injuries," by Paul R. Haller.

178 ANKLE AND FOOT INJURIES

Michael C. Wadman

ANKLE INJURIES

PATHOPHYSIOLOGY

- Ankle joint injuries are due to abnormal movement of the talus within the mortise and the resultant stress on the malleoli and ligaments.
- Injuries resulting in disruption of both sides of the joint (malleoli fracture and ruptured ligament, fracture of both malleoli, or disruption of both ligaments) are unstable.

ANKLE SPRAINS

CLINICAL FEATURES

- Sprains result from abnormal motion of the talus within the mortise, leading to stretching or disruption of the ligaments.
- Typically, the patient is able to bear weight immediately after the injury, with subsequent increase in pain and swelling as the patient continues to ambulate.
- Physical examination reveals tenderness and swelling over the involved ligament with a corresponding lack of tenderness over the bony prominences of the ankle.
- The lateral ankle is injured more frequently, with the anterior talofibular ligament the most commonly injured ligament.
- Isolated sprain of the medial deltoid ligament is rare, and an associated fibular fracture or syndesmotic ligament injury may be present.

DIAGNOSIS AND DIFFERENTIAL

- To exclude other injuries, evaluation of the injured ankle begins with examination of the joints above and below the injury.
- The Achilles tendon should be palpated for tenderness or a defect, and the Thompson test (squeezing the calf while observing for resultant plantar flexion) performed.
- The proximal fibula should be palpated for tenderness resulting from a Maisonneuve fracture or fibulotibialis ligament tear.
- The fibula should be squeezed toward the tibia to evaluate for syndesmotic ligament injury.
- Also, the calcaneus, tarsals, and the base of the fifth metatarsal should be palpated to evaluate for foot fractures causing ankle pain that may not readily be apparent on standard ankle radiography.
- The posterior aspects of the medial and lateral malleoli should be palpated from 6 cm proximally to the distal tips. If tenderness is isolated to the posterior aspect of the lateral malleolus, then a peroneal tendon subluxation may be present.
- The Ottawa Ankle Rules (Fig. 178-1) are simple guidelines that have been extensively validated in numerous clinical trials. When applied properly, they can help the emergency physician identify a subset of patients who can be safely treated without undergoing radiographic studies.[1,2]
- The determination of ankle instability by radiography is made by any asymmetry in the gap between the talar dome and the malleoli on the talus view.

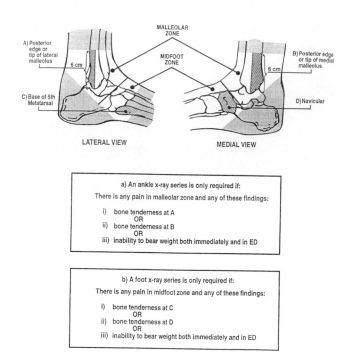

FIG. 178-1. Ottawa Ankle Rules for ankle and midfoot injuries.

EMERGENCY DEPARTMENT CARE AND DISPOSITION

- Initial treatment consists of **r**est, **i**ce, **c**ompression, and **e**levation (RICE) for 24 to 72 hours and analgesics.
- The patient with a stable joint and the ability to easily bear weight needs only analgesics, an elastic compression bandage, and a one-week follow-up if the pain persists.
- If unable to bear weight, the patient with a stable joint may benefit from an ankle brace (allowing dorsoplantar flexion while preventing eversion or inversion) and a 1-week follow-up for repeat examination.
- Patients with unstable joints should be immobilized in a posterior splint and referred to an orthopedist.[3,4]

ANKLE FRACTURES

- Emergency department decision making is facilitated by Henderson's scheme that groups ankle fractures into three classifications based on radiologic appearance: unimalleolar, bimalleolar, and trimalleolar.
- Bimalleolar and trimalleolar fractures usually require open reduction and internal fixation. Emergency department care includes posterior splinting, elevation, and ice application while initiating appropriate consultation for definitive treatment.
- Unimalleolar fractures are usually treated with posterior splinting, no weight bearing, and orthopedic follow-up.

Minimally displaced, small (<3 mm) avulsion fractures of the fibula are treated like ankle sprains.
- Open fractures require wet sterile dressing coverage, splinting, and administration of tetanus toxoid, as necessary, and a first-generation cephalosporin (eg, cefazolin).
- If gross contamination is noted, tetanus immunoglobulin and an aminoglycoside should be added to the treatment regimen.

ANKLE DISLOCATIONS

- Ankle dislocations most commonly occur in the posterior plane and frequently involve associated fractures.
- Most dislocations are treated urgently by an orthopedist, but the absence of dorsalis pedis or posterior tibial pulses and a cool, dusky foot require immediate reduction by the examining physician.
- Reduction is performed by applying longitudinal traction on the heel and foot and rotation opposite that of the mechanism of injury while an assistant stabilizes the proximal leg. Longitudinal traction is then applied with rotation in the direction opposite of the mechanism of injury.
- Postreduction, patients require neurovascular examination to ensure restoration of perfusion, and orthopedic consultation and admission.

FOOT INJURIES

PATHOPHYSIOLOGY

- Foot injuries most commonly result from direct or twisting forces, with twisting type mechanisms resulting in more minor avulsion-type injuries.
- The first metatarsal bears twice the weight of any other metatarsal, necessitating a more conservative approach to fracture management.
- The base of the second metatarsal is an important component of the Lisfranc complex and any sign of injury warrants caution.
- Major fractures of the talus and subtalar dislocations are at risk for avascular necrosis because of the tenuous blood supply of the foot.

HINDFOOT INJURIES

- Small avulsion fractures of the talus are usually treated with posterior splinting and orthopedic follow-up.
- Major fractures of the talar neck and body as well as subtalar dislocations require immediate orthopedic consultation.

- Calcaneus fractures frequently result when a patient falls from a height and may accompany other fractures of the lower extremities and vertebral column.
- Compression fractures of the calcaneus may result in subtle radiographic findings that require the measurement of Bohler's angle (formed at the intersection of a line along the superior cortex of the body of the calcaneus with a line from the dome to the anterior tubercle on the lateral view) to improve diagnostic accuracy; an angle less than 20 degrees increases the likelihood of fracture.
- Treatment consists of posterior splinting, elevation, analgesics, and orthopedic consultation.

MIDFOOT INJURIES

- Tarsal bone fractures are uncommon and treated conservatively.
- Isolated fractures of the cuboid and cuneiforms suggest injury to the Lisfranc joint (the ligamentous tarsometatarsal complex).[5]
- Most Lisfranc joint injuries are associated with a fracture, especially of the base of the second metatarsal. Point tenderness over the midfoot and laxity between the first and second metatarsal in a dorsal to plantar direction suggest the diagnosis.
- On the plain anteroposterior radiograph of the foot, a gap of more than 1 mm between the bases of the first and second metatarsals is diagnostic of Lisfranc joint injury, but computed tomography is the imaging modality of choice.[6]
- All Lisfranc joint injuries require orthopedic consultation for possible open reduction and internal fixation.

FOREFOOT INJURIES

- Most nondisplaced metatarsal shaft fractures need only conservative management, with the exception of keeping fractures of the first metatarsal from bearing weight.
- Displaced shaft fractures of the middle metatarsals are treated with closed reduction and cast immobilization, while displaced fracture of the first metatarsal usually requires open reduction and internal fixation.
- Fifth metatarsal fractures, including the pseudo-Jones avulsion fractures at the tuberosity of the metatarsal base, are likewise treated conservatively.
- The true Jones fracture (transverse fracture at the fifth metatarsal base) is frequently complicated by nonunion and is treated in a non–weight bearing cast and orthopedic follow-up.

- Phalangeal fractures, if nondisplaced, are easily treated with buddy taping and a stiff-soled cast shoe.
- Displaced fractures and dislocations are treated with digital block, reduction by manual traction, and buddy taping.

CRUSH INJURY AND COMPARTMENT SYNDROME

- A crushed foot that becomes tensely swollen and is associated with complaints of pain out of proportion to physical examination findings suggests the possibility of compartment syndrome.
- Typically, pain is not relieved by elevation of the foot and is increased with passive dorsiflexion of the great toe.
- Distal neurovascular examination may yield normal results.
- Diagnosis is made by measurement of intracompartmental pressure.

REFERENCES

1. Stiell IG, Greenberg GH, McKnight RD, et al: Decision rules for the use of radiography in acute ankle injuries. *JAMA* 269:1127, 1993.
2. Stiell IG, Mc Knight RD, Greenberg GH, et al: Implementation of the Ottawa Ankle Rules. *JAMA* 271:827, 1994.
3. Kerkhoffs GM, Rowe BH, Assendelft WJ, et al: Immobilisation for ankle sprains. A systematic review. *Arch Orthop Trauma Surg* 121:462, 2001.
4. Kerkhoffs GM, Struijs PA, Marti RK, et al: Different functional treatment strategies for acute lateral ligament injuries in adults. *Cochrane Database Syst Rev* 3:CD002938, 2002.
5. Englanoff G, Anglin D, Hutson HR: Lisfranc fracture-dislocation: A frequently missed diagnosis in the emergency department. *Ann Emerg Med* 26:229, 1995.
6. Preidler KW, Peicha L, Lajtai G, et al: Conventional radiography, CT, and MR imaging in patients with hyperflexion injuries to the foot: Diagnostic accuracy in detection of bony and ligamentous changes. *AJR Am J Roentgenol* 173:1673, 1999.

For further reading in *Emergency Medicine: A Comprehensive Study Guide*, 6th ed., see Chap. 276, "Ankle Injuries," and Chap. 277, "Foot Injuries," by John A. Michael and Ian G. Stiell.

179 COMPARTMENT SYNDROMES

Gary M. Gaddis

PATHOPHYSIOLOGY

- Compartment syndromes are caused by increased hydrostatic pressure that compromises blood flow to muscles and nerves within a closed tissue space.
- Normal tissue pressure measures 0 to 10 mm Hg.
- Capillary blood flow is compromised at pressures greater than 20 mm Hg and muscle and nerves become at risk for injury.
- Necrosis of nerve and muscle is likely at pressures of 30 to 40 mm Hg or greater. Nerves are more sensitive than muscle because they are reliant on nutrient capillaries.[1]
- There are two causes that lead to compartment syndromes: (1) extrinsic compression of a compartment, which either limits compartment size or distensibility; and (2) intrinsic volume increase within a closed compartment, such as that caused by hematoma or postischemic reperfusion edema.
- Compartments that are bordered by bone or dense connective tissue are more prone to compartment syndromes than compartments with relatively elastic borders.

CLINICAL FEATURES

- Conscious patients who develop compartment syndromes usually experience deep, severe, constant, poorly-localized pain over the involved muscle compartment.
- Pain is the earliest symptom, and is almost universally present.
- Palpation of the affected compartment, active contraction, or passive stretching of muscles in the affected compartments will exacerbate the pain.
- Hypesthesia can appear shortly after the onset of pain when elevated compartment pressures compromise neurologic function.
- Sensory changes precede motor weakness or paralysis.
- Paralysis requires prolonged ischemia and occurs late.
- Absent pulses, pallor, and excessive coolness are unlikely to appear until well after occurrence of pain and neurologic compromise.
- Muscle necrosis and permanent posttraumatic muscle contracture (Volkmann's ischemia) are the end result of an untreated compartment syndrome.
- Any muscle mass enclosed by fascia is at risk for compartment syndrome.
- Tables 179-1 and 179-2 review the anatomical structures involved in acute compartment syndromes.[2]

TABLE 179-1   Anatomy of the Forearm

COMPARTMENT	MUSCLES	VESSELS	NERVES
Volar forearm	Wrist & fnger flexors	Radial artery Ulnar artery	Median & ulnar
Dorsal forearm	Wrist & finger extenders		Radial

DIAGNOSIS AND DIFFERENTIAL

- Patients who present with compression injuries, fractures, penetrating wounds, or hemorrhage should prompt a high index of suspicion.
- The mainstay of diagnosis is measuring compartment pressures.
- Compartment pressures can easily be measured hydrostatically in the emergency department with a Stryker STIC Monitor or ACE Intracompartmental Pressure Monitor.[3]
- Most muscle compartments normally have pressures of less than 10 mm Hg, and such pressures are often normally near 0 mm Hg. The presence of an abnormally elevated pressure confirms the diagnosis.

EMERGENCY DEPARTMENT CARE AND DISPOSITION

- Initial stabilization of injuries and measurement of compartment pressures dictate subsequent treatment and disposition.
- Patients with compartment pressures under 10 mm Hg do not require further therapy.
- Compartment pressures of 10 to 20 mm Hg require re-evaluation in 12 to 24 hours, with serial compartment pressure measurements in persistently symptomatic patients. Clinical judgment must be exercised regarding whether to discharge patients based on their likelihood to follow discharge instruction and return for close follow-up.
- Compartment pressures greater than 20 mm Hg can compromise capillary blood flow; these patients require hospital admission or surgical consultation, as persistent pressures in this range can damage nerve and muscle.
- Compartment pressures over 30 to 40 mm Hg place nerve and muscle at risk for necrosis and are grounds for immediate fasciotomy.
- Ice cooling and limb elevation should be avoided since both techniques can decrease perfusion to muscle.
- Bedrest and serial neurovascular checks are the conservative treatments when immediate fasciotomy is not indicated.
- The goal of treatment is the avoidance of muscle necrosis, rhabdomyolysis, and nerve damage in the affected area(s).[4]

REFERENCES

1. Mubarak SJ, Hargens AR: *Compartment Syndromes and Volkman's Contracture.* Philadelphia: Saunders, 1981, p. 47.
2. Whitesides TE, Haney TC, Morimoto K, Harada H: Tissue pressure measurements as a determinant for the need of fasciotomy. *Clin Orthop* 113:43, 1975.
3. Heppenstall RB, Sapega AA, Scott R, et al: The compartment syndrome: An experimental and clinical study of muscular energy metabolism using phosphorus nuclear magnetic resonance spectroscopy. *Clin Orthop* 226:138, 1988.
4. Moore RE, Friedman RJ: Current concepts and pathophysiology in the diagnosis of compartment syndromes. *J Emerg Med* 7:657, 1989.

For further reading in *Emergency Medicine: A Comprehensive Study Guide,* 6th ed., see Chap. 278, "Compartment Syndromes," by Paul R. Haller.

TABLE 179-2   Anatomy of the Leg

COMPARTMENT	MUSCLES	VESSELS	NERVES	SENSORY DISTRIBUTION
Anterior	Extensor muscles of toes	Anterior tibial artery	Deep peroneal nerve	Web space of first & second toes
Deep posterior	Deep flexor muscles	Posterior tibial artery	Tibial nerve Peroneal nerve	Heel
Superficial posterior	Superficial flexor muscles (gastrocnemius and soleus)			
Lateral	Peroneal muscles		Superficial peroneal nerve	Lateral dorsum of foot

180 RHABDOMYOLYSIS

Gary M. Gaddis

EPIDEMIOLOGY

- Alcohol and drugs of abuse play a role in up to 80% of cases of rhabdomyolysis in adults.[1-3]
- Rhabdomyolysis is very uncommon among pediatric patients.[4]

PATHOPHYSIOLOGY

- Rhabdomyolysis syndromes involve skeletal muscle injury and necrosis, followed by release of intracellular contents, most notably myoglobin (which leads to nephrotoxicity) and skeletal muscle biomarker enzymes, such as creatine phosphokinase (CPK).
- Ferrihemate, a breakdown product of myoglobin, is directly nephrotoxic.
- The common cellular event involves disruption of the Na^+-K^+-ATPase pump and calcium transport. The result is increased intracellular calcium and muscle cell necrosis via several mechanisms.[5]
- In addition to alcohol and drug abuse, rhabdomyolysis is strongly associated with trauma, strenuous physical activity, heat-related illness, toxin ingestion, and certain infections.
- Chronic malnutrition and hypophosphatemia, commonly found among alcoholics, increases the risk for rhabdomyolysis.
- The drugs of abuse most commonly involved with rhabdomyolysis include cocaine, amphetamines, lysergic acid diethylamide (LSD), heroin, and phencyclidine (PCP).
- Medications most commonly associated with rhabdomyolysis include diuretics, statin lipid-lowering agents, narcotics, theophylline, corticosteroids, benzodiazepines, phenothiazines, and tricyclic antidepressants.
- Influenza is the most frequent infectious cause of rhabdomyolysis and *Legionella* infection is the most common bacterial cause.[6]

CLINICAL FEATURES

- A patient history compatible with risk factors for this illness should increase suspicion for rhabdomyolysis syndromes because classic signs of rhabdomyolysis may be absent in up to 50% of cases.[1]
- Historical clues that strongly suggest that the patient may be at risk for rhabdomyolysis include:
  - Recent immobility with probable prolonged muscle compression or abnormally increased muscular activity due to drug intoxication (such as after alcohol, cocaine, amphetamine, or PCP use).
  - Unaccustomed muscular activity. Examples include strenuous exercise by those with poor fitness (especially when done in the heat), seizures, dystonia, or delirium tremens.
  - Electrical or lightning injury.
  - Injuries that might cause compartment syndromes and/or prolonged muscular compression, such as traumatic crush injuries, heat stroke, and acutely casted long-bone fractures.
  - Diseases such as sickle cell disease, dermatomyositis, and polymyositis.
- Classically, rhabdomyolysis syndromes are of acute onset and patients present with myalgias, muscle stiffness, weakness, malaise, and low-grade fever.
- Dark, tea-colored urine is expected when significant myoglobinuria occurs.
- Most cases of rhabdomyolysis are associated with the presence of myoglobinuria.
- Nonspecific symptoms such as nausea, vomiting, abdominal pain, palpitations, and mental status changes due to acute uremia may be present.
- The most common muscles involved are the postural muscles of the calves, thighs, and lower back. Involved muscles are often tender to palpation, but observable swelling of these muscles may be subtle or absent until the patient is rehydrated.
- Acute renal failure (ARF), which may be oliguric (most commonly) or nonoliguric, is the most serious complication of rhabdomyolysis. Up to 10% of ARF may be due to rhabdomyolysis.[1,7,8]
- The probability of developing ARF with rhabdomyolysis is not directly related to the degree of elevation of CPK or to the degree of myoglobinuria. However, the degree of elevation of CPK correlates with the extent of muscular injury.
- Hypovolemia and aciduria (pH <5.6) potentiate ARF.
- Hyperkalemia may be present, which is due to myonecrosis or ARF.
- Other early complications can include hypocalcemia, hyperuricemia, and hyperphosphatemia.
- Late complications include hypercalcemia, hypophosphatemia, disseminated intravascular coagulation, and compartment syndrome with peripheral neuropathy.
- Risk factors for developing ARF include myoglobinuria, hypovolemia, acidemia, and renal tubular obstruction.

DIAGNOSIS AND DIFFERENTIAL

- A fivefold or greater increase of serum CPK above the upper limit of normal is the hallmark for the diagnosis of rhabdomyolysis.
- The CPK-MB fraction, originating primarily in car-

diac muscle, should not exceed 5% of the total CPK value.

- In general, serum CPK levels rise from 2 to 12 hours after muscle injury. Peak levels occur in 24 to 72 hours and then decline about 39% per day thereafter. If CPK levels fail to fall in this manner, ongoing muscular necrosis should be suspected.
- Myoglobin released after muscle necrosis will be present in the urine if plasma concentrations exceed 1.5 mg/dL. Reddish-brown urine is observed at or above about 100 mg/dL of myoglobinuria.
- Myoglobin contains the heme ring, so it causes positive urine dipstick tests in the absence of microhematuria. Whenever the urine dipstick test is positive and very few or no blood cells are present on microscopic examination, rhabdomyolysis should be suspected.
- Radioimmunoassays are sensitive for the presence of myoglobinuria, but are not required for the diagnosis.
- Serum myoglobin levels may return to normal within 1 to 6 hours of injury, so the absence of myoglobinuria or myoglobinemia does not rule out the diagnosis of rhabdomyolysis.
- The differential diagnosis includes other causes of muscle ischemia or pain, such as sickle cell disease, toxin exposures, inflammatory myopathies, and infectious myalgias.

EMERGENCY DEPARTMENT CARE AND DISPOSITION

- Rehydration is the mainstay of therapy. Volume deficits should be corrected by IV normal saline to maintain a urine output of at least 2 mL/kg/h. This requires approximately 2.5 mL/kg/h of crystalloid infusion after an initial 1- to 2-L bolus of crystalloid.
- Solutions containing potassium or lactate should be avoided.
- Cardiac monitoring is required. Electrolyte derangements are common, especially hyperkalemia and hypocalcemia.
- Invasive hemodynamic monitoring to prevent fluid overload may be prudent for patients with significant cardiac or renal disease.
- A Foley catheter is required to monitor urine output.
- Serial measurements of urinary pH, venous pH, electrolytes, CPK, calcium, phosphorus, blood urea nitrogen, and creatinine must be performed.
- The use of sodium bicarbonate should be considered. A bicarbonate infusion can be prepared by adding two or three ampules of sodium bicarbonate to 1 L of 5% dextrose in water (D_5W), then initiating an infusion rate of 100 mL/h.
- A urine pH above 6.5 is the target of bicarbonate therapy. This may be associated with decreased renal injury via decreased ferrihemate production; however,

hypocalcemia can be exacerbated by bicarbonate administration.

- Diuresis can be enhanced by 20% mannitol after fluid replacement, although no controlled studies exist to support its theoretical benefit.
- Mannitol should only be administered after sufficient volume replacement has occurred and oliguria is absent.
- Use of loop diuretics such as furosemide has become controversial, as loop diuretics acidify the urine while mannitol does not.
- Hyperkalemia should be treated using standard regimens (eg, sodium bicarbonate, calcium chloride, sodium polystyrene sulfonate, and glucose and insulin therapy) to prevent cardiac dysrhythmia complications.
- Hypocalcemia, hypercalcemia, hyperphosphatemia, and hypophosphatemia also should be treated using standard regimens.
- All patients with rhabdomyolysis require hospital admission to a monitored bed.
- Along with treatment of the underlying etiology of the disease, a nephrology consultation should be obtained for all cases of renal insufficiency or ARF.
- Magnetic resonance imaging with gadolinium enhancement may occasionally be useful to localize the site of rhabdomyolysis and to direct treatment of underlying causes when the site of myonecrosis may be unclear.[9]

REFERENCES

1. Gabow PA, Kaehny WD, Kelleher SP: The spectrum of rhabdomyolysis. *Medicine* 61:141, 1982.
2. Richards JR: Rhabdomyolysis and drugs of abuse. *J Emerg Med* 19:51, 2000.
3. Warren JD, Blumbergs PC, Thompson PD: Rhabdomyolysis: A review. *Muscle Nerve* 25:332, 2002.
4. Ng Y-T, Johnson HM: Clinical rhabdomyolysis. *J Paediatr Child Health* 36:39, 2000.
5. Vanholder R, Sever MS, Ekrem E, et al: Rhabdomyolysis. *J Am Soc Nephrol* 11:1553, 2000.
6. David WS: Myoglobinuria. *Neurol Clin* 18:215, 2000.
7. Moore RE, Friedman RJ: Current concepts and pathophysiology in diagnosis of compartment syndromes. *J Emerg Med* 7:657, 1989.
8. Curry SC, Chang D, Connor D: Drug- and toxin-induced rhabdomyolysis. *Ann Emerg Med* 18:1068, 1989.
9. Kakuda W, Naritomi H, Miyashita K, et al: Rhabdomyolysis lesions showing magnetic resonance contrast enhancement. *J Neuroimaging* 9:182, 1999.

For further reading in *Emergency Medicine: A Comprehensive Study Guide,* 6th ed., see Chap. 279, "Rhabdomyolysis," by Francis L. Counselman.

181 NECK AND THORACOLUMBAR PAIN

Thomas K. Swoboda

EPIDEMIOLOGY

- In most cases of neck pain, no specific cause can be identified.[1]
- Cervical disc prolapse is more common in males and is most common during the fourth decade of life. Levels C5 and C6 (C6 root: 20%) and C6 and C7 (C7 root: 70%) are most commonly involved.[2]
- Incidence of spinal spondylosis and stenosis increases with age.
- Thoracic compression fractures are commonly seen in patients with advanced age, especially in elderly females with osteoporosis.
- Thoracic and lumbar spine fractures are most common at levels T11 to L2. They result from direct trauma or from severe flexion such as trunk flexion about a seat belt.[3]
- Lumbar pain is the most common cause of work-related disability in those younger than 45 years, and it is the second most common cause of temporary disability in all age groups.[4,5]
- Sixty to ninety percent of persons will experience back pain at some time. In 85%, no definite source of the pain can be diagnosed.[5,6]

PATHOPHYSIOLOGY

- A radiculopathy is segmental motor or sensory signs and symptoms associated with a nerve root injury.
- A myelopathy, which is signs and symptoms due to a spinal cord lesion, stenosis, or compression, has more generalized symptoms than a radiculopathy.
- Neck trauma may cause soft tissue hemorrhage or edema between any of the seven fascial planes of the neck, resulting in limited range of motion, pain, or swelling. Inflammation develops in the soft tissues within several hours, resulting in delayed neck stiffness and pain after initial trauma.
- Rear-end motor vehicle crashes often cause hyperextension of the neck, associated with atlas fractures, extension teardrop fractures, posterior arch fractures, laminar fractures, hyperextension dislocations, and traumatic spondylolisthesis.
- Head-on motor vehicle crashes cause hyperflexion of the neck, associated with anterior subluxations, unilateral or bilateral facet dislocations, vertebral compression fractures, and spinous process avulsions.
- Direct posterior cervical disc herniations or rupture can produce progressive myelopathy. The more common posterolateral herniations can cause acute cervical radiculopathy.
- Cervical spondylosis, a progressive, degenerative condition, can present with loss of cervical range of motion, neck pain, occipital pain, or radicular pain. Osteophytic spurs can develop leading to cervical stenosis.
- Myelopathy due to cervical stenosis becomes more frequent as the spinal canal diameter is reduced to less than 13 mm by the anterior osteophytes and posterior buckling ligamentum flavum in a congenitally narrowed spinal canal.
- The spinal canal and the canals for the paired segmental nerve roots are narrowest in the thoracic spine, which is most prone to neurologic compromise from compressing or space-occupying lesions.

- Thoracic vertebral compression fractures seldom cause neurologic compromise, but are extremely painful. Fractures may be due to direct trauma, osteoporosis, or hyperflexion.
- Pathologic thoracic fractures associated with metastatic lesions are likely to present with myelopathy and long tract signs.
- Since the spinal cord ends at the first or second lumbar vertebra in adults and the size of the spinal canal is larger than in the thoracic region, the rate of neurologic compromise observed with lumbar bony injuries is decreased.
- Spinal canal hemorrhage, tumors of the epidural space or spinal column, infection, and massive midline disc herniation in the lumbar region can result in myelopathy.

CLINICAL FEATURES

- Most patients with neck and back pain often complain of localized stiffness and limited range of motion. Commonly, they have one position that will exacerbate symptoms and another position that relieves symptoms. Localized tenderness to palpation may be absent.
- Neck pain radiating in a dermatomal pattern suggests a cervical radiculopathy. Radiculopathies may present with neurogenic signs such as sensory abnormalities, weakness, muscle hypertonicity, reflex changes, or incoordination.
- Neck extension and lateral flexion should exacerbate radicular neck pain. Flexion and distraction usually relieve radicular neck pain.

- Signs and symptoms of cervical radiculopathy are summarized in Table 181-1.
- Spinal cord dysfunction is associated with a myelopathy. Myelopathies are often seen with long tract signs, such as lower extremity hyperreflexia, positive Babinski's sign (extensor toe sign), loss of sphincter control, or sexual dysfunction.
- Myofascial pain syndrome (MPS) causes chronic neck pain with symptoms similar to those of cervical radiculopathy. MPS patients have pain in the neck, scapula, and shoulder in a nondermatomal distribution ("trigger point").
- MPS patients frequently have psychological distress and personality characteristics, causing conversion of emotional distress into complaints of pain.[7]
- In thoracic pain syndromes, localized pain and tenderness may not be present during examination. Resulting radicular pain in the chest or abdomen is more common. This pain is worsened by reclining and improved by upright positioning.
- Herpes zoster neuralgia and diabetic radiculopathy may affect any spinal level.
- Pain from zoster may precede the development of rash. Both may cause radicular pain symptoms at the chest, abdomen, or hip.
- Osteoarthritis can cause localized stiffness, radicular pain, or spinal stenosis.
- Spinal stenosis is more common in the thoracic spine, where the spinal canal has its most narrow diameter.
- Lumbar radiculopathies are summarized in Table 181-2.
- A straight leg raising sign (SLR) is radicular pain in the symptomatic leg elicited by elevation of that leg, commonly noted in patents with a lumbar radiculopathy.
- A crossed straight leg raising sign (radicular pain in

TABLE 181-1 Symptoms and Signs of Cervical Radiculopathies

DISK SPACE	NERVE ROOT	PAIN COMPLAINT	SENSORY CHANGE	MOTOR WEAKNESS	ALTERED REFLEX
C1–2	C1–2	Neck, scalp	Scalp	None	None
C4–5	C5	Neck, shoulder, upper arm	Shoulder, thumb	Spinati, deltoid, biceps	Biceps
C5–6	C6	Neck, shoulder, upper scapula, proximal forearm, thumb	Thumb, index finger, lateral forearm	Deltoid, biceps, pronator teres, wrist extensors	Biceps, brachioradialis
C6–7	C7	Neck, posterior arm, dorsal and proximal forearm, chest, medical scapula, middle finger	Middle finger, forearm	Triceps, pronator teres	Triceps
C7–T1	C8	Neck, posterior arm, proximal forearm, medial scapula, medial hand, ring and little fingers	Ring, little fingers	Triceps, flexor carpi ulnaris, hand intrinsic muscles	Triceps

TABLE 181-2   Symptoms and Signs of Lumbar Radiculopathies

DISK SPACE	NERVE ROOT	PAIN COMPLAINT	SENSORY CHANGE	MOTOR WEAKNESS	ALTERED REFLEX
L2–3	L3	Medial thigh, knee	Medial thigh, knee	Hip flexors	None
L3–4	L4	Medial lower leg	Medial lower leg	Quadricepts	Knee jerk
L4–5	L5	Anterior tibia, great toe	Medial foot	Extensor hallucis longus	Biceps femoris
L5–S1	S1	Calf, little toe	Lateral foot	Foot plantar flexors	Achilles

the affected leg when lifting the asymptomatic leg) is more specific for nerve root compression than a SLR.[5,8]

• Patients with lumbar radiculopathy tend to lean backward to relieve tension on the nerve. They often complain more about the symptoms associated with the radiculopathy than any pain in the back.

• In contrast to adults, back pain in children is more likely to result from a serious etiology. An investigation for signs of infection, neurofibromatosis, or spinal abnormalities such as spina bifida, should be made.

DIAGNOSIS AND DIFFERENTIAL

• Large spinal disk herniations, significant spinal stenosis, epidural hematomas, epidural abscesses, and spinal or epidural neoplasms can present with similar neurologic findings of radiculopathy and/or myelopathy at any level of the spine.

• At all spinal levels, magnetic resonance imaging (MRI) is the diagnostic test of choice in the work-up of suspected radiculopathy or myelopathy, especially when compressive or neoplastic lesions are suspected. The presence of long tract signs infers that intrinsic or extrinsic spinal cord pathology must be suspected.

• Patients with new or progressing signs or symptoms require emergent MRI imaging and prompt treatment for optimal outcome.[9]

• Plain radiographs are useful for selected trauma patients, especially if they are elderly or if the mechanism of injury leads to suspicion of fracture. Radiographs are not useful to diagnose small or even large disk herniations.

• Techniques to test for cervical radiculopathy such as Spurling's sign (gentle pressure applied to the patient's head during extension with lateral rotation) and abduction relief sign (relief of symptoms by having the patient place the hand of the affected extremity on top of the head) should also be utilized.[10]

• Immunocompromised patients with cancer, organ transplants, diabetes, or injection drug abuse are at highest risk for spinal infection. Fever is not always present with these infections, but back pain is often present for more than 3 months prior to eventual diagnosis.[11]

• Patients with spinal infection often have vertebral body tenderness to percussion and an elevated erythrocyte sedimentation rate. MRI imaging is required to confirm this diagnosis.

• Low back pain may be the presenting symptom of several serious intra-abdominal conditions, including pyelonephritis, peptic ulcer disease, pancreatic disease, diverticulitis, abdominal aortic aneurysm, and pelvic inflammatory disease. All patients with back pain require spinal, neurologic, vascular, abdominal, and lower extremity evaluations.

• Epidural compression syndrome (ECS) encompasses spinal cord compression, cauda equina syndrome, and conus medullaris syndrome.

• Patients with ECS usually have a history of incontinence, sciatica, and associated neurologic deficits of relatively rapid progression.

• Physical examination findings of ECS can include lower extremity weakness or stiffness, paresthesias, anesthesias, gait disturbances, and abnormal SLR. The finding of urinary retention with overflow incontinence is highly sensitive and specific for cauda equina syndrome.[12]

• Patients with ECS require urgent imaging with MRI, early treatment, and admission.

• Lumbosacral radiographs should be utilized for both trauma patients and the elderly with acute back pain, but are not indicated for most cases of lumbar pain.

• Low back and lower extremity pain that occurs with walking and is relieved with rest can be caused by either spinal stenosis or arterial insufficiency secondary to peripheral vascular disease. An MRI of the lumbar spine and possibly arteriography are often needed to determine the diagnosis.

EMERGENCY DEPARTMENT CARE AND DISPOSITION

• Any patient with significant trauma or a life- and limb-threatening condition requires aggressive and urgent evaluation, resuscitation, and treatment as appropriate.

• Patients with a progressing neurologic deficit or myelopathy that suggests ECS should be immediately treated with IV dexamethasone before any imaging tests are done. Prompt consultation with appropriate specialists should be obtained.

- Any ECS patient with intractable pain, progression of neurologic deficits, or myelopathy should be admitted.
- The vast majority of patients with neck and back pain can be sent home with medications for symptomatic relief. Treatment with nonsteroidal anti-inflammatory drugs for a period of 5 to 7 days can be started. Elderly patients and patients with renal disease or peptic ulcer disease should be treated with acetaminophen instead.
- A muscle relaxant such as diazepam may help relieve neck and back pain. A limited amount of opioid analgesic can be provided for patients with moderate to severe pain.
- Discharged patients should be encouraged to resume normal activities as quickly as possible.[13]
- Close follow-up with a primary physician is suggested for any further evaluation and treatment and to monitor for any new neurologic findings.

REFERENCES

1. Tsang I: Rheumatology: Pain in the neck. *CMAJ* 164:1182, 2001.
2. Kriss TC, Kriss VM: Neck pain—primary care work-up of acute and chronic symptoms. *Geriatrics* 55:47, 2000.
3. Weeks Jandreau S, Gibbs MA: Vertebral injuries, in Ferrera PC, Colucciello SA, Marx JA, Verdile VP, Gibbs MA (eds.): *Trauma Management: An Emergency Medicine Approach.* St. Louis: Mosby, 2001, p. 163.
4. Mazanec D: Back pain: Medical evaluation and therapy. *Cleve Clin J Med* 62:163, 1995.
5. Deyo R, Weinstein J: Primary care: Low back pain. *N Engl J Med* 344:363, 2001.
6. Deyo RA, Tsui-Wu YJ: Descriptive epidemiology of low back pain and its related medical care in the United States. *Spine* 12:264, 1987.
7. Pawl RP: Chronic neck syndromes: An update. *Comp Ther* 25:278, 1999.
8. Deyo RA, Losser JD, Bigos SJ: Herniated intervertebral disk. *Ann Intern Med* 112:598, 1990.
9. Helwig-Larsen S: Clinical outcome in metastatic spinal cord compression: A prospective study of 153 patients. *Acta Neurol Scand* 94:269, 1996.
10. Levy HI: Cervical pain syndromes: Primary care diagnosis and management. *Comp Ther* 26:82, 2000.
11. Rothman S: The diagnosis of infections of the spine by modern imaging techniques. *Orthop Clin North Am* 27:15, 1996.
12. Deyo RA, Rainville J, Kent DL: What can the history and physical examination tell us about low back pain? *JAMA* 286:760, 1992.
13. Malmivaara A, Hakkinen U, Aro T, et al: The treatment of acute low back pain—bed rest, exercise, or ordinary activity. *N Engl J Med* 332:321, 1995.

For further reading in *Emergency Medicine: A Comprehensive Study Guide,* 6th ed., see Chap. 281, "Neck Pain," by William J. Frohna; and Chap. 282, "Thoracic and Lumbar Pain Syndromes," by David Della-Giustina and Marco Coppola.

182 SHOULDER PAIN

Andrew D. Perron

EPIDEMIOLOGY

- Rotator cuff impingement injury is the most common cause of intrinsic shoulder pain.[1] This injury continuum ranges from subacromial bursitis, through rotator cuff tendinitis, to partial- and full-thickness rotator cuff tears.
- Patients younger than 25 years are most susceptible to subacromial bursitis. Patients older than 40 years are unlikely to have rotator cuff tears.
- Adhesive capsulitis ("frozen shoulder") is most common in postmenopausal, diabetic women younger than 70 years. It is rarely associated with rotator cuff tears and is frequently associated with prior immobilization, trauma, or cervical disc disease.

PATHOPHYSIOLOGY

- The muscles of the rotator cuff (supraspinatus, infraspinatus, teres minor, and subscapularis) are dynamic stabilizers of the glenohumeral joint and provide much of the power for shoulder movement.[2]
- The muscles of the rotator cuff must function within the coracoacromial arch, between the humeral head and the coracoid, acromion, and acromioclavicular ligament. They also function beneath the deltoid muscle and subacromial bursa. The rotator cuff is therefore prone to compression and impingement.
- The biceps tendon inserts on the glenoid labrum after passing between the subscapularis and supraspinatus tendons, and assists with rotator cuff function. The long head of the biceps can become impinged due to its location.
- The biceps tendon can rupture or become subluxed or dislocated out of the bicipital groove of the humerus.
- Activities that cause repeated compression of these structures can cause impingement syndromes.[3]
- The supraspinatus muscle or its tendon is the most commonly injured rotator cuff structure.
- Calcific tendinitis, associated with reversible calcium hydroxyapatite deposition within one or more rotator

cuff tendons, is most common in the supraspinatus tendon.

- Adhesive capsulitis is associated with idiopathic fibrosis and scarring of the shoulder joint capsule.

CLINICAL FEATURES

- Decreased range of motion, crepitus, weakness, or atrophy of shoulder muscles may accompany various causes of shoulder pain, especially the more severe impingement syndromes.
- Neer's test involves compressing the rotator cuff and subacromial bursa as the examiner forcibly but smoothly fully abducts the straightened arm. Pain is associated with a positive test.
- Hawkins' test involves inward rotation of an arm previously placed in 90 degrees of abduction and 90 degrees of elbow flexion. Inward rotation of the arm across the front of the body compresses the rotator cuff and bursa between the coracoacromial ligament and the humeral head. Pain is associated with a positive test.
- Speed's and Yergason's tests are used to identify biceps tendon pathology.
- A positive Speed's test finds pain in the anterior shoulder with resisted forward flexion of the shoulder when the elbow is extended and forearm supinated.
- A positive Yergason's test finds pain in the anterior shoulder with the elbow flexed to 90 degrees when forearm supination is resisted.
- Subacromial bursitis is commonly associated with positive impingement tests and tenderness at the lateral proximal humerus or in the subacromial space.
- Rotator cuff tendinitis is more common between ages 25 and 40 and is associated with signs of impingement, tenderness of the rotator cuff, and rotator cuff muscular weakness.
- Acute injuries to the rotator cuff generally involve acute traumatic forced hyperabduction or hyperextension of the shoulder.
- Rotator cuff tears may be partial or full thickness.
- Commonly associated findings of rotator cuff tears are muscular weakness, especially with abduction and external rotation, cuff tenderness, muscular atrophy, and impingement signs. Crepitus suggests more chronic injury.
- Calcific tendinitis causes sudden onset of shoulder pain, usually at rest, and is exacerbated by any shoulder motion. It is usually worse at night and coincides with resorption of the calcium deposit.
- The onset of calcific tendinitis is usually over a very short time period and more severe than pain associated with rotator cuff tendinitis. The pain generally is self-limited after 2 weeks.
- Some patients with calcific tendinitis have calcific

deposits on shoulder radiographs long before they develop shoulder pain, and over 60% of people with calcifications never develop pain.

- Adhesive capsulitis often follows periods of immobilization of the shoulder, and causes diffuse aching, especially at night, and limited passive and active range of motion. Pain is reproduced at the limits of motion, but not by palpation.
- Primary osteoarthritis is associated with degenerative disease in other joints. Osteoarthritis of the shoulder is rare, as it is not a weight-bearing joint.
- Osteoarthritis is often present in multiple joints, but is especially likely in a previously injured shoulder.
- Osteoarthritis causes pain with activity, and is relieved with rest.

DIAGNOSIS AND DIFFERENTIAL

- The most specific radiographic sign for large rotator cuff tears is a narrowing of the acromiohumeral space (<7 mm).[3]
- Radiographs are rarely diagnostic, but help detect abnormal calcifications with calcific bursitis, osteophytes, or other arthritic changes, or subtle glenohumeral dislocations, which can be mistaken for adhesive capsulitis.[3]
- Extrinsic causes of shoulder pain should be considered in the differential diagnosis, and these include acute cardiac, pulmonary, aortic, and abdominal pathology.
- Cervical spine radiculopathy, brachial plexus disorders, Pancoast's tumor, and axillary artery thrombosis must be considered in the evaluation of shoulder pain.

EMERGENCY DEPARTMENT CARE AND DISPOSITION

- Reduction of pain and inflammation are the goals of emergency department care. This usually involves nonsteroidal anti-inflammatory drugs, "relative rest," cryotherapy (icing), and immobilization. "Relative rest" means avoidance of painful activities.
- Gentle range-of-motion exercises should begin as soon as pain allows.
- A potential complication of local steroid injection is tendon rupture.

REFERENCES

1. Stevenson JH, Trojan T: Evaluation of shoulder pain. *J Fam Pract* 51:605, 2002.

2. Blake R, Hoffman J: Emergency department evaluation and treatment of the shoulder and humerus. *Emerg Med Clin North Am* 17:859, 1999.

3. Resnick D (ed.): *Diagnosis of Bone and Joint Disorders.* Philadelphia: Saunders, 2002, p. 387.

For further reading in *Emergency Medicine: A Comprehensive Study Guide,* 6th ed., see Chap. 283, "Shoulder Pain," by David Della-Giustina, Benjamin Harrison, and D. Monte Hunter.

183 ACUTE DISORDERS OF THE JOINTS AND BURSAE

Andrew D. Perron

SEPTIC ARTHRITIS

- Bacterial infection of the joint space presents as a monarticular arthritis that can destroy the joint in a few hours to days.
- Patients may lack fever, chills, and malaise.
- While an elevated erythrocyte sedimentation rate is insensitive for septic arthritis in adults, it is 90% sensitive in children and infants with septic arthritis.[1,2]
- The white blood cell count lacks sensitivity and specificity in both adults and children with septic arthritis.
- Synovial fluid analysis usually reveals cloudy fluid with white blood cell count greater than 50,000/mm^3 and cultures that are positive more than 50% of the time (Table 183-1).
- Septic arthritis requires admission to the hospital for parenteral antibiotics, generally a combination of nafcillin and a third-generation cephalosporin, and orthopedic consultation for possible surgical drainage.
- Specific patient demographics can help guide empiric antibiotic therapy in septic arthritis (Table 183-2).

GONOCOCCAL ARTHRITIS

- Gonococcal arthritis is the most common cause of septic arthritis in adolescents and young adults and usually presents with fever, chills, and migratory arthralgias or tenosynovitis preceding a monarthritis.[3]
- Vesiculopustular lesions may be present distal to the involved joint.
- Synovial fluid cultures are often negative. However, cultures of the posterior pharynx, urethra, cervix, and rectum may increase the yield of isolating the organism.[3]

TRAUMATIC HEMARTHROSIS

- Hemarthrosis has a high association with intraarticular fracture and ligamentous injury.
- The synovial fluid aspirate may show fat droplets if an intra-articular fracture is present.
- Spontaneous hemarthrosis should prompt an investigation for a coagulopathy.

CRYSTAL-INDUCED SYNOVITIS

- Gout, caused by uric acid crystal deposition, is the most common cause of inflammatory joint disease in men over the age of 40 years, and typically affects the great toe, tarsal joints, or knee.[4]
- Up to 30% of patients with acute gout will have normal serum uric acid levels making this test of little utility in diagnosing gout.[4]

TABLE 183-1   Examination of Synovial Fluid

	NORMAL	NONINFLAMMATORY	INFLAMMATORY	SEPTIC
Clarity	Transparent	Transparent	Cloudy	Cloudy
Color	Clear	Yellow	Yellow	Yellow
WBC/μL	<200	<200–2000	200–50,000	>50,000
PMNs (%)*	<25	<25	>50	>50
Culture	Negative	Negative	Negative	>50% positive
Crystals	None	None	Multiple or none	None
Associated conditions		Osteoarthritis, trauma, rheumatic fever	Gout, pseudogout, spondyloarthropathies, RA, Lyme disease, SLE	Nongonococcal or gonococcal septic arthritis

*The white blood cell count (WBC) and percent polymorphonuclear leukocytes (PMNs) are affected by a number of factors, including disease progression, affecting organism, and host immune status. The joint aspirate WBC and PMNs should be considered part of a continuum for each disease, particularly septic arthritis, and should be correlated with other clinical information.

ABBREVIATIONS: RA = rheumatoid arthritis; SLE = systemic lupus erythematosus.

TABLE 183-2 Commonly Encountered Organisms in the Septic Arthritis Patient

PATIENT/ CONDITION	EXPECTED ORGANISMS	ANTIBIOTIC CONSIDERATIONS
Neonates and infants	Staphylococcus, gram-negative bacteria, group B Streptococcus, Candida	Nafcillin* plus aminoglycoside or third-generation cephalosporin, ampicillin-sulbactam
Children <5 years	Staphylococcus, Streptococcus, Haemophilus influenzae	Nafcillin* plus cefuroxime, ampicillin-sulbactam
Older children and healthy adults	Staphylococcus, Neisseria gonorrhoeae, Streptococcus	Nafcillin* plus third-generation cephalosporin, ampicillin-sulbactam
Involvement of the foot	Staphylococcus, Pseudomonas	Nafcillin* plus ceftazidime or aminoglycoside
Intravenous drug users	Staphylococcus, gram-negative bacilli	Nafcillin* plus aminoglycoside, ampicillin-sulbactam
Sickle-cell patients	Salmonella	Ciprofloxacin, ofloxacin, or ceftriaxone

*First-generation cephalosporin may be substituted for penicillinase-resistant penicillin. Vancomycin should be employed for treatment of suspected methicillin-resistant staphylococci.

- Pseudogout, calcium pyrophosphate crystal deposition, typically affects the knee, wrist, ankle, or elbow. Onset is usually slower than with gout (onset over a day or more with pseudogout compared to an onset over hours with gout).
- Either gout or pseudogout may be precipitated by trauma, surgery, significant illness, dietary or alcohol indiscretions, or certain medications.
- Synovial fluid analysis will reveal negative birefringent needle-shaped uric acid crystals in gout and weakly positive birefringent rhomboid calcium pyrophosphate crystals in pseudogout.
- Determining the number and distribution of joints affected can help narrow the differential diagnosis (Table 183-3).
- Acute treatment is with nonsteroidal anti-inflammatory drugs (NSAIDs) such as indomethacin. Opioid narcotics may also be required for effective analgesia.
- Colchicine, although often not necessary, can be prescribed at 0.6 mg/h orally until efficacy ensues or the patient experiences intolerable gastrointestinal side effects.

OSTEOARTHRITIS

- Osteoarthritis is a chronic, often symmetric, arthritis lacking constitutional symptoms, that is caused by destruction of the articular hyaline cartilage.
- Radiographs may show joint space narrowing, sclerosis, or osteophyte formation.
- Acute pain is treated with NSAIDs and resting the affected joint.

LYME ARTHRITIS

- Lyme arthritis is the result of a tick bite that infects the host with the spirochete *Borrelia burgdorferi*.
- Lyme arthritis manifests as a monarticular or symmetric oligoarticular arthritis, primarily affecting the large joints, with alternating periods of exacerbation and complete remission.
- Synovial fluid cultures are usually negative.[5]
- Treatment of Lyme arthritis consists of 3 to 4 weeks of doxycycline, penicillin, amoxicillin, or erythromycin.

REITER'S SYNDROME

- Reiter's syndrome is a seronegative spondyloarthropathy that manifests as an acute, asymmetric oligoarthritis with a predilection for the lower

TABLE 183-3 Classification of Arthritis by Number of Affected Joints

NUMBER OF JOINTS	DIFFERENTIAL CONSIDERATIONS
1 = Monarthritis	Trauma-induced arthritis Infection/septic arthritis Crystal-induced (gout, pseudogout) Osteoarthritis (acute) Lyme disease Avascular necrosis Tumor
2–3 = Oligoarthritis	Lyme disease Reiter syndrome Ankylosing spondylitis Gonococcal arthritis Rheumatic fever
>3 = Polyarthritis	Rheumatoid arthritis Systemic lupus erythematosus Viral arthritis Osteoarthritis (chronic)

extremities, that may be preceded 2 to 6 weeks earlier by an infectious illness, usually urethritis (*Ureaplasma* or *Chlamydia*) or enteritis (*Salmonella* or *Shigella*).[6]

- The classic triad of urethritis, conjunctivitis, and arthritis is not mandatory for diagnosis.
- NSAIDs should be used for the symptomatic treatment of joint pain. Antibiotics are of no proven benefit.

ANKYLOSING SPONDYLITIS

- Ankylosing spondylitis is a seronegative spondyloarthropathy primarily affecting the spine and pelvis, that is characterized by morning stiffness as well as constitutional symptoms such as fatigue, weakness, and malaise.
- Ankylosing spondylitis is associated with HLA-B27 antigen positivity.
- Classic radiographic findings include sacroiliitis and squaring of the vertebral bodies (eg, bamboo spine).
- Joint pain should be treated symptomatically with NSAIDs.

RHEUMATOID ARTHRITIS

- Rheumatoid arthritis is a chronic, symmetric, polyarticular synovial joint disease, pathologically characterized by synovial pannus formation.
- This disease is also associated with morning stiffness, depression, fatigue, and myalgias.
- Pericarditis, myocarditis, pleural effusion, pneumonitis, and mononeuritis multiplex may occur.
- Articular involvement is noted for symmetric, painful, tender joints, with sparing of the distal interphalangeal joints.
- Acute exacerbations of joint pain are treated with immobilization of the affected joint, NSAIDs, and corticosteroids.

BURSITIS

- Bursitis is an inflammatory process involving any bursae, that can be caused by infection, trauma, rheumatologic disorders, crystal deposition, or idiopathic.
- Commonly affected bursae include the prepatellar bursa (eg, carpet layer's knee) and the olecranon bursa.
- Septic and aseptic bursitis cannot reliably be differentiated by physical examination alone, so aspiration of bursal fluid is required for cell count and differential, Gram's stain, and culture.[7–10]
- Septic bursal fluid characteristically is purulent in appearance, with greater than 15,000 white blood cells/mm^3 and culture positive.
- Treatment entails resting the affected joint, a com-

pressive dressing, analgesics, and antistaphylococcal antibiotics for 10 to 14 days if there is evidence of infection.

REFERENCES

1. Malleson PN: Management of childhood arthritis: Part I. Acute arthritis. *Arch Dis Child* 76:460, 1997.
2. Del Beccaro MA, Champoux AN, Bockers T, Mendelman PM: Septic arthritis versus transient synovitis of the hip: The value of screening laboratory tests. *Ann Emerg Med* 21:1418, 1992.
3. Shaw BA, Kasser JR: Acute septic arthritis in infancy and childhood. *Clin Orthop* 257:212, 1990.
4. Joseph J, McGrath H: Gout or pseudogout: How to differentiate crystal induced arthropathies. *Geriatrics* 50:33, 1995.
5. Gerber MA, Zemel LS, Shapiro ED: Lyme arthritis in children: Clinical epidemiology and long-term outcomes. *Pediatrics* 102:905, 1998.
6. Pinals RS: Polyarthritis and fever. *N Engl J Med* 330:769, 1994.
7. McAfee JH, Smith DL: Olecranon and prepatellar bursitis: Diagnosis and treatment. *West J Med* 149:607, 1988.
8. Smith DL, McAfee JH, Lucas LM, et al: Septic and nonseptic olecranon bursitis: Utility of the surface temperature probe in the early differentiation of septic and nonseptic cases. *Arch Intern Med* 149:1581, 1989.
9. Ho G, Tice AD, Kaplan SR: Septic bursitis in the prepatellar and olecranon bursae: An analysis of 25 cases. *Ann Intern Med* 89:21, 1978.
10. Smith DL, McAfee JH, Lucas LM, et al: Treatment of nonseptic olecranon bursitis: A controlled, blinded prospective trial. *Arch Intern Med* 149:2527, 1989.

For further reading in *Emergency Medicine: A Comprehensive Study Guide,* 6th ed., see Chap. 286, "Acute Disorders of the Joints and Bursae," by John H. Burton.

184 EMERGENCIES IN SYSTEMIC RHEUMATIC DISEASES

Michael P. Kefer

RHEUMATIC EMERGENCIES ASSOCIATED WITH RISK OF MORTALITY

RESPIRATORY SYSTEM

- Death may result from airway obstruction, respiratory muscle failure, or pulmonary tissue involvement.

- Relapsing polychondritis presents with the abrupt onset of pain, redness, and swelling of the ears or nose. The tracheobronchial cartilage is involved in approximately 50% of cases. Hoarseness and throat tenderness over the cartilage are noted. Repeated attacks can lead to airway collapse.
- Treatment of a relapsing polychondritis exacerbation involves administering high-dose steroids and hospital admission for observation.
- Rheumatoid arthritis (RA) may involve the cricoarytenoid joints, causing pain with speaking, hoarseness, or stridor. The cricoarytenoid joints may fix in a closed position, which may mandate emergency tracheostomy.
- Dermatomyositis and polymyositis may lead to respiratory failure from respiratory muscle involvement in poorly controlled disease.
- Pulmonary hemorrhage complicates Goodpasture's disease, systemic lupus erythematosus (SLE), Wegener's granulomatosis, and other vasculitic conditions.
- Pulmonary fibrosis occurs in ankylosing spondylitis, scleroderma, and other conditions.
- Pleural effusion occurs in RA and SLE.

CARDIAC

- Pericarditis occurs in RA and SLE.
- Myocardial infarction may occur from coronary artery involvement in Kawasaki's disease or polyarteritis nodosa.
- Pancarditis occurs in acute rheumatic fever.
- Valvular heart disease occurs in ankylosing spondylitis, relapsing polychondritis, and rheumatic fever. Involvement may extend into the conduction system.

ADRENAL

- Glucocorticoids are often used in the treatment of rheumatic conditions. Doses required may result in adrenal suppression. As a result, these patients may be unable to respond to the physiologic stress of an acute illness or injury and proceed to develop adrenal insufficiency.
- In this situation, treatment with stress-dose steroids is indicated.

RHEUMATIC PRESENTATIONS ASSOCIATED WITH RISK OF MORBIDITY

CERVICAL SPINE AND SPINAL CORD

- Patients with rheumatologic involvement of the cervical spine may be at high risk for serious cervical spine

or spinal cord injury from otherwise trivial trauma. This includes manipulation during endotracheal intubation if extreme caution is not exercised.
- Ligamentous destruction of the transverse ligament of C2, with resultant symptoms of cord compression, may complicate RA.
- Cervical spine inflexibility from ankylosing spondylitis predisposes to injury out of proportion to the mechanism.
- Anterior spinal artery syndrome may result from rheumatologic conditions causing vasculitis, aortic dissection, or embolism.

OPHTHALMIC

- Temporal arteritis is a cause of sudden blindness and should be considered in any patient older than 50 years who presents with new-onset headache, visual change, or jaw or tongue claudication.
- Laboratory investigation of temporal arteritis reveals an elevated erythrocyte sedimentation rate (>50 mm/h) and C-reactive protein (>2.45 mg/dL).
- Treatment with prednisone 60 mg/day should be initiated immediately based on clinical and laboratory findings of temporal arteritis.
- Temporal artery biopsy for definitive diagnosis must be obtained within the first week of treatment to be accurate.
- Dry eyes (and dry mouth) from Sjögren's syndrome may occur alone or coexist with many rheumatologic conditions.
- Episcleritis is a self-limited, painless injection of the episcleral vessels. It is in the differential diagnosis of the red eye in patients with RA.
- Scleritis is also seen in patients with RA and presents with marked ocular tenderness. The eye has a purple discoloration. The potential for visual impairment and scleral rupture mandate emergent ophthalmologic consult and high-dose steroids.

HYPERTENSION

- Hypertension can complicate any rheumatologic condition that affects the kidneys, either directly, as in polyarteritis nodosa, scleroderma, or SLE, or indirectly, from nephrotoxic drugs used to treat the underlying disorder.

RENAL

- Renal insult is due either to the primary disease process, the drugs used to treat the disease, or both.

- Nephritis is a common complication of SLE, Wegener's granulomatosis, and systemic vasculitis.
- Renal dysfunction from malignant hypertension occurs with scleroderma.
- Nephrotic syndrome in patients with SLE predisposes to renal vein thrombosis.
- Renal insufficiency from prostaglandin inhibition by nonsteroidal anti-inflammatory drugs is more frequent in the elderly.
- Renal insufficiency may result from rhabdomyolysis in the patient with florid myositis or sclerosis in the patient with scleroderma.

BIBLIOGRAPHY

Halla J: Rheumatology emergencies. *Bull Rheum Dis* 46:4, 1997.

Kelley WN, Harris ED Jr, Ruddy S, Sledge CB: *Textbook of Rheumatology.* Philadelphia: Saunders, 1997, p. 216.

Klippel JH (ed.): *Primer on Rheumatic Diseases,* 11th ed. Atlanta: Arthritis Foundation, 1997, p. 157.

Salvarani C, Hunder GG: Giant cell arteritis with low erythrocyte sedimentation rate: Frequency of occurrence in a population-based study. *Arthritis Rheum* 45:140, 2001.

For further reading in *Emergency Medicine: A Comprehensive Study Guide,* 6th ed., see Chap. 284, "Emergencies in Systemic Rheumatic Diseases," by Richard C. Chandler and Mary Chester Morgan Wasko.

185 INFECTIOUS AND NONINFECTIOUS DISORDERS OF THE HAND

Michael P. Kefer

HAND INFECTION

- Hand infections most commonly occur from injury to the dermis. Skin organisms, *Staphylococcus* and *Streptococcus* species, are the most common pathogens. Infection rarely may result from a hematogenous source.[1-3]
- Infections from animal bite wounds may be infected with *Pasteurella multocida* and human bite wounds with *Eikenella corrodens.*
- Abscesses always require surgical drainage.
- A history of chronic illness or immunodeficiency in-

creases the risk of hand infection by atypical pathogens.[2,3]
- Table 185-1 summarizes the common infections of the hand, the likely organisms involved, and recommended antibiotic therapy.
- Injection drug abusers may present with infection secondary to *Staphylococcus aureus* by direct needle inoculation or from hematogenous spread from endocarditis.
- Rest and elevation are the mainstays of treatment for many inflammatory conditions of the hand. This helps to decrease inflammation, avoid secondary injury, and prevent spread of any existing infection.
- The optimal position for splinting of the hand is the position of function: wrist in 15 degrees of extension, metacarpophalangeal (MCP) joint in 50 to 90 degrees of flexion, proximal interphalangeal (PIP) joint in 10 to 15 degrees of flexion, and distal interphalangeal (DIP) joint in 10 to 15 degrees of flexion.

CELLULITIS

- Cellulitis is a superficial infection presenting with localized warmth, erythema, and edema.
- The examiner must exclude the involvement of deeper structures by demonstrating absence of tenderness on deep palpation and range of motion of the hand.
- Emergency department (ED) care consists of antibiotics, splinting in the position of function, elevation, and close follow-up.

FLEXOR TENOSYNOVITIS

- Flexor tenosynovitis is diagnosed by the presence of the four cardinal signs: (1) tenderness over the flexor tendon sheath; (2) symmetric swelling of the finger; (3) pain with passive extension; and (4) flexed position of the involved digit.[3]
- ED care consists of splinting, elevation, IV antibiotics, and orthopedic consultation for drainage.

DEEP SPACE INFECTION

- Deep space infections involve the web or midpalmar space. Web space infection occurs after penetrating injury to the web space.
- Clinically, dorsal and volar swelling of the web space with separation of the affected digits is noted.
- Midpalmar space infection occurs from spread of a flexor tenosynovitis or penetrating wound to the palm, causing infection of the radial or ulnar bursa of the hand.

TABLE 185-1   Initial Antibiotic Coverage for Common Hand Infections

INFECTION	INITIAL ANTIBIOTIC	LIKELY ORGANISMS	COMMENTS
Cellulitis	First-generation cephalosporin (cephalexin) *or* antistaphylococcal penicillin (amoxicillin-clavulanate, dicloxacillin)	*Streptococcus pyogenes, Staphylococcus aureus*	Consider vancomycin for intravenous drug abusers
Felon/paronychia	First-generation cephalosporin (cephalexin) *or* antistaphylococcal penicillin (amoxicillin-clavulanate, dicloxacillin)	Polymicrobial, *S. aureus,* anaerobes	Antibiotics indicated for infections with associated localized cellulitis
Flexor tenosynovitis	Aminopenicillin with a β-lactamase inhibitor (ampicillin-sulbactam) *or* first-generation cephalosporin (cefazolin) and penicillin	*S. aureus,* streptococci, anaerobes, gram-negatives	Parenteral antibiotics are indicated; consider ceftriaxone for *Neissera gonorrhoeae*
Deep space infection	Aminopenicillin with a β-lactamase inhibitor (ampicillin-sulbactam) *or* first-generation cephalosporin (cefazolin) and penicillin	*S. aureus,* streptococci, anaerobes, gram-negatives	Inpatient management
Animal bites (including human)	Aminopenicillin with a β-lactamase inhibitor (ampicillin-sulbactam) *or* first-generation cephalosporin (cefazolin) and penicillin	*S. aureus,* streptococci, *Eikenella corrodens* (human), *Pasteurella multocida* (cat), anaerobes and gram-negatives	All animal bite wounds should receive prophylactic oral antibiotics
Herpetic whitlow	None, unless secondary bacterial contamination is present	Herpes simplex	Consider acyclovir, no surgical drainage is indicated

- ED care of deep space infections consists of splinting, elevation, IV antibiotics, and orthopedic consultation for drainage.

CLOSED FIST INJURY

- Closed fist injury is essentially a human bite wound to the MCP joint that results from punching an individual in the teeth.
- Risk of infection spreading along the extensor tendons is high.
- Wounds penetrating the skin should be explored, irrigated, and allowed to heal by secondary intention.
- When inspecting for extensor tendon injury, it is essential to consider the position of the hand at the time of injury.
- ED care consists of IV antibiotics, splinting, and hand surgery consultation for disposition.
- Extensor tendon repair should be delayed until the risk of infection has passed.

PARONYCHIA

- Paronychia is an infection of the lateral nail fold.
- ED care of a small paronychia consists of inserting a #11 blade into the nail fold, parallel to the nail, to drain the abscess.
- In an advanced infection, or one in which pus is seen beneath the nail, the corner of the perionychium should be incised and the nail fold lifted. A portion of the nail may have to be removed and packing placed for adequate drainage. Injury to the nail bed should be avoided.

- The wound should be rechecked in 24 to 48 hours; the packing should be pulled and warm soaks initiated.
- Chronic paronychia may be due to atypical organisms such as *Candida albicans,* especially in immunocompromised hosts.[4]

FELON

- Felon is an infection of the pulp space of the fingertip. Pain results from the accumulation of pus in the fibrous septae of the finger pad.
- ED care consists of drainage by the lateral approach to protect the neurovascular bundle. An incision should begin 5 mm distal to the DIP joint crease and continue just palmar to and parallel with the perionychium, stopping distally at the phalangeal tuft. The incision should be deep enough to extend across the entire finger pad to divide the septae at the bony insertions.
- Unless there is a pointing abscess, the radial aspect of the index and middle fingers and the ulnar aspect of the thumb and small finger should be avoided.
- The wound should be packed loosely. The hand should be splinted in the position of function.
- The wound should be rechecked in 24 to 48 hours; the packing should be pulled and warm soaks initiated.

HERPETIC WHITLOW

- Herpetic whitlow is a viral infection of the fingertip involving intracutaneous vesicles.
- Clinically, it may present similarly to a felon.
- ED care consists of immobilization, elevation, and

protection with a dry dressing to prevent autoinoculation and transmission. Antiviral agents may shorten the duration.[5]

NONINFECTIOUS CONDITIONS

TENDINITIS

- Tendinitis is usually due to overuse.
- Examination reveals tenderness over the involved tendon.
- ED care consists of immobilization and nonsteroidal anti-inflammatory drugs (NSAIDs).

TRIGGER FINGER

- Trigger finger is a tenosynovitis of the flexor sheath of the digit and may result in stenosis of the sheath.
- Impingement and snap release of the tendon occurs as the finger is extended from a flexed position.
- Steroid injection may be effective in early stages. Definitive treatment is surgery.

DEQUERVAIN'S TENOSYNOVITIS

- DeQuervain's tenosynovitis involves the extensor pollicis brevis and abductor pollicis tendons. Pain occurs at the radial aspect of the wrist and radiates into the forearm.
- The Finkelstein test is diagnostic: the patient grasps the thumb in the fist and deviates the hand ulnarly, reproducing the pain.
- ED care consists of a thumb spica splint, NSAIDs, and referral.

CARPAL TUNNEL SYNDROME

- Carpal tunnel syndrome results from compression of the median nerve by the transverse carpal ligament.
- The cause is usually edema secondary to overuse, pregnancy, or congestive heart failure.
- Pain in the median nerve distribution of the hand tends to be worse at night.
- On examination, pain may be reproduced by tapping over the nerve at the wrist (Tinel's sign) or by holding the wrist flexed maximally for >1 minute (Phalen's sign).[6]
- Treatment consists of a wrist splint and NSAIDs. Advanced cases require surgical decompression.

DUPUYTREN'S CONTRACTURE

- Dupuytren's contracture results from fibrous changes in the subcutaneous tissues of the palm, which may lead to tethering and joint contractures.
- Referral to a hand surgeon is indicated.

GANGLION CYST

- Ganglion cyst is a cystic collection of synovial fluid within a joint or tendon sheath.
- Treatment consists of NSAIDs and referral.

REFERENCES

1. Hausman MR, Lisser SP: Hand infections. *Orthop Clin North Am* 5:171, 1992.
2. Kour AK, Looi KP, Phone MH, et al: Hand infections in patients with diabetes. *Clin Orthop* 331:238, 1996.
3. Moran GJ, Talan DA: Hand infections *Emerg Med Clin North Am* 11:601, 1993.
4. Brook I: Aerobic and anaerobic microbiology of paronychia. *Ann Emerg Med* 19:994, 1990.
5. Laskin OL: Acyclovir and suppression of frequently recurring herpetic whitlow. *Ann Emerg Med* 102:494, 1985.
6. Novak M: Carpal tunnel syndrome. *Primary Care Pract* 4:642, 2000.

For further reading in *Emergency Medicine: A Comprehensive Study Guide,* 6th ed., see Chap. 285, "Nontraumatic Disorders of the Hand," by Mark W. Fourre.

186 SOFT TISSUE PROBLEMS OF THE FOOT

Mark B. Rogers

PLANTAR WARTS

- Plantar warts are contagious and caused by the human papillomavirus.
- The diagnosis is clinical and treatment options exist; however, many lesions spontaneously resorb within 2 years.[1]

ONYCHOCRYPTOSIS (INGROWN TOENAIL)

- Ingrown toenails occur when part of the nail plate penetrates the nail sulcus, usually involving the great toe.
- Patients with diabetes, arterial insufficiency, cellulitis, ulceration, or necrosis are at risk for toe amputation.
- If infection is not present, elevation with a wisp of cotton between the nail plate and skin, daily foot soaks, and avoiding pressure on the area is often sufficient.
- If granulation tissue or infection is present, partial removal of the nail is indicated and débridement is indicated with a wound check in 24 to 48 hours.[2]

BURSITIS

- Noninflammatory bursae are pressure-induced over the bony prominences.
- Inflammatory bursae are due to gout, syphilis, or rheumatoid arthritis.
- Diagnosis and treatment is dependent on aspirated bursa fluid. Fluid should be sent for cell count, crystal analysis, Gram's stain, culture, protein, glucose, and lactate levels.
- Suppurative bursae are due to pyogenic organisms, usually from adjacent wounds. Nafcillin or oxacillin is the therapy of choice.[3]

PLANTAR FASCIITIS

- Plantar fasciitis usually is caused by overuse or may affect those unaccustomed to activity.
- Patients have point tenderness over the anterior-medial calcaneus that is worse upon arising and after activity.
- Plantar fasciitis is usually self-limited; the treatment includes rest, ice, and nonsteroidal anti-inflammatory drugs (NSAIDs). Severe cases may need a short-leg walking cast and podiatric referral.[4]

TARSAL TUNNEL SYNDROME

- Tarsal tunnel syndrome involves compression of the posterior tibial nerve as it courses inferior to the medial malleolus.
- The causes include running, restrictive footwear (eg, ski boots or skates), edema of pregnancy, posttraumatic fibrosis, ganglion cysts, osteophytes, and tumors.
- Pain is worse at night and located at the medial malleolus, heel, sole, and distal calf. Tinel's sign is positive and eversion and dorsiflexion worsen symptoms.
- Ultrasound, computed tomography, or magnetic resonance imaging aid with the diagnosis.

- Differential diagnosis includes plantar fasciitis and Achilles tendinitis; however, the pain of tarsal tunnel syndrome involves the more medial heel and arch and worsens with activity.
- Treatment includes NSAIDs, rest, and orthopedic referral.[5]

GANGLION CYST

- A ganglion is a benign synovial cyst attached to a joint capsule or tendon sheath.
- The anterolateral ankle is a typical site. A firm, usually nontender, cystic lesion is seen on examination.
- Treatment includes aspiration and injection of glucocorticoids, but most require surgical excision.[6]

TENDON LESIONS

- Tenosynovitis or tendinitis usually occur due to overuse and present with pain over the involved tendon. Treatment includes ice, rest, and NSAIDs.
- Tendon lacerations should require orthopedic consultation due to the high complication rate. After repair, extensor tendons are immobilized in dorsiflexion and flexor tendons in equinus.
- Achilles tendon rupture presents with pain, a palpable defect in the area of tendon, inability to stand on tiptoes, and absence of plantar flexion with squeezing of the calf (Thompson's sign). Treatment is generally surgical in younger patients and conservative (casting in equinus) in the elderly.
- Anterior tibialis tendon rupture results in a palpable defect and mild foot drop. Surgery is usually not necessary.
- Posterior tibialis tendon rupture is usually chronic and insidious. Findings include a flattened arch, weakness on inversion, a palpable defect, and inability to stand on tiptoes.
- Flexor hallucis longus rupture presents with loss of plantar flexion of the great toe and must be surgically repaired in athletes.
- Disruption of the peroneal retinaculum occurs with a direct blow during dorsiflexion, causing localized pain behind the lateral malleolus and clicking while walking as the tendon subluxes. The treatment is surgery.[7]

PLANTAR INTERDIGITAL NEUROMA (MORTON'S NEUROMA)

- Neuromas are thought to occur from entrapment of the plantar digital nerve due to tight-fitting shoes, typically women's.

- Patients present with burning, cramping, or aching over the area of the metatarsal head that improves after shoe removal.
- The diagnosis is clinical and conservative treatment includes wide shoes with inserts and glucocorticoid injections.[8]

IMMERSION FOOT (TRENCH FOOT)

- Immersion foot results from prolonged exposure to a moist, nonfreezing (<60°F or <15°C) and occlusive environment. It is classically seen in military recruits and in the homeless.
- The foot initially becomes pale, anesthetic, pulseless, and immobile, but not frozen. With rewarming, one sees hyperemia (lasting up to weeks) with severe burning pain and return of sensation. Edema, bullae, and hyperhidrosis may develop.
- Treatment includes admission for bedrest, leg elevation, and air drying at room temperature. Normally, antibiotics are not indicated.[9]

PLANTAR FIBROMATOSIS

- Plantar fibromatosis (Dupuytren's contracture of the plantar fascia) involves small, asymptomatic, palpable, slowly growing, firm masses on the non–weight bearing plantar surface of the foot.
- Toe contractures do not occur, lesions tend to reabsorb spontaneously, and treatment is conservative.[10]

FOOT ULCERS

- Ischemic ulcers are due to vascular compromise of the larger vessels. The examination shows a cool foot; dependent rubor; pallor on elevation; atrophic, shiny skin; and diminished pulses. Treatment is vascular surgery.[11]
- Neuropathic ulcers are pressure ulcers due to poor sensation. The ulcers appear well demarcated with surrounding white callus-like material. The foot (in the absence of severe vascular disease) is normal except with regard to sensation. Treatment is relief of pressure and referral to a podiatrist.[12]
- Diabetics may have both ischemic and neuropathic ulcers.
- Infected ulcers require débridement, pressure relief via bedrest or total contact casting, and broad-spectrum IV antibiotics (eg, ampicillin-sulbactam). Cultures of the drainage and radiographs should be obtained. Vascular surgery consultation and admission are often warranted.[13]

- Palpation of bone in an infected ulcer strongly correlates with osteomyelitis.[14]

MALIGNANT MELANOMA

- Melanoma can present as a pigmented or nonhealing lesion of the foot or nail. It may imitate a fungal infection or plantar wart.
- Acral lentiginous melanoma, a particularly aggressive form, tends to affect non-Caucasian persons and the plantar surface of the foot.[15]
- Suspicious lesions should be referred for biopsy.

REFERENCES

1. Glover MG: Plantar warts. *Foot Ankle* 11:172, 1990.
2. Malusky LP: Podiatric procedures, in Roberts JR, Hedges JR (eds.): *Clinical Procedures in Emergency Medicine,* 3rd ed. Philadelphia: Saunders, 1998, p. 23.
3. Hernandez PA, Hernandez WA, Hernandez A: Clinical aspects of bursae and tendon sheaths of the foot. *J Am Podiatr Med Assoc* 81:366, 1991.
4. Young CC, Rutherford DS, Niedfeldt MW: Treatment of plantar fasciitis. *Am Fam Physician* 64:570, 2001.
5. Reade BM, Longo DC, Keller MC: Tarsal tunnel syndrome. *Clin Podiatr Med Surg* 18:395, 2001.
6. Wu KK: Ganglions of the foot. *J Foot Ankle Surg* 32:343, 1993.
7. Coughlin MJ: Disorders of tendons, in Coughlin MJ, Mann RA (eds.): *Surgery of the Foot and Ankle,* 7th ed. St. Louis: Mosby, 1999, p. 786.
8. Wu KK: Morton neuroma and metatarsalgia. *Curr Opin Rheumatol* 12:131, 2000.
9. Pedowitz WJ: Soft tissue disorders of the foot, in Coughlin MJ, Mann RA, (eds.): *Surgery of the Foot and Ankle,* 7th ed. St. Louis: Mosby, 1999, p. 1373.
10. Lee TH, Wapner KL, Hecht PJ: Plantar fibromatosis. *J Bone Joint Surg* 75A:1080, 1993.
11. Sumpio BE: Foot ulcers. *N Engl J Med* 343:787, 2000.
12. Kantor J, Margolis DJ: Treatment options for diabetic neuropathic foot ulcers: A cost-effectiveness analysis. *Dermatol Surg* 27:347, 2001.
13. Temple ME, Nahata MC: Pharmacotherapy of lower limb diabetic ulcers. *J Am Geriatr Soc* 48:822, 2000.
14. Grayson ML, Gibbons GW, Balogh K, et al: Probing to bone in infected pedal ulcers: A clinical sign of underlying osteomyelitis in diabetic patients. *JAMA* 273:7221, 1995.
15. Franke W, Neumann NJ, Ruzicka T, et al: Plantar malignant melanoma—a challenge for early recognition. *Melanoma Res* 10:571, 2000.

For further reading in *Emergency Medicine: A Comprehensive Study Guide,* 6th edition, see Chap. 287, "Soft Tissue Problems of the Foot," by Frantz R. Melio.

Section 23
PSYCHOSOCIAL DISORDERS

187 CLINICAL FEATURES OF BEHAVIORAL DISORDERS

Lance H. Hoffman

DEMENTIA

- Dementia is a disorder consisting of a pervasive disturbance in cognition, which impairs memory, abstraction, judgment, personality, and higher critical functions such as language.
- The first and second most common causes of dementia are Alzheimer's disease and multi-infarct dementia, respectively.
- Its onset is typically gradual, and the patient's normal level of consciousness is maintained.
- Individuals familiar with the affected person usually notice memory disturbances prior to impairment in other cognitive areas.
- Medical illnesses, adverse drug effects, or a change in the patient's environment may all contribute to acutely diminished functioning in a patient with dementia.
- Metabolic and endocrine disorders, adverse drug effects and interactions, and depression are potentially reversible causes of dementia.

DELIRIUM

- Delirium is characterized by a global impairment in cognitive functioning that is usually acute in onset with a fluctuating severity of symptoms.
- The patient experiences a diminished level of consciousness, inattention, and sensory misperceptions.

- Visual hallucinations are common and typically result in a strong emotional response.
- Most causes of delirium are reversible and include infection, electrolyte abnormalities, toxic ingestions, and head injury
- Treatment should be directed toward correcting the underlying cause.

SUBSTANCE-INDUCED DISORDERS

- Intoxication is an exogenous substance-induced syndrome that results in maladaptive behavior and impaired cognitive functioning and psychomotor activity.
- The individual's judgment, perception, attention, and emotional control may be affected.
- Repeated use of such a substance is defined as substance abuse and may lead to physical or psychological dependence on the substance.

WITHDRAWAL

- Substance withdrawal entails a collection of abuse-specific symptoms that result from the reduction or cessation of use of that substance.
- The symptoms of substance withdrawal are typically opposite those initiated by ingesting the substance, and the withdrawal symptoms quickly subside with ingestion of the substance.

SCHIZOPHRENIA

- Schizophrenia affects just under 1% of the world's population and is the most common psychotic disorder, with symptoms usually beginning in late adolescence or early adulthood.

- Schizophrenia is a chronic disease characterized by functional deterioration; the presence of hallucinations, delusions, disorganized speech or behavior, or catatonic behavior ("positive symptoms"); the presence of blunted affect, emotional withdrawal, lack of spontaneity, anhedonia, or impaired attention ("negative symptoms"); cognitive impairment expressed as loose associations or incoherence; and the relative absence of a mood disorder.
- Patients may present to the emergency department for worsening psychosis, suicidal ideations, bizarre or violent behavior, or adverse effects of medications.
- Older antipsychotic medications such as haloperidol effectively treat the positive symptoms, while newer antipsychotic medications, such as olanzapine and clozapine, effectively treat both positive and negative symptoms.

BRIEF PSYCHOTIC DISORDER

- A brief psychotic disorder is a psychosis of less than 4 weeks' duration that begins acutely as a result of a recent traumatic life experience.

MAJOR DEPRESSION

- Major depression consists of a persistent dysphoric mood or a pervasive loss of interest and pleasure in usual activities (anhedonia) lasting more than 2 weeks.
- Associated psychological symptoms include feelings of guilt over past events, self-reproach, worthlessness, hopelessness, and recurrent thoughts of death or suicide.
- Vegetative symptoms affecting physiological functioning include a loss of appetite and weight, sleep disturbances, fatigue, inability to concentrate, and psychomotor agitation or retardation.
- The diagnosis should be entertained in any patient presenting with multiple vague complaints.
- The lifetime risk of suicide in patients with this disorder is 15%.
- All patients suspected of having major depression should be questioned about suicidal thoughts, and an appropriate psychiatric consultation and referral are mandatory for those with suicidal thoughts.

DYSTHYMIC DISORDER

- Dysthymic disorder is a chronic, less severe form of depression that does not impair daily functioning,

with a depressed mood being present more days than not for at least 2 years.

BIPOLAR DISORDER

- Bipolar disorder is characterized by recurrent, cyclic episodes of manic and depressive symptoms, with depressive episodes being more common than manic episodes.
- Manic individuals experience an elated mood that can quickly deteriorate to irritability and hostility should their expectations not be met.
- They tend to act energetic and expansive, while demonstrating a decreased need for sleep, poor impulse control, racing thoughts, and pressured speech.
- Complications of this disorder include suicide, substance abuse, and marital and occupational disruptions.
- Valproic acid and lithium salts are commonly prescribed as chronic mood stabilizers.

PANIC DISORDER

- Panic disorder is more common in women and tends to manifest in late adolescence to the mid-30s.[1]
- Individuals with panic disorder experience recurrent episodes of intense anxiety or fear accompanied by autonomic symptoms including palpitations, dyspnea, chest pain or tightness, dizziness, and tremulousness.[1]
- The symptoms of the panic attack generally peak in approximately 10 minutes and last no more than 1 hour.
- Patients should be screened for domestic violence, sexual abuse or assault, and suicidal thoughts.
- Effective treatment modalities include cognitive-behavioral therapy and pharmacotherapy with selective serotonin reuptake inhibitors, tricyclic antidepressants, monoamine oxidase inhibitors, or benzodiazepines.[2]

GENERALIZED ANXIETY DISORDER

- Individuals with generalized anxiety disorder experience chronic anxiety without discrete panic attacks for at least 6 months.
- Symptoms include apprehensive worrying, muscle tension, insomnia, irritability, restlessness, and distractibility.

SPECIFIC PHOBIA

- A specific phobia exists when exposure to, or anticipated exposure to, a specific stimulus (eg, height, insects, enclosed spaces, etc) results in excessively anxious symptoms that are recognized by the individual as being irrational.

POSTTRAUMATIC STRESS DISORDER

- Posttraumatic stress disorder is an anxiety reaction to experiencing a severe psychosocial stressor that is usually life threatening, such as rape, military combat, or a natural disaster.
- Symptoms include the repetitive and intrusive memories of the event, nightmares, emotional numbing, survivor guilt, depression, and autonomic hyperactivity associated with anxiety.

CONVERSION DISORDER

- Conversion disorder is a diagnosis of exclusion that involves a psychologically produced, unconscious loss of function in response to a recent psychological stressor.
- Serious organic conditions develop later in 25 to 50% of individuals with conversion disorder.[3,4]
- Physical disorders with nonspecific symptoms such as systemic lupus erythematosus, multiple sclerosis, polymyositis, Lyme disease, and drug toxicity should be considered as possible causes for the loss of function.
- Patients should be reassured that no serious medical condition is present and that their symptoms will resolve.

SOMATIZATION DISORDER

- Somatization disorder affects women more often than men and begins in late adolescence or early adulthood.
- Somatization disorder is characterized by the presence of symptoms that do not have an identifiable organic etiology involving multiple organ systems.

HYPOCHONDRIASIS

- Hypochondriasis is a preoccupation with the fear that an organic medical illness is present despite normal results of an appropriate medical evaluation and reassurance to the contrary.

REFERENCES

1. American Psychiatric Association: *Diagnostic and Statistical Manual of Mental Disorders,* 4th ed. Washington: American Psychiatric Association, 1994.

2. American Psychiatric Association: Practice guideline for the treatment of patients with panic disorder. *Am J Psychiatry* 155:1, 1998.
3. Kaplan HI, Sadock BJ (eds.): Conversion disorder, in *Comprehensive Textbook of Psychiatry,* 6th ed, Vol. 1. Baltimore: Williams & Wilkins, 1995, p. 1252.
4. Hafeiz HV: Hysterical conversion: A prognostic study. *Br J Psychiatry* 136:548, 1980.

For further reading in *Emergency Medicine: A Comprehensive Study Guide,* 6th ed., see Chap. 288, "Behavioral Disorders: Clinical Features," by Douglas A. Rund.

188 EMERGENCY ASSESSMENT AND STABILIZATION OF BEHAVIORAL DISORDERS
Lance H. Hoffman

CLINICAL FEATURES

- Emergency stabilization is required of those patients demonstrating suicidal behavior, homicidal or violent behavior, and abnormal behavior secondary to an acute medical condition.[1]
- The goal of the emergency department evaluation is to distinguish between a medical and psychiatric cause of the abnormal behavior.
- Patients with schizophrenia, substance abuse, and depression are at higher risk of being suicidal.
- Additional suicidal risk factors include advanced age, male gender, divorced or widowed, unemployed, chronic medical illness, prior suicide attempt (especially if the attempt is violent or highly lethal), and poor social support with social isolation.
- Medication overdose is the most common type of suicide attempt.
- Homicidal or violent patients tend to pose little diagnostic dilemma to the clinician. These patients may openly assert their harmful intentions.
- Mannerisms suggestive of a potentially violent patient include restlessness, pacing in the exam room, clenched fists, acts of violence directed toward inanimate objects in the room, and hypervigilance.
- Patients possessing a rapidly progressive medical condition as the etiology of their abnormal behavior may present to the emergency department as suicidal, homicidal, acutely psychotic, or with altered level of consciousness.

- Individuals over the age of 40 years presenting with an acute alteration of behavior without a prior psychiatric diagnosis have a higher likelihood of possessing a medically reversible etiology for their altered behavior.

DIAGNOSIS AND DIFFERENTIAL

- The emergency evaluation should include a detailed history (confirmed by a third party if possible), physical examination, and mental status examination guiding the appropriate use of laboratory and radiographic studies.[2-5]
- Life-threatening disorders that should be excluded during the emergency evaluation include hypoglycemia, hypoxemia, infections (especially those of the central nervous system), intracranial hemorrhage or mass, stroke, substance poisoning or withdrawal, adverse medication effects or drug-drug interactions, acute organ failure, and endocrinopathies.[6,7]
- All abnormal vital signs should be investigated for a medical etiology and corrected prior to discharging a patient from the emergency department.
- A medical etiology of the patient's altered behavior is supported by the presence of an acute behavioral change in a patient over 40 years of age without a prior psychiatric diagnosis, abnormal vital signs, impaired language performance, difficulty with serial subtraction, visual hallucinations, and the inability of the patient to draw a clock face reading a specific time.
- Auditory hallucinations favor a psychiatric cause of the patient's behavioral disturbance.
- Potentially useful ancillary studies include capillary glucose measurement, pulse oximetry, complete blood count, serum electrolytes and creatinine, serum ammonia and hepatic transaminases, free T_4 and thyroid-stimulating hormone, ethanol level, salicylate and acetaminophen levels, urine drug screen, pregnancy test, arterial blood gas analysis, cerebrospinal fluid analysis, electrocardiogram, and computed tomography or magnetic resonance imaging of the brain.

EMERGENCY DEPARTMENT CARE AND DISPOSITION

- Patients demonstrating violent behavior toward themselves or others in the emergency department should be immediately restrained by physical and chemical means.
- Lorazepam is a safe and effective benzodiazepine sedative that can be titrated to the desired effect.

- Haloperidol is a neuroleptic sedating agent that can be used alone or with benzodiazepines. Cardiac dysrhythmias resulting in cardiac arrest have rarely been described with this class of medication when used on patients with a prolonged QT interval by electrocardiogram (ECG) or sympathomimetic intoxication.
- Suicidal and homicidal or violent patients should be disrobed, gowned, and searched for potentially dangerous items.
- Suicidal patients should be approached in an empathetic and nonthreatening manner, clarifying that the physician's goal is to help the individual.
- Enforceable limits as to what constitutes acceptable behavior by the patient must be set by the clinician.
- After an appropriate history, mental status examination, physical examination, and laboratory evaluation have excluded a medical cause as an individual's altered behavior, a psychiatric consultation should be obtained.
- Patients judged to be at high risk to themselves or others or who are unable to effectively care for themselves should be admitted to a psychiatric facility for definitive care.
- Patients whose evaluation demonstrates a medical etiology for their behavioral change should receive appropriate medical therapy specific to the disorder, whether it mandates hospital admission or outpatient treatment.
- Hospital admission is necessary if the disorder is not readily reversible, is likely to recur or progress, or if the patient's behavior remains such that independent living would be dangerous.

REFERENCES

1. Centers for Disease Control and Prevention: Nonfatal self-inflicted injuries treated in hospital emergency departments—United States, 2000. *MMWR* 51:429, 2002.
2. Tintinalli JE, Peacock FW, Wright MA: Emergency medical evaluation of psychiatric patients. *Ann Emerg Med* 22:859, 1994.
3. Reeves RR, Pendarvis EJ, Kimble R: Unrecognized medical emergencies admitted to psychiatric units. *Am J Emerg Med* 18:391, 2000.
4. Marsh C: Psychiatric presentations of medical illness. *Psychiatr Clin North Am* 20:181, 1997.
5. Korn CS, Currier GW, Henderson SO: Medical clearance of psychiatric patients without medical complaints in the emergency department. *J Emerg Med* 18:173, 2000.
6. Drugs that may cause psychiatric symptoms. *Med Lett* 44:59, 2002.
7. D'Onofrio GD, Degutis LC: Preventive care in the emergency department: Screening and brief intervention for alcohol problems in the emergency department, a systematic review. *Acad Emerg Med* 9:627, 2002.

For further reading in *Emergency Medicine: A Comprehensive Study Guide,* 6th ed., see Chap. 289, "Behavioral Disorders: Emergency Assessment," by Douglas A. Rund and Jeffrey C. Hutzler.

189 PANIC AND CONVERSION DISORDERS
Lance H. Hoffman

PANIC DISORDER

EPIDEMIOLOGY

- Panic disorder has a national lifetime prevalence of 3.5%.[1]
- Women are two to three times more likely than men to be afflicted with this disorder. Symptoms usually begin in the second to fourth decades of life.

PATHOPHYSIOLOGY

- The etiology of panic disorder is unknown; however, a combination of genetic, behavioral, and biological factors have been postulated as contributing to the disease.[2,3]

CLINICAL FEATURES

- Individuals with panic disorder suffer from recurrent, unexpected episodes of intense anxiety or fear, resulting in a variety of somatic and cognitive symptoms that typically peak in approximately 10 minutes and persist for approximately an hour.
- Somatic symptoms include dyspnea, chest pain or tightness, palpitations, generalized weakness, dizziness, nausea, and paresthesias.
- Cognitive symptoms include feelings of derealization and depersonalization and a fear of losing control or dying.

DIAGNOSIS AND DIFFERENTIAL

- In order to diagnose panic disorder, the patient must experience recurrent, unexpected panic episodes followed by at least 1 month of persistent fear of having additional attacks, worry about the implications of the attacks, or a significant change in behavior because of the attacks.[4]
- Panic disorder is a diagnosis of exclusion as its signs and symptoms overlap with multiple life-threatening cardiopulmonary medical illnesses and several psychiatric illnesses.
- A high index of suspicion should be maintained for intimate partner violence, sexual abuse or assault, and depression with suicidal ideation.

EMERGENCY DEPARTMENT CARE AND DISPOSITION

- Evaluation and treatment of acute life-threatening conditions are of primary importance in the initial management of a patient with symptoms suggestive of panic disorder.
- Benzodiazepines, such as alprazolam or lorazepam, are the drugs of choice in acutely controlling the anxiety of a panic attack.
- The patient should be screened for depression and specifically questioned about suicidal thoughts.
- An emergent psychiatric consultation should be obtained if the patient's symptoms are poorly controlled or the patient is at risk of suicide. Otherwise, outpatient psychiatric referral is indicated for further evaluation and treatment with cognitive-behavioral therapy and pharmacotherapy, usually using a selective serotonin reuptake inhibitor.

CONVERSION DISORDER

EPIDEMIOLOGY

- Conversion disorder is rare, but affects women approximately four times more commonly than men.

PATHOPHYSIOLOGY

- The etiology is uncertain; however, the symptoms of conversion disorder are believed to be psychiatric exertions of control on the patient's environment, allowing the patient to avoid confronting uncomfortable feelings triggered by the patient's environment.

CLINICAL FEATURES

- The patient with conversion disorder unconsciously produces a symptom suggestive of a physical disorder that results in a change or loss of physical function in response to a recent psychological stressor.[4]

- The symptom is typically isolated, neurologic, and of acute onset. Classic symptoms include focal paralysis, pseudoseizures, coma, paresthesias, or blindness; motor complaints are more common than sensory complaints.[5–7]

DIAGNOSIS AND DIFFERENTIAL

- Conversion disorder is a diagnosis of exclusion; acutely disabling or life-threatening disorders must be eliminated through a careful history, physical examination, and appropriate use of laboratory and imaging studies.
- A careful neurologic examination is necessary to document inconsistencies in known neuroanatomic pathways.
- A high index of suspicion should be maintained for systemic lupus erythematosus, polymyositis, multiple sclerosis, Lyme disease, and drug toxicities.

EMERGENCY DEPARTMENT CARE AND DISPOSITION

- Acute disabling or life-threatening organic illness should be excluded as the cause of the patient's symptom.
- The patient should be reassured that a serious medical disorder is not present. It should be suggested to the patient that the symptom will likely spontaneously resolve. Confronting the patient directly that the symptom is not organic may worsen the symptom.
- Psychiatric consultation in the emergency department is needed if the symptom does not resolve and precludes discharging the patient.

REFERENCES

1. Kessler RC, McGonagle KA, Zhao S, et al: Lifetime and 12-month prevalence of the DSM-III-R psychiatric disorders in the United States. Results from the National Comorbidity Survey. *Arch Gen Psychiatry* 51:8, 1994.
2. George DT, Landenheim JA, Nutt D: Effect of pregnancy on panic attacks. *Am J Psychiatry* 44:1078, 1987.
3. Bourin M, Baker GB, Bradwejn J: Neurobiology of panic disorder. *J Psychosom Res* 44:163, 1998.
4. American Psychiatric Association: *Diagnostic and Statistical Manual of Mental Disorders,* 4th ed. Washington: American Psychiatric Association, 1994, p. 347.
5. Sadock BS, Sadock VA: Conversion disorder, in Sadock, BJ, Sadock VA (eds.): *Kaplan and Sadock's Comprehensive Textbook of Psychiatry,* 7th ed. Baltimore: Lippincott Williams & Wilkins, 2000, p. 213.
6. Binzer M, Andersen PM, Kullgren G: Clinical characteristics of patients with motor disability due to conversion disorder: A prospective control group study. *J Neurol Neurosurg Psychiatry* 63:83, 1997.
7. Dula DJ, DeNaples L: Emergency department presentation of patients with conversion disorder. *Acad Emerg Med* 2:120, 1995.

For further reading in *Emergency Medicine: A Comprehensive Study Guide,* see Chap. 292, "Panic Disoder," by Linda M. Nicholas, Ann E. Maloney, and Susan L. Siegfried; and Chap. 293, "Conversion Disorder," by Gregory P. Moore and Kenneth C. Jackimczyk.

Section 24
ABUSE AND ASSAULT

190 CHILD AND ELDER ABUSE

Kristine L. Bott

CHILD ABUSE

EPIDEMIOLOGY

- Young children are more likely than older children to become victims of physical violence. Two thirds of victims of physical abuse are under the age of 3 years, and one third of the victims are under the age of 6 months.
- Children who are diagnosed with sexual abuse in the emergency department (ED) present with an unrelated complaint such as abdominal pain, asthma, or sore throat in 15% of cases.
- Ninety percent of victims of sexual abuse know their abusers.

CLINICAL FEATURES

- Neglect in infancy results in the condition of failure to thrive (FTT). This syndrome usually affects children younger than 3 years of age.
- Infants with FTT exhibit distinct behavioral characteristics, such as wariness, avoidance of eye contact, and irritability with interpersonal interaction.
- Overall physical care and hygiene in infants with FTT is frequently poor. There is little subcutaneous tissue, the ribs are prominent, and the skin of the buttocks hangs in loose folds.
- Neglected children over the age of 3 years are termed psychosocial dwarfs. They exhibit the classic triad of short stature, bizarre voracious appetite, and dis-turbed home situation. They are frequently hyperactive and have delayed speech.
- Munchausen syndrome by proxy (MSBP) is an uncommon form of child abuse in which a caretaker fabricates an illness in a child to secure the prolonged attention of health care providers. These cases are often medically perplexing, and result in the child being seen at multiple hospitals and subjected to many unnecessary tests.
- Children with MSBP may arrive at the ED with bleeding, seizures, altered mental status, apnea, diarrhea, vomiting, fever, rash, or multiple organ system involvement. These symptoms may result from the administration of warfarin, ipecac, or other substances.[1,2]
- Children who have been sexually abused may have vaginal or urethral discharge, vaginal bleeding, dysuria, urinary tract infection, or urethral discharge. They may exhibit excessive masturbation, genital fondling, encopresis, nightmares, or sexually oriented or provocative behavior.[3]
- Normal children in nonabusive situations, especially toddlers, will have multiple ecchymoses over the anterior shins, forehead, and other bony prominences. Most falls result in bruises on only one body surface. Bruises over multiple areas, especially the low back, buttocks, thighs, cheeks, ear pinnae, neck, ankles, wrists, corners of the mouth, and lips suggest physical abuse.
- The examiner may observe handprints or other bizarre bruises that are caused by belt buckles, cords, or blunt instruments.[4] Bites produce a characteristic oval pattern.
- Lacerations of the frenulum and oral mucosa may be seen in infants who have been force fed.
- Several burn patterns should be recognized as characteristic for abuse. Scald burns do not follow a typical splash configuration but rather a "glove and stocking"

distribution with sharp demarcation of the borders caused by immersion in hot water.

- The buttocks may be burned during toilet training "punishment." Typically, the anterior thighs, feet, and portions of the abdomen are spared while the genitalia and buttocks are scalded.
- Cigarette burns leave small 5-mm circumferential scab-covered injuries, often resembling impetigo.
- Children with skeletal injuries may have unexplained swelling of an extremity, refusal to walk, or refusal to use an extremity.
- Spiral fractures caused by twisting of the bone and metaphyseal chip fractures suggest abuse, especially when present in patients less than 6 months of age.
- Head injuries can be a potentially lethal form of child abuse.[5] These patients may appear well or may have vomiting, irritability, apnea, or seizures. They may have swelling of the scalp or bruising around the eyes, ears, or cheeks.
- Shaken baby or shaken impact syndrome is caused by vigorous shaking of an infant or from thrusting the infant down onto a surface, resulting in intracranial hemorrhage and retinal hemorrhage.
- Abdominal injuries can be severe and are a common cause of death from child abuse. Symptoms include recurrent vomiting, abdominal pain and distention, and diminished bowel sounds.
- Abused children may be overly affectionate with medical staff, may be compliant and submissive, and often do not resist painful medical procedures, such as blood draws.

DIAGNOSIS AND DIFFERENTIAL

- A history that is inconsistent with the nature or extent of the injury, keeps changing as to the circumstances surrounding the injury, or a discrepancy between the story the child gives and the story the caretaker gives should raise the index of suspicion for child abuse.
- Any serious injury in a child younger than 5 years should be viewed with suspicion, especially if unwitnessed by a third party.
- Children younger than 6 months are unlikely to induce accidents or accidentally ingest drugs or poisons.
- Weights and lengths should be plotted on a growth chart. FTT may be reflected in a body mass index below the fifth percentile.
- In MSBP, the parent (the mother in 98% of cases) encourages the staff to do more diagnostic procedures and seems inappropriately happy with a positive result.
- Children with suspected sexual abuse should have a careful genital and perianal examination. The examination of the hymen is typically unreliable. Notches or clefts in the hymen, especially at the 6 o'clock position, are suggestive of previous trauma.

- Children with multiple bruises or injuries should have a complete blood cell count and coagulation studies checked.
- When head injury is suspected, a computed tomography scan should be obtained. Funduscopic examination should evaluate for retinal hemorrhages.[6,7]

EMERGENCY DEPARTMENT CARE AND DISPOSITION

- Abused children should be treated medically according to the nature of their injuries.
- A full social services consultation should be obtained.
- Infants and children with FTT and MSBP should be admitted.
- All states mandate that suspected cases of child abuse or neglect be reported. A verbal report should be made to law enforcement and/or the child protection agency. Failure to report can result in misdemeanor charges and lead to a fine or imprisonment.
- The child may then be admitted, placed in protective custody, taken to a juvenile facility, placed temporarily with other relatives, or placed in a foster shelter home. The final disposition is dependent on the outcome of a court hearing.

ELDER ABUSE

EPIDEMIOLOGY

- By the year 2020, about 20% of the U.S. population will be 65 years of age and older.
- About 3% of the elderly population experiences abuse or neglect.[8]

CLINICAL FEATURES

- Elderly victims frequently live with their abuser, who may be dependent upon them financially, socially, and emotionally. They are often isolated from other family and friends.
- The caretaker may have a history of mental illness, substance abuse, or personality disorders.
- Abuse is associated more with personality problems of the caregiver than with situational stress.[9]
- Abused patients may have poor personal hygiene, inappropriate or soiled clothing, malnutrition, and worsening decubiti. They may be abusing alcohol or drugs.
- Specific injuries suggestive of abuse include unexplained fractures or dislocations, unexplained lacerations or abrasions, burns in unusual locations or of unusual shapes, unexplained injuries to the head or face, and the presence of sexually transmitted diseases.

- Abused patients have been found to have significantly greater cognitive impairment than nonabused elderly patients. There is often a history of problematic behavior such as incontinence, nocturnal shouting, wandering, or paranoia.[8]

DIAGNOSIS AND DIFFERENTIAL

- Most mistreatment of elderly patients occurs in residential settings and can be difficult to recognize. This is confounded by the fact that patients are often reluctant to disclose their abuse due to embarrassment, fear of abandonment, fear of retaliation, and fear of nursing home placement.
- The following findings during the examination are suggestive of an abusive relationship between the patient and their caretaker:
  - The patient appears fearful of his or her companion.
  - There are conflicting accounts of the injury or illness between the patient and caretaker.
  - There is an absence of assistance from the caretaker.
  - The caretaker displays an attitude of anger or indifference toward the patient.
  - The caretaker is overly concerned with the cost of treatment.
  - The caretaker denies the patient the opportunity to interact privately with the physician.
- Whenever suspected, the patient must be directly questioned about potential abuse.

EMERGENCY DEPARTMENT CARE AND DISPOSITION

- A complete physical examination should be performed and the patient should be worked up and treated medically according to his or her injuries.
- Detection of elder abuse must be aimed at intervention. All 50 states have passed legislation aimed at protecting elderly victims of abuse and neglect and establishing adult protective services programs.[10] Forty-two states have mandatory reporting laws directed towards health care and social service professionals.
- Patients should be admitted if medically necessary. They may also require admission if they cannot be safely discharged with their caretaker or to their nursing home.

REFERENCES

1. Rosenberg DA: Web of deceit: A literature review of Munchausen syndrome by proxy: *Child Abuse Negl* 11:547, 1987.

2. Ayoub CC, Schreier HA, Alexander R: Munchausen by proxy: Special focus issue. *Child Maltreat* 7:103, 2002.
3. Seidel JS, Elvik SL, Berkowitz CD, et al: Presentation and evaluation of sexual misuse in the emergency department. *Pediatr Emerg Care* 2:157, 1986.
4. Berkowitz CD: Pediatric abuse: New patterns of injury. *Emerg Med Clin North Am* 13:321, 1995.
5. Alexander R, Sato Y, Smith W, Bennett T: Incidence of impact trauma with cranial injuries ascribed to shaking. *Am J Dis Child* 144:724, 1990.
6. Levin AV: Retinal hemorrhages and child abuse. *Recent Adv Paediatr* 18:151, 2000.
7. Budenz DL, Faber MG, Mirchandani HG, et al: Ocular and optic nerve hemorrhages in abused infants with intracranial injuries. *Ophthalmology* 101:559, 1994.
8. Jones JS, Holstege H: Elder abuse and neglect: Understanding the causes and potential risk factors. *Am J Emerg Med* 15:579, 1997.
9. Lachs MS, Williams C, O'Brian, S et al: Risk factors for reported elder abuse and neglect: a nine year observational cohort study. *Gerontologist* 37:469, 1997.
10. Jones J, Dougherty, J, Schelble D, et al: Emergency department protocol for the diagnosis and evaluation of geriatric abuse. *Ann Emerg Med* 17:1006, 1988.

For further reading in *Emergency Medicine: A Comprehensive Study Guide,* 6th ed., see Chap. 297, "Child Abuse and Neglect," by Carol D. Berkowitz; and Chap. 300, "Abuse in the Elderly and Impaired," by Ellen H. Taliaferro.

191 SEXUAL ASSAULT AND INTIMATE PARTNER VIOLENCE AND ABUSE

Stefanie R. Ellison

EPIDEMIOLOGY

SEXUAL ASSAULT

- Sexual assault accounts for 1% of all violent crimes reported.[1]
- Most episodes of sexual assault are committed by a person known to the victim.
- Only one in three cases of sexual assault is reported to law enforcement.[2]
- Until recently male sexual assault was underrecognized and underreported. The incidence in men is estimated to be 10% of all sexual assaults.[2]

INTIMATE PARTNER VIOLENCE AND ABUSE

- Intimate partner violence and abuse (IPVA) is defined as a pattern of assaultive behavior that may include physical injury, sexual assault, psychological abuse, stalking, deprivation, intimidation, and threats.
- IPVA occurs in people of every race, ethnicity, culture, geographic region, and religious affiliation.[3,4]
- IPVA occurs in gay, lesbian, and heterosexual relationships with equal frequency.
- Risk factors include female gender, age 16 to 24 years, low socioeconomic status, separated relationship status, and children under 3 years of age in the home.[5,6]
- Between 4 and 15% of women are seen in emergency departments (ED) because of symptoms related to IPVA.[7,8]

CLINICAL FEATURES

SEXUAL ASSAULT

- A brief, tactfully obtained history should include the following elements:
  - Who (whether the assailant was known and the number of attackers).
  - What happened (including physical assault and injuries).
  - When (time since assault).
  - Where (actual or attempted vaginal, oral, or anal penetration and whether ejaculation occurred; use of condoms or foreign bodies).
  - Whether the patient has showered, douched, or changed clothes since the attack.
  - Suspicion of drug-facilitated sexual assault (whether there was a period of amnesia, intoxication greater than expected for the amount of alcohol consumed, or history of waking in a different location with genital pain).
- Past medical history pertinent to the sexual assault victim should include last menstrual period, birth control method, and last consensual intercourse (this may affect laboratory analysis of evidence).
- Allergies and prior medical history should be obtained for sexually transmitted disease (STD) and pregnancy prophylaxis, and prior sexual assault.
- General trauma is present in 45 to 67% of sexual assault cases, with genital injury in 9 to 45%.[9–12]
- A speculum examination should note vaginal discharge, abrasions, cervical abrasions, and lacerations. Colposcopy increases documentation of subtle injuries.[12]
- The rectum should also be examined for injuries, especially in the male victim. Anoscopy is more sensitive in detecting rectal trauma.[13]

- Toluidine blue can detect small lacerations by staining the deeper dermis.
- Evidence collection in sexual assault is only possible within the first 72 hours following the sexual assault.

INTIMATE PARTNER VIOLENCE AND ABUSE

- When a victim reveals a history of IPVA it should be documented in the patient's own words.
- Recent and remote abuse including dates, locations, details of abuse, and witnesses should be documented.
- Many experts recommend routine screening for IPVA in all adolescent and adult women who present to the ED.[14–18]
- Injuries characteristic of IPVA are fingernail scratches, bite marks, cigarette burns, rope burns, and forearm bruising or nightstick fractures.
- Central injuries to the head, neck, face, and thorax may be seen, and abdominal injury is common in the pregnant victim.

DIAGNOSIS AND DIFFERENTIAL

- Sexual assault is a legal determination, not a medical diagnosis.
- The legal definition contains three elements: carnal knowledge, lack of consent, and compulsion or fear of harm.[19,20]
- Informed consent should be obtained for the sexual assault evaluation, and a system to preserve the chain of evidence maintained.
- A prepackaged sexual assault or rape kit with directions for sample collection should be used.
- If a sexual assault kit is not available, smears from the vagina and cervix are made, labeled, and air dried.
- A wet mount from the same areas should be microscopically examined for sperm. A vaginal aspirate using 5 to 10 mL of normal saline should be obtained and tested for acid phosphatase.
- A Wood's lamp should be used to examine for areas where semen may be collected on the body. If anal penetration occurred, a rectal aspirate and rectal swab should be taken and slides made, labeled, and air dried in the same manner as for the vaginal swabs.
- Additional forensic laboratory evaluation may include glycoprotein p30 testing and genetic typing.
- Injuries inconsistent with the patient's history, multiple injuries in various stages of healing, delay between the time of injury and presentation, a visit for vague complaints without evidence of injury, or suicide attempts should trigger suspicions of IPVA.[21]

EMERGENCY DEPARTMENT CARE AND DISPOSITION FOR THE SEXUAL ASSAULT VICTIM

PREGNANCY PROPHYLAXIS

- A pregnancy test should be obtained. Approximately 5% of all sexual assault victims will become pregnant as a result of the assault.
- Oral pregnancy prophylaxis options include levonorgestrel (Plan B) 1 tablet initially followed by 1 tablet in 12 hours; ethinyl estradiol and levonorgestrel (Preven) 2 tablets initially followed by 2 tablets in 12 hours; or ethinyl estradiol and norgestrel (Ovral) 2 tablets initially followed by 2 tablets in 12 hours.[22]

STD PROPHYLAXIS

- The 2002 Centers for Disease Control's guidelines for gonorrhea prophylaxis are a single dose of ceftriaxone 125 mg IM, cefixime 400 mg orally, ciprofloxacin 500 mg orally, or ofloxacin 400 mg orally. Ceftriaxone 125 mg IM is recommended in pregnancy.[23]
- Recommended regimens for chlamydia prophylaxis are a single dose of azithromycin 1 g orally, doxycycline 100 mg orally bid for 7 days, erythromycin base 500 mg orally qid for 7 days, or amoxicillin 500 mg orally tid for 7 days.
- Recommended regimens for trichomoniasis and bacterial vaginosis prophylaxis are a single dose of metronidazole 2 g orally, metronidazole 250 mg tid for 7 days, or clindamycin 300 mg orally bid for 7 days. If pregnant and symptomatic, metronidazole 2 g orally may be used along with close follow-up.
- The recommended treatment regimen for hepatitis B prophylaxis is vaccination at the time of initial evaluation, and follow-up doses at 1 to 2 months and 4 to 6 months.

HIV PROPHYLAXIS OR COUNSELING

- HIV rates from receptive, unprotected anal intercourse are 0.008 to 0.032%, and from vaginal intercourse are 0.005 to 0.0015% with HIV-positive assailants.[24]
- Circumstances should guide treatment with known assailant HIV positivity, high viral load exposures, vaginal trauma, and ejaculate on membranes, which represent a moderate to high risk for HIV seroconversion.
- The decision about postexposure prophylaxis should also take into account expense and side effects of the medications, and the need to arrange follow-up with a primary physician with experience in HIV treatment.[24]
- Treatment is currently only recommended for victims with moderate- and high-risk exposures. Routine prophylaxis is not recommended and counseling and follow-up should be provided.

EMERGENCY DEPARTMENT CARE AND DISPOSITION FOR THE IPVA VICTIM

- The first goal of treatment should be to address any life-threatening injuries to the patient while simultaneously ensuring the safety of the victim and any children involved while they are in the ED.
- Safety assessment should identify indicators of a potentially lethal situation. Risk indicators include increasing frequency or severity of violence, the threat or use of weapons, obsession with the victim, hostage-taking, stalking, homicidal or suicidal threats, and substance abuse by the assailant, especially with crack cocaine or amphetamines.
- The most dangerous period for victims is during the time of abuse disclosure and during an attempt to leave the relationship.
- Hospital admission is an option in high-risk situations if a safe location cannot be established before discharge.
- Victims should also be asked about suicidal or homicidal ideation. If a plan is revealed, then psychiatric consultation should be obtained.

REFERENCES

1. U.S. Department of Justice, Federal Bureau of Investigation, Uniform Crime Reports: *Crime in the United States, 2001.* Washington: U.S. Government Printing Office, 2001.
2. U.S. Department of Justice, Bureau of Justice Statistics: *Rape and Sexual Assault: Reporting to the Police and Medical Attention, 1992–2000.* Washington: U.S. Government Printing Office, NCJ 194530, 2002.
3. Rennison CM, Welchans S: *Intimate Partner Violence.* Bureau of Justice Statistics Special Report, NCJ 178247. May 2000, revised January 31, 2002.
4. Watts C, Zimmerman C: Violence against women: Global scope and magnitude. *Lancet* 359:1232, 2002.
5. Rennison CM: *Intimate Partner Violence and Age of Victim, 1993–1999.* Bureau of Justice Statistics Special Report, NCJ 187635. October 2001, revised November 28, 2001.
6. Duffy SJ, McGrath ME, Becker BM, Linakis JG: Mothers with histories of domestic violence in a pediatric emergency department. *Pediatrics* 103:1007, 1999.
7. Abbott J: Domestic violence against women: incidence and prevalence in an emergency department population. *JAMA* 273:1763, 1995.
8. Ernst AA, Weiss SJ: Intimate partner violence from the emergency medicine perspective. *Women Health* 35:71, 2002.

9. Riggs N, Houry D, Long G, et al: Analysis of 1076 cases of sexual assault. *Ann Emerg Med* 35:358, 2000.

10. Gray-Eurom K, Seaberg DC, Wears RL: The prosecution of sexual assault cases: correlation with forensic evidence. *Ann Emerg Med* 39:39, 2002.

11. Lincoln C: Genital Injury: Is it significant? A review of the literature. *Med Sci Law* 41:206, 2001.

12. Slaughter L, Brown CR, Crowley S, et al: Patterns of genital injury in female sexual assault victims. *Am J Obstet Gynecol* 176:609, 1997.

13. Ernst AA, Green E, Ferguson MT, et al: The utility of anoscopy and colposcopy in the evaluation of male sexual assault victims. *Ann Emerg Med* 36:432, 2000.

14. Duffy SJ, McGrath ME, Becker BM, Linakis JG: Mothers with histories of domestic violence in a pediatric emergency department. *Pediatrics* 103:1007, 1999.

15. Bureau of Justice Statistics, U.S. Department of Justice: *Homicide Trends in the U.S.: Intimate Homicide.* Available at: http://www.ojp.usdoj.gov/jbs/homicide/intimates.htm. Updated January 4, 2001.

16. Kellerman A, Heron S: Firearms and family violence. *Emerg Clin North Am* 17:699, 1999.

17. Abbott J: Injuries and illnesses of domestic violence. *Ann Emerg Med* 29:781, 1997.

18. Fanslow JL, Norton RN, Spinola CG: Indicators of assault-related injuries among women presenting to the emergency department. *Ann Emerg Med* 32:341, 1998.

19. DeLahunta EA, Baram DA: Sexual assault. *Clin Obstet Gynecol* 40:648, 1997.

20. Patel M, Minshall L: Management of sexual assault. *Emerg Med Clin North Am* 19:817, 2001.

21. Preventing Domestic Violence: Clinical Guidelines on Routine Screening. San Francisco: Family Violence Prevention Fund, 1999.

22. Mendez MN: Emergency contraception: A review of current oral options. *West J Med* 176:188, 2002.

23. Centers for Disease Control and Prevention: Sexually transmitted diseases treatment guidelines 2002. *MMWR* 51 (RR-6):1, 2002.

24. Moran GJ: Pharmacologic management of HIV/STD exposure. *Emerg Med Clin North Am* 18:829, 2000.

For further reading in *Emergency Medicine: A Comprehensive Study Guide,* 6th ed., see Chap. 298, "Female and Male Sexual Assault," by Kim M. Feldhaus; and Chap. 299, "Intimate Partner Violence and Abuse," by Patricia R. Salber.

192 PRINCIPLES OF EMERGENCY DEPARTMENT USE OF COMPUTED TOMOGRAPHY AND MAGNETIC RESONANCE IMAGING

Matthew C. Gratton

COMPUTED TOMOGRAPHY

- Computed tomography (CT) creates a cross-sectional image of a patient by placing an x-ray source and a detector on a gantry that rotates around a patient. An image is displayed after computer reconstruction.
- Spiral (helical) scanning, an important technological advance, allows for continuous image acquisition by continuously rotating the gantry around a continuously moving patient table.[1]
- The major advantages of spiral CT scanning over conventional CT scanning are: (1) rapid data acquisition, (2) less contrast material needed due to decreased scanning time, (3) retrospective image reconstruction at different slice thicknesses without rescanning, (4) decreased respiratory, cardiac, and other motion artifacts, and (5) high-quality three-dimensional and multiplanar reconstruction.
- The major disadvantages of spiral scanning over conventional scanning are: (1) image resolution may be lost due to processing constraints (scans are obtained at an oblique angle and are converted to transverse slices by computerized data averaging), (2) weight limitation of 400 to 450 pounds, (3) timing of contrast injection must be precise, and (4) sedation and close observation are needed for children and uncooperative adults.

GENERAL USES AND LIMITATIONS OF CT

- Head CT is the primary study for screening emergency department (ED) patients for acute intracranial bleeding, trauma, and stroke.
- CT is the imaging study of choice for many disorders of the abdomen, pelvis, retroperitoneum, and thoracic cavity.
- Fractures and other bony abnormalities are usually well demonstrated by CT, especially cervical spine, facial, and pelvic fractures.
- Spiral CT is the primary modality for visualizing acute appendicitis and ureteral stones at many institutions.[2]
- Body areas that are poorly visualized with CT include the posterior cranial fossa and the pituitary fossa; the spinal cord cannot be well differentiated from cerebrospinal fluid without contrast (CT myelogram).

USE OF CONTRAST

- Contrast material can be administered by the oral, intravenous, rectal, intra-arterial, intra-articular, or intrathecal route.
- Oral contrast for abdominal CT scanning improves the likelihood of detecting bowel wall abnormalities, including hematoma, edema, mass, or laceration.
- If contrast is to be administered to trauma patients, a water soluble agent should be used to avoid the extravasation of barium-containing agents.

MAGNETIC RESONANCE IMAGING

- Magnetic resonance imaging (MRI) takes advantage of the fact that the nuclei of hydrogen atoms in water and fat molecules act like spinning magnets. When placed in a strong magnetic field, these "magnets" align with the field, and when a short pulse of a radio wave of specific frequency is applied, the magnets change alignment and then realign with the external magnetic field. The resultant small voltage can be measured and displayed as an image.

- The major advantages of MRI over other imaging modalities are: (1) it does not use ionizing radiation and no short- or long-term side effects have been demonstrated, (2) it can produce image slices of any orientation through the body, and (3) in many body areas, it produces better contrast resolution and tissue discrimination than x-rays or ultrasound.

MRI SAFETY AND OTHER CONSIDERATIONS

- In some cases the large static magnetic field can be a health hazard:[3-5]
  - Internal cardiac pacemakers may be converted to the asynchronous mode.
  - Certain (ferromagnetic) aneurysm clips may be affected, causing brain injury.
  - Steel slivers in the eye (asymptomatic in some metal workers) may injure the retina.
  - Cochlear implants may be damaged or cause injury.
  - Other implanted devices (implantable defibrillators, neurostimulators, bone growth stimulators, etc) may malfunction or cause injury.
  - Some prosthetic heart valves are subjected to strong forces (likely less than the stress placed by the heart itself), and so these valves are a relative contraindication to MRI.
- Life support equipment containing steel is attracted to the magnetic field and could injure the patient and the system.
- Any ferromagnetic object carried into the room can also become a potential missile.
- The examination can take from 30 to 60 minutes and there must be no motion (except breathing).

APPLICATIONS

- MRI of the brain and spinal cord provides better diagnostic quality images than CT. Special intravenous contrast agents (that are less toxic than agents used for CT) are sometimes required.
- Because of recent developments in echo planar and diffusion imaging MRI, it is possible to diagnose cytotoxic cerebral edema earlier than with conventional MRI or CT. This may have implications in the early treatment of ischemic stroke.

- MRI has a major role in imaging the musculoskeletal system[6] because it visualizes soft tissue with better resolution than CT and because it is sensitive to marrow and trabecular bone changes.
- MRI is particularly useful in the diagnosis of rotator cuff injury, internal derangement of the knee, tendon or soft tissue injury of small joints, soft tissue injury of the spine, and posttraumatic avascular necrosis, but is not indicated for most acute fractures.
- MRI is also useful in evaluation of other soft tissue musculoskeletal trauma such as muscle or tendon tears, hemorrhage, and edema, and injuries to medium sized nerves and the brachial plexus.[7,8]
- MRI can detect metastatic disease with high sensitivity and specificity.
- Because it is fast, readily available, and compatible with life-support equipment, CT is still the imaging technique of choice for suspected head, spine, and abdominal injuries.

MRI SCANNING IN THE EMERGENT SETTING

- In the ED setting, MRI is the imaging modality of choice for: (1) evaluation of suspected spinal cord compression of any cause, (2) evaluation of radiographically occult femoral intertrochanteric and femoral neck fractures, and (3) evaluation of posterior cranial fossa pathology.
- Potential uses include: (1) evaluation of aortic dissection (MRI is better than CT and possibly transesophageal echo in visualizing an intimal flap, but this indication will await the availability of MRI-compatible life support equipment) and (2) evaluation of pediatric fractures potentially involving open growth plates.[9]

REFERENCES

1. Brink JA: Technical aspects of helical (spiral) CT. *Radiol Clin North Am* 33:825, 1995.
2. Rao PM, Rhea JT, Novelline RA, et al: Effect of computed tomography of the appendix on treatment of patients and the use of hospital resources. *N Engl J Med* 338:141, 1998.
3. Kanal E (ed.): *Practical MR Safety Considerations for Physicians, Physicists, and Technologists.* Oak Brook, IL: Radiological Society of North America, 2001, p. 17.
4. Shellock FG: *Pocket Guide to MR Procedures and Metallic Objects: Update 1999.* Philadelphia: Lippincott Williams & Wilkins, 1999, p. 125.
5. Kanal E, Borgstede JP, Barkovich AJ, et al: American College of Radiology White Paper of MR Safety. *AJR Am J Roentgenol* 178:1335, 2002.

6. Stoller DW (ed.): *Magnetic Resonance Imaging in Orthopedics and Sports Medicine.* Philadelphia: Lippincott-Raven, 1997, p. 351.
7. Wittenberg KH, Adkins MC: MR imaging of nontraumatic brachial plexopathies: Frequency and spectrum of finding. *Radiographics* 20:1023, 2000.
8. Kneeland JB, Kellman GM, Middleton WD, et al: Diagnosis of diseases of the supraclavicular region by use of MR imaging. *AJR Am J Roentgenol* 148:1149, 1887.
9. Jaramillo D, Shapiro F: Musculoskeletal trauma in children. *MRI Clin North Am* 6:521, 1998.

For further reading in *Emergency Medicine: A Comprehensive Study Guide,* 6th ed., see Chap. 304, "Principles of Emergency Department Use of Computed Tomography," by Stephanie Abbuhl; and Chap. 305, "Magnetic Resonance Imaging: Principles and Some Applications," by Irwin D. Weisman.

193 PRINCIPLES OF EMERGENCY DEPARTMENT ULTRASONOGRAPHY

J. Christian Fox

FUNDAMENTALS

- A perfect reflector of ultrasound waves appears white and is referred to as hyperechoic.
- A perfect transmitter of ultrasound waves appears black and is referred to as anechoic.
- Structures on the left side of the monitor correspond to the marker on the probe. This marker is generally oriented toward the patient's head in sagittal planes and towards the patient's right in transverse planes.
- Structures toward the top of the monitor correspond to structures closest (more superficial) to the probe. There are 1 cm hash-marks on the screen that correspond to increasing depths.

PRIMARY INDICATIONS FOR EMERGENCY DEPARTMENT ULTRASONOGRAPHY

ABDOMINAL AORTIC ANEURYSM

- Ultrasonography is as accurate as computed tomography (CT) in measuring the diameter of an abdominal aortic aneurysm.
- An ultrasound examination that images the aorta from the diaphragm to its distal bifurcation is extremely accurate in the evaluation for an abdominal aortic aneurysm.
- Any abdominal aortic diameter greater than 3 cm is abnormal. Transverse images measured horizontally from outside wall to outside wall are the most reliable in determining the true size of the aorta.
- The indications for performing ultrasonography of the aorta in the emergency department (ED) include hypotensive patients or elderly patients with unexplained back, flank, or abdominal pain.

RENAL COLIC

- The renal sinus appears as an extremely echogenic region within the center of the kidney and includes the collecting system. The renal cortex occupies the periphery of the kidney and has an echogenicity slightly less than that of the liver or spleen.
- Obstruction of urine outflow from a calculus will result in hydronephrosis, which appears as anechoic fluid collection within the renal sinus. Hydronephrosis can be graded from mild (minimal separation of the sinus) to severe (extensive communicating anechoic regions in the sinus).
- Both longitudinal and transverse images must be obtained of both kidneys.
- Renal cysts are thin-walled, round, anechoic structures located within the cortex of the kidney.
- Ureteral calculi are visualized on ultrasound in only 19% of patients with documented kidney stones.[1]
- Hydronephrosis is identified in 73% of patients with ureteral calculi. The calculus causing the obstruction typically lodges at the ureterovesicular junction, the ureteropelvic junction, or the pelvic brim.

GALLBLADDER DISEASE

- Ultrasound is the imaging modality of choice in evaluating biliary disease.[2]
- Gallstones appear as echolucent structures lying within the gallbladder and move with position changes.
- A sonographic Murphy's sign is positive when the point of maximal tenderness to transducer pressure is directly over the sonographically located gallbladder. This sign, in the presence of gallstones, is reported to have a 92% positive predictive value for symptomatic gallbladder disease.
- Gallbladder wall thickening, defined as proximal gallbladder wall thickness greater than 3 mm, occurs in 50 to 75% of patients with acute cholecystitis.
- Other ultrasound findings suggestive of biliary disease include gallbladder sludge and pericholecystic fluid.

FOCUSED ASSESSMENT WITH SONOGRAPHY IN TRAUMA

• Because the focused assessment with sonography in trauma (FAST) examination has an accuracy rate similar to diagnostic peritoneal lavage (DPL), but with fewer complications, it has replaced DPL as the initial imaging modality of choice in patients who are unstable for CT scan.[3] The FAST examination has a sensitivity of 90% and a specificity of 99%.[4]

• The standard views on FAST examination[4] include: (1) the subxiphoid view for the evaluation of pericardial fluid; (2) Morison's pouch, the potential space between the right kidney and the liver; (3) splenorenal recess, the potential space between the left kidney and the spleen; and (4) the pouch of Douglas and rectovesical space.

• In addition, the upper abdominal views are useful in the evaluation of the patient for hemothorax.[5]

• Hemodynamically unstable blunt trauma patients with a positive FAST examination for free intraperitoneal fluid should be taken directly to the operating room for exploratory laparotomy.

• The advantages of the FAST examination are that it is rapid, portable, accurate, repeatable, noninvasive, and inexpensive.

EVALUATION OF FIRST-TRIMESTER PREGNANCY

• In the ED, ultrasound detection of an intrauterine pregnancy greatly reduces the possibility of ectopic pregnancy. The incidence of heterotopic (simultaneous intrauterine and extrauterine pregnancies) is less than 1 in 30,000.[6]

• When ED patients present with abdominal pain, adnexal mass, and vaginal bleeding, the incidence of ectopic pregnancy is greater than 10%.

• The current recommendation is that all first-trimester pregnant patients presenting to the ED with any abdominal or pelvic pain, vaginal bleeding, or risk factors for ectopic pregnancy should have an ultrasound evaluation for the location of the pregnancy.

• Pelvic ultrasound by emergency physicians has been shown to decrease the length of stay in the ED.[7]

• The earliest sonographic finding of a pregnancy is the gestational sac. This appears as a round or oval anechoic area within the uterus. True gestational sacs have two concentric echogenic rings surrounding the gestation sac (double decidual sign).

• Endovaginal ultrasound can detect a gestational sac as early as 4.5 weeks after the last menstrual period (LMP), while transabdominal scanning can detect a gestational sac at 5.5 to 6 weeks after the LMP. An intrauterine pregnancy should be detectable on endovaginal scanning if the beta-human chorionic gonadotropin (β-hCG) is greater than 2000 mIU/mL (termed the discriminatory zone).[8]

• Patients with a β-hCG greater than the discriminatory zone who do not have evidence of an intrauterine pregnancy on ultrasound are at high risk for an ectopic pregnancy; immediate obstetric consultation is indicated.

CARDIAC ULTRASONOGRAPHY

• The major applications for ED cardiac ultrasonography are in the evaluation of pulseless electrical activity, cardiac trauma, and pericardial tamponade. Key sonographic findings are pericardial fluid collections and myocardial wall activity.

• Pericardial effusions appear as echo-free areas within the pericardial sac. A small pericardial effusion ($<$100 mL) will occupy a dependent position, while a larger effusion ($>$300 mL) will present both anteriorly and posteriorly.

• Sonographic localization of the pericardial sac is the best approach for a pericardiocentesis.

MISCELLANEOUS EMERGENCY DEPARTMENT APPLICATIONS

• Compression ultrasound has been used by emergency physicians to diagnose deep venous thrombosis (DVT) in ED patients.[9] Compression ultrasound has a sensitivity and specificity of 95% in venographically proven acute DVT of the proximal leg.

• Ultrasonography helps guide the emergency physician in performing thoracentesis for small pleural effusions.

• Ultrasonography assists physicians in identifying small foreign bodies in soft tissue.[10]

• Ultrasound use in the placement of central venous catheters decreases failure rates and complications.[11]

REFERENCES

1. Henderson SO, Hoffner RJ, Aragona JL, et al: Bedside emergency department ultrasonography plus radiography of the kidneys, ureters, and bladder vs intravenous pyelography in the evaluation of suspected ureteral colic. *Acad Emerg Med* 5:666, 1998.
2. Simmons MZ: Pitfalls in ultrasound of the gallbladder and biliary tract. *Ultrasound Q* 14:2, 1998.

3. Thomas B, Falcone RE, Vasquez D, et al: Ultrasound evaluation of blunt abdominal trauma: Program implementation, initial experience, and learning curve. *J Trauma* 42:384, 1997.

4. Ma OJ, Mateer JR, Ogata M, et al: Prospective analysis of a rapid trauma ultrasound examination performed by emergency physicians. *J Trauma* 38:879, 1995.

5. Ma OJ, Mateer JR: Trauma ultrasound evaluation versus chest radiograph in the detection of hemothorax. *Ann Emerg Med* 29:312, 1997.

6. Stovall TG, Kellerman AL, Ling FW, Buster JE: Emergency department diagnosis of ectopic pregnancy. *Ann Emerg Med* 19:1098, 1990.

7. Shih C: Effect of emergency physician-performed pelvic sonography on length of stay in the emergency department. *Ann Emerg Med* 29:348, 1997.

8. Mateer JR, Valley VT, Aiman EJ, et al: Outcome analysis of a protocol including bedside endovaginal sonography in patients at risk for ectopic pregnancy. *Ann Emerg Med* 27:283, 1996.

9. Jolly BT, Massarin CVT, Pigman EC: Color Doppler ultrasonography by emergency physicians for the diagnosis of acute venous thrombosis. *Acad Emerg Med* 4:129, 1997.

10. Jacobson JA, Powell A, Craig JG, et al: Wooden foreign bodies in soft tissue: Detection at US. *Radiology* 206:45, 1998.

11. Randolph AG, Cook DJ, Gonzales CA, Pribble CG: Ultrasound guidance for placement of central venous catheters: A meta-analysis of the literature. *Crit Care Med* 24:2053, 1996.

For further reading in *Emergency Medicine: A Comprehensive Study Guide,* 6th ed., see Chap. 303, "Principles of Emergency Department Sonography," by Scott W. Melanson and Michael B. Heller.

194 EMERGENCY MEDICAL SERVICES

Matthew C. Gratton

GENERAL CONSIDERATIONS

- In 1973, Public Law 93-154, designed to improve emergency medical services (EMS) nationwide, defined 15 elements of an EMS system: (1) personnel, (2) training, (3) communications, (4) transportation, (5) facilities, (6) critical care units, (7) public safety agencies, (8) consumer participation, (9) access to care, (10) transfer of care, (11) standardization of patients' records, (12) public information and education, (13) independent review and evaluation, (14) disaster linkage, and (15) mutual aid agreements.
- The Department of Transportation (DOT) has defined four levels of EMS providers:
  - First Responder: Designed for individuals who may be first to respond to an emergency; their training includes cardiopulmonary resuscitation (CPR), spinal immobilization, bleeding control, and other basic emergency procedures.
  - Emergency Medical Technician Basic (EMT-B): Their training includes CPR, use of an automatic external defibrillator (AED), and the safe extrication, immobilization, and transport of victims. Also, EMT-Bs are trained to help patients self-administer nitroglycerin, epinephrine, and inhalers.
  - Emergency Medical Technician Intermediate (EMT-I): The training includes the above plus intravenous therapy, defibrillation, basic electrocardiogram (ECG) interpretation, and the ability to give some medications.
  - Emergency Medical Technician Paramedic (EMT-P): The training includes all the above plus increased education about anatomy, physiology, and pharmacology; patient assessment; and the ability to administer additional medications.
- Citizen access to the EMS system has been improved by the adoption of a universal emergency telephone number (911 in the United States). Many 911 answering centers have equipment that allows the call taker to identify the calling number and location.
- In a process called priority dispatch, EMS call takers collect information from callers in a structured manner and then direct the most appropriate EMS response. In addition, they provide basic first aid instructions to callers, which are termed prearrival instructions.
- As a general rule, patients are transported to the closest appropriate hospital or the hospital of the patient's choice. In some states or regions, specialty hospitals are designated to receive certain types of patients (eg, trauma, cardiac, burn, etc).

MEDICAL CONTROL

- Considerable physician (medical director) input is required for a safe and effective EMS system.[1]
- In online medical control, the medical director directs field personnel actions in person, or more often, via radio or telephone communication. The medical director may allow the EMT to use standing orders to direct actions under some circumstances.
- Offline medical control consists of three main components: (1) protocol development, (2) medical accountability (quality assurance), and (3) ongoing educational program development. The medical director should also approve the medical devices and equipment used in the system.

MEDICAL BASIS FOR EMERGENCY MEDICAL SERVICES

EMERGENCY CARDIAC CARE

- Rapid defibrillation of cardiac arrest patients in ventricular fibrillation (VF) is the most effective treatment for cardiac arrest.[2] Some communities successfully resuscitate over 20% of out-of-hospital cardiac arrest patients.
- AEDs have been developed to allow individuals with minimal training to administer a countershock to patients with VF.
- Studies with publicly accessible AEDs in casinos and airports have found survival rates of over 50% when used by bystanders or trained security personnel.[3,4]
- Time to reperfusion of patients with acute myocardial infarction (AMI) can be reduced by identifying AMI patients in the field with 12-lead ECG and notifying the receiving hospital in advance to allow time for preparation.[5]
- Use of out-of-hospital aspirin and nitroglycerine may improve patient's symptoms and decrease hospital use.[6]

TRAUMA CARE

- The delivery of critically injured trauma patients to trauma centers is thought to improve outcome.[7] Trauma triage protocols based on the mechanism of injury or the patient's physiologic status direct patient routing.
- Treatment is focused on rapid transport and appropriate airway management; intravenous fluid administration is frequently recommended, but controversial.[8]

ADULT MEDICAL CARE

- Paramedics are able to obtain definitive airway control by endotracheal intubation with a high success rate and low complication rate.
- Respiratory distress can be evaluated and treated with pulse oximetry, β_2-agonists, ipratropium, and devices that deliver continuous positive airway pressure.[9]
- Glucose and/or naloxone can be used to treat altered mental status, and diazepam or lorazepam can be used for seizures.

PEDIATRIC CARE

- About 5 to 10% of EMS calls are for pediatric cases; the most common involve trauma, respiratory problems, and seizures.

- The success rates for endotracheal intubation and intravenous access are lower for infants and small children; the benefits of intubation have recently been challenged by a study in Los Angeles County that showed there was no improvement in survival of patients who were intubated as compared to those who were managed with bag-valve-mask ventilation.[10]

RURAL EMERGENCY MEDICAL SERVICES

- Challenges faced by rural EMS include: long distances involved; need for specialized search and rescue and off-road capabilities; low population density making the likelihood of the event being witnessed less than in urban areas; population tends to be older and less affluent; universal emergency phone number may not be implemented, or if implemented, may not be "enhanced"; call volume is too low to allow for employment of full-time providers; relatively few paramedic level providers; and decreased training opportunities.

MASS GATHERINGS

- Any voluntary and temporary collection of greater than 1000 people at one site for a common purpose is defined as a mass gathering.[11]
- Mass gatherings present challenges to typical out-of-hospital care: (1) densely clustered crowds, (2) physical barriers to access to patients, (3) exposure to climatic elements and/or risk of intentional injury, (4) distances between or within venues, and (5) potential for a large number of casualties.
- Sporting events have an incidence of medical problems ranging from 0.12 to 17 per 1000 spectators and cardiac arrest ranging from 0.3 to 4.0 per 1,000,000 spectators; spectator medical problems can be 3 to 10 times higher at major rock concerts.[12,13]
- The responsibility to provide for the safety and security of participants, spectators, and workers belongs to the owner or promoter of an event. The event medical director is responsible for the actual provision of medical care.
- The goal of the medical director should to be to supply the same level of medical care that is found in the community at large outside the venue. Personnel that can provide basic life support and AED treatment should be placed within 3 minutes of everyone in the venue.
- Medical planning for the event must take into account the type of event, the type of venue, the expected population of spectators as well as participants, and the possible hazards.

- Planning must involve close coordination with local fire, EMS, rescue, HAZMAT, law enforcement, and public health authorities.
- Training for event medical personnel should include: (1) locations of command center, medical care facilities, ambulance, radio-equipped staff, and ingress and egress; (2) coverage areas; (3) communication plans and equipment; (4) medical care report issues; and (5) request for outside help.

DISASTER MEDICAL SERVICES

- The future will likely continue to produce disasters with mass casualties, perhaps at an even higher rate due to: (1) increased population in flood-, earthquake-, and hurricane-prone areas, (2) continued transportation of toxic and hazardous materials, (3) risks of accidents at fixed-site industrial facilities, and (4) increased likelihood of terrorism with nuclear, explosive, chemical, or biological agents.[14]
- The World Health Organization defines a disaster as an ecological phenomenon of such a magnitude as to require external assistance. From the emergency department perspective, a disaster occurs when the number of patients presenting in a given time is such that even minimal care cannot be given without external help.
- Disasters that produce a large number of casualties are called mass casualty incidents.[15]
- External disasters occur physically outside the hospital, while internal disasters occur physically within the facility.
- Hospital disaster plan difficulties include: (1) delayed or improper notification, (2) command structure not well defined, (3) inadequate communications network, (4) inadequate identification, (5) lack of supplies, and (6) lack of public relations.[16]
- After a mass casualty incident, most patients do not arrive by EMS. Patients with minor injuries make their way to the ED rapidly by private means, and those with more severe injury may arrive later, so without planning the patients with minor injuries may be treated first.[17,18]

DISASTER PLANNING

- Different types of disasters can cause different patterns of morbidity and mortality and have different health care requirements; therefore, the hospital plan must anticipate disasters likely to occur in its community.[19,20]
- The Joint Commission on Accreditation of Healthcare Organizations (JCAHO) requires hospitals to have a written plan for, and conduct exercises in, both internal and external disasters.[21]

- The hospital disaster plan must be coordinated with community agencies that are involved in disaster planning and management, which include the local fire department, the regional EMS system, and local emergency management and civil defense agencies.[19]
- Other organizations to consider for coordination include: the military, American Red Cross, local emergency planning committee, other volunteer agencies, and state and federal agencies.
- The Metropolitan Medical Response System (sponsored by the Office of Emergency Preparedness) coordinates the local response to weapons of mass destruction incidents.
- The National Disaster Medical System coordinates the sharing of resources between the Federal Emergency Management Agency, the Department of Defense, the Veterans Health Administration, and public and private organizations.
- Disaster medical assistance teams are composed of physicians, nurses, and other personnel who respond to federally-declared disasters to support the local community response.
- The Centers of Disease Control and Prevention (CDC), the main federal resource for responding to bioterrorism, administers a number of resources:[22]
  - Rapid Response Teams: Consists of epidemiologists and others who investigate outbreaks.
  - Laboratory Response Network: a program to link state and local public health laboratories.
  - Rapid Response and Advanced Technology Lab: Provides laboratory support to terrorism response teams.
  - National Electronic Disease Surveillance System: Attempts to integrate disease surveillance systems.
  - Health Alert Network: Internet connection between CDC and local health departments to allow for early dissemination of information.
  - National Pharmaceutical Stockpile: System designed to allow rapid delivery of medications and equipment in the event of a chemical or biological event.

HOSPITAL DISASTER PLAN

- Activation of the Disaster Plan: Situations that warrant activation of the plan, as well as those individuals who can declare the plan to be activated, must be delineated.
- Assessment of the Hospital's Capacity: The hospital must be inspected to determine if it is structurally and functionally capable of receiving casualties, and then it must be determined how many casualties can be cared for.
- Establishment of Disaster Command: A site and command personnel structure must be delineated.

- Communication: Intra- and interhospital communications must be planned for and multiple modalities can be considered: CB radios, cell phones, blackboards, e-mail, intercoms, closed circuit television, shortwave radio, radio equipped individuals, and messenger and courier services.
- Supplies: Must be available for rapid distribution within the hospital.
- Hospital Disaster Administration and Treatment Areas: A number of areas should be pre-designated for specific functions: (1) disaster control center, (2) triage area, (3) patient care areas for both major (usually in the ED) and minor injuries, (4) presurgical holding area, (5) operating rooms, (6) morgue, (7) decontamination area, (8) psychiatry area, (9) family waiting and discharge area, and (10) area to receive and assign volunteers.
- Training must be carried out on the plan and the plan must be exercised. JCAHO requires two drills per year.

CATASTROPHIC CASUALTY MANAGEMENT: DISASTER OPERATIONS

- Field medical personnel initially assess respirations, perfusion, and mental status as part of the simple triage and rapid treatment (START) technique.[23]
- The incident command system (ICS) is used to provide command, control, and organization to complex on-scene responses to disasters.[24] ICS has five components: (1) incident command, (2) operations, (3) planning, (4) logistics, and (5) finance. ICS principles can be used within the hospital to manage disasters (hospital incident command system).[25]
- Hospitals should notify the emergency communications center about: (1) bed availability, (2) number of patients received, (3) number of additional patients that the hospital can receive, and (4) specific supply issues. This information will allow the communications center to attempt to equitably distribute patients between hospitals.
- On-site disaster medical teams from hospitals may be useful depending on the number of victims and requirements for prolonged extrication. Since most physicians and nurses are not trained to function in the field, response teams should be developed only as part of a hospital disaster plan.

TRIAGE

- Triage is defined as the sorting of patients into groups according to priority for treatment using the severity of illness/injury, prognosis, and availability of resources.
- At the hospital, triage should be performed by a team consisting of a physician (emergency physician or surgeon), ED nurse, and a clerk.
- As patients are triaged they should be assigned to appropriate treatment areas. In some cases, very basic treatment may be initiated (eg, oral airway insertion, external hemorrhage control).
- In the United States, the most common triage system uses four color-coded categories:
  - Red: First priority for treatment, most urgent; includes life-threatening shock or hypoxia, but the patient has a good possibility of survival with immediate care.
  - Yellow: Second priority for treatment, urgent; includes injuries with systemic implications, but no shock or hypoxia as yet. The patient can probably wait 45 to 60 minutes without treatment and still survive.
  - Green: Third priority for treatment, nonurgent; the injuries are localized, without systemic implications.
  - Black: Dead; some patients with catastrophic injuries who have a very poor chance for survival also may be placed into this category.

REFERENCES

1. Alonso-Serra H, Blanton D, O'Connor RE: Physician medical direction in EMS. *J Prehosp Care* 2:153, 1998.
2. Eisenberg MS, Pantridge JF, Cobb LA, Geddes JS: The revolution and evolution of prehospital cardiac care. *Arch Intern Med* 156:1611, 1996.
3. Valenzuela TD, Roe DJ, Nichol G, et al: Outcome of rapid defibrillation by security officers after cardiac arrest in casinos. *N Engl J Med* 343:1206, 2000.
4. Caffery SL, Willoughby PJ, Pepe PE, Becker LB: Public use of automated external defibrillators. *N Engl J Med* 347:1242, 2002.
5. Patel RJ, Vilke GM, Chan TC: The prehospital electrocardiogram. *J Emerg Med* 21:35, 2001.
6. Ferrazzi S, Waltner-Toews D, Abernathy T, et al: The effects of prehospital advanced life support drug treatment on patient improvement and in-hospital utilization. *Prehosp Emerg Care* 5:252, 2001.
7. Mann NC, Mullins RJ, MacKenzie EJ, et al: Systemic review of published evidence regarding trauma system effectiveness. *J Trauma* 47:S25, 1999.
8. Pepe PE, Mosesso VN, Falk JL: Prehospital fluid resuscitation of the patient with major trauma. *Prehosp Emerg Care* 6:81, 2002.
9. Kosowsky JM, Stephanides SL, Branson RD, Sayre MR: Prehospital use of continuous positive airway pressure (CPAP) for presumed pulmonary edema: A preliminary case series. *Prehosp Emerg Care* 5:190, 2001.
10. Gausche M, Lewis RJ, Stratton SJ, et al: A prospective,

randomized study of the effect of out-of-hospital pediatric intubation on patient outcome. *JAMA* 283:783, 2000.

11. DeLorenzo RA: Mass gathering medicine: A review. *Prehospital Disaster Med* 12:68, 1997.

12. Michael JA, Barbera JA: Mass gathering medical care: A twenty-five year review. *Prehospital Disaster Med* 12:305, 1997.

13. Arbon P, Bridgewater FH, Smith C: Mass gathering medicine: A predictive model for patient presentation and transport rates. *Prehospital Disaster Med* 16:150, 2001.

14. Noji EK: Progress in disaster management. *Lancet* 343:1239, 1994.

15. Koenig KL, Dinerman N, Kuehl AE: Disaster nomenclature: A functional impact approach. *Acad Emerg Med* 3:723, 1996.

16. Auf der Heide A: *Disaster Response: Principles of Preparation and Coordination.* St Louis: CV Mosby, 1989, p. 178.

17. Orr M, Robinson A: The Hyatt Regency skywalk collapse: An EMS-based disaster response. *Ann Emerg Med* 12:601, 1983.

18. Oklahoma State Health Department: *Injury Update: Investigation of Death and Injuries Resulting from the May 3, 1999, Tornados.* Oklahoma City. Injury Prevention Service of the Oklahoma State Health Department, July 21, 2000.

19. Auf der Heide E: Community hospital and medical disaster planning guidelines, in *ACEP Handbook-Disaster Preparedness.* Dallas: American College of Emergency Physicians, 1993.

20. Noji EK, Sivertson KT: Injury prevention in natural disasters: A theoretical framework. *Disasters* 11:290, 1987.

21. Joint Commission on Accreditation of Healthcare Organizations (JCAHO): *Emergency Management Standard.* Oak Brook Terrace, IL: JCAHO, 2001.

22. Centers for Disease Control and Prevention: *Public Health Emergency Preparedness and Response: Bioterrorism. What has the CDC Accomplished?* Available from: http://www.bt.cdc.gov/Documents/BTInitiative.asp, accessed August 1, 2002.

23. Super G, Groth S, Hook R, et al: *START: Simple Triage and Rapid Treatment Plan.* Newport Beach, CA: Hoag Memorial Hospital Presbyterian, 1994.

24. Koenig KL, Schultz CH: Disaster medicine: Advances in local catastrophic disaster-response. *Acad Emerg Med* 1:133, 1994.

25. State of California Emergency Medical Services Authority: *Hospital Emergency Incident Command System.* Sacramento, CA: Emergency Medical Services Authority, 2002.

For further reading in *Emergency Medicine: A Comprehensive Study Guide,* 6th ed., see Chap 1, "Emergency Medical Services," by C. Patrick Lilja; Chap. 5, "Mass Gatherings," by Eric W. Ossmann and Arthur H. Yancey II; and Chap. 6, "Disaster Medical Services," by Eric K. Noji and Gabor D. Kelen.

195 EMERGENCY MEDICINE ADMINISTRATION
David M. Cline

NEGLIGENCE AND MEDICAL MALPRACTICE

• Negligence is defined as the omission to do something that a reasonable practitioner, guided by those ordinary considerations that ordinarily regulate human affairs, would do, or the doing of something that a reasonable and prudent practitioner would not do.[1]

• The four components of negligence are duty, breach of duty, damages, and causation. The plaintiff (injured or complaining party) must prove all four elements existed in order to find the defendant guilty of negligence.[2]

• Duty is considered a contract created by formation of a physician-patient relationship whereby the physician must act in accordance with "standards of care" to protect the patient from unreasonable risk.[2] In general, by contract with the hospital, emergency physicians have a duty to see all patients that present themselves to the emergency department to be seen.

• The standard of care is that which a similarly trained, "reasonable and prudent physician" would exercise under similar circumstances.[2] The emergency physician is not required to exercise the optimally highest degree of skill and care possible, but must use the degree of skill and care ordinarily exercised by physicians within the same specialty.

• Breach of duty occurs if the physician with an established duty fails to act in accordance with these standards of care by commission or omission of a certain act.[2] Emergency physicians are held to a national standard of care for a specialist in emergency medicine.

• Damages encompass any actual loss, injury, or deterioration sustained by the plaintiff due to the breach of duty.[2] A plaintiff must prove that the damage occurred because of the physician's negligence.

• Legal causation theoretically consists of two branches: causation in fact and foreseeability.[2] Causation in fact means that "an event A is the cause of another event B, if and only if B would not have occurred when and as it did but for event A." The concept of foreseeability is fulfilled if the patient's damages must be the foreseeable result of the defendant's substandard practice, as compared with the standard of the reasonable physician. A bad result without proof of violation of the standard of care does not constitute negligence.

• Failure to diagnose myocardial infarction represents the largest single category of monetary settlements for emergency medicine physicians.[3] Other high-risk areas for emergency physicians include: abdominal pain, wounds, fractures, pediatric fever/meningitis, airway obstruction, central nervous system bleeding, and abdominal aortic aneurysms.[3]

CONSENT

- Informed consent is considered ideal—the patient knows and understands the risks, benefits, and consequences of accepting or refusing treatment.[4] Specific, informed consent should be sought and obtained by the emergency physician whenever an invasive, risky, or complicated treatment or procedure is proposed. Examples include nonemergent thoracentesis, tube thoracostomies, paracentesis, and incision and drainage of a complex abscess.[5]
- Elements of informed consent include the following: (1) a concise statement of the patient's medical condition or problem; (2) an understandable statement of the nature and purpose of the proposed test, treatment, or procedure; (3) a description of the risks, consequences, and benefits of the proposed test, treatment, or procedure; (4) a statement regarding any viable alternatives to the test, treatment, or procedure; and (5) a statement regarding the patient's prognosis if the proposed test, treatment, or procedure is not given.[5]
- Express consent entails an awareness of the proposed care and an overt agreement (eg, in oral or written form) to proceed. An example would be the patient who comes to the emergency department, requests assistance for a problem, and signs a registration form authorizing evaluation and treatment of the problem.[5]
- Implied consent is invoked if an emergency exists and the patient is incompetent (eg, a minor or someone with an altered mental status). Simple procedures such as minor wound suturing, phlebotomy, injections, and peripheral IVs are allowed under express or implied consent.[4] An exception to this is testing for human immunodeficiency virus (HIV), which requires written informed consent.[6]
- Emergency consent bypasses normal consent standards due to the rapid need to treat a clinically ill patient. Implied consent is inferred by the patient's actions, but without specific agreement. Emergency consent covers actions such as emergent intubation or placement of central lines in a critical patient when there is no other access.[5]
- Failure to obtain appropriate consent can leave the emergency physician vulnerable to a legal action based on battery (intentional, unauthorized touching).[5]

MINORS AND CONSENT

- The law always implies consent for treatment of a child in the event of an emergency. Parental consent is not needed—it is implied.[7]
- All states without a general consent statute for minors have provisions that specifically permit the physician to treat any minor for venereal disease.[7]
- Most states have treatment statutes for minors (usually 16 years or older), which enable them to consent for medical care. Many states also specifically permit treatment of minors for drug or alcohol problems, pregnancy, and psychiatric conditions.[7]
- "Mature minor" statutes vary from state to state, but allow a minor (usually between 14 and 18 years of age) to give informed consent when he or she understands the risks and benefits of a treatment. This generally applies to treatments that do not pose a serious risk.[7]
- A parent with sole custody of a child has the legal right to provide consent for medical treatment. Obtain this permission prior to treatment whenever possible. On a practical basis however, if a medical necessity exists and a delay could be deleterious, the EP may need to assume that a parent in possession of a child has the authority to provide consent.[7]

REFUSAL OF CONSENT AND PATIENTS LEAVING AGAINST MEDICAL ADVICE

- On general principle, adult patients may ethically and legally refuse treatment totally or in part.[8]
- A patient does not require a global decision-making ability to refuse treatment, but rather enough for a given situation (ie, a relative decision-making capacity). Clinical circumstances require the use of the term **capacity,** whereas **competence** is a legal term, which can only be determined by a court ruling.
- Multiple components are required for a decision-making capacity. These include: understanding the options, awareness of the consequences of each option, and appreciation of the costs and benefits of the options in relation to relatively stable values and preferences.[9,10]
- Informed refusal should be carefully documented on the chart of a patient who leaves against medical advice (AMA).[11] The following five issues can be problematic and should be addressed in the chart:
  - Capacity: Document the patient's mental status. Ideally, a patient should be awake and alert, able to carry on a reasonable conversation, and possess the mental ability to discuss the problem and act with self-interest.
  - Discussion: Use and document clear terms that a layperson can understand; avoid euphemisms and technical jargon. If death is a possibility, say so.

- Offer of alternative treatment: Document whether or not alternative treatments are available and are offered.
- Family involvement: Document efforts to involve family or friends in the decision process. If the patient forbids family involvement, document this accordingly.
- Patient's signature: The physician is not legally protected if the patient signs a standard AMA form devoid of the other four elements. However, if a patient refuses to sign after an appropriate informed discussion, simply document the refusal to sign.

RESUSCITATION AND DO NOT RESUSCITATE ORDERS

- Current standards suggest that when the possibility exists that the brain is viable and there are no compelling medical or legal reasons to act otherwise, resuscitation should be initiated.[12]
- The current medical standard used to terminate resuscitations should be brain death or cardiovascular unresponsiveness. This principle is well founded in the standard references and well supported ethically.[13]
- Medically and ethically, it is important to remember that there is no obligation to deliver treatment that is futile.[14] When a person with a terminal illness is expected to die within a few hours or days, further aggressive diagnostic or therapeutic care would not benefit the patient and would be considered medically futile (and thus an ethical reason to withhold or cease resuscitation).[15]
- It is prudent to stabilize the patient first and then seek further clarification of his wishes, either from the patient directly or with the family or physician. Appropriate, ethical reasons to withhold or cease resuscitation include irreversible cessation of cardiac function, brain death, competent patient refusal, or an advance directive such as "DNR."[16]
- Even with a valid DNR order, conditions such as pain, infection, dehydration, and respiratory difficulty should be addressed. A patient with a DNR deserves respectful and compassionate care, which can maximize comfort and possibly improve the remaining quality of life.[16]

PHYSICIAN TELEPHONE ADVICE

- Even brief, seemingly straightforward advice is potentially a high-risk action when given over the telephone. A legally binding relationship (duty—the first element of a negligence tort) is established once advice is given.[11] Since one cannot see the patient and

further information may not be forthcoming, an accurate assessment truly cannot be made.[11]
- It is acceptable, however, to give basic first aid advice if one includes a rejoinder to come immediately to the emergency department.[11]
- Medical facilities with formal telephone advice programs should use specific guidelines, track outcomes, provide close follow-up, and complete the calls with a patient reminder to come to the emergency department.[11]

THE EMERGENCY MEDICAL TREATMENT AND ACTIVE LABOR ACT (EMTALA)

- In 1986 Congress enacted the Comprehensive Omnibus Budget Reconciliation Act (COBRA) to combat widespread patient-dumping practices. The Emergency Medical Treatment and Active Labor Act (EMTALA) is the section of COBRA that applies to emergency departments.[17,18]
- According to EMTALA regulations, a medically unstable patient can be transferred to another facility only if the transferring physician certifies the transfer is medically necessary and the receiving facility agrees to accept the patient.[18]
- A patient with an illness or injury who presents to an emergency department (whose hospital has a Medicare contract) must receive a medical screening examination, regardless of the patient's ability to pay or insurance coverage.[18]
- If the medical screening exam determines that an emergency medical condition exists, the patient must have that condition stabilized. Stabilization should take place prior to transfer to another facility, up to the full capacity of that the admitting facility.[18]
- The patient must understand the risks and benefits, and sign informed consent for the transfer.[18]
- EMTALA also applies to patients who are not being transferred, as all ED patients must receive a screening examination and be stabilized according to the standard procedures of the emergency department.[19] The patient's condition may preclude successful stabilization, and failure to stabilize the patient alone is not an EMTALA violation. However, the physician and hospital may be subject to an EMTALA investigation if it can be established that standard procedures including specialty consultation were not implemented in the attempt to stabilize the patient.

MEDICAL ETHICS

- There are five basic principles that should guide ethical decision making in medical practice.[20,21]

- Veracity is telling the truth. It forms the basis of maintaining an open health care provider–patient relationship and of keeping promises.
- Patient autonomy is based on a person's right and freedom to make an informed choice about what will and will not be done; it also acknowledges the patient's right to privacy.
- Beneficence is the principle of doing good; it involves promoting the well being of others, and responding to those in need.
- Nonmaleficence is the principle of "do no harm," which obliges the physician (or other health care provider) to protect others from danger, pain, and suffering. This concept stems from the Hippocratic Oath as well as other ancient medical traditions.
- Justice involves fairness, respect for human equality, and the equitable allocation of scarce resources.

REFERENCES

1. *Black's Law Dictionary,* 7th ed. St. Paul, MN: West Group, 1999.
2. Wood CL: Historical perspectives on law, medical malpractice and the concept of negligence. *Emerg Med Clin North Am* 11:819, 1993.
3. Karcz A, Korn R, Burke MC, et al: Malpractice claims against emergency physicians in Massachusetts: 1975-1993. *Am J Emerg Med* 14:341. 1996.
4. Flannery F, et al: Consent to treatment, in *Legal Medicine, American College of Legal Medicine.* St. Louis: Mosby, 1988.
5. Siegel DM: Consent and refusal of consent. *Emerg Med Clin North Am* 11:833, 1993.
6. Derse AR: Legal and ethical issues in the emergency department. *Emerg Med Clin North Am* 3:213, 1995.
7. Sullivan DJ: Minors and emergency medicine. *Emerg Med Clin North Am* 11:841, 1993.
8. Schwartz M: The patient who refuses medical treatment: a dilemma for hospitals and physicians. *Am J Law Med* 11:147, 1985.
9. Drane JF: Competency to give an informed consent. *JAMA* 252:925, 1984.
10. Buchanan AE: The question of competence, in Iserson KV et al (eds.): *Ethics in Emergency Medicine,* Tucson, AZ: Galen Press, 1995.
11. Henry GL: Risk management and high-risk issues in emergency medicine. *Emerg Med Clin North Am* 11:905, 1993.
12. McIntyre KM: Medicolegal aspects of cardiopulmonary resuscitation (CPR) and emergency cardiac care (ECC). *JAMA* 244:511, 1980.
13. Curtis RJ, et al: Use of the medical futility rationale—do not attempt resuscitation orders. *JAMA* 273:124, 1995.
14. Tomlinson T, Brady H: Futility and the ethics of resuscitation. *JAMA* 264:1276, 1990.
15. American College of Emergency Physicians: Policy statement: Nonbeneficial ("futile") emergency medical interventions, Irving, TX. ACEP, 1998.
16. American Medical Association Council on Ethical and Judicial Affairs: Guidelines for the appropriate use of do-not-resuscitate orders. *JAMA* 265:1241, 1990.
17. Frew S, Roush W, LaGreca K: COBRA: implications for emergency medicine. *Ann Emerg Med* 17:835, 1988.
18. Bitterman RA: Explaining the EMTALA paradox. *Ann Emerg Med* 40:470, 2002.
19. Kaszynski SB: EMTALA: Duty extends to even non-transferring emergency patients. *J Law Med Ethics* 29:102, 2001.
20. American Medical Association: *AMA Code of Ethics.* Chicago, 1997.
21. American Collage of Emergency Physicians: *ACEP Code of Ethics.* Irving, TX, 1997.

INDEX

Page numbers followed by italic *f* or *t* denote figures or tables, respectively.

A

Abominal aortic aneurysm, 118–119, 637
Abdominal distension, neonates, 237
Abdominal pain, acute. *See also* Pelvic pain
  causes, 144*t*
  clinical features, 143–144
  diagnosis and differential, 144–145
  in elderly patients, 144, 144*t*
  emergency department care and disposition, 145
  epidemiology, 143
  pathophysiology, 143
  in pediatric patients, 261–264, 262*t*
Abdominal trauma
  clinical features, 572
  diagnosis and differential, 572–573
  emergency department care and disposition, 573, 574*t*
  epidemiology, 571
  pathophysiology, 571
  in pregnancy, 551–552
Abdominal wall
  hernias, 158–159
  pain, 145
Abduction relief sign, 611
ABEM. *See* American Board of Emergency Medicine (ABEM)
Abortion, 217, 228
Abruptio placentae, 218, 551
Abscess
  anorectal, 167
  cutaneous, 336–337
  odontogenic, 531
  parapharyngeal, 530
  peritonsillar, 280, 529
  retropharyngeal, 280, 530
Absinthe, toxicology, 404
Abuse and assault. *See* Child abuse; Intimate partner violence; Sexual abuse; Sexual assault

Accelerated idioventricular rhythm (AIVR), 19–20, 20*f*
Acetabular fractures, 597
Acetaminophen, 58
  toxicology, 348*t*, 350*t*, 375–377, 376*f*
Achilles tendon rupture, 601
Acid-base disorders
  clinical features, 41
  diagnosis and differential, 41–42
  metabolic acidosis, 42–43, 43*t*
  metabolic alkalosis, 43–44
  respiratory acidosis, 44
  respiratory alkalosis, 44
Acid burns, 434–436
Acidosis, metabolic. *See* Metabolic acidosis
Acidosis, respiratory. *See* Respiratory acidosis
Acquired immune deficiency syndrome (AIDS), 309–311, 309*t*. *See also* Human immunodeficiency virus (HIV) infection
Acromioclavicular joint injuries, 592
Activated partial prothrombin time (aPTT), 457*t*
Acute angle closure glaucoma, 518
Acute chest syndrome, 293–294, 464–465
Acute coronary syndromes. *See* Myocardial infarction (MI)
Acute intermittent porphyria, 503–504
Acute mountain sickness (AMS), 425–427
Acute myocardial infarction (AMI). *See* Myocardial infarction (MI)
Acute pain
  analgesia, 58–59
  clinical features, 57
  emergency department care and disposition, 57–60
  local and regional anesthesia, 59–60
  pathophysiology, 57
  procedural sedation, 57–59
Acute respiratory distress syndrome (ARDS), 49
Adenosine, 18, 29, 34
ADH. *See* Vasopressin
Adhesive tapes, for wound closure, 70
Administration, emergency medical services. *See* Emergency medical services
Adrenal insufficiency, 452–453, 479

African eye worm, 325

Agonal rhythm, 25

AIDS. *See* Acquired immune deficiency syndrome (AIDS)

Airway obstruction
  acute, 532
  tumor-related, 476

Airway support
  bag-valve-mask ventilation, 9–10
  cricothyrotomy, 10
  nasotracheal intubation, 9
  pathophysiology, 7–8, 7*f*
  in pediatric patients, 32
  in shock, 48
  tracheal intubation, 8–9, 8*t*, 9*t*

AIVR. *See* Accelerated idioventricular rhythm (AIVR)

Albuterol
  for asthma, 253
  for bronchiolitis, 254
  for hyperkalemia, 39

Alcoholic ketoacidosis, 448–449

Alcoholic liver disease, 178–179

Alcohols, toxicology, 364–367

Alkali burns, 434–436

Alkalosis, metabolic. *See* Metabolic alkalosis

Alkalosis, respiratory. *See* Respiratory alkalosis

Allergic reactions, 53–54

Alopecia, 540–541

Alpha-adrenergic receptor antagonists, toxicology, 384

ALS. *See* Amyotrophic lateral sclerosis (ALS)

ALTE. *See* Apparent life-threatening event (ALTE)

Altered mental status
  diagnosis and differential, 269, 269*t*
  in pediatric patients, 268–269, 269*t*

Alternobaric vertigo, 428

Altitude-related syndromes, 425–427

Amanita mushrooms, 441

Amantadine, for influenza, 307

American Board of Emergency Medicine (ABEM)
  Certification Exam, 1–2
  Continuous Certification, 2–3
  In-Training Exam, 3
  Lifelong Learning and Self-Assessment test, 2–3, 3*t*

American Osteopathic Board of Emergency Medicine (AOBEM), 1, 3

AMI. *See* Myocardial infarction (MI)

Aminoglycosides, 406

Amiodarone, 28
  for atrial fibrillation, 17
  for atrial flutter, 16
  for ventricular fibrillation, 21
  for ventricular tachycardia, 20

Amniotic fluid embolism, 219–220

Amphetamines, toxicology, 370–371

AMS. *See* Acute mountain sickness (AMS)

Amyotrophic lateral sclerosis (ALS), 505–506

Anal fissure, 166–167

Anal fistula, 168

Analgesia, 57–59

Analgesics, toxicology, 373–378

Anaphylaxis, 53–54

Ancylostoma duodenale, 324

Anemia(s)
  acquired hemolytic, 466–468, 466*t*, 467*t*
  clinical features, 455
  diagnosis and differential, 455, 456*f*, 456*t*
  emergency department care and disposition, 458
  hereditary hemolytic, 464–466

Anesthesia, local and regional, 59–60

Aneurysm, abdominal aortic, 118–119, 637

Angioedema, 53, 532

Angiography, in aortic dissection, 120

Angiotensin-converting enzyme inhibitors, 385

Angiotensin II receptor antagonists, 385

Animal bites, 85–87, 619*t*

Anion gap, 42, 367*t*. *See also* Metabolic acidosis

Ankle-brachial index, 580

Ankle injuries, 80, 601–603

Ankylosing spondylitis, 616

Anorectal disorders
  abscess, 167
  cryptitis, 166
  fissure, 166–167
  fistula, 168
  foreign bodies, 169
  hemorrhoids, 165–166, 166*f*
  pilonidal sinus, 167
  procidentia, 168
  prolapse, 168
  pruritus, 169
  tumors, 168–169

Anterior cord syndrome, 559*t*

Anterior cruciate ligament injuries, 600

Anthrax, 331, 339*t*

Antiarrhythmics, 28, 29. *See also specific drugs*

Antibiotics
  for cat bite wounds, 87
  for cellulitis, 248–249
  for cholecystitis, 182
  for diarrhea, 172
  for dog bite wounds, 86
  for human bite wounds, 85
  for meningitis, 232*t*, 511*t*
  for otitis media, 243
  for pharyngitis, 245
  for pneumonia, 131
  for puncture wounds, 84
  for sepsis, 232*t*
  for septic shock, 51
  for ulcerative colitis, 162
  for urinary tract infections, 196
  in wound management, 66, 88

Anticholinergics, toxicology, 348*t*, 350*t*, 351–353, 352*t*

Anticoagulants
  bleeding and, 461–462
  oral, 472–473
  parenteral, 473

Anticonvulsants, 502*t*

Antidepressants
  for chronic pain, 62
  toxicology, 353–360

Antidiarrheals, 172
Antidiuretic hormone (ADH). *See* Vasopressin
Antidotes, poison, 350*t*
Antidysrhythmics, 26. *See also specific classes and drugs*
Antiemetics, 172
Antiepileptics, 258
Antihistamines, 54
Antihypertensives, toxicology, 383–385
Antimalarials, toxicology, 405–406
Antimicrobials, toxicology, 405–406
Antiplatelets, 95*t*, 473
Antipsychotics, toxicology, 358–360
Antithrombotics. *See* Fibrinolytic agents
Anxiety disorder, 624
AOBEM. *See* American Osteopathic Board of Emergency
    Medicine (AOBEM)
Aortic aneurysm, abdominal, 118–119, 637
Aortic dissection, 117, 119–120
Aortic incompetence, 102*t*, 104–105
Aortic rupture, 570–571
Aortic stenosis, 104
Aphthous stomatitis, 526
Apnea, in neonates, 237–238
Apparent life-threatening event (ALTE), 238
Appendicitis. *See also* Abdominal pain, acute
    clinical features, 154–155, 154*t*
    diagnosis and differential, 155
    emergency department care and disposition, 155
    epidemiology, 154
    pathophysiology, 154
    in pediatric patients, 263
    white blood cell count, 155
APTT. *See* Activated partial prothrombin time (aPTT)
Arborviruses, 512
ARDS. *See* Acute respiratory distress syndrome (ARDS)
Arnold-Chiari malformation, 277
Aronen technique, 593
Arsenic, toxicology, 399
Arterial occlusion, 123–124
Arthritis
    classification, 615*t*
    juvenile rheumatoid, 290
    Lyme, 615
    poststreptococcal, 291
    rheumatoid, 616
    septic. *See* Septic arthritis
Articular back pain, 61*t*, 62*t*
Ascaris lumbricoides, 323
Aspiration
    foreign body, 279–280
    pneumonitides, 132
Aspirin
    for acute coronary syndromes, 96, 474
    as antiplatelet, 473
    Reye's syndrome and, 58
    toxicology, 348*t*, 373–375
Asthma
    clinical features, 139, 253
    diagnosis and differential, 139, 253
    emergency department care and disposition, 139–140, 253

epidemiology, 138, 252
pathophysiology, 138–139, 252–253
in pediatric patients, 252–254
in pregnancy, 214
Asystole, 25
Ataxia, 495–496, 495*t*
Atenolol, 95*t*
Atracurium, 9*t*
Atrial fibrillation, 16–17, 16*f*
Atrial flutter, 15–16, 16*f*
Atrioventricular (AV) block
    second-degree Mobitz I, 22
    second-degree Mobitz I (Wenckebach), 22*f*
    second-degree Mobitz II, 22–23, 22*f*
    third-degree (complete), 23, 23*f*
Atrioventricular (AV) node, 11
Atropine, 29–30
    in atrioventricular block, 23
    in pediatric intubation, 32
    for pulseless electrical activity, 25
    for sinus pause, 22
AV block. *See* Atrioventricular (AV) block
AV node. *See* Atrioventricular (AV) node

B
B-type natriuretic peptide (BNP), 52
Bacillus anthracis, 331, 339*t*
Back pain, chronic, 61, 61*t*
Bacteremia
    occult, 231
    in pediatric patients, 229, 231–232
    predisposing factors, 49
Bacterial vaginosis, 300*t*. *See also* Vulvovaginitis
Bag-valve-mask (BVM) ventilation, 9–10, 23
Balanoposthitis, 200
Balloon tamponade, 147
Bankard lesion, 593
Barbiturates, toxicology, 360–361
Barotitis media, 428
Barotrauma, 428–430
Battle's sign, 554, 560
Beck's triad, 568
Bedbugs, 420–421
Bee stings, 418
Beef tapeworm, 326
Behavioral disorders
    clinical features, 623–625
    diagnosis and differential, 626
    emergency assessment and stabilization, 625–626
Bell's palsy, 504–505
Benign paroxysmal positional vertigo (BPPV), 496–499
Benzodiazepines (BNZ)
    for conscious sedation, 59
    toxicology, 362
Beta-adrenergic antagonists, 27–28
    for asthma, 140
    for chronic obstructive pulmonary disease, 140
    in myocardial infarction, 97
    for premature atrial contractions, 14

Beta-adrenergic antagonists (*Continued*)
   for premature ventricular contractions, 19
   toxicology, 350*t*, 381–382
Beta-lactams, toxicology, 406
Biceps rupture, 590–591
Bicycle spoke injuries, 79
Bifascicular block, 24
Biliary colic, 181–182
Biological agents, 339*t*
Bioterrorism, 338–340, 339*t*
Bipolar disorder, 624
Bites and stings
   ant, 418
   bedbug, 420
   bee, 418
   blister beetle, 420
   cat, 86–87
   chigger, 420
   coral snake, 422
   dog, 85–86
   flea, 420
   Gila monster, 422
   human, 85, 619, 619*t*
   Hymenoptera, 418
   kissing bug, 420
   lice, 420
   marine animals, 423–425
   pit viper, 420–421
   puss caterpillar, 420
   rodent, 86–87
   scabies, 420
   scorpion, 419–420
   spider, 419
   wasp, 418
Black cohosh, 404
Black widow spider bite, 419
Blackwater fever, 320
Bladder, traumatic injury, 578
Bleeding
   diagnosis and differential, 457
   gastrointestinal. *See* Gastrointestinal bleeding
Bleeding disorders
   acquired, 458–462
   clinical features, 455
   diagnosis and differential, 457*t*
   emergency department care and disposition, 458
Bleeding time, 457*t*
Blister beetle, 421
Blowout fractures, 517, 562
Blue spells, in neonates, 238
BNP. *See* B-type natriuretic peptide (BNP)
BNZ. *See* Benzodiazepines (BNZ)
Body lice, 420
Boerhaave's syndrome, 149
Bone metastases, 474–475
Bordetella pertussis, 129
Borrelia burgdorferi, 327
Botulism, 339*t*, 340, 503
Boutonnière deformity, 585
Bowel obstruction. *See* Intestinal obstruction

BPPV. *See* Benign paroxysmal positional vertigo (BPPV)
Brachial neuritis, 504
Bradycardia, in pediatric patients, 34
Bradydysrhythmia, 13. *See also* specific dysrhythmias
Brain abscess, 512–513
Brain tumor, 484
Braxton-Hicks contractions, 220
Breast surgery complications, 186
Breech presentation, 222
Bronchiolitis, in pediatric patients, 254
Bronchitis, 129–130
   chronic. *See* Chronic obstructive pulmonary disease (COPD)
   high altitude, 427
Bronchopulmonary dysplasia, 238
Brown recluse spider bite, 419
Brown-Séquard syndrome, 559*t*
Brudzinski's sign, 510
Brugia malayi, 325
Bullous myringitis, 523
Bullous pemphigoid, 538–539
Bundle-branch block, 23
Bupropion, toxicology, 355
Burns
   chemical, 434–436, 518
   thermal, 432–434, 432–434*f*
Bursitis, 616, 621
Buspirone, tox, 363
Buttocks, traumatic injury, 575–576
Button battery ingestion, 151–152
BVM ventilation. *See* Bag-valve-mask (BVM) ventilation

C
Calcitonin
   for hypercalcemia, 40
   for reflex sympathetic dystrophy, 62
Calcium channel blockers, 28–29
   toxicology, 350*t*, 382–383
Cancer pain, 62*t*, 481–482
Candidal intertrigo, 541–542
Candidal vaginitis. *See* Vulvovaginitis
Candidiasis, oral, 238, 311, 526
Capitate fracture, 587
Capnocytophaga canimorsus, 86
Captopril, 118
Carbamazepine
   complications, 258
   properties, 502*t*
Carbon monoxide poisoning, 439–441, 441*t*
Carbonic anhydrase inhibitors, toxicology, 383–384
Carcinomas
   bone complications, 474–475
   spinal cord compression, 475
Cardiac arrest, in pediatric patients, 32
Cardiac conduction system, 11
Cardiac dysrhythmias, 12–13, 12–13*f. See also specific dysrhythmias*
Cardiac tamponade
   in end-stage renal disease, 193
   nontraumatic, 110–111

Cardiac tamponade (*Continued*)
  traumatic, 568
Cardiac transplant patients, 343–344
  immunosuppressive complications, 342–343, 343*t*
  infectious complications, 341–342, 341*t*
Cardiac ultrasonography, 638
Cardiogenic shock, 51–52
Cardiomyopathy
  dilated, 107–108
  hypertrophic, 108
  restrictive, 108–109
  right ventricular, 109
Cardiothoracic trauma, 565–571
Cardioversion
  in atrial fibrillation, 17
  in atrial flutter, 16
  in pediatric patients, 34–35
  in supraventricular tachycardia, 17
  in ventricular tachycardia, 20
  for Wolff-Parkinson-White syndrome, 26
Carnett's sign, 145
Carotid sinus hypersensitivity, 98
Carotid sinus massage
  for supraventricular tachycardia, 17–18
  in ventricular dysrhythmias, 19
Carpal tunnel syndrome, 620
Catastrophic casualty management, 644
Cauda equina, 559*t*
Caustics, ingestion, 392–394
Cellulitis, 335–336, 520
  hand, 618, 619*t*
  orbital, 516
  in pediatric patients, 248–249
  periorbital, 516
Central cord syndrome, 559*t*
Central retinal artery occlusion, 519
Central retinal vein occlusion, 519
Cephalic tetanus, 316
Cerebral edema
  in diabetic ketoacidosis, 265–266, 447
  high altitude, 425–427
Cerebral perfusion pressure, 553
Cerebrospinal fluid rhinorrhea, 561
Cerebrotonsillar herniation, 555
Certification Examination, American Board of Emergency
    Medicine, 1–2, 2*t*
Cervical disc prolapse, 609
Cervical spine fracture
  characteristics, 558*t*
  diagnosis and differential, 558*t*
  in elderly patients, 549
  in head injury, 555
Cervical spondylosis, 609
Cesarean section, in maternal trauma, 552
Cestodes, 325–326
CFI. *See* Clenched fist injury (CFI)
Chalazion, 515
Chamomile, toxicology, 404
Chancroid, 300*t*, 302
Chaparral, 404

Cheeks, wound repair, 73–74, 74*f*
Chemical burns, 434–436, 518
Chemical pneumonitis, 390–391
Chest pain
  in acute pericarditis, 110
  in aortic dissection, 120
  causes, 92*t*, 93*t*
  clinical features, 91–92
  diagnosis and differential, 92, 92*f*, 92*t*
  emergency department care and disposition, 93
  pathophysiology, 91, 91*f*
  prognosis, 93*t*
Chest wall injury, 566–567
Chickenpox. *See* Varicella
Chigger bites, 420
Chilblains, 414
Child abuse, 236
  clinical features, 629–630
  diagnosis and differential, 630
  emergency department care and disposition, 630
  epidemiology, 629
  injury patterns, 288, 629–630
Children. *See* Pediatric patients
Chlamydia pneumoniae, 129, 130
Chlamydia trachomatis, 299, 300*t*
Chloral hydrate
  for conscious sedation, 59
  toxicology, 363
Chloroquine
  for malaria, 320–321, 321*t*
  toxicology, 405–406
Cholangitis, 181
Cholecystitis
  clinical features, 181
  diagnosis and differential, 181–182
  emergency department care and disposition, 182
  epidemiology, 180–181
  postsurgical, 187
Cholelithiasis, 181
Chondromalacia patellae, 601
Christmas disease. *See* Hemophilia
Chronic obstructive pulmonary disease (COPD)
  clinical features, 139
  diagnosis and differential, 139
  emergency department care and disposition, 139–140
  epidemiology, 138
  pathophysiology, 138–139
Chronic pain
  clinical features, 61, 61*t*
  diagnosis and differential, 61
  emergency department care and disposition, 61–62, 62*t*
  epidemiology, 60
  pathophysiology, 61
Chvostek's sign, 40
Cingulate herniation, 555
Ciprofloxacin, 135*t*
Cirrhosis
  clinical features, 178
  diagnosis and differential, 178–179
  emergency department care and disposition, 179–180

Cirrhosis (*Continued*)
  pathophysiology, 178
Clavicle, fractures, 288, 591–592
Clenched fist injury (CFI), 85, 619, 619*t*
Clonazepam, complications, 258
Clonidine
  for hypertensive emergencies, 118
  toxicology, 384
Clonorchis sinensis, 325
Clopidogrel, 96
Closed fist injury. *See* Clenched fist injury
Clostridial myonecrosis, 333–334
Clostridium botulinum, 339*t*, 340
Clostridium difficile, 162–163
Clostridium tetani. See Tetanus
Cluster headache, 484, 485
CMV. *See* Cytomegalovirus (CMV) infections
Cocaine
  ingestion, 152
  toxicology, 369–371
Coin ingestion, 151
Cold injury, 413–415, 414*t*
Colitis
  pseudomembranous, 162–163
  ulcerative, 161–162
Colles' fracture, 588
Colorado tick fever, 330
Coma, 493–494, 494*t*
Compartment syndrome, 586, 604–605, 605*t*
Complex regional pain type I, 61, 61*t*, 62*t*
Complex regional pain type II, 61, 61*t*, 62*t*
Complications
  assisted reproductive technology, 228
  conization, 228
  dialysis, 194
  end-stage renal disease, 193–194
  endoscopic, 227
  induced abortion, 228
  nephrostomy tubes, 204
  pancreatitis, 184*t*
  postsurgical. *See* Postsurgical complications
  ureteral stents, 205
  urinary catheters, 204
  vascular access, 194
Computed tomography (CT)
  in abdominal trauma, 573
  in appendicitis, 155
  in buttock trauma, 576
  emergency department use, 635
  in flank trauma, 575
  for pulmonary embolism, 113–114
  for renal colic, 203
ConCert. *See* Continuous Certification
Conduction disturbances. *See* specific conditions
Congenital heart disease, 240–241
Congestive heart failure
  causes, 100*t*
  clinical features, 100
  diagnosis and differential, 100
  emergency department care and disposition, 100–101

  in end-stage renal disease, 193
  epidemiology, 99
  pathophysiology, 99–100
  in pediatric patients, 241–242, 241*t*
Conization, complications, 228
Conjunctival abrasion, 516
Conjunctivitis, 515
  in pediatric patients, 246–247
Consent, 646–647
Constipation, 173–174, 173*t*
  in neonates, 237
Contact dermatitis, 540
Continuous Certification, American Board of Emergency
    Medicine, 2–3
Conversion disorder, 625, 627–628
Coombs test, 456*t*
COPD. *See* Chronic obstructive pulmonary disease (COPD)
Coral snake bites, 422
Cord prolapse, 221–222
Corneal abrasion, 516–517
Corneal ulcer, 516
Corticosteroids
  for asthma, 140, 253
  for chronic obstructive pulmonary disease, 140
Cramps, heat-related, 417
Creatine kinase-MB (CK-MB), 92, 92*f*, 92*t*
Cricothyrotomy, 10
Crohn's disease, 159–161
  ulcerative colitis and, 161
Crotalidae, 350*t*, 421
Crush injury, 604
Crying, conditions associated with, 236*t*
Cryoprecipitate transfusion therapy, 469
Cryptitis, 166
CT. *See* Computed tomography (CT)
Cuff cellulitis, 227
Cullen's sign, 183
Cushing reflex, 553
Cutaneous abscess, 336–337
Cyanide poisoning, 350*t*, 407–408, 408*t*
Cyanoacrylate adhesives
  in eye, 518
  for wound closure, 70
Cyanosis, 128–129, 128*t*
  in neonates, 238
  in pediatric patients, 240–241
Cytomegalovirus (CMV) infections
  in AIDS, 310–311
  in transplant patients, 341–342

D
D-dimer testing
  for deep venous thrombosis, 122
  for pulmonary embolism, 113
Debridement, 66
Decompression sickness, 428–430
Decontamination, 400–401
Deep venous thrombosis (DVT)
  clinical features, 121

Deep venous thrombosis (DVT) (*Continued*)
  diagnosis and differential, 121–122
  emergency department care and disposition, 122–123
  epidemiology, 121
  pathophysiology, 121
  risk factors, 121, 122*t*
DEET, toxicology, 395
Defibrillation
  in pediatric patients, 35
  in ventricular fibrillation, 21
Dehydration
  clinical features, 274*t*
  diagnosis and differential, 259, 274
  pathophysiology, 273
Delirium
  causes, 491, 492*t*, 623
  clinical features, 491*t*
  diagnosis and differential, 491
  emergency department care and disposition, 492
  epidemiology, 491
  pathophysiology, 491
Delivery, emergency
  breech presentation, 222
  clinical features, 220
  cord prolapse, 221–222
  diagnosis and differential, 220
  epidemiology, 220
  postpartum care, 222
  procedure, 221
  shoulder dystocia, 222
Dementia
  in AIDS, 310–311
  causes, 493*t*, 623
  clinical features, 491*t*, 492
  diagnosis and differential, 492
  emergency department care and disposition, 493
  pathophysiology, 492
Demerol, Phenergan, Thorazine (DPT) cocktail, 58
Dental fractures, 527–528
Department of Transportation, 641
Depression, major, 624
DeQuervain's tenosynovitis, 620
Dermatitis
  contact, 540
  exfoliative, 535–536
  schistosomal, 325
Dermatomyositis, 503
Diabetes insipidus, 38
Diabetes mellitus
  clinical features, 264–265
  epidemiology, 264
  pathophysiology, 264
  in pediatric patients, 264
  in pregnancy, 214
Diabetic ketoacidosis, 446–447
  in pediatric patients, 264–266
Diagnostic peritoneal lavage, 572–573
Dialysis
  for acute renal failure, 191–192
  complications, 194

Diaphragmatic injuries, 568, 572
Diarrhea
  agents causing, 260*t*
  in AIDS, 311
  clinical features, 171, 259, 260*t*
  in Crohn's disease, 161
  diagnosis and differential, 171–172, 259–260
  emergency department care and disposition, 172, 261
  epidemiology, 169–170, 259
  in neonates, 237
  pathophysiology, 170, 259
  in pediatric patients, 259–261, 260*t*
  treatment, 260*t*
DIC. *See* Disseminated intravascular coagulation (DIC)
Digitalis glycosides, toxicology, 380–382
Digoxin
  for atrial fibrillation, 17
  for atrial flutter, 16
  for supraventricular tachycardia, 18
  toxicology, 350*t*, 380–382
Diltiazem, 29
  for atrial fibrillation, 17
  for atrial flutter, 16
  for multifocal atrial tachycardia, 15
  for supraventricular tachycardia, 18
Diphyllobothrium, 326
Disaster medical services, 643–644
Dislocation(s)
  ankle, 603
  elbow, 588
  finger and hand, 583–586
  glenohumeral joint, 592–593
  hip, 597–598
  knee, 600
  mandible, 522
  shoulder, 592–593
  temporomandibular, 563
  wrist, 586–587
Disseminated intravascular coagulation (DIC)
  bleeding and, 460–461
  conditions associated with, 460*t*
  laboratory results, 461*t*
  septic shock and, 50
Diuretics
  for congestive heart failure, 101
  toxicology, 383–384
Diverticulitis, 163–164
Diving, complications, 428–430
Diving reflex, 18
Dizziness, 496–499
Do not resuscitate orders, 647
Dobutamine, 30, 48
Dog bites, 85–86
Domestic violence. *See* Intimate partner violence
Donovanosis, 300*t*, 303
Dopamine, 30
  for congestive heart failure, 101
  for septic shock, 50
  for shock, 48
  for sinus bradycardia, 14

Dopamine agonists, toxicology, 385
Doxacurium, 9t
DPT. *See* Demerol, Phenergan, Thorazine (DPT) cocktail
Dracunculus medinensis, 325
Dressings, 87
Drowning, 430
Drug Abuse Warning Network, 63
Drug dosages, pediatric, 34
Drug-seeking behavior, 63, 63t
Dry drowning, 430
Dumping syndrome, 187
Dupuytren's contracture, 620
DVT. *See* Deep venous thrombosis (DVT)
Dysbarism, 428–430
Dysdiadochokinesia, 496
Dysequilibrium, 497–498
Dysphagia, 148
Dyspnea
    in aortic incompetence, 105
    in aortic stenosis, 104
    causes, 125t
    clinical features, 125
    diagnosis and differential, 125
    emergency department care and disposition, 126
    in mitral stenosis, 102
    pathophysiology, 125
Dysrhythmias, 12–13, 13f. *See also specific dysrhythmias*
    with acute myocardial infarction, 94
    in pediatric patients, 34
    in pregnancy, 214
Dyssynergia, 496
Dysthymic disorder, 624

E
Ear
    trauma to, 524
    wound repair, 74, 74f
Ebola virus, 340
ECG. *See* Electrocardiogram (ECG)
Echinacea, toxicology, 404
Ectopic pregnancy
    clinical features, 212
    diagnosis and differential, 212–213
    emergency department care and disposition, 213
    epidemiology, 212
    pathophysiology, 212
Ehrlichiosis, 329–330
Elbow injuries, 588–589. *See also* Upper extremity
Elderly patients
    abdominal pain, 144, 144t
    abuse, 630–631
    falls, 549
    trauma, 548–550
Electrical injuries, 436–438, 437–438t
Electrocardiogram (ECG)
    in acute pericarditis, 110
    in dilated cardiomyopathy, 107
    in myocardial infarction, 95t
    normal, 11–12, 11f, 12f

in syncope, 98
Electrolyte disorders. *See* Fluid and electrolyte disorders
Elephantiasis, 325
Emergency medical services
    administration, 645–648
    catastrophic casualty, 644
    Department of Transportation definitions, 641
    disaster-related, 643–644
    at mass gatherings, 642–643
    medical control, 641–642
    rural, 641
    triage, 644
Emergency Medical Treatment and Active Labor Act, 647
Emphysema. *See* Chronic obstructive pulmonary disease (COPD)
Encephalitis, 511–512
Encephalopathy
    hypertensive, 117
    metabolic, 268
    uremic, 193
End-stage renal disease
    complications, 193–194
    epidemiology, 192–193
    pathophysiology, 193
Endocarditis, infective, 313–314, 314t
Endometriosis, 209
Endometritis, postpartum, 219
Endotracheal intubation, 8–9, 8t, 9t
    in pediatric patients, 32, 33t
Enemas, 173
Enterobius vermicularis, 323–324
Enteroviral infections, 283
Entrapment neuropathies, 504
Ephedra, toxicology, 404
Epicondyle fracture, 589
Epidermal necrolysis, 536–537
Epididymitis, 199–200
Epidural compression syndrome, 611–612
Epidural hematoma, 554
Epiglottitis, 530–531
    in pediatric patients, 277–278
Epinephrine, 30
    for anaphylaxis, 54
    for bronchiolitis, 254
    for idioventricular rhythm, 25
    in neonatal resuscitation, 35
    in pediatric patients, 34
    for pulseless electrical activity, 25
    for sinus bradycardia, 14
Epistaxis, 525
Epley maneuver, 499
Epstein-Barr virus, 245
Erysipelas, 336, 520
    in pediatric patients, 282
Erythema chronicum migrans, 327
Erythema infectiosum, 283, 284f
Erythema multiforme, 536
Erythema nodosum, 285
Escherichia coli, 195, 195t
Esmolol, 27

Esophageal bleeding, 149–150
Esophageal injury, 149, 571
Ethambutol, 135*t*
Ethanol, toxicology, 364–365, 448–449
Ethchlorvynol, toxicology, 363
Ethosuximide, complications, 258
Ethylene glycol, toxicology, 366–367
Etomidate, 8*t*
  for conscious sedation, 59
  in pediatric intubation, 33
Exam preparation, 4–5
Exanthem subitum. *See* Roseola infantum
Exfoliative dermatitis, 535–536
Extensors, forearm, 76*t*
External rotation technique, 593
Extracorporeal shock wave lithotripsy, 203
Eyelids, wound repair, 72, 72*f*

F
Facial infections, 519–520
Facial pain, 485–487
Factor level assays, 457*t*
Falls, in elderly patients, 549
False labor, 220
Fascicular block, 23
Fasciola hepatica, 325
Fasciolopsis buski, 325
Febrile seizures, 257
Felon, 619, 619*t*
Femoral condyle fractures, 599
Femoral epiphysis, slipped capital, 289
Femoral shaft fracture, 598
Fenoldopam, 117
Fentanyl, 8*t*, 58
Fever
  pathophysiology, 229
  in pediatric patients, 229–230, 236
  postoperative, 185
FFP. *See* Fresh frozen plasma (FFP)
Fibrin degradation products, 457*t*
Fibrinolytic agents
  bleeding and, 459
  contraindications, 474*t*
  for deep venous thrombosis, 123, 474
  for ischemic stroke, 474
  for myocardial infarction, 95, 95*t*, 473–474, 474*t*
Fibromyalgia, 61*t*, 62*t*
Fibular fractures, 599–600
Finger
  anatomy, 78*f*
  injuries, 585–586
  wound repair, 77, 78*f*
Fire worm, 325
Fish handler's disease, 423
Fissure, anal, 166–167
Fistula, anal, 168
Flank trauma, 574–575
Flatworms, 325–326
Flea bites, 420

Flexor tenosynovitis, 618, 619*t*
Fluid and electrolyte disorders
  diagnosis and differential, 36, 274, 274*t*
  emergency department care and disposition, 274–275
  fluid replacement, 36
  hypercalcemia, 40
  hyperkalemia, 39, 39*t*
  hypermagnesemia, 41
  hypernatremia, 37–38, 38*t*
  hypocalcemia, 39–40
  hypokalemia, 38–39, 38*t*
  hypomagnesemia, 40–41
  hyponatremia, 37
  pathophysiology, 273
  in pediatric patients, 273–275
  in septic shock, 50
  in shock, 48
Flukes, 325
Flumazenil, 58
Food-borne illnesses, 170, 171*t*
Food impaction, 151
Foot. *See also* Lower extremity
  injuries, 80–81, 603–604
  malignant melanoma, 622
  puncture wounds, 83–84
  soft tissue problems, 620–622
  ulcers, 622
Forearm. *See also* Upper extremity
  anatomy, 76*t*, 605*t*
  fractures, 589–590
  wound repair, 75–76, 76*f*
Forehead, wound repair, 71*f*, 72
Foreign bodies
  aspiration, 279–280, 532
  conjunctival, 517
  corneal, 517
  nasal, 525
  rectal, 169
  soft tissue, 81–83
  swallowed, 150–152
  urethral, 201
  vaginal, 211
Fosphenytoin toxicology, 386–387, 387*t*
Fournier's gangrene, 200
Fracture(s)
  acetabular, 597
  ankle, 602–603
  capitate, 587
  cervical spine, 549, 555, 558*t*
  classification of, 287, 287*f*
  clavicle, 288, 591–592
  clinical features, 583–584
  Colles', 588
  dental, 527–528
  elbow, 588–589
  emergency department care and disposition, 584
  epicondyle, 589
  femoral condyle, 599
  femoral shaft, 598
  fibula, 599–600

Fracture(s) (*Continued*)
  forearm, 589–590
  frontal sinus, 562
  greenstick, 287
  hamate, 587
  hand, 584–586
  hip, 597
  humerus, 594
  knee, 599–600
  LeFort, 560, 561*f*
  lunate, 587
  mandible, 563
  maxilla, 563
  metacarpal, 586
  nasoethmoidal-orbital, 562
  nose, 525, 562
  orbital blowout, 517, 562
  pathophysiology, 583
  pelvic, 594–597, 595*t*
  phalanx, 586
  physeal, 287, 287*f*
  pisiform, 587
  radial head, 588–589
  radial styloid, 587
  rib, 566
  scaphoid, 587
  scapula, 593–594
  Smith's, 588
  supracondylar, 288–289
  tibia, 599
  torus, 287
  trapezium, 587
  trapezoid, 587
  triquetrum, 587
  ulnar styloid, 587–588
  wrist, 587–588
  zygomatic, 562
Francisella tularensis, 329
Fresh frozen plasma (FFP)
  in shock, 48
  transfusion therapy, 469
Frontal sinus fractures, 562
Frostbite, 413–415, 414*t*
Furosemide
  for hypercalcemia, 40
  for hypermagnesemia, 41

G
Gabapentin
  for chronic pain, 62
  complications, 258
Gait disturbances, 495–495, 495*t*
Galeazzi's fracture-dislocation, 480
Gallstones
  diagnosis and differential, 637
  epidemiology, 180–181
  pathophysiology, 181
Gamekeeper's thumb, 585
Gamma-hydroxybutyrate (GHB), toxicology, 363

Ganglion cyst, 620, 621
Garlic, toxicology, 404
Gas gangrene, 333–335
Gastritis, 152–153
Gastroenteritis, viral, 170
Gastrointestinal bleeding
  clinical features, 146
  emergency department care and disposition, 147
  epidemiology, 146
  pathophysiology, 146
  in pediatric patients, 262
Gastrointestinal reflux disease (GERD), 148–149
Gastrointestinal surgery complications, 186–187
Gastrostomy tube replacement, 187
Genital warts, 301
Genitourinary trauma, 576–579
GERD. *See* Gastrointestinal reflux disease (GERD)
Giant cell arteritis, 519
Giardia lamblia, 259
Gila monster bites, 422
Gingivostomatitis, 526
Ginkgo, toxicology, 404
Ginseng, toxicology, 404
Glasgow Coma Scale, 553, 553*t*
Glaucoma, acute angle closure, 518
Glenohumeral joint dislocation, 592–593
Glucagon, for allergic reactions, 54
Glucose-6–phosphate dehydrogenase deficiency, 464
Glutethimide, toxicology, 363
Glycoprotein IIb/IIIa inhibitors, for myocardial infarction, 95*t*, 97
Gonococcal infections, 299–301, 300*t*
  arthritis, 614
  conjunctivitis, 246–247
  disseminated, 539
  pharyngitis, 245
Gonorrhea. *See* Gonococcal infections
Gout, 614–615
Granuloma inguinale. *See* Donovanosis
Great vessels
  blunt trauma, 570–571
  penetrating trauma, 569–570
Greenstick fractures, 287
Grey Turner's sign, 183
Groin hernias, 158–159
Guillain-Barré syndrome, 503

H
H$_1$-blockers, for allergic reactions, 54
H$_2$-blockers, for allergic reactions, 54
H$_2$-receptor antagonists, for peptic ulcer disease, 153
HACE. *See* High altitude cerebral edema (HACE)
Haemophilus ducreyi. See Chancroid
Haemophilus influenzae, 130
  in cellulitis, 520
  in meningitis, 509, 511*t*
  in parotitis, 521
Hair-thread tourniquet syndrome, 81
Hallpike test, 498

Hallucinogens, toxicology, 371–372, 372*t*

Halo sign, 561

Hamate fracture, 587

Hammon's crunch, 149

Hand. *See also* Upper extremity
    infection, 618–620, 619*t*
    injuries, 584–586
    noninfectious conditions, 620
    wound repair, 76–77, 77*f*, 78*f*

Hand-foot-and-mouth disease, 283

Hantavirus, 330–331

HAPE. *See* High altitude pulmonary edema (HAPE)

Hawkins' test, 613

Hazardous materials exposure
    decontamination, 400–401
    emergency department care and disposition, 401–403

Head injury
    clinical features, 553–555, 553*t*
    diagnosis and differential, 555
    emergency department care and disposition, 555–556
    epidemiology, 553
    pathophysiology, 553
    seizures and, 257

Head-thrust test, 498

Headache
    chronic, 61*t*
    clinical features, 483–484
    diagnosis and differential, 484, 485*t*, 486*t*
    emergency department care and disposition, 485
    epidemiology, 483
    pathophysiology, 483
    in pediatric patients, 269–270

Hearing loss, 524–525

Heart
    blunt injuries, 568–569
    murmurs, 102*t*
    penetrating injuries, 568
    sounds, 102*t*

Heat-related illnesses, 415–417

Heel-to-shin test, 496

Helicobacter pylori, 152–153

Heliox
    for asthma, 140, 253
    for bronchiolitis, 254

HELLP syndrome, 219, 466*t*, 467

Helminth infections, 322, 322*t*, 323–326

Hemarthrosis, 614

Hematemesis, 146

Hematuria, 197–198

Hemoglobinopathies, hereditary, 464–466

Hemolytic crises, 295

Hemolytic-uremic syndrome, 263, 466–468, 466*t*

Hemophilia, 462–463

Hemoptysis, 137–138

Hemorrhoids, 165–166, 165*f*, 166*f*

Hemostasis, 66

Henoch-Schönlein purpura, 263, 290

Heparin, 474
    for atrial fibrillation, 17
    for atrial flutter, 16

    bleeding and, 459
    for deep venous thrombosis, 122–123, 474
    for myocardial infarction, 97
    for pulmonary embolism, 114

Hepatitis
    clinical features, 176–177
    diagnosis and differential, 177
    emergency department care and disposition, 177–178
    epidemiology, 176
    pathophysiology, 176

Herbal agents, toxicology, 404

Herbicides, toxicology, 395–397

Hernias, 158–159, 159*f*
    in pediatric patients, 262

Herpangina, 526–527

Herpes simplex virus (HSV) infections, 300*t*, 302, 307
    ocular, 515–516

Herpes zoster, 307–308, 542–543
    ophthalmicus, 516

Herpetic whitlow, 619–620, 619*t*

High altitude cerebral edema (HACE), 425–427

High altitude pulmonary edema (HAPE), 425–427

High-pressure injection injuries, 84–85

Hip injuries, 597–598

Hip pain, 292

Hippocratic technique, 593

Hirudin, 473

HIV infection. *See* Human immunodeficiency virus (HIV) infection

Hobo spider bite, 419

Hockey skate injuries, 79

Homan's sign, 121

Hookworm, 324

Hordeolum, 515

Household cleaners
    burns, 434–436
    ingestion, 392–394

HSV infections. *See* Herpes simplex virus (HSV) infections

Human bites, 85, 619, 619*t*

Human immunodeficiency virus (HIV) infection
    bleeding in, 462
    clinical features, 309–311
    diagnosis and differential, 311
    emergency department care and disposition, 312
    epidemiology, 309
    pathophysiology, 309
    peripheral nerve disorders in, 504
    in pregnancy, 216
    prophylaxis, 633
    tuberculosis and, 134

Human papillomaviruses, 301

Humerus fractures, 594

Hydralazine, toxicology, 384–385

Hydrocarbons, ingestion, 390–391, 391*t*

Hydromorphone, 58

Hymenolepis nana, 326

Hymenoptera stings, 418

Hyperbaric oxygen, 441*t*

Hyperbilirubinemia, 174–175

Hypercalcemia

Hypercalcemia (*Continued*)
  clinical features, 40
  diagnosis and differential, 40
  emergency department care and disposition, 40
  of malignancy, 478
  pathophysiology, 40
Hypercapnia, 126–127, 127*t*
Hypercyanotic episodes, 240
Hyperkalemia, 39, 39*t*
Hypermagnesemia, 41
Hypernatremia, 37–38, 38*t*
Hyperosmolar hyperglycemic state, 447–448
Hyperoxaluria, in Crohn's disease, 160
Hypertension
  emergencies, 115–118
  in end-stage renal disease, 193
  headache in, 484
  in pediatric patients, 117
  in pregnancy, 117
Hyperthyroidism, 450
  in pregnancy, 214
Hyperviscosity syndrome, 480–481
Hyphema, 517
Hypobaric hypoxemia, 425–427
Hypocalcemia, 39–40
Hypochondriasis, 625
Hypoglycemia, 445–446
    in pediatric patients, 266–267, 267*t*
Hypoglycemic agents, toxicology, 410–411
Hypokalemia, 38–39, 38*t*
Hypomagnesemia, 40–41
Hyponatremia, 37, 37*t*, 273
Hypotension. *See* Shock
Hypothermia, 413–415, 414*t*
Hypothyroidism, 451
Hypoxemia, hypobaric, 425–427
Hypoxia, 126
Hysterectomy, complications, 227
Hysteroscopy, complications, 227

I

Ibutilide, 28
  for atrial flutter, 16
  contraindications, 16
Idioventricular rhythm, 25
Immersion foot, 622
Immune reconstitution illness to MAC, 310
Immunoglobulins, intravenous, 470
Immunosuppression, complications, 343*t*
Immunosuppression, complications, 342–343
Impetigo, 519–520
  in pediatric patients, 281–282, 281*f*
Induction agents, 8*t*
Infantile spasms, 257
Infants. *See* Pediatric patients
Infection(s)
  hand, 618–620, 619*t*
  ocular, 515–516
  posttransplantation, 341–342, 341*t*

Inflammatory bowel disease
  in Crohn's disease, 160
  in pregnancy, 216
Infliximab, for Crohn's disease, 161
Influenza, 306–307
Inguinal hernias, 158–159, 159*f*
Inhibitor screens, 457*t*
Injury patterns, pediatric, 286–288
INR. *See* International normalized ratio (INR)
Insecticides, ingestion, 394–397
Insulin
  for diabetic ketoacidosis, 265, 447
  toxicology, 348*t*
International normalized ratio (INR), 457*t*
Intestinal colic, 236
Intestinal obstruction
  causes, 156*t*
  clinical features, 156
  diagnosis and differential, 157, 157*f*
  emergency department care and disposition, 157
  epidemiology, 156
  pathophysiology, 156
  in pediatric patients, 262
  postsurgical, 186
Intimate partner violence
  clinical features, 632
  emergency department care and disposition, 633
  epidemiology, 632
  in pregnancy, 216
Intracranial pressure, elevated, 553, 555–556
Intraosseous cannulation, 33–34
Intravenous pyelogram, 203
Intussusception, 263
Ipratropium, for asthma, 253
Iron poisoning, 350*t*, 388–389
Ischemia
  mesenteric, 145
  vs. myocardial infarction, 94
Isoniazid (INH)
  dosage and side effects, 135*t*
  toxicology, 405
Isopropanol, toxicology, 365–366

J

Jaundice
  causes, 175*t*
  clinical features, 175
  diagnosis and differential, 175–176
  emergency department care and disposition, 176
  in neonates, 238
  pathophysiology, 174–175
Jellyfish stings, 423–425
Jock itch, 541
Junctional rhythms, 18, 18*f*
Juniper, toxicology, 404

K

Kaposi's sarcoma, 311

Kawasaki's disease, 286
Kehr's sign, 572
Keratitis, ultraviolet, 427
Kernig's sign, 510
Ketamine, 8t
   for analgesia, 59
   in pediatric intubation, 33
Ketoacidosis
   alcoholic. *See* Alcoholic ketoacidosis
   diabetic. *See* Diabetic ketoacidosis
Kidney, traumatic injury, 578
Kidney transplant patients, 344–345
   immunosuppressive complications, 342–343
   infectious complications, 341–342, 341t
Kissing bug, 420–421
Knee injuries, 80
   dislocations, 600
   fractures, 599–600
   ligamentous, 600
   meniscal, 600
   overuse, 601
   radiographic evaluation, 598–599
   tendon, 600–601

L
Labetalol, 27, 117, 118
Lambert-Eaton myasthenic syndrome, 507–508
Lamotrigine, complications, 258
Laparoscopy, complications, 227
Laparotomy, exploratory, 573, 574t
Laplace's law, 119
Large bowel obstruction. *See* Intestinal obstruction
Laryngeal mask airway, 10
Laryngeal trauma, 532–533
Laryngomalacia, in neonates, 276–277
Laryngotracheobronchitis. *See* Viral croup
Lateral sinus thrombosis, 524
Lawn mower injuries, 79
Laxatives, 173
Lead poisoning, 398, 398t
LeFort fractures, 560, 561f
Left ventricular outlet flow obstruction, 241
Leg. *See* Lower extremity
Legg-Calvé-Perthes' disease, 290–291
Legionella, 130–131
Lid lacerations, 517
Lidocaine, 26–27
   in pediatric intubation, 32
   for ventricular fibrillation, 21
Lifelong Learning and Self-Assessment (LLSA) test, 2–3, 3t
Lightning injuries, 438–439, 439t
Lips, wound repair, 73, 73f
Lithium, toxicology, 359–360
Liver, in septic shock, 50
Liver disease, bleeding and, 459
Liver transplant patients, 345–346
   immunosuppressive complications, 342–343
   infectious complications, 341–342, 341t
Livestock bites, 87

LLSA test. *See* Lifelong Learning and Self-Assessment (LLSA) test
LMA. *See* Laryngeal mask airway
Loa loa, 325
Lobelia, toxicology, 404
Loop diuretics, hypokalemia and, 38
Lorazepam, 316
Lower extremity
   anatomy, 605t
   penetrating trauma, 579–580
   peripheral nerve testing, 79t
   wound repair, 80–81
   wounds, 79–80
Ludwig's angina, 531
Lumbar plexopathy, 504
Lumbar puncture, 256
Lunate fracture, 587
Lung injuries, 567
Lung transplant patients, 344
   immunosuppressive complications, 342–343
   infectious complications, 341–342, 341t
Lyme disease, 327, 505
Lymphogranuloma venereum, 300t, 303

M
MAC. *See Mycobacterium avium* complex
Magnesium sulfate, 29
   for asthma, 140, 253
   for multifocal atrial tachycardia, 15
   for torsades de pointes, 21
Magnetic resonance imaging
   emergency department use, 635–636
   in radiculopathy, 611
   in seizure disorders, 256
Malaria, 319–321, 321t
Malignant melanoma, 622
Mallet finger, 585
Mallory-Weiss tears, 150
Malrotation of the gut, 262
Mandibular dislocation, 522
Mandibular fractures, 563
Mantoux testing, 134
MAOIs. *See* Monoamine oxidase inhibitors (MAOIs)
MAP. *See* Mean arterial pressure (MAP)
Marburg virus, 340
Marcus Gunn pupil, 506, 561
Marfan's syndrome, 119
Marine animals, trauma from, 423–425
Masticator space abscess, 521–522
Mastitis, 220
Mastoiditis, 523–524
Maxillary fractures, 563
Maxillofacial trauma, 527–528, 560–563
Mean arterial pressure (MAP), 47
Mean corpuscular hemoglobin, 456t
Measles, 284
Meconium aspiration, 35
Medical ethics, 647–648
Medical malpractice, 645–646

Ménière's disease, 498–499
Meningitis
    antibiotics for, 232*t*
    clinical features, 230, 510
    diagnosis and differential, 510, 510*t*
    emergency department care and disposition, 510–511, 511*t*
    epidemiology, 509
    headache from, 483
    organisms causing, 233*t*, 234
    pathophysiology, 509–510
    in pediatric patients, 233–234
Meningococcemia, 539
Meniscal injuries, 600
Menometrorrhagia, 208
Menorrhagia, 208
Menstrual cycle, 207*f*
Meperidine, 58
Meprobamate, toxicology, 363
Mercury poisoning, 399–400
Mesenteric ischemia, 145
Metabolic acidosis
    causes, 42*t*, 43*t*
    clinical features, 42
    diagnosis and differential, 42–43, 367*t*
    emergency department care and disposition, 43, 43*t*
    in shock, 48
Metabolic alkalosis, 43
Metacarpal fractures, 586
Metalloids, toxicology, 398–400
Metals, toxicology, 398–400
Metastases, emergency complications, 474–477
Metformin, toxicology, 410–411
Methanol, toxicology, 350*t*, 366–367
Methaqualone, toxicology, 363
Methemoglobinemia, 408–409
Methohexital, 8*t*, 59
Metoprolol, 27
    for atrial flutter, 16
    for myocardial infarction, 95*t*
    for premature atrial contractions, 14
    for premature ventricular contractions, 19
Metrorrhagia, 208
MI. *See* Myocardial infarction (MI)
Midazolam
    for conscious sedation, 59
    in pediatric intubation, 33
    for tetanus, 316
Middle ear squeeze, 428
Migraine headache, 61, 61*t*, 62*t*
    clinical features, 483–484
    emergency department care and disposition, 485
    in pregnancy, 216
    treatment, 486*t*
Milch technique, 593
Milrinone, for cardiogenic shock, 52
Minoxidil, toxicology, 384–385
Mirtazapine, toxicology, 356
Mitral incompetence, 102–103
Mitral stenosis, 102, 102*t*
Mitral valve prolapse, 102*t*, 103–104

Mittelschmerz, 209
Monoamine oxidase inhibitors (MAOIs)
    drug-drug interactions, 357*t*
    toxicology, 348*t*, 356–357, 358*t*
Mononeuritis multiplex, 504
Mononucleosis, infectious, 284
Monteggia's fracture-dislocation, 590
Morphine
    for analgesia, 58
    for myocardial infarction, 95*t*
Morton's neuroma, 621–622
Multifocal atrial tachycardia (MAT)
    clinical features, 15, 15*f*
    emergency department care and disposition, 15*f*
Multiple sclerosis, 506
Mumps, 520–521
Munchausen syndrome by proxy, 629–630
Mushrooms, poisonous, 441–443, 443*t*
Myasthenia gravis, 506–507, 507*t*
Mycobacterium avium complex, 310
Mycobacterium tuberculosis, 133
Mycoplasma pneumoniae
    in bronchitis, 129
    in pediatric patients, 282
    in pneumonia, 130–131
Myocardial infarction (MI)
    cardiogenic shock and, 50
    clinical features, 94
    diagnosis and differential, 95, 95*t*
    emergency department care and disposition, 95–97, 95*t*, 96*f*, 96*t*
    epidemiology, 94
    pathophysiology, 94
Myocardial injury, 569
Myocardial ischemia, 117
Myocarditis, 109
    in pediatric patients, 242
Myofascial back pain, 61*t*, 62*t*
Myofascial chest pain, 61*t*, 62*t*
Myofascial headache, 61*t*, 62*t*
Myofascial pain syndrome, 610
Myonecrosis, 333–335
Myopathies, 503
Myxedema coma, 451–452

N
Naloxone
    in neonatal resuscitation, 35
    as reversal agent, 58
Nasal emergencies, 525–526
Nasal fractures, 525, 562
Nasoethmoidal-orbital fractures, 562
Nasotracheal intubation, 9
Natriuretic peptides, 100
Nausea
    cancer-related, 481
    in pregnancy, 217–218
Near drowning, 430–431
Near syncope, 497

Necator americanus, 324
Neck pain, 609–612, 610*t*, 611*t*
Neck trauma, 563–565, 563*t*, 564*t*
Necrolysis, toxic epidermal, 536–537
Necrotizing fasciitis, 335
Needlestick injuries, 84
Neer's test, 613
Nefazodone, toxicology, 355
Negligence, 645–646
Neisseria gonorrhoeae. See Gonococcal infections
Neisseria meningitidis, 509, 511*t*
Nematodes, 323–325
Neonatal resuscitation, 35
Neonatal tetanus, 316
Neonates. *See also* Pediatric patients
  apparent life-threatening events, 238–239
  bacteremia, 231
  cyanosis, 240–241
  fever, 229–230, 236
  gastrointestinal symptoms, 236–237
  jaundice, 238
  laryngomalacia, 276–277
  meningitis, 234
  nonspecific symptoms, 235*t*
  normal functions, 235–236
  oral thrush, 238
  respiratory symptoms, 237–238
  seizures, 257
  sepsis, 236
  unexplained crying, 236, 236*t*
  vocal cord paralysis, 277
Nephrostomy tubes, complications, 204
Nesiritide, 31, 101
Neurogenic back pain, 61, 62*t*
Neurogenic shock, 54–55
Neuromuscular blockade, 8–9, 9*t*
Neuromuscular junction disorders, 503
Neuropathies, peripheral, 503–505
Neutropenic fever, 480
Nifedipine, for hypertensive emergencies, 118
Nikolsky's sign, 537
Nitroglycerin, 31
  for cardiogenic shock, 52
  for congestive heart failure, 101
  for myocardial infarction, 95*t*
Nitroprusside, 31
  for cardiogenic shock, 52
  for hypertensive emergencies, 117
Nitrous oxide (N_2O), for analgesia, 58
Nonclostridial myonecrosis, 334–335
Nonketotic hyperosmolar coma, 447
Nonopiates, 58
Nonsteroidal anti-inflammatory drugs (NSAIDs), 58
  toxicology, 377–378
Norepinephrine, 30
  for cardiogenic shock, 52
  for septic shock, 50
  for shock, 48
Nose, wound repair, 72–73
NSAIDs. *See* Nonsteroidal anti-inflammatory drugs (NSAIDs)

Nursemaid's elbow, 289
Nystagmus, 497

O
Octopus stings, 424
Octreotide, for gastrointestinal bleeding, 147
Ocular emergencies, 515–519
Odontogenic abscess, 531
Ogilvie's syndrome, 157
Onchocerca volvulus, 325
Onychocryptosis, 621
Opioids
  for analgesia, 58
  for chronic pain, 61–62
  toxicology, 348*t*, 350*t*, 368–369
Optic neuritis, 519
Oral cavity, soft tissue lesions, 526–527
Oral hemorrhage, 528
Oral thrush, 526
  in AIDS, 311
  in neonates, 238
Orbit
  blowout fractures, 517, 562
  cellulitis, 249, 516
Orchitis, 199–200
Organochlorines, toxicology, 394–397
Organophosphates, toxicology, 348*t*, 394–397, 397*t*
Orofacial pain, 526
Orofacial trauma, 527–528, 560–563
Osgood Schlatter's disease, 291
Osmolarity, calculation, 37
Osmotic agents, toxicology, 383–384
Osteoarthritis, 615
Otalgia, 524
Otitis externa, 522–523
  in pediatric patients, 244
Otitis media, 523
  in pediatric patients, 243–244
Otologic emergencies, 522–525
Ottawa Ankle Rules, 602, 602*f*
Ovarian cysts, 209

P
P. multocida, 86
P-QRS-T complex, 12, 12*f*
Pacemaker, malfunctions, 24–25
Packed red blood cells, 468–469
PACs. *See* Premature atrial contractions (PACs)
Pain. *See* Acute pain; Chronic pain
Palm, wound repair, 76
Pancreatic injury, 572
Pancreatitis
  causes, 183*t*
  clinical features, 183
  complications, 184*t*
  diagnosis and differential, 183–184
  emergency department care and disposition, 184
  epidemiology, 183

Pancreatitis (*Continued*)
 gallstones and, 181
 pathophysiology, 183
 in pediatric patients, 263
Panic disorder, 624, 627
Paragonimus westermani, 325
Parapharyngeal abscess, 530
Paraphimosis, 200
Paraquat, toxicology, 395
Parkinson's disease, 508
Paronychia, 619, 619*t*
Parotitis, 520–521
Patellar injuries, 599–601
PEA. *See* Pulseless electrical activity (PEA)
Peak expiratory flow rate, in asthma, 253
Pediatric patients. *See also* Neonates
 abdominal pain, 261–264, 262*t*
 altered mental status, 268–269, 269*t*
 appendicitis, 263
 asthma, 252–254
 bacteremia, 231–232
 bacterial tracheitis, 278–279
 bronchiolitis, 254
 cellulitis, 248–249
 congestive heart failure, 241–242, 241*t*
 conjunctivitis, 246–247
 cyanosis, 240–241
 diabetes mellitus, 264–266
 diabetic ketoacidosis, 264–266
 diarrhea, 259–261, 260*t*
 epiglottitis, 277–278
 exanthems, 281–286
 fever, 229–230
 fluid and electrolyte disorders, 273–275
 foreign body aspiration, 279–280
 gastrointestinal bleeding, 262
 headache, 269–270
 heart disease, 239–242, 239*t*
 hernias, 262
 hypertensive emergencies, 117
 hypoglycemia, 266–267, 267*t*
 intestinal obstruction, 262
 intussusception, 263
 meningitis, 233–234
 normal functions of, 235–236
 otitis externa, 244
 otitis media, 243–244
 peritonsillar abscess, 280
 pharyngitis, 244–245
 pneumonia, 250–252, 251
 pyloric stenosis, 262–263
 retropharyngeal abscess, 280
 seizure disorders, 255–258
 sepsis, 232–233
 sickle cell anemia, 292–296
 sinusitis, 247–248
 sudden cardiac death, 271*t*
 syncope, 270–272, 271*t*
 trauma, 547–548
 urinary tract infections, 296–297

 viral croup, 278
 vomiting, 259–261
Pediculosis, 542
Pelvic abscess, 227
Pelvic inflammatory disease, 225–226, 226*t*
Pelvic injuries
 avulsion, 596, 596*t*
 fractures, 594–597, 595*t*
 in pregnancy, 551–552
Pelvic pain, 209–210, 210*t*. *See also* Abdominal pain, acute
Pemphigus vulgaris, 538–539
Penicillin, toxicology, 406
Penile injuries, 200
Penis, traumatic injury, 578–579
Peptic ulcer disease, 152–153
Pericardial effusion, cancer-related, 476–477
Pericardial inflammation syndrome, 569
Pericarditis
 acute, 109–110
 constrictive, 111
 in end-stage renal disease, 193
 in pediatric patients, 242
Periorbital cellulitis, 516
 in pediatric patients, 249
Peripheral artery disease, 123–124
Peripheral blood smear, 456*t*
Peripheral nerve testing, 75*t*, 79*t*
Peripheral neuropathy, 503–505
 in end-stage renal disease, 193
Peritoneal lavage, diagnostic, 572–573
Peritonitis
 in abdominal trauma, 572
 in dialysis patients, 194
Peritonsillar abscess, 280, 529
Pesticides, toxicology, 394–397, 397*t*
Peyronie's disease, 200–201
Phalanx fractures, 586
Phantom limb pain, 61*t*, 62*t*
Pharyngitis, 528–529
 high altitude, 427
 in pediatric patients, 244–245
Phenobarbital
 complications, 258
 properties, 502*t*
 toxicology, 360–361
Phenytoin
 complications, 258
 properties, 502*t*
 toxicology, 386–387, 387*t*
Phimosis, 200
Phobia, 624–625
Photosensitivity, 540
Physeal fractures, 287, 287*f*
Physician telephone advice, 647
Pilonidal sinus, 167
Pinworm, 323–324
Pisiform fracture, 587
Pit viper bites, 421–422
Pityriasis rosea, 286
Placenta previa, 218, 221

Placental abruption, 221
Plague, 331–332, 339*t*
Plantar fasciitis, 621
Plantar fibromatosis, 622
Plantar interdigital neuroma, 621–622
Plantar warts, 620
Plants, poisonous, 441–443
Plasmodium, 319–321, 321*t*
Platelet(s)
    abnormalities, 458
    count, 457*t*
    inhibitors, 473
    in shock, 48
    transfusion therapy, 469
Pleural effusion, in tuberculosis, 134
Pneumococcus, 130
Pneumocystis carinii, 310
Pneumonia
    in AIDS patients, 310
    aspiration, 132
    clinical features, 130–131, 250–251
    diagnosis and differential, 131, 251
    emergency department care and disposition, 131–132,
        251–252
    epidemiology, 130, 250
    etiologic agents, 250*t*
    pathophysiology, 130, 250
    in pediatric patients, 250–252, 251
    treatment, 251*t*
Pneumothorax, 136
    tension, 567
Poisoning. *See also* specific substances
    antidotes, 350*t*
    clinical features, 347, 349*t*
    diagnosis and differential, 347
    emergency department care and disposition, 347–351, 348*t*
    epidemiology, 347
    pathophysiology, 347
Poliomyelitis, 508–509
Polycythemia, chronic mountain, 427
Polymyositis, 503
Polyps, colonic, 263
Pork tapeworm, 326
Portal hypertension, 263
Portuguese man-of-war, 423
Postherpetic neuralgia, 61*t*, 62*t*
Postpartum hemorrhage, 219
Postpolio syndrome, 508–509
Postsurgical complications
    breast surgery, 186
    clinical features, 185
    diagnosis and differential, 186
    emergency department care and disposition, 186
    gastrointestinal surgery, 186–187
Posttraumatic stress disorder, 625
Potassium chloride
    for diabetic ketoacidosis, 265, 447
    for hypokalemia, 39
PR interval, 12
Pre-eclampsia, 218–219, 219*t*

Pre-excitation syndromes, 25–26
Prednisone, for ulcerative colitis, 162
Pregnancy. *See also* Delivery, emergency
    comorbid diseases, 214–216
    diagnostic imaging, 216, 638
    drug use, 215*t*
    emergencies during, 217–218
    high altitude effects, 426
    hypertensive emergencies, 117, 218–219, 219*t*
    nausea and vomiting, 217–218
    postpartum emergencies, 219–220
    pre-eclampsia, 218–219, 219*t*
    prophylaxis after sexual assault, 633
    threatened abortion, 217
    trauma, 550–552
    ultrasonography, 638
    vaginal bleeding, 218
Premature atrial contractions (PACs), 14–15, 15*f*
Premature rupture of membranes, 218
Premature ventricular contractions (PVCs), 19, 19*f*
Preterm labor, 218
Priapism, 201
Prickly heat, 417
Primidone, 502*t*
Procainamide, 26
    for ventricular fibrillation, 21
    for ventricular tachycardia, 20
    for Wolff-Parkinson-White syndrome, 26
Procedural sedation and analgesia (PSA), 58. *See also specific
        agents*
Procidentia, 168
Propofol, 8*t*, 33
Propranolol, 27
Prosthetic valve disease, 105–106
Prothrombin time (PT), 457*t*
Proton pump inhibitors, 153
Pruritus ani, 169
PSA. *See* Procedural sedation and analgesia (PSA)
Pseudocyanosis, 128
Pseudohyperkalemia, 39
Pseudomembranous colitis, 162–163
Psoriasis, 542
Psychosis, 491*t*
PT. *See* Prothrombin time (PT)
Pubic lice, 420
Pulmonary angiography, 112–113
Pulmonary edema
    causes, 100*t*
    clinical features, 100
    diagnosis and differential, 100
    emergency department care and disposition, 100–101
    high altitude, 425–427
    with hypertensive emergency, 117
Pulmonary embolism
    cancer-related, 477–478
    clinical features, 112
    diagnosis and differential, 112–114, 113*t*
    emergency department care and disposition, 114, 474
    epidemiology, 112
    pathophysiology, 112

Pulseless electrical activity (PEA), 25
Puncture wounds, 83–84
Puss caterpillar, 421
PVCs. *See* Premature ventricular contractions (PVCs)
Pyelonephritis, 199–197
Pyloric stenosis, in pediatric patients, 262–263
Pyrazinamide, 135*t*
Pyrethrins, toxicology, 394–397

Q

Q waves, 12
QRS complex, 12
QT interval, 12
Quadriceps tendon rupture, 601
Quinine
    for malaria, 320–321, 321*t*
    toxicology, 405–406

R

Rabies, 316–318
Radial head fracture, 588–589
Radial head subluxation, 289
Radial styloid fracture, 587
Radiculopathy, 609–612
    cervical, 610*t*
    lumbar, 611*t*
Ramsay Hunt syndrome, 505
Rapid sequence intubation (RSI), 8–9, 8*t*, 9*t*
    in pediatric patients, 32–33
Rebound tenderness, 143–144
Recombinant tissue-type plasminogen activator (rt-PA), 489, 490*t*
Rectal foreign bodies, 169
Rectal prolapse, 168
Reflex sympathetic dystrophy (RSD), 61, 61*t*
Regurgitation, in neonates, 237
Reiter's syndrome, 615–616
Renal colic
    clinical features, 202–203
    diagnosis and differential, 203, 637
    emergency department care and disposition, 203
    epidemiology, 202
    pathophysiology, 202
Renal failure, acute. *See also* End-stage renal disease
    causes, 190*t*
    clinical features, 190
    diagnosis and differential, 190, 191*t*
    emergency department care and disposition, 190–192
    epidemiology, 189
    pathophysiology, 189
Renal system injury, 577*t*, 578–579
Renal transplant patients, 344–345
    immunosuppressive complications, 342–343
    infectious complications, 341–342, 341*t*
Reproductive technology, complications, 228
Respiratory acidosis, 44
Respiratory alkalosis, 44, 47
Respiratory syncytial virus, 254

Resuscitation
    neonatal, 35
    standards for, 647
Reteplase, for myocardial infarction, 95*t*, 96
Reticulocyte count, 456*t*
Retinitis, cytomegalovirus, 311
Retinopathy, high altitude, 427
Retropharyngeal abscess, 280, 530
Rhabdomyolysis, 606–607
Rheumatic emergencies, 616–618
Rheumatic fever, 291
Rheumatoid arthritis, emergencies, 616–618
Rib fractures, 566
Ricin, 340
Rickettsia rickettsii, 327
Rifampin, 135*t*
Rimantadine, for influenza, 307
Ring removal, string technique, 78*f*
Ring tourniquet syndrome, 78, 78*f*
River blindness, 325
Rocky Mountain spotted fever, 327–328
    in pediatric patients, 282–283
Rocuronium, 9*t*, 33
Rodent bites, 87
Rodenticides, toxicology, 395–397, 397*t*
Romberg test, 496
Roseola infantum, 285, 285*f*
Rotator cuff impingement injury, 610–611
Roundworms, 323–324
RSD. *See* Reflex sympathetic dystrophy (RSD)
RSI. *See* Rapid sequence intubation (RSI)
Rt-PA. *See* Recombinant tissue-type plasminogen activator (rt-PA)
Rubella, 284
Rule of sixes, 34

S

SA block. *See* Sinoatrial (SA) block
SA node. *See* Sinoatrial (SA) node
Salicylates, toxicology, 348*t*, 373–375
Salivary gland disorders, 520–522
Salter-Harris classification, 287*f*
SARS. *See* Severe acute respiratory syndrome (SARS)
Scabies, 420, 542
Scalp, wound repair, 71–72, 71*f*
Scaphoid fracture, 587
Scapula injuries, 593–594
Scapular manipulation technique, 593
Scarlet fever, 282, 283*f*
Schistosomiasis, 325
Schizophrenia, 623–624
Scorpion bite, 419–420
Scrotal abscess, 200
Scrotum, traumatic injury, 578
Sea snake bites, 424–425
Sea urchin stings, 424
Sedation, 57–59
Sedative-hypnotics, toxicology, 360–364
Seizure disorders

Seizure disorders (*Continued*)
   classification, 500*t*
   clinical features, 255–256, 500
   complications of drug therapy, 258
   diagnosis and differential, 256, 500–501, 501*t*
   emergency department care and disposition, 256–258,
      501–502, 501*f*, 502*t*
   epidemiology, 255, 499
   neonatal, 257
   pathophysiology, 255, 499–500
   in pediatric patients, 255–258
   in pregnancy, 216
Selective serotonin reuptake inhibitors (SSRIs), toxicology,
   348*t*, 356
Sellick's maneuver, 9
Sepsis. *See* Septic shock
Septic arthritis, 614, 614*t*, 615*t*
   in pediatric patients, 289–290
Septic shock
   antibiotics for, 232*t*
   clinical features, 49–50
   diagnosis and differential, 50
   emergency department care and disposition, 50–51
   epidemiology, 49
   in neonates, 236
   organisms causing, 233*t*
   pathophysiology, 49
   in pediatric patients, 232–233
Sequestration crises, 294
Serotonin syndrome, 348*t*, 353
Serum ketone testing, 43
Severe acute respiratory syndrome (SARS), 132
Sexual abuse, 629–630
Sexual assault, 631–632
Sexually transmitted disease, prophylaxis, 633
Shaken baby syndrome, 630
Sharp object ingestion, 152
Shingles. *See* Herpes zoster
Shock
   cardiogenic. *See* Cardiogenic shock
   causes, 48
   classification, 47
   clinical features, 47
   diagnosis and differential, 48
   in dialysis patients, 194
   emergency department care and disposition, 48
   epidemiology, 47
   neurogenic, 54–55
   pathophysiology, 47
   septic. *See* Septic shock
Shoulder
   dystocia, 222
   injuries, 591–594
   pain, 612–613
SIADH. *See* Syndrome of inappropriate secretion of antidiuretic
      hormone (SIADH)
Sialolithiasis, 521
Sickle cell disease
   acute chest syndrome, 293–294
   aplastic episodes, 294–295

   blood transfusions, 295
   central nervous system events, 294
   epidemiology, 292, 464
   hematological crises, 294–295
   hospital admission, 295
   infections, 295
   pain crises, 293
   pathophysiology, 292, 464–465
   in pregnancy, 216
   variants of, 295–296
Sinoatrial (SA) block, 21
Sinoatrial (SA) node, 11
Sinus bradycardia, 14, 14*f*
Sinus dysrhythmia, 13, 13*f*
Sinus pause, 22
Sinus tachycardia, 14, 14*f*
Sinusitis, 525–526
   in pediatric patients, 247–248
Slipped capital femoral epiphysis, 289
Small bowel obstruction. *See* Intestinal obstruction
Smallpox, 339–340, 339*t*
Smith's fracture, 588
Snake bites, 421–422
Snow blindness, 427
Sodium bicarbonate
   in hypermagnesemia, 41
   in metabolic acidosis, 43, 43*t*, 447
   in neonatal resuscitation, 35
Sodium-channel blockers, 26–27. *See also* specific drugs
Sodium nitroprusside, toxicology, 384–385
Sodium polystyrene sulfonate, 39
Soft tissue
   foreign body injury, 81–83
   infections, 333–338
Somatization disorder, 625
Somatostatin, 147
Sotalol, 27–28
   toxicology, 382
Speed's test, 613
Spider bites, 419
Spinal cord compression, 475
Spinal cord injury
   clinical features, 557
   diagnosis and differential, 557–559, 557*t*, 558*t*
   emergency department care and disposition, 559–560
   epidemiology, 556
   pathophysiology, 556
   in pediatric trauma, 547
   syndromes, 559*t*
Spinal shock, 559*t*
Spleen, traumatic injury, 572
Spontaneous bacterial peritonitis, 178–179
Sporotrichosis, 337–338
Sprains, ankle, 602
Spurling's sign, 611
SSRIs. *See* Selective serotonin reuptake inhibitors (SSRIs)
St. John's wort, toxicology, 404
ST segment, 12
Staphylococcal scalded-skin syndrome, 537–538
Staphylococcus aureus

Staphylococcus aureus (*Continued*)
  in cellulitis, 335–336, 520
  in parotitis, 521
  in pneumonia, 130
Stapling, for wound closure, 70
Status epilepticus, 258
  emergency department care and disposition, 501*t*
  pathophysiology, 500
Sternoclavicular joint injuries, 591
Stevens-Johnson syndrome, 536
Stimson technique, 593
Stinging ants, 418
Stingray stings, 423–425
Stool culture, 172
Streptococcal toxic shock syndrome, 305, 305*t*, 537–538
Streptococcus
  in cellulitis, 335–336
  in meningitis, 509, 511*t*
  in pharyngitis, 245, 529
Streptokinase, for myocardial infarction, 95, 95*t*
Streptomycin, dosage and side effects, 135*t*
Stridor
  in neonates, 237
  in pediatric patients, 276
String technique, ring removal, 78*f*
Stroke
  clinical features, 487–488, 488*f*
  diagnosis and differential, 488–489, 489*t*
  emergency department care and disposition, 474, 489–490, 490*t*
  epidemiology, 487
  hemorrhagic, 488*t*
  ischemic, 488*t*
  pathophysiology, 487
Strongyloides stercoralis, 324
Study techniques, 4
Stye, 515
Subarachnoid hemorrhage
  emergency department care and disposition, 485
  headache from, 483
Subconjunctival hemorrhage, 516
Subdural hematoma
  in end-stage renal disease, 193
  in head injury, 554
  headache from, 483
Substance abuse, 623
  in pregnancy, 216
Subtentorial mass lesions, 268
Succinylcholine, 9*t*
  in pediatric intubation, 33
Sudden cardiac death, in pediatric patients, 271
Sulfasalazine
  for Crohn's disease, 160
  for ulcerative colitis, 162
Sulfhemoglobinemia, 409–410
Sulfonylureas, toxicology, 348*t*, 410–411
Sunburn, 540
Superior vena cava syndrome, 477
Supracondylar fractures, 288–289
Supratentorial mass lesions, 268

Supraventricular tachycardia (SVT)
  clinical features, 17, 17*f*
  emergency department care and disposition, 17–18
  in pediatric patients, 34
  in Wolff-Parkinson-White syndrome, 26
Sutures
  continuous percutaneous, 68, 68*f*
  deep dermal, 68–69, 69*f*
  horizontal mattress, 69, 69*f*
  interrupted percutaneous, 67–68, 68*f*
  vertical mattress, 69, 69*f*
SVT. *See* Supraventricular tachycardia (SVT)
Swimmers itch, 325
Syncope, 97–99
  causes, 271*t*
  clinical features, 271–272
  diagnosis and differential, 272, 272*t*
  emergency department care and disposition, 272
  epidemiology, 270–271
  heat-related, 417
  pathophysiology, 271
  in pediatric patients, 270–272, 271*t*
  risk factors, 271*t*
Syndrome of inappropriate secretion of antidiuretic hormone (SIADH), 479–480
Synovitis, crystal-induced, 614–615
Syphilis, 300*t*, 301–302
Systemic lupus erythematosus, 616–618

T
T wave, 12
Tachycardia-bradycardia syndrome, 24
Tachydysrhythmia, 12–13, 13*f. See also* specific dysrhythmias
  in Wolff-Parkinson-White syndrome, 26
Taenia saginata, 326
Taenia solium, 326
Tapeworm, 326
Tarantula bite, 419
Tarsal tunnel syndrome, 621
TCT. *See* Thrombin clotting time (TCT)
TEE. *See* Transesophageal echocardiogram (TEE)
Telephone advice, physician, 647
Telogen effluvium, 541
Temporal arteritis, 484, 485, 519
Temporomandibular dislocation, 563
Temporomandibular disorder, 485–486, 522
Tendinitis
  foot, 621
  hand, 620
Tendon function
  forearm, 76*t*
  hand, 77, 77*f*
  lower extremities, 80*t*
Tendon injuries, hand, 585
Tenecteplase
  for myocardial infarction, 95*t*, 96
Tenosynovitis
  DeQuervain's, 620
  foot, 621

Tenosynovitis (*Continued*)
   hip pain, 292
Tensilon test, 507
Tension headache, 484, 485
Tension pneumothorax, 567
Test performance, 4–5
Testicles, traumatic injury, 578
Testicular torsion, 199
Tet spells, 240
Tetanus
   clinical features, 315–316
   diagnosis and differential, 316
   emergency department care and disposition, 316
   epidemiology, 315
   pathophysiology, 315
   prophylaxis, 66, 88, 317t
Tetralogy of Fallot, 240
Thalassemias, 464–465
Theophylline, toxicology, 379–380, 380t
Thermal burns, 432–434, 432–434f
Thiazides, toxicology, 383–384
Thiazolidinediones, toxicology, 411
Thiocyanate, toxicology, 384–385
Thiopental, 8t, 33
Thompson's test, 80, 590, 602
Threadworm, 324
Thrombin clotting time (TCT), 457t
Thromboembolism
   cancer-related, 477–478
   in pregnancy, 214
Thrombophlebitis, 121–123
Thrombotic thrombocytopenia purpura (TTP), 466–468, 466t
Thumbprint sign, 531
Thyroid storm, 450–451, 451t
Tiagabine, complications, 258
Tibial fractures, 599
Tic douloureux, 486–487
Tick paralysis, 328–329
Tinea capitis, 540–541
Tinea cruris, 541
Tinea pedis, 541
Tinnitus, 524
Tongue lesions, 527
Tongue size, 7f
Torsades de pointes, 20–21, 20f
Torus fractures, 287
Toxic epidermal necrolysis, 536–537
Toxic megacolon, 160
Toxic shock syndrome, 303–305, 304t, 305t, 537–538
Toxins, emergency department care and disposition, 401–403.
      See also specific toxins
Tracheal intubation. *See* Endotracheal intubation
Tracheitis, bacterial, 278–278
Tracheobronchial injuries, 567–568
Transcutaneous cardiac pacing
   for atrioventricular block, 22–23
   for junctional rhythms, 18
   for pacemaker failure, 24
   in pediatric patients, 34–35
   for sinus bradycardia, 14

Transesophageal echocardiogram (TEE)
   in atrial fibrillation, 17
   in atrial flutter, 16
Transformed migraine, 61, 61t, 62t
Transfusion therapy
   administration, 472
   albumin, 470
   antithrombin III, 470
   complications, 471, 471t
   cryoprecipitate, 469
   emergency, 471–472
   fresh frozen plasma, 469
   immunoglobulins, 470
   massive, 472
   packed red blood cells, 468–469
   platelets, 469
   specific factor replacement, 470t
   whole blood, 468
Transient ischemic attack, 487–488
Transplant patients
   cardiac, 343–344
   immunosuppressive complications, 342–343, 343t
   infectious complications, 341–342, 341t
   liver, 345
   lung, 344
   renal, 344–345
Transposition of the great vessels, 240–241
Transtentorial herniation, 554–555
Transvenous cardiac pacing, 22–23
Trapezium fracture, 587
Trapezoid fracture, 587
Trauma. *See also* Dislocation(s); Fracture(s); Wounds
   abdominal, 571–574, 574t
   approach to the patient, 545–546
   brain, 553–556
   buttock, 575–576
   cardiothoracic, 565–571
   in elderly patient, 548–550
   extremities, 579–580
   flank, 574–575
   focused assessment with sonography, 638
   genitourinary, 576–579
   head, 553–556
   laryngeal, 532–533
   maxillofacial, 560–563
   neck, 563–565
   in pediatric patient, 547–548
   in pregnancy, 550–552
   spinal, 556–560, 557–559t
Traumatic brain injury. *See* Head injury
Trazodone, toxicology, 355
Trematodes, 325
Trench foot, 414, 622
Treponema pallidum. See Syphilis
Triage, 644
Triceps rupture, 590–591
Trichinella spiralis, 324
Trichinosis, 324
Trichomonas vaginalis. See Trichomoniasis
Trichomoniasis, 300t, 301. *See also* Vulvovaginitis

Trichuris trichiura, 324
Tricyclic antidepressants, toxicology, 354–355
Trifascicular block, 24
Trigeminal neuralgia, 486–487
Trigger finger, 620
Triquetrum fracture, 587
Trousseau's sign, 40
TTP. *See* Thrombotic thrombocytopenia purpura (TTP)
Tuberculosis
    in AIDS, 310
    clinical features, 133–134
    diagnosis and differential, 134
    emergency department care and disposition, 134–135
    epidemiology, 133
    pathophysiology, 133
    pharmacologic treatment, 134–135, 135*t*
Tularemia, 329, 339*t*
Tumor lysis syndrome, 478–479
Tympanic membrane perforation, 524

U
U wave, 12
Ulcerative colitis, 161–162
Ulnar styloid fracture, 587–588
Ultrasonography
    in abdominal trauma, 573
    in appendicitis, 155
    emergency department use, 637–638
Ultraviolet keratitis, 427, 518
Umbilical vein catheterization, 35
Unifascicular block, 23–24
Upper extremity. *See also* Hand
    elbow injuries, 588–589
    penetrating trauma, 579–580
    peripheral nerve testing, 75*t*
    shoulder injuries, 591–594
    shoulder pain, 612–613
    wound repair, 75–78
    wounds, 74–75
Upper respiratory emergencies, 275–276
Ureter(s)
    stents, 205
    traumatic injury, 578
Urethra
    foreign bodies, 201
    stricture, 201
    traumatic injury, 578
Urinary catheters, complications, 204
Urinary retention, 201–202
Urinary stones. *See* Renal colic
Urinary tract infections
    causes, 195*t*
    clinical features, 196
    diagnosis and differential, 196
    emergency department care and disposition, 196–197
    epidemiology, 195
    pathophysiology, 195
    in pediatric patients, 296–297
    in pregnancy, 214–215

Urticaria, 53

V
V/Q scanning. *See* Ventilation-perfusion (V/Q) scanning
Vaginal bleeding, abnormal
    clinical features, 208
    diagnosis and differential, 208
    emergency department care and disposition, 208–209
    epidemiology, 207
    pathophysiology, 207
    in pregnancy, 218
    in prepubertal children, 210–211
Vaginal obstruction, 211
Valproate, complications, 258
Valproic acid, properties, 502*t*
Valsalva maneuver, 18
Valvular heart disease
    aortic incompetence, 104–105
    aortic stenosis, 104
    mitral incompetence, 102–103, 102*t*
    mitral stenosis, 102, 102*t*
    mitral valve prolapse, 103–104
    prosthetic valve, 105–106
Varicella, 284–285, 285*f*
Variola major, 339*t*
Vascular access
    complications, 194
    in pediatric patients, 33–34
Vaso-occlusive crisis, 464–465
Vasoactive drugs, 29–31
Vasodilators, 31
    toxicology, 384–385
Vasopressin, 30–31
Vasopressors, for shock, 48
Vaughn-Williams classification, 26
Vecuronium, 9*t*
    in pediatric intubation, 33
Venlafaxine, toxicology, 356
Ventilation-perfusion (V/Q) scanning, 113
Ventricular fibrillation (VF)
    clinical features, 21, 21*f*
    emergency department care and disposition, 21
    in pediatric patients, 35
Ventricular tachycardia (VT)
    clinical features, 18–19, 20, 20*f*
    emergency department care and disposition, 20–21
Verapamil, 28–29
    for atrial fibrillation, 17
    for atrial flutter, 16
    for multifocal atrial tachycardia, 15
    for supraventricular tachycardia, 18
Vertebrobasilar insufficiency (VBI), 498–499
Vertigo, 496–499, 497*t*
Vesicovaginal fistulas, 228
VF. *See* Ventricular fibrillation (VF)
Viral croup, 278
Viral hemorrhagic fevers, 339*t*, 340
Vitamin K
    bleeding and, 458

Vitamin K (*Continued*)
toxicology, 403–404
Vitamins, toxicology, 403–404
Vocal cord paralysis, in neonates, 277
Volatile substances, toxicology, 390–391, 391*t*
Volkmann's ischemia, 604
Volume overload, 36
Volume status, assessment, 36
Vomiting
cancer-related, 481
clinical features, 170–171, 259
diagnosis and differential, 171–172, 259–260
emergency department care and disposition, 172, 260–261
epidemiology, 169–170, 259
in neonates, 237
pathophysiology, 170, 259
in pediatric patients, 259–261
in pregnancy, 217–218
Von Willebrand's disease, 463–464
VT. *See* Ventricular tachycardia (VT)
Vulvovaginitis, 223–224
in prepubertal children, 211

W
Wallenberg's syndrome, 498
Warfarin, 472–473, 458, 459*t*
Warm-type antibody hemolytic anemia, 466–468, 467*t*
Wasp stings, 418
Water deficit, calculation, 38
West Nile virus encephalitis, 332–333, 312
Wet drowning, 430
Wheezing, 127–128, 127*t*. *See also* Asthma
Whipworm, 324
Whole blood transfusion, 468
Wide complex tachycardia, 18–19
Wolff-Parkinson-White (WPW) syndrome, 25–26, 25*f*
Wound closure
adhesive tape, 70

delayed, 69
staples, 69–70, 70*f*
suturing techniques, 67–69, 68–69*f*
tissue adhesives, 70
Wounds
animal bite, 85–87
clinical features, 65
closure. *See* Wound closure
diagnosis and differential, 65
drains, 88
emergency department care and disposition, 66
epidemiology, 65
face and scalp, 71–74, 71–74*f*
foreign bodies in, 81–83
high-pressure-injection, 84–85
human bite, 85
lower extremity, 79–81
pathophysiology, 65
postrepair care, 87–89
puncture, 83–84
upper extremity, 74–78
WPW syndrome. *See* Wolff-Parkinson-White (WPW) syndrome
Wrist, injuries, 586–588. *See also* Upper extremity
Wuchereria bancrofti, 325

Y
Yergason's test, 613
Yersinia pestis, 331–332, 339*t*
Yohimbine, toxicology, 404

Z
Zaleplon, toxicology, 363
Zolpidem, 363
Zonisamide, complications, 258
Zoonotic infections, 326–333
Zygomatic fractures, 562